BMA
The British
Medical Association

ILLUSTRATED
MEDICAL
DICTIONARY

London, New York, Munich,
Melbourne, and Delhi

BRITISH MEDICAL ASSOCIATION
Chairman of Council Mr James Johnson
Treasurer Dr David Pickersgill
Chairman of the Representative Body Dr Michael Wilks

MEDICAL EDITORS AND CONSULTANTS
BMA Consulting Medical Editor Dr Michael Peters
Medical Consultants Dr Ian Beider, Dr Susanna Kahtan, Dr Dina Kaufman, Ann Peters SRN HV

DORLING KINDERSLEY
Editor Tom Broder
Senior Art Editor Nicola Rodway
Executive Managing Editor Adèle Hayward
Managing Art Editor Nick Harris
DTP Designer Traci Salter
Production Controller Stuart Masheter
Art Director Peter Luff
Publishing Director Jackie Douglas
Publisher Corinne Roberts

DK INDIA
Manager Aparna Sharma
Project Editor Dipali Singh
Editors Shinjini Chatterjee, Ankush Saikia, Rohan Sinha
Project Art Editor Kavita Dutta
DTP Designers Harish Aggarwal, Govind Mittal, Pushpak Tyagi

Edited for Dorling Kindersley by Martyn Page

First published in the United Kingdom in 2002 by Dorling Kindersley Limited, 80 Strand, London
WC2R 0RL
A Penguin Company
Second edition 2007

2 4 6 8 10 9 7 5 3 1

A CIP catalogue record for this book is available from the British Library.

ISBN 978-1-4053-1997-3

Colour reproduction by Colourscan, Singapore
Printed and bound in Singapore by Star Standard Industries (Pte.) Ltd

See our complete catalogue at
www.dk.com

BMA
The British
Medical Association

ILLUSTRATED
MEDICAL
DICTIONARY

BMA Consulting Medical Editor Dr Michael Peters

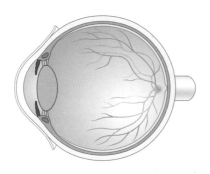

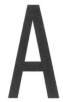

abdomen The region of the body between the chest and the pelvis. The abdominal cavity is bounded by the ribs and diaphragm above, and by the pelvis below, with the spine and abdominal muscles forming the back, side, and front walls. It contains the liver, stomach, intestines, spleen, pancreas, and kidneys. In the lower abdomen, enclosed by the pelvis, are the bladder, rectum, and, in women, the uterus and ovaries.

ABDOMEN

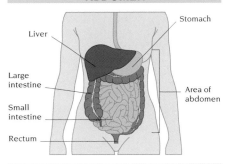

Liver

Large intestine

Small intestine

Rectum

Stomach

Area of abdomen

abdomen, acute Persistent, severe abdominal pain of sudden onset, usually associated with spasm of the abdominal muscles, vomiting, and fever.

The most common cause of an acute abdomen is *peritonitis*. Other causes include *appendicitis*, abdominal injury, perforation of an internal organ due to disorders such as *peptic ulcer* or *diverticular disease*. Acute abdominal pain commonly begins as a vague pain in the centre but then becomes localized.

An acute abdomen requires urgent medical investigation that may involve a *laparoscopy* or a *laparotomy*. Treatment depends on the underlying cause.

abdominal pain Discomfort in the abdomen. Mild abdominal pain is common and is often due to excessive alcohol intake, eating unwisely, or an attack of *diarrhoea*. Pain in the lower abdomen is common during menstruation but is occasionally due to a gynaecological disorder such as *endometriosis*. *Cystitis* is a common cause of pain or discomfort in the abdomen. Bladder distension as a result of urinary obstruction may also cause abdominal pain.

Abdominal colic is pain that occurs every few minutes as one of the internal organs goes into muscular spasm in an attempt to overcome an obstruction such as a stone or an area of inflammation. The attacks of colic may become more severe and may be associated with vomiting (see *abdomen, acute*).

Peptic ulcer often produces recurrent gnawing pain. Other possible causes of abdominal pain are infection, such as *pyelonephritis*, and *ischaemia* (lack of blood supply), as occurs when a *volvulus* (twisting of the intestine) obstructs blood vessels. Tumours affecting an abdominal organ can cause pain. Abdominal pain can also result from anxiety.

For mild pain, a wrapped hot-water bottle is often effective. Pain due to peptic ulcer can be temporarily relieved by food or by taking *antacid drugs*. Abdominal pain that is not relieved by vomiting, persists for more than 6 hours, or is associated with sweating or fainting requires urgent medical attention. Urgent attention is also necessary if pain is accompanied by persistent vomiting, vomiting of blood, or passing of bloodstained or black faeces. Unexplained weight loss or changes in bowel habits should always be investigated.

Investigation of abdominal pain may include the use of imaging tests such as *ultrasound scanning*, and endoscopic examination in the form of *gastroscopy*, *colonoscopy*, or *laparoscopy*.

abdominal swelling Enlargement of the abdomen. Abdominal swelling is a natural result of *obesity* and growth of the uterus during pregnancy. Wind in the stomach or intestine may cause uncomfortable, bloating distension of the abdomen. Some women experience abdominal distension due to temporary water retention just before menstruation. Other causes may be more serious.

For instance, *ascites* (accumulation of fluid between organs) may be a symptom of cancer or disease of the heart, kidneys, or liver; swelling may also be due to intestinal obstruction (see *intestine, obstruction of*) or an *ovarian cyst*.

Diagnosis of the underlying cause may involve *abdominal X-rays*, *ultrasound scanning*, *laparotomy*, or *laparoscopy*. In ascites, some fluid between organs may be drained for examination.

abdominal thrust A first-aid treatment for choking, in which sharp upward pressure is applied to the upper abdomen to dislodge a foreign body obstructing the airway. The technique is also known as the *Heimlich manoeuvre.*

abdominal X-ray An X-ray examination of the abdominal contents. X-rays can show whether any organ is enlarged and can detect swallowed foreign bodies in the digestive tract. They also show patterns of fluid and gas: distended loops of bowel containing fluid often indicate an obstruction (see *intestine, obstruction of*); gas outside the intestine indicates intestinal *perforation.*

Calcium, which is opaque to X-rays, is present in most kidney stones (see *calculus, urinary tract*) and in some *gallstones* and aortic *aneurysms*; these can sometimes be detected on an abdominal X-ray.

abducent nerve The 6th *cranial nerve.* It supplies the lateral rectus muscle of each eye, which is responsible for moving the eyeball outwards. The nerve originates in the pons (part of the *brainstem*) and passes along the base of the brain, entering the back of the eye socket through a gap between the skull bones.

abduction Movement of a limb away from the central line of the body, or of a digit away from the axis of a limb. Muscles that carry out this movement are called abductors. (See also *adduction*.)

ablation Removal or destruction of diseased tissue by excision (cutting away), *cryosurgery* (freezing), *radiotherapy, diathermy* (burning), *laser treatment*, or *radiofrequency ablation.*

abnormality A physical deformity or malformation, a behavioural or mental problem, or a variation from normal in the structure or function of a cell, tissue, or organ in the body.

ABO blood groups See *blood groups.*

abortifacient An agent that causes *abortion.* In medical practice, abortion is induced using *prostaglandin drugs*, often given as vaginal pessaries.

abortion In medical terminology, either spontaneous abortion (see *miscarriage*) or medically induced termination of pregnancy (see *abortion, induced*).

abortion, induced Medically induced termination of pregnancy. Abortion may be performed if the pregnancy threatens the woman's physical or emotional health or if tests show a severe fetal abnormality.

Depending on the stage of pregnancy, termination may be induced by using drugs or by the surgical technique of vacuum suction curettage, under either a general or local anaesthetic, during which the fetal and placental tissues are removed. Complications are rare.

abrasion Also called a graze, a *wound* on the skin surface that is caused by scraping or rubbing.

abrasion, dental The wearing away of tooth enamel, often accompanied by the erosion of dentine (the layer beneath the enamel) and cementum (the bone-like tissue that covers the tooth root), usually through too-vigorous brushing. Abraded areas are often sensitive to cold or hot food or drink, and a desensitizing toothpaste and/or protection with a bonding (see *bonding, dental*) agent or *filling* may be needed.

abreaction In *psychoanalysis*, the process of becoming consciously aware of repressed (buried) thoughts and feelings. In Freudian theory, abreaction ideally occurs by way of *catharsis.*

abscess A collection of *pus* formed as a result of infection by microorganisms, usually bacteria. Abscesses may develop in any organ and in the soft tissues beneath the skin in any area. Common sites include the armpit, breast (see *breast abscess*), groin, and gums (see *abscess, dental*). Rarer sites include the liver (see *liver abscess*) and the brain (see *brain abscess*).

Common bacteria, such as staphylococci, are the usual cause of abscesses, although fungal infections can cause them, and *amoebae* are an important cause of liver abscesses (see *amoebiasis*).

Infectious organisms usually reach internal organs via the bloodstream, or they penetrate tissues under the skin through a wound.

An abscess may cause pain, depending on where it occurs. Most larger abscesses cause fever, sweating, and malaise. Those close to the skin often cause obvious redness and swelling.

Antibiotics, antifungal drugs, or *amoebicides* are usually prescribed as appropriate. Most abscesses also need to be drained (see *drain, surgical*), and in some cases a tube may be left in place to allow continuous drainage. Some abscesses burst and drain spontaneously. Occasionally, an abscess within a vital organ damages enough surrounding tissue to cause permanent loss of normal function, or even death.

abscess, dental A pus-filled sac in the tissue around the root of a tooth. An abscess may occur when bacteria invade the pulp (the tissues in the central cavity of a tooth) as a result of dental *caries*, which destroys the tooth's enamel and dentine, allowing bacteria to reach the pulp. Bacteria can also gain access to the pulp when a tooth is injured. The infection in the pulp then spreads into the surrounding tissue to form an abscess. Abscesses can also result from *periodontal disease*, in which bacteria accumulate in pockets that form between the teeth and gums.

The affected tooth aches or throbs, and biting or chewing is usually extremely painful. The gum around the tooth is tender and may be red and swollen. An untreated abscess eventually erodes a sinus (channel) through the jawbone to the gum surface, where it forms a swelling known as a gumboil. As the abscess spreads, the glands in the neck and the side of the face may become swollen, and fever may develop.

Treatment may consist of draining the abscess, followed by *root-canal treatment* of the affected tooth, but in some cases *extraction* of the tooth is necessary. *Antibiotics* are prescribed if the infection has spread beyond the tooth. An abscess in a periodontal pocket can usually be treated by the dentist scraping away infected material.

ABSCESS, DENTAL

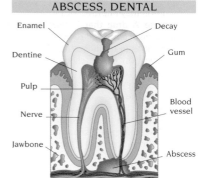

absence In medical terms, a temporary loss or impairment of consciousness that occurs in some forms of *epilepsy,* typically generalized absence (petit mal) seizures in childhood.

absorption The process by which fluids or other substances are taken up by body tissues. The term is commonly applied to the uptake of the nutrients from food into blood and lymph from the digestive tract. The major site of absorption is the small intestine, which is lined with microscopic finger-like projections called villi (see *villus*). The villi greatly increase the surface area of the intestine, thereby increasing the rate of absorption.

acamprosate A drug used to help those who are dependent on alcohol maintain abstinence. Possible side effects include diarrhoea, nausea, and abdominal pain. Acamprosate is not generally advised for those with kidney or severe liver damage.

acanthosis nigricans A rare condition in which thickened dark patches of skin appear in the groin, armpits, neck, and other skin folds. The condition may occur in young people as a genetic disorder or as the result of an endocrine disorder such as *Cushing's syndrome*. It also occurs in people with carcinomas of the lung and other organs.

Pseudoacanthosis nigricans is a much more common condition, usually seen in dark-complexioned people who are overweight. In this form, the skin in fold areas is both thicker and darker than the surrounding skin, and there is usually excessive sweating in affected areas. The condition may improve with weight loss.

acarbose A drug that is used to treat type 2 *diabetes mellitus*. Acarbose acts on enzymes in the intestines, inhibiting the digestion of starch and therefore slowing the rise in *blood glucose* levels after a carbohydrate meal.

accessory nerve The 11th *cranial nerve*. Unlike other cranial nerves, most of the accessory nerve originates from the spinal cord. The small part of the nerve that originates from the brain supplies many muscles of the palate, pharynx (throat), and larynx (voice box). Damage to this part of the nerve may cause difficulty in speaking and swallowing. The spinal part of the nerve supplies large muscles of the neck and back, notably the sternomastoid and trapezius. Damage to the spinal fibres of the nerve paralyses these muscles.

accidental death Death that occurs as a direct result of an accident. A high proportion of deaths in young adults, particularly among males, are accidental. Many of these deaths are due to road traffic accidents, drowning, or drug overdose. Falls in the home and burning or asphyxiation due to fire are common causes of accidental death in elderly people. Fatal accidents at work have become less common with the introduction of effective safety measures.

accommodation Adjustment, especially the process by which the eye adjusts itself to focus on near objects. At rest, the eye is focused for distant vision, when its lens is thin and flat. To make focusing on a nearer object possible, the ciliary muscle of the eye contracts, which reduces the pull on the outer rim of the lens, allowing it to become thicker and more convex.

With age, the lens loses its elasticity. This makes accommodation more and more difficult and results in a form of longsightedness called *presbyopia*.

acebutolol A *beta-blocker drug* used to treat *hypertension, angina pectoris*, and certain types of *arrhythmia* in which the heart beats too rapidly.

ACE inhibitor drugs A group of *vasodilator drugs* used to treat *heart failure, hypertension*, and diabetic *nephropathy*. ACE (*angiotensin converting enzyme*) inhibitors are often prescribed with other drugs such as *diuretic drugs* or *beta-blocker drugs*. Possible side effects include nausea, loss of taste, headache, dizziness, and dry cough.

acetaminophen An *analgesic drug* more commonly known as *paracetamol*.

acetazolamide A drug that is used in the treatment of *glaucoma* and, occasionally, to prevent or treat symptoms of *mountain sickness*. Possible adverse effects include lethargy, nausea, diarrhoea, and erectile dysfunction.

acetic acid The colourless, pungent, organic acid that gives vinegar its sour taste. In medicine, acetic acid is an ingredient of preparations that are used for certain ear infections.

acetylcholine A type of *neurotransmitter* (a chemical that transmits messages between nerve cells or between nerve and muscle cells). It is the neurotransmitter found at all nerve-muscle junctions and at many other sites in the nervous system. The actions of acetylcholine are called cholinergic actions, and these can be blocked by *anticholinergic drugs*.

acetylcholinesterase inhibitors A group of drugs used in the treatment of mild to moderate *dementia* due to *Alzheimer's disease*, in which there is a deficiency of the neurotransmitter *acetylcholine* in the brain. Drugs such as *donepezil* and *rivastigmine* work by

ACCOMMODATION

Light rays from near object

Point of focus

Ciliary muscle

Rounded lens bends the light

NEAR FOCUS

Light rays from distant object

Point of focus

Ciliary muscle

Flattened lens

DISTANT FOCUS

blocking the action of acetylcholinesterase, the enzyme in the brain responsible for the breakdown of acetylcholine. This raises acetylcholine levels, and, in half of all patients, the drugs slow the rate of progression of dementia. They have no effect on dementia due to other causes, such as stroke or head injury, however. Common side effects include nausea, diarrhoea, dizziness, and headache. Rarely, difficulty in passing urine may occur. Those taking acetylcholinesterase inhibitors require regular medical monitoring.

acetylcysteine A drug used in the treatment of *paracetamol* overdose. When the drug is taken in large doses, vomiting or rash may occur as rare side effects.

achalasia A rare condition of unknown cause in which the muscles at the lower end of the *oesophagus* and the sphincter (valve) between the oesophagus and the stomach fail to relax to let food into the stomach after swallowing. As a result, the lowest part of the oesophagus is narrowed and becomes blocked with food, while the part above widens. Symptoms include difficulty and pain with swallowing and pain in the lower chest and upper abdomen.

A barium swallow (a type of *barium X-ray examination*) and *gastroscopy* may be performed to investigate achalasia. *Oesophageal dilatation* allows the oesophagus to be widened for long periods. Surgery to cut some of the muscles at the stomach entrance may be necessary.

ACHILLES TENDON

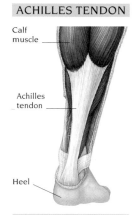

Calf muscle

Achilles tendon

Heel

Achilles tendon The tendon that raises the heel. The Achilles tendon is formed from the calf muscles (gastrocnemius, soleus, and plantar muscles) and is attached to the *calcaneus* (heel-bone). Minor injuries to this tendon are common and can result in inflammation (*tendinitis*). Violent stretching of the tendon can cause it to rupture; in such cases, surgical repair may be necessary.

achlorhydria Absence of stomach acid secretions. This may be due to chronic atrophic *gastritis* or to an absence or malfunction of acid-producing parietal cells in the stomach lining. Achlorhydria may not produce symptoms but is associated with *stomach cancer*, however, and is a feature of pernicious anaemia (see *anaemia, megaloblastic*).

achondroplasia A rare genetic disorder of bone growth that leads to *short stature*. The condition is caused by a dominant gene (see *genetic disorders*) but often arises as a new *mutation*. The long bones of the arms and legs are affected mainly. The cartilage that links each bone to its epiphysis (the growing area at its tip) is converted to bone too early, preventing further limb growth. Those affected have short limbs, a well-developed trunk, and a head of normal size except for a protruding forehead.

aciclovir An *antiviral drug* that can be taken by mouth, used topically, or given intravenously to reduce the severity of viral infections including *herpes simplex* and *herpes zoster*. Local adverse reactions commonly occur after topical use. Other side effects are uncommon but can include nausea and vomiting.

acid A substance defined as a donor of hydrogen ions (hydrogen atoms with positive electrical charges). Acid molecules, when mixed with or dissolved in water, split up to release their constituent ions; all acids release hydrogen as the positive ion. (See also *acid–base balance*; *alkali*.)

acid–base balance A combination of mechanisms that ensures that the body's fluids are neither too *acid* nor too alkaline (*alkalis* are also called bases).

The body has three mechanisms for maintaining normal acid–base balance: buffers, breathing, and the activities of the kidneys. Buffers are substances in the blood that neutralize acid or alkaline wastes. Rapid breathing results in the blood becoming less acidic; slow breathing has the opposite effect. The kidneys regulate the amounts of acid or alkaline wastes in the urine.

Disturbances of the body's acid–base balance result in either *acidosis* (excessive blood acidity) or *alkalosis* (excessive blood alkalinity).

acidosis A disturbance of the body's *acid–base balance* in which there is an accumulation of acid or loss of *alkali* (base). There are two types of acidosis: metabolic and respiratory.

One form of metabolic acidosis is ketoacidosis, which occurs in uncontrolled *diabetes mellitus* and starvation. Metabolic acidosis may also be caused by loss of bicarbonate (an alkali) as a result of severe diarrhoea. In *kidney failure*, there is insufficient excretion of acid in the urine.

Respiratory acidosis occurs if breathing fails to remove enough carbon dioxide from the lungs. The excess carbon dioxide remains in the bloodstream, where it dissolves to form carbonic acid. Impaired breathing leading to respiratory acidosis may be due to chronic obstructive pulmonary disease (see *pulmonary disease, chronic obstructive*), bronchial *asthma*, or *airway obstruction*.

acid reflux See *gastro-oesophageal reflux disease.*

acitretin A retinoid drug (see *vitamin A*) used to treat severe *psoriasis* and rare skin conditions such as *ichthyosis*. Possible side effects include headaches, skin problems such as blistering and *dermatitis*, and kidney damage. Acitretin should not be used during pregnancy because of the risk of damage to the fetus. Women should avoid becoming pregnant for at least a month before starting acitretin, while taking the drug, and for at least two years after stopping it.

acne A chronic skin disorder caused by inflammation of the hair follicles and sebaceous glands in the skin. The most common type is acne vulgaris, which almost always develops during puberty. However, acne can occur at any age.

Acne spots are caused by the obstruction of hair follicles by sebum (the oily substance secreted by the sebaceous glands). Bacteria multiply in the follicle, causing inflammation. The change in sebum secretion at puberty seems to be linked with increased levels of *androgen hormones* (male sex hormones).

Acne may be brought on or aggravated by drugs such as *corticosteroids* and *androgens*. Exposure to certain chemicals

and oils in the workplace can cause a type of acne. Heredity may also play a part in some cases.

Acne develops in areas of skin with a high concentration of sebaceous glands, mainly the face, chest, upper back, shoulders, and around the neck. Milia (whiteheads), comedones (blackheads), nodules (firm swellings beneath the skin), and cysts (larger, fluid-filled swellings) are the most commonly occurring spots. Some, particularly cysts, leave scars after they heal, which may cause emotional distress in some people.

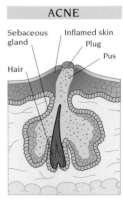

ACNE

Sebaceous gland
Inflamed skin
Plug
Pus
Hair

ACNE SPOT

There is no instant cure for acne, but washing the affected areas twice daily may help to keep it under control. Topical drug treatments, such as benzoyl peroxide or retinoic acid, unblock the pores and promote healing. If topical treatment has failed, oral drug treatment with *antibiotics*, hormones, or *isotretinoin* may be given. Acne improves slowly over time, often clearing up by the end of the teenage years. Any severe residual scarring may be treated by cosmetic surgery.

acoustic nerve The part of the *vestibulocochlear nerve* (the 8th *cranial nerve*) that is concerned with hearing. It is also known as the auditory nerve.

acoustic neuroma A rare, noncancerous tumour arising from supporting cells that surround the 8th cranial nerve (see *acoustic nerve*), usually within the internal auditory meatus (the canal in the skull through which the nerve passes from the inner ear to the brain). Usually, the cause of an acoustic neuroma is unknown. However, tumours that affect the nerves on both sides of the head simultaneously may be part of a condition known as *neurofibromatosis*. Acoustic neuroma can cause *deafness, tinnitus,* loss of balance, and pain in the face and the affected ear.

Diagnosis is made by *hearing tests* followed by *X-rays, CT scanning,* or *MRI*. Surgery may be needed, but treatment with radiotherapy to shrink the tumour is also effective.

acrocyanosis A circulatory disorder in which the hands and feet turn blue, may become cold, and sweat excessively. It is caused by spasm of the small blood vessels and is often aggravated by cold weather. It is related to *Raynaud's disease*.

acrodermatitis enteropathica A rare inherited disorder in which areas of the skin (most commonly the fingers, toes, scalp, and the areas around the anus and mouth) are reddened, ulcerated, and covered with *pustules*. The disorder is due to an inability to absorb enough zinc from food. Zinc supplements usually help.

acromegaly A rare disease characterized by abnormal enlargement of the skull, jaw, hands, feet, and also of the internal organs. It is caused by excessive secretion of *growth hormone* from the anterior pituitary gland at the base of the brain and is the result of a *pituitary tumour*. A tumour that develops before puberty results in *gigantism*. Acromegaly is diagnosed by measuring blood levels of growth hormone, followed by *CT scanning* or *MRI*.

acromioclavicular joint The joint that lies between the outer end of the *clavicle* (collarbone) and the acromion (the bony prominence at the top of the *scapula* (shoulderblade).

ACROMIOCLAVICULAR JOINT

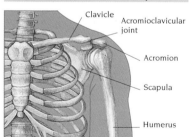

Clavicle
Acromioclavicular joint
Acromion
Scapula
Humerus

acromion A bony prominence at the top of the *scapula* (shoulderblade). The acromion articulates with the end of the *clavicle* (collarbone) to form the *acromioclavicular joint*.

acroparaesthesia A medical term used to describe tingling in the fingers or toes (see *pins-and-needles*).

ACTH The common abbreviation for adrenocorticotrophic hormone (also called corticotrophin). ACTH is produced by the anterior *pituitary gland* and stimulates the adrenal cortex (outer layer of the *adrenal glands*) to release various *corticosteroid hormones*, most importantly *hydrocortisone* (cortisol) but also *aldosterone* and *androgen hormones*.

ACTH production is controlled by a feedback mechanism involving both the *hypothalamus* and the level of hydrocortisone in the blood. ACTH levels increase in response to stress, emotion, injury, infection, burns, surgery, and decreased blood pressure.

A tumour of the pituitary gland can cause excessive ACTH production which leads to overproduction of hydrocortisone by the adrenal cortex, resulting in *Cushing's syndrome*. Insufficient ACTH production results in decreased production of hydrocortisone, causing low blood pressure. Synthetic ACTH is occasionally given to treat *arthritis* or *allergy*.

actin A *protein* involved in *muscle* contraction, in which microscopic filaments of actin and another protein, myosin, slide in between each other.

acting out Impulsive actions that may reflect unconscious wishes. The term is most often used by psychotherapists to describe behaviour during analysis when the patient "acts out" rather than reports fantasies, wishes, or beliefs. Acting out can also occur as a reaction to frustrations encountered in everyday life, often taking the form of antisocial, aggressive behaviour.

actinic Pertaining to changes caused by the ultraviolet rays in sunlight, as in actinic *dermatitis* (inflammation of the skin) and actinic *keratosis* (roughness and thickening of the skin).

actinomycosis An infection caused by *ACTINOMYCES ISRAELII* or related actinomycete bacteria. The most common form of actinomycosis affects the jaw area. A painful swelling appears and pus discharges through small openings that develop in the skin. Another form of actinomycosis affects the pelvis in women, causing lower abdominal pain and bleeding between periods. This form was associated with a type of *IUD*, no longer in use, that did not contain copper. Rarely, forms of the disorder affect the appendix or lung. Actinomycosis is treated with *antibiotics*.

acuity, visual See *visual acuity.*

acupressure A derivative of *acupuncture* in which pressure is applied instead of needles.

acupuncture A branch of *Chinese medicine* in which needles are inserted into a patient's skin as therapy for various disorders or to induce anaesthesia.

Traditional Chinese medicine maintains that the chi (life-force) flows through the body along channels called meridians. A blockage in one or more of these meridians is thought to cause ill health. Acupuncturists aim to restore health by inserting needles at appropriate sites along the affected meridians. The needles are stimulated by rotation or by an electric current. Acupuncture has been used successfully as an anaesthetic for surgical procedures and to provide pain relief after operations and for chronic conditions.

acute A term often used to describe a disorder or symptom that develops suddenly. Acute conditions may or may not be severe, and they are usually of short duration. (See also *chronic.*)

Adam's apple A projection at the front of the neck, just beneath the skin, that is formed by a prominence on the thyroid cartilage, which is part of the *larynx* (voice box). The Adam's apple enlarges in males at puberty.

ADD The abbreviation for attention deficit disorder, more commonly known as *attention deficit hyperactivity disorder.*

addiction Dependence on, and craving for, a particular drug, for example alcohol, diazepam (a tranquillizer), or heroin. Reducing or stopping intake of the drug may lead to characteristic physiological or psychological symptoms (see *withdrawal syndrome*), such as tremor or anxiety. (See also *alcohol dependence; drug dependence.*)

Addison's disease A rare chronic disorder in which there is a deficiency of the corticosteroid hormones *hydrocortisone* and *aldosterone*, normally produced by the adrenal cortex (the outer part of the *adrenal glands*). Excessive amounts of *ACTH* are secreted by the pituitary gland in an attempt to increase output of the corticosteroid hormones. Secretion and activity of another hormone, melanocyte stimulating hormone (MSH), is also increased.

Addison's disease can be caused by any disease that destroys the adrenal cortices. The most common cause is an *autoimmune disorder* in which the immune system produces antibodies that attack the adrenal glands.

Symptoms generally develop gradually over months or years, and include tiredness, weakness, abdominal pain, and weight loss. Excess MSH may cause darkening of the skin in the creases of the palms, pressure areas of the body, and the mouth. Acute episodes, called Addisonian crises, brought on by infection, injury, or other stresses, can also occur. The symptoms of these include extreme muscle weakness, dehydration, *hypotension* (low blood pressure), confusion, and coma. *Hypoglycaemia* (low blood glucose) also occurs.

Life-long *corticosteroid drug* treatment is needed. Treatment of Addisonian crises involves rapid infusion of saline and glucose, and supplementary doses of corticosteroid hormones.

adduction Movement of a limb towards the central line of the body, or of a digit towards the axis of a limb. Muscles that carry out this movement are often called adductors. (See also *abduction.*)

adenitis Inflammation of *lymph nodes.* Cervical adenitis (swelling and tenderness of the lymph nodes in the neck) occurs in certain bacterial infections, especially *tonsillitis*, and glandular fever (see *infectious mononucleosis*). Mesenteric lymphadenitis is inflammation of the lymph nodes inside the abdomen and is usually caused by viral infection. Treatment of adenitis may include *analgesic drugs*, and *antibiotic drugs* if there is a bacterial infection.

adenocarcinoma The technical name for a *cancer* of a gland or glandular tissue, or for a cancer in which the cells form gland-like structures. An adenocarcinoma arises from epithelium (the layer of cells that lines the inside of organs). Cancers of the

A

colon, breast, pancreas, and kidney are usually adenocarcinomas, as are some cancers of the cervix, oesophagus, salivary glands, and other organs. (See also *breast cancer; colon, cancer of; kidney cancer; pancreas, cancer of.*)

adenoidectomy Surgical removal of the *adenoids*. An adenoidectomy is usually performed on a child with abnormally large adenoids that are causing recurrent infections of the middle ear or air sinuses. The operation may be performed together with *tonsillectomy*.

adenoids A mass of glandular tissue at the back of the nasal passage above the tonsils. The adenoids are made up of *lymph nodes*, which form part of the body's defences against upper respiratory tract infections; they tend to enlarge during early childhood, a time when such infections are common.

ADENOIDS

Adenoids

Nasal cavity

Opening of eustachian tube

Pharynx

Tongue

Tonsils

In most children, adenoids shrink after the age of about 5 years, disappearing altogether by puberty. In some children, however, they enlarge, causing a blocked nose and blocking the eustachian tubes, which connect the middle ear to the throat. This results in recurrent infections and deafness. Infections usually respond to *antibiotic drugs*, but if they recur frequently, adenoidectomy may be recommended.

adenoma A noncancerous tumour or cyst that resembles glandular tissue and arises from the epithelium (the layer of cells that lines the inside of organs). Adenomas of *endocrine glands* can cause excessive hormone production, leading to disease. For example,

pituitary gland adenomas can result in *acromegaly* or *Cushing's syndrome*.

adenomatosis An abnormal condition of glands in which they are affected either by *hyperplasia* (overgrowth) or the development of numerous *adenomas* (noncancerous tumours). Adenomatosis may simultaneously affect two or more different *endocrine glands*.

ADH The abbreviation for antidiuretic hormone (also called vasopressin), which is released from the posterior part of the *pituitary gland* and acts on the kidneys to increase their reabsorption of water into the blood. ADH reduces the amount of water lost in the urine and helps to control the body's overall water balance. ADH production is controlled by the *hypothalamus*. Various factors can affect ADH production and thus disturb the body's water balance, including drinking alcohol, the disorder *diabetes insipidus*, or a major operation.

ADHD The abbreviation for *attention deficit hyperactivity disorder*.

adhesion The joining of normally unconnected body parts by bands of fibrous tissue. Adhesions are sometimes present from birth, but they most often develop as a result of scarring after inflammation. Adhesions are most common in the abdomen, where they often form after *peritonitis* (inflammation of the abdominal lining) or surgery. Sometimes, loops of intestine are bound together by adhesions, causing intestinal obstruction (see *intestine, obstruction of*). In such cases, surgery is usually required to cut the bands of tissue.

adipose tissue A layer of fat just beneath the skin and around various internal organs. Adipose tissue is built up from fat deposited as a result of excess food intake, thus acting as an energy store; excessive amounts of adipose tissue produce *obesity*. The tissue insulates against loss of body heat and helps absorb shock in areas subject to sudden or frequent pressure, such as the buttocks or feet.

In men, superficial adipose tissue accumulates around the shoulders, waist, and abdomen; in women, it occurs on the breasts, hips, and thighs.

adjuvant A substance that enhances the action of another substance in the body.

The term is usually used to describe an ingredient added to a *vaccine* to increase the production of antibodies by the immune system, thus enhancing the vaccine's effect. Adjuvant chemotherapy is the use of *anticancer drugs* in addition to surgical removal of a tumour.

Adlerian theory The psychoanalytical ideas set forth by the Austrian psychiatrist Alfred Adler. Also called individual psychology, Adler's theories were based on the idea that everyone is born with feelings of inferiority. Life is seen as a constant struggle to overcome these feelings; failure to do so leads to neurosis. (See also *psychoanalytic theory*.)

adolescence The period between childhood and adulthood, which broadly corresponds to the teenage years. Adolescence commences and overlaps with, but is not the same as, *puberty*.

ADP The abbreviation for adenosine diphosphate, the chemical that takes up energy released during biochemical reactions to form *ATP* (adenosine triphosphate), the body's main energy-carrying chemical. When ATP releases its energy, ADP is reformed. (See also *metabolism*.)

adrenal failure Insufficient production of hormones by the adrenal cortex (the outer part of the *adrenal glands*). It can be acute or chronic. Adrenal failure may be caused by a disorder of the adrenal glands, in which case it is called *Addison's disease*, or by reduced stimulation of the adrenal cortex by *ACTH*, a hormone produced by the *pituitary gland*.

adrenal glands A pair of small, triangular *endocrine glands* located above the kidneys. Each adrenal gland has two distinct parts: the outer cortex and the smaller, inner medulla.

The cortex secretes *aldosterone*, which, together with hydrocortisone and corticosterone and small amounts of *androgen hormones* helps to maintain blood pressure. Hydrocortisone controls the body's use of fats, proteins, and carbohydrates and is also important in helping the body to cope with stress. Hydrocortisone and corticosterone also suppress inflammatory reactions and some activities of the *immune system*. Production of adrenal cortical hormones is controlled by *ACTH*, which is produced in the pituitary gland.

The adrenal medulla is part of the sympathetic *autonomic nervous system*. In response to stress, it secretes the hormones *adrenaline* (epinephrine) and *noradrenaline* (norepinephrine), which increase heart-rate and blood flow.

ADRENAL GLANDS

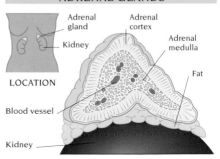

LOCATION

STRUCTURE OF ADRENAL GLAND

adrenal gland disorders A range of uncommon but sometimes serious disorders due to deficient or excessive production of hormones by one or both of the *adrenal glands*.

A genetic defect causes congenital *adrenal hyperplasia*, in which the adrenal cortex is unable to make sufficient hydrocortisone and *aldosterone*, and *androgens* are produced in excess. In *adrenal failure*, there is also deficient production of hormones by the adrenal cortex; if due to disease of the adrenal glands, it is called *Addison's disease*. *Adrenal tumours* are rare and generally lead to excess hormone production.

In many cases, disturbed activity of the adrenal glands is caused, not by disease of the glands themselves, but by an increase or decrease in the blood level of hormones that influence the action of the adrenal glands. For example, hydrocortisone production by the adrenal cortex is controlled by *ACTH*, which is secreted by the pituitary gland. Pituitary disorders can disrupt production of hydrocortisone.

adrenal hyperplasia, congenital An uncommon *genetic disorder* in which an *enzyme* defect blocks the production of corticosteroid hormones from the adrenal glands. Excessive amounts of *androgens* (male sex hormones) are produced, which can result in abnormal genital development in an affected fetus.

Other effects include dehydration, weight loss, low blood pressure, and *hypoglycaemia*. Hyperplasia (enlargement) of the adrenal glands occurs and there is excessive skin pigmentation in skin creases and around the nipples.

In severe cases, the disorder is apparent soon after birth. In milder cases, symptoms appear later, sometimes producing premature puberty in boys and delayed menstruation, *hirsutism*, and potential infertility in girls.

Congenital adrenal hyperplasia is confirmed by measuring corticosteroid hormones in blood and urine. Treatment is by hormone replacement. If this is started early, normal sexual development and fertility usually follow.

adrenaline A hormone, also called epinephrine, released by the adrenal glands in response to signals from the sympathetic *autonomic nervous system*. These signals are triggered by stress, exercise, or by an emotion such as fear.

Adrenaline increases the speed and force of the heartbeat. It widens the airways to improve breathing and narrows blood vessels in the skin and intestine so that an increased flow of blood reaches the muscles.

Synthetic adrenaline is sometimes given by injection as an emergency treatment for *cardiac arrest* or *anaphylactic shock*. Adrenaline eye drops may be used to treat *glaucoma*, but regular use can cause a burning pain in the eye.

adrenal tumours Cancerous or noncancerous tumours in the *adrenal glands*, usually causing excess secretion of hormones. Adrenal tumours are rare. Tumours of the adrenal cortex may secrete *aldosterone*, causing primary *aldosteronism*, or hydrocortisone, causing *Cushing's syndrome*. Tumours of the *medulla* may cause excess secretion of *adrenaline* and *noradrenaline*. Two types of tumour affect the medulla: *phaeochromocytoma* and *neuroblastoma*, which affects children. These tumours cause intermittent *hypertension* and sweating attacks. Surgical removal of a tumour usually cures these conditions.

adrenocorticotrophic hormone See *ACTH*.

adrenogenital syndrome See *adrenal hyperplasia, congenital*.

aerobic Requiring oxygen to live, function, and grow. Humans and many other forms of life are dependent on oxygen for "burning" foods to produce energy (see *metabolism*). In contrast, many bacteria thrive without oxygen and are described as *anaerobic*.

aerobics Exercises, such as swimming and cycling, that allow muscles to work at a steady rate with a constant, adequate supply of oxygen-carrying blood, and that can therefore be sustained for long periods. Oxygen is used to release energy from the body's stores. To fuel aerobic exercise, the muscles use fatty acid, burning it completely to produce energy, carbon dioxide, and water.

When performed regularly, aerobic exercises improve stamina and endurance. They encourage the growth of capillaries, improving blood supply to the cells. Aerobic exercises also improve body cells' capacity to use oxygen and increase the amount of oxygen the body can use in a given time. The condition of the heart also improves. (See also *exercise; fitness*).

aerodontalgia Sudden pain in a tooth brought on by a change in surrounding air pressure. Flying at a high altitude in a lowered atmospheric pressure can cause a pocket of air in the dental pulp to expand and irritate the nerve in the root. Aerodontalgia is more likely if there are improperly fitting fillings or poorly filled root canals.

aerophagy Excessive swallowing of air, which may occur during rapid eating or drinking or be caused by anxiety.

aetiology The cause of a disease or the study of the various factors involved in causing a disease.

affect A term used to describe a person's mood. The two extremes of affect are elation and depression. A person who has extreme moods or changes in moods may have an *affective disorder*. Shallow or reduced affect may be a sign of *schizophrenia* or of an organic *brain syndrome*.

affective disorders Mental illnesses characterized predominantly by marked changes in *affect*. Mood may vary over a period of time between *mania* (extreme elation) and severe *depression*. (See also *bipolar disorder*.)

affinity A term used to describe the attraction between chemicals that causes them to bind together, as, for example, between an antigen and an antibody (see *immune response*). In microbiology, affinity describes physical similarity between organisms. In psychology, it refers to attraction between two people.

aflatoxin A poisonous substance produced by ASPERGILLUS FLAVUS moulds, which contaminate stored foods, especially grains, peanuts, and cassava. Aflatoxin is believed to be one of the factors responsible for the high incidence of liver cancer in tropical Africa.

afterbirth The common name for the tissues that are expelled from the uterus after delivery of a baby. The afterbirth includes the *placenta* and the membranes that surrounded the fetus.

afterpains Contractions of the uterus that continue after childbirth. Afterpains are normal and are experienced by many women, especially during breast-feeding. They usually disappear a few days following the birth but may require treatment with *analgesic drugs*.

agammaglobulinaemia A type of *immunodeficiency disorder* in which there is almost complete absence of *B-lymphocytes* and *immunoglobulins* in the blood.

agar An extract of certain seaweeds with similar properties to gelatine. It is used as a gelling agent in media for bacterial *cultures*.

age The length of time a person has existed. Of medical significance in diagnosis and in deciding treatment, a person's age is usually measured chronologically, but can also be measured in terms of physical, mental, or developmental maturity.

The age of a fetus is measured in terms of gestational age, which can be assessed accurately by *ultrasound scanning*. In children, the most useful measure of physical development is bone age (degree of bone maturity as seen on an *X-ray*) because all healthy individuals reach the same adult level of skeletal maturity, and each bone passes through the same sequence of growth. Dental age, another measure of

physical maturity, can be assessed by the number of teeth that have erupted (see *eruption of teeth*) or by the amount of dental calcification (as seen on an X-ray) compared with standard values.

In adults, physical age is difficult to assess other than by physical appearance. It can be estimated after death by the state of certain organs.

Mental age can be assessed by comparing scores on *intelligence tests* with standards for chronological age. A young child's age can be expressed in terms of the level of developmental skills, manual dexterity, language, and social skills.

agenesis The complete absence at birth of an organ or bodily component, caused by failure of development in the embryo.

agent Any substance or force capable of bringing about a biological, chemical, or physical change. (See also *reagent*.)

Agent Orange A herbicide of which the major constituent is the phenoxy acid herbicide 2,4,5 T. This substance may be contaminated in manufacture with the highly toxic TCDD, commonly known as dioxin (see *defoliant poisoning*).

age spots Blemishes that appear on the skin with increasing age. Most common are seborrhoeic *keratoses*, which are brown or yellow, slightly raised spots that can occur at any site. Also common in elderly people are freckles, solar keratoses (small blemishes caused by overexposure to the sun), and *De Morgan's spots*, which are red, pinpoint blemishes on the trunk. Treatment is usually unnecessary for any of these, apart from solar keratoses, which may eventually progress to skin cancer.

ageusia The lack or an impairment of the sense of taste (see *taste, loss of*).

aggregation, platelet The clumping together of platelets (small, sticky blood particles). Aggregation is the first stage of *blood clotting* and helps to plug injured vessels. Inappropriate aggregation can have adverse effects; for example, if aggregation occurs in an artery, it may result in a *thrombosis*.

aggression A general term for a wide variety of acts of hostility. A number of factors, including human evolutionary survival strategies, are thought to be involved in aggression. *Androgen* *hormones*, the male sex hormones, seem to promote aggression, whereas *oestrogen hormones*, the female sex hormones, actively suppress it. Age is another factor; aggression is more common among teenagers and young adults. Sometimes, a brain tumour or head injury leads to aggressive behaviour.

Psychiatric conditions associated with aggressive outbursts are *schizophrenia*, *antisocial personality disorder*, *mania*, and abuse of amphetamines or alcohol. *Temporal lobe epilepsy*, *hypoglycaemia*, and *confusion* due to physical illnesses are other, less common, medical causes.

aging The physical and mental changes that occur with the passing of time. Aging is associated with degenerative changes in various organs and tissues, such as loss of elasticity in the skin and a progressive decline in organ function. Mechanical wear and tear causes cumulative damage to the joints, and the muscles lose bulk and strength. Wound healing and resistance to infection also decline. Gradual loss of nerve cells can lead to reduced sensory acuity and difficulties with learning and memory. However, *dementia* occurs in only a minority of elderly people.

Heredity is an important determinant of life expectancy, but physical degeneration may be accelerated by factors such as smoking, excessive alcohol intake, poor diet, and insufficient exercise.

agitation Restless inability to keep still, usually as a result of anxiety or tension. Agitated people engage in aimless, repetitive behaviour, such as pacing up and down or wringing their hands, and they often start tasks without completing them. Persistent agitation is seen in *anxiety disorders*, especially if there is an underlying physical cause such as alcohol withdrawal. *Depression* may be accompanied by agitation.

agnosia An inability to recognize objects despite adequate sensory information about them reaching the brain via the eyes or ears or through touch. Agnosia is caused by damage to areas of the brain that are involved in interpretative and recall functions. The most common causes of this kind of damage are *stroke* or *head injury*.

Agnosia is usually associated with just one of the senses of vision, hearing, or touch and is described as visual, auditory, or tactile respectively. Some people, after a stroke that damages the right cerebral hemisphere, seem unaware of any disability in their affected left limbs. This is called anosognosia or sensory inattention. There is no specific treatment for agnosia, but some interpretative ability may return eventually.

agonist Having a stimulating effect. An agonist drug, sometimes known as an activator, is one that binds to a sensory nerve cell (*receptor*) and triggers or increases a particular activity in that cell.

agoraphobia Fear of going into open spaces or public places. Agoraphobia (see *phobia*) may occur with *claustrophobia*. If sufferers do venture out, they may have a *panic attack*, which may lead to further restriction of activities. People with agoraphobia may eventually become housebound. Treatment with *behaviour therapy* is usually successful. *Antidepressant drugs* may be helpful.

agraphia Loss of, or impaired, ability to write, despite normal functioning of the hand and arm muscles, caused by brain damage. Agraphia can result from damage to any of the various parts of the *cerebrum* concerned with writing and can therefore be of different types and degrees of severity. Such damage is most commonly due to *head injury*, *stroke*, or a *brain tumour*. Agraphia is often accompanied by *alexia* (loss of the ability to read) or may be part of an expressive *aphasia* (general disturbance in the expression of language). There is no specific treatment for agraphia, but some lost writing skills may return in time.

AIDS Acquired immune deficiency syndrome, a deficiency of the *immune system* due to infection with *HIV* (human immunodeficiency virus). In most countries, illness and death from AIDS is a major health problem, and there is, as yet, no cure or vaccine.

AIDS does not develop in all people infected with HIV. The interval between infection and the development of AIDS is highly variable. Without treatment, around half of those people infected will develop AIDS within 8–9 years.

HIV is transmitted in body fluids, including semen, blood, vaginal secretions, and breast milk. The major methods of transmission are sexual contact (vaginal, anal, or oral), blood to blood (via transfusions or needle-sharing in drug users), and mother to fetus. HIV has also been transmitted through blood products given to treat *haemophilia*, artificial insemination by donated semen, and kidney transplants; but improved screening has greatly reduced these risks. HIV is not spread by everyday contact, such as hugging or sharing crockery.

The virus enters the bloodstream and infects cells that have a particular receptor, known as the CD4 receptor, on their surface. These cells include a type of white blood cell (a CD4 lymphocyte) responsible for fighting infection, and cells in other tissues such as the brain. The virus reproduces within the infected cells, which then die, releasing more virus particles into the blood. If the infection is left untreated, the number of CD4 lymphocytes falls, resulting in greater susceptibility to certain infections and some types of cancer.

Some people experience a short-lived illness similar to infectious *mononucleosis* when they are first infected with HIV. Many individuals have no obvious symptoms (but are still infectious); some have only vague complaints, such as weight loss, fevers, sweats, or unexplained diarrhoea, known as AIDS-related complex.

Minor features of HIV infection include skin disorders such as seborrhoeic *dermatitis*. More severe features include persistent *herpes simplex* infections, oral *candidiasis* (thrush), *shingles*, *tuberculosis*, and *shigellosis*. HIV may also affect the brain, causing a variety of neurological disorders, including *dementia*.

AIDS-defining illnesses are conditions typical of full-blown AIDS. These include cancers (*Kaposi's sarcoma* and lymphoma of the brain), and various infections (*pneumocystis pneumonia*, tuberculosis, *human papillomavirus, cytomegalovirus* infection, *toxoplasmosis*, diarrhoea due to *CRYPTOSPORIDIUM* or *ISOSPORA*, candidiasis, disseminated *strongyloidiasis*, and *cryptococcosis*), many of which are described as *opportunistic infections*.

Confirmation of HIV infection involves testing a blood sample for the presence of antibodies to HIV. Diagnosis of full-blown AIDS is based on a positive HIV test along with the presence of an AIDS-defining illness or a reduced CD4 count.

The risk of infection with HIV can be reduced by practising *safer sex*. Intravenous drug users should not share needles. There is a small risk to health workers handling infected blood products or needles, but this risk can be minimized by safe practices.

Treatment of HIV infection with a combination of antiviral drugs can slow the disease's progress, and may prevent the development of full-blown AIDS by reducing the amount of virus in the bloodstream. The two main types of antiviral drug used are *protease inhibitors*, such as indinavir, and *reverse transcriptase inhibitors* such as zidovudine. Other drugs, such as tenofovir and nevirapine, may be given in addition to protease inhibitors and reverse transcriptase inhibitors to prevent viral replication. The emergence of resistant strains of HIV has led to the development of fusion inhibitor drugs, such as enfuvirtide, which prevent the virus from infecting cells. Treatment is also available for AIDS-defining illnesses.

AIDS-related complex A combination of weight loss, fever, and enlarged lymph nodes in a person who has been infected with *HIV* (the *AIDS* virus), but does not have AIDS itself. Many people with AIDS-related complex will eventually develop the features of AIDS.

air The colourless, odourless mixture of gases that forms the Earth's atmosphere. Air consists of 78 per cent *nitrogen*, 21 per cent *oxygen*, small quantities of *carbon dioxide* and other gases, and some water vapour.

air conditioning A system that controls the purity, humidity, and temperature of the air in a building. Contaminated air conditioning systems may cause *legionnaires' disease* and humidifier fever (a lung disease causing coughing and breathing difficulty).

air embolism Blockage of a small artery by an air bubble carried in the blood. Air embolism is rare. In most cases, it is caused by air entering the circulation through a vein, either due to injury or surgery. Air embolism can also occur during diving or air travel accidents, in which lung tissue ruptures, releasing bubbles into the bloodstream.

air pollution See *pollution*.

air swallowing See *aerophagy*.

airway A collective term for the passages through which air enters and leaves the lungs (see *respiratory system*). The term is also applied to a tube inserted into the mouth of an unconscious person to prevent the tongue from obstructing breathing.

airway obstruction Narrowing or blockage of the respiratory passages. The obstruction may be due to a foreign body, such as a piece of food, that becomes lodged in part of the upper airway and may result in *choking*. Certain disorders, such as *diphtheria* and *lung cancer*, can cause obstruction. Additionally, spasm of the muscular walls of the airway, as occurs in *bronchospasm* (a feature of *asthma*), results in *breathing difficulty*.

akathisia An inability to sit still, occasionally occurring as a side effect of an *antipsychotic drug* or, less commonly, as a complication of *Parkinson's disease*.

akinesia Complete or almost complete loss of movement. It may be a result of damage to part of the brain due, for example, to a *stroke* or *Parkinson's disease*.

albinism A rare *genetic disorder* characterized by a lack of the pigment *melanin*, which gives colour to the skin, hair, and eyes. In oculocutaneous albinism (the most common type), the hair, skin, and eyes are all affected. Less often, only the eyes are affected. In both forms, skin cannot tan and ages prematurely, and *skin cancers* may develop on areas exposed to the sun. Visual problems of people with albinism include *photophobia*, *nystagmus*, *squint*, and *myopia*. Glasses are usually needed from an early age; and tinted glasses help to reduce photophobia.

albumin The most abundant protein in the *blood* plasma. Albumin is made in the liver from amino acids. It helps to retain substances (such as calcium, some hormones, and certain drugs) in the circulation by binding to them to prevent them from being filtered out by

the kidneys and excreted. Albumin also regulates the movement of water between tissues and the bloodstream by *osmosis*. (See also *albuminuria*.)

albuminuria The presence of the protein *albumin* in the urine; a type of *proteinuria*. Normally, the glomeruli (the filtering units of the kidneys) do not allow albumin to pass into the urine Albuminuria therefore usually indicates that there is damage to the kidneys' filtering mechanisms. Such damage may be due to a kidney disorder, such as *glomerulonephritis* or *nephrotic syndrome*, or may be a sign that the kidneys have been affected by *hypertension*. Albuminuria can be detected by a simple urine test.

alcohol A colourless liquid produced from the fermentation of carbohydrates by yeast. Also known as ethanol, alcohol is the active constituent of drinks such as beer and wine. In medicine, it is used as an antiseptic and solvent. *Methanol* is a related, highly toxic substance.

Alcohol is a drug and produces a wide range of mental and physical effects. The effect of alcohol on the *central nervous system* is as a depressant, decreasing its activity and thereby reducing anxiety, tension, and inhibitions. In moderate amounts, alcohol produces a feeling of relaxation, confidence, and sociability. However, alcohol slows reactions, and the more that is drunk, the greater is the impairment of concentration and judgement. Excessive consumption of alcohol results in poisoning or acute *alcohol intoxication*, with effects ranging from euphoria to unconsciousness.

Short-term physical effects of alcohol include peripheral *vasodilation* (widening of the small blood vessels), which causes the face to flush, and increased flow of gastric juices, which stimulates the appetite. Alcohol increases sexual confidence, but high levels can cause *erectile dysfunction*. Alcohol also acts as a diuretic, increasing urine output.

In the long term, regular excessive alcohol consumption can cause *gastritis* (inflammation and ulceration of the stomach lining), and lead to *alcohol-related disorders*. Binge drinking can cause similar problems. Heavy drinking in the long term may also lead to *alcohol dependence*. However, people who drink regular, small amounts of alcohol (an average of 1–2 units a day) seem to have lower rates of *coronary heart disease* and *stroke* than total abstainers. The recommended upper limit is 3–4 units a day for men and 2–3 units a day for women. (A unit is half a pint of beer, a small glass of wine, or a single measure of spirits.)

alcohol dependence An illness characterized by habitual, compulsive, long-term, heavy consumption of alcohol and the development of withdrawal symptoms when drinking is suddenly stopped.

Three causative factors interact in the development of the illness: personality, environment, and the addictive nature of alcohol. Environmental factors are important, especially the ready availability, affordability, and social acceptance of alcohol. Genetic factors may play a part in causing dependence in some cases, but it is now widely believed that anyone, irrespective of personality, environment, or genetic background, can become an alcoholic. Stress is often a major factor in precipitating heavy drinking.

Behavioural symptoms of alcohol dependence are varied and can include furtive, aggressive, or grandiose behaviour; personality changes (such as irritability, jealousy, or uncontrolled anger); neglect of food intake and personal appearance; and lengthy periods of intoxication.

Physical symptoms may include nausea, vomiting, or shaking in the morning; abdominal pain; cramps; numbness or tingling; weakness in the legs and hands; irregular pulse; enlarged blood vessels in the face; unsteadiness; confusion; memory lapses; and incontinence. After sudden withdrawal from alcohol, *delirium tremens* may occur.

Alcohol-dependent persons are more susceptible than others to a variety of physical and mental disorders (see *alcohol-related disorders*).

Many alcoholics require detoxification followed by long-term treatment. Different methods of treatment may be combined. Psychological treatments involve *psychotherapy* and are commonly carried out as *group therapy*. Social treatments may offer practical help and tend to include family members in the process. Physical treatment generally includes the use of disulfiram, a drug that sensitizes the drinker to alcohol so that he or she experiences unpleasant side effects when drinking. Other treatments may include *benzodiazepine drugs* to help control withdrawal symptoms and vitamins to treat any deficiency. *Acamprosate* may also be given to help maintain abstinence. *Alcoholics Anonymous* and other self-help organizations can provide support and advice.

Alcoholics Anonymous A worldwide, independent, self-help organization that is operated locally by people working on a voluntary basis to overcome *alcohol dependence*. Regular group meetings are held in which members are encouraged to help one another stay sober by sharing their experiences openly and offering support and advice.

alcohol intoxication The condition that results from consuming an excessive amount of *alcohol*, often over a relatively short period. The effects of a large alcohol intake depend on many factors, including physical and mental state, body size, social situation, and acquired tolerance. The important factor, however, is the blood alcohol level. Mild intoxication promotes relaxation and increases social confidence. Alcohol causes acute poisoning if taken in sufficiently large amounts, however. It depresses the activity of the *central nervous system*, leading to loss of normal mental and physical control. In extreme cases, intoxication may lead to loss of consciousness and even death.

In most cases, recovery from alcohol intoxication takes place naturally as the alcohol is gradually broken down in the liver. Medical attention is required if the intoxication has resulted in coma. For the chronic mental, physical, and social effects of long-term heavy drinking, see *alcohol dependence* and *alcohol-related disorders*.

alcoholism See *alcohol dependence*.

alcohol-related disorders A wide variety of physical and mental disorders associated with heavy, prolonged consumption of alcohol.

High alcohol consumption increases the risk of cancers of the mouth, tongue, pharynx (throat), larynx (voice box), and oesophagus, especially if combined with smoking. Incidence of *liver cancer*, as well as the liver diseases alcoholic *hepatitis* and *cirrhosis*, is higher among alcoholics. High alcohol consumption increases the risk of *cardiomyopathy*, *hypertension*, *atrial fibrillation*, and *stroke*. Alcohol irritates the digestive tract and may cause *gastritis* and *pancreatitis*. Heavy drinking in pregnancy increases the risk of miscarriage and *fetal alcohol syndrome*. Alcoholics are more likely to suffer from *anxiety*, *depression*, and personality changes, and to develop *dementia*.

Many alcoholics have a poor diet and are prone to diseases caused by nutritional deficiency, particularly of thiamine (see *vitamin B complex*). Severe thiamine deficiency, called *beriberi*, disturbs nerve function, causing cramps, numbness, and weakness in the legs and hands. Its effects on the brain can cause confusion, disturbances of speech and gait, and eventual coma (see *Wernicke–Korsakoff syndrome*). Severe thiamine deficiency can also cause *heart failure*.

A prolonged high level of alcohol in the blood and tissues can disturb body chemistry, resulting in *hypoglycaemia* (reduced glucose in the blood) and *hyperlipidaemia* (increased fat in the blood). These may damage the heart, liver, blood vessels, and brain; irreversible damage may cause premature death.

aldosterone A hormone secreted by the adrenal cortex (the outer part of the *adrenal glands*). Aldosterone acts on the kidneys to regulate the concentrations of sodium and potassium in the blood and tissues and control blood pressure. Production of aldosterone is stimulated mainly by the action of *angiotensin* II, a chemical produced by a series of reactions involving the enzymes *renin* and *angiotensin-converting enzyme*. Aldosterone production is also stimulated by the action of *ACTH*, which is produced by the pituitary gland.

aldosteronism A disorder that results from the excessive production of the hormone *aldosterone* from one or both *adrenal glands*. Aldosteronism caused by an *adrenal tumour* is known as Conn's syndrome. Aldosteronism may also be caused by disorders, such as *heart failure* or liver damage, that reduce the flow of blood through the kidneys. Reduced blood flow through the kidneys leads to overproduction of *renin* and *angiotensin*, which, in turn, leads to excessive aldosterone production.

Symptoms are directly related to the actions of aldosterone. Too much sodium is retained in the body, leading to a rise in blood pressure, and excess potassium is lost in the urine. Low potassium causes tiredness and muscle weakness and impairs kidney function, leading to thirst and overproduction of urine.

Treatment in all cases includes restriction of dietary salt and use of the diuretic drug *spironolactone*. If the cause of aldosteronism is an adrenal tumour, this may be surgically removed.

alendronate sodium See *alendronic acid*.

alendronic acid A *bisphosphonate drug* used in the treatment of *osteoporosis* and *Paget's disease* of bone. The most common side effect is inflammation of the oesophagus, which causes heartburn or difficulty in swallowing. Other side effects can include headache and abdominal pain.

Alexander technique A therapy that aims to improve health by teaching people to stand and move more efficiently. It is based on the belief that bad patterns of body movement interfere with the proper functioning of the body and contribute to the development of disease.

alexia Word blindness; inability to recognize and name written words. Alexia is caused by damage to part of the cerebrum (the main mass of the brain) by a *stroke*, for example. It severely disrupts the reading ability of a person who was previously literate. (See also *dyslexia*.)

alienation Feeling like a stranger, even when among familiar people or places, and being unable to identify with a culture, family, or peer group. Alienation is common in adolescents and also occurs in people who are isolated by cultural or language differences. In some people, it may be an early symptom of *schizophrenia* or a *personality disorder*.

alignment, dental The movement of teeth by using either fixed or removable *orthodontic appliances* (braces) to correct *malocclusion* (incorrect bite).

alimemazine An *antihistamine drug*, also known as trimeprazine, that is used mainly to relieve itching in allergic conditions such as *urticaria* and atopic *eczema*. Alimemazine often causes drowsiness.

alimentary tract The tube-like structure that extends from the mouth to the anus (see *digestive system*).

alkali Also known as a base, an alkali is chemically defined as a donor of hydroxyl ions (each of which comprises an atom of hydrogen linked to an atom of oxygen and has an overall negative electrical charge). *Antacid drugs*, such as sodium bicarbonate, are alkalis. Some alkalis, such as sodium hydroxide, are corrosive. (See also *acid; acid–base balance*.)

alkaloids A group of nitrogen-containing substances obtained from plants. *Morphine, codeine, nicotine*, and strychnine (see *strychnine poisoning*) are examples.

alkalosis A disturbance of the body's *acid–base balance* in which there is an accumulation of alkali or a loss of acid. There are two types: metabolic and respiratory. In metabolic alkalosis, the increase in alkalinity may be caused by taking too much of an *antacid drug* or by losing a large amount of stomach acid as a result of severe vomiting. In respiratory alkalosis, there is a reduction in the blood level of carbonic acid (derived from carbon dioxide). This reduction is a consequence of *hyperventilation*, which may occur during a panic attack or at high altitudes due to lack of oxygen. (See also *acidosis*.)

alkylating agents A class of *anticancer drugs*.

allele One of two or more different forms of a gene that occupies a specific position on a *chromosome* (see *gene; inheritance*).

allergen A normally harmless substance that causes an allergic reaction (see *allergy*) in people who have become sensitized to it. Allergens can include foods (for example, nuts, eggs, and shellfish); inhaled substances such as pollen, house dust, and fur; and some drugs.

allergy Various conditions caused by inappropriate or exaggerated reactions of the *immune system* (known as hypersensitivity reactions) to a variety of substances. Many common illnesses, such as *asthma* and allergic *rhinitis* (hay fever), are caused by allergic reactions to substances that in the majority of people cause no symptoms.

Allergic reactions occur only on second or subsequent exposure to the *allergen*, once first contact has sensitized the body.

The function of the immune system is to recognize *antigens* (foreign proteins) on the surfaces of microorganisms and to form *antibodies* (also called immunoglobulins) and sensitized *lymphocytes* (white blood cells). When the immune system next encounters the same antigens, the antibodies and sensitized lymphocytes interact with them, leading to destruction of the microorganisms.

A similar immune response occurs in allergies, except that the immune system forms antibodies or sensitized lymphocytes against harmless substances because these *allergens* are misidentified as potentially harmful antigens.

The inappropriate or exaggerated reactions seen in allergies are termed *hypersensitivity* reactions and can have any of four different mechanisms (termed Types I to IV hypersensitivity reactions). Most well known allergies are caused by Type I (also known as anaphylactic or immediate) hypersensitivity in which allergens cause immediate symptoms by provoking the immune system to produce specific antibodies, belonging to a type called immunoglobulin E (IgE), which coat cells (called mast cells or basophils). When the allergen is encountered for

ALLERGY

TYPE I HYPERSENSITIVITY

the second time, it binds to the IgE antibodies and causes the granules in mast cells to release various chemicals, which are responsible for the symptoms of the allergy.

Among the chemicals released is histamine, which causes widened blood vessels, leakage of fluid into tissues, and muscle spasm. Symptoms can include itching, swelling, sneezing, and wheezing. Particular conditions associated with Type I reactions include asthma, hay fever, *urticaria* (nettle rash), *angioedema*, *anaphylactic shock* (a severe, generalized allergic reaction), possibly atopic *eczema*, and many food allergies.

Types II to IV reactions are less often implicated in allergies. However, contact dermatitis, in which the skin reacts to substances such as nickel, is due to a Type IV hypersensitivity reaction.

It is not known why certain individuals and not others get allergies, but about 1 in 8 people seem to have an inherited predisposition to them (see *atopy*).

Whenever possible, the most effective treatment for allergy of any kind is avoidance of the relevant allergen.

Drug treatment for allergic reactions includes the use of *antihistamine drugs*, which relieve the symptoms. Some antihistamine drugs have a sedative effect, which is useful in treating itching at night due to eczema. Many antihistamines do not cause drowsiness, making them more suitable for daytime use.

Other drugs, such as *sodium cromoglicate*, *montelukast*, and *corticosteroid drugs*, can be used regularly to prevent symptoms from developing.

Hyposensitization can be valuable for a minority of people who suffer allergic reactions to specific allergens such as bee stings. Treatment involves gradually increasing doses of the allergen, but must be carried out under close supervision because a severe allergic reaction can result.

allopathy The practice of conventional medicine. (See also *homeopathy*.)

allopurinol A drug treatment for *gout*. Taken long term, it reduces the frequency of attacks by decreasing production of *uric acid*. Possible adverse reactions include itching, rashes, and nausea.

alopecia Loss or absence of *hair*, which may occur at any hair-bearing site on the body but which is usually noticeable only on the scalp.

Male-pattern baldness, the most common form of alopecia, is hereditary and most often affects men. Normal hair is lost initially from the temples and crown and is replaced by fine, downy hair; the affected area gradually widens. Other hereditary forms are rare. They may be due to an absence of hair roots or abnormalities of the hair shaft.

In generalized alopecia, the hair falls out in large amounts. Causes include various forms of stress, such as surgery, prolonged illness, or childbirth. Many *anticancer drugs* cause temporary alopecia. The hair regrows when the underlying cause is corrected.

Localized alopecia may be due to permanent skin damage (for example, by burns or *radiotherapy*) or trauma to the hair roots by styling or, rarely, *trichotillomania*. The most common type of localized hair loss is alopecia areata, which is an *autoimmune disorder*. There is no specific treatment, but the hair usually regrows within a few months. Alopecia universalis is a rare, permanent form of alopecia areata that causes loss of all the hair on the scalp and body, including the eyelashes and eyebrows. Skin diseases such as scalp ringworm (see *tinea*), *lichen planus*, *lupus erythematosus*, and *skin tumours* may also cause localized hair loss.

Treatments for male-pattern baldness include hair transplants or drug treatments with *minoxidil* or *finasteride*.

alpha$_1$-antitrypsin deficiency A rare *genetic disorder* in which a person is missing the enzyme alpha$_1$-antitrypsin, which protects the body from damage by other enzymes. The disease mainly affects tissues in the lungs, resulting in *emphysema*, and the liver, causing *cirrhosis*. The effects of alpha$_1$-antitrypsin deficiency may not become apparent until after the age of 30. There is no cure, but symptoms can be relieved by drug treatment. In severe cases, a *liver transplant* may be a possibility.

alpha-blocker drugs A group of drugs used to treat *hypertension* (high blood pressure) and urinary symptoms due to enlargement of the *prostate gland*. Alpha-blockers are also used to treat urinary retention caused by an enlarged prostate gland (see *prostate, enlarged*). Side effects of the drugs may include dizziness and fatigue due to a sudden drop in blood pressure, nausea, dry mouth, and drowsiness.

alpha-fetoprotein A protein that is produced in the liver and gastrointestinal tract of the fetus and by some abnormal tissues in adults.

Alpha-fetoprotein (AFP) can be measured in the maternal blood from the latter part of the first trimester of pregnancy, and its concentration rises between the 15th and 20th weeks. Raised levels of AFP are associated with fetal *neural tube defects*, such as *spina bifida* or *anencephaly*, and certain kidney abnormalities. High levels of AFP also occur in multiple pregnancies (see *pregnancy, multiple*) and threatened or actual *miscarriage*. AFP levels may be unusually low if the fetus has *Down's syndrome*. For this reason, measurement of blood AFP is included in blood tests, which are used to screen pregnant women for an increased risk of Down's syndrome.

AFP levels are commonly raised in adults with hepatoma (see *liver cancer*), cancerous *teratoma* of the testes or ovaries, or, less commonly, cancer of the pancreas, stomach, or lung. For this reason, AFP is known as a tumour marker. AFP levels can be used to monitor the results of treatment of certain cancers; increasing levels after surgery or chemotherapy may indicate tumour recurrence. However, AFP levels are also raised in some noncancerous conditions, including viral and alcoholic *hepatitis* and *cirrhosis*.

alprazolam A *benzodiazepine drug* used in the treatment of *anxiety, panic attacks*, and *phobias*.

alprostadil A *prostaglandin drug* used, prior to surgery, to minimize the effects of congenital heart defects in newborn babies. Alprostadil is also used as a treatment for erectile dysfunction. It is administered by self-injection into the penis or as a gel introduced into the *urethra* to produce an erection.

alternative medicine Any medical system based on a theory of disease or method of treatment other than the orthodox science of Western medicine. (See also *complementary medicine*.)

altitude sickness See *mountain sickness*.

aluminium A light, metallic element found in bauxite and various other minerals. Aluminium compounds are used in *antacid* medications and in *antiperspirants*. Most of the aluminium taken into the body is excreted. Excessive amounts are toxic and are stored in the lungs, brain, liver, and thyroid gland, where they may result in organ damage.

Certain industrial processes give off fumes containing aluminium into the air. These fumes can cause *fibrosis* of lung tissue. Drugs containing aluminium may interfere with the absorption of other drugs and, therefore, should not be taken at the same time.

alveolectomy See *alveoloplasty*.

alveolitis Inflammation and thickening of the walls of the alveoli (tiny air sacs) in the lungs. Alveolitis reduces the elasticity, and therefore the efficiency, of the lungs. It is most commonly due to an allergic reaction to inhaled dust of animal or plant origin, as in *farmer's lung, bagassosis*, and pigeon fancier's lung (due to particles from bird droppings).

Fibrosing alveolitis is an *autoimmune disorder*. In some cases, it occurs with other autoimmune disorders such as *rheumatoid arthritis* or systemic *lupus erythematosus*. Radiation alveolitis is caused by irradiation of the lungs and may occur as a rare complication of *radiotherapy* for lung or breast cancer.

Alveolitis usually causes a dry cough and breathing difficulty on exertion. A chest X-ray, blood tests, *pulmonary function tests*, or a lung *biopsy* may be needed to diagnose alveolitis.

For most types of alveolitis, a short course of *corticosteroid drugs* relieves symptoms, but for fibrosing alveolitis these may need to be taken indefinitely. If the cause of allergic alveolitis is recognized and avoided before lung damage occurs, the effects are not permanent. In fibrosing alveolitis, damage progresses despite treatment, causing increasing breathing difficulty and, sometimes, *respiratory failure*.

alveoloplasty Dental surgery to remove protuberances and smooth out uneven areas from bone in the jaw before the fitting of dentures.

alveolus, dental The bony cavity or socket supporting each tooth in the jaw.

alveolus, pulmonary One of a large number of tiny, balloon-like sacs at the end of a bronchiole (one of many small air passages in the lungs) where gases are exchanged during *respiration*.

ALVEOLUS, PULMONARY

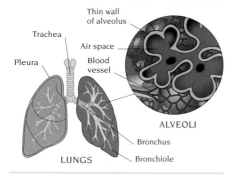

Thin wall of alveolus
Trachea
Air space
Pleura
Blood vessel
ALVEOLI
Bronchus
LUNGS
Bronchiole

Alzheimer's disease A progressive condition in which nerve cells in the brain degenerate and the brain shrinks. Alzheimer's disease is the most common cause of *dementia*. Onset is uncommon before the age of 60.

In most cases, Alzheimer's disease occurs without an identifiable cause. However, early onset Alzheimer's disease, in which symptoms develop before age 60, may rarely be inherited as a *dominant* disorder, and late onset Alzheimer's disease is sometimes associated with various genes, including three that are responsible for the production of the blood protein *apolipoprotein* E. These genes also result in the deposition of a protein called beta amyloid in the brain. Other chemical abnormalities may include deficiency of the *neurotransmitter* acetylcholine.

The features of Alzheimer's disease vary, but there are three broad stages. At first, the person becomes increasingly forgetful, and problems with memory may cause *anxiety* and *depression*. In the second stage, loss of memory, particularly for recent events, gradually becomes more severe, and there may be disorientation as to time or place. The person's concentration and numerical ability decline, and there is noticeable *dysphasia* (inability to find the right word). Anxiety increases, mood changes are unpredictable, and personality changes may occur. Finally, confusion becomes profound. There may be symptoms of *psychosis*, such as *hallucinations* and *delusions*. Signs of nervous system disease, such as abnormal *reflexes* and faecal or urinary *incontinence*, begin to develop.

Alzheimer's disease is usually diagnosed from the symptoms, but tests including blood tests and *CT scanning* or *MRI* of the brain may be needed to exclude treatable causes of dementia.

There is no cure for Alzheimer's disease. The most important aspect of treatment is the provision of suitable nursing and social care for sufferers and support for their relatives. *Tranquillizer drugs* can often improve difficult behaviour and help with sleep. Treatment with drugs such as *donepezil*, *rivastigmine*, and memantine may slow the progress of the disease for a time, but side effects such as nausea and dizziness may occur.

amalgam, dental A material, consisting of an alloy of mercury with other metals, that is used as fillings for teeth (see *filling, dental*).

amantadine An *antiviral drug* used in the prevention and treatment of *influenza* A and to help relieve symptoms of *Parkinson's disease*.

amaurosis fugax Brief loss of vision, lasting for seconds or minutes, usually affecting one eye and caused by the temporary blockage of a small blood vessel in the eye by *emboli* (particles of solid matter such as cholesterol or clotted blood). These are carried in the bloodstream from diseased arteries in the neck or, rarely, the heart. Attacks may be infrequent or they may occur many times a day. This symptom indicates an increased risk of *stroke* and requires medical investigation.

ambidexterity The ability to perform manual skills equally well with either hand because there is no definite *handedness*. Ambidexterity is an uncommon and often familial trait.

amblyopia A permanent defect of visual acuity in which there is usually no structural abnormality in the eye. In many cases, there is a disturbance of the visual pathway between the retina and the brain. The term is sometimes applied to toxic or nutritional causes of decreased visual acuity, as in tobacco-alcohol amblyopia.

Amblyopia will develop if there is a marked discrepancy between the images received by the brain from each eye while vision is developing during early childhood. The most common cause is *squint*. Failure to form normal retinal images may also result from congenital *cataract*, and severe, or unequal, focusing errors, such as when one eye is normal and there is an uncorrected large degree of *astigmatism* in the other. Toxic and nutritional amblyopia may result from damage to the retina and/or the optic nerve.

To prevent amblyopia due to squint, patching (covering up the good eye to force the deviating eye to function properly) is the usual treatment. Surgery to place the deviating eye in the correct position may be necessary. Glasses may be needed to correct severe focusing errors. Cataracts may be removed surgically. After the age of 8, amblyopia cannot usually be remedied.

ambulance A vehicle for transporting sick or injured people that is staffed by trained personnel who can provide emergency treatment during the journey.

ambulatory ECG In ambulatory ECG (*electrocardiography*), a wearable device called a *Holter monitor* is used to record the electrical activity of the heart by means of electrodes attached to the chest. The monitor is usually worn for 24 hours or longer and detects intermittent *arrhythmias* (abnormal heart rates and rhythms). The wearer can press a button on the monitor to mark the recording whenever symptoms occur. The recording can be analysed to see if the periods of arrhythmia coincide with the symptoms.

amelogenesis imperfecta An inherited condition of the teeth in which the enamel is either abnormally thin or is deficient in calcium. Affected teeth may be pitted and discoloured (see *discoloured teeth*) and more susceptible to dental *caries* (tooth decay) and wear

amenorrhoea The absence of menstrual periods. Primary amenorrhoea is defined as failure to start menstruating by the age of 16. Secondary amenorrhoea is the temporary or permanent cessation of periods in a woman who has menstruated regularly in the past.

The main cause of primary amenorrhoea is delayed *puberty*. The delay may not indicate a disorder, but, rarely, it may result from a disorder of the *endocrine system*, such as a *pituitary tumour*, *hypothyroidism*, an *adrenal tumour*, or *adrenal hyperplasia*. Another rare cause of delayed puberty is *Turner's syndrome*. In some cases, menstruation fails to take place because the vagina or the uterus has been absent from birth, or because there is no perforation in the hymen to allow blood to escape.

The most common cause of temporary secondary amenorrhoea is *pregnancy*. Periods may also cease temporarily after a woman has stopped taking *oral contraceptives*. Secondary amenorrhoea may also result from hormonal changes due to stress, *depression*, *anorexia nervosa*, or certain drugs. Another possible cause is a disorder of the ovary such as polycystic ovary (see *ovary, polycystic*) or an ovarian tumour. Amenorrhoea occurs permanently following the *menopause* or after a *hysterectomy*.

amfetamine drugs See *amphetamine drugs*.

amiloride A potassium-sparing *diuretic drug*. Combined with loop or thiazide diuretics, amiloride is used to treat *hypertension* and fluid retention due to *heart failure* or *cirrhosis* of the liver.

amino acids A group of chemical compounds that form the basic structural units of all *proteins*. Each amino acid molecule consists of amino and carboxyl groups of atoms linked to a variable chain or ring of carbon atoms.

Individual amino acid molecules are linked together by chemical bonds called *peptide* bonds to form short chains of molecules called *polypeptides*. Hundreds of polypeptides are, in turn, linked together, also by peptide bonds, to form a protein molecule. What differentiates one protein from another is the sequence of the amino acids.

There are 20 different amino acids that make up all the proteins in the body. Of these, 12 can be made by the body; they are known as nonessential amino acids because they do not need to be obtained from the diet. The other eight, known as the essential amino acids, cannot be made by the body and must therefore be obtained from the diet.

aminoglutethimide An *anticancer drug* used to treat certain types of breast cancer, prostate cancer, and some endocrine gland tumours.

aminoglycoside drugs A type of *antibiotic drug*. Aminoglycoside drugs are given by injection and are generally reserved for the treatment of serious infections because their use can damage the inner ear or kidneys. Important examples are *gentamicin* and *streptomycin*, which are also used topically for eye and ear infections.

aminophylline A bronchodilator drug used to treat chronic *bronchitis* and *asthma*. Nausea, vomiting, headache, dizziness, and palpitations are possible side effects.

amiodarone An *antiarrhythmic drug* used in the treatment of various types of *arrhythmia* (irregular heartbeat). Long-term use of amiodarone may result in inflammation of the liver, thyroid problems, and eye and lung damage.

amitriptyline A tricyclic *antidepressant drug* with a sedative effect. It is useful in the treatment of *depression* accompanied by *anxiety* or *insomnia*. Possible adverse effects include blurred vision, dizziness, and drowsiness.

amlodipine A *calcium channel blocker* drug used to prevent *angina* and to treat *hypertension*. Possible side effects are headaches and dizziness.

ammonia A colourless, pungent gas that dissolves in water to form ammonium hydroxide, an alkaline solution (see *alkali*). Ammonia is produced in the body and helps to maintain the *acid–base balance*. In severe liver damage, the ability of the liver to convert ammonia to *urea* is reduced. This leads to a high level of ammonia in the blood, which is thought to be a cause of the impaired consciousness that occurs in *liver failure*.

amnesia Loss of ability to memorize information and/or to recall information stored in *memory*. Possible causes of amnesia are *head injury*; degenerative disorders such as *Alzheimer's disease* and other forms of *dementia*; infections such as *encephalitis*; thiamine deficiency in alcoholics, leading to *Wernicke–Korsakoff syndrome*; *brain tumours*; *strokes*; and *subarachnoid haemorrhage*. Amnesia can also occur in some forms of psychiatric illness.

In retrograde amnesia, the loss of memory extends back for some time before the onset of the disorder. In anterograde amnesia, there is an inability to store new information in the period following the onset of illness.

amniocentesis A diagnostic procedure in which a small amount of *amniotic fluid* is withdrawn, using a syringe and guided by ultrasound scanning, from the *amniotic sac* that surrounds the *fetus* in the *uterus*. This fluid contains fetal cells that can be subjected to *chromosome analysis* to identify chromosomal defects such as *Down's syndrome* or genetic analysis to look for *genetic disorders* such as *haemophilia*, *cystic fibrosis*, and *Tay-Sachs disease*. Chemical analysis of amniotic

AMNIOCENTESIS

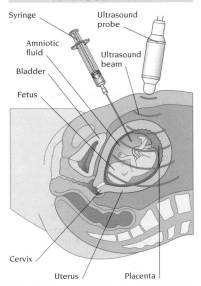

Syringe, Ultrasound probe, Amniotic fluid, Ultrasound beam, Bladder, Fetus, Cervix, Uterus, Placenta

fluid can help to diagnose developmental abnormalities such as *spina bifida*. *Rhesus incompatibility* and maturity of the fetal lungs can also be checked.

Amniocentesis is usually performed in the 15th–20th week of pregnancy. It slightly increases the risk of *miscarriage* or early rupture of the membranes and is therefore recommended only when the fetus is thought to be at increased risk of an abnormality. (See also *antenatal care*, *chorionic villus sampling*.)

amnion One of the membranes that surrounds the *fetus* in the *uterus*. The outside of the amnion is covered by another membrane called the *chorion*.

amniotic fluid The clear, watery fluid (popularly called the "waters") that surrounds the *fetus* in the *uterus*. The fluid is contained within the *amniotic sac*. It cushions the fetus, allowing movement.

Amniotic fluid is produced by cells lining the amniotic sac and is constantly circulated. It appears in the first week after conception and gradually increases in volume until the 10th week, when the increase becomes very rapid. Occasionally, excessive fluid is formed (see *polyhydramnios*); less frequently, insufficient amniotic fluid is formed (see *oligohydramnios*).

amniotic sac The membranous bag that surrounds the *fetus* and is filled with *amniotic fluid* as pregnancy advances. The sac is made up of two membranes, the inner *amnion* and the outer *chorion*.

amniotomy Artificial rupture of the amniotic membranes (breaking the "waters") performed for *induction of labour*.

amoeba A type of protozoon (see *protozoa*). An amoeba is a microscopic single-celled organism with an irregular, changeable shape. Amoebae live in moist environments, such as fresh water and soil. Some types are parasites of humans, causing diseases such as *amoebiasis*.

amoebiasis An infection caused by the amoeba ENTAMOEBA HISTOLYTICA, a tiny single-celled parasite that lives in the human large intestine. Amoebiasis is spread through drinking water or eating food contaminated by human excreta containing cysts of the amoeba.

Some people carry the amoeba in their intestines and excrete cysts but have no symptoms. However, some strains invade and ulcerate the intestinal wall, causing diarrhoea and abdominal pain, which may develop into full-blown *dysentery*. The amoebae may spread via the bloodstream to the liver, or, rarely, the brain or lung, where they cause abscesses. Symptoms of an amoebic liver abscess are chills, fever, weight loss, and painful enlargement of the liver.

Treatment of all forms of amoebiasis is with drugs such as *metronidazole* or diloxanide, which kill the parasite within a few weeks, leading to full recovery.

amoebic dysentery See *amoebiasis*.

amoebicides A group of drugs used to treat *amoebiasis*. Examples are diloxanide and *metronidazole*.

amoxapine An *antidepressant drug* related to the tricyclics. Possible adverse effects include blurred vision, dizziness, drowsiness, abnormal muscular movements, menstrual irregularities, and breast enlargement.

amoxicillin A *penicillin drug* commonly used to treat a variety of infections, including *bronchitis*, *cystitis*, and ear and skin infections. Allergy to amoxicillin causes a blotchy rash and, rarely, fever, swelling of the mouth and tongue, itching, and breathing difficulty.

amoxycillin See *amoxicillin*.

amphetamine drugs A group of *stimulant drugs* used mainly in the treatment of *narcolepsy* (a rare disorder characterized by excessive sleepiness). In high doses, amphetamines can cause tremors, sweating, anxiety, and sleeping problems. Delusions, hallucinations, high blood pressure, and seizures may also occur. Prolonged use may produce *tolerance*, symptoms of *psychosis*, and *drug dependence*. Amphetamines may be abused for their stimulant effect and as appetite suppressants.

amphotericin B A drug used to treat fungal infections. Lozenges are used for *candidiasis* of the mouth. Life-threatening infections, such as *cryptococcosis* and *histoplasmosis*, are treated by injection. Adverse effects may occur with injection and include vomiting, fever, headache, and, rarely, seizures.

ampicillin A *penicillin drug* commonly used to treat *cystitis*, *bronchitis*, and ear infections. Diarrhoea is a common adverse effect of ampicillin. Some people are allergic to it and suffer from rash, fever, swelling of the mouth and tongue, itching, and breathing difficulty.

ampulla An enlarged, flask-shaped area at the end of a tubular structure or canal. There are several ampullae in the body, including at the end of the fallopian tubes, at the opening of the bile duct into the intestine, and on each of the semicircular canals of the inner ear.

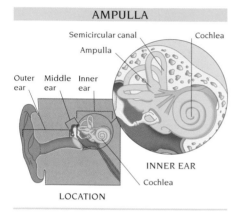

AMPULLA

Semicircular canal — Cochlea
Ampulla
Outer ear   Middle ear   Inner ear
INNER EAR
Cochlea
LOCATION

amputation Surgical removal of part or all of a limb. Amputation is necessary if *peripheral vascular disease* as a result of *atherosclerosis* or *diabetes mellitus* has impaired the blood supply to a limb. If blood supply cannot be restored, amputation is carried out to prevent the development of *gangrene*. Amputation may also be needed if a limb has been irreparably damaged in an accident.

For some time after amputation, there may be an unpleasant sensation that the limb is still present, a phenomenon known as "phantom limb". A prosthesis (see *limb, artificial*) is usually fitted when the stump has healed.

amputation, congenital The separation of a body part (usually a limb, finger, or toe) from the rest of the body, as a result of the part's blood supply being blocked by a band of *amnion* (fetal membrane) in the uterus. The affected part may be completely separated or show the marks of the "amniotic band" after birth. (See also *limb defects*.)

amputation, traumatic Loss of a finger, toe, or limb through injury. (See also *microsurgery*.)

amylase An *enzyme* found in *saliva* and pancreatic secretions (see *pancreas*). It helps to digest dietary starch, breaking it down into smaller components such as the sugars *glucose* and maltose.

amyl nitrite A *nitrate drug* formerly prescribed to relieve *angina*. Because amyl nitrite frequently causes adverse effects, it has been superseded by other drugs. It is sometimes abused for its effect of intensifying pleasure during orgasm.

amyloidosis An uncommon disease in which a substance called amyloid, composed of fibrous protein, accumulates in tissues and organs, including the liver, kidneys, tongue, spleen, and heart. Amyloidosis may occur for no known reason, in which case it is called primary; more commonly, it is a complication of some other disease, and in such cases it is called secondary. Conditions that may lead to amyloidosis include *multiple myeloma* (a cancer of bone marrow), *rheumatoid arthritis*, *tuberculosis*, and some other longstanding infections, such as chronic *osteomyelitis*.

The symptoms of amyloidosis vary, depending on the organs affected and the duration of the condition. Deposits of amyloid in the kidneys may cause *kidney failure*, which may be fatal.

There is no treatment, but secondary amyloidosis can be halted if the underlying disorder is treated.

amyotrophic lateral sclerosis See *motor neuron disease*.

amyotrophy Shrinkage or wasting away of a muscle, leading to weakness. Amyotrophy is usually due to poor nutrition, reduced use of the muscle (as when a limb is immobilized for a long period), or disruption of the blood or nerve supply to the muscle (as can occur in *diabetes mellitus* or *poliomyelitis*).

anabolic steroids See *steroids, anabolic*.

anabolism The manufacture of complex molecules, such as *fats* and *proteins*, from simpler molecules by metabolic processes in living cells. (See also *catabolism*; *metabolism*.)

anaemia A condition in which the concentration of the oxygen-carrying pigment *haemoglobin* in the blood is below normal. Haemoglobin molecules are carried inside red *blood cells* and transport oxygen from the lungs to the tissues. Normally, stable haemoglobin concentrations in the blood are maintained by a balance between red-cell production in the bone marrow and red-cell destruction in the spleen. Anaemia may result if this balance is upset.

Anaemia is not a disease but a feature of many different disorders. There are various types, which can be classified into those due to decreased or defective red-cell production by bone marrow (see *anaemia, aplastic*; *anaemia, megaloblastic*; *anaemia, iron-deficiency*) and those due to decreased survival of the red cells in the blood (see *anaemia, haemolytic*).

The severity of symptoms depends on how low the haemoglobin concentration has become. Slightly reduced levels can cause headaches, tiredness, and lethargy. Severely reduced levels can cause breathing difficulty on exercise, dizziness, *angina*, and palpitations. General signs include pallor, particularly of the skin creases, the lining of the mouth, and the inside of the eyelids.

Anaemia is diagnosed from the symptoms and by blood tests (see *blood count*; *blood film*). A *bone marrow biopsy* may be needed if the problem is with red blood cell production.

anaemia, aplastic A rare but serious type of *anaemia* in which the red cells, white cells, and platelets in the blood are all reduced in number. Aplastic anaemia is caused by a failure of the *bone marrow* to produce stem cells, the initial form of all blood cells.

Treatment of cancer with *radiotherapy* or *anticancer drugs* can temporarily interfere with the cell-producing ability of bone marrow, as can certain viral infections and other drugs. Long-term exposure to toxic chemicals may cause more persistent aplastic anaemia, and a moderate to high dose of nuclear radiation is another recognized cause. An *autoimmune disorder* is responsible for about half of all cases. Aplastic anaemia sometimes develops for no known reason.

A low level of red blood cells may cause symptoms common to all types of anaemia, such as fatigue and breathlessness. White-cell deficiency increases susceptibility to infections; platelet deficiency may lead to a tendency to bruise easily, bleeding gums, and nosebleeds.

The disorder is usually suspected from blood-test results, particularly a *blood count*, and is confirmed by a *bone marrow biopsy*. Blood and platelet transfusions can control symptoms. Immunosuppression is used to treat anaemia due to an autoimmune process. Severe persistent aplastic anaemia may be fatal unless a *bone marrow transplant* or *stem cell transplant* is carried out.

anaemia, haemolytic A form of *anaemia* caused by premature destruction of red cells in the bloodstream (haemolysis). Haemolytic anaemias can be classified according to whether the cause of haemolysis is inside or outside the red cells.

When haemolysis is due to a defect inside the red cells, the underlying problem is abnormal rigidity of the cell membrane. This causes the cells to become trapped, at an early stage of their life-span, in the small blood vessels of the spleen, where they are destroyed by macrophages (cells that ingest foreign particles). Abnormal rigidity may result from an inherited defect of the cell membrane (as in hereditary *spherocytosis*), a defect of the *haemoglobin* in the cell (as in *sickle-cell anaemia*), or a defect of one of the cell's enzymes. An inherited deficiency of the glucose-6-phosphate dehydrogenase enzyme (see *G6PD deficiency*) may result in episodes of haemolytic anaemia since the red cells are prone to damage by infectious illness or certain drugs or foods.

Haemolytic anaemias due to defects outside the red cells fall into three main groups. First are disorders in which red cells are destroyed by buffeting (by artificial surfaces such as replacement heart valves, abnormal blood-vessel linings, or a blood clot in a vessel, for example). In the second group, the red cells are destroyed by the *immune system*. Immune haemolytic anaemias may occur if foreign blood cells enter the bloodstream, as occurs in an incompatible blood transfusion, or they may be due to an *autoimmune disorder*. In *haemolytic* disease of the newborn, the baby's red cells are destroyed by the mother's antibodies crossing the placenta. Thirdly, the red cells may be destroyed by microorganisms; the most common cause is *malaria*.

People with haemolytic anaemia may have symptoms common to all types of anaemia, such as fatigue and breathlessness, or symptoms specifically due to haemolysis, such as *jaundice*.

Diagnosis is made by examination of the blood (see *blood film*). Some inherited anaemias can be controlled by removing the spleen (see *splenectomy*). Others, such as G6PD deficiency, can be prevented by avoiding the drugs or foods that precipitate haemolysis. Anaemias due to immune processes can often be controlled by *immunosuppressant drugs*. Transfusions of red cells are sometimes needed for emergency treatment of life-threatening anaemia.

anaemia, iron-deficiency The most common form of *anaemia* caused by a deficiency of iron, an essential constituent of *haemoglobin*. The main cause of iron-deficiency anaemia is iron loss due to heavy or persistent bleeding; the most common cause in women of childbearing age is menstruation. Other causes include blood loss from the digestive tract due to disorders such as erosive *gastritis*, *peptic ulcer*, *stomach cancer*, *inflammatory bowel disease*, *haemorrhoids*, and bowel tumours (see *colon, cancer of*). Prolonged use of aspirin and other *nonsteroidal antiinflammatory drugs* (NSAIDs) can cause gastrointestinal bleeding. In some countries, *hookworm infestation* of the digestive tract is an important cause of anaemia. Rarely, bleeding may also occur as a result of disorders of the urinary tract (such as *kidney tumours* or *bladder tumours*).

Iron deficiency may also be caused or worsened by lack of iron in, or its poor absorption from, the diet.

The symptoms are those of the underlying cause, along with a sore mouth or tongue, and those common to all forms of anaemia, such as fatigue and breathlessness. The diagnosis is made from blood tests and tests to look for an underlying cause. Treatment is given for the cause, along with a course of iron tablets or, very rarely, injections.

anaemia, megaloblastic An important type of *anaemia* caused by a deficiency of vitamin B_{12} or another vitamin, folic acid. Either of these deficiencies seriously interferes with production of red blood cells in the bone marrow. An excess of cells called megaloblasts appears in the marrow. Megaloblasts give rise to enlarged and deformed red blood cells known as macrocytes.

Vitamin B_{12} is found only in foods of animal origin, such as meat and dairy products. It is absorbed from the small intestine after first combining with intrinsic factor, a chemical produced by the stomach lining. The most common cause of vitamin B_{12} deficiency is failure of the stomach lining to produce intrinsic factor, usually due to an *autoimmune disorder*; this is called pernicious anaemia. Total *gastrectomy* (removal of the stomach) prevents production of intrinsic factor, and removal of part of the small intestine prevents B_{12} absorption, as does the intestinal disorder *Crohn's disease*. In a minority of cases, vitamin B_{12} deficiency is due to a vegan diet.

Folic acid is found mainly in green vegetables and liver. The usual cause of deficiency is a poor diet, but it can be caused by anything that interferes with the absorption of folic acid from the small intestine (for example Crohn's disease or *coeliac disease*). Folic acid requirements are greater than normal in pregnancy.

Many people with mild megaloblastic anaemia have no symptoms. Others may experience tiredness, headaches, a sore mouth and tongue, and mild *jaundice*. If B_{12} deficiency continues for a long time, additional symptoms due to nerve damage, including numbness and tingling in the feet, may develop.

Megaloblastic anaemia is diagnosed by *blood tests* and a *bone marrow biopsy*. Megaloblastic anaemia due to poor diet can be remedied with a short course of vitamin B_{12} injections or folic acid tablets and the introduction of a normal diet. A lifelong course of vitamin B_{12} injections or folic acid tablets is required if the underlying cause of malabsorption is untreatable.

anaemia, pernicious See *anaemia, megaloblastic.*

anaerobic Capable of living, functioning, and growing without oxygen. Many bacteria are anaerobic. Some human body cells are capable of limited anaerobic activity. When muscular exertion is so strenuous that oxygen is used faster than the blood circulation can supply it, such as during sprinting, muscle cells temporarily work anaerobically. When this happens, lactic acid is produced as waste (instead of the carbon dioxide from *aerobic* activity), sometimes causing muscle fatigue and pain.

anaesthesia Absence of all sensation; insensibility. The term most commonly refers to anaesthesia that is induced artificially for medical purposes. Two types of anaesthesia are used: local (see *anaesthesia, local*) and general (see *anaesthesia, general*).

Damage to nerve tissues by injury or disease can produce anaesthesia in a localized area.

anaesthesia, dental Loss of sensation induced in a patient to prevent pain during dental treatment.

For minor procedures, a local anaesthetic (see *anaesthesia, local*) is injected either into the gum at the site being treated or into the nerve a short distance away (called a peripheral *nerve block*). In addition, topical anaesthetics are often used on the gums. For more complicated procedures, such as periodontal (gum) surgery and multiple tooth extractions, general anaesthesia is carried out (see *anaesthesia, general*).

anaesthesia, general Reversible loss of sensation and consciousness induced to prevent the perception of pain throughout the body during surgery. General anaesthesia is usually induced by intravenous injection of propofol or a *barbiturate drug* and maintained by inhalation of anaesthetic gases such as *halothane* or isoflurane, which may be introduced into the lungs via an *endotracheal tube*. During the anaesthetic, the pulse, blood pressure, blood oxygenation, and other vital signs are continuously monitored.

General anaesthetics have become much safer, and serious complications are rare. However, severe pre-existing diseases such as lung or heart disorders increase the risks. Minor after-effects such as nausea and vomiting are usually controlled effectively with *antiemetic drugs.*

ANAESTHESIA, GENERAL

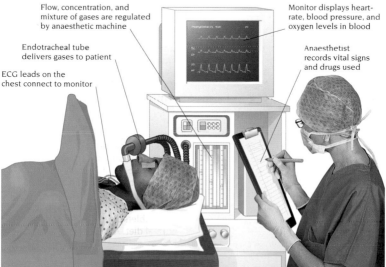

Flow, concentration, and mixture of gases are regulated by anaesthetic machine

Monitor displays heart-rate, blood pressure, and oxygen levels in blood

Endotracheal tube delivers gases to patient

Anaesthetist records vital signs and drugs used

ECG leads on the chest connect to monitor

anaesthesia, local Loss of sensation induced in a limited region of the body to prevent pain during examinations, diagnostic or treatment procedures, and surgical operations. Local anaesthesia is produced by the administration of drugs that temporarily interrupt the action of pain-carrying nerve fibres.

Local anaesthetics applied topically before injections or blood tests include sprays and skin creams and ointments. These are often used for children. For minor surgical procedures, such as stitching of small wounds, local anaesthesia is usually produced by direct injection into the area to be treated. To anaesthetize a large area, or when an injection would not penetrate deeply enough into body tissues, a *nerve block* may be used. Nerves can also be blocked where they branch off from the spinal cord, as in *epidural anaesthesia*, which is widely used in childbirth, and spinal anaesthesia, which is used for surgery on the lower limbs and abdomen.

Serious reactions to local anaesthetics are uncommon. Repeated use of topical preparations may cause allergic rashes.

anaesthetics A term for the group of drugs that produce *anaesthesia* and for the medical discipline concerned with their administration.

anal dilatation A procedure for enlarging the anus. Anal dilatation is used to treat conditions in which the anus becomes too tight, such as *anal stenosis* and *anal fissure*. It is also used to treat *haemorrhoids*. Anal dilatation is usually performed under general anaesthesia. Reflex anal dilatation, in which the anus dilates in response to local contact, may occur in certain anal disorders or after repeated anal penetration.

anal discharge The loss of mucus, pus, or blood from the anus. Causes include *haemorrhoids, anal fissures*, and *proctitis* (inflammation of the rectum). Rarely, cancer may be a cause.

analeptic drugs Drugs that stimulate breathing. Replaced by *ventilation*, they are seldom used now.

anal fissure A common anal disorder caused by an elongated ulcer or tear that extends upwards into the anal canal from the anal sphincter. A fissure may be caused by the passage of hard,

dry faeces. There is usually pain during defaecation and the muscles of the anus may go into spasm. There may be a small amount of bright red blood on faeces or toilet paper.

The tear often heals naturally over a few days. Treatment of recurrent or persistent fissures is by *anal dilatation* and a high-fibre diet, which helps soften the faeces. Surgery to remove the fissure is occasionally necessary.

anal fistula An abnormal channel connecting the inside of the anal canal with the skin surrounding the anus.

An anal fistula may be an indication of *Crohn's disease, colitis*, or cancer of the colon or rectum (see *colon, cancer of*; *rectum, cancer of*). In most cases, it results from an *abscess* that develops for unknown reasons in the anal wall. The abscess discharges pus into the anus and out on to the surrounding skin.

An anal fistula is treated surgically by opening the abnormal channel and removing the lining. The wound is then left to heal naturally.

analgesia Loss or reduction of pain sensation. Analgesia differs from *anaesthesia* in that sensitivity to touch is still preserved. (See also *analgesic drugs*.)

analgesic drugs Drugs used to relieve pain. The two main types are nonopioid and *opioid*. Nonopioids, which include *aspirin, paracetamol*, and *nonsteroidal anti-inflammatory drugs* (NSAIDs), are useful in the treatment of mild to moderate pain. Combinations of a weak opioid, such as *codeine*, with a nonopioid relieve more severe pain. Potent opioids such as *morphine* can produce *tolerance* and *drug dependence* and are therefore used only when other preparations would be ineffective.

Adverse effects are uncommon with paracetamol. Aspirin and NSAIDs may irritate the stomach lining and cause nausea, abdominal pain, and, rarely, a *peptic ulcer*. Nausea, drowsiness, constipation, and breathing difficulties may occur with opioid analgesics. Do not give aspirin to children under 16, except on the advice of a doctor, because it increases the risk of *Reye's syndrome*. Aspirin should also not be taken by women who are breast-feeding.

anal stenosis A tightness of the anus, sometimes referred to as anal stricture. Anal stenosis prevents the normal passage of faeces, causing constipation and pain during defaecation. The condition may be present from birth, or may be caused by a number of conditions in which scarring has occurred, such as *anal fissure, colitis*, or cancer of the anus. Anal stenosis sometimes occurs after surgery on the anus (for example, to treat *haemorrhoids*). The condition is treated by *anal dilatation*.

anal stricture See *anal stenosis*.

anal tag A type of *skin tag*.

analysis, chemical Determination of the identity of a substance or of the individual chemical constituents of a mixture. Analysis may be qualitative, as in determining whether a particular substance is present, or it may be quantitative, that is, measuring the amount or concentration of one or more constituents. (See also *assay*.)

analysis, psychological See *psychoanalysis*.

anaphylactic shock A rare, life-threatening allergic reaction that occurs in people with an extreme sensitivity to a particular substance (allergen), often insect venom, a food item, or a drug (see *allergy*). When the allergen enters the bloodstream, massive amounts of *histamine* and other chemicals are released, causing sudden, severe lowering of blood pressure and constriction of the airways. Other symptoms may include abdominal pain, diarrhoea, swelling of the tongue and throat, and itchy rash.

Anaphylactic shock requires emergency medical treatment. An injection of *adrenaline* may be life-saving. *Antihistamine drugs* and *corticosteroid drugs* may also be given.

anastomosis A natural or artificial communication between two blood vessels or tubular cavities that may or may not normally be joined. Natural anastomoses usually occur when small *arteries* are attached directly to *veins* without passing through capillaries. They occur in the skin and are used to help control temperature regulation. Surgical anastomoses are used to create a bypass around a blockage in an artery or in the intestine. They are also used to rejoin cut ends of the bowel or blood vessels. (See also *bypass surgery*.)

anatomy The structure of the body of any living thing, and its scientific study. Human anatomy, together with *physiology* (the study of the functioning of the body), forms the foundation of medical science. Anatomy is subdivided into many branches. These include comparative anatomy (the study of the differences between human and animal bodies), surgical anatomy (the practical knowledge required by surgeons), *embryology* (the study of structural changes that occur during the development of the embryo and fetus), systematic anatomy (the study of the structure of particular body systems), and *cytology* and *histology* (the microscopic study of cells and tissues respectively).

ancylostomiasis See *hookworm infestation*.

androgen drugs Natural or synthetic *androgen hormones* used as drugs; one of the most important is *testosterone*. These drugs are used in the treatment of male *hypogonadism* (underactivity of the testes) to stimulate the development of sexual characteristics.

Androgen drugs are occasionally used to treat certain types of *breast cancer*. They have been used by sportsmen wishing to increase muscle bulk and strength, a practice that is dangerous to health (see *steroids, anabolic*).

Adverse effects include fluid retention, weight gain, increased blood cholesterol, and, rarely, liver damage. When taken by women, the drugs can cause male characteristics, such as facial hair, to develop.

androgen hormones A group of hormones that stimulate the development of male sexual characteristics.

Androgens are produced by specialized cells in the testes in males and in the adrenal glands in both sexes. The ovaries secrete very small quantities of androgens until the menopause. The most active androgen is *testosterone*, which is produced in the testes. The production of androgens by the testes is controlled by pituitary hormones called *gonadotrophins*. Adrenal androgens are controlled by *ACTH*, another pituitary hormone.

Androgens stimulate male secondary sexual characteristics at *puberty*, such as the growth of facial hair and deepening of the voice. They have an anabolic effect (they raise the rate of protein synthesis and lower the rate at which it is broken down). This increases muscle bulk and accelerates growth. At the end of puberty, androgens cause the long bones to stop growing. They stimulate sebum secretion, which, if excessive, causes *acne*. In early adult life, androgens promote male-pattern baldness.

Androgen deficiency may occur if the testes are diseased or if the pituitary gland fails to secrete gonadotrophins. Typical effects include decreased body and facial hair, a high-pitched voice, underdevelopment of the genitalia, and poor muscle development.

Overproduction of androgens may be the result of adrenal disorders (see *adrenal tumours*; *adrenal hyperplasia, congenital*), of testicular tumours (see *testis, cancer of*), or, rarely, of androgen-secreting ovarian tumours (see *ovary, cancer of*). In men, excess androgens accentuate male characteristics; in boys, they cause premature sexual development. In women, excess androgens cause *virilization*, the development of masculine features such as an increase in body hair, deepening of the voice, clitoral enlargement, and *amenorrhoea*.

anencephaly Absence of the brain and cranial vault (top of the skull) at birth. Most infants with anencephaly are stillborn or survive only a few hours. Anencephaly is detectable early in pregnancy by measurement of the maternal *alpha-fetoprotein*, by *ultrasound scanning*, by *amniocentesis*, or by *fetoscopy*; if anencephaly is detected, termination of the pregnancy may be considered. Anencephaly is due to a failure in the development of the neural tube, which is the nerve tissue in the embryo that normally develops into the spinal cord and brain. (See also *neural tube defects*.)

aneurysm Abnormal dilation (ballooning) of an *artery* caused by the pressure of blood flowing through a weakened area. Aneurysms most commonly affect the *aorta* and arteries supplying the brain.

The most common cause of an aneurysm is *atherosclerosis*, a condition in which fatty deposits weaken the artery wall. The aorta is the usual site of atherosclerotic aneurysms.

Less commonly, aneurysms may be due to a congenital weakness of the artery walls. Most cerebral aneurysms, known as berry aneurysms because of their appearance, are congenital. *Marfan's syndrome*, an inherited disorder in which the muscular layer of the aorta is defective, is often associated with aneurysms just above the heart. The arterial wall can also be weakened by inflammation, as occurs in *polyarteritis nodosa*.

ANEURYSM

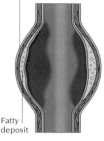

Weakened, bulging artery wall

Fatty deposit

Most aneurysms are symptomless and remain undetected, but if the aneurysm expands rapidly and causes pain, or it is very large, the symptoms are due to pressure on nearby structures.

Aneurysms may eventually rupture, cause fatal blood loss, or, in the case of a cerebral aneurysm, loss of consciousness (see *subarachnoid haemorrhage*).

In some cases, only the inner layer of the artery wall ruptures, which allows blood to track along the length of the artery and block any branching arteries. There is usually severe pain and high risk of rupture occurring.

Aneurysms sometimes develop in the heart wall due to weakening of an area of heart muscle as a result of *myocardial infarction*. Such aneurysms seldom rupture but interfere with the pumping action of the heart.

Aneurysms of the aorta may be detected by *ultrasound scanning*, and cerebral aneurysms by *CT scanning* or *MRI*. *Angiography* provides information on all types of aneurysm. Ruptured or enlarged aneurysms require immediate surgery (see *arterial reconstructive surgery*).

angina A strangling or constrictive pain. Angina has become synonymous with the heart disorder *angina pectoris*. Other types of angina include abdominal angina (abdominal pain after eating caused by poor blood supply to the intestines) and Vincent's angina, pain caused by inflammation of the mouth (see *Vincent's disease*).

angina pectoris Pain in the chest due to insufficient oxygen being carried to the heart muscle in the blood.

Inadequate blood supply to the heart is usually due to *coronary artery disease*. Other causes include coronary artery spasm, in which the blood vessels narrow suddenly for a short time, *aortic stenosis*, in which the aortic valve in the heart is narrowed, and *arrhythmias*. If the pain of angina pectoris continues, it may be due to *myocardial infarction*. Rare causes include severe *anaemia* and *polycythaemia*, which thickens the blood, causing its flow through the heart muscle to slow.

The pain usually starts in the centre of the chest but can spread to the throat, upper jaw, back, and arms (usually the left one) or between the shoulder-blades. The pain usually comes on when the heart is working harder and requires more oxygen, for example during exercise. Angina developing during sleep or without provocation is known as unstable angina. Other symptoms may include nausea, sweating, dizziness, and breathing difficulty.

Diagnostic tests usually include an *ECG*, which may register normal between attacks, and a *cardiac stress test*. Blood tests and coronary *angiography* may also be performed.

Preventive measures include controlling high blood pressure and reducing raised blood cholesterol levels; daily aspirin may also be recommended. To help control the symptoms, it is important to stop smoking and to lose weight if necessary. Attacks of angina pectoris may be prevented and treated by *nitrate drugs*. However, if nitrates are not effective or are causing side effects, *beta-blocker drugs*, *potassium channel activators*, or *calcium channel blockers* may be used.

Drug treatment can control the symptoms for many years. If attacks become more severe or more frequent, despite treatment, *coronary artery bypass* surgery or *angioplasty* may be necessary.

angioedema A type of reaction caused by *allergy*. Angioedema is characterized by large, well-defined swellings, of sudden onset, in the skin, larynx (voicebox), and other areas.

The most common cause is a sudden allergic reaction to a food. Less commonly, it results from allergy to a drug (such as *penicillin*), a reaction to an insect bite or sting, or from infection, emotional stress, or exposure to animals, moulds, pollens, or cold conditions. There is also a hereditary form of the disease.

Angioedema may cause sudden difficulty in breathing, swallowing, and speaking, accompanied by swelling of the lips, face, and neck, depending on the area of the body affected. Angioedema that affects the throat and the larynx is potentially life-threatening because the swelling can block the airway, causing *asphyxia*.

Severe cases are treated with injections of *adrenaline* (epinephrine) and may require intubation (passage of a breathing tube via the mouth into the windpipe) or *tracheostomy* (surgical creation of a hole in the windpipe) to prevent suffocation. *Corticosteroid drugs* may also be given. In less severe cases, *antihistamine drugs* may relieve symptoms.

angiogenesis The growth of new blood vessels. Angiogenesis is the process that enables tumours to grow; cancerous cells produce chemicals (called *growth factors*) that stimulate new blood vessels to form near the tumour, supplying it with nutrients.

angiography An imaging procedure that enables blood vessels to be seen clearly on X-ray film following the injection of a *contrast medium* (a substance that is opaque to X-rays). Angiography is used to detect conditions that alter the appearance of blood vessels, such as *aneurysm*, and narrowing or blockage of blood vessels by *atherosclerosis*, or by a *thrombus* or *embolus*. It is also used to detect changes in the pattern of blood vessels that supply organs injured or affected by a tumour.

Carotid angiography (of the arteries in the neck) may be used to investigate *transient ischaemic attacks*. Cerebral angiography can be used to detect an aneurysm in the brain or pinpoint the position of a brain tumour. Coronary angiography, often combined with cardiac *catheterization*, can identify the sites of narrowing or blockage in *coronary artery disease*. Digital subtraction angiography uses computer techniques to process images and remove unwanted background information.

Angiographic techniques have been adapted to allow certain treatments that, in some cases, eliminate the need for surgery (see *angioplasty, balloon; embolization*). (See also *aortography*.)

angioma A noncancerous tumour made up of blood vessels (see *haemangioma*) or lymph vessels (see *lymphangioma*).

angioplasty, balloon A technique for treating a narrowed or blocked section of blood vessel by introducing a catheter with a balloon into the constricted area. The balloon is inflated to widen the narrowed area, deflated again, and then removed. Usually, a *stent* is inserted into the artery to keep it open. Balloon angioplasty is used to restore blood flow in *peripheral vascular disease* and *coronary artery disease*.

Coronary balloon angioplasty is usually successful, but the narrowing may recur in the affected vessel, requiring repeat treatment. However, stents have been developed that are coated with slow-release drugs that reduce the risk of arterial renarrowing. Angioplasty of peripheral vessels is most successful in treating the iliac and femoral arteries in the legs.

angiotensin The name of two related proteins involved in regulating blood pressure. The first, angiotensin I, is inactive and is formed when renin, which is produced by the kidneys, acts on the substance angiotensinogen. Angiotensin I is then converted to the second, active, form, angiotensin II, by angiotensin-converting enzyme. Angiotensin II causes narrowing of the small blood vessels in tissues, resulting in increased blood pressure. It also stimulates release (from the adrenal cortex, the outer part of each *adrenal gland*) of the hormone *aldosterone*, which also increases blood pressure.

Certain kidney disorders can increase the production of angiotensin II, causing *hypertension*. Whatever the cause of hypertension, it may be treated with drugs called *ACE inhibitors*, which work by reducing angiotensin II formation.

angiotensin converting enzyme A substance that converts angiotensin I to its active form, angiotensin II. Drugs that reduce the action of this enzyme are known as *ACE inhibitor drugs* and are used in the treatment of *hypertension* and *heart failure*.

angiotensin II antagonists A group of drugs used in the treatment of *hypertension* (high blood pressure). They have a similar action to *ACE inhibitors* but do not cause a dry cough. Examples are losartan and valsartan.

anhedonia Total loss of the feeling of pleasure from activities that would normally give pleasure. Anhedonia is often a symptom of *depression*.

anhidrosis Complete absence of sweating. (See also *hypohidrosis*.)

animal experimentation The use of animals in research to obtain information on animal biology or, by inference, human physiology or behaviour. Animal

ANGIOPLASTY, BALLOON

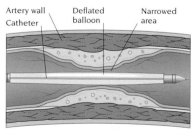

Artery wall — Deflated balloon — Narrowed area
Catheter

BALLOON IN POSITION

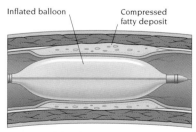

Inflated balloon — Compressed fatty deposit

BALLOON INFLATED

research has contributed to the development of drugs, such as vaccines, and surgical techniques, such as transplant surgery. However, because of ethical concerns, alternatives such as cell cultures are now used wherever possible.

animals, diseases from See *zoonosis*.

anisometropia Unequal focusing power in the two eyes, usually due to a difference in size and/or shape of the eyes, that causes visual discomfort. For example, one eye may be normal and the other affected by *myopia* (shortsightedness), *hypermetropia* (longsightedness), or *astigmatism* (uneven curvature of the cornea). Glasses or contact lenses correct the problem in most cases.

ankle joint The hinge joint between the foot and the leg. The talus (uppermost bone in the foot) fits between the two protuberances formed by the lower ends of the tibia (the shinbone) and the fibula (the outer bone of the lower leg). Ligaments on either side of the ankle joint give it support. The ankle allows the foot to move up and down.

ANKLE JOINT

- Tibia
- Fibula
- Ankle joint
- Talus
- Calcaneus

An ankle *sprain* is one of the most common injuries. It is usually caused by twisting the foot over on to its outside edge, causing overstretching and bruising of the ligaments. Violent twisting of the ankle can cause a combined fracture and dislocation known as *Pott's fracture*.

ankylosing spondylitis An uncommon inflammatory disease affecting joints between the vertebrae of the spine and the sacroiliac joints (joints between the spine and pelvis).

The cause of ankylosing spondylitis is usually unknown, but in some cases the disease may be associated with *colitis* (inflammation of the colon) or *psoriasis* (a skin disease). Ankylosing spondylitis may run in families; and about 90 percent of people with the condition have the genetically determined *histocompatibility antigen* (HLA-B27).

Ankylosing spondylitis usually starts with pain and stiffness in the hips and lower back, which are worse after resting and are especially noticeable in the early morning. Other, less common, symptoms include chest pain, painful heels due to additional bone formation, and redness and pain in the eyes due to *iritis*. In time, inflammation in the spine can lead to *ankylosis* (permanent stiffness and limited movement) and *kyphosis* (curvature of the spine).

The condition is diagnosed by *X-rays* and *blood tests*. There is no cure but treatment with exercises, physiotherapy, and *anti-inflammatory drugs* can reduce the pain and limitation of movement.

ankylosis Complete loss of movement in a joint caused by fusion of the bony surfaces. Ankylosis may be due to degeneration as a result of inflammation, infection, or injury, or be produced surgically by surgery to fuse a diseased joint to correct deformity or to alleviate persistent pain (see *arthrodesis*).

anodontia Failure of some or all of the teeth to develop. It may be due to absence of tooth buds at birth or the result of damage to developing tooth buds by infection or other widespread disease. If only a few teeth are missing, a *bridge* can fill the gap; if all the teeth are missing, a *denture* is needed.

anomaly A deviation from what is accepted as normal, especially a birth defect such as a limb malformation.

anorexia The medical term for loss of appetite (see *appetite, loss of*).

anorexia nervosa An eating disorder characterized by severe weight loss and altered self-image that leads sufferers to believe they are fat when they are, in fact, dangerously underweight. Anorexia nervosa most often affects teenage girls and young women, but the incidence in young men is rising.

The causes of anorexia are unclear, but the condition may be linked to a lack of self-worth that leads to excessive concern over physical appearance. Normal dieting may develop into starvation.

In the early stages, sufferers may be overactive and exercise excessively. They are obsessed with food, and often make complicated meals for their families, but are reluctant to eat socially and manage to avoid eating the meals themselves. As weight loss continues, they become tired and weak, the skin becomes dry, lanugo hair (fine, downy hair) grows on the body, and normal hair becomes thinner. Starvation leads to *amenorrhoea* in many women. Some anorexics sometimes make themselves vomit or take *laxative drugs* or *diuretic drugs* to promote weight loss (see *bulimia*). Chemical imbalances as a result of starvation with or without vomiting can cause potentially fatal cardiac *arrhythmias*.

Hospital treatment is often necessary and is usually based on a closely controlled feeding programme, combined with *psychotherapy* or *family therapy*. For some people, *antidepressant drugs* may be helpful. Many sufferers relapse after treatment, and long-term psychotherapy is required.

anorgasmia Inability to achieve orgasm (see *orgasm, lack of*).

anosmia Loss of the sense of *smell*.

anoxia A complete absence of oxygen in a body tissue. Anoxia causes disruption of cell *metabolism* and cell death unless corrected within a few minutes. Anoxia occurs during cardiopulmonary arrest or asphyxiation and will cause permanent organ damage or even death if not corrected. (See also *hypoxia*.)

antacid drugs Drugs taken to relieve the symptoms of *indigestion*, *heartburn*, *oesophagitis*, *gastro-oesophageal reflux disease*, and *peptic ulcer*. Antacids usually contain compounds of *magnesium* or *aluminium*, which neutralize stomach acid. Some also contain alginates, which protect the lining of the oesophagus from stomach acid, or dimeticone, an antifoaming agent, which helps to relieve flatulence.

Aluminium may cause constipation and magnesium may cause diarrhoea; but these effects may be avoided if a preparation contains both ingredients. Antacids interfere with the absorption of many drugs and should not be taken at the same time as other drugs.

antagonist Having an opposing effect. For example, antagonist drugs counteract the effects of naturally occurring chemicals in the body. (see also *agonist*.)

antenatal care The care of a pregnant woman and her unborn baby throughout a pregnancy. Such care involves regular visits to a doctor or midwife, who performs abdominal examinations, blood and urine tests, and monitoring of blood pressure and fetal growth to detect disease or potential problems.

Ultrasound scanning is carried out to assess the age of the fetus and help identify any abnormalities. *Chorionic villus sampling* or *amniocentesis* may be performed if the baby is thought to be at increased risk of a *chromosomal abnormality* or a *genetic disorder*. The woman is also advised on general aspects of pregnancy, such as diet, exercise, lifestyle, feeding, and techniques to help her with childbirth. (See also *childbirth, natural.*)

antepartum haemorrhage Bleeding from the vagina after the 28th week of pregnancy. Antepartum haemorrhage is most commonly due to a problem with the placenta, such as *placenta praevia* or *placental abruption*. Bleeding can also be caused by *cervical ectopy* or other disorders of the cervix or vagina.

Admission to hospital is necessary for investigation and treatment. *Ultrasound scanning* is used to diagnose problems with the placenta. If the bleeding is severe, the woman is given a *blood transfusion*, and the baby is delivered immediately by *caesarean section*.

anterior Relating to the front of the body. In human *anatomy*, the term is synonymous with *ventral*.

anthelmintic drugs A group of drugs that are used to eradicate *worm infestations*. Possible side effects include nausea, abdominal pain, rash, headache, and dizziness.

anthracosis An outdated term for coal worker's *pneumoconiosis*. Anthracosis is a lung disease caused by the inhalation of large amounts of coal dust over a period of many years.

anthrax A serious bacterial infection of livestock that occasionally spreads to humans. In humans, the most common form of the infection is cutaneous anthrax, which affects the skin. Another form, pulmonary anthrax, affects the lungs. Anthrax is caused by BACILLUS ANTHRACIS. This microorganism produces spores that can remain dormant for years in soil and animal products and are capable of reactivation. Animals become infected by grazing on contaminated land. People may become infected via a scratch or sore if they handle materials from infected animals. Pulmonary anthrax occurs as a result of inhaling spores from animal fibres.

In cutaneous anthrax, a raised, itchy, area develops at the site of entry of the spores, progressing to a large blister and finally a black scab, with swelling of the surrounding tissues. This is treatable with *antibiotic drugs* in its early stages. Without treatment, the infection may spread to lymph nodes and the bloodstream, and may be fatal. Pulmonary anthrax causes severe breathing difficulty and is fatal in most cases.

antiallergy drugs Drugs that are used to treat or prevent allergic reactions (see *allergy*). There are several groups, including *corticosteroids*, *antihistamines*, *leukotriene receptor antagonists*, and *sodium cromoglicate*.

antianxiety drugs A group of drugs used to relieve the symptoms of *anxiety*. *Benzodiazepine drugs* and *beta-blocker drugs* are the two main types, although *antidepressant drugs* may occasionally be used. Benzodiazepine drugs promote mental and physical relaxation; they can also be used to treat insomnia, but their use for this purpose is avoided because they are addictive. Beta-blockers reduce only the physical symptoms of anxiety, such as shaking and palpitations, and are not addictive.

antiarrhythmic drugs A group of drugs used to prevent or treat *arrhythmia* (irregular heartbeat). This group includes those given intravenously in hospital to treat arrhythmias that are causing symptoms such as breathlessness or chest pain. Adenosine is an example of a drug used only in hospital. A number of drugs are used to prevent intermittent arrhythmias or to slow the rate if an arrhythmia is persistent. These include *amiodarone*, *beta-blocker drugs*, *calcium channel blockers*, *digitalis drugs*, *disopyramide*, *flecainide*, *lidocaine* (lignocaine), *mexiletine*, and *procainamide*. Side effects are common and often include nausea and

rash. Some antiarrhythmics can result in tiredness or breathlessness because they reduce the heart's pumping ability.

antibacterial drugs A group of drugs used to treat infections caused by *bacteria*. The term antibacterial was once used to describe antibiotics that had been produced synthetically rather than naturally. The terms are now used interchangeably. (See also *antibiotic drugs*.)

antibiotic drugs A group of drugs used to treat infections caused by *bacteria* and to prevent bacterial infection in cases of *immune system* impairment.

Most of the commonly used antibiotic drugs belong to one of the following classes: *penicillins*, *quinolones*, *aminoglycosides*, *cephalosporins*, *macrolides*, and *tetracyclines*. Some antibiotics are effective against only certain types of bacteria; others, which are known as broad-spectrum antibiotics, are effective against a wide range.

Some bacteria develop resistance to a previously effective antibiotic drug. This is most likely to occur during long-term treatment. Some alternative antibiotics are available to treat bacteria that have become resistant to the more commonly prescribed drugs.

Most antibiotic drugs can cause nausea, diarrhoea, or a rash. Antibiotics may disturb the normal balance between certain types of bacteria and fungi in the body, leading to proliferation of the fungi that cause *candidiasis* (thrush). Some people experience a severe allergic reaction to the drugs, resulting in facial swelling, itching, or breathing difficulty.

antibody A protein that is made by certain lymphocytes (white blood cells) to neutralize an *antigen* (foreign protein) in the body. Bacteria, viruses, and other microorganisms contain many antigens; antibodies that are formed against these antigens help the body to neutralize or destroy the invading microorganisms. Antibodies may be formed in response to *vaccines*, thereby giving immunity. Antibodies are also known as *immunoglobulins*.

Inappropriate or excessive formation of antibodies may lead to illness, as in an *allergy*. Antibodies against antigens in organ transplants may result in rejection of the transplanted organ. In some disorders, antibodies are formed against the body's own tissues, resulting in an *autoimmune disorder.*

antibody, monoclonal An artificially produced *antibody* that neutralizes only one specific *antigen* (foreign protein).

Monoclonal antibodies are produced in a laboratory by stimulating the growth of a large number of antibody-producing cells that are genetically identical. In effect, this process enables antibodies to be tailor-made so that they will react with a particular antigen.

Monoclonal antibodies are used in the study of human cells, hormones, microorganisms, and in the development of vaccines. They are also being used in the diagnosis and treatment of some forms of cancer, such as *lymphoma.*

anticancer drugs Drugs that are used to treat many forms of *cancer.* They are particularly useful in the treatment of *lymphomas, leukaemias, breast cancer,* cancer of the testis (see *testis, cancer of*), and *prostate cancer* and are often used together with surgery or *radiotherapy.*

Most anticancer drugs are cytotoxic (kill or damage rapidly dividing cells), but some act by slowing the growth of hormone-sensitive tumours. Anticancer drugs are often prescribed in combination to maximize their effects.

Treatment with cytotoxic drugs is often given by injection in short courses repeated at intervals. Some drugs cause nausea and vomiting and may result in hair loss and increased susceptibility to infection. Others, such as tamoxifen, which is used for breast cancer, are given continuously by mouth for months or years and generally cause few side effects.

anticholinergic drugs A group of drugs that block the effects of *acetylcholine,* a chemical released from nerve endings in the parasympathetic *autonomic nervous system.* Acetylcholine stimulates muscle contraction, increases secretions in the mouth and lungs, and slows the heartbeat.

Anticholinergic drugs are used in the treatment of *irritable bowel syndrome,* urinary *incontinence, Parkinson's disease,* asthma, and *bradycardia* (abnormally slow heartbeat). They are also used to dilate the pupil before eye examination or surgery. Anticholinergic drugs are used as a *premedication* before general *anaesthesia* and to treat *motion sickness.* They may cause dry mouth, constipation, urinary retention, and confusion.

anticoagulant drugs A group of drugs used to treat and prevent abnormal *blood clotting,* to treat *thrombosis,* and occasionally to prevent or treat *stroke* and *transient ischaemic attack.* Anticoagulant drugs are also given to prevent abnormal blood clotting after major surgery (especially heart-valve replacement) or during haemodialysis (see *dialysis*). The most common anticoagulants are *heparin* and the newer heparin-derived drugs, such as tinzaparin, all of which have to be given by injection, and *warfarin,* which is taken orally.

Excessive doses of anticoagulant drugs increase the risk of unwanted bleeding, and regular monitoring is needed.

anticonvulsant drugs A group of drugs used to treat or prevent seizures. They are used mainly in the treatment of *epilepsy* but are also given to prevent seizures following serious *head injury* or some types of brain surgery. They may be needed to control seizures in children with a high fever (see *convulsions, febrile*).

Anticonvulsants may produce various side effects, including impaired memory, reduced concentration, poor coordination, and fatigue. If the side effects are severe, they can often be minimized by use of an alternative anticonvulsant.

antidepressant drugs Drugs used in the treatment of *depression.* Most of the commonly used antidepressant drugs belong to one of the following groups: *tricyclic* drugs, *selective serotonin reuptake inhibitors* (SSRIs), and *monoamine oxidase inhibitors* (MAOIs). These drugs are usually successful at relieving the symptoms of depression but often take 2–3 weeks before benefit is felt. Treatment usually lasts for at least 6 months, and the dosage is reduced gradually before being stopped altogether.

Tricyclics may cause drowsiness, dry mouth, constipation, blurred vision, urinary difficulty, and irregular heartbeat. SSRIs may cause nausea, indigestion, insomnia, agitation, or allergic reactions but are less dangerous in overdose than other antidepressants. MAOIs may interact with foods containing tyramine (for example, cheese) and other drugs to cause a dangerous rise in blood pressure, although one MAOI, *moclobemide*, is less likely to cause problems. Antidepressants are not addictive, but abrupt withdrawal of some types can result in physical symptoms and should be avoided. SSRIs are generally not advised for those under 18.

antidiabetic drugs A group of drugs used to treat *diabetes mellitus*, in which a lack of *insulin*, or resistance to its actions, results in raised *blood glucose levels*. A wide range of antidiabetics are used to keep the blood glucose level as close to normal as possible, and consequently reduce the risk of complications such as vascular (blood vessel) disease. Antidiabetic drugs include insulin, which is administered by injection, infusion, or inhalation, and oral *hypoglycaemics* such as gliclazide and *metformin*. *Acarbose* reduces or slows absorption of carbohydrate from the intestines after meals. *Repaglinide* stimulates insulin release from the pancreas for a short time and may be taken directly before meals. *Rosiglitazone* reduces resistance to the effects of insulin in the tissues and may be used together with other hypoglycaemics.

antidiarrhoeal drugs Drugs used to reduce or stop diarrhoea and to help regulate bowel action in people with a *colostomy* or *ileostomy*. In most acute cases of diarrhoea, the only treatment recommended is *oral rehydration therapy*. Antidiarrhoeal drugs include adsorbents such as kaolin, bulk-forming agents, and antimotility drugs (including the opioid drugs, *morphine* and *codeine*, and loperamide), which slow movement through the intestine. None of these drugs are suitable for children.

antidiuretic hormone See *ADH*.

antidote A substance that neutralizes or counteracts the effects of a poison.

anti-D(Rh$_0$) immunoglobulin An *antiserum* that contains antibodies against Rhesus (Rh) D factor (a substance present on the red blood cells of people with Rh-positive blood). Anti-

D(Rh$_0$) immunoglobulin is given routinely at intervals during normal pregnancy and at delivery. An additional dose is also given after an amniocentesis, miscarriage, or any event in which the baby's blood may enter the mother's circulation. The injected antibodies prevent the woman from forming her own antibodies against Rh-positive blood, which might adversely affect a subsequent pregnancy. (See also *haemolytic disease of the newborn*; *Rhesus incompatibility*.)

antiemetic drugs A group of drugs used to treat *nausea* and *vomiting*. Antihistamine drugs and anticholinergic drugs reduce vomiting in *motion sickness*, vertigo, and *Ménière's disease*. The most powerful antiemetics are used to control nausea and vomiting associated with *radiotherapy* or *anticancer drugs*. These drugs include *serotonin antagonists* such as *ondansetron* and *nabilone*. Antiemetics are not normally used in the treatment of food poisoning because the body needs to rid itself of harmful substances. Rarely, an antiemetic such as *promethazine* may be used to treat severe vomiting in pregnancy. Many antiemetics cause drowsiness.

antifreeze poisoning Most antifreeze in the UK contains ethylene glycol, which is poisonous. Drinking antifreeze initially produces effects similar to *alcohol intoxication*, but vomiting, stupor, seizures, and coma may follow; acute *kidney failure* may occur within 24–36 hours. Antifreeze poisoning requires immediate medical attention.

antifungal drugs A group of drugs used to treat infections caused by *fungi*. Antifungal drugs are commonly used to treat different types of *tinea*, including *athlete's foot* and scalp ringworm. They are also used for *candidiasis* (thrush) and rare fungal infections, such as *cryptococcosis*, that affect internal organs. Antifungal preparations are available in various forms, including tablets, injection, creams, and pessaries. Prolonged treatment of serious fungal infections can result in side effects that include liver or kidney damage.

antigen A substance that can trigger an *immune response*, resulting in production of an *antibody* as part of the body's defence against infection and disease.

Many antigens are foreign proteins (not found naturally in the body) such as parts of microorganisms and toxins or tissues from another person that have been used in organ transplants. Sometimes, harmless substances (pollen, for example) are misidentified by the immune system as potentially harmful antigens, which results in an allergic response (see *allergy*).

antihistamine drugs A group of drugs that block the effects of *histamine*, a chemical released in allergic reactions (see *allergy*). Antihistamines are used to treat rashes such as *urticaria* and to relieve sneezing and a runny nose in allergic *rhinitis*. They are also sometimes included in *cough remedies* and *cold remedies* and are used as *antiemetic drugs*. Antihistamines are usually taken by mouth but may be given by injection for *anaphylactic shock*. Some antihistamines cause drowsiness, but newer drugs have little sedative effect. Other possible side effects include loss of appetite, nausea, dry mouth, blurred vision, and difficulty in passing urine.

antihypertensive drugs A group of drugs used in the treatment of *hypertension* (high blood pressure) to prevent complications such as *stroke*, *myocardial infarction*, *heart failure*, and kidney damage. There are several types, including *angiotensin II antagonists, beta-blocker drugs, ACE inhibitor drugs, calcium channel blockers, alpha-blocker drugs, vasodilator drugs,* and *diuretic drugs*. Side effects depend on the type of antihypertensive drugs used, but all can cause dizziness if the blood pressure falls excessively.

anti-inflammatory drugs Drugs that reduce *inflammation*. The main groups of these drugs are *nonsteroidal anti-inflammatory drugs* and *corticosteroid drugs*. (See also *analgesic drugs*.)

antimalarial drugs Drugs used to treat *malaria*. One antimalarial drug, *chloroquine*, also works as a *disease-modifying antirheumatic drug* and can be used to treat *rheumatoid arthritis*; it may also be used to treat systemic *lupus erythematosus*.

antioxidant A type of chemical that neutralizes potentially damaging oxidizing molecules known as *free radicals*. Some antioxidants occur naturally in the body; others (vitamin C, vitamin E, and beta-carotene, for example) are obtained through food intake or from dietary supplements.

antiperspirant A substance applied to the skin in the form of a lotion, cream, or spray to reduce sweating. High concentrations are sometimes used to treat *hyperhidrosis* (abnormally heavy sweating). Antiperspirants may cause skin irritation, particularly if they are used on broken skin. (See also *deodorants*.)

antiplatelet drugs Drugs that reduce the tendency of *platelets* to stick together to form blood clots when blood flow in the arteries is disrupted. This action reduces the risk of *thromboembolism*, which can cause potentially fatal disorders such as a *myocardial infarction* or *stroke*. Aspirin and *clopidogrel* are commonly used antiplatelet drugs. Others, such as tirofiban, are used specifically to protect against blood clots forming in the *coronary arteries* of people with *angina pectoris*.

antipruritic drugs Drugs that are used to relieve persistent itching (*pruritus*). Antipruritics may be applied as creams and *emollients* and may contain *corticosteroid drugs, antihistamine drugs,* or *local anaesthetics*. Oral antihistamines may also be used to relieve itching.

antipsychotic drugs A group of drugs used to treat *psychoses* (mental disorders involving loss of contact with reality), particularly *schizophrenia* and *mania* in *bipolar disorder*. Antipsychotic drugs may also be used to sedate people who have other mental disorders (such as *dementia*) and who are very agitated or aggressive. Antipsychotics include *phenothiazine drugs*, butyrophenones, such as *haloperidol*, and several newer drugs including *risperidone*.

Antipsychotics can cause drowsiness, lethargy, *dyskinesia*, and *parkinsonism*. Other possible side effects include dry mouth, blurred vision, and difficulty in passing urine. However, newer drugs may have fewer side effects when used in the long term.

antipyretic drugs Drugs that reduce fever. Examples of antipyretic drugs include *paracetamol, aspirin*, and other *nonsteroidal anti-inflammatory drugs*

antiretroviral drugs Drugs that are used to slow or halt the spread of viruses in people with *HIV* infection and *AIDS*. There are three main groups: reverse transcriptase inhibitors, protease inhibitors, and non-nucleoside reverse transcriptase inhibitors. Drugs from different groups are often used in combination. New antiretroviral drugs, such as fusion inhibitors, are being developed to treat resistant forms of HIV. Antiretroviral drugs can have a range of side effects, including nausea, vomiting, diarrhoea, tiredness, and a range of effects on blood chemistry, particularly involving fats.

antirheumatic drugs A group of drugs used to treat *rheumatoid arthritis* and types of arthritis that are caused by other *autoimmune disorders* such as systemic *lupus erythematosus*. Antirheumatic drugs modify the disease process by affecting the body's immune response. They may limit joint damage, unlike *nonsteroidal anti-inflammatory drugs*, which only relieve pain and stiffness. The main antirheumatic drugs are *immunosuppressant drugs, chloroquine, gold, penicillamine,* and *sulfasalazine.* Many of these drugs can have serious side effects and treatment must be under specialist supervision.

antiseptics Chemicals applied to the skin in order to destroy bacteria and other microorganisms, thereby preventing infection. Common antiseptics are *chlorhexidine, cetrimide,* and compounds containing *iodine*. (See also *disinfectants; aseptic technique.*)

antiserum A preparation containing *antibodies* (also known as *immunoglobulins*) that combine with specific *antigens* (foreign proteins), usually components of microorganisms, leading to deactivation or destruction of the microorganisms. Antiserum is usually used, along with *immunization*, as an emergency treatment when someone has been exposed to a dangerous infection such as *rabies* and has not previously been immunized.

antisocial personality disorder Impulsive, destructive behaviour that often disregards the feelings and rights of others. People who have an antisocial personality lack a sense of guilt and cannot tolerate frustration. They may have problems with relationships and are frequently in trouble with the law. *Behaviour therapy*, and various forms of *psychotherapy*, may help to improve integration. In general, the effects of this disorder decrease with age.

antispasmodic drugs A group of drugs that relax spasm in smooth muscle in the wall of the intestine or bladder. These drugs are used to treat *irritable bowel syndrome* and *irritable bladder*. Possible side effects include dry mouth, blurred vision, and difficulty in passing urine. (See also *anticholinergic drugs.*)

antithyroid drugs Drugs used to treat *hyperthyroidism*, in which the thyroid gland is overactive. They may be used as the sole treatment or before thyroid surgery. *Carbimazole* and *propylthiouracil* interfere with the production of thyroid hormone by the gland.

antitoxin Any of a variety of commercially prepared substances containing *antibodies* that can combine with and neutralize the effect of a specific *toxin* released into the bloodstream by particular bacteria. Antitoxins are usually given by injection into a muscle. Occasionally, an antitoxin may cause an allergic reaction (see *allergy*).

antitussive drugs Drugs that suppress or relieve a *cough* (see *cough remedies*).

antivenom A specific treatment for bites or stings inflicted by venomous animals such as snakes, spiders, and scorpions. Antivenoms are given by intravenous injection and may cause allergic reactions.

antiviral drugs Drugs used in the treatment of infection by *viruses*. No drugs have been developed that can eradicate viruses, and at present *immunization* is the most effective way of preventing serious viral infections.

However, antiviral drugs can reduce the severity of some viral infections (most notably *herpes, influenza,* viral *hepatitis*, and *cytomegalovirus* infections), particularly in people who have reduced immunity. Advances have also been made in the treatment of HIV infection (see *antiretroviral drugs*).

antral irrigation Irrigation of the maxillary antrum, one of the nasal sinuses. More commonly known as sinus washout, this procedure is used to diagnose and treat persistent *sinusitis*. Antral irrigation is performed less often since the introduction of nasal *endoscopy*.

anuria Complete cessation of urine output. Anuria may be caused by a severe malfunction of the kidneys, but a more common cause is a complete blockage of urine flow, due to enlargement of the prostate gland (see *prostate, enlarged*), a *bladder tumour*, or a stone (see *calculus, urinary tract*). Failure of the kidneys to produce urine may be due to oxygen depletion as a result of reduced blood flow through the kidneys, as occurs in *shock*, or to severe kidney damage caused by a disease such as *glomerulonephritis*. Anuria requires urgent investigation. Treatment of the cause may restore urine production, but any delay can result in permanent kidney damage, leading to *uraemia*.

anus The end of the alimentary tract through which faeces are expelled from the body. The orifice at the end of the anal canal is open only during defaecation; at other times it is kept closed by the muscles of the anal sphincter. (See also *digestive system*.)

anus, cancer of A rare cancer of the skin of the anus. Possible early signs are development of swelling or an ulcer at the anus accompanied by bleeding and discomfort. Treatment is by surgical removal and/or *radiotherapy*.

anus, disorders of Most anal disorders affect adults and are minor, but they may cause discomfort. Rarely, the anus may fail to develop normally and surgical treatment is needed (see *anus, imperforate*). In *anal stenosis*, the anus is too narrow to allow the passage of faeces. *Anal fissures* originate from tears in the lining of the anus, usually as a result of straining to pass faeces. Cancer of the skin around the anus is rare (see *anus, cancer of*). *Haemorrhoids* are enlarged blood vessels under the anal lining. An *anal fistula* is an abnormal channel connecting the anal canal with the skin surrounding the anus. *Itching* of the anus is common and may be due to haemorrhoids or other disorders such as *threadworm* infestation.

anus, imperforate A rare *congenital* abnormality in which the anal opening is missing or covered over. The severity of the condition varies from complete absence of the anal canal to only a layer of skin covering the anal opening.

Treatment involves surgery. A *colostomy* may be needed initially before definitive surgery to construct an anus.

anxiety An unpleasant emotional state ranging from mild unease to intense fear. Various physical symptoms are associated with anxiety; the most common include palpitations, chest pains, a feeling of tightness in the chest, and a tendency to overbreathe (see *hyperventilation*). Muscle tension leads to headaches and back pains. Gastrointestinal symptoms include dry mouth, bloating, diarrhoea, nausea, and difficulty in swallowing. Other symptoms include sweating, blushing, pallor, lightheadedness, and a frequent need to urinate or defaecate. Anxiety is a normal response to stressful situations and prepares the mind and body to respond effectively. However, anxiety that occurs without reason may be a symptom of an *anxiety disorder* or another psychological disorder such as *depression*.

anxiety disorders A group of mental illnesses, including several specific syndromes, in which symptoms of *anxiety* are the main feature. These disorders are common and mainly affect young adults.

In *generalized anxiety disorder*, there is persistent tension and apprehension that has no specific focus or cause, together with physical or psychological symptoms that disrupt normal activity. *Panic disorders* are characterized by sudden attacks of extreme, unreasonable anxiety. *Phobias* are irrational fears, such as the fear of open spaces or spiders, that lead to avoidance of certain situations or objects.

Counselling, psychotherapy, and group or individual cognitive-behaviour therapy are used to treat anxiety disorders. *Antianxiety drugs* may be used for short-term treatment but some are addictive.

anxiolytics See *antianxiety drugs*.

aorta The body's main *artery*, which supplies oxygenated blood to all other parts. The aorta arises from the left ventricle (the main pumping chamber of the *heart*) and arches up over the heart before descending, behind it, through the chest cavity. It terminates in the abdomen by dividing into the two common iliac arteries of the legs.

The aorta is thick-walled and has a large diameter in order to cope with the high pressure and large volume of blood passing through it. (See also *arteries, disorders of*; *circulatory system*.)

AORTA

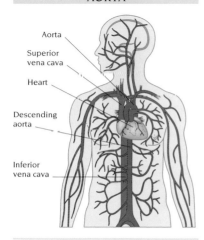

- Aorta
- Superior vena cava
- Heart
- Descending aorta
- Inferior vena cava

aortic incompetence Leakage of blood through the aortic valve (one of the *heart valves*), resulting in a backflow of blood from the aorta into the left ventricle (the heart's main pumping chamber).

Failure of the aortic valve to close properly may be due to a *congenital* abnormality in which the valve has two flaps rather than three. The valve leaflets can be destroyed by infective *endocarditis*. Long-term *hypertension* can sometimes cause the root of the aorta to stretch so that the valve does not close properly. Aortic incompetence is associated with *ankylosing spondylitis* and *Marfan's syndrome*. *Atherosclerosis* may damage the valve, causing incompetence combined with *aortic stenosis*. Incompetence is also found in untreated *syphilis*.

Aortic incompetence may not cause symptoms and is sometimes found during a routine medical examination. The heart compensates for the backflow of blood into the left ventricle by working harder, which may eventually lead to *heart failure*; this causes breathing difficulty and *oedema* (fluid accumulation).

Chest X-ray, *ECG*, and *echocardiography* may be carried out to diagnose aortic incompetence. A cardiac catheter may be used to show the degree of incompetence (see *catheterization, cardiac*). Heart failure can be treated with *diuretic drugs*. *Heart-valve surgery* to replace the damaged valve may eventually be necessary.

aortic stenosis Narrowing of the opening of the aortic valve (one of the *heart valves*). The narrowing obstructs the flow of blood into the circulation; this makes the heart work harder and causes the muscle in the wall of the left ventricle (the main pumping chamber) to thicken. It also reduces the amount of blood flowing into the coronary arteries.

The most common cause of aortic stenosis is deposition of calcium on the aortic valve, usually associated with *atherosclerosis*. Aortic stenosis may also be caused by a *congenital* abnormality.

Aortic stenosis may not cause symptoms. When symptoms do occur, they include fainting, lack of energy, chest pain on exertion due to *angina*, and breathing difficulty.

Chest X-ray, *ECG*, and *echocardiography* may be carried out to diagnose aortic stenosis. A cardiac catheter can be used to demonstrate the degree of stenosis (see *catheterization, cardiac*). *Heart-valve surgery* may be needed to widen or replace the damaged valve.

AORTIC STENOSIS

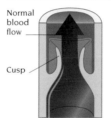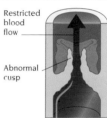

- Normal blood flow
- Cusp
- Restricted blood flow
- Abnormal cusp

NORMAL AORTA   **STENOSED AORTA**

aortitis Inflammation of the *aorta* (the main artery of the body). Aortitis is a rare condition that occurs in people with *arteritis* or untreated *syphilis* and in some people with *ankylosing spondylitis*.

Aortitis may cause part of the aorta to widen and its walls to become thinner. This may lead to an *aneurysm* (ballooning of the artery). Aortitis may damage the ring around the aortic valve in the heart, leading to *aortic incompetence*.

aortography An imaging technique that enables the *aorta* (the main artery of the body) and its branches to be seen clearly on X-ray film following injection of a *contrast medium* (a substance that is opaque to X-rays). Aortography is used if surgery is needed to treat an *aneurysm* (ballooning of the aorta).

aperient A mild *laxative drug*.

apex The uppermost surface of a structure, for example the top, end, or tip of an organ such as a lung or the heart.

apex beat A normal heartbeat felt through the chest wall. As the heart contracts, its tip hits the chest wall and can be felt between the fifth and sixth ribs on the left side of the chest. The apex beat is displaced when the heart is enlarged.

Apgar score A system designed to assess the condition of a newborn baby. Five features are scored 1 minute and again 5 minutes after birth. These are breathing, heart-rate, colour, muscle tone, and response to stimulation.

focusing in the affected eye and requires correction by implanting a lens or with contact lenses or glasses.

aphasia A complete absence of previously acquired language skills, caused by a brain disorder affecting the ability to speak and write, and/or the ability to comprehend and read. Related disabilities that may occur in aphasia are *alexia* (word blindness) and *agraphia* (writing difficulty).

Language function in the brain lies in the dominant cerebral hemisphere (see *cerebrum*). Two particular areas in this hemisphere, Broca's and Wernicke's areas, and the pathways connecting the two, are important in language skills. Damage to these areas, which most commonly occurs as a result of stroke or head injury, can lead to aphasia.

Some recovery from aphasia is usual following a stroke or head injury, although the more severe the aphasia, the less the chances of recovery. *Speech therapy* is the main treatment. (See also *dysphasia; speech; speech disorders*.)

apheresis A procedure in which blood is withdrawn from a donor and is reinfused after one or more selected components have been separated and removed. In plasmapheresis, antibodies causing a disease are removed; and in leukapheresis, white blood cells are removed.

aphonia Complete loss of the voice, which may result from surgery to the *larynx*, or it may be sudden in onset and due to emotional stress. (See also *dysphonia*.)

aphrodisiac Any substance that is thought to stimulate erotic desire and enhance sexual performance. For centuries, various substances (most notably oysters and rhinoceros horn) have been used as aphrodisiacs. In fact, no

APGAR SCORE

SIGN	SCORE 0	SCORE 1	SCORE 2
Heart-rate	None	Below 100 beats per minute	Over 100 beats per minute
Breathing	None	Weak cry; irregular breathing	Strong cry; regular breathing
Muscle tone	Limp	Some muscle tone	Active movement
Response to stimulation	None	Grimace or whimpering	Cry, sneeze or cough
Colour	Pale; blue	Blue extremities	Pink

aphakia The absence of the *lens* from the eye. Aphakia may be congenital, may result from surgery (for example, *cataract surgery*), or may be due to a penetrating injury. Aphakia causes severe loss of

substance has a proven aphrodisiac effect.

aphthous ulcer See *ulcer, aphthous*.

apicectomy Surgical removal of the tip of a tooth root. Apicectomy may be performed as part of *root-canal treatment*.

aplasia Absent or severely reduced growth and development of any organ or tissue. For example, in bone marrow aplasia, the rate of cell division in the bone marrow is reduced, leading to insufficient blood-cell production (see *anaemia, aplastic*). Some birth defects, such as stunted limbs (see *phocomelia*), occur as a result of incomplete tissue formation during prenatal development.

aplastic anaemia See *anaemia, aplastic.*

apnoea Cessation of breathing, either temporarily or for a prolonged period.

Breathing is an automatic process controlled by the respiratory centre in the brainstem. Failure of this centre to maintain normal breathing is known as central apnoea. It may occur in babies, particularly those who are premature, and can be detected by an apnoea alarm. Central apnoea can also result from brainstem damage, for example following a *stroke* or *head injury*.

In obstructive apnoea, breathing is prevented by a blockage in the airway. The most common type is *sleep apnoea*, in which blockage of the upper airway occurs repeatedly during sleep.

Deliberate temporary apnoea occurs in *breath-holding attacks*. Another type of apnoea occurs in *Cheyne–Stokes respiration*, in which cycles of deep, rapid breathing alternate with episodes of breathing stoppage.

Treatment of apnoea depends on the cause. In newborn babies, it resolves as they mature. In stroke or head injury, artificial ventilation may be needed temporarily until recovery occurs.

apocrine gland A gland that discharges cellular material in addition to the fluid it secretes. The term is usually applied to the type of *sweat glands* that appear in hairy body areas after puberty. (See also *eccrine gland*.)

apolipoprotein A group of proteins that are constituents of *lipoproteins*, the carriers of fat in the bloodstream. Apolipoproteins are also involved in the growth and repair of nerve tissues.

aponeurosis A wide sheet of tough, fibrous tissue that acts as a tendon, attaching a muscle to a bone or a joint.

apophysis An outgrowth of bone at the site of attachment of a tendon to bone.

Inflammation may also occur, as in *Osgood–Schlatter disease.*

apoplexy An outdated term for a *stroke*.

apoptosis The natural process of programmed cell death. Apoptosis occurs in embryonic development, when the shaping of body parts is taking place and continues throughout life in the constant cycle of death and renewal of body cells. Failure of apoptosis is implicated in the development of cancers.

apothecary An old term for a *pharmacist.*

appendicectomy Surgical removal of the appendix to treat acute *appendicitis*.

appendicitis Acute inflammation of the appendix. The cause is usually not known, but appendicitis is sometimes caused by obstruction of the appendix by a lump of faeces. The first symptom is usually vague discomfort around the navel. Within a few hours, this develops into severe, more localized pain, which is usually most intense in the lower right-hand side of the abdomen. Symptoms may differ if the appendix is not in the most common position. For example, if the appendix impinges on the ureter, the urine may become bloodstained.

The usual treatment for appendicitis is *appendicectomy*, which is often performed endoscopically (see *minimally invasive surgery*). If the treatment is delayed, an inflamed appendix may burst, releasing its contents into the abdomen. This leads to *peritonitis* and, in some cases, an *abscess.*

appendix A small, narrow tube that projects out of the caecum (the first part of the colon) at the lower right-hand side of the abdomen. It may lie behind or below the caecum, or in front of or behind the

APPENDIX

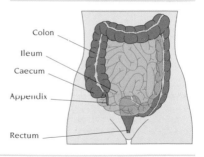

Colon
Ileum
Caecum
Appendix
Rectum

ileum (part of the small intestine). The appendix has no known function, but it contains a large amount of lymphoid tissue which provides a defence against local infection. The position of an individual's appendix partly determines the set of symptoms produced by acute *appendicitis* (inflammation of the appendix).

appetite A desire for food; a pleasant sensation felt in anticipation of eating. Appetite, which is regulated by two parts of the *brain* (the *hypothalamus* and the cerebral cortex), is learned by enjoying a variety of foods that smell, taste, and look good. It combines with *hunger* to ensure that the right amount of a wide range of foods is eaten to stay healthy. (See also *appetite, loss of.*)

appetite, loss of Loss of appetite is usually temporary and due to an emotional upset or minor illness. Persistent loss of appetite may have a more serious underlying cause, such as chronic infection or cancer.

appetite stimulants Various tonics and remedies traditionally prescribed to stimulate the appetite. None are proven to be effective. Some drugs such as *corticosteroids* may stimulate the appetite when used to treat unrelated disorders.

appetite suppressants Drugs that reduce the desire to eat. Appetite suppressants may be used in the treatment of severe *obesity*, along with diet and exercise. *Sibutramine* is the main appetite suppressant drug.

apraxia An inability to carry out purposeful movements despite normal muscle power and coordination. Apraxia is caused by damage to nerve tracts in the *cerebrum* (the main mass of the brain) that translate the idea for a movement into an actual movement. Damage to the cerebrum may be caused by a *head injury*, infection, *stroke*, or *brain tumour*.

There are various forms of apraxia, each related to damage in different parts of the brain. A person with ideomotor apraxia is unable to carry out a spoken command to make a particular movement, but at other times can make the same movement unconsciously. In sensory apraxia, a person may not be able to use an object due to loss of ability to recognize its purpose.

APUD cell tumour A growth composed of cells that produce various hormones. These cells, amine precursor uptake and decarboxylation (APUD) cells, occur in different parts of the body. Some tumours of the thyroid gland, pancreas, and lungs are APUD cell tumours, as are a carcinoid tumour (see *carcinoid syndrome*) and *phaeochromocytoma* (a type of adrenal tumour).

aqueous cream An *emollient* preparation that is commonly used to treat dry, scaly, or itchy skin in conditions such as *eczema*.

aqueous humour A watery fluid that fills the front chamber of the *eye*, behind the *cornea*.

arachidonic acid One of the fatty acids in the body that are essential for growth.

arachis oil Peanut oil, mostly used in *enemas*, to soften faeces and make bowel movements easier. It may also be applied to the scalp, followed by shampooing, in the treatment of *cradle cap*.

arachnodactyly Long, thin, spider-like fingers and toes that sometimes occur spontaneously but are characteristic of *Marfan's syndrome*, an inherited connective tissue disease.

arachnoiditis A rare condition that is characterized by chronic inflammation and thickening of the arachnoid mater, which is the middle of the three *meninges* (the membranes that cover the brain and spinal cord).

arachnoid mater The middle of the three layers of membrane (*meninges*) that cover the *brain*.

arbovirus Any of the many viruses transmitted by a member of the arthropod group of animals, including insects, mites, and ticks. (See also *insects and disease; mites and disease; ticks and disease*).

ARC An abbreviation for *AIDS-related complex*. (See also *AIDS*.)

arcus senilis A grey-white ring near the edge of the *cornea* overlying the iris (the coloured part of the eye). Arcus senilis is caused by degeneration of fatty material in the cornea and develops gradually during adult life. The ring does not affect eyesight. Development of the condition in early adult life may be associated with an abnormality of fats in the blood (see *hyperlipidaemia*).

areola The pigmented circular area surrounding the *nipple*. The term is also used to describe an inflamed area around a pimple (see *pustule*).

aromatherapy A form of *complementary medicine* that uses aromatic oils extracted from plants. The oil is applied in small quantities through massage; or it is inhaled, incorporated into creams or lotions, or, very occasionally, taken internally. There is no conclusive scientific evidence of the benefits.

arousal The awakening of a person from unconsciousness or semiconsciousness. The term is also used to describe any state of heightened awareness, such as that caused by sexual stimulation or fear. Arousal is regulated by the reticular formation in the *brainstem*.

arrhenoblastoma A rare tumour of the ovary that occurs in young women. The tumour is noncancerous but secretes *androgen hormones* (male sex hormones) that cause *virilization* (the development of male characteristics). Treatment is by surgical removal of the affected ovary.

arrhythmia, cardiac An abnormality of the rhythm or rate of the *heartbeat*. Arrhythmias, which are caused by a disturbance in the electrical impulses in the *heart*, can be divided into two main groups: tachycardias, in which the rate is faster than normal, and bradycardias, in which the rate is slower.

In *sinus tachycardia*, the rate is raised, the rhythm is regular, and the beat originates in the sinoatrial node (see *pacemaker*). *Supraventricular tachycardia* is faster and the rhythm is regular. It may be caused by an abnormal electrical pathway that allows an impulse to circulate continuously in the heart and take over from the sinoatrial node. Rapid, irregular beats that originate in the ventricles are called *ventricular tachycardia*. In *atrial flutter*, the atria (see *atrium*) beat regularly and very rapidly, but not every impulse reaches the ventricles, which beat at a slower rate. Uncoordinated, fast beating of the atria is called *atrial fibrillation* and produces totally irregular ventricular beats. *Ventricular fibrillation* is a form of *cardiac arrest* in which the ventricles twitch very rapidly in a disorganized manner.

Sinus bradycardia is a slow, regular beat. In *heart block*, the conduction of electrical impulses through the heart muscle is partially or completely blocked, leading to a slow, irregular heartbeat. Periods of bradycardia may alternate with periods of tachycardia due to a fault in impulse generation (see *sick sinus syndrome*).

A common cause of arrhythmia is *coronary artery disease*, particularly after *myocardial infarction*. Some tachycardias are due to a *congenital* defect in the heart's conducting system. *Caffeine* can cause tachycardia in some people. *Amitriptyline* and some other *antidepressant drugs* can cause serious arrhythmias if they are taken in high doses.

An arrhythmia may be felt as palpitations, but in some cases arrhythmias

ARRHYTHMIA, CARDIAC

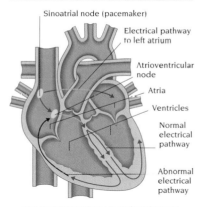

Sinoatrial node (pacemaker)

Electrical pathway to left atrium

Atrioventricular node

Atria

Ventricles

Normal electrical pathway

Abnormal electrical pathway

SUPRAVENTRICULAR TACHYCARDIA

can cause fainting, dizziness, chest pain, and breathlessness, which may be the first symptoms.

Arrhythmias are diagnosed by an *ECG*. If they are intermittent, a continuous recording may need to be made using an *ambulatory ECG*.

Treatments for arrhythmias include *antiarrhythmic drugs*, which prevent or slow tachycardias. With an arrhythmia that has developed suddenly, it may be possible to restore normal heart rhythm by using electric shock to the heart (see *defibrillation*). Abnormal conduction pathways in the heart can be treated using *radiofrequency ablation* during cardiac catheterization (see *catheterization, cardiac*). In some cases, a pacemaker can be fitted to restore normal heartbeat by overriding the heart's abnormal rhythm.

arsenic A poisonous metallic element that occurs naturally in its pure form and in various compounds. Arsenic poisoning, which is now rare, used to occur as a result of continuous exposure to industrial pesticides.

arterial reconstructive surgery An operation to repair *arteries* that are narrowed, blocked, or weakened. Arterial reconstructive surgery is most often performed to repair arteries that have been narrowed by *atherosclerosis*. It is also used to repair *aneurysms* and arteries damaged as a result of injury. (See also *angioplasty, balloon*; *coronary artery bypass*; *endarterectomy*.)

arteries, disorders of Disorders of the arteries may take the form of abnormal narrowing (which reduces blood flow and may cause tissue damage), complete obstruction (which may cause tissue death), or abnormal widening and thinning of an artery wall (which may cause rupture of the blood vessel).

Atherosclerosis, in which fat deposits build up on artery walls, is the most common arterial disease. It can involve arteries throughout the body, including the brain (see *cerebrovascular disease*), heart (see *coronary artery disease*), and legs (see *peripheral vascular disease*). Atherosclerosis is the main type of *arteriosclerosis*, a group of disorders that cause thickening and loss of elasticity of artery walls. *Hypertension* is another common cause of thickening and narrowing of arteries, and it increases the risk of a *stroke* or *kidney failure*. Arteritis is inflammation of artery walls that causes narrowing and sometimes blockage. *Aneurysm* is ballooning of an artery wall caused by the pressure of blood flowing through a weakened area. *Thrombosis* occurs when a blood clot forms in a blood vessel, causing obstruction of the blood flow. Blockage of an artery by a fragment of blood clot or other material travelling in the circu-

lation is called an *embolism*. *Raynaud's disease* is a disorder involving intermittent spasm of small arteries in the hands and feet, usually due to cold.

arteriography An alternative name for *angiography*, an X-ray technique for imaging arteries.

arteriole A blood vessel that branches off an *artery*. Arterioles branch to form *capillaries*. They have muscular walls, and their nerve supply enables them to be narrowed or widened to meet the blood-flow needs of tissues they supply.

arteriopathy Any disorder of an artery (see *arteries, disorders of*).

arterioplasty Surgical repair of an artery (see *arterial reconstructive surgery*).

arteriosclerosis A group of disorders that cause thickening and loss of elasticity of artery walls. *Atherosclerosis* is the most common type, and the two terms are often used synonymously. Other types are medial arteriosclerosis (in which muscle and elastic fibres in larger arteries are replaced by fibrous tissue, as occurs in *Marfan's syndrome*) and Monckeberg's arteriosclerosis (in which there are calcium deposits in the arterial lining).

arteriovenous fistula An abnormal communication directly between an artery and a vein. An arteriovenous fistula may be present at birth or result from injury. A fistula can also be created surgically for easy access to the bloodstream in *dialysis*.

arteritis Inflammation of an artery wall, causing narrowing or complete blockage of the affected artery, reduced blood flow, and, in some cases, *thrombosis* and tissue damage. There are several types, including *Buerger's disease*, an arteritis that affects the limbs, causing pain, numbness, and, in severe cases, *gangrene*. Polyarteritis nodosa, a serious *autoimmune disorder*, can affect arteries in any part of the body, especially the heart and kidneys. *Temporal arteritis* affects arteries in the scalp and may affect the eyes. A rare type of arteritis is Takayasu's arteritis, which is thought to be an autoimmune disorder. This usually affects young women and involves the arteries that branch from the *aorta* into the neck and arms.

artery A blood vessel that carries blood away from the *heart*. Systemic arteries carry blood pumped from the left ventricle of the heart to all parts of the body except the lungs. The largest systemic artery is the *aorta*, which emerges from the left ventricle; other major systemic arteries branch off from the aorta. The pulmonary arteries carry blood from the right ventricle to the lungs.

Arteries are tubes with thick, elastic, muscular walls able to withstand the high pressure of blood flow. The structure of arteries helps to even out the peaks and troughs of blood pressure caused by the heartbeat, so that the blood is kept flowing at a relatively constant pressure. (See also *arteries, disorders of.*)

ARTERY

Outer layer
Muscle layer
Elastic layer
Inner lining

arthralgia Pain in the joints or a single joint. (See also *arthritis; joint.*)

arthritis Inflammation of one or more joints, with pain, swelling, and stiffness.

There are several different types of arthritis, each having different characteristics. The most common form is *osteoarthritis*, which most often involves the knees, hips, and hands and usually affects middle-aged and older people. *Cervical osteoarthritis* is a form of osteoarthritis that affects the joints in the neck. *Rheumatoid arthritis* is a damaging condition that causes inflammation in the joints and other body tissues such as the membranous heart covering, blood vessels, lungs, and eyes. The disorder has different effects in children (see *juvenile chronic arthritis*). Ankylosing spondylitis is another persistent form of arthritis that initially affects the spine and the joints between the base of the spine and the pelvis. Other tissues, such as the eyes, may also be affected.

Eventually, the disorder may cause the vertebrae (bones of the spine) to fuse. *Reactive arthritis* typically develops in susceptible people following an infection, most commonly of the genital tract or intestines. *Gout* and *pseudogout* are types of arthritis in which crystals are deposited in a joint, causing swelling and pain. *Septic arthritis* is a relatively rare condition that can develop when infection enters a joint either through a wound or from the bloodstream.

Diagnosis of particular types of arthritis is by *blood tests* and, in some cases, microscopic examination of fluid from the affected joint. *X-rays* or *MRI* can indicate the type and extent of joint damage.

Physiotherapy and exercises can help to minimize the effects of arthritis, and there are specific treatments for some types, such as *antibiotic drugs* for septic arthritis. *Analgesic drugs, nonsteroidal anti-inflammatory drugs, disease-modifying antirheumatic drugs,* and *corticosteroids* may be used to relieve the symptoms and/or affect the course of the arthritis. In severe cases, one or more joints may need *arthroplasty* (replacement with an artificial substitute) or *arthrodesis* (fusion of the bones)

arthrodesis A surgical procedure in which the bones in a diseased joint are fused to prevent the joint from moving, which relieves pain. Arthrodesis is performed if a joint is painful or unstable and other treatments such as drugs or *arthroplasty* have failed or are inappropriate.

arthrogryposis See *contracture.*

arthropathy Disease of the *joints.*

arthroplasty Replacement of a joint or part of a joint by metal or plastic components. A *hip replacement* is one of the most common operations of this type, as is *knee-joint replacement*. Replacement of other joints, such as the finger (see *finger-joint replacement*), shoulder, and elbow, is also common.

arthroscopy Inspection through an *endoscope* (viewing tube) of the interior of a joint. Arthroscopy is most often used to diagnose disorders of the knee joint but can also be used in other joints such as the shoulder, hip, or wrist. It allows the surgeon to see the surface of the bones, the ligaments, the cartilages, and

artificial insemination A form of assisted conception in which semen is introduced artificially into the uterus, instead of by sexual intercourse, with the aim of inducing pregnancy.

the synovial membrane. Specimens can be taken for examination. Some surgical procedures, such as removal of damaged cartilage, repair of ligaments, and shaving of the patella (kneecap), are usually performed arthroscopically.

There are two types of artificial insemination: AIH, artificial insemination with the semen of the woman's male partner; and AID, insemination with a donor's sperm. AIH is usually used for couples who are unable to have intercourse, or if the man has a low sperm count or a low volume of ejaculate. It is also used when semen has been stored from a man prior to treatment (such as chemotherapy) that has made him sterile. AID is available to couples if the man is infertile or is a carrier of a genetic disease. It may also be used by a woman who wants children but has no male partner.

Insemination is timed to coincide with natural ovulation or may be combined with treatment to stimulate ovulation.

artificial kidney The common name for the machine used in *dialysis*.

artificial respiration Forced introduction of air into the lungs of someone who has stopped breathing (see *respiratory arrest*) or whose breathing is inadequate. As emergency first aid, artificial respiration (rescue breathing) can be given mouth-to-mouth or mouth-to-nose, which can prevent brain damage due to oxygen deprivation; a delay in breathing for more than about 3 minutes can cause death. Cardiac compressions may be necessary if poor respiration has led to cessation of the heartbeat (see *cardiopulmonary resuscitation*). Artificial respiration can be continued by use of a ventilator (see *ventilation*).

artificial rupture of membrane See *amniotomy*.

artificial sweeteners Synthetic substitutes for sugar that are used by people on slimming diets and by the food industry; examples include aspartame and saccharin. Sorbitol is an artificial sweetener that is useful for diabetics,

but it can cause diarrhoea and bloating when consumed in large quantities.

arytenoid One of two pyramid-shaped cartilages that form part of the *larynx*.

asbestos-related diseases A variety of diseases caused by inhalation of asbestos fibres. Asbestos is a fibrous mineral formerly used as a heat- and fire-resistant insulating material. There are three main types of asbestos fibre: white, which is widely used; blue; and brown, the most dangerous. The use of all types is now carefully controlled.

In asbestosis, widespread fine scarring occurs in the lungs. The disease causes breathlessness and a dry cough, eventually leading to severe disability and death. It develops mostly in industrial workers who have been heavily exposed to asbestos. The period from initial exposure to development of the disease is usually at least 20 years. Diagnosis is by *chest X-ray*. Asbestosis increases the risk of *lung cancer*.

Mesothelioma is a cancerous tumour of the *pleura* (the membrane surrounding the lungs) or the *peritoneum* (the membrane lining the abdominal cavity). In the pleura, mesotheliomas cause pain and breathlessness; in the peritoneum they cause enlargement of the abdomen and intestinal obstruction. The condition cannot be treated and usually leads to death within 1 or 2 years. The average interval between initial exposure to asbestos and death is 20–30 years. Mesothelioma affects people who have worked with blue or brown asbestos.

In diffuse pleural thickening, the outer and inner layers of the pleura become thickened, and excess fluid may accumulate in the cavity between them. This combination restricts the ability of the lungs to expand, resulting in shortness of breath. The condition may develop even after short exposure to asbestos.

asbestosis See *asbestos-related diseases*.

ascariasis Infestation with the roundworm *ASCARIS LUMBRICOIDES*, which lives in the small intestine of its human host. Ascariasis is common worldwide, especially in the tropics. The disease is spread by ingestion of worm eggs, usually from food grown in soil that has been contaminated by human faeces.

Light infestation may cause no symptoms, but mild nausea, abdominal pain, and irregular bowel movements may occur. A worm may be passed via the rectum or vomited. A large number of worms may compete with the host for food, leading to malnutrition and *anaemia*, which in children can retard growth. Treatment is with *anthelmintic drugs*, such as *levamisole*, which usually produce complete recovery.

ascites Excess fluid in the peritoneal cavity, the space between the two-layered membrane that lines the inside of the abdominal wall and which covers the abdominal organs.

Ascites may occur in any condition that causes generalized *oedema,* such as congestive *heart failure, nephrotic syndrome,* and *cirrhosis* of the liver. Ascites may occur in *cancer* if metastases (secondary growths) from a cancer elsewhere in the body develop in the peritoneum. The condition also occurs if *tuberculosis* affects the abdomen.

Ascites causes abdominal swelling and discomfort. It may cause breathing difficulty due to pressure on the diaphragm. The underlying cause is treated if possible. *Diuretic drugs,* particularly *spironolactone,* are often used to treat ascites associated with cirrhosis.

ascorbic acid The chemical name for *vitamin C.*

ASD See *atrial septal defect.*

aseptic technique Creation of a germ-free environment to protect a patient from infection. Aseptic technique is used during surgery and when caring for people suffering from diseases, such as *leukaemia,* in which the *immune system* is suppressed. All people who come in contact with the patient must scrub their hands and wear pre-sterilized gowns and disposable gloves and masks. Surgical instruments are sterilized in an *autoclave.* The patient's skin is cleaned with *antiseptic* solutions. A special ventilation system in the operating theatre purifies the air. (See also *isolation.*)

aspartame An *artificial sweetener* used in some foods and drugs.

Asperger's syndrome A developmental disorder that is usually first recognized in childhood because of dif-

ficulties with social interactions and very specialized interests. It is more common in boys than in girls. Intelligence is normal or high. Asperger's syndrome is considered to be an *autism spectrum disorder* and is also known as pervasive developmental disorder. Special educational support may be needed, often within mainstream education. The condition is lifelong.

aspergillosis An infection caused by inhalation of spores of aspergillus, a fungus that grows in decaying vegetation. Aspergillus is harmless to healthy people but may proliferate in the lungs of people with *tuberculosis,* worsen the symptoms of *asthma,* and produce serious, even fatal, infection in people with reduced immunity, such as those taking *immunosuppressant drugs.*

aspermia See *azoospermia.*

asphyxia The medical term for suffocation. Asphyxia may be caused by the obstruction of a large airway, usually by a foreign body (see *choking*), by insufficient oxygen in the surrounding air (as occurs when a closed plastic bag is put over the head), or by poisoning with a gas such as carbon monoxide that interferes with the uptake of oxygen into the blood. First-aid treatment is by *artificial respiration* after clearing the airway of obstruction. Untreated asphyxia leads to death within a few minutes.

aspiration The withdrawal of fluid or cells from the body by suction. The term also refers to the act of accidentally inhaling a foreign body, usually food or drink. If consciousness is impaired, for example by a head injury or excess

ASPIRATION

Normal breast tissue — Fat layer — Breast lump — Needle — Syringe draws cells into needle

ASPIRATION OF A BREAST LUMP

alcohol intake, aspiration of the stomach contents is common.

Aspiration *biopsy* is the removal of cells or fluid for examination using a needle and syringe. The procedure is commonly used to obtain cells from a fluid-filled cavity (such as a *breast lump* or *breast cyst*). It is also used to obtain cells from the bone marrow (see *bone marrow biopsy*), or from internal organs, when a fine needle is guided into the site of the biopsy by *CT scanning* or *ultrasound scanning*.

aspirin A nonopioid *analgesic drug* and *nonsteroidal anti-inflammatory drug* used to treat disorders such as headache, menstrual pain, and muscle discomfort. Aspirin has an anti-inflammatory action and is particularly useful for joint pain in *arthritis*. It reduces fever and is included in some *cold remedies*. In small doses, it reduces the stickiness of platelets (blood particles involved in clotting). This has led to its use in preventing *thrombosis* in people at risk of developing *stroke* or *myocardial infarction* and as initial treatment of chest pain that may be due to myocardial infarction.

Aspirin may cause irritation of the stomach lining, resulting in indigestion or nausea. Prolonged use of the drug may cause bleeding from the stomach due to *gastric erosion* or *peptic ulcer*. Aspirin should therefore not be used by people who have or have had a peptic ulcer. Aspirin should also not be used by people who have had a previous reaction to it (for example, *asthma*, *rhinitis*, or *rash*) or to any other nonsteroidal anti-inflammatory drug, such as ibuprofen. Do not give aspirin, or aspirin-containing medications, to children under the age of 16, except on the advice of a doctor, because it increases the risk of *Reye's syndrome*, a rare but serious brain and liver disorder. Aspirin should also not be taken by women who are breast-feeding.

assay Analysis or measurement of a substance to determine its presence or effects. Biological assays (bioassays) measure the responses of an animal or organ to particular substances. They can be used to assess the effects of a drug or to measure hormone levels. (See also *immunoassay*; *radioimmunoassay*.)

assisted conception Treatment for *infertility* involving techniques that assist the fertilization and implantation of eggs.

association area One of a number of areas in the outer layer (cortex) of the *brain* that are concerned with higher levels of mental activity. Association areas interpret information received from sensory areas and prompt appropriate responses such as voluntary movement.

astereognosis An inability to recognize objects by touch when they are placed in the hand, even though there is no defect of sensation in the fingers or difficulty in holding the object. Astereognosis is either left- or right-sided; tactile recognition is normal on the other side. If both sides are affected, the condition is called tactile *agnosia*. Astereognosis and tactile agnosia are caused by brain damage, often from a *stroke* or *head injury*.

asthma A lung disease in which there is intermittent narrowing of the *bronchi* (airways), causing shortness of breath, wheezing, and cough. The illness often starts in childhood but can develop at any age. At least one child in seven suffers from asthma, and the number affected has increased dramatically in recent years. Childhood asthma may be outgrown in about half of all cases.

During an asthma attack, the muscle in the walls of the airways contracts, causing narrowing. The linings of the airways also become swollen and inflamed, producing excess mucus that can block the smaller airways.

In some people, an allergic response triggers the airway changes. This allergic type of asthma tends to occur in childhood and may develop in association with eczema or certain other allergic conditions such as hay fever (see *rhinitis, allergic*). Susceptibility to these conditions often runs in families.

Some substances, called *allergens*, are known to trigger attacks of allergic asthma. They include pollen, house-dust mites, mould, and *dander* and saliva from furry animals such as cats and dogs. Rarely, certain foods, such as milk, eggs, nuts, and wheat, provoke an allergic asthmatic reaction. Some people with asthma are sensitive to *aspirin*, and taking it may trigger an attack.

When asthma starts in adulthood, there are usually no identifiable allergic triggers. The first attack is sometimes brought on by a respiratory infection.

Factors that can provoke attacks in a person with asthma include cold air, exercise, smoke, and occasionally emotional factors such as stress and anxiety. Although industrial pollution and exhaust emission from motor vehicles do not normally cause asthma, they do appear to worsen symptoms in people who already have the disorder. Pollution in the atmosphere may also trigger asthma in susceptible people.

In some cases, a substance inhaled regularly in the workplace can cause a previously healthy person to develop asthma. This is called occupation asthma and is one of the few occupational lung diseases still increasing in incidence.

There are currently about 200 substances used in the workplace that are known to trigger symptoms of asthma, including glues, resins, latex, and some chemicals such as isocyanates used in spray painting. However, occupational asthma can be difficult to diagnose because a person may be regularly exposed to a particular trigger substance for weeks, months, or years before symptoms begin to appear.

Asthmatic attacks can vary in severity from mild breathlessness to *respiratory failure*. The main symptoms are wheezing, breathlessness, dry cough, and tightness in the chest. In a severe attack, breathing becomes increasingly difficult, resulting in a low level of oxygen in the blood. This causes *cyanosis* (bluish discoloration) of the face, particularly the lips. Untreated, such attacks may be fatal.

There is no cure for asthma, but attacks can be prevented to a large extent if a particular allergen can be identified.

Treatment involves inhaled *bronchodilator drugs* (also known as relievers) to relieve symptoms. When symptoms occur frequently, or are severe, inhaled *corticosteroids* are also prescribed. These drugs are used continuously to prevent attacks by reducing inflammation in the airways and are also known as preventers.

Other drug treatments include *sodium cromoglicate* and nedocromil sodium, which are useful in preventing exercise-

ASTHMA

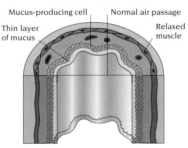

Mucus-producing cell   Normal air passage
Thin layer of mucus   Relaxed muscle

NORMAL AIRWAY

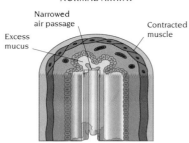

Narrowed air passage   Contracted muscle
Excess mucus

AIRWAY DURING ASTHMA ATTACK

induced asthma. A group of drugs called *leukotriene receptor antagonists* may reduce the dose of corticosteroid needed to control the condition. *Theophylline* or the inhaled anticholinergic drug *ipratropium* may also be used as bronchodilators. An asthma attack that has not responded to treatment needs immediate medical attention.

asthma, cardiac Breathing difficulty in which *bronchospasm* and wheezing are caused by accumulation of fluid in the lungs (*pulmonary oedema*). This is usually due to reduced pumping efficiency of the left side of the heart (see *heart failure*) and is not true asthma. Treatment is with *diuretic drugs*.

astigmatism A condition in which the front surface of the *cornea* does not conform to the normal "spherical" curve, although the eye is perfectly healthy. Because the cornea is unevenly curved, it refracts (bends) the light rays that strike it to differing degrees. The *lens* is then unable to bring all the rays into focus on the light-sensitive *retina*.

A minor degree of astigmatism is normal and does not require correction. More severe astigmatism causes blurring of lines at a particular angle and requires correction, which be achieved by special "cylindrical" glasses that can be framed at a precise angle, contact lenses that can give an even spherical surface for focusing, or laser surgery.

astringent A substance that causes tissue to dry and shrink by reducing its ability to absorb water. Astringents are widely used in *antiperspirants* and to promote healing of broken or inflamed skin. They are also used in some eye or ear preparations. Astringents may cause burning or stinging when applied.

astrocytoma A type of cancerous *brain tumour*. Astrocytomas are the most common type of *glioma*, a tumour arising from the glial (supporting) cells in the nervous system. They most commonly develop in the cerebrum (the main mass of the brain). Astrocytomas are classified in four grades (I-IV) according to their rate of growth and malignancy. The most severe and common type is called *glioblastoma multiforme*. Symptoms are similar to those of other types of brain tumour. Diagnostic tests include *CT scanning* or *MRI*. Treatment is with surgery and, in some cases, *radiotherapy* and/or *chemotherapy*.

asylum An outdated term for an institution providing care for the mentally ill.

asymptomatic A medical term meaning without *symptoms*. For example, *hypertension* is often asymptomatic and is usually discovered during a routine blood pressure test.

asystole A term meaning absence of the heartbeat (see *cardiac arrest*).

ataxia Incoordination and clumsiness that affects balance and gait, limb or eye movements, and/or speech. Ataxia may be caused by damage to the *cerebellum* or to nerve pathways in the *brainstem* and spinal cord. Possible causes include injury to the brain or spinal cord. In adults, ataxia may be caused by *alcohol intoxication*, a *stroke* or a *brain tumour* affecting the cerebellum or the brainstem, a disease of the balance organ in the ear, or *multiple sclerosis* or other types of nerve degeneration. In children,

causes include acute infection, brain tumours, and the inherited condition *Friedreich's ataxia*.

Symptoms of ataxia depend on the site of damage, although a lurching, unsteady gait is common to most forms. In addition, damage to certain parts of the brain may cause *nystagmus* and slurred speech. *CT scanning* or *MRI* may be used to determine the cause of ataxia. Treatment of the condition depends on the cause.

atelectasis Collapse of part or all of a *lung* caused by obstruction of one or more air passages in the lung. Obstruction may be caused by accumulation of mucus, by an accidentally inhaled foreign body, by a tumour in the lung, or by enlarged lymph nodes exerting pressure on the airway.

The main symptom is shortness of breath. There may also be a cough and chest pain. The condition can be diagnosed by *chest X-ray*. Treatment is aimed at removing the cause of the blockage and may include *physiotherapy* or *bronchoscopy*. If the obstruction can be removed, the lung should reinflate normally.

atenolol A *beta-blocker drug* used to treat *hypertension*, *angina*, and certain types of *arrhythmia*.

atheroma Fatty deposits on the inner lining of an artery that occur in *atherosclerosis* and restrict blood flow.

atherosclerosis Accumulation of *cholesterol* and other fatty substances (lipids) in the walls of arteries, causing them to narrow. Atherosclerosis can affect arteries in any area of the body and is a major cause of *stroke*, heart attack (see *myocardial infarction*), and poor circulation in the legs. The arteries become narrowed when fatty substances, such as cholesterol, that are carried in the blood accumulate on the inside lining of the arteries and form yellow deposits called atheroma. These deposits restrict blood flow through the arteries. In addition, the muscle layer of the artery wall becomes thickened, narrowing the artery even more. Platelets (tiny blood cells responsible for clotting) may collect in clumps on the surface of the deposits and initiate the formation of blood clots.

ATHEROSCLEROSIS

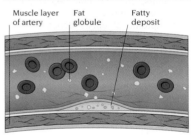

Muscle layer of artery | Fat globule | Fatty deposit

EARLY ATHEROSCLEROSIS

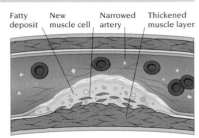

Fatty deposit | New muscle cell | Narrowed artery | Thickened muscle layer

ADVANCED ATHEROSCLEROSIS

A large clot may completely block the artery, resulting in the organ it supplies being deprived of oxygen.

There are usually no symptoms in the early stages of atherosclerosis. Later, symptoms are caused by reduced or total absence of a blood supply to the organs supplied by the affected arteries. If the coronary arteries, which supply the heart muscle, are partially blocked, symptoms may include the chest pain of *angina*. If there is complete blockage in a coronary artery, a sudden, often fatal, heart attack may occur. Many strokes are a result of atherosclerosis in the arteries that supply blood to the brain. If atherosclerosis affects the leg arteries, the first symptom may be cramping pain when walking due to poor blood flow to the leg muscles. If the condition is associated with an inherited lipid disorder (see *hyperlipidaemias*), fatty deposits may develop on tendons or under the skin in visible lumps.

Major risk factors for the development of artherosclerosis are raised blood lipid levels and *hypertension*. Atherosclerosis is most common in Western countries, where most people eat a diet high in fat. Some disorders such as diabetes mellitus can be associated with a high cholesterol level regardless of diet.

Blood flow through an artery can be investigated by *angiography* or *Doppler* ultrasound scanning.

The best treatment for atherosclerosis is to prevent it from progressing by following a healthy lifestyle. This includes eating a low-fat diet, not smoking, exercising regularly, and maintaining the recommended weight for height. These measures lead to a lower-than-average risk of developing significant atherosclerosis. People found to have high blood cholesterol but who are otherwise in good health will be advised to adopt a low-fat diet. They may also be given drugs that decrease blood cholesterol levels (see *lipid-lowering drugs*). For people who have had a heart attack, research has shown that there may be a benefit in lowering blood cholesterol levels, even if the level is within the average range for healthy people. People with diabetes can help reduce their risk of artherosclerosis by careful control of their blood sugar levels. For those with hypertension, reducing their blood pressure to within recommended limits can help reduce the risk of artherosclerosis.

People who have atherosclerosis and are experiencing symptoms of the condition may be prescribed a drug such as *aspirin* to reduce the risk of blood clots forming on the damaged artery lining.

Surgical treatment such as coronary angioplasty (see *angioplasty, balloon*) may be recommended for those people thought to be at high risk of severe complications. If blood flow to the heart is severely obstructed, a *coronary bypass* operation to restore blood flow may be carried out.

athetosis A disorder of the nervous system that is characterized by slow, writhing, involuntary movements, most often of the face, head, neck, and limbs. These movements commonly include facial grimacing, with contortions of the mouth. There may also be difficulty in balancing and walking. Athetosis tends to be combined with *chorea* (jerky involuntary movements). Both athetosis and chorea arise from damage to the *basal ganglia*, clusters of nerve cells in the brain that control movement. Causes of athetosis include brain damage prior to or at birth (see *cerebral palsy*), *encephalitis* (brain infection), degenerative disorders such as *Huntington's disease*, or as a side effect of *phenothiazine drugs* or *levodopa*.

athlete's foot A common condition in which the skin between the toes becomes itchy and sore, and may crack, peel, or blister. It is due to a fungal infection but may also be caused by bacteria. Because the fungi thrive in humid conditions, athlete's foot is more common in people with particularly sweaty feet and with shoes and socks made from synthetic fibres, which do not absorb sweat. Self-treatment with topical *antifungal drugs* is usually effective and should be combined with careful washing and drying of the feet.

atlas The topmost cervical *vertebra* in the human *spine*. The atlas is attached to and supports the skull. A pivot joint attaching the atlas to the second cervical vertebra, the *axis*, allows the atlas to rotate and therefore the head to turn from side to side.

atony Loss of tension in a muscle, so that it is completely flaccid. Atony can occur in some nervous system disorders or after injury to nerves. For example, the arm muscles may become atonic after injury to the *brachial plexus* (nerve roots in the neck passing into the arm).

atopic eczema The most common form of *eczema*. It usually begins in infancy but may flare up during adolescence and adulthood. The cause is unknown, but people with *atopy* are more susceptible.

atopy A predisposition to various allergic reactions (see *allergy*). Atopic individuals have a tendency to suffer from one or more allergic disorders, such as *asthma*, *eczema*, *urticaria*, and allergic *rhinitis* (hay fever). The mechanism that underlies the predisposition is unclear, but atopy does seem to run in families.

ATP An abbreviation for the compound adenosine triphosphate, the principal energy-carrying chemical in the body. (See also *ADP*; *metabolism*.)

atresia *Congenital* absence or severe narrowing of a body opening or tubular organ, due to a failure of development in the uterus. Examples are *biliary atresia*, in which the bile duct between the liver and duodenum are absent; *oesophageal atresia*, in which the oesophagus comes to a blind end; and anal atresia (see *anus, imperforate*), in which the anal canal is shut off. Most forms of atresia require surgical correction early in life.

atrial fibrillation A type of abnormality of the heartbeat (see *arrhythmia, cardiac*) in which the atria (see *atrium*) of the heart beat irregularly and rapidly. The ventricles (lower chambers) also beat irregularly. The heart's pumping ability is reduced as a result. Atrial fibrillation can occur in almost any longstanding heart disease but is most often associated with *heart-valve* disorders or *coronary artery disease*.

Sudden onset of atrial fibrillation can cause *palpitations, angina,* or breathlessness. The heart's inefficient pumping action reduces the output of blood into the circulation. Blood clots may form in the atria and may enter the bloodstream and lodge in an artery (see *embolism*).

Diagnosis of atrial fibrillation is confirmed by *ECG*. *Digoxin, beta-blocker drugs*, or *calcium channel blockers* may be given to control the heart-rate. Alternatively, a *pacemaker* may be inserted to regulate the heart rhythm. Atrial fibrillation of recent onset may be treated by *cardioversion*. In some cases, *radiofrequency ablation* (in which the heart tissue that triggers the abnormal rhythms is destroyed) may be recommended. In most cases, *anticoagulant drugs* are given to reduce the risk of embolism.

atrial flutter A type of abnormality of the heartbeat (see *arrhythmia, cardiac*) in which the atria beat regularly and very rapidly. Symptoms and treatment are the same as for *atrial fibrillation*.

atrial natriuretic peptide A substance produced in special cells in the muscular wall of the atria (see *atrium*) of the heart. Atrial natriuretic peptide is released into the bloodstream in response to swelling of the atrial muscle due, for example, to *heart failure*, *kidney failure*, or *hypertension*. It lowers blood pressure by increasing the amount of sodium excreted in the urine, which reduces blood volume.

atrial septal defect (ASD) A congenital heart abnormality (see *heart disease, congenital*) in which there is a hole in the dividing wall (see *septal defect*) between the heart's two upper chambers, or atria (see *atrium*).

atrioventricular node A small knot of specialized muscle cells in the right atrium of the *heart*. Electrical impulses from the *sinoatrial node* pass through the atrioventricular node and along conducting fibres to the *ventricles*, causing them to contract.

atrium Either of the two (right and left) upper chambers of the *heart* that collect blood from the body and lungs respectively. The atria open directly into the *ventricles*.

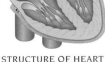

ATRIUM

Right atrium of heart

Left atrium of heart

STRUCTURE OF HEART

atrophy Wasting away or shrinkage of a normally developed tissue or organ due to a reduction in the size or number of its cells. Atrophy is commonly caused by disuse or inadequate cell nutrition due to poor blood circulation. It may also occur during prolonged illness, when the body needs to use up protein reserves in muscles. In some circumstances, atrophy is a normal process, as in ovarian atrophy in women who have passed the *menopause*.

atropine An *anticholinergic drug* derived from *belladonna*. Atropine is used to dilate the pupil in eye conditions such as *iritis* (inflammation of the iris) and *corneal ulcer*. It is also used in children before eye examination. Atropine may be included in a *premedication* before general *anaesthesia* to reduce respiratory secretions and is also used as an emergency treatment for *bradycardia* (abnormally slow heartbeat). It is sometimes combined with an *antidiarrhoeal drug* to relieve abdominal cramps accompanying diarrhoea.

Adverse effects include dry mouth, blurred vision, retention of urine, and, in the elderly, confusion. Atropine eyedrops are rarely given to adults because they cause disturbance of vision lasting 2–3 weeks and may precipitate acute *glaucoma* in susceptible people.

attachment An affectionate bond between individuals, especially between a parent and child (see *bonding*), or a person and an object, as in a young child and a security blanket. The term is also used to refer to the site at which a muscle or tendon is attached to a bone.

attention deficit hyperactivity disorder (ADHD) A behavioural disorder in which a child has a consistently high level of activity and/or difficulty in attending to tasks. Attention deficit hyperactivity, or hyperkinetic, disorder affects up to 1 in 20 children in the UK. The disorder, which is more common in boys, should not be confused with the normal boisterous conduct of a healthy child. Children with ADHD consistently show abnormal patterns of behaviour over a period of time. An affected child is likely to be restless, unable to sit still for more than a few moments, inattentive, and impulsive.

The causes of ADHD are not fully understood, but the disorder often runs in families, which suggests that genetic factors may be involved. ADHD is not, as popularly believed, a result of poor parenting or abuse.

Symptoms develop in early childhood, usually between the ages of 3 and 7, and may include inability to finish tasks; short attention span; inability to concentrate in class; difficulty in following instructions; a tendency to talk excessively, frequently interrupting other people; difficulty in waiting or taking turns; inability to play quietly alone; and physical impulsiveness. Children with ADHD may have difficulty in forming friendships. Self-esteem is often low because an affected child is frequently scolded and criticized.

Treatment includes behaviour modification techniques, both at home and at school. In some children, avoidance of certain foods or food additives seems to reduce symptoms. In severe cases, *stimulant drugs*, usually *methylphenidate*, may be prescribed. Other medications that may be prescribed include *amphetamine drugs* and atomoxetine. Paradoxically, the use of stimulants in ADHD reduces hyperactivity and improves concentration. In general, the condition improves by adolescence but may be followed by antisocial behaviour and *drug abuse* or *substance abuse.*

audiogram A graph produced as a result of *audiometry* that shows the hearing threshold (the minimum audible decibel level) for each of a range of sound frequencies.

audiology The study of hearing, especially of impaired hearing that cannot be corrected by drugs or surgery.

audiometry Measurement of the sense of hearing. The term often refers to *hearing tests* in which a machine is used to produce sounds of a defined intensity and frequency and in which the hearing in each ear is measured over the full range of normally audible sounds.

auditory nerve The part of the *vestibulocochlear nerve* (the 8th *cranial nerve*) concerned with hearing.

aura A peculiar "warning" sensation that precedes or marks the onset of a *migraine* attack or of a seizure in *epilepsy.* A migraine attack may be preceded by a feeling of elation, excessive energy or drowsiness, thirst, or a craving for sweet foods. Migraine may be heralded by flashing light before the eyes, blurred or tunnel vision, or difficulty in speaking. There may also be weakness, numbness, or tingling in one half of the body.

An epileptic aura may be a distorted perception, such as a hallucinatory smell or sound. One type of attack (in people with *temporal lobe epilepsy*) is often preceded by a vague feeling of discomfort in the upper abdomen and followed by a sensation of fullness in the head.

auranofin A *gold preparation* used as a *disease-modifying antirheumatic drug* in the treatment of active, progressive *rheumatoid arthritis.* Unlike other gold preparations, auranofin is taken orally.

auricle Another name for the pinna, the external flap of the *ear.* The term is also used to describe ear-like appendages of the atria (see *atrium*) of the heart.

auriscope An instrument for examining the ear, also called an *otoscope.*

auscultation The procedure of listening to sounds within the body by using a *stethoscope.* Some organs make sounds during normal functioning, such as the movement of fluid through the stomach and intestine, the opening and closing of heart valves (see *heart sounds*), and the flow of air through the lungs. Abnormal sounds may indicate disease.

autism A condition in which a child is unable to relate to people and situations. Autism is more common in boys. It is by definition evident before the age of 30 months and is usually apparent in the first year of life. The precise causes of autism are unknown. Often, autistic children seem normal for the first few months of life before becoming increasingly unresponsive to parents or other stimuli. Extreme resistance to change of any kind is an important feature. The child reacts with distress to alteration in routine or interference with activities. Rituals develop in play, and there is often attachment to unusual objects or obsession with one particular idea. Delay in speaking is common and most autistic children have a low *IQ.* Behavioural abnormalities may include rocking, self-injury, screaming fits, and *hyperactivity.*

Despite these symptoms, appearance and muscular coordination are normal. Some autistic people have an isolated special skill, such as an outstanding rote memory or musical ability.

There is no effective treatment for autism, which is lifelong. Special schooling, support and *counselling* for families, and sometimes *behaviour therapy* can be helpful. Medication is useful only for specific problems, such as hyperactivity. The majority of autistic people need special, sometimes institutional, care.

autism spectrum disorders A range of developmental disorders, usually first diagnosed in childhood, that are characterized by obsessive behaviour and impaired communication and social skills (see *autism; Asperger's syndrome*).

autoantibody An *antibody* that reacts against the body's own cells (see *autoimmune disorders*).

autoclave An apparatus that produces steam at high pressure within a sealed chamber. Autoclaving is used in hospitals for the sterilization of surgical equipment (see *sterilization*).

autoimmune disorders Any of a number of disorders caused by a reaction of the *immune system* against the body's own cells and tissues. Bacteria, viruses, and drugs may play a role in initiating an autoimmune disorder, but in most cases the trigger is unknown.

Autoimmune disorders are classified into organ-specific and non-organ-specific types. In organ-specific disorders, the autoimmune process is directed mainly against one organ. Examples include *Hashimoto's thyroiditis* (thyroid gland), pernicious *anaemia* (stomach), *Addison's disease* (adrenal glands), and type I *diabetes mellitus* (pancreas). In non-organ-specific disorders, autoimmune activity is towards a tissue, such as connective tissue, that is widespread in the body. Examples of non-organ-specific disorders are systemic *lupus erythematosus* and *rheumatoid arthritis*.

Initial treatment for any autoimmune disorder is to reduce the effects of the disease, for example by replacing hormones that are not being produced. In cases in which the disease is having widespread effects, treatment is also directed at diminishing the activity of the immune system while maintaining the body's ability to fight disease. *Corticosteroid drugs* are most commonly used but may be combined with other *immunosuppressant drugs*.

automatism A state in which behaviour is not controlled by the conscious mind. The individual carries out activities without being aware of doing so, and later has no clear memory of what happened. Automatism is uncommon and may be a symptom of *temporal lobe epilepsy*, *dissociative disorders*, drug or *alcohol intoxication*, or *hypoglycaemia*.

autonomic nervous system The part of the *nervous system* that controls the involuntary activities of a variety of body tissues. The autonomic nervous system is divided into the sympathetic and parasympathetic nervous systems.

The sympathetic nervous system comprises two chains of nerves that pass from the spinal cord throughout the body tissues. Into these tissues, the nerve endings release the *neurotransmitters adrenaline* (epinephrine) and *noradrenaline* (norepinephrine). The system also stimulates adrenaline release from the adrenal glands. In general, the actions of the sympathetic nervous system heighten activity in the body, quickening the heartbeat and breathing rate, widening blood vessels, and inducing sweating.

The parasympathetic nervous system is composed of a chain of nerves that passes from the brain and another that leaves the lower spinal cord. The nerves are distributed to the same tissues that are supplied by the sympathetic nerves. The parasympathetic nerves release the neurotransmitter *acetylcholine*, which has the opposite effect to adrenaline and noradrenaline. The parasympathetic system is mainly concerned with everyday functions such as digestion and excretion.

The two systems act in conjunction and normally balance each other. During exercise or at times of stress, the sympathetic system predominates, however, during sleep the parasympathetic system exerts more control.

autopsy A postmortem examination of the body, including the internal organs, usually to determine cause of death

autosome Any chromosome that is not a sex chromosome. Of the 23 pairs of *chromosomes* in each human cell, 22 pairs are autosomes.

autosuggestion Putting oneself into a receptive hypnotic-like state as a means of stimulating the body's ability to heal itself. For example, in one method used to control anxiety symptoms, people are taught muscular relaxation (*biofeedback*) techniques and learn to summon up calming imagery or pleasant thoughts.

avascular necrosis The death of cells in body tissue caused by damage to blood vessels supplying the area

aversion therapy An outdated form of *behaviour therapy* in which unpleasant stimuli, such as electric shocks, are administered at the same time as an unwanted behaviour in an attempt to alter behavioural patterns.

avian influenza Commonly known as bird flu, avian influenza is a highly infectious disease of birds, especially poultry, that can occasionally infect people who are in close contact with infected birds. There are many strains of avian influenza but the strain caused by the H5N1 virus is particularly virulent. People infected with this strain may develop symptoms including fever, sore throat, muscle aches, headaches, breathing problems, and chest pains. In some cases, infection with the H5N1 strain may be fatal. There is concern that this strain may develop the ability to pass from one person to another, instead of only from birds to birds or from birds to humans. If this occurs, there is the possibility of a global epidemic (pandemic). Normal influenza vaccines do not protect against the H5N1 virus, although drugs such as *oseltamivir* may be effective.

aviation medicine The medical speciality concerned with the physiological effects of air travel and with the causes and treatment of medical problems that may occur during a flight.

avulsed tooth A tooth that has become completely dislodged from its socket following an injury. If the tooth is kept moist, and treatment is sought immediately, reimplantation may be possible (see *reimplantation, dental*).

avulsion The tearing away of a body structure from its point of attachment. For example, excessive contraction of a *tendon* may avulse a small piece of bone at its attachment point. Avulsion may be due to an injury or be performed as part of a surgical procedure.

axilla The medical name for the armpit.

axis The second cervical *vertebra* in the human *spine*. The axis is attached by a pivot joint to the *atlas*, the topmost vertebra, which in turn is attached to the base of the skull. The pivot joint allows the head to turn to either side.

axon The thin, elongated part of a *neuron* (nerve cell) that conducts nerve impulses. Many axons in the body are covered with a fatty *myelin* sheath.

Ayurvedism See *Indian medicine*.

azathioprine A *disease-modifying antirheumatic drug* and *immunosuppressant drug* used to treat active, progressive *rheumatoid arthritis* and other *autoimmune disorders*. It is also used to prevent organ rejection after *transplant surgery*.

Increased susceptibilty to infection is a side effect.

azelaic acid A *topical* drug used to treat mild to moderate *acne*.

azithromycin A macrolide *antibiotic drug* used to treat infections of the skin, chest, throat, and ears. Azithromycin is also used to treat genital infections due to chlamydia (see *chlamydial infections*).

azoospermia The absence of sperm from semen, causing *infertility* in males. Azoospermia may be caused by a disorder present at birth or that develops later in life or after *vasectomy*.

Congenital azoospermia may be due to a *chromosomal abnormality* such as *Klinefelter's syndrome*; failure of the testes to descend into the scrotum; absence of the vasa deferentia (ducts that carry sperm from the testes to the seminal vesicles); or *cystic fibrosis*.

In some males, azoospermia may be the result of hormonal disorders affecting the onset of puberty. Another cause is blockage of the vasa deferentia, which may follow a *sexually transmitted infection*, *tuberculosis*, or surgery on the groin. Azoospermia can also be the result of damage to the testes. This can follow *radiotherapy*, treatment with certain drugs, or the effects of occupational exposure to toxic chemicals.

If the cause is treatable, sperm production may restart. However, in some cases, the testes will have been permanently damaged.

AZT The abbreviation for azidothymidine, the former name for *zidovudine*.

aztreonam An *antibiotic* used to treat some types of *meningitis* and infections by certain types of bacteria, including PSEUDOMONAS.

AXON

NERVE CELL

B

Babinski's sign A reflex movement in which the big toe bends upwards when the outer edge of the sole of the foot is scratched. In adults, Babinski's sign indicates damage or disease of the brain or the spinal cord. In babies, Babinski's sign is a normal reflex.

baby blues A common name for a mild form of depression that sometimes occurs in women after childbirth. Baby blues almost always disappears without treatment but can occasionally develop into a more serious depressive illness (see *postnatal depression*).

bacilli Rod-shaped *bacteria*. The singular term is bacillus.

back The area between the shoulders and the buttocks. The back is supported by the spinal column (see *spine*), which is bound together by ligaments and supported by muscles that also control posture and movement. Disorders that affect the bones, muscles, ligaments, tendons, nerves, and joints in the spine may cause *back pain*. (See also *spine, disorders of*.)

back pain Pain affecting the back, often restricting movement. The pain usually lasts for only a week or so but can recur in some people. Rarely, persistent back pain causes long-term disability.

Back pain is usually caused by minor damage to the ligaments and muscles in the back. The lower back is especially vulnerable to these problems because it supports most of the body's weight and is under continual stress from movements such as bending, twisting, and stretching. Less commonly, lower back pain may result from an underlying disorder such as a prolapsed intervertebral disc (see *disc prolapse*) in the spine.

In most cases, back pain can be treated with over-the-counter painkillers (see *analgesic drugs*) such as *aspirin* and related drugs, *nonsteroidal anti-inflammatory drugs*, or *muscle-relaxant drugs*. If the pain persists, a heat pad, a wrapped hot-water bottle or, sometimes, an ice-pack, may provide additional relief. Generally, it is advisable to remain as active as the pain permits. People whose pain worsens or is still too severe to allow normal movement after several days should consult a doctor.

Investigations for back pain, such as *X-rays*, *CT scanning*, *MRI*, or *bone imaging*, sometimes reveal abnormalities, such as disc prolapse, that require surgical treatment and can be treated by a *microdiscectomy*.

Other treatments for back pain include *acupuncture*, spinal injection, exercise, *TENS*, or spinal *manipulation*.

baclofen A *muscle-relaxant drug* that is used to relieve muscle spasm and stiffness due to brain or spinal cord injury, *stroke*, or neurological disorders such as *multiple sclerosis*. Adverse effects of baclofen include drowsiness and muscle weakness; these side effects can be limited, however, by increasing the dose of the drug gradually.

bacteraemia The presence of *bacteria* in the bloodstream. Bacteraemia occurs briefly after many minor surgical operations and dental treatment. The *immune system* usually prevents the bacteria from multiplying and causing damage. However, in people who have abnormal heart valves, the bacteria may settle on the valve and cause *endocarditis*. If the immune system is damaged or suppressed, *septicaemia* (an infection of the blood) may develop.

bacteria Single-celled *microorganisms* that are invisible to the naked eye. The singular form of the term is bacterium. Abundant in the air, soil, and water, most bacteria are harmless to humans. Some bacteria, such as those that live in the intestine, are beneficial and help to break down food for digestion. Bacteria that cause disease are known as pathogens and are classified by shape into three main groups: cocci (spherical); bacilli (rod-shaped); and spirochaetes or spirilla (spiral-shaped). Many bacteria have whip-like threads called flagella, which enable them to move in fluids, and pili, which anchor them to other cells.

Aerobic bacteria require oxygen to grow and multiply; in the body, these are most commonly found on the skin or in the respiratory system. Anaerobic bacteria thrive where there is no oxygen, deep within tissue or wounds. They reproduce by simple division, which can take place every 20 minutes. Some bacteria also produce spores that can survive high temperatures, dry conditions, and lack of nourishment; and some produce poisons (either endotoxins or exotoxins) that are harmful to human cells.

BACTERIA

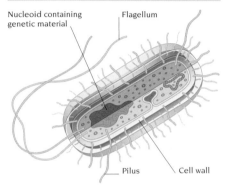

Nucleoid containing genetic material

Flagellum

Pilus

Cell wall

A ROD-SHAPED BACTERIUM

The body's *immune system* attacks invading bacteria, but in some cases treatment with *antibiotic drugs* is necessary and will speed recovery. Superficial inflammation and infected wounds may be treated with *antiseptics*. Immunity to invading bacterial diseases, such as some types of *meningitis*, can be acquired by active *immunization*. (See also *infectious disease*.)

bacterial vaginosis An infection of the *vagina* that causes a greyish-white discharge and itching. The disorder is due to excessive growth of bacteria that normally live in the vagina. It is more common in sexually active women and is treated with *antibiotic drugs*.

bactericidal A term used to describe any substance that kills bacteria. (See also *antibacterial drugs*; *antibiotic drugs*.)

bacteriology The study of *bacteria*, particularly of the types that cause disease.

Bacteriology includes techniques used to isolate and identify bacteria from specimens such as a throat swab or urine. Bacteria are identified by their appearance under a microscope, including their response to stains (see *staining*) and the use of *culture*. Testing for sensitivity to antibiotics may be performed.

bacteriostatic A term used to describe a substance that stops the growth or multiplication of *bacteria* but does not kill them. (See also *antibacterial drugs*; *antibiotic drugs*.)

bacteriuria The presence of *bacteria* in the urine that is abnormal.

bad breath See *halitosis*.

bagassosis A rare disease affecting the lungs of workers who handle mouldy bagasse (the fibrous residue of sugarcane after juice extraction). Bagassosis is one cause of allergic *alveolitis*. Symptoms develop 4–5 hours after inhaling dust and include shortness of breath, wheezing, fever, headache, and cough. Repeated dust exposure may lead to permanent lung damage.

Baker's cyst A fluid-filled lump behind the knee. A Baker's cyst is caused by increased pressure in the knee joint due to a buildup of fluid in a disorder such as *rheumatoid arthritis*. Most Baker's cysts are painless, and some disappear spontaneously. Occasionally, a cyst may rupture, producing pain and swelling in the calf that can mimic a deep vein thrombosis (see *thrombosis, deep vein*). Diagnosis of a Baker's cyst is confirmed by *ultrasound scanning*. Treatment is rarely needed.

balance The ability to remain upright and move without falling over. Information on body position is relayed to the brain by many parts of the body: the eyes; proprioceptors (sense organs) in the skin, muscle, and joints; and the labyrinth of the inner *ear*. The *cerebellum* (part of the brain) integrates the information and sends instructions to enable various parts of the body to perform adjustments needed to maintain balance.

Disorders affecting the ear, brain, or spinal cord commonly affect balance. Ear disorders include *labyrinthitis* and *Ménière's disease*. Less commonly, *otitis media* may affect balance.

B

Damage to nerve tracts in the spinal cord, which carry information from position sensors in the joints and muscles, can also impair balance. This damage may result from spinal tumours, circulatory disorders, nerve degeneration due to deficiency of vitamin B_{12}, or, rarely, tabes dorsalis (a complication of *syphilis*). A tumour or stroke that affects the cerebellum may cause clumsiness of the arms and legs and other features of impaired muscular coordination.

balanitis Inflammation of the foreskin and glans (head) of the penis. Balanitis causes pain and/or itchiness, and the entire area may be red and moist. Causes include infection or chemical irritation to contraceptive creams or laundry products. Treatment is usually with *antibiotic* or *antifungal drugs* (as creams or taken orally) and careful washing of the penis and foreskin. Phimosis, in which the foreskin is overly tight, makes balanitis more likely to recur. In such cases, *circumcision* may be recommended.

baldness See *alopecia*.

balloon catheter A flexible tube with a balloon at its tip, which, when inflated, keeps the tube in place or applies pressure to an organ or vessel. One type is used to drain urine from the bladder (see *catheterization, urinary*). Balloon catheters are sometimes used to expand narrowed arteries (balloon *angioplasty*). They may also be used to control bleeding *oesophageal varices* before surgery.

balm A soothing or healing medicine applied to the skin.

bambuterol A *bronchodilator drug* that is converted to *terbutaline* in the liver. Bambuterol can only be taken orally.

bandage A strip or tube of fabric used to keep *dressings* in position, to apply pressure, to control bleeding, or to support a sprain or strain. Roller bandages are the most widely used. Tubular gauze bandages require a special applicator and are used mainly for areas that are awkward to bandage, such as a finger. Triangular bandages are used to make slings. (See also *wounds*.)

barber's itch See *sycosis barbae*.

barbiturate drugs A group of *sedative drugs* that work by depressing activity within the brain. They include *thiopental*

and *phenobarbital*. In the past, barbiturates were widely used as *antianxiety drugs* and *sleeping drugs* but have been largely replaced by *benzodiazepine drugs* and other nonbarbiturates. Barbiturates are now strictly controlled because they are habit-forming and widely abused. An overdose can be fatal, particularly in combination with alcohol, which dangerously increases the depressant effect on the brain (including suppression of the respiratory centre). However, phenobarbital is still commonly used as an *anticonvulsant drug* in the treatment of *epilepsy*. Thiopental is very short acting and is used to induce anaesthesia (see *anaesthesia, general*).

barium X-ray examinations Procedures that are used to detect and follow the progress of some gastrointestinal tract disorders. Because X-rays do not pass through barium, it is used to outline organs, such as the stomach, that are not normally visible on an X-ray. In some cases, barium X-rays are an alternative to *endoscopy* (although the latter is now often the preferred form of investigation). Barium sulphate mixed with water is passed into the part of the tract requiring examination, and X-rays are taken. Barium X-rays may be single- or double-contrast. In single-contrast X-rays, the barium fills the area and provides an outline image that shows up prominent abnormalities. In double-contrast X-rays, the barium forms a thin film over the inner surface of the tract, and the tract is filled with air so that small surface abnormalities can be seen.

Different types of barium X-ray examination are used to investigate different parts of the gastrointestinal tract. Barium swallow involves drinking a barium solution and is used to investigate the *oesophagus*. A barium meal is carried out to look at the lower oesophagus, stomach, and *duodenum*. Barium follow-through is used to investigate disorders of the small intestine; X-rays are taken at intervals as the barium reaches the intestine. A barium enema is used to investigate disorders of the large intestine and rectum; barium is introduced through a tube inserted in the rectum. Barium remaining in the intestine may

BARIUM X-RAY EXAMINATIONS

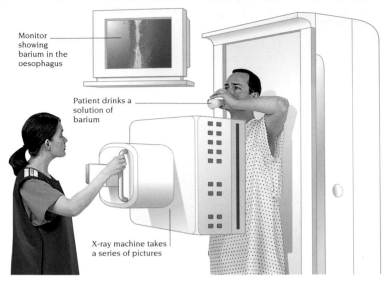

Monitor showing barium in the oesophagus

Patient drinks a solution of barium

X-ray machine takes a series of pictures

BARIUM SWALLOW

cause constipation. Therefore, it is important to have a high-fibre diet and drink plenty of water after a barium examination, until all the barium has passed through.

barotrauma Damage or pain, mainly affecting the middle *ear* and facial *sinuses*, that is caused by changes in surrounding air pressure. Air travellers are at the greatest risk, but scuba divers face similar problems (see *scuba-diving medicine*).

Aircraft cabin pressure decreases as the plane ascends and increases as it descends. As the aircraft ascends, the ears may "pop" as the air in the middle ear expands and is expelled via the eustachian tubes, which connect the middle ear to the back of the throat. On descent, the higher pressure may push the eardrum inwards and cause pain. Minor pressure damage in the middle ear may cause pain, hearing loss, and *tinnitus* for a few days; damage within the facial sinuses may also cause pain, and possibly a discharge of mucus or blood. Symptoms usually wear off within hours or days, but treatment may be needed if they worsen or persist. Large

pressure changes can rupture the eardrum (see *eardrum, perforated*).

Barotrauma can be avoided by vigorous swallowing or by forcibly breathing out with the mouth closed and the nose pinched (the Valsalva manoeuvre). This action equalizes the internal and external pressures in the middle ear and sinuses. If the eustachian tubes are blocked, as commonly occurs with a cold, use of a nasal spray containing a *decongestant drug* is recommended shortly before the descent of the aircraft. Infants should be breast- or bottle-fed during descent to encourage swallowing.

barrier cream A cream used to protect the skin against the effects of irritant substances and of excessive exposure to water. (See also *sunscreens*.)

barrier method A method of preventing pregnancy by blocking the passage of sperm to the uterus, for example by using a condom or a diaphragm. (See also *contraception, barrier methods of*.)

barrier nursing The nursing technique by which a patient with an infectious disease is prevented from infecting other people (see *isolation*). In reverse barrier nursing, a patient with reduced ability to fight infections is protected against outside infection. (See also *aseptic technique*.)

bartholinitis An infection of *Bartholin's glands*, at the entrance to the *vagina*, that may be due to a *sexually transmitted infection* such as *gonorrhoea* or chlamydia (see *chlamydial infections*). It causes an intensely painful red swelling at the opening of the ducts. Treatment is with *antibiotic drugs*, *analgesic drugs*, and warm baths. Bartholinitis sometimes leads to an *abscess* or a painless cyst (called a Bartholin's cyst), which may become infected. Abscesses are drained under general *anaesthesia*. Recurrent abscesses or infected cysts may need surgery to convert the duct into an open pouch (see *marsupialization*) or to remove the gland completely

Bartholin's glands A pair of oval, pea-sized glands whose ducts open into the vulva (the folds of flesh that surround the opening of the vagina). During sexual arousal, these glands secrete a fluid to lubricate the vulval region. Infection of the glands causes *bartholinitis*.

basal cell carcinoma A type of skin cancer, also known as a rodent ulcer or BCC, that occurs most commonly on the face or neck. It starts as a small, flat nodule and grows slowly, eventually forming a shallow ulcer with raised pearly edges. Basal cell carcinoma is caused by skin damage from the ultraviolet radiation in sunlight. Fair-skinned people over 50 are the most commonly affected; dark and black-skinned people are protected by the larger amount of the skin pigment *melanin*. The risk is reduced by avoiding overexposure to strong sunlight, using *sunscreens*, and wearing protective clothing and sun hats. Without treatment, the carcinoma gradually invades and destroys surrounding tissues but virtually never spreads to other parts of the body. Treatment is usually with surgery (or in some cases *radiotherapy*) and is often completely successful. Plastic surgery may also be needed, however, depending on the size and site of the tumour. People who have had a basal cell carcinoma may develop new tumours and should be alert to any changes in their skin. (See also *melanoma, malignant*; *squamous cell carcinoma*; *sunlight, adverse effects of*.)

basal ganglia Paired nerve cell clusters deep within the cerebrum (the main mass of the *brain*) and upper part of the brainstem. The basal ganglia play a vital part in producing smooth, continuous muscular actions and in stopping and starting movement. Any disease or degeneration affecting the basal ganglia and their connections may lead to the appearance of involuntary movements, trembling, and weakness, as occur in *Parkinson's disease*.

base see *alkali*.

basophil A type of white *blood cell* that plays a part in inflammatory and allergic reactions.

B-cell See *lymphocyte*.

BCG vaccination A vaccine that provides immunity against *tuberculosis*. BCG is prepared from an artificially weakened strain of bovine (cattle) tubercle bacilli, the microorganisms responsible for the disease. BCG stands for "bacille Calmette–Guérin", after the two Frenchmen who developed the vaccine in 1906.

BCG is given to people at risk of tuberculosis and for whom a *tuberculin test* is negative. These people include health workers, contacts of people who have tuberculosis, and immigrants (including children) from countries with a high rate of tuberculosis. Infants born to immigrants in this category are immunized, without having a tuberculin test, within a few weeks of birth.

beclometasone A *corticosteroid drug* that is used in the treatment of *asthma*

BASAL CELL CARCINOMA

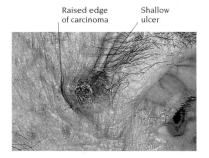

Raised edge of carcinoma   Shallow ulcer

B

and hay fever (see *rhinitis, allergic*). Beclometasone, which is prescribed as an inhaler or nasal spray, controls the symptoms by reducing inflammation and mucus production in the lining of the nose or, in asthma, inflammation of the airways. The drug is often given with *bronchodilator drugs* in the management of asthma. A severe asthma attack may require the dose to be increased. The action of beclometasone is slow, however, and its full effect takes several days to occur. Adverse effects of the drug may include hoarseness, throat irritation, and, on rare occasions, fungal infections in the mouth. Beclometasone is also prescribed in the form of a cream or ointment to treat inflammation of the skin caused by *eczema*.

becquerel A unit of radioactivity (see *radiation units*).

bed bath A method of washing a person who is confined to bed.

bedbug A flat, wingless, brown insect about 5 mm long and 3 mm wide. Bedbugs live in furniture, especially beds and carpets, emerging at night to feed on humans by sucking blood. They are not known to transmit disease, but their bites are itchy and may become infected.

bedpan A metal, plastic, or fibre container into which a patient can defaecate or urinate without getting out of bed.

bed rest A term used to describe periods spent in bed. Bed rest may be a part of treatment in certain illnesses, such as *rheumatic fever*, and for some types of injury, such as a fractured vertebra. Prolonged bed rest carries risks such as muscle wasting, weakness, and increased risk of blood clots developing in the legs. Bed rest was once considered an essential part of the treatment of many common conditions but is now avoided whenever possible. Patients are now encouraged to be mobile as soon as possible after surgery.

bedridden A term used to describe a person who is unable to leave their bed due to illness or injury. People most likely to be bedridden are the very elderly, the terminally ill, and those paralysed as the result of an accident.

bedsores See *pressure sores*.

bed-wetting The common name for poor bladder control at night (see *enuresis*).

bee stings See *insect stings*.

behavioural problems in children - Behavioural problems range from mild, short-lived periods of unacceptable behaviour, which are common in most children, to more severe problems such as conduct disorders and refusal to go to school. Behavioural problems may occasionally occur in any child; specialist management is called for when the problems become frequent and disrupt school and/or family life. Some behavioural problems can occur whatever the family or home situation. In some cases, however, stressful external events, such as moving home or divorce, may produce periods of problem behaviour.

Behavioural problems that are common in babies and young children include feeding difficulties (see *feeding, infant*) and sleeping problems, such as waking repeatedly in the night. In toddlers, *breath-holding attacks*, *tantrums*, separation anxiety, and *head-banging* are problems best dealt with by a consistent and appropriate approach. Problems with *toilet-training* are usually avoided if the training is delayed until the child is physically and emotionally ready.

Between the ages of 4 and 8, behavioural problems such as nail-biting and *thumb-sucking*, clinginess, *nightmares*, and bed-wetting (see *enuresis*) are so common as to be almost normal. They are best dealt with by a positive approach that concentrates on rewarding good behaviour. In most cases, the child grows out of the problem, but sometimes medical help may be needed.

behaviourism An American school of *psychology* founded by John Broadus Watson early in the 20th century. He argued that, because behaviour, rather than experience, was all that could be observed in others, it should constitute the sole basis of psychology.

behaviour therapy A collection of techniques, based on psychological theory, for changing abnormal behaviour or treating anxiety. The treatment relies on two basic ideas: that exposure to a feared experience under safe conditions will render it less threatening, and that desirable behaviour can be encouraged by using a system of rewards.

Specific behaviour therapy techniques include exposure therapy (also called desensitization), response prevention, flooding, and modelling. Exposure therapy is commonly used to treat phobic disorders such as *agoraphobia*, animal phobias, and flying phobias. It consists of exposing the patient in stages to the cause of the anxiety. The patient is taught to cope with anxiety symptoms by using relaxation techniques. In flooding, the patient is confronted with the anxiety-provoking stimulus all at once, but with the support of the therapist. In response prevention, the patient is prevented from carrying out an obsessional task; the technique is used in combination with other methods. In modelling, the therapist acts as a model for the patient, performing the anxiety-provoking activity first, in order that the patient may copy.

Behçet's syndrome A rare, multisystem disorder with recurrent *mouth ulcers* and *genital ulcers* and inflammation of the eyes, skin joints, blood vessels, brain, and intestines. The cause of Behçet's syndrome is unknown, but it is strongly associated with a genetically determined *histocompatability antigen*, HLA-B51. Treatment is difficult and may require *corticosteroid* and *immunosuppressant drugs*. The condition often becomes long-term.

belching The noisy return of air from the stomach through the mouth. Swallowing air is usually an unconscious habit, which may result from eating or drinking too much too quickly. Sometimes, belching alleviates discomfort caused by indigestion.

belladonna An extract of the deadly nightshade plant that has been used medicinally since ancient times. It contains *alkaloids*, including *atropine*, that are used as *antispasmodic drugs* in treating gastrointestinal disturbances. (See also *anticholinergic drugs*.)

Bell's palsy The most common form of *facial palsy* (facial muscle weakness).

bendrofluazide An alternative name for *bendroflumethiazide*.

bendroflumethiazide A thiazide *diuretic drug* used to treat *hypertension* and *heart failure*.

bends The nonmedical term for *decompression sickness*.

benign A term used to describe a disease that is relatively harmless. When used to refer to tumours, benign means noncancerous tumours that do not invade or destroy local tissues and do not spread to other sites within the body.

benign prostatic hyperplasia (BPH) A medical term for enlargement of the prostate gland (see *prostate, enlarged*).

benzalkonium chloride A widely used preservative in eye drops and products such as cosmetics and mouth washes.

benzodiazepine drugs A group of drugs given for short periods as *sleeping drugs* for *insomnia* and to control the symptoms of *anxiety* or *stress* (see *tranquillizer drugs*). Common benzodiazepines include *diazepam*, which is used as a tranquillizer, and *nitrazepam*, which is sometimes used for insomnia. Benzodiazepines are also used in the management of alcohol withdrawal and in the control of *epilepsy*.

Minor adverse effects of benzodiazepines include daytime drowsiness, dizziness, and forgetfulness. Unsteadiness and slowed reactions may also occur. Regular users may become psychologically and physically dependent; for this reason, the drugs are usually given for courses of 2–3 weeks or less. When the drugs are stopped suddenly, withdrawal symptoms, such as anxiety, restlessness, and nightmares may occur. Benzodiazepine drugs are sometimes abused for their sedative effect.

benzoyl peroxide An *antiseptic* agent used in the treatment of acne and fungal skin infections (see *fungal infections*). In acne, benzoyl peroxide also acts by removing the surface layer of skin, unblocking sebaceous glands.

benzylpenicillin A type of *penicillin drug* that is given by injection.

bereavement The emotional reaction following the death of a loved relative or friend. The expression of grief is individual to each person, but there are recognized stages of bereavement, each characterized by a particular attitude. In the first stage, which may last from three days to three months, there is numbness and an unwillingness to recognize the death.

B

Hallucinations, in which the dead person is seen, are a common experience. Once the numbness wears off, the person may be overwhelmed by feelings of anxiety, anger, and despair that can develop into a depressive illness (see *depression*).

Insomnia, malaise, agitation, and tearfulness are also common. Gradually, but usually within two years, the bereaved person adjusts to the loss.

Family and friends can often provide support. Outside help may be required and may be given by a social worker, health visitor, member of the clergy, or self-help group. For some people, when depression, apathy, and lethargy impede any chance of recovery, specialized *counselling* or *psychotherapy* is necessary. (See also *stillbirth*.)

beriberi A nutritional disorder resulting from a lack of *thiamine* (vitamin B_1) in the diet. Without thiamine, the brain, nerves, and muscles (including the heart muscle) are unable to function properly. In developed countries, the illness is seen only in people who are starving or on an extremely restricted diet, such as alcoholics. There are two forms of the illness. In dry beriberi, thiamine deficiency mainly affects the nerves and skeletal muscles. Symptoms include numbness, a burning sensation in the legs, and muscle wasting. In severe cases, the patient becomes virtually paralysed, emaciated, and bedridden. In wet beriberi, the main problem is *heart failure*, which leads to *oedema* in the legs, and sometimes also in the trunk and face. Other symptoms of wet beriberi include poor appetite, rapid pulse, and breathlessness. Beriberi is treated with thiamine.

berry aneurysm An abnormal swelling that occurs at the junction of *arteries* supplying the brain. Berry aneurysms, which are usually due to a *congenital* weakness, can sometimes rupture, resulting in a *subarachnoid haemorrhage*. (See also *aneurysm*.)

berylliosis An occupational disease that is caused by the inhalation of dust or fumes containing beryllium, a metallic element which is used in some high-technology industries. Short exposure to high concentrations of beryllium may lead to an episode of severe *pneumonitis*. Exposure over a number of years to smaller concentrations may lead to permanent damage to lungs and liver. Treatment with *corticosteroid drugs* can reduce damage to the lungs. In most cases, the introduction of safe working practices prevents exposure to dangerous levels of berylliosis.

beta-blocker drugs A group of drugs, also known as beta-adrenergic blocking agents, prescribed principally to treat heart and circulatory disorders such as *angina* and cardiac *arrhythmias*. They may also be used to treat *hypertension*, although they are not usually recommended as first-line treatment. Beta-blockers block the effects of the *sympathetic nervous system*, which releases *adrenaline* (epinephrine) and *noradrenaline* (norepinephrine) at nerve endings known as beta receptors.

There are two types of beta receptor: beta 1 and beta 2. Beta 1 receptors are present in the heart and blood vessels, and beta 2 in the lungs. Some beta-blockers (such as acebutolol, atenolol, and metoprolol) are termed cardio-selective and, because they act mostly on beta 1 receptors, are used mainly to treat heart disease such as angina, and cardiac arrhythmias; they may also be used to treat hypertension. The drugs are sometimes given after a *myocardial infarction* to reduce the likelihood of further damage to the heart.

Other types of beta-blocker, such as oxprenolol, propranolol, and timolol, may be given to prevent *migraine* attacks by acting on blood vessels in the head; reduce the physical symptoms of *anxiety*; or control the symptoms of *thyrotoxicosis*. Beta-blocker drugs such as timolol are sometimes given in the form of eye drops to treat *glaucoma* and work by lowering the fluid pressure in the eyeball.

Beta-blockers may reduce an individual's capacity for strenuous exercise. The drugs may worsen the symptoms of *asthma*, *bronchitis*, or other forms of lung disease. They may also reduce the flow of blood to the limbs, causing cold hands and feet. In addition, sleep disturbance and depression can be side effects of beta-blockers.

betahistine A drug used to treat *Ménière's disease*, reducing the frequency and severity of the attacks of nausea and vertigo.

betamethasone A *corticosteroid drug* used to treat inflammation. Betamethasone is applied to the skin as cream to treat contact *dermatitis* and *eczema*. It is also prescribed as nasal spray to treat allergic *rhinitis*.

Betamethasone is taken by mouth to treat some cases of *asthma* and *arthritis*. Adverse effects are unlikely with short-term use. However, prolonged topical use of the drug can cause thinning of the skin and may aggravate any infection. Taken orally for a prolonged period or in high doses, betamethasone can cause adverse effects typical of other corticosteroid drugs.

bezoar A ball of food and mucus, vegetable fibre, hair, or other indigestible material, in the stomach. Trichobezoars, which are composed of hair, may form in children or emotionally disturbed adults who nibble at, or pull out and swallow, their hair. Symptoms include loss of appetite, constipation, nausea and vomiting, and abdominal pain. If trichobezoars pass into the intestines, they may cause obstruction (see *intestine, obstruction of*). Bezoars can be removed endoscopically or surgically.

bi- The prefix meaning two or twice, as in bilateral (two-sided).

bicarbonate of soda See *sodium bicarbonate*.

biceps muscle The name given to a muscle originating as two separate parts, which then fuse. It is the commonly used name for the biceps brachii muscle of the upper arm, which bends the arm at the elbow and rotates the forearm. The biceps femoris at the back of the thigh bends the leg at the knee and extends the thigh.

bicuspid A term meaning to have two cusps (curved, pointed structures). Bicuspid describes certain *heart valves* and is used as an alternative name for a premolar tooth (see *teeth*).

bifocal A spectacle lens with two different focal lengths. Glasses with bifocal lenses make corrections for both close and distant vision.

bilateral A term that means affecting both sides of the body, or affecting both organs if they are paired (for example, both ears in bilateral deafness).

bile A greenish-brown alkaline liquid secreted by the *liver*. Bile carries away waste products formed in the liver and also helps to break down fats in the small intestine for digestion.

The waste products in bile include the pigments *bilirubin* and biliverdin, which give bile its greenish-brown colour; bile salts, which aid in the breakdown and absorption of fats; and *cholesterol*. Bile passes out of the liver through the *bile ducts* and is then concentrated and stored in the gallbladder. After a meal, bile is expelled and enters the duodenum (the first section of the small intestine) via the common bile duct. Most of the bile salts are later reabsorbed into the bloodstream to be recycled by the liver into bile. Bile pigments are excreted in the faeces. (See also *biliary system*; *colestyramine*.)

bile duct Any of the ducts by which *bile* is carried from the liver, first to the gallbladder and then to the duodenum (the first section of the small intestine). The bile duct system forms a network of tubular canals. Canaliculi (small canals) surround the liver cells and collect the bile. The canaliculi join together to form ducts of increasing size. The ducts emerge from the liver as the two hepatic ducts, which join within or just outside

BICEPS MUSCLE

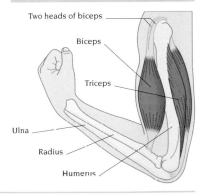

Two heads of biceps

Biceps

Triceps

Ulna

Radius

Humerus

the liver to form the common hepatic duct. The cystic duct branches off to the gallbladder; from this point the common hepatic duct becomes the common bile duct and leads into the duodenum. (See also *biliary system*.)

BILE DUCT

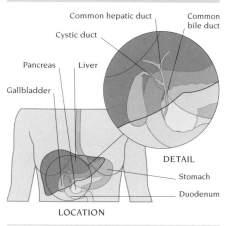

Common hepatic duct
Cystic duct
Common bile duct
Pancreas   Liver
Gallbladder

DETAIL
Stomach
Duodenum

LOCATION

bile duct cancer See *cholangiocarcinoma*.
bile duct obstruction A blockage or constriction of a bile duct (see *biliary system*). Bile duct obstruction results in accumulation of bile in the liver (*cholestasis*) and *jaundice* due to a build-up of *bilirubin* in the blood. Prolonged obstruction of the bile duct can lead to secondary *biliary cirrhosis*. The most common cause of obstruction is *gallstones*. Other causes include a tumour affecting the pancreas (see *pancreas, cancer of*), where the bile duct passes through it, or cancer that has spread from elsewhere in the body. *Cholangiocarcinoma* (cancer of the bile ducts) is a very rare cause of blockage. Bile duct obstruction is a rare side effect of certain drugs. It may also be caused by *cholangitis* (inflammation of the bile ducts), trauma (such as injury during surgery), and rarely by *flukes* or worms.

Bile duct obstruction causes "obstructive" jaundice, which is characterized by pale-coloured faeces, dark urine, and a yellow skin colour. There may also be itching. Other symptoms may include abdominal pain (with gallstones) or weight loss (with cancer). Treatment depends on the cause, but surgery may be necessary. Gallstones may be removed with an endoscope (see *ERCP*).

bilharzia Another name for the tropical parasitic disease *schistosomiasis*.

biliary atresia A rare disorder, present from birth, in which some or all of the *bile ducts* fail to develop or have developed abnormally. As a result, *bile* is unable to drain from the liver (see *cholestasis*). Unless the atresia can be treated, secondary *biliary cirrhosis* will develop and may prove fatal. Symptoms include deepening *jaundice*, usually beginning a week after birth, and the passing of dark urine and pale faeces. Treatment is by surgery to bypass the ducts. If this fails, or if the jaundice recurs, a *liver transplant* is the only possible treatment.

biliary cirrhosis An uncommon form of liver *cirrhosis* that results from problems with the bile ducts, either due to an *autoimmune disorder* known as primary biliary cirrhosis, or a longstanding blockage. Primary biliary cirrhosis affects mainly middle-aged women and seems to be linked with a malfunction of the *immune system*. Secondary biliary cirrhosis results from prolonged *bile duct obstruction* or *biliary atresia*. In both types, liver function is impaired due to *cholestasis* (accumulation of bile in the liver). In primary biliary cirrhosis, the bile ducts within the liver become inflamed and are destroyed. Symptoms include itching, *jaundice*, an enlarged liver, and sometimes abdominal pain, fatty diarrhoea, and *xanthomatosis*. *Osteoporosis* may develop. Symptoms of liver cirrhosis and *liver failure* may occur after several years. Drugs can minimize complications and relieve symptoms such as itching. A *liver transplant* is the only long-term cure. The symptoms and signs of secondary biliary cirrhosis include abdominal pain and tenderness, liver enlargement, fevers and chills, and sometimes blood abnormalities. Treatment is the same as for bile duct obstruction.

biliary colic A severe pain in the upper right quadrant of the abdomen that is usually caused by the gallbladder's attempts to expel *gallstones* or by the movement of a stone in the bile ducts.

The pain may be felt in the right shoulder (see *referred pain*) or may penetrate to the centre of the back. Episodes of biliary colic often last for several hours and may recur, particularly after meals.

Injections of an *analgesic drug* and an *antispasmodic drug* may be given to relieve the colic. Tests such as *cholecystography* or *ultrasound scanning* can confirm the presence of gallstones, in which case *cholecystectomy* (surgical removal of the gallbladder) is possible.

biliary system The organs and ducts by which *bile* is formed, concentrated, and carried from the *liver* to the duodenum (the first part of the small intestine). Bile is secreted by the liver cells and collected by a network of *bile ducts* that carry the bile out of the liver by way of the hepatic duct. A channel called the cystic duct branches off the hepatic duct and leads to the gallbladder where bile is concentrated and stored. Beyond this junction, the hepatic duct becomes the common bile duct and opens into the duodenum at a controlled orifice called the ampulla of Vater. The presence of fat in the duodenum after a meal causes secretion of a hormone, which opens the ampulla of Vater and makes the gallbladder contract, squeezing stored bile into the duodenum.

The main disorders affecting the biliary system are *gallstones*, congenital *biliary atresia* and *bile duct obstruction*. (See also *gallbladder, disorders of.*)

biliousness A condition in which bile is brought up to the mouth from the stomach. It is also used as a nonmedical term for nausea and vomiting.

bilirubin The main pigment found in *bile*. It is produced by the breakdown of *haemoglobin*, the pigment in red blood cells. Excessively high levels of bilirubin cause the yellow pigmentation associated with *jaundice*.

Billings' method Also called the mucus inspection method, a technique in which a woman notes changes in the characteristics of mucus produced by the cervix in order to predict ovulation for the purposes of *contraception* or *family planning*.

Billroth's operation A type of partial *gastrectomy* in which the lower part of the stomach is removed. Once used as a surgical treatment for *peptic ulcers*, it has now largely been replaced by treatment with *antibiotic drugs*.

Binet test The first *intelligence test* that attempted to measure higher mental functions, devised in 1905.

binge-purge syndrome An alternative term for *bulimia*.

bio- A prefix describing a relationship to life, as in biology, the science of life.

bioavailability The proportion of a drug that reaches the target organs and tissues, usually expressed as a percentage of the dose administered. Intravenous administration results in 100 per cent bioavailability because the drug is injected directly into the bloodstream. Drugs taken orally have a much lower bioavailability. Preparations that have equal bioavailabilities are described as bioequivalent. (See also *drug*.)

biochemistry A science that studies the chemistry of living organisms. It includes the chemical processes involved in the maintenance and reproduction of body cells and the chemical reactions carried out inside cells that make up the *metabolism* of the body. Overall regulation of these chemical processes is a function of *hormones*, whereas regulation of individual reactions is carried out by *enzymes*. A constant interchange occurs between cell fluids and blood and urine. Biochemists can therefore learn about the chemical changes going on inside cells from measurements of the various minerals, gases, enzymes, hormones, and proteins in blood, urine, and other body fluids. Such tests are used to make diagnoses and to screen for a disease and to monitor its progress. The most common biochemical tests are performed on *blood*, and they include *liver function tests* and *kidney function tests*. Biochemical tests can also be performed on urine (see *urinalysis*) and other body fluids.

bioengineering See *biomechanical engineering*.

biofeedback training A technique in which a person uses information about a normally unconscious body function to gain conscious control over that function. Biofeedback training may help in the treatment of stress-related conditions, including certain types of *hypertension, anxiety,* and *migraine.*

The patient is connected to a recording instrument that measures one of the unconscious body activities, such as blood pressure, heart-rate, or the quantity of sweat on the skin. The patient receives information (feedback) on the changing levels of these activities from changes in the instrument's signals. Using *relaxation techniques,* the patient learns to change the signals by conscious control of the body function. Once acquired, this control can be exercised without the instrument.

BIOFEEDBACK TRAINING

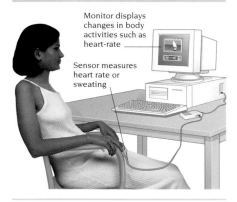

Monitor displays changes in body activities such as heart-rate

Sensor measures heart rate or sweating

biological clock A popular term for the inherent timing mechanism that supposedly controls physiological processes and cycles in living organisms. (See also *biorhythms.*)

biomechanical engineering A discipline that applies engineering methods and principles to the body to explain how it functions and to treat disorders. Practical applications include the design of artificial joints and heart valves, plaster casts, and kidney dialysis machines.

biopsy A diagnostic test in which a small amount of tissue or cells are removed from the body for microscopic examination. It is an accurate method of diagnosing many illnesses, including cancer. Microscopic examination of tissue (*histology*) or of cells (*cytology*) usually gives a correct diagnosis.

There are several types of biopsy. In excisional biopsy, the whole abnormal area is removed for study. Incisional biopsy involves cutting away a small sample of skin or muscle for analysis. In a needle biopsy, a needle is inserted through the skin and into the organ or tumour to be investigated. Aspiration biopsy uses a needle and syringe to remove cells from a solid lump. A guided biopsy uses *ultrasound scanning* or *CT scanning* to locate the area of tissue to be biopsied and to follow the progress of the needle. In endoscopic biopsy, an *endoscope* is passed into the organ to be investigated and an attachment is used to take a sample from the lining of accessible hollow organs and structures, such as the lungs, stomach, colon, and bladder. In an open biopsy, a surgeon opens a body cavity to reveal a diseased organ or tumour and removes a sample of tissue. Prompt analysis, in some cases by *frozen section,* can enable the surgeon to decide whether to remove the entire diseased area immediately.

Biopsy samples are analysed by *staining,* in which dyes are used to to show up structures or identify constituents such as *antibodies* or *enzymes.* A tissue sample may be tested with specific antibodies in the investigation of infection and inflammation. In some cases, a tissue *culture* may be required.

biorhythms Physiological functions that vary in a rhythmic way. Most biorhythms are based on a daily, or circadian (24-hour), cycle. Our bodies are governed by an internal clock, which is itself regulated by *hormones.* Periods of sleepiness and wakefulness may be affected by the level of *melatonin* secreted by the pineal gland in the brain. Melatonin release is stimulated by darkness and suppressed by light. Cortisol, secreted by the adrenal

BIOPSY

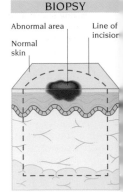

Abnormal area

Line of incision

Normal skin

EXCISIONAL SKIN BIOPSY

glands, also reflects the sleeping and waking states, being low in the evening and high in the morning.

biotechnology The use of living organisms such as *bacteria* in industry and science (for example, in drug production).

biotin A vitamin of the B complex (see *vitamin B complex*) that is essential for the breakdown of fats.

biphosphonate drugs See *bisphosphonate drugs*.

bipolar disorder An illness, also known as manic-depressive illness, characterized by swings in mood between the opposite extremes of severe *depression* and overexcitability (*mania*). Initially, the mood disturbance may consist of depression or mania but eventually it alternates between the two. In a severe form that is sometimes referred to as manic-depressive psychosis, there may also be grandiose ideas or negative delusions.

Abnormalities in brain biochemistry or in the structure and/or function of certain nerve pathways in the brain may be the underlying cause of bipolar disorder. An inherited tendency may also be a causative factor.

Bipolar disorder is almost always treated with drugs, often in combination with other therapies. *Antidepressant drugs* are used to treat depression; *ECT* may also be used if depression is severe. *Antipsychotic drugs* are given to control manic symptoms. *Lithium* or *carbamazepine* are used to prevent relapses. In severe cases, bipolar disorder often needs hospital treatment. *Group therapy*, *family therapy*, and individual *psychotherapy* may be useful in treatment. *Cognitive-behavioural therapy* may also be helpful. With treatment, most patients improve or remain stable. Even those with severe illness may be restored to near-normal health with lithium.

bird flu See *avian influenza*.

birth See *childbirth*.

birth canal The passage through the pelvis from the cervix (neck of the womb) to the vaginal opening through which the baby passes during *childbirth*.

birth control Limitation of the number of children born, either to an individual or within a population *Family planning* allows men and women to choose if and

when to have children; *contraception* can prevent unwanted pregnancies.

birth defects Abnormalities that are obvious at birth or detectable early in infancy. Also called congenital defects, they encompass both minor abnormalities, such as *birthmarks*, and serious disorders such as *spina bifida*.

Causes include *chromosomal abnormalities*, genetic defects, drugs taken during pregnancy, exposure to radiation, and infections. In some cases, the cause of a defect is unknown. Defects that are due to chromosomal abnormalities include *Down's syndrome*. Some defects, such as *achondroplasia* and *albinism*, are usually inherited from one or both parents (see *gene*; *genetic disorders*). Certain drugs and chemicals (called *teratogens*) can damage the fetus if the mother takes or is exposed to them during early pregnancy. Teratogenic drugs include *thalidomide* (now rarely prescribed) and *isotretinoin*, which is used in the treatment of severe *acne*. Alcohol can affect the development of the brain and face (see *fetal alcohol syndrome*).

Irradiation of the embryo in early pregnancy can cause abnormalities. Very small doses of radiation increase the child's risk of developing *leukaemia* later in life (see *radiation hazards*).

Certain illnesses, such as *rubella* (German measles) and *toxoplasmosis*, can cause birth defects if they are contracted during pregnancy.

Brain and spinal cord abnormalities, such as spina bifida and *hydrocephalus*, and congenital heart disorders (see *heart disease, congenital*) result from interference with the development of particular groups of cells. Other common defects include *cleft lip and palate*.

Ultrasound scanning and blood tests during pregnancy can identify women at high risk of having a baby with a birth defect. Further tests such as *chorionic villus sampling*, *amniocentesis*, or *fetoscopy* may then be carried out.

birth injury Damage sustained during birth. Minor injuries, such as bruising and swelling of the scalp during a vaginal delivery (see *cephalhaematoma*) are common. More serious injury can occur, particularly if the baby is excessively

B

large and has difficulty in passing through the birth canal. A *breech delivery* may result in injury to nerves in the shoulder, causing temporary paralysis in the arm. The face may be paralysed temporarily if the facial nerve is traumatized by forceps. Fractured bones are another hazard of difficult deliveries, but the bones usually heal easily. (See also *birth defects; brain damage.*)

birthmark An area of discoloured skin present from birth, or very soon afterwards, such as *moles*, freckles, and other types of melanocytic *naevus* (various flat, brown to blue-grey skin patches), strawberry marks, and port-wine stains. The last two are types of *haemangioma* (malformation of blood vessels). Strawberry marks often increase in size in the first year, but most disappear after the age of about 9 years. Port-wine stains seldom fade, but *laser treatment* performed in adulthood can make some of them fade.

birthpool A pool of warm water in which a woman can sit to help relieve pain during labour.

birth rate A measurement of the number of births in a year in relation to the population.

birthweight A baby's weight at birth that usually ranges from 2.5–4.5 kg. Birthweight depends on a number of factors, including the size and ethnic origin of the parents. Babies who weigh less than 2.5 kg at birth are classified as being of low birthweight. Causes of low birthweight include *prematurity* and undernourishment in the uterus (for example, because the mother had *pre-eclampsia*). Abnormally high birthweight is often due to unrecognized or poorly controlled *diabetes mellitus* in the mother.

bisexuality Sexual interest in members of both sexes that may or may not involve sexual activity.

bismuth A metal, salts of which are used in tablets to treat *peptic ulcer* and in suppositories and creams to treat *haemorrhoids*. Bismuth preparations taken by mouth may colour the faeces black. The tongue may darken and occasional nausea and vomiting may occur.

bisphosphonate drugs Drugs used in the prevention or treatment of *osteo-porosis*. They are also used to slow bone metabolism (for example, in *Paget's disease*) and to reduce the high calcium levels in the blood associated with destruction of bone by secondary cancer growths.

bite See *occlusion*.

bites, animal Any injury inflicted by the mouthparts of an animal, from the puncture wounds of bloodsucking insects to the massive injuries caused by shark or crocodile attacks. Teeth, especially those of carnivores, can inflict severe and widespread mechanical injury. Severe injuries and lacerations to major blood vessels can lead to severe blood loss and physiological *shock*. Serious infection may occur due to bacteria in the animal's mouth; and *tetanus* is a particular hazard. In countries where *rabies* is present, any mammal may potentially harbour the rabies virus and transmit it via a bite. Medical advice should be sought for all but minor injuries or if there is a possibility of rabies. Treatment usually includes cleaning and examination of the wound. The wound will usually be left open and dressed. Preventive *antibiotic drug* treatment and an antitetanus injection may also be given. Antirabies vaccine is given, with *immunoglobulin*, if there is any possibility that the animal is infected with the rabies virus. (See also *bites, human; insect bites; snake bites; spider bites; venomous bites and stings.*)

bites, human Wounds caused by one person biting another. Human bites rarely cause serious tissue damage or blood loss, but infection is likely, particularly if the bite is deep. There is a risk of *tetanus* infection. Transmission of *hepatitis B, hepatitis C, herpes simplex,* and *AIDS* by a bite is a hazard.

black death The medieval name for bubonic *plague*, which killed 50 per cent of its victims. One feature of the disease is bleeding beneath the skin, causing dark blue or black bruises, hence the name 'black death'.

black eye The bruised appearance of the skin around the eye, usually following an injury. The discoloration is due to blood collecting under the skin.

blackhead A semi-solid, black-capped plug of greasy material, also known as a comedo, blocking the outlet of a sebaceous (oil-forming) gland in the skin. Blackheads occur most commonly on the face, chest, shoulders, and back and are associated with increased sebaceous gland activity. They are one of the features of most types of *acne*.

blackout A common term for loss of consciousness (see *fainting*).

black teeth See *discoloured teeth*.

blackwater fever An occasional and life-threatening complication of falciparum *malaria* (the most dangerous form of malaria). Symptoms include loss of consciousness, fever, and vomiting, and very dark urine (due to pigment from destroyed red blood cells being filtered into the urine), which gives the condition its name.

bladder The hollow, muscular organ in the lower abdomen that acts as a reservoir for *urine*. It lies within, and is protected by, the pelvis. An adult bladder can hold about 0.5 litres of urine before the need to pass urine is felt

The bladder walls consist of muscle and an inner lining. Two ureters carry urine to the bladder from the kidneys. At the lowest point of the bladder is the opening into the urethra, which is known as the bladder neck. This is normally kept tightly closed by a ring of muscle (the urethral sphincter). The function of the bladder is to collect and store urine until it can be expelled. Defective bladder function, leading to problems such as *incontinence* and *urinary retention*, can have a variety of causes. (See also *bladder, disorders of; enuresis*).

bladder cancer See *bladder tumours.*

bladder, disorders of A group of disorders affecting the bladder, including inflammation (*cystitis*) usually caused by a bacterial infection; *calculi* (stones); impairment of the nerve supply; and tumours. In men, obstruction to urine flow from the bladder by an enlarged prostate gland may cause *urinary retention*. Tumours of, or injury to, the spinal cord may affect the nerves controlling the bladder, leading either to retention or *incontinence*. Bladder stones are caused by the precipitation of substances that are present in the urine. Injury to the bladder is uncommon but may occur if the pelvis is fractured when the bladder is full.

Disturbed bladder control can also result from nerve degeneration in conditions such as *diabetes mellitus*, *multiple sclerosis*, or *dementia*. An unstable or *irritable bladder* is a common condition and is sometimes associated with a *urinary tract infection* or prolapse of the uterus. Tension or anxiety can cause frequent urination. In children, delayed bladder control (see *enuresis*) most often results from delayed maturation of the nervous system.

bladder tumours Growths originating in the inner lining of the bladder. Many are *papillomas* (small wart-like growths), which tend to recur and will eventually become cancerous. Other, more malignant growths may extend not only into the bladder cavity but may also spread through the bladder wall to involve nearby organs such as the colon, rectum, prostate gland, or uterus.

BLADDER

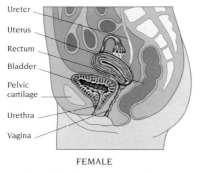

Ureter
Uterus
Rectum
Bladder
Pelvic cartilage
Urethra
Vagina

FEMALE

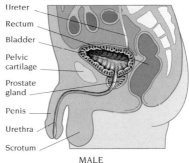

Ureter
Rectum
Bladder
Pelvic cartilage
Prostate gland
Penis
Urethra
Scrotum

MALE

B

Bladder cancer is more common in smokers and workers in the dye and rubber industries. *Haematuria* (blood in the urine) is the main symptom of bladder cancer. A tumour may obstruct the entry of a ureter into the bladder, causing back pressure and pain in the kidney region, or may obstruct the urethral exit, causing difficulty in passing, or retention of, urine.

Bladder tumours are diagnosed with urine tests, *cystoscopy*, and biopsy of the abnormal area. If small, they can be treated by heat or surgically during cystoscopy; in such cases, chemotherapeutic drugs may also be inserted into the bladder. Bladder tumours tend to recur at the same or other sites within the bladder, so that regular follow-up cystoscopy or urine testing is needed. Bladder tumours that have spread through the bladder wall may be treated by *radiotherapy* or by surgical removal of part or all of the bladder.

blastocyst A cell cluster that develops from a fertilized *ovum* and grows into an *embryo* (see *fertilization*).

blastomycosis A type of *fungal infection* that can affect the lungs and other internal organs.

bleaching, dental A cosmetic procedure for lightening certain types of *discoloured teeth*, including nonvital 'dead' teeth. The surface of the affected tooth is painted with oxidizing agents and then exposed to ultraviolet light.

bleeding Loss of blood from the *circulatory system* caused by damage to the blood vessels or by a *bleeding disorder*. Bleeding may be visible (external) or concealed (internal). Rapid loss of more than 10 per cent of the blood volume can cause symptoms of *shock*, with fainting, pallor, and sweating.

The speed with which blood flows from a cut depends on the type of blood vessel damaged: blood usually oozes from a capillary, flows from a vein, and spurts from an artery. If an injury does not break open the skin, blood collects around the damaged blood vessels close under the skin to form a *bruise*.

Any lost blood that mixes with other body fluids such as sputum (phlegm) or urine will be noticed quite readily; bleeding in the digestive tract may make vomit or faeces appear darker than usual. Internal bleeding may not be discovered until severe *anaemia* develops.

bleeding disorders A group of conditions characterized by bleeding in the absence of injury or by abnormally prolonged and excessive bleeding after injury. The disorders result from defects in mechanisms by which bleeding is normally stopped: blood coagulation, plugging of damaged blood vessels by platelets, and constriction of blood vessels (see *blood clotting*).

Coagulation disorders are usually due a deficiency or abnormality in the *enzymes* (coagulation factors) involved in blood clotting. Defects may be *congenital* or acquired later in life. The main congenital coagulation defects are *von Willebrand's disease*, *haemophilia*, and *Christmas disease*.

Acquired defects of coagulation factors may develop at any age due to severe liver disease, digestive system disorders that prevent the absorption of *vitamin K* (needed to make certain coagulation factors), or the use of *anticoagulant drugs*. Disseminated intravascular coagulation (DIC) is an acquired disorder that is both complex and serious. It may be the result of underlying infection or cancer. In this condition, platelets accumulate and clots form within small blood vessels; coagulation factors are used up faster than they can be replaced, and severe bleeding may result.

Coagulation disorders are treated by replacement of the missing factor, factors extracted from fresh blood, or fresh frozen plasma. Genetically engineered factors may be used. Anticoagulants are sometimes used to suppress excess clotting activity in DIC.

Thrombocytopenia, which results from insufficient platelets in the blood, produces surface bleeding into the skin and gums and multiple small bruises. Platelet defects may be inherited, associated with the use of certain drugs (including *aspirin*), or a complication of certain bone marrow disorders such as myeloid *leukaemia*. Treatment consists of platelet transfusions. Rarely, abnormal bleeding is caused by a blood vessel defect or scurvy. Elderly people and patients on long-term courses of *corticosteroid drugs* may suffer mild abnormal bruising due to loss of skin support to the smallest blood vessels. Treatment is rarely required.

bleeding gums See *gingivitis*.

blepharitis Inflammation of the eyelids, with redness, irritation, and scaly skin at the lid margins. Blepharitis may cause burning and discomfort in the eyes and flakes or crusts on the lashes. The condition is common, tends to recur, and is sometimes associated with dandruff of the scalp or *eczema*. Severe blepharitis may lead to *corneal ulcers*. In many cases, treatment of associated dandruff with an antifungal shampoo will result in improvement of the blepharitis.

blepharoplasty A cosmetic operation to remove wrinkled, drooping skin from the upper and/or lower eyelids.

blepharospasm Prolonged, involuntary, contraction of one of the muscles controlling the eyelids, causing them to close. It may be due to *photophobia*, damage to the *cornea*, or *dystonia*, for which *botulinum toxin* (a muscle relaxant) treatment is highly effective.

blind loop syndrome A condition in which a redundant area or dead end (blind loop) in the small intestine becomes colonized with bacteria. This results in abnormal faeces and poor absorption of nutrients. The syndrome may result from surgery or a *stricture* (narrowing) in the intestine due to a disorder such as *Crohn's disease*. It is characterized by *steatorrhoea* (pale yellow, foul-smelling, fatty, bulky faeces that are difficult to flush away), tiredness, and weight loss. *Antibiotic drug* treatment usually cures the condition.

blindness Inability to see. Definitions of blindness and partial sight vary. In the UK, blindness is defined as a corrected *visual acuity* of 3/60 or less in the better eye, or a *visual field* of no more than 20 degrees in the better eye. Blindness may result from injury to, or disease or degeneration of, the eyeball; the optic nerve or nerve pathways connecting the eye to the brain; or the brain itself. Clouding of the cornea may result from *Sjögren's syndrome*, vitamin

A deficiency, chemical damage, infections, and injury. *Corneal ulcers* can cause blindness due to scarring of the cornea. *Uveitis* and *cataracts* are other common causes of blindness. *Diabetes mellitus*, *hypertension*, or injury can all cause bleeding into the cavity of the eyeball and subsequent loss of vision. Bleeding into the fluid in front of the lens *(hyphaema)* or behind the lens *(vitreous haemorrhage)* can also result in loss of vision. Other conditions that may cause blindness include *glaucoma*; *retinal artery occlusion* or *retinal vein occlusion*; age-related *macular degeneration*; *retinopathy*; *retinal detachment*; tumours such as *retinoblastoma* and malignant *melanoma* of the eye; and *retinal haemorrhage*.

Loss of vision may be due to nerve conduction problems. These problems may be the result of pressure caused by a tumour; reduced blood supply to the optic nerve; *optic neuritis*; or toxic or nutritional deficiencies. Blindness can result if there is pressure on the visual cortex from a *brain tumour* or *brain haemorrhage*, or if the blood supply to the cortex is reduced following a *stroke*.

Treatment depends on the underlying cause. If the loss of vision cannot be corrected, the patient may then be registered as legally blind or partially sighted. (See also *eye*; *vision, loss of*.)

blind spot The small, oval-shaped area on the retina of the eye where the optic nerve leaves the eyeball. The area is not sensitive to light because it has no light receptors (nerve endings responsive to light). The blind spot can also be used to describe the part of the *visual field* in which objects cannot be detected.

blister A collection of fluid beneath the outer layer of the skin that forms a raised area. A blister contains fluid that has leaked from blood vessels in underlying skin layers after minor damage and protects the damaged tissue. Common causes are *burns* and friction. Blisters may also occur with *pemphigus*, *pemphigoid*, *dermatitis herpetiformis*, some types of *porphyria*, and some skin diseases. These include *eczema*, *epidermolysis bullosa*, *impetigo*, and *erythema multiforme*. Small blisters develop in the viral infections *chickenpox*, *herpes zoster* (shingles), and *herpes simplex*. Generally, blisters are best left intact, but large or unexplained blisters need medical attention.

bloating Distension of the abdomen, commonly due to wind in the stomach or intestine (see *abdominal swelling*).

blocked nose See *nasal congestion*; *nasal obstruction*.

blocking Inability to express true feelings or thoughts, usually as a result of emotional or mental conflict. In Freudian-based psychotherapies, blocking is regarded as originating from repression of painful emotions in early life. A very specific form of thought blocking occurs in *schizophrenia*: trains of thought are persistently interrupted involuntarily to be replaced by unrelated new ones. (See also *psychotherapy*.)

blood The red fluid that circulates in the body's veins, arteries, and capillaries. Blood is pumped by the heart via the arteries to the lungs and all other tissues and is then returned to the heart in veins (see *circulatory system*). Blood is the body's transport system and plays an important role in the defence against infection. An average adult has about 5 litres of blood.

Almost half of the volume of blood consists of *blood cells*; these include red blood cells (erythrocytes), which carry oxygen to tissues; white blood cells (leukocytes), which fight infection; and platelets (thrombocytes), which are involved in *blood clotting*. The remainder of the blood volume is a watery, straw-coloured fluid called plasma, which contains dissolved proteins, sugars, fats, salts, and minerals. Nutrients are transported in the blood to the tissues after absorption from the intestinal tract or after release from storage depots such as the liver. Waste products, including *urea* and *bilirubin* are carried in the plasma to the kidneys and liver respectively.

Plasma proteins include fibrinogen, which is involved in blood clotting; *immunoglobulins* (also called *antibodies*) and *complement*, which are part of the *immune system*; and *albumin*. Hormones are also transported in the blood to their target organs.

blood cells Cells, also called blood corpuscles, present in blood for most or part of their lifespan. They include red blood cells, which make up about 45 per cent by volume of normal blood, white blood cells, and *platelets*. Blood cells are made in the bone marrow by a series of divisions from *stem cells*.

Red blood cells (also known as RBCs, red blood corpuscles, or erythrocytes) transport oxygen from the lungs to the tissues (see *respiration*). Each RBC is packed with *haemoglobin*, *enzymes*, minerals, and sugars. Abnormalities can occur in the rate at which RBCs are either produced or destroyed, in their numbers, and in their shape, size, and haemoglobin content, causing forms of *anaemia* and *polycythaemia* (see *blood, disorders of*).

White blood cells (also called WBCs, white blood corpuscles, or leukocytes) help to protect the body against infection and fight infection when it occurs. The three main types of WBC are granulocytes (also called polymorphonuclear leukocytes), monocytes, and *lymphocytes*. Granulocytes are further classified as neutrophils, eosinophils, or basophils, and each type of granulocyte has a role in either fighting infection or in inflammatory or allergic reactions. Monocytes and lymphocytes also play an important part in the *immune system*. Lymphocytes are usually formed in the lymph nodes. One type, a T-lymphocyte, is responsible for the delayed hypersensitivity reactions (see *allergy*) and is also involved in protection against cancer. T-lymphocytes manufacture chemicals, known as lymphokines, which affect the function of other cells. In addition, the T-cells moderate the activity of B-lymphocytes, which form the *antibodies* that can prevent a second attack of

BLOOD CELLS

Red blood cell

White blood cell (neutrophil)

White blood cell (lymphocyte)

Platelet

Plasma

certain infectious diseases. Platelets (also known as thrombocytes), are the smallest blood cells and are important in *blood clotting*.

The numbers, shapes, and appearance of the various types of blood cell are of great value in the diagnosis of disease (see *blood count; blood film*).

blood clotting The process of blood solidification. Clotting is important in stemming bleeding from damaged blood vessels. However, unwanted blood clotting can occur inside major blood vessels and cause a *myocardial infarction* (heart attack) or stroke (see *thrombosis*).

When a blood vessel is damaged, it constricts immediately to reduce blood flow to the area. The damage sets off a series of chemical reactions that lead to the formation of a clot to seal the injury. First, *platelets* around the injury site are activated, becoming sticky and adhering to the blood-vessel wall. Then, the activated platelets release chemicals, which, in turn, activate blood clotting factors. These factors, together with vitamin K, act on *fibrinogen* and convert it to *fibrin*. Strands of fibrin form a meshwork, which traps red blood cells to form a clot.

There are several anticlotting mechanisms to prevent the formation of unwanted clots. These include prostacyclin (a *prostaglandin*), which prevents platelet aggregation, and plasmin, which breaks down fibrin (see *fibrinolysis*). Blood flow washes away active coagulation factors; and the liver deactivates excess coagulation factors.

Defects in blood clotting may result in *bleeding disorders*. Excessive clotting (thrombosis) may be due to an inherited increase or defect in a coagulation factor (see *factor V*), the use of oral contraceptives, a decrease in the level of enzymes that inhibit coagulation, or sluggish blood flow through a particular area. Treatment is usually with *anticoagulant drugs,* such as heparin or warfarin, or *thrombolytic drugs*, such as *streptokinase*.

blood-clotting tests Tests to screen for and diagnose *bleeding disorders*, usually resulting from deficiencies or abnormalities of blood coagulation factors or of platelets (see *blood clotting*). Tests are also used to monitor treatment with *anticoagulant drugs*.

blood count A test, also called full blood count, that measures *haemoglobin* concentration and the numbers of red blood cells, white blood cells, and platelets in 1 cu. mm of blood. The proportion of various white blood cells is measured and the size and shape of red and white cells is noted. It is the most commonly performed blood test and is important for diagnosing *anaemia* or confirming the presence of an infection to which the blood has responded. It is also used to diagnose disorders such as *leukaemia* and *thrombocytopenia*.

blood culture See *culture*.

blood, disorders of Disorders resulting from abnormalities in any of the components of blood or from infection. Disorders include types of *anaemia*, *polycythaemia*, *bleeding disorders, and* unwanted clot formation (*thrombosis*),

BLOOD CLOTTING

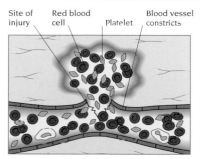

Site of injury Red blood cell Platelet Blood vessel constricts

PLATELETS ACTIVATED

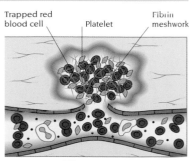

Trapped red blood cell Platelet Fibrin meshwork

BLOOD CLOT FORMS

hypoalbuminaemia (*albumin* deficiency) and agammaglobulinaemia (deficiency of *gamma-globulin*). Blood disorders such as *sickle cell anaemia, thalassaemia,* and *haemophilia* are inherited. Bone marrow cancers that affect production of blood components include *leukaemia,* polycythaemia vera, and *multiple myeloma*. Blood poisoning is usually due to *septicaemia* or a toxin such as carbon monoxide. Some drugs can cause blood abnormalities as a side effect. (See also *anaemia, haemolytic; anaemia, iron-deficiency; anaemia, megaloblastic; malaria; hyperbilirubinaemia.*)

blood donation The process of giving blood for use in *blood transfusion*. Donated blood is tested for a range of infectious agents such as *hepatitis B* and *hepatitis C* and antibodies to *HIV*. After being classified into *blood groups*, the blood is stored in a blood bank, either whole or separated into its different components (see *blood products*). Apheresis is a type of blood donation in which only a specific blood component, such as plasma, platelets, or white cells, is withdrawn from the donor.

blood film A test that involves smearing a drop of blood on to a glass slide for examination under a microscope. The blood film is stained with dyes to make the blood cells show up clearly.

The test allows the shape and appearance of blood cells to be checked for any abnormality, such as the sickle-shaped red blood cells characteristic of *sickle cell anaemia*. The relative proportions of the different types of white blood cells can also be counted. This examination, called a differential white cell count, may be helpful in diagnosing infection or *leukaemia*. Blood films are also used in diagnosing infections, such as *malaria*, in which the parasites can be seen inside the red blood cells. Blood films are usually carried out together with a full *blood count.*

blood gases A test for determining the acidity-alkalinity (pH) and the concentrations of oxygen, carbon dioxide, and bicarbonate in the blood. The test is carried out on a sample of blood taken from an artery, usually at the wrist or groin. It is useful in diagnosing and monitoring *respiratory failure*. Bicarbonate and acidity reflect the *acid-base balance* of the body, which may be disturbed in conditions such as diabetic ketoacidosis, aspirin poisoning, hyperventilation, or repeated vomiting. Blood oxygen can also be measured without taking a blood sample by using an *oximeter.*

blood glucose The level of *glucose* in the blood. Abnormally high blood glucose (sometimes called sugar) levels are an indication of *diabetes mellitus*. (See also *hyperglycaemia; hypoglycaemia.*)

blood groups Systems of classifying blood according to the different marker proteins (*antigens*) on the surface of red blood cells and antibodies in the plasma. These antigens affect the ability of the red blood cells to provoke an *immune response*. There are two main blood grouping systems: the ABO system and the rhesus system.

In the ABO system, the presence or absence of two types of antigen (named A and B) on the surface of the red blood cells determine whether a person's blood group is A, B, AB (which

BLOOD GROUPS

BLOOD GROUP A

BLOOD GROUP B

BLOOD GROUP AB

BLOOD GROUP O

has both A and B), or O (which has neither A nor B). People with the A antigen (group A) have anti-B antibodies; people with the B antigen (group B) have anti-A antibodies; those with both antigens (blood group AB) have neither; and those with neither antigen (group O) have both.

The rhesus system involves several antigens, the most important of which is factor D. People with this factor are Rh positive; those without it are Rh negative. The importance of the Rh group relates mainly to pregnancy in Rh-negative women, since, if the baby is Rh positive, the mother may form antibodies against the baby's blood (see *rhesus incompatibility*).

A person's blood group is inherited and may be used in paternity testing. Genetic analysis allows identification of the blood of a person with virtual certainty (see *genetic fingerprinting*).

blood level The concentration of a given substance in the blood plasma or serum that may be measured by *blood tests*.

blood poisoning A common name for *septicaemia* with *toxaemia*, a life-threatening illness caused by multiplication of bacteria and formation of toxins in the bloodstream. Septicaemia may be a complication of an infection in an organ or tissue. In some infective conditions, *septic shock* may be caused by toxins released by bacteria. Treatment is with *antibiotic drugs* and intensive therapy for shock. (See also *bacteraemia*.)

blood pressure The pressure exerted by the flow of blood through the main arteries. The pressure at two different phases is measured. Systolic, the higher pressure, is created by the contraction of the *heart*. Diastolic, the lower, is recorded during relaxation of the ventricles between heartbeats; it reflects the resistance of all the small arteries in the body and the load against which the heart must work. The pressure wave that is transmitted along the arteries with each heartbeat is easily felt as the *pulse*.

Blood pressure is measured using a *sphygmomanometer* and is expressed as millimetres of mercury (mmHg). Blood pressure varies with age, between individuals, and at different times in the same individual but a healthy young adult usually has a blood pressure reading, at rest, of about 120/80 (that is 120 mmHg systolic and 80 mmHg diastolic). Abnormally high blood pressure is called *hypertension*; abnormally low pressure is termed *hypotension*.

blood products Donated blood that is separated into its various components: red cells, white cells, platelets, and plasma (see *blood donation*). Each blood product has a specific lifespan and use. Leukodepleted red cells (blood with the plasma removed) are used to treat patients with acute bleeding or some forms of chronic *anaemia* and babies with *haemolytic disease of the newborn*.

Platelets may be given in transfusions for people with blood-clotting disorders. Patients who have life-threatening infections may be treated with granulocytes, a type of white blood cell. Fresh frozen plasma is used to correct many types of *bleeding disorder* because it contains all the clotting factors. Purified *albumin* preparations are used to treat *nephrotic syndrome* and chronic liver disease.

Concentrates of blood clotting factors VIII and IX are used in the treatment of *haemophilia* and *Christmas disease*. *Immunoglobulins* (also called antibodies), which are extracted from blood plasma, can be given by injection (see *immunoglobulin injection*) to protect people who are unable to produce their own antibodies or have already been exposed to an infectious agent, or to provide short-term protection against *hepatitis A*. Immunoglobulins are given in large doses to treat certain *autoimmune disorders*.

blood smear See *blood film*.

blood spot screening tests A series of tests carried out in the first week of birth on a small sample of a baby's blood to check for several rare but potentially serious disorders. The blood sample is obtained by pricking the baby's heel and collecting the blood on a special card, which is then tested for various disorders, including *phenylketonuria*, congenital *hypothyroidism*, *cystic fibrosis*, *sickle cell anaemia*, and, occasionally, *thalassaemia*.

B

blood sugar See *blood glucose*.

blood tests Analysis of a sample of blood to give information on its cells and proteins and any of the chemicals, antigens, antibodies, and gases that it carries. Such tests can be used to check on the health of major organs, as well as on respiratory function, hormonal balance, the immune system, and metabolism. Blood tests may look at numbers, shape, size, and appearance of blood cells and assess the function of clotting factors. The most important tests are *blood count* and *blood group* tests if transfusion is needed. Biochemical tests measure chemicals in the blood (see *acid-base balance; kidney function tests; liver function tests*). Microbiological tests (see *immunoassay*) look for microorganisms that are in the blood, as in septicaemia. Microbiology also looks for antibodies in the blood, which may confirm immunity to an infection.

blood transfusion The infusion of large volumes of blood or *blood products* directly into the bloodstream to remedy severe blood loss or to correct chronic *anaemia*. In an exchange transfusion, nearly all of the recipient's blood is replaced by donor blood. Before a transfusion, a sample of the recipient's blood is taken to identify the *blood groups*, and it is matched with suitable donor blood. The donor blood is transfused into an arm vein through a plastic cannula. Usually, each unit (about 500 ml) of blood is given over 1–4 hours; in an emergency, 500 ml may be given in a couple of minutes. The blood pressure, temperature, and pulse are monitored during the procedure.

If mismatched blood is accidentally introduced into the circulation, anti-bodies in the recipient's blood may cause donor cells to burst, leading to *shock* or *kidney failure*. Less severe reactions can produce fever, chills, or a rash. Reactions can also occur as a result of an allergy to transfused blood components. All blood used for transfusion is carefully screened for a number of infectious agents, including *HIV* (the *AIDS* virus), *hepatitis B*, and *hepatitis C*.

In elderly or severely anaemic patients, transfusion can overload the circulation, leading to heart failure. In patients with chronic anaemia who need regular transfusion over many years, excess iron may accumulate (haemosiderosis) and damage organs such as the heart, liver, and pancreas. Treatment with *desferrioxamine* to remove excess iron may be needed.

blood transfusion, autologous The use of a person's own blood, donated earlier, for *blood transfusion*. Autologous transfusion eliminates the slight but serious risk of contracting a serious infectious illness from contaminated blood. There is no risk of a transfusion reaction occurring as a result of incompatibility between donor and recipient blood. Up to 3.5 litres of blood can be removed and stored in several sessions at least 4 days apart and up to 3 days before planned surgery. Blood may be salvaged during surgery, filtered and returned to the circulation, reducing the need for transfusion of donated blood.

blood vessels A general term given to arteries, veins, and capillaries (see *circulatory system*).

blue baby An infant with a cyanotic (bluish) complexion, especially of the lips and tongue, caused by a relative lack of oxygen in the blood. This is usually due to a structural defect of the heart or the major arteries leaving the heart. Such defects may need to be corrected surgically (see *heart disease, congenital*).

blurred vision Indistinct or fuzzy visual images. Blurred vision, which should not be confused with *double vision* (diplopia), can occur in one *eye* or both, for episodes of varying lengths of time, and can develop gradually or suddenly. The usual cause of longstanding blurred vision is a refractive error such as *astigmatism* (unequal curvature of the front of the eye), *hypermetropia* (longsightedness), or *myopia* (shortsightedness), all of which can be corrected by glasses or contact lenses. After the age of 40, *presbyopia* (reduced ability to focus on near objects) becomes more common.

Vision may also be impaired or blurred as a result of damage, disease, or abnormalities of parts of the eye or its connections to the brain. The most common causes of blurred vision as a result of disease are *cataract* and *retinopathy*.

blushing Brief reddening of the face and sometimes the neck caused by widening of the blood vessels close to the skin's surface. Blushing is usually an involuntary reaction to embarrassment. In some women, blushing is a feature of the *hot flushes*, which occur during the *menopause*. Flushing of the face occurs in association with *carcinoid syndrome*.

BMI The abbreviation for *body mass index*.

body contour surgery Surgery performed to remove excess fat, skin, or both, from various parts of the body, especially the abdomen, thighs, and buttocks. Abdominal wall reduction, also known as abdominoplasty, involves removing excess skin and fat from the abdomen. With all of these procedures, there is a risk of complications, and the wound may become infected.

In suction lipectomy (liposuction), a rigid hollow tube is inserted through a small skin incision and use to break up large areas of fat, which can then be sucked out through the instrument. Minor irregularities and dimpling of the skin commonly occur after surgery.

body dysmorphic disorder A psychiatric disorder in which a person suffers intense anxiety about an imagined defect in part of his or her body.

body image A person's perception of the different parts of his or her own body.

body mass index (BMI) An indicator of healthy body *weight*. BMI is calculated by dividing the weight in kilograms by the square of the height in metres. A BMI of 18.4 or less is classed as underweight; a BMI of 18.5–24.9 is classed as an ideal weight; a BMI of 25–29.9 is classed as overweight; a BMI of 30–39.9 is classed as obese; and a BMI over 40 is classed as very obese. These figures are general ones that apply to most healthy adults under the age of 60. They are not applicable to children or people over 60; people with chronic health problems; pregnant or breast-feeding women; or athletes, weight-trainers, or similar groups of people with a high proportion of body muscle.

body odour The smell caused by the action of *bacteria* on sweat. It is most noticeable in the armpits and around the genital area, where the *apocrine glands* contain proteins and fatty materials favourable to bacterial growth.

boil An inflamed, pus-filled area of skin, usually an infected hair follicle. A more severe and extensive form of a boil that involves several hair follicles is a *carbuncle*. The usual cause of a boil is infection with the bacterium STAPHYLOCOCCUS AUREUS. Recurrent boils may occur in people with known or unrecognized *diabetes mellitus* or with other conditions in which general resistance to infection is impaired. Treatment may be with *antibiotic drugs* but, if pus is released surgically, the boil will usually heal without antibiotics.

bolus A soft mass of chewed food that is produced by the action of the tongue, teeth, and saliva. The term bolus is also used to describe a single dose of a drug that is rapidly injected into a vein.

bonding The process by which a strong tie, both psychological and emotional, is established between a parent and newborn child.

bonding, dental Dental techniques that use plastic resins and acrylic or porcelain veneers and inlays to repair, restore, or improve the appearance of damaged or defective *teeth*. It is sometimes used as an alternative to crowning (see *crown, dental*) and may also be used as a preventive technique to protect the teeth.

bone The structural material of the *skeleton* that provides a rigid framework for the muscles and protects certain body organs. Bone consists of several layers: a thin outer covering (the periosteum), which contains blood vessels and nerves; an inner shell of hard (compact or cortical) bone composed of columns of bone cells (osteoclasts and osteoblasts), each with a central hollow (haversian canal) that is important for the nutrition, growth, and repair of the bone; and a central, mesh-like structure (known as spongy, cancellous, or trabecular bone). The cavity in the centre of some bones, and the spaces in spongy bone, contain *bone marrow*.

Bone is continuously reabsorbed by osteoclasts and replaced by osteoblasts. Osteoblasts encourage deposition of calcium phosphate on the protein framework of the bone, and osteoclasts remove it. The actions of these cells are controlled by hormones, which also maintain the calcium level in the blood.

BONE

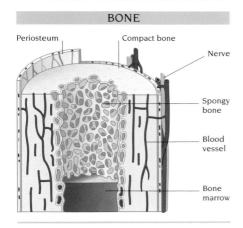

Periosteum
Compact bone
Nerve
Spongy bone
Blood vessel
Bone marrow

At birth, many bones consist mainly of cartilage, which ossifies later (see *ossification*). The *epiphyses* (growing ends of the long bones) are separated from the bone shaft (*diaphysis*) by the epiphyseal plate. Some bones, such as certain skull bones, do not develop from cartilage and are known as membranous bones.

bone abscess A localized collection of pus in a bone (see *osteomyelitis*).

bone age A measure of skeletal maturity used to assess physical development in children. *X-rays*, which show how much bones have grown in a particular body area, are used to determine bone age. (See also *age*.)

bone cancer *Malignant* growth in bone, which may originate in the bone itself (primary bone cancer) or, more commonly, occur as a result of cancer spreading from elsewhere in the body (secondary, or metastatic, bone cancer). Primary bone cancers are rare. The type that occurs most often is *osteosarcoma*. Other types include *chondrosarcoma* and *fibrosarcoma*. Bone cancer can also start in the bone marrow (see *multiple myeloma* and *leukaemia*). The treatment of primary bone cancer depends on the extent to which the disease has spread.

If it remains confined to bone, amputation may be recommended; but it may be possible to remove the cancer and fill the defect with a *bone graft* or prosthesis. *Radiotherapy* or *chemotherapy*, or both, may also be needed.

The cancers that spread readily to form secondary bone cancer are those of the breast, lung, prostate, thyroid, and kidney. These bone metastases occur commonly in the spine, pelvis, ribs, and skull. Pain is usually the main symptom. Affected bones are abnormally fragile and may easily fracture. Bone cancer that affects the spine may cause collapse or crushing of vertebrae, damaging the spinal cord and causing weakness or paralysis of one or more limbs. Secondary bone cancers from the breast and prostate often respond to treatment with *hormone antagonists*. Other treatments that may be used include radiotherapy, chemotherapy, and surgery.

bone cyst An abnormal cavity in a bone. Bone cysts typically develop at one end of a long bone and maybe discovered only by chance after a bone fracture at the site of the cyst. Minor surgery to scrape out the cyst and fill the the cavity with bone chips usually cures the condition, although many small cysts do not need treatment.

bone density The compactness of *bone* tissue in relation to its volume. A decrease in bone density is a normal part of aging. However, in some people, excessive loss of density (see *osteoporosis*) can lead to fractures. Less commonly, an increase in bone density (see *osteosclerosis*) occurs in certain disorders (see *osteopetrosis; Paget's disease*). Bone density can be measured by a technique known as *densitometry*, which uses low-dose X-rays.

bone, disorders of Any of the group of disorders that affects the bones, including *fractures*; bone infections such as *osteomyelitis* or a *bone abscess*; inherited conditions such as *achondroplasia* and *osteogenesis imperfecta*; and metabolic disorders such as *osteomalacia, osteoporosis*, and *rickets*. Tumours and cysts (see *bone cancer* and *bone tumour*) are another, uncommon, group of bone disorders.

bone graft An operation in which several small pieces of bone are taken from one part of the body and used to repair or replace abnormal or missing bone elsewhere. The bone graft eventually dies, but it acts as a scaffold upon which strong new bone grows.

Bone is most commonly taken from the iliac crests (upper part of the hipbones), which contain a large amount of the inner, spongy bone that is especially useful for getting grafts to "take". Other sources are the ribs (for curved bone), and the ulna (in the forearm).

bone imaging Techniques for providing pictures that show the structure or function of bones. *X-ray* images are the most commonly used technique for diagnosing fractures and injuries. More detailed information is provided by *tomography*, *CT scanning*, or *MRI*, which can show tumours and infections and the effect of diseased bone on the surrounding tissues. *Radionuclide scanning* detects areas throughout the skeleton in which there is high bonecell activity. This type of scanning is used mainly to determine whether or not cancer has spread to the bones.

bone marrow The soft fatty tissue that is found in bone cavities; it may be red or yellow. Red bone marrow is present in all bones at birth and is the factory for most of the *blood cells*. During the teens, red bone marrow is gradually replaced in some bones by less active yellow marrow. In adults, red marrow is confined chiefly to the spine, sternum, (breastbone), ribs, pelvis (hipbones), scapulae (shoulder-blades), clavicles (collarbones), and bones of the skull.

Stem cells within the red marrow are stimulated to form blood cells by the hormone erythropoietin. Yellow bone marrow is composed mainly of connective tissue and fat. If the body needs to increase its rate of blood formation, some of the yellow marrow will be replaced by red. Sometimes marrow fails to produce sufficient numbers of normal blood cells, as occurs in aplastic anaemia (see *anaemia, aplastic*) or when marrow has been displaced by tumour cells. In other cases, marrow may overproduce certain blood cells, as occurs in *polycythaemia* and *leukaemia*.

bone marrow biopsy A procedure to obtain a sample of cells from the bone marrow (aspiration biopsy) or a small core of bone with marrow inside (trephine biopsy). The sample is usually taken, under local *anaesthesia*, from the sternum (breastbone) or iliac crests (upper part of the hip-bones). Microscopic examination gives information on the development of the blood components and on the presence of cells foreign to the marrow. It is useful in the diagnosis of many blood disorders, including *leukaemia* and *anaemia*. It can also show whether bone marrow has been invaded by *lymphoma* or cells from other tumours.

bone marrow transplant The technique of using normal red *bone marrow* to replace cancerous or defective marrow in a patient. In allogeneic bone marrow transplantation (BMT), healthy bone marrow is taken from a donor who has a very similar tissue-type to the recipient's (usually a brother or sister). In autologous BMT, the patient's own

BONE MARROW BIOPSY

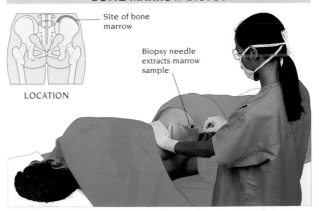

Site of bone marrow

Biopsy needle extracts marrow sample

LOCATION

B

healthy bone marrow is harvested while his or her disease is in remission and is reinfused later. BMT is used only in the treatment of serious, mostly potentially fatal, blood and immune system disorders, including severe aplastic anaemia (see *anaemia, aplastic*), *sickle cell anaemia*, and *leukaemia*. Increasingly, *stem-cell* transplantation is used as an alternative to BMT.

Before BMT, all of the recipient's marrow is destroyed by *cytotoxic drugs* or radiation in order to prevent rejection of the donated cells and to kill any cancer cells present. The donor bone marrow is transfused into the circulation from where cells find their way to the bone marrow cavities and start to grow. In autologous BMT, the patient's bone marrow is stored by *cryopreservation*. Before being frozen, the marrow is usually treated to eliminate any undetected cancerous cells. If the patient's disease recurs, the stored marrow can then be reinfused.

The major risks with BMT are infection during the recovery period and rejection (known as *graft-versus-host disease*, or GVHD). *Immunosuppressant drugs* are used to prevent and treat rejection. The risk of GVHD may be reduced by removing the *T-cells* from the bone marrow using monoclonal antibodies (see *antibody, monoclonal*) before reinfusion. GVHD does not occur with autologous BMT or stem-cell transplantation.

bone tumour A bone swelling that may be cancerous (see *bone cancer*) or noncancerous. The most common type of noncancerous bone tumour is an *osteochondroma*. Other types are *osteoma* and chondroma (see *chondromatosis*). Treatment is only necessary if the tumour becomes very large or causes symptoms by pressing on other structures. In such cases, the tumour can be removed by surgery. Osteoclastoma (also called a giant cell tumour), which usually occurs in the arm or leg of a young adult, is tender and painful and has to be removed.

booster A follow-up dose of *vaccine*, given to reinforce or prolong immunity after an initial course of *immunization*.

borborygmi See *bowel sounds*.

borderline personality disorder A personality disorder that falls between

neurotic and psychotic levels. Mood changes are often rapid and inappropriate. Angry outbursts are common, as are impulsive, self-damaging acts such as gambling or suicide attempts.

Bornholm disease One of the names for epidemic *pleurodynia*, an infectious viral disease that is characterized by severe chest pains and fever.

bottle-feeding Infant feeding using a milk preparation usually based on modified cow's milk. Formula milk contains similar proportions of protein, fat, lactose (milk sugar), and minerals as those in human milk, but it lacks the protective antibodies that are present in breast milk. Vitamins are added. Bottle-fed babies are at higher risk of gastrointestinal infections than breast-fed babies and may be more likely to develop allergic disorders. (See also *feeding, infant*.)

botulinum toxin A potentially lethal toxin produced by the bacterium CLOSTRIDIUM BOTULINUM (see *botulism*). In tiny doses, botulinum toxin is used as a drug to control muscle spasms in some disorders (see *blepharospasm; facial spasm; torticollis*). It is also sometimes injected into facial muscles to reduce visible wrinkles temporarily and injected into the skin as a treatment for severe *hyperhidrosis*.

botulism A rare but serious form of poisoning caused by eating improperly canned or preserved food contaminated with a toxin produced by the bacterium CLOSTRIDIUM BOTULINUM. The toxin causes progressive muscular paralysis as well as other disturbances of the central and peripheral nervous system. CLOSTRIDIUM BOTULINUM produces spores that resist boiling, salting, smoking, and some forms of pickling. These spores, which multiply only in the absence of air, thrive in canned or improperly preserved food. Ingestion of even minute amounts of toxin can lead to severe poisoning. Symptoms first occur within 8–36 hours and include difficulty in swallowing and speaking, vomiting, and double vision. Prompt treatment is vital. In infants, the toxin can form within the body after the ingestion of foods contaminated with the bacterium, such as honey. (See also *food poisoning*.)

bovine spongiform encephalopathy (BSE) A neurological disorder in cattle that can be transmitted to humans through consumption of infected meat, causing *Creutzfeldt–Jakob disease*. (See also *encephalopathy*.)

bowel A common name for the large and/or small *intestines*.

bowel movements, abnormal See *faeces, abnormal*.

bowel sounds Sounds made by the passage of air and fluid through the *intestine*. Absent or abnormal bowel sounds may indicate a disorder. Those that are audible without a stethoscope are known as borborygmi and are a normal part of the digestive process, but they may be exaggerated by anxiety and some disorders of the intestine.

Bowen's disease A rare skin disorder that sometimes becomes cancerous. A flat, regular-shaped, patch of red, scaly skin forms, most commonly on the face or hands. The diseased skin is removed surgically or destroyed by freezing or *cauterization*.

bowleg An outward curving of bones in the legs that results in wide separation of the knees when the feet are together. Bowlegs are common in very young children and are a normal part of development. In most cases, the curve straightens as the child grows. If the bowing is severe, is on one side only, or persists beyond the age of 6, a doctor should be consulted. Surgery may be needed. Rarely, leg deformity is a result of bone disease, particularly *rickets* (a vitamin D deficiency) in children.

brace, dental See *orthodontic appliances*.

brace, orthopaedic An appliance worn to support part of the body or hold it in a fixed position. It may be used to correct or halt the development of a deformity, to aid mobility, or to relieve pain. (See also *caliper splint; splint*.)

brachial artery The *artery* that runs down the inner side of the upper arm, between the armpit and the elbow.

brachialgia Pain or stiffness in the arm that is often accompanied by pain, tingling and/or numbness of the hands or fingers, and weak hand grip. It may be a symptom of underlying disorders such as *frozen shoulder* or nerve compression from *cervical osteoarthritis*.

brachial plexus A collection of large nerve trunks that are formed from nerve roots of the lower part of the cervical spine (in the neck) and the upper part of the thoracic spine (in the chest). These nerve trunks divide into the musculocutaneous, axillary, median, ulnar, and radial nerves, which control muscles in and receive sensation from the arm and hand. Injuries to this plexus can cause loss of movement and sensation in the arm.

In severe injuries, there may be damage to both the upper and the lower nerve roots of the brachial plexus, producing complete paralysis of the arm. Paralysis may be temporary if the stretching was not severe enough to tear nerve fibres. Nerve roots that have been torn can be repaired by nerve grafting, a *microsurgery* procedure. If a nerve root has become separated from the spinal cord, surgical repair will not be successful. Apart from injuries, the brachial plexus may be compressed by the presence of a *cervical rib* (extra rib).

brachytherapy A form of *radiotherapy* in which radioactive material is placed in or near the area or tissue being treated (often a tumour). *Interstitial radiotherapy* and intracavitary radiotherapy (see *intracavitary therapy*) are types of brachytherapy.

bradycardia An abnormally slow heart-rate. Most people have a heart-rate of between 60 and 100 beats per minute. Many athletes and healthy people who exercise regularly and vigorously have slower rates. In others, bradycardia may indicate an underlying disorder such as *hypothyroidism* or *heart block*. Bradycardia may also occur as a result of taking *beta-blocker drugs*. Profound or sudden bradycardia may cause a drop in blood pressure that results in fainting (see *vasovagal attack*).

Braille A system of embossed dots, now accepted for all written languages, that enables blind people to read and write. The system is based on six raised dots, which can be combined in different ways. There are two types of Braille. In grade I, each symbol represents an individual letter or punctuation mark. In grade II, which is the more widely used, symbols represent common letter combinations or words.

brain The major organ of the *nervous system*, located in the *cranium* (skull). The brain receives, sorts, and interprets sensations from the nerves that extend from the *central nervous system* (brain and spinal cord) to the rest of the body; it initiates and coordinates nerve signals involved in activities such as speech, movement, thought, and emotion.

An adult brain weighs about 1.4 kg and has three main structures: the largest part, the *cerebrum*, consisting of left and right hemispheres; the *brainstem*; and the *cerebellum*. Each hemisphere in the cerebrum has an outer layer called the cortex, consisting of grey matter, which is rich in nerve-cell bodies and is the main region for conscious thought, sensation, and movement. Beneath the cortex are tracts of nerve fibres called white matter, and, deeper within the hemispheres, the *basal ganglia*. The surface of each hemisphere is divided by fissures (sulci) and folds (gyri) into distinct lobes (occipital, frontal, parietal, and temporal lobes), named after the skull bones that overlie them. A thick band of nerve fibres called the corpus callosum connects the hemispheres.

The cerebrum encloses a central group of structures that includes the *thalami* and the *hypothalamus*, which has close connections with the *pituitary gland*. Encircling the thalami is a complex of nerve centres called the *limbic system*. These structures act as links between parts of the cerebrum and the brainstem lying beneath the thalami.

The brainstem is concerned mainly with the control of vital functions such as breathing and blood pressure. The cerebellum at the back of the brain controls balance, posture, and muscular coordination. Both of these regions operate at a subconscious level.

The brain and spinal cord are encased in three layers of membranes, known as *meninges*. *Cerebrospinal fluid* circulates between the layers and within the four main brain cavities called *ventricles*. This fluid helps to nourish and cushion the brain. The brain receives about 20 per cent of the blood from the heart's output.

BRAIN

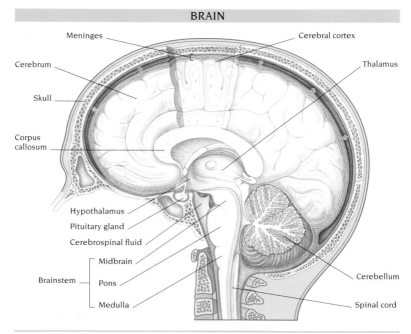

Meninges — Cerebral cortex
Cerebrum — Thalamus
Skull —
Corpus callosum —
Hypothalamus —
Pituitary gland —
Cerebrospinal fluid —
Midbrain —
Brainstem — Pons — Cerebellum
Medulla — Spinal cord

brain abscess A collection of pus, surrounded by inflamed tissues, within the brain or on its surface. The most common sites are the frontal and temporal lobes of the *cerebrum* in the fore brain.

Brain abscesses may occur after a head injury, but most cases result from the spread of infection from elsewhere in the body, such as the middle ear or sinuses. Another cause is an infection following a penetrating brain injury. Multiple brain abscesses may occur as a result of blood-borne infection, most commonly in patients with a heart-valve infection (see *endocarditis*). Symptoms include headache, drowsiness, vomiting, visual disturbances, fever, seizures, and symptoms, such as speech disturbances, that are due to local pressure. Treatment is with *antibiotic drugs* and surgery. A *craniotomy* may be needed to open and drain the abscess. Untreated, brain abscesses can cause permanent damage or can be fatal. Despite treatment, scarring can cause *epilepsy* in some cases.

brain damage Degeneration or death of nerve cells and tracts within the brain that may be localized to a particular area of the brain or diffuse. Diffuse damage most commonly results from prolonged cerebral *hypoxia* (which may occur in a baby during a difficult birth), *cardiac arrest*, *respiratory arrest*, or causes such as poisoning or *status epilepticus* (prolonged convulsions). The damage may also occur gradually due to environmental pollutants such as lead or mercury compounds (see *Minamata disease*) or if nerve-cell poisons build up in the brain, as in untreated *phenylketonuria*. Other possible causes include brain infections such as *encephalitis*.

Localized brain damage may occur as a result of a *head injury*, *stroke*, *brain tumour*, or *brain abscess*. At birth, a raised blood level of bilirubin (in *haemolytic disease of the newborn*) causes local damage to the *basal ganglia* deep within the brain. This leads to a condition called *kernicterus*. Brain damage that occurs before, during, or after birth may result in *cerebral palsy*.

Damage to the brain may result in disabilities such as *learning difficulties* or disturbances of movement or speech. Nerve cells and tracts in the brain and spinal cord cannot repair themselves once they have been damaged, but some return of function may be possible.

brain death The irreversible cessation of all functions of the brain, including the brainstem. (See also *death*.)

brain, disorders of Defects and disorders of the brain, which may have one of numerous causes, including infection, injury, *brain tumour*, or a lack of blood or oxygen (*hypoxia*). Because the brain is encased in the skull, any space-occupying tumour, *brain abscess*, or *haematoma* creates raised pressure, which impairs the function of the whole brain. Brain disorders that are localized in a small region may affect a specific function such as speech (see *aphasia*). More often, damage is more diffuse and the symptoms can be varied and numerous.

Some brain disorders are *congenital* due to genetic or chromosomal disorders, as in *Down's syndrome*. Structural defects that arise during the development of the fetus in the womb include *hydrocephalus and anencephaly*.

Reduced oxygen supply may occur at birth, causing *cerebral palsy*. Later in life, cerebral hypoxia can result from choking or from arrest of breathing and heartbeat. From middle age onwards, *cerebrovascular disease* is the most important cause of brain disorder. If an artery within the brain becomes blocked or ruptures, leading to haemorrhage, the result is a *stroke*. The brain may also be damaged by a blow to the head (see *head injury*).

Infection within the brain (*encephalitis*) may be due to viral infection. Infection of the membranes surrounding the brain (*meningitis*) is generally due to bacterial infection. *Creutzfeldt–Jakob disease* is a rare, fatal brain disease associated with an infective agent called a prion which, in some cases, has been linked with BSE (*bovine spongiform encephalopathy*), a disease in cattle.

Multiple sclerosis is a progressive disease of the brain and spinal cord. Degenerative brain diseases include

B

Alzheimer's disease and *Parkinson's disease*. Emotional or behavioural disorders are generally described as psychiatric illnesses; but the distinction between neurological and psychiatric disorders is not clear-cut.

brain failure See *brain syndrome, organic.*

brain haemorrhage Bleeding within or around the brain that is caused either by injury or by spontaneous rupture of a blood vessel. There are four possible types of brain haemorrhage: *subdural, extradural, subarachnoid,* and *intracerebral.* Extradural and subdural haemorrhages are usually the result of a blow to the head (see *head injury*). Subarachnoid and intracerebral haemorrhages usually occur spontaneously due to rupture of *aneurysms* or small blood vessels in the brain.

brain imaging Techniques that provide pictures of the brain; they are used to detect injury or disease and include *X-rays, angiography, CT scanning, MRI, PET* (positron emission tomography) scanning, and *SPECT* (single photon emission CT). X-ray films can show changes in the skull caused by a fracture or, rarely, by a *brain tumour* or *aneurysm.* Angiography shows up the blood vessels in the brain, and is used to investigate *subarachnoid haemorrhage,* aneurysms, abnormalities of the blood vessels, and other circulatory disorders.

CT scanning gives images of the brain substance; it gives clear pictures of the ventricles (fluid-filled cavities) and can reveal tumours, blood clots, strokes, aneurysms, and abscesses. MRI is especially helpful in showing tumours of the posterior fossa (back of the skull). PET and SPECT scanning are specialized forms of *radionuclide scanning* that use small amounts of radioactive material to give information about brain function as well as structure. They enable blood flow and metabolic activity in the brain to be measured. A type of MRI called functional MRI (fMRI) can reveal areas of neural activity in the brain.

Ultrasound scanning is used only in premature or very young babies since ultrasound waves cannot penetrate the bones of a mature skull.

brainstem A stalk of nerve tissue that forms the lowest part of the brain and links with the spinal cord. The brainstem acts partly as a highway for messages travelling between other parts of the brain and spinal cord. It also connects with 10 of the 12 pairs of *cranial nerves* (which emerge directly from the underside of the brain) and controls basic functions such as breathing, vomiting, and eye reflexes. Brainstem activities are below the level of consciousness, and they operate mainly on an automatic basis.

The brainstem is composed of three main parts: the midbrain, pons, and medulla. The midbrain contains the nuclei (nerve-cell centres) of the 3rd and 4th cranial nerves. It also contains cell groups involved in smooth coordination of limb movements. The pons contains nerve fibres that connect with the *cerebellum.* It also houses the nuclei for the 5th–8th cranial nerves. The medulla contains the nuclei of the 9th–12th cranial nerves. It also contains the "vital centres" or groups of nerve cells that regulate the heartbeat, breathing, blood pressure, and digestion, information on which is relayed via the 10th cranial nerve (see *vagus nerve*). Nerve-cell groups in the brainstem, known collectively as the reticular formation, alert the higher brain centres to sensory stimuli that may require a conscious response. Our sleep/wake cycle is controlled by the reticular formation.

BRAINSTEM

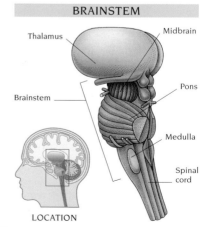

Thalamus

Midbrain

Pons

Brainstem

Medulla

Spinal cord

LOCATION

The brainstem is susceptible to the same disorders that afflict the rest of the central nervous system (see *brain, disorders of*). Damage to the medulla's vital centres is rapidly fatal; damage to the reticular formation may cause *coma*. Damage to specific cranial nerve nuclei can sometimes lead to specific effects. For example, damage to the 7th cranial nerve (the facial nerve) leads to *facial palsy*. Degeneration of the substantia nigra in the midbrain is thought to be a cause of *Parkinson's disease*.

brain syndrome, organic Disorder of consciousness, intellect, or mental functioning that is of organic (physical), as opposed to psychiatric, origin. Causes include degenerative diseases, such as *Alzheimer's disease*; infections; certain drugs; or the effects of injury, stroke, or tumour. Symptoms range from mild confusion to stupor or *coma*. They may also include disorientation, memory loss, hallucinations, and delusions (see *delirium*). In the chronic form, there is a progressive decline in intellect, memory, and behaviour (see *dementia*). Treatment is more likely to be successful with the acute form. In chronic cases, irreversible brain damage may already have occurred. (See also *psychosis*.)

brain tumour An abnormal growth in or on the brain. Tumours may be primary growths arising directly from tissues within the skull or metastases (secondary growths) that have spread from tumours elsewhere in the body. The cause of primary brain tumours is not known. About 60 per cent are *gliomas* (frequently cancerous), which arise from the brain tissue. Other primary tumours include *meningiomas, acoustic neuromas*, and *pituitary tumours*. Most of these tumours are noncancerous, but their size can cause local damage. Certain types of primary brain tumour mainly affect children. These include two types of glioma called *medulloblastoma* and cerebellar *astrocytoma*. Primary brain tumours virtually never spread (metastasize) outside the central nervous system.

Symptoms include muscle weakness, loss of vision, or other sensory disturbances, speech difficulties, and epileptic seizures. Increased pressure within the skull can cause headache, visual disturbances, nausea, vomiting, and impaired mental functioning. *Hydrocephalus* may occur.

When possible, primary tumours are removed by surgery after opening the skull (see *craniotomy*). In cases where a tumour cannot be completely removed, as much as possible of it will be cut away to relieve pressure. For primary and secondary tumours, *radiotherapy*, hormone therapy, or *anticancer drugs* may also be given. *Corticosteroid drugs* are often prescribed temporarily to reduce the size of a tumour and associated brain swelling.

bran The fibrous outer covering of grain that cannot be digested. The fibre is used as a bulk-forming *laxative* to prevent constipation (see fibre, *dietary*)

branchial disorders Disorders due to abnormal development, in an embryo, of the branchial arches (paired segmented ridges of tissue in each side of the throat). They include branchial cyst and branchial *fistula*. A branchial cyst is a soft swelling, containing a pus-like or clear fluid, that appears on the side of the neck in early adulthood. Treatment is by surgical removal. A branchial fistula occurs between the back of the throat and the external surface of the neck, where it appears as a small hole, usually noted at birth. A hole in the neck that does not extend to the back of the throat is a branchial cleft sinus. A branchial fistula or cleft sinus may discharge mucus or pus and may be removed surgically.

brash, water See *waterbrash*.

Braxton Hicks' contractions Short, relatively painless contractions of the uterus during pregnancy. They may be felt in late pregnancy and are sometimes mistaken for labour pains.

breakbone fever A tropical viral illness, also called *dengue*, that is spread by mosquitoes.

breakthrough bleeding Bleeding or staining ("spotting") from the vagina between periods in women taking an oral contraceptive. The bleeding is most common during the first few months of taking the pill and is caused by incomplete suppression of the *endometrium*. (See also *vaginal bleeding*.)

B

breast Either one of the two mammary glands, which, in women, provide milk to nourish a baby and are secondary *sexual characteristics*. In males, the breast is an immature version of the female breast. At puberty, a girl's breasts begin to develop: the areola (the circular area of pigmented skin around the nipple) swells and the nipple enlarges. This is followed by an increase in glandular tissue and fat. The adult female breast consists of 15–20 lobes of milk-secreting glands embedded in fatty tissue. The ducts of these glands have their outlet in the nipple. Bands of fine ligaments determine the breast's height and shape. The areolar skin contains sweat glands, sebaceous glands, and hair follicles.

The size and shape and general appearance of the breasts may vary during the menstrual cycle, during pregnancy and lactation, and after the menopause.

BREAST

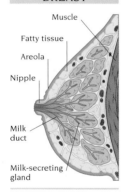

Muscle
Fatty tissue
Areola
Nipple
Milk duct
Milk-secreting gland

During pregnancy, *oestrogen* and *progesterone*, secreted by the ovary and placenta, cause the milk-producing glands to develop and become active and the nipple to become larger. Just before and after childbirth, the glands in the breast produce a watery fluid known as *colostrum*. This fluid is replaced by milk a few days later. Milk production and its release is stimulated by the hormone *prolactin*, which is produced by the pituitary gland.

breast abscess A collection of pus in the mammary gland, usually in a woman who is lactating (producing milk). Breast abscesses develop if acute *mastitis* (infection of the breast tissue) is not treated promptly. They occur most commonly during the first month after a woman's first delivery. The initial symptoms are of acute mastitis. The abscess develops in one area, which becomes very firm, red, and extremely painful. The treatment usually includes *antibiotic drugs* and repeated *aspiration* of the pus

with a needle and syringe. Rarely, surgical drainage may be needed.

breast awareness See *breast self-examination*.

breastbone The common name for the *sternum*, the front part of the *thorax*.

breast cancer A cancerous tumour of the breast. The incidence is raised in women whose menstrual periods began at an early age and whose menopause was late; in those who had no children or had their first child later in life; in those with mothers or sisters who had breast cancer; and in those who are obese. The risk of breast cancer is also increased in postmenopausal women using *hormone replacement therapy* (*HRT*); the risk increases with duration of HRT use. Breast cancer is also more common in countries in which the typical diet contains a lot of fat. One form of breast cancer has a genetic component; two genes, called BRCA1 and BRCA2, appear to be involved in this type of breast cancer.

The first sign of breast cancer may be a painless lump. Other symptoms may include a dark discharge from the nipple, retraction (indentation) of the nipple, and an area of dimpled, creased skin over the lump. In 90 per cent of the cases, only one breast is affected. The cancer may be suspected after discovering a lump during *breast self-examination* or *mammography*.

If a lump is detected, cells will be collected from it by *needle aspiration* or surgical *biopsy*. If the lump is cancerous, the treatment given depends on the woman's age, the size of the tumour, whether or not there are signs of spread to the *lymph nodes*, and the sensitivity of the tumour cells to hormones, as assessed in the laboratory.

A small tumour, with no evidence of having spread outside the breast, is removed by surgery. Lymph nodes in the armpit may be removed at the same time and examined for any signs of cancer. Surgery may be combined with *radiotherapy* and/or *anticancer drugs*. Drugs are also usually given to prevent recurrence of the tumour. Secondary tumours in other parts of the body are treated with anticancer drugs and hormones.

B

Regular check-ups are required to detect recurrence or the development of a new cancer in the other breast. if the cancer recurs, it can be controlled, in some cases for years, by drugs and/or radiotherapy.

Drugs such as *trastuzumab* may be used to treat advanced cancer.

breast cyst A fluid-filled lump that forms within the milk-producing tissue of the breast. Breast cysts most commonly affect women in their 40s and 50s, especially in the years around the *menopause*. A lump can be diagnosed as a cyst by *ultrasound scanning*, a *mammography*, or by withdrawing fluid from it with a syringe and needle (see *aspiration*), which usually results in the lump disappearing. About half of all women who have a breast cyst will develop future cysts. Any new breast lump should be seen by a doctor to confirm the diagnosis.

breast, disorders of the Disorders affecting the breast that are mostly minor and respond readily to treatment. The most important causes of problems are infection, such as *mastitis*, tumours, and hormonal changes. *Breast cysts, fibroadenomas*, other noncancerous tumours, or, more rarely, *breast cancer* may occur. Breast pain and tenderness is common just before *menstruation* or when a woman is taking hormones. Before menstruation, breasts may become bigger and lumpy. Such lumps shrink when menstruation is over. Hormonal disorders may, rarely, cause *galactorrhoea* (abnormal milk production). In men, *gynaecomastia* may result from hormonal disturbance or treatment with certain drugs.

breast enlargement surgery A type of *mammoplasty*.

breast-feeding The natural method of infant feeding from birth to weaning. Human milk contains the ideal balance of nutrients for a baby and provides valuable *antibodies* against infections. For the first few days after birth, the breasts produce *colostrum*. Milk flow is stimulated by the baby's sucking and is usually established within 3-4 days.

Breast-feeding problems may occur as a result of engorged breasts and cracked nipples or if the baby has problems sucking; a breast-feeding advisor may be able to help with these difficulties. Breast-feeding can sometimes cause an infection that leads to a *breast abscess*. In such cases, treatment with *antibiotic drugs* may mean that it is possible to continue breast-feeding.

breast implant An artificial structure surgically introduced into the breast to increase its size (see *mammoplasty*). Breast implants consist of a filler material inside a silicone elastomer shell. In the UK, the fillers available are silicone gel and saline liquid (salt water).

breast lump Any mass, swelling, or cyst that can be felt in the breast tissue. About 85 per cent of lumps are noncancerous; the rest are *breast cancer*. Many women have generally lumpy breasts, with the lumps more obvious in the days before a period. Once known as *fibrocystic disease* or *fibroadenosis*, this is now considered to be a variation of normal. Lumpy breasts do not increase the risk of developing breast cancer. However, any new, distinct, or separate lump should be assessed by a doctor. In a young woman, a single lump is most likely to be a *fibroadenoma*. This noncancerous growth is usually round, firm, and rubbery, causes no pain, and can be moved about beneath the skin using the fingertips. In an older woman, a lump is more likely to be a noncancerous, fluid-filled *breast cyst*.

Treatment depends on the cause and type of lump. Cysts can be drained in a simple outpatient procedure. Other lumps can be removed surgically.

breast pump A device used to draw milk from the breasts in order to relieve overfull breasts during lactation, to express milk for future use, or to feed a baby who is unable to suckle.

breast reconstruction See *mammoplasty*.

breast reduction See *mammoplasty*.

breast self-examination Visual and manual examination of the breasts carried out by a woman to detect lumps and other changes that might be early indications of *breast cancer*. The object of self-examination is to make a woman familiar with the appearance and feel of her breasts so that she will notice any changes. One possible way of doing a self-examination is to stand in front of a mirror and check for any dimpling of the skin or changes in the nipples or breast size and shape. Then, with one arm behind the head, and using small circular movements, gently but firmly press each breast. The entire breast, armpit area, and nipple should be examined. Any changes should be reported to a doctor without delay.

BREAST SELF-EXAMINATION

AREA TO BE EXAMINED

Entire breast and armpit are felt

Hand is held flat and the breast pressed gently with the fingertips

breast tenderness Soreness or tenderness of the breasts, often with a feeling of fullness. Breast tenderness is an extremely common problem. In most women it is cyclical, varying in severity in response to the hormonal changes of the menstrual cycle. It is usually most severe before a period (see *premenstrual syndrome*). It tends to affect both breasts and may be aggravated by stress or caffeine in drinks. Breast tenderness can also be noncyclical and may be caused by muscle strain or *mastitis*. During lactation, it may be due to engorgement with milk. Rarely, tenderness may be due to a *breast cyst* or *breast cancer*. However, examination by a doctor will exclude any underlying problems. Women with large breasts are more likely to suffer from both cyclical and noncyclical breast tenderness.

Cyclical tenderness may be relieved by reduced caffeine intake, taking over-the-counter painkillers, relaxation exercises for stress, a well-fitting bra, or weight loss to reduce breast size. If these measures do not work, hormonal treatment may be recommended.

breath-holding attacks Periods during which a toddler holds his or her breath, usually as an expression of pain, frustration, or anger. The child usually becomes red or even blue in the face after a few seconds, and may faint. Breathing quickly resumes as a natural reflex, ending the attack. Attacks cause no damage and are usually outgrown.

breathing The process by which air passes into and out of the lungs to allow the blood to take up oxygen and dispose of carbon dioxide. Breathing is controlled by the respiratory centre in the *brainstem*. When air is inhaled, the diaphragm contracts and flattens. The intercostal

BREATHING

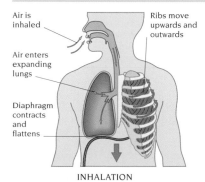

Air is inhaled

Ribs move upwards and outwards

Air enters expanding lungs

Diaphragm contracts and flattens

INHALATION

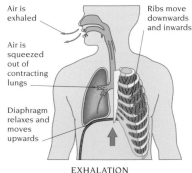

Air is exhaled

Ribs move downwards and inwards

Air is squeezed out of contracting lungs

Diaphragm relaxes and moves upwards

EXHALATION

muscles (muscles between the ribs) contract and pull the ribcage upwards and outwards. The resulting increase in chest volume causes the lungs to expand, and the reduced pressure draws air into the lungs. When air is exhaled, the chest muscles and diaphragm relax, causing the ribcage to sink and the lungs to contract, squeezing air out.

In normal, quiet breathing, only about a tenth of the air in the lungs passes out to be replaced by the same amount of fresh air (tidal volume). This new air mixes with the stale air (residual volume) already held in the lungs. The normal breathing rate for an adult at rest is 13–17 breaths per minute. (See also *respiration*.)

breathing difficulty Laboured or distressed breathing that includes a change in the rate and depth of breathing or a feeling of breathlessness. Some degree of breathlessness is normal after exercise, particularly in unfit or overweight people. Breathlessness at rest is always abnormal and is usually due to disorders that affect the airways (see *asthma*), lungs (see *pulmonary disease, chronic obstructive*), or cardiovascular system (see *heart failure*). Severe anxiety can result in breathlessness, even when the lungs are normal (see *hyperventilation*). Damage to the breathing centre in the brainstem due to a *stroke* or *head injury* can affect breathing. This may also happen as a side effect of certain drugs. *Ventilator* assistance is sometimes needed.

At high altitudes, the lungs have to work harder in order to provide the body with sufficient oxygen (see *mountain sickness*). Breathlessness may occur in severe anaemia because abnormal or low levels of the oxygen-carrying pigment *haemoglobin* means that the lungs need to work harder to supply the body with oxygen. Breathing difficulty that intensifies on exertion may be caused by reduced circulation of blood through the lungs. This may be due to *heart failure*, *pulmonary embolism*, or *pulmonary hypertension*. Breathing difficulty due to air-flow obstruction may be caused by chronic *bronchitis*, asthma, an allergic reaction, or *lung cancer*. Breathing difficulty may also be due to inefficient transfer of oxygen from the lungs into the bloodstream. Temporary damage to lung tissue may be due to *pneumonia*, *pneumothorax*, *pulmonary oedema*, or *pleural effusion*. Permanent lung damage may be due to *emphysema*.

Chest pain (for example, due to a broken rib) that is made worse by chest or lung movement can make normal breathing difficult and painful, as can *pleurisy*, which is associated with pain in the lower chest and often in the shoulder tip of the affected side.

Abnormalities of the skeletal structure of the thorax (chest), such as severe *scoliosis* or *kyphosis*, may cause difficulty in breathing by impairing normal movements of the ribcage.

breathing exercises Techniques for learning to control the rate and depth of breathing. They aim to teach people to inhale through the nose, while expanding the chest, and then to exhale fully through the mouth, while contracting the abdominal muscles. They are used after chest surgery and for people with chronic obstructive pulmonary disease (see *pulmonary disease, chronic obstructive*). Breathing exercises can also help people with *anxiety disorders* and may help to relieve symptoms in some people with *asthma*.

In *yoga*, deep rhythmic breathing is used to achieve a state of relaxation. During *childbirth*, breathing exercises relax the mother and also help to control contractions and reduce pain. (See also *physiotherapy*.)

breathlessness A feeling of laboured breathing. Breathlessness is a normal response to exercise or exertion but may also be caused by some underlying disorders (see *breathing difficulty*).

breech delivery A birth in which the fetus presents buttocks first. Many fetuses lie in a breech position before week 32 of pregnancy, but most of them turn by week 36. The 3 per cent that do not turn are in one of three types of breech presentation. A complete breech is one in which the fetus is curled up. In a frank breech, the legs are extended and the feet are close to the face. In a footling breech, one or both feet are positioned over the cervix. Sometimes, a mother with a fetus in a breech presentation is

B

offered a procedure to turn the fetus at around the 36th weeek of pregnancy. Often, one twin fetus is a breech. In some breech deliveries, a *caesarean section* may be recommended.

bridge, dental False teeth that are attached to natural teeth on either side of a gap left by a missing tooth or teeth. (See also *denture*.)

Bright's disease Another name for *glomerulonephritis*.

brittle bones Bones with an increased tendency to fracture. They are a feature of *osteoporosis* and may occur in people who are taking *corticosteroid drugs*, are immobile, or have certain hormonal disorders. In *osteomalacia*, the bones are soft and have an increased tendency both to become deformed and to fracture. The inherited disorder *osteogenesis imperfecta* is a rare cause of brittle bones and frequent fractures and is usually detected in infancy.

Broca's area An area of the cerebral cortex (the outer layer of the *brain*) that is responsible for speech origination.

broken tooth See *fracture, dental*.

broken veins See *telangiectasia*.

bromides Substances formerly used as *sedative drugs* or as *anticonvulsant drugs* in the treatment of *epilepsy*. They are no longer prescribed because of their side effects.

bromocriptine A drug used to suppress production of the hormone *prolactin* to treat conditions such as noncancerous pituitary tumours (see *prolactinomas* and *acromegaly*). Bromocriptine can be used to suppress lactation after childbirth. The drug may also be used as a treatment for *Parkinson's disease*. Side effects of bromocriptine include nausea and vomiting. High doses may cause drowsiness and confusion.

bronchiectasis A lung disorder in which one or more bronchi (the air passages leading from the trachea) are abnormally widened, distorted, and have damaged linings. Bronchiectasis most often develops during childhood and was once commonly associated with infections such as *measles* and *pertussis* (whooping cough). The condition is also a complication of *cystic fibrosis*. It results in pockets of long-term infection within the airways and the continuous production of large volumes of green or yellow sputum (phlegm). Extensive bronchiectasis causes shortness of breath. The symptoms are usually controlled with *antibiotic drugs* and *postural drainage*. If the condition is confined to one area of the lung, surgical removal of the damaged area may be recommended.

bronchiole One of many small airways of the *lungs*. Bronchioles branch from larger airways (bronchi) and subdivide into progressively smaller tubes before reaching the alveoli (see *alveolus, pulmonary*), where gases are exchanged.

bronchiolitis An acute viral infection of the lungs, mainly affecting babies and young children, in which the bronchioles (the smaller airways branching off from the bronchi in the lungs) become inflamed. The most common cause is the respiratory syncytial virus (RSV).

Symptoms include rapid breathing, a cough, and fever. Sometimes no treatment is necessary but, in more severe cases, hospital admission is needed so that *oxygen therapy* and *physiotherapy* (to clear the mucus) can be given. With prompt treatment, sufferers usually recover within a few days. *Antibiotic drugs* may be prescribed to prevent any secondary bacterial infection.

bronchitis A disorder in which the bronchi, the airways connecting the trachea (windpipe) to the lungs, are inflamed. Bronchitis results in a cough that may produce considerable quantities of sputum (phlegm) and may be acute or chronic. Both types are more common in smokers and in areas with high atmospheric pollution. (See also *bronchitis, acute*; *bronchitis, chronic*.)

bronchitis, acute A form of *bronchitis* that develops suddenly but usually clears up within a few days. It is usually due to a viral infection. Bacterial infection of the airways may occur as a complication. Smokers, babies, elderly people, and those with lung disease are particularly susceptible. The main symptoms are wheezing, shortness of breath, and a cough that produces yellow or green sputum. There may also be pain behind the sternum (breastbone) and fever. Symptoms may be relieved by drinking plenty of fluids and inhaling steam or using a humidifier. Most cases clear up without further treatment, but acute bronchitis may be serious in people who already have lung damage.

bronchitis, chronic Inflammation of the airways, as a result of smoking, that is always associated with emphysema. The combination of chronic bronchitis and emphysema are now known as chronic obstructive pulmonary disease (see *pulmonary disease, chronic obstructive*).

bronchoconstrictor A substance that causes constriction (narrowing) of the airways in the lungs. Bronchoconstrictors, such as *histamine*, are released during an *allergic* reaction. They may provoke an *asthma* attack. The effect can be reversed by a *bronchodilator drug*.

bronchodilator drugs A group of drugs that widen the bronchioles (small airways in the lungs) to increase air flow and improve breathing, especially in the treatment of *asthma* and chronic obstructive pulmonary disease (see *pulmonary disease, chronic obstructive*). There are three main types of bronchodilator: sympathomimetic drugs (such as *salbutamol*), *anticholinergic drugs*, and xanthine drugs (such as *aminophylline*). Sympathomimetic drugs are used primarily for the rapid relief of *breathing difficulty*. Anticholinergic and xanthine drugs are more often used for the long-term prevention of attacks of breathing difficulty. Drugs can be given by *inhaler*, in tablet form, or, in severe cases, by *nebulizer* or injection.

The main side effects of sympathomimetics are palpitations and trembling. Anticholinergics may cause dry mouth, blurred vision, and, rarely, difficulty in passing urine. Xanthines may cause headaches, nausea and palpitations.

bronchography A rarely used *X-ray* procedure for examining the bronchi, the main air passages of the lungs. Once used to diagnose *bronchiectasis*, it has now been largely replaced by other imaging techniques, such as *CT scanning*, and by the use of *bronchoscopy*.

bronchopneumonia The most common form of *pneumonia*; it differs from the other main type of pneumonia (lobar pneumonia) in that the inflammation is spread throughout the lungs in small patches around the airways, rather than being confined to one lobe.

bronchoscopy Examination of the bronchi, which are the main airways of the lungs, by means of an *endoscope* known as a bronchoscope. There are two types of bronchoscope: rigid and flexible. The rigid type is a hollow viewing tube that is passed into the bronchi via the mouth and requires anaesthesia. The flexible fibre-optic endoscope (a narrower tube formed from light-transmitting

BRONCHOSCOPY

Bronchoscope with fibre-optic cable
Eyepiece to view bronchi
Flexible bronchoscope
Bronchus
ROUTE OF BRONCHOSCOPE

fibres) can be inserted through either the mouth or nose. It can reach farther into the lungs and requires only a mild sedative and/or local anaesthesia.

Bronchoscopy is performed to inspect the bronchi for abnormalities, such as *lung cancer* and *tuberculosis*, to collect samples of mucus, to obtain cells, and for taking *biopsy* specimens from the airways or samples of lung tissue. Bronchoscopy is used in treatments such as removing inhaled foreign bodies, destroying abnormal growths, and sealing off damaged blood vessels. The last two are carried out by *laser treatment*, *diathermy*, or *cryosurgery* by means of bronchoscope attachments.

bronchospasm Temporary narrowing of the bronchi (airways into the lungs) due to contraction of the muscles in the walls of the bronchi, by inflammation of the lining of the bronchi, or by a combination of both. Contraction may be triggered by the release of substances during an allergic reaction (see *allergy*). When the airways are narrowed, the air is reduced, causing wheezing or coughing. *Asthma* is the most common cause of bronchospasm. Other causes include respiratory infection, chronic obstructive pulmonary disease (see *pulmonary disease, chronic obstructive*), *anaphylactic shock*, or allergic reaction to chemicals.

bronchus A large air passage in a lung. Each lung has one main bronchus, originating at the end of the trachea (windpipe). This main bronchus divides into smaller branches known as segmental bronchi, which further divide into bronchioles.

bronchus, cancer of See *lung cancer*.

brown fat A special type of fat, found in infants and some animals. Brown fat is located between and around the scapulae (shoulderblades) on the back. It is a source of energy and helps infants to maintain a constant body temperature.

brucellosis A rare bacterial infection, caused by various strains of *BRUCELLA*, which may be transmitted to humans from affected cattle, goats, and pigs. Brucellosis may also be transmitted in unpasteurized dairy products. Initially, it causes a single bout of high fever, aches, headache, backache, poor appetite, weakness, and depression. Rarely, untreated severe cases may lead to *pneumonia* or *meningitis*. In long-term brucellosis, bouts of the illness recur over months or years; and depression can be severe. The disease is treated by *antibiotic drugs*.

bruise A discoloured area under the skin caused by leakage of blood from damaged capillaries (tiny blood vessels). At first, the blood appears blue or black; then the breakdown of *haemoglobin* turns the bruise yellow. If a bruise does not fade after a week, or if bruises appear for no apparent reason or are severe after only minor injury, they may be indications of a *bleeding disorder*. (See also *black eye*; *purpura*.)

bruits The sounds made in the heart, arteries, or veins when blood circulation becomes turbulent or flows at an abnormal speed. This happens when blood vessels become narrowed by disease (as in *arteriosclerosis*), when heart valves are narrowed or damaged (as in *endocarditis*), or if blood vessels dilate (as in an *aneurysm*). Bruits are usually heard through a *stethoscope*.

bruxism Rhythmic grinding or clenching of the teeth that usually occurs during sleep. The chief underlying causes are emotional stress and minor discomfort when the teeth are brought together.

BSE The abbreviation for *bovine spongiform encephalopathy*.

bubonic plague The most common form of *plague*, characterized by the development of a bubo (swollen lymph node) in the groin or armpit.

buccal An anatomical term, from the Latin word for cheek, that means relating to the cheek or mouth. Some drugs are available as buccal preparations, which are placed between the cheek and gum, where they dissolve and are absorbed directly into the circulation.

buck teeth Prominent upper incisors (front teeth), which protrude from the mouth. Orthodontic treatment involves repositioning the teeth with a removable brace (see *brace, dental*) or a fixed *orthodontic appliance*.

Budd–Chiari syndrome A rare disorder in which the veins draining blood from the liver become blocked or narrowed. Blood accumulates in the liver, which swells. *Liver failure* and *portal hypertension* result. Treatment is aimed at removing the cause of the obstruction: this may be a blood clot, pressure on the veins from a liver tumour, or a congenital abnormality of the veins. In most cases, treatment has only a limited effect and, unless a *liver transplant* can be done, the disease is fatal within two years.

budesonide An inhaled *corticosteroid drug* used in the treatment of bronchial *asthma* to prevent asthma attacks. It is administered using an *inhaler*. Side effects of budesonide, which include hoarseness, throat irritation and, rarely, fungal infections, can be reduced by rinsing the mouth after administration.

Buerger's disease A rare disorder, also called thromboangiitis obliterans, in which the arteries, nerves, and veins in the legs, and sometimes those in the arms, become severely inflamed. Blood supply to the toes and fingers becomes cut off, eventually causing *gangrene*. The disease is most common in men under the age of 45 who smoke heavily.

bulimia An illness that is characterized by bouts of overeating usually followed by self-induced vomiting or excessive laxative use. Most sufferers are girls or women between the ages of 15 and 30. In some cases, the symptoms coexist with those of *anorexia nervosa*. Repeated vomiting can lead to dehydration and loss of potassium, causing weakness and cramps, and tooth damage due to the gastric acid in vomit. Treatment includes supervision and regulation of eating habits, and sometimes, *antidepressant drugs* and/or *psychotherapy*.

bulk-forming agent A substance that makes stools less liquid by absorbing water: a type of *antidiarrhoeal drug*.

bulla A large air- or fluid-filled bubble, usually in the lungs or skin. Lung bullae in young adults are usually *congenital*. In later life, lung bullae develop in patients with *emphysema*. Skin bullae are large, fluid-filled *blisters* with a variety of causes, including the bullous disease *pemphigus*.

bumetanide A powerful, short-acting loop *diuretic drug* used to treat oedema (fluid retention) resulting from *heart failure*, *nephrotic syndrome*, or liver *cirrhosis*. It may be given by injection for emergency treatment of *pulmonary oedema*. Adverse effects can include rash and muscle pain.

bundle branch block See *heart block*.

bunion A thickened pad of tissue or a fluid-filled bursa overlying a deformed big-toe joint. The underlying cause is an abnormal outward projection of the big toe called a *hallux valgus*. Small bunions are remedied by wearing well-fitting shoes and a special toe pad to straighten the big toe. Large bunions may require surgery to realign the joint and relieve the pressure.

buphthalmos A large, prominent eyeball in an infant as a result of increased pressure inside the eyeball due to congenital *glaucoma*. Treatment of the condition usually involves surgery to reduce the pressure, otherwise the child's sight is progressively damaged.

bupivacaine A long-acting local anaesthetic often used as a *nerve block*, particularly during *labour* and in *epidural anaesthesia* and *spinal anaesthesia*. Side effects of bupivacaine are uncommon, but high doses may cause blood pressure to fall excessively.

bupropion Also known as amfebutamone, a drug used, in combination with self-help measures, as an aid to stopping smoking. Taken as tablets, the drug has a number of side effects, including dry mouth, gastrointestinal disturbances, and headache. Some people may find impairment in their ability to undertake activities such as driving. Bupropion is not usually prescribed for those who have had seizures or an eating disorder.

Burkitt's lymphoma A cancer of lymph tissues that is characterized by tumours within the jaw and/or abdomen. It is confined almost exclusively to children living in low-lying, moist, tropical regions of Africa and New Guinea. *Anticancer drugs* or *radiotherapy* give complete or partial cure in about 80 per cent of cases.(See also *lymphoma*.)

burns Tissue damage resulting from contact with heat, electricity, chemicals or radiation. Burns are classified according to the severity of damage to the skin. A 1st-degree burn causes reddening of the skin and affects only the epidermis, the top layer of the skin. A 2nd-degree burn damages the skin more deeply, extending into the dermis and causing blister formation. A 3rd-degree burn destroys the full skin thickness and may extend to the muscle layer beneath the skin. Specialist treatment, and possibly skin grafts, is necessary for 3rd-degree burns. Electrical burns can cause extensive tissue damage with minimal external skin damage. A 2nd- or 3rd-degree burn that affects more than 10 per cent of the body surface causes *shock* due to massive fluid loss.

BURNS

A 1st-degree burn affects the epidermis

A 2nd-degree burn extends to the dermis

A 3rd-degree burn extends to the fatty layer

A 3rd-degree burn may also extend to the muscle layer

CLASSIFICATION OF BURNS

A burn is covered with a non-stick dressing to keep the area moist. If necessary, *analgesic drugs* are given, and *antibiotic drugs* are prescribed if there is any sign of infection. For extensive 2nd-degree burns, when there may be slow healing or a risk of infection, a topical *antibacterial* agent such as silver sulfadiazine is used. *Skin grafts* are used early in treatment to minimize scarring. 3rd-degree burns always require skin grafting. Extensive burns may require repeated plastic surgery.

burping Another term for *belching*.

burr hole A hole made in the skull by a special drill with a rounded tip (burr). A hole is made to relieve the pressure on the brain that often results from bleeding inside the skull, usually following a *head injury*. Burr holes may be made as part of a *craniotomy* and may be life-saving procedures.

bursa A fluid-filled sac that acts as a cushion at a pressure point in the body, often near a joint, where a tendon or muscle crosses bone or other muscles. The important bursae are around the knee, elbow, and shoulder.

bursitis Inflammation of a *bursa*, causing pain and swelling. Bursitis may result from pressure, friction, or slight injury to the membrane surrounding the joint, or to infection. For example, prepatellar bursitis ("housemaid's knee") is caused by prolonged kneeling on a hard surface. Avoiding further pressure and taking *nonsteroidal anti-inflammatory drugs* are usually all the treatment needed. Occasionally, *antibiotic drugs* may be needed if the bursa is infected.

bypass operations Procedures to bypass the blockage or narrowing of an artery or vein or any part of the digestive system. Arteries can become blocked or narrowed in *atherosclerosis*. Obstructions can be bypassed using sections of healthy artery or vein from elsewhere in the body or using synthetic tubing. Veins are bypassed most often in patients with diseases of the liver that cause portal hypertension and bleeding oesophageal varices. This kind of bypass is called a *shunt*. Intestinal bypasses are employed most commonly in patients with cancer in which tumour growth is too extensive to be removed. An obstructed bile duct can be bypassed by constructing a new opening into the digestive tract. (See also *coronary artery bypass*.)

byssinosis A lung disease caused by an unknown agent in the dust produced during the processing of flax, cotton, hemp, or sisal. Byssinosis produces a feeling of tightness in the chest and shortness of breath that may become chronic if exposure continues. *Bronchodilator drugs* and other drugs used to treat asthma may relieve symptoms, but adequate ventilation and personal protective equipment such as dust masks will reduce the risk.

C

cachexia A condition of severe weight loss and decline in health caused by a serious underlying disease, such as cancer or tuberculosis, or by starvation.

cadaver A dead human body used as a source of transplant organs or for anatomical study and dissection.

cadmium poisoning The toxic effects of cadmium, a tin-like metal. Poisoning due to the inhalation of cadmium dust or fumes is an industrial hazard. Short-term exposure may lead to *pneumonitis*. Exposure over a long period can lead to urinary tract *calculi* (stones), *kidney failure*, or *emphysema*. Eating vegetables grown in cadmium-rich soil, or food or drink stored in cadmium-lined containers, can also cause poisoning

caecum The first section of the large intestine, joining the *ileum* (the end of the small intestine) to the *colon*. The *appendix* projects from the caecum. (See also *digestive system*).

caesarean section An operation to deliver a baby from the uterus through a horizontal or, less commonly, a vertical incision in the abdomen. A caesarean section is performed when it is difficult or dangerous to deliver a baby vaginally. The procedure is performed using *epidural* or general *anaesthesia*.

café au lait spots Patches of coffee-coloured skin that may occur anywhere on the body. Café au lait spots are usually oval in shape and may measure several centimetres across. Generally, a few spots are not significant; larger numbers may be a sign of *neurofibromatosis*.

caffeine A *stimulant drug* found in coffee, tea, cocoa, and cola drinks. Caffeine reduces fatigue, improves concentration, makes the heart pump blood faster, and has a diuretic effect. Large quantities may produce side effects such as agitation and tremors. A regular high intake may lead to increased *tolerance* and *withdrawal* symptoms, such as headaches and tiredness, after a few hours without caffeine. Caffeine is used in some drug preparations, particularly in combination with *analgesics* and with *ergotamine* in preventive treatments for migraine.

caisson disease An alternative term for *decompression sickness*.

calamine A preparation of zinc oxide and iron oxide applied as an ointment, lotion, or dusting powder to relieve skin irritation and itching. Calamine may be combined with a local anaesthetic (see *anaesthesia, local*), a *corticosteroid drug*, or an *antihistamine drug*.

CAESAREAN SECTION

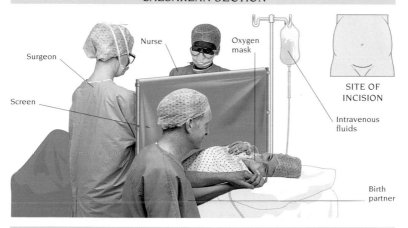

Surgeon
Nurse
Oxygen mask
Screen
SITE OF INCISION
Intravenous fluids
Birth partner

C

calcaneus The heel bone. It is one of the tarsal bones and is the largest bone in the *foot*. The *Achilles tendon* is attached to the back of the calcaneus.

calciferol An alternative name for vitamin D$_2$, also known as ergocalciferol (see *vitamin D*).

calcification The deposition of *calcium* salts in body tissues that is part of the normal process of bone and teeth formation and the healing of fractures. Calcification also occurs in injured muscles, in arteries affected by *atherosclerosis*, and when blood calcium levels are raised by disorders of the *parathyroid glands*.

calcification, dental The deposition of *calcium* salts in developing teeth. Primary teeth begin to calcify in a fetus at between 3 and 6 months gestation; calcification of permanent teeth (other than the wisdom teeth) begins between birth and 4 years. Abnormal calcification occurs in amelogenesis imperfecta, an inherited disorder of the enamel (see *hypoplasia, enamel*), and can also result from the absorption of high levels of fluoride (see *fluorosis*).

calcinosis The abnormal deposition of *calcium* salts in the skin, muscles, or *connective tissues*, forming *nodules*. The condition occurs in connective tissue disorders such as *scleroderma* or *dermatomyositis*. (See also *calcification*.)

calcipotriol A derivative of *vitamin D*, used in topical preparations for treating the skin disorder *psoriasis*.

calcitonin A *hormone* produced by the *thyroid gland* that helps to control blood *calcium* levels by slowing loss of calcium from the bones. A synthetic form of calcitonin is used in the treatment of *Paget's disease*. Calcitonin is also used to reduce high blood levels of calcium in *hypercalcaemia*.

calcium The body's most abundant mineral, essential for cell function, muscle contraction, the transmission of nerve impulses, and *blood clotting*. Calcium phosphate is the hard basic constituent of teeth and bones. Dietary sources of calcium include dairy products, eggs, and green, leafy vegetables. Calcium uptake is facilitated by *vitamin D*.

The body's calcium levels are controlled by *parathyroid* hormone and *calcitonin*. Abnormally high levels in the blood (*hypercalcaemia*) or abnormally low levels (*hypocalcaemia*) may seriously disrupt cell function, particularly in muscles and nerves. (See also *mineral supplements*.)

calcium channel blockers Drugs used to treat *angina pectoris, hypertension*, and types of cardiac *arrhythmia*. Side effects such as headaches, swollen ankles, flushing, and dizziness may occur, but tend to diminish with continued treatment.

calculus A deposit on the teeth (see *calculus, dental*) or a small, hard, crystalline mass that is formed in a body cavity from certain substances in fluids such as bile, urine, or saliva. Calculi can occur in the gallbladder and bile ducts (see *gallstones*), the kidneys, ureters, or bladder (see *calculus, urinary tract*), or in the salivary ducts.

calculus, dental A hard, crust-like deposit (also known as tartar) found on the crowns and roots of the teeth. Calculus forms when mineral salts in saliva are deposited in existing *plaque*. Supragingival calculus is a yellowish or white deposit that forms above the gum margin, on the crowns of teeth near the openings of *salivary gland* ducts. Subgingival calculus forms below the gum margin and is brown or black. Toxins in calculus cause gum inflammation (see *gingivitis*), which may progress to destruction of the supporting tissues (see *periodontitis*). Calculus is removed by professional *scaling*. Attention to *oral hygiene* reduces recurrence.

calculus, urinary tract A stone in the kidneys, ureters, or bladder formed from substances in urine.

Most urinary tract stones are composed of calcium oxalate or other salts crystallized from the urine. These may be associated with a diet rich in oxalic acid (found in leafy vegetables and coffee); high levels of *calcium* in the blood as a result of *hyperparathyroidism*; or chronic dehydration. Other types of stone are associated with *gout* and some cancers. An infective stone is usually a result of chronic *urinary tract infection*.

In developing countries, bladder stones usually occur as a result of dietary deficiencies. In developed countries, they are usually caused by an obstruction to urine flow from the bladder and/or a longstanding urinary tract infection.

The most common symptom of a stone in the kidney or ureter is renal colic (a severe pain in the loin) that may cause nausea and vomiting. There may be *haematuria* (blood in the urine). A bladder stone is usually indicated by difficulty in passing urine. The site of the stone can usually be confirmed by intravenous or retrograde *urography*.

Renal colic is treated with bed rest and an opioid *analgesic* (painkiller). With an adequate fluid intake, small stones are usually passed in the urine without problems. The first line of treatment for larger stones is *lithotripsy*, which uses ultrasonic or shock waves to disintegrate the stones. Alternatively, *cytoscopy* can be used to crush and remove stones in the bladder and lower ureter. In some cases, surgery may be needed.

calendar method A method of *contraception*, also called the rhythm method, based on abstaining from sexual intercourse around the time of *ovulation* (calculated by a woman's menstrual cycles). The method is unreliable because the menstrual cycle may vary (see *contraception, natural methods*).

calf muscles The muscles extending from the back of the knee to the heel. The gastrocnemius muscle starts behind the knee and forms the bulky part of the calf; under it is the soleus muscle which starts at the back of the *tibia* (shin). The two muscles join to form the *Achilles tendon*, which connects them to the heel. Contraction of the calf muscles pulls the heel up and is important in walking, running, and jumping. Pain in these muscles occurs because of *cramp*, *sciatica*, or, more rarely, deep vein *thrombosis*. The calf muscles may be affected by *claudication* (pain caused by walking and relieved by rest).

caliper splint An *orthopaedic* device that corrects or controls a deformed leg or supports a leg weakened by a muscular disorder, allowing a person to stand and walk.

callosity See *callus, skin*.

callus, bony A diffuse growth of new, soft bone that forms as part of the healing process in a *fracture*. As healing continues, the callus is replaced by harder bone, and the original shape of the bone is restored.

callus, skin An area of thickened skin, usually on the hands or feet, caused by regular or prolonged pressure or friction. A *corn* is a callus on a toe. If corns are painful, the thickened skin can be pared away by a chiropodist using a scalpel.

caloric test A method of finding out whether the *labyrinth* in the inner ear is diseased. It is performed as part of investigations into *vertigo* (dizziness) and hearing loss. The outer-ear canal of the ear is briefly flooded with water at different temperatures. If the labyrinth is normal, *nystagmus* (rapid reflex flickering of the eyes) occurs for a predictable period. If the labyrinth is diseased, the response is absent or reduced.

calorie A unit of energy. One calorie is the amount of energy needed to raise the temperature of 1 gram of water by 1°C. However, the term calorie is also used in medicine and *dietetics* to mean kilocalorie, a larger unit equal to 1,000 calories. Normally, when calorie intake matches the amount of energy expended, body weight remains constant. If intake exceeds expenditure, weight is usually gained; if expenditure exceeds intake, weight is usually lost. In general, fats contain the most calories. Energy can also be measured in joules: 1 calorie equals 4.2 joules. (See also *calorimetry; diet and disease*.)

calorie requirements See *energy requirements*.

calorimetry The measurement of the *calorie* value of foodstuffs or the energy expenditure of a person. In direct calorimetry, a small measure of food is burned up inside a sealed container, which is immersed in water. The rise in water temperature that results is used to calculate the calorie value.

Energy production in humans is measured by *oxygen* uptake. Every litre of oxygen taken into the body produces 4.8 kilocalories of energy. Energy production is calculated by comparing the percentage of oxygen in air inhaled and exhaled.

campylobacter A group of bacteria that are among the most common causes of gastrointestinal disorders. The bacteria are harboured by animals and can be passed to humans in contaminated food,

C

especially poultry, causing *food poisoning*. The bacteria also cause a form of the inflammatory colon disease *colitis*.

cancer A group of diseases characterized by the abnormal and unrestrained growth of cells in body organs or tissues. Tumour-forming cells develop when the *oncogenes* (genes controlling cell growth and multiplication) in a cell or cells undergo a series of changes. A small group of abnormal cells develop that divide more rapidly than normal, lack *differentiation* (they no longer perform their specialized task), and may escape the normal control of hormones and nerves. Cancers differ from benign *neoplasms* (abnormal growths, such as *warts*) in that they spread and infiltrate surrounding tissue and may cause blockages, destroy nerves, and erode bone. Cancer cells may also spread via the blood vessels and lymphatic system to form secondary tumours (see *metastasis*).

Causes of cancer include factors like sunlight, smoking, pollutants, alcohol consumption, and dietary factors. These factors may cause critical changes in body cells in susceptible people. Susceptibility to some cancers may be inherited.

Many cancers are now curable, usually by combinations of surgery, *radiotherapy*, and *anticancer drugs*. For information on particular cancers, refer to the organ in question (for example *lung cancer*; *stomach cancer*).

cancerphobia An intense fear of developing cancer, out of proportion to the actual risk, that significantly affects the sufferer's life. Patterns of behaviour typical of *obsessive–compulsive disorder* (for example, prolonged washing rituals) may be adopted in an attempt to reduce the risk of cancer. *Psychotherapy* including *behaviour therapy* may be of benefit.

cancer screening Tests to detect early signs of cancer in groups of people who are susceptible to cancer because of their age, occupation, lifestyle, or genetic predisposition. Tests for cancers of the cervix (see *cervical smear test*), breast (see *mammography*), bladder, and colon (see *colon, cancer of*) have proven to be effective.

cancrum oris See *noma*.

candidiasis Infection by the fungus *CANDIDA ALBICANS*, also known as thrush or moniliasis. Candidiasis affects areas of mucous membrane in the body, most commonly the vagina and the inside of the mouth. In infants, it can occur in conjunction with *nappy rash*.

The fungus is normally present in the mouth and vagina but may multiply excessively if *antibiotic drugs* destroy the harmless bacteria that control its growth, or if the body's resistance to infection is lowered. Certain disorders, notably *diabetes mellitus*, and hormonal changes due to pregnancy may also encourage its growth. Candidiasis can be contracted by sexual intercourse with an infected partner. The infection is far more common in women than in men. Symptoms of vaginal infection include a thick, white discharge, genital irritation, and discomfort when passing urine. Less commonly, the penis is infected in men, usually causing *balanitis*. Oral candidiasis produces sore, creamy-yellow, raised patches in the mouth. Candidiasis may spread to other moist body areas and may also affect the gastrointestinal tract, particularly in people with impaired immune systems. Treatment for candidiasis is with topical preparations such as creams, pessaries, or lozenges, or with oral *antifungal drugs*.

canine tooth See *teeth*.

cannabis Preparations that are derived from the hemp plant *CANNABIS SATIVA*, which produce euphoria and hallucinations (see *marijuana*).

cannula A smooth, blunt-ended tube inserted into a blood vessel, lymphatic vessel, or body cavity, in order to introduce or withdraw fluids. Cannulas are used for *blood transfusions* and *intravenous infusions* and for draining *pleural effusions*. They may be left in place for several days if continuous testing of, or introduction of, fluids is required.

cap, cervical A flexible contraceptive device placed directly over the *cervix* to prevent sperm from entering (see *contraception, barrier methods of*).

Capgras' syndrome The delusion that a relative or friend has been replaced by an identical impostor. Also known as the "illusion of doubles", the syndrome is seen most frequently in paranoid *schizophrenia*, but also occurs in organic brain disorders (see *brain syndrome, organic*) and *affective disorders*.

capillary Any of the vessels that carry blood between the smallest arteries, or arterioles, and the smallest veins, or venules (see *circulatory system*). Capillaries form a fine network throughout the body's organs and tissues. Their thin walls are permeable and allow blood and cells to exchange constituents such as oxygen, glucose, carbon dioxide, and water (see *respiration*). Capillaries open and close to blood flow according to the requirements of different organs. The opening and closing of skin capillaries helps to regulate *temperature*.

A direct blow to the body may rupture the thin capillary walls, causing bleeding under the surface of the skin, which in turn causes swelling and bruising. Increasing age, high doses of *corticosteroid drugs*, and *scurvy* (vitamin C deficiency) make capillaries more fragile; a tendency to *purpura* (small areas of bleeding under the skin) may develop.

CAPILLARY

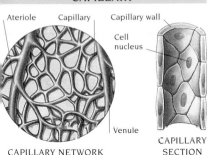

Ateriole Capillary Capillary wall

Cell nucleus

Venule

CAPILLARY NETWORK

CAPILLARY SECTION

capping, dental See *crown, dental*.

capsule An anatomical structure enclosing an organ or body part: for example, capsules enclose the liver, kidneys, joints, and eye lenses.

The term capsule is also used to describe a soluble, elongated shell, usually made of gelatine, containing a drug to be taken by mouth. The coating of some capsules prevents a drug that may have an irritant effect being released into the stomach, or allows a drug to be released slowly so it can be taken less frequently.

capsulitis Inflammation of a *capsule* around an organ or joint, for example as occurs in *frozen shoulder*.

captopril A drug belonging to the category *ACE inhibitors*, which are used in the treatment of *hypertension*, *heart failure*, and diabetic *nephropathy*.

caput Latin for "head". The term is used to refer to the caput succedaneum, a soft, temporary swelling in the scalp of newborn babies, caused by pressure during labour. Caput is also used to refer to the face, skull, and associated organs, to the origin of a muscle, or to any enlarged extremity, such as the caput femoris, the head of the femur (thigh bone).

carbamazepine An *anticonvulsant drug*, chemically related to the *tricyclic antidepressants*. It is mainly used in the long-term treatment of *epilepsy*. It is also used to treat *neuralgia* and psychological disorders, such as *bipolar disorder*.

carbaryl An insecticide used to treat head *lice* and *crab lice*. Carbaryl is applied topically as a liquid, avoiding contact with the eyes or broken skin.

carbenoxolone A drug used to treat mouth ulcers.

carbimazole A drug that is used to treat *hyperthyroidism* (overactivity of the thyroid gland). Carbimazole is slow to take effect, so *beta-blockers* may be given to relieve symptoms in the interim. Possible adverse effects of carbimazole include headaches, dizziness, joint pain, and nausea. Carbimazole may also reduce the production of blood cells, so people taking the drug should report promptly to their doctor any symptoms of infection, especially a sore throat.

carbohydrates A group of compounds composed of carbon, hydrogen, and oxygen, which supply the body with its main source of energy. Carbohydrates are found in fruits, cereals, and root crops and fall into two groups. These are available carbohydrates, which are metabolized into glucose for the body's use, and unavailable carbohydrates, such as cellulose, which cannot be broken down by digestive *enzymes* and make up the bulk of dietary fibre (see *fibre, dietary*).

Available carbohydrates are predominantly starches (complex carbohydrates) and sugars (simple carbohydrates). In carbohydrate metabolism, the monosaccharides (simple sugars) glucose, galactose, and fructose are absorbed into

C

the bloodstream unchanged. The disaccharides (double sugars) sucrose, maltose, and lactose are broken down into simple sugars before they are absorbed. Starches also have to be broken down into simple sugars.

Some glucose is burned up immediately (see *metabolism*) in order to generate energy for cells, such as brain cells, that need a constant supply. Galactose and fructose have to be converted to glucose in the liver before they can be used by body cells. Surplus glucose is conveyed to the liver, muscles, and fat cells where it is converted into *glycogen* and fat for storage. When blood glucose levels are high, glucose storage is stimulated by *insulin*, a hormone that is secreted by the *pancreas*. When the blood glucose level becomes low, insulin secretion diminishes and *glucagon*, which is another hormone produced by the pancreas, stimulates the conversion of stored glycogen to glucose for release into the bloodstream. Although fat cannot be converted to glucose, it can be burned as a fuel in order to conserve glucose. In the disorder *diabetes mellitus*, carbohydrate metabolism is disturbed by a deficiency of insulin.

carbon A nonmetallic element present in all the fundamental molecules of living organisms, such as *proteins*, *fats*, and *carbohydrates*, and in some inorganic molecules such as *carbon dioxide*, *carbon monoxide*, and *sodium bicarbonate*. Pure carbon is the major constituent of diamond, coal, charcoal, and graphite.

carbon dioxide (CO_2) A colourless, odourless gas. Carbon dioxide is present in small amounts in the air and is a by-product of *metabolism* in cells. It is produced by the breakdown of substances such as carbohydrates and fats to produce energy, and is carried in the blood to the lungs and exhaled. Carbon dioxide helps to control the rate of respiration: when a person exercises, CO_2 levels in the blood rise, causing the person to breathe more rapidly to expel carbon dioxide and take in more *oxygen*.

When it is compressed and cooled to -75°C, carbon dioxide becomes solid *dry ice*, which is used in *cryosurgery*.

carbon monoxide (CO) A colourless, odourless, poisonous gas present in

motor exhaust fumes and produced by inefficient burning of coal, gas, or oil. Carbon monoxide binds with *haemoglobin* and prevents the transportation of oxygen to body tissues. The initial symptoms of acute high-level carbon monoxide poisoning are dizziness, headache, nausea, and faintness. Continued inhalation of the gas may lead to loss of consciousness, permanent brain damage, and even death. Low-level exposure to carbon monoxide over a period of time may cause fatigue, nausea, diarrhoea, abdominal pain, and general malaise.

carbon tetrachloride (CCl_4) A colourless, poisonous, volatile chemical with a characteristic odour that is present in some dry-cleaning fluids and industrial solvents. It can cause dizziness, confusion, and liver and kidney damage if it is inhaled or swallowed.

carbuncle A cluster of interconnected boils, usually caused by the bacterium STAPHYLOCOCCUS AUREUS. The back of the neck and the buttocks are common sites. Carbuncles mainly affect people with reduced immunity, particularly those with *diabetes mellitus*. Treatment is usually with an *antibiotic* and hot *compresses*. Incision and drainage may be necessary if a carbuncle is persistent.

carcinogen Any agent capable of causing *cancer*. Chemicals are the largest group of carcinogens. Major types include polycyclic aromatic hydrocarbons (PAHs), which occur in tobacco smoke, pitch, tar fumes, and soot. Exposure to PAHs may lead to cancer of the respiratory system or skin. Certain aromatic amines used in the chemical and rubber industries may cause bladder cancer after prolonged exposure.

The best-known physical carcinogen is high-energy *radiation*, such as nuclear radiation and X-rays. Exposure may cause cancerous changes in cells, especially in cells that divide quickly: for example, changes in the precursors of white blood cells in the bone marrow cause *leukaemia*. The risk depends on the dosage and duration of exposure. Over many years, exposure to ultraviolet radiation in sunlight can cause skin cancer. Another known physical carcinogen is asbestos (see *asbestos-related diseases*).

Only a few biological agents are known to cause cancer in humans. SCHISTOSOMA HAEMATOBIUM, one of the blood flukes responsible for schistosomiasis, can cause cancer of the bladder; and ASPERGILLUS FLAVUS, a fungus that produces the poison aflatoxin in stored peanuts and grain, is believed to cause liver cancer. Viruses associated with cancer include strains of the human papillomavirus, which are linked to cancer of the cervix; the hepatitis B virus, which is linked to liver cancer; and a type of herpes virus which is associated with Kaposi's sarcoma.

carcinogenesis The development of a cancer caused by the action of carcinogens (cancer-causing factors) on normal cells. Carcinogens are believed to alter the DNA in cells, particularly in oncogenes (genes that control the growth and division of cells). An altered cell divides abnormally fast, passing on the genetic changes to all offspring cells. A group of cells is established that is not affected by the body's normal restraints on growth.

carcinoid syndrome A rare condition caused by an intestinal or lung tumour, called a carcinoid, which secretes excess amounts of the hormone serotonin. Carcinoid syndrome is marked by bouts of facial flushing, diarrhoea, and wheezing, but symptoms usually occur only if the tumour has spread to the liver or has arisen in a lung. Sometimes tumours in the intestine, lung, and, rarely, the liver are removed surgically, but, in most cases, surgery is unlikely to be of benefit. However, symptoms may be relieved by drugs that block the action of serotonin.

carcinoma Any cancerous tumour (see cancer) arising from cells in the covering surface layer or lining membrane of an organ. The most common cancers of the lungs, breast, stomach, skin, cervix, colon, and rectum are carcinomas.

carcinoma in situ The earliest, usually curable, stage of a cancer in which it has not yet spread from the surface layer of cells of an organ.

carcinomatosis The presence of cancerous tissue in different sites of the body due to the spread of cancer cells from a primary (original) cancerous tumour. Symptoms depend on the site of the metastases (secondary tumours). Carcinomatosis may be confirmed by X-rays or by radionuclide scanning of the bones and lungs, by biochemical tests, or during an operation. The condition is not improved by removing the primary tumour unless the tumour is producing a hormone that stimulates the growth of metastases. Anticancer drugs or radiotherapy may be given to treat metastases.

cardiac arrest A halt in the pumping action of the heart that occurs when its rhythmic muscular activity ceases. The most common cause is a myocardial infarction (heart attack). Other causes include respiratory arrest, electrical injury, loss of blood, hypothermia, drug overdose, and anaphylactic shock. Cardiac arrest causes sudden collapse, loss of consciousness, and absence of pulse and breathing.

The diagnosis is confirmed by monitoring the electrical activity of the heart by ECG. This distinguishes between ventricular fibrillation and asystole, the two abnormalities of heart rhythm that cause cardiac arrest. Ventricular fibrillation may be corrected by defibrillation. Asystole, the complete absence of heart muscle activity, is more difficult to reverse but may respond to injection of adrenaline.

cardiac cycle The sequence of events, lasting for less than a second, that make up each beat of the heart. A heartbeat has three phases. In diasystole, the heart relaxes. During atrial systole, the atria contract, and in ventricular systole, the ventricles contract. The sinoatrial node (the heart's pacemaker) regulates the timing of the phases by sending electrical impulses to the atria and ventricles.

cardiac massage See cardiopulmonary resuscitation.

cardiac neurosis Excessive anxiety about the condition of the heart, usually after a myocardial infarction (heart attack) or heart surgery, but sometimes occurring when there is no previous heart trouble. The person experiences symptoms, such as breathlessness and chest pain, that are typical of heart disease, and may be reluctant to exercise or work for fear of an attack. Medical investigation reveals no physical cause. Psychotherapy may be helpful.

cardiac output The measured volume of blood pumped by the heart each minute,

C

used to assess how efficiently the heart is working. At rest, a healthy adult's heart pumps 2.5–4.5 litres of blood per minute; during exercise this figure may be as much as 30 litres per minute. A low output during exercise indicates damage to the heart muscle or major blood loss.

cardiac stress test Also known as an exercise *ECG*, one of a group of tests used to assess the function of the heart in people who experience chest pain, breathlessness, or palpitations during exercise. The test establishes whether the patient has *coronary artery disease*. An ECG machine records the patterns of the heart's electrical activity while the heart is stressed. This is usually achieved by the patient exercising on a treadmill or cycling. Specific changes in the electrical pattern as exercise levels increase indicate *angina*. Cardiac stress testing may be used in conjunction with *radionuclide scanning* or *angiography* to identify damaged areas of heart muscle.

cardiology The study of the function of the heart and the investigation, diagnosis, and medical treatment of disorders of the heart and blood vessels.

cardiomegaly Enlargement of the *heart*. Cardiomegaly may take the form of *hypertrophy* (thickening) of the heart muscle or of dilatation (increase in volume) of one or more of the heart chambers. Hypertrophy occurs in conditions in which the heart has to work harder than normal to pump blood around the body. These include *hypertension*, *pulmonary hypertension*, thyroid disease, severe *anaemia*, and one type of *cardiomyopathy*. Dilatation of a heart chamber may be due to heart valve incompetence (failure of a valve to close properly after a contraction) such as occurs in *aortic insufficiency*.

Symptoms may not occur until the heart has enlarged to the point where it cannot cope with additional stress. Its reduced pumping efficiency leads to *heart failure*, with symptoms of breathlessness and ankle swelling. Cardiomegaly is diagnosed by physical examination, *chest X-ray*, and *echocardiography*. Treatment is directed at the underlying cause.

cardiomyopathy Any disease of the heart muscle that weakens the force of cardiac contractions, thereby reducing the efficiency of blood circulation. Cardiomyopathies may have an infectious, metabolic, nutritional, toxic, autoimmune, or degenerative cause. However, in many cases the cause is unknown.

There are three main types. In hypertrophic cardiomyopathy, which is usually inherited, the heart muscle is abnormally thickened. In dilated cardiomyopathy, *metabolism* of the heart muscle cells is abnormal and the walls of the heart tend to balloon out under pressure. Restrictive cardiomyopathy is caused by scarring of the endocardium (the inner lining of the heart) or by *amyloidosis*.

Symptoms of cardiomyopathy include fatigue, chest pain, and palpitations. The condition may lead to *heart failure*, symptoms of which include breathing difficulty and *oedema*. A *chest X-ray* may show enlargement of the heart, and *echocardiography* may show thickened heart muscle. A *biopsy* of heart muscle may reveal muscle cell abnormalities.

Symptoms may be treated with *diuretic drugs* to control heart failure and *antiarrhythmic drugs* to correct abnormal heart rhythm. In many cases, heart muscle function deteriorates, and the only remaining option is a *heart transplant*.

cardiopulmonary bypass The method by which the circulation of blood around the body is maintained while the heart is stopped during heart surgery. A *heart-lung machine* is used to maintain the supply of oxygenated blood to the body.

cardiopulmonary resuscitation The administration of life-saving measures to a person who has suffered a *cardiac arrest*. A person in cardiac arrest is not breathing and has no detectable pulse or heartbeat. First, mouth-to-mouth resuscitation (see *artificial respiration*) is given; if this fails to restart breathing, repeated chest compressions, using the heel of the hand, are applied to the lower breastbone until trained help arrives. Both these measures are used to restore blood circulation to the brain. Brain damage or death is likely if the brain is starved of oxygen for about 3 minutes.

cardiotocography See *fetal heart monitoring*.

cardiovascular Pertaining to the heart and blood vessels.

cardiovascular disorders Disorders of the heart, blood vessels, and blood circulation (see *heart disorders*; *arteries, disorders of*; *veins, disorders of*).

cardiovascular surgery The branch of surgery concerned with the heart and blood vessels. Cardiovascular surgery includes operations to prevent or repair damage caused, for example, by congenital heart disease (see *heart disease, congenital*), *atherosclerosis*, or a *myocardial infarction* (heart attack). Procedures include *heart valve surgery*, *coronary artery bypass*, and *heart transplant*.

cardioversion The restoration of normal heart rhythm, usually by applying an electric shock to the chest. Cardioversion is also sometimes known as *defibrillation*.

carditis A general term for inflammation of any part of the heart or its linings. There are three types of carditis: *myocarditis* (inflammation of the heart muscle), which is usually caused by a viral infection; *endocarditis* (inflammation of the internal lining of the heart), which is usually due to a bacterial infection; and *pericarditis* (inflammation of the outer covering of the heart), which is usually due to a viral or bacterial infection but may be associated with a *myocardial infarction* or an autoimmune disorder, such as systemic *lupus erythematosus*.

caries, dental Tooth decay; the gradual erosion of enamel (the covering of the tooth) and dentine (the substance beneath the enamel). Initial decay usually occurs on the grinding surfaces of the back teeth and areas around the gum line. The main cause is *plaque*, a sticky substance consisting of food deposits, dead cells from the lining of the mouth, saliva by-products, and bacteria that collects on the teeth. The breakdown of food deposits by bacteria creates an acid that eats into the enamel to form cavities. Unchecked decay spreads to the dentine, and as the cavity enlarges, bacteria may invade and destroy the pulp at the tooth's core. Advanced decay causes toothache and bad breath.

Treatment consists of drilling away the area of decay and filling the cavity (see *filling, dental*). In advanced decay, it may be necessary to remove the infected pulp (see *extraction, dental*).

Water *fluoridation* and the use of fluoride toothpaste helps prevent caries. The risk of caries is also reduced by cutting sugar consumption, practising good *oral hygiene*, and visiting the dentist regularly.

carotenaemia A harmless condition in which the blood level of the orange pigment *carotene*, found in carrots and other vegetables, is excessively high. The condition may cause temporary yellowing of the skin.

carotene An orange pigment found in carrots, tomatoes, and leafy green vegetables. The most important form, called beta-carotene, is an *antioxidant* that is converted in the intestines into *vitamin A*, which is essential for vision and the health of the skin and other organs. Excessive intake of foods containing carotene may result in *carotenaemia*.

carotid artery Any of the main arteries of the neck and head. There are two common carotid arteries (left and right), each of which divides into two main branches (internal and external).

The left carotid arises from the *aorta* and runs up the neck on the left side of the *trachea* (windpipe). The right carotid arises from the subclavian artery (which branches off the aorta) and follows a similar route on the right side of the neck. Just above the level of the *larynx* (voice-box), each carotid artery divides to form an external carotid artery and an internal carotid artery. The external arteries have multiple branches that supply most tissues in the face, scalp, mouth, and jaws; the internal arteries enter the skull to

CAROTID ARTERY

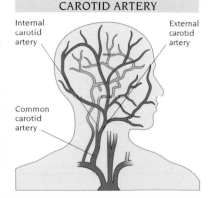

Internal carotid artery

External carotid artery

Common carotid artery

C

supply the brain and eyes. At the base of the brain, branches of the two internal carotids and the basilar artery join to form a ring of vessels called the circle of Willis. Narrowing of these vessels may be associated with *transient ischaemic attack (TIA)*; obstruction of them causes a *stroke*.

carpal tunnel syndrome Numbness, tingling, and pain in the thumb, index finger, and middle fingers caused by compression of the *median nerve* at the wrist. Symptoms may be worse at night. The condition results from pressure on the nerve where it passes into the hand via a gap (the "carpal tunnel") under a ligament at the front of the wrist. It is common among keyboard users. It also occurs without obvious cause in middle-aged women, and is associated with pregnancy, initial use of *oral contraceptives*, *premenstrual syndrome*, *rheumatoid arthritis*, *myxoedema*, and *acromegaly*.

The condition often disappears without treatment. Persistent symptoms may be treated with a *corticosteroid drug* injected under the ligament, or the ligament may be cut to relieve pressure on the nerve.

carpus The eight bones of the *wrist*.

carrier A person who is able to pass on an infectious or inherited disease without actually suffering from it.

car sickness See *motion sickness*.

cartilage A type of *connective tissue* made up of varying amounts of the gel-like substance *collagen*. Cartilage forms an important structural component of various parts of the skeletal system, including the *joints*. There are three main types. Hyaline cartilage is a tough, smooth tissue that lines the surfaces of joints. Fibrocartilage is solid and strong; it makes up the intervertebral discs between the bones of the spine and the shock-absorbing pads in joints. Elastic cartilage is soft and rubbery and found in structures such as the outer ear and the *epiglottis*.

CARTILAGE

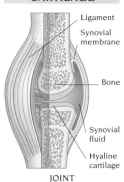

- Ligament
- Synovial membrane
- Bone
- Synovial fluid
- Hyaline cartilage

JOINT

cast A rigid casing for a limb or other body part to hold a broken bone or dislocated joint immobile as it heals. Most casts are made of bandages impregnated with *plaster of Paris* or polyurethane resin; they are applied wet and harden as they dry.

castration Removal of the testes (see *orchidectomy*). The term is sometimes used for removal of the ovaries (see *oophorectomy*). Castration is performed when organs are diseased, or to reduce the level of testosterone or of oestrogen in people with certain types of cancer that are stimulated by these hormones.

catabolism A chemical process by which constituents of food stored in the body (for example, fats) are broken down, releasing energy into body cells (see *biochemistry*; *metabolism*).

catalepsy A physical state in which the muscles of the face, body, and limbs are maintained in a semi-rigid, statue-like position for minutes, hours, or even days. Catalepsy occurs in people with *schizophrenia* or *epilepsy*, but may also be caused by brain disease or some drugs.

cataplexy A sudden loss of muscle tone, causing an involuntary collapse without loss of consciousness. Cataplexy is triggered by intense emotion, particularly laughter, and occurs almost exclusively in those suffering from *narcolepsy* and other sleep disorders.

cataract Loss of transparency of the crystalline *lens* of the eye, due to changes in its delicate protein fibres. At an advanced stage, the front part of the lens becomes densely opaque, but the cataract never causes total blindness.

Almost everyone over 65 has some degree of cataract. Regular exposure to *ultraviolet* light increases the risk. Other causes include injury to the eye, particularly if a foreign body enters the lens. Cataract is common in people who have *diabetes mellitus*. Long-term use of *corticosteroid drugs* may contribute to cataract development. *Congenital* cataract may be due to an infection of the mother in early pregnancy, especially with *rubella*, or to the toxic effects of certain drugs in pregnancy; it may also be associated with *Down's syndrome* or with *galactosaemia*.

Onset of symptoms is almost imperceptible, although night driving may be affected early on. There is slow, progressive loss of visual acuity. The person may become shortsighted and notice disturbances in colour perception. When vision has become seriously impaired, *cataract surgery* is performed to remove the lens.

cataract surgery Removal of the *lens* from the eye, performed to restore sight in people whose vision is impaired by a *cataract*. The lens is usually replaced with a plastic implant during the operation, although for young people and those with other eye disorders, a contact or spectacle lens fitted after the operation may be preferable.

catarrh Excessive secretion of mucus by the *mucous membranes* lining the nose (see *rhinitis*), sinuses (see *sinusitus*), or upper air passages, due to inflammation.

catatonia A state in which a person becomes mute or adopts a bizarre, rigid pose. It is seen in a rare form of *schizophrenia* and some types of brain disease.

catharsis A term meaning purification or cleansing. Catharsis is used to refer to the process of cleaning out the bowels. Sigmund Freud used the term in *psychoanalytic theory* to describe the expression of repressed feelings and memories.

cathartic A term that means having the power to purify or cleanse. A cathartic drug stimulates movement of the bowels (see *laxative drugs*).

catheter A flexible tube inserted into the body to drain or introduce fluids or carry out other functions. Catheters are commonly used to drain urine from the bladder (see *catheterization, urinary*). Other types are used to investigate the condition of the heart (see *catheterization, cardiac*), to widen obstructed blood vessels, or to control bleeding. (See also *balloon catheter*.)

catheterization, cardiac A diagnostic test in which a fine, sterile *catheter* is introduced into the heart via a blood vessel. It is used to diagnose and assess the extent of congenital heart disease (see *heart disease, congenital*) and *coronary artery disease*, and to diagnose and treat some disorders of the heart valves (see *valvuloplasty*). During the procedure, the pressure within the heart's chambers can be measured, samples of blood and tissue can be taken, and a *radiopaque*

substance can be injected to allow the heart's cavities to be X-rayed.

catheterization, urinary Insertion of a sterile *catheter* into the *bladder* to drain urine. The procedure is used when a person is unable to empty the bladder normally or is incontinent (see *incontinence, urinary*). Urinary catheterization is also used during operations, in bladder function tests such as *cystometry* and *cystourethrography*, and to monitor urine production in the critically ill.

CAT scanning An abbreviation for computerized axial tomographic scanning, commonly known as *CT scanning*.

cat-scratch fever An uncommon disease that develops after a scratch or bite by a cat. Three quarters of cases occur in children. The fever is due to infection with a small bacterium called *ROCHALIMAEA HENDELAE*. The main symptom, appearing after 3–10 days, is a swollen lymph node near the bite or scratch. The node may become painful and tender, and an infected blister may develop at the site of the injury. A fever, rash, and headache may occur. Diagnosis is confirmed by *biopsy* of the swollen lymph node and a skin test. *Analgesic drugs* (painkillers) may be used to relieve the fever and headache.

cats, diseases from Various parasites and infectious organisms can spread from cats to humans. The most serious disease is *rabies*. *Cat-scratch fever* is an uncommon illness caused by infection with the bacterium *ROCHALIMAEA HENDELAE* following a cat scratch or bite. Cats commonly carry the *protozoan TOXOPLASMA GONDII*, which causes *toxoplasmosis*. Infection, usually from contact with cat's faeces, is not generally serious but has serious consequences if a woman is infected during pregnancy. Cat faeces may also carry eggs of the cat roundworm, a possible cause of *toxocariasis*. Rarely, a larva from an ingested roundworm egg migrates to and lodges in an eye, causing deterioration of vision or even blindness. Children who have been playing in sand or soil contaminated by cat faeces are most commonly affected. Other cat-related disorders in humans include *tinea* (ringworm), fungal infections of the skin, bites from cat fleas, and allergic reactions to dander that may cause *asthma* or

C

urticaria. Diseases from cats can be avoided by good hygiene, veterinary care for animals that are ill, and regular worming and flea treatment of cats.

cauda equina A "spray" of nerve roots resembling a horse's tail that descends from the lower *spinal cord* and occupies the lower third of the spinal canal.

caudal Relating to the lower end of the *spine*. Caudal means "of the tail".

caudal block A type of *nerve block*, in which a local anaesthetic is injected into the lower part of the spinal canal. Caudal block may be used for *obstetric* and gynaecological procedures.

cauliflower ear A painful, swollen distortion of the pinna (ear flap) resulting from blows or friction that have caused bleeding in the soft *cartilage*. Immediate treatment after an injury is with ice-packs to reduce the swelling. In severe cases, a doctor may drain blood from the ear and apply a pressure bandage.

causalgia A persistent, burning pain, usually in an arm or leg, most often as a result of injury to a nerve by a deep cut, limb *fracture*, or gunshot wound. The skin overlying the painful area may be red and tender, or blue, cold, and clammy. Causalgia may be aggravated by light sensations, such as touch, or emotional factors. In some cases, treatment with *antidepressant drugs* or *anticonvulsant drugs* may be effective. A few people benefit from *sympathectomy*, an operation in which nerves are severed.

caustic A term used for any substance that has a burning or corrosive action on body tissues or has a burning taste. Caustic agents such as silver nitrate are used to destroy warts.

cauterization The application of a heated instrument to destroy tissues, to stop bleeding, or to promote healing, used in conditions such as *haemorrhoids* and *cervical ectopy*. Cauterization has been largely replaced by *electrocoagulation*.

cavernous sinus thrombosis Blockage of a venous *sinus* (a channel for venous blood deep in the skull behind an eye socket) by a *thrombus* (abnormal blood clot). The condition is usually a complication of a bacterial infection in an area drained by the veins entering the sinus. Such infections include *cellulitis* of the face, infections of the mouth, eye, or middle ear, *sinusitis*, and *septicaemia*.

Symptoms include severe headache, high fever, pain and loss of sensation in and above the affected eye, and *proptosis* (protrusion of the eyeball). Vision may become blurred and eye movements paralysed due to pressure on the *optic nerve* and other cranial nerves. Treatment with *antibiotic drugs* and *anticoagulant drugs* can save vision. Left untreated, blindness results, and the infection may prove fatal.

cavity, dental A hole in a tooth, commonly caused by dental caries (see *caries, dental*).

CD4 count A blood test used to monitor *HIV infection* and *AIDS*. The procedure counts the number of CD4 *lymphocytes* (white blood cells that fight infection) in a blood sample. CD4 lymphocytes are destroyed by HIV, and reduced levels of these cells indicate the progression of HIV and the eventual development of AIDS. A CD4 count can also be used to monitor the effectiveness of treatment.

cefaclor A common antibiotic, one of the *cephalosporin drugs*.

cefadroxil A *cephalosporin drug*, used to treat bacterial infections.

cefalexin A *cephalosporin drug*, used to treat bacterial infections.

cefotaxime A *cephalosporin drug*, used to treat bacterial infections.

cefuroxime A *cephalosporin drug*, used to treat bacterial infections.

celecoxib A *COX-2 inhibitor drug* (a type of *nonsteroidal anti-inflammatory drug*) used to relieve the pain and inflammation of *rheumatoid arthritis* and *osteoarthritis*. Possible side effects include nausea and diarrhoea. Abdominal discomfort may also occur, but can be minimized by taking the drug with food. Celecoxib is associated with an increased risk of heart disease and is therefore not generally recommended for people who have had a heart attack or stroke or who are at risk of these conditions.

cell The basic structural unit of all living organisms. The human body consists of billions of cells, structurally and functionally integrated to perform the complex tasks necessary for life. In spite of variation in size and function, most human cells have a similar basic structure.

Each cell is an invisibly small bag containing liquid cytoplasm, surrounded by a cell membrane that regulates the passage of useful substances (such as oxygen and nutrients) into the cell; and waste materials (such as carbon dioxide) and manufactured substances (such as hormones) out of the cell. Some cells, such as those lining the small intestine, have microvilli, projections that increase the cells' surface area to facilitate absorption.

All cells, except red blood cells, have a *nucleus*, a control centre that governs all major cell activities by regulating the amount and types of *proteins* made in the cell. Inside the nucleus are the *chromosomes*, which are made of the nucleic acid *DNA*. This contains the instructions for *protein synthesis*, which are carried into the cytoplasm by a type of *RNA*, another nucleic acid, and are decoded in particles called ribosomes. The nucleus also contains a spherical structure called the nucleolus, which plays a role in the production of ribosomes.

The cell also contains various organelles, each with a specific role. Energy is generated from the breakdown of sugars and fatty acids by mitochondria. Substances that would damage the cell if they came into contact with the cyto-plasm are contained in particles called lysosomes and peroxisomes. A system of membranes in the cytoplasm called the endoplasmic reticulum transports materials through the cell. Flattened sacs called the Golgi complex receive and process proteins dispatched by the endoplasmic reticulum. Products for export, such as enzymes and hormones, are secreted by vesicles at the cell surface. Other materials, water, and waste products are transported and stored in the cytoplasm by vacuoles. The cyto-plasm itself has a network of fine tubes (microtubules) and filaments (microfilaments) known as the cytoskeleton, which gives the cell a definite shape.

cell division The processes by which cells multiply. *Mitosis* is the most common form of cell division, giving rise to daughter cells identical to the parent cells. *Meiosis* produces egg (see *ovum*) and *sperm* cells that differ from their parent cells in that they have only half the normal number of *chromosomes*.

cellulitis A bacterial infection of the skin and the tissues beneath it, usually affecting the face, neck, or legs. Cellulitis is most commonly caused by streptococci bacteria, which enter the skin via a wound. The affected area is hot, tender,

CELL

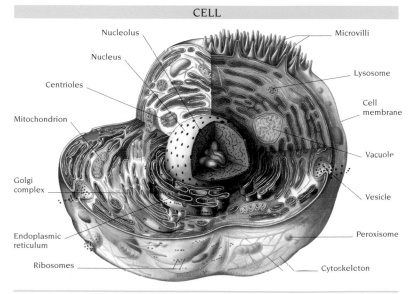

Nucleolus
Nucleus
Centrioles
Mitochondrion
Golgi complex
Endoplasmic reticulum
Ribosomes
Microvilli
Lysosome
Cell membrane
Vacuole
Vesicle
Peroxisome
Cytoskeleton

C

and red, and there may be fever and chills. Untreated cellulitis at the site of a wound may progress to *bacteraemia* and *septicaemia* or, occasionally, to *gangrene*. Cellulitis is usually more severe in people with reduced immune response, such as those with *diabetes mellitus* or an *immunodeficiency disorder*. Treatment is with an *antibiotic* such as a *penicillin* drug or *erythromycin*. (See also *erysipelas*.)

celsius scale A temperature scale in which the melting point of ice is zero degrees (0°C) and the boiling point of water is 100 degrees (100°C). On this scale, normal body temperature is 37°C. (See also *Fahrenheit scale*.)

cementum Bone-like tissue surrounding the root of a tooth (see *teeth*).

centigrade scale The obsolete name for the *celsius scale*.

central nervous system The anatomical term for the *brain* and *spinal cord*, often abbreviated as CNS. The central nervous system is made up of neurons (nerve cells) and works in tandem with the *peripheral nervous system* (PNS), which carries signals between the CNS and the rest of the body. The CNS is responsible for receiving sensory information from organs such as the eyes and ears, analysing it, and then initiating an appropriate motor response. (See also *nervous system*.)

centrifuge A machine that separates the different components of a body fluid for analysis. When a fluid such as blood is spun at high speed around a central axis, groups of particles of varying density, for example red and white blood cells, are separated by centrifugal force.

cephalexin An alternative spelling of cefalexin, a common *cephalosporin drug*.

cephalhaematoma An extensive, soft swelling on the scalp of a newborn infant, which is caused by bleeding into the space between the *cranium* and its fibrous covering due to pressure on the baby's head during delivery. The swelling is not serious and gradually subsides.

cephalic Relating to the head, as in cephalic presentation, the head-first position of a baby in the birth canal.

cephalopelvic disproportion A complication of childbirth (see *childbirth, complications of*) in which the mother's pelvis is too narrow in proportion to the size of the baby's head.

cephalosporin drugs A large group of *antibiotic drugs* derived from the fungus CEPHALOSPORIUM ACREMONIUM, which are effective against a wide range of infections. Cephalosporins are used to treat ear, throat, and respiratory tract infections, and conditions, such as *urinary tract infections* and *gonorrhoea*, in which the causative bacteria are resistant to other types of antibiotics. Occasionally, the drugs cause allergic reactions, such as rash, itching, and fever. Rarely, *anaphylactic shock* occurs. Other side effects include diarrhoea and *blood disorders*.

cerebellar ataxia Jerky, staggering gait and other uncoordinated movements caused by a disease of or damage to the *cerebellum*. Other features include *dysarthria* (slurred speech), hand tremor, and *nystagmus* (abnormal jerky eye movements). Possible causes include *stroke*, *multiple sclerosis*, a *brain tumour*, damage caused by *alcohol dependence*, and degeneration of the cerebellum due to an inherited disorder.

cerebellum A region of the brain behind the *brainstem* concerned with maintaining posture and balance and coordinating movement. The cerebellum has two hemispheres. From the inner side of each hemisphere arise three nerve fibre stalks, which link up with different parts of the brainstem and carry signals between the cerebellum and the rest of the brain. Nerve fibres from these stalks fan out towards the deep folds of the *cortex* (outer part) of each brain hemisphere, which consists of layers of *grey matter*. Information about the body's posture and the state of contraction or relaxation in its muscles is conveyed from muscle tendons and the labyrinth in the inner ear via the brainstem to the cerebellum. Working with the basal ganglia (nerve cell clusters deep within the brain), the cerebellum uses this data to fine tune messages sent to muscles from the motor cortex in the *cerebrum*.

cerebral haemorrhage Bleeding within the brain due to a ruptured blood vessel (see *intracerebral haemorrhage*; *stroke*.)

cerebral palsy A disorder of posture and movement resulting from damage to a child's developing brain before, during, or immediately after birth, or in early childhood. Cerebral palsy is non-progressive and varies in degree from slight clumsiness of hand movement and gait to complete immobility.

A child with cerebral palsy may have *spastic paralysis* (abnormal stiffness of muscles), *athetosis* (involuntary writhing movements), or *ataxia* (loss of coordination and balance). Other nervous system disorders, such as hearing defects or epileptic seizures, may be present. About 70 per cent of affected children have mental impairment, but the remainder are of normal or high intelligence.

In most cases, damage occurs before or at birth, most commonly as a result of an inadequate supply of oxygen to the brain. More rarely, the cause is a maternal infection spreading to the baby in the uterus. In rare cases, cerebral palsy is due to *kernicterus*. Possible causes after birth include *encephalitis*, *meningitis*, *head injury*, or *intracerebral haemorrhage*.

Cerebral palsy may not be recognized until well into the baby's 1st year. Initially, the infant may have hypotonic (floppy) muscles, be difficult to feed, and show delay in sitting without support.

Although there is no cure for cerebral palsy, much can be done to help affected children using specialized *physiotherapy*, *speech therapy*, and techniques and devices for nonverbal communication.

cerebral thrombosis The formation of a *thrombus* (blood clot) in an artery in the brain. The clot may block the artery, cutting off the supply of blood, nutrients, and oxygen to a region of the brain, causing a *stroke*.

cerebrospinal fluid A clear, watery fluid that circulates between the ventricles (cavities) within the *brain*, the central canal in the *spinal cord*, and the space between the brain and spinal cord and their protective coverings, the *meninges*. Cerebrospinal fluid functions as a shock-absorber, helping to prevent or reduce damage to the brain and spinal cord after a blow to the head or back. It contains glucose, proteins, salts, and white blood cells. Examination of the fluid, usually obtained by *lumbar puncture*, is used to diagnose disorders such as *meningitis*.

cerebrovascular accident Sudden rupture or blockage of a blood vessel in the brain, causing serious bleeding and/or local obstruction to blood circulation, and leading to a *stroke*. Blockage may be due to *thrombosis* or *embolism*. Rupture of vessels may cause *intracerebral haemorrhage* or *subarachnoid haemorrhage*.

cerebrovascular disease Any disease affecting an artery in, and supplying blood to, the brain: for example, *atherosclerosis* (narrowing of the arteries) or defects or weaknesses in arterial walls causing *aneurysm* (a balloon-like swelling in an artery). The disease may eventually cause a *cerebrovascular accident*, which commonly leads to a *stroke*. Extensive narrowing of blood vessels throughout the brain can be a cause of *dementia*.

cerebrum The largest and most developed part of the *brain*, the site of most conscious and intelligent activities. Its main components are two large cerebral hemispheres that grow out from the upper part of the *brainstem*. Their surface is made up of a series of folds called gyri, separated by fissures called sulci, with a deep longitudinal fissure separating the two hemispheres. The four main surface regions of each hemisphere – the frontal, parietal, temporal, and occipital lobes – are named after their overlying bones. Each hemisphere has a central cavity, called a *ventricle*, filled with *cerebrospinal fluid*. This is surrounded by an inner layer, consisting of clusters of nerve cells called the basal ganglia. A middle layer of white matter is composed mainly of nerve fibres, which carry information between specific areas of the *cortex* and between areas of the cortex, central brain, and the brainstem. A thick band of fibres called the corpus callosum carries nerve signals between the two hemispheres.

The outer surface layer of each hemisphere is the cerebral cortex – the grey matter, where much of the sensory information from organs such as the eyes and ears is processed. Specific sensory processing takes place in separate regions. For example, visual perception is located in a part of the occipital lobe called the visual cortex.

The cortex also contains motor areas concerned with the initiation of signals

C

for movement by the skeletal muscles. Linked to the sensory and motor areas of the cortex are association areas, which integrate information from various senses and also perform functions such as comprehension and recognition, memory storage and recall, thought and decision making. Some of these cortical functions are localized to one dominant hemisphere (the left in almost all right-handed and many left-handed people). Two clearly defined areas in the dominant hemisphere are Wernicke's area, responsible for the comprehension of words, and Broca's area, which is concerned with language expression.

CEREBRUM

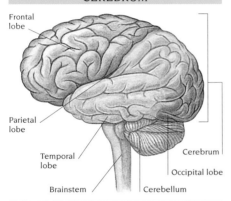

Frontal lobe

Parietal lobe

Temporal lobe

Brainstem

Cerebrum

Occipital lobe

Cerebellum

certification An old term for procedures to commit a person to be compulsorily detained for mental health treatment.

cerumen The substance commonly called *earwax*.

cervical Relating to the neck or the *cervix*.

cervical cancer See *cervix, cancer of*.

cervical dysplasia The former term for *cervical intraepithelial neoplasia*.

cervical ectopy Formerly known as cervical erosion, a benign condition affecting the *cervix* in which a layer of mucus-forming cells more characteristic of those found in the inner lining of the cervix appear on its outside surface. The affected cervix has a fragile, reddened area on the surface. Usually, there are no symptoms, but some women experience bleeding at unexpected times and may have a vaginal discharge.

Cervical ectopy may be present from birth. Other causes include pregnancy and long-term use of *oral contraceptives*. The condition is often detected during a routine *cervical smear test*. Only women who have symptoms need treatment. Abnormal tissue may be destroyed using *cauterization*, *cryosurgery*, *diathermy*, or *laser treatment*.

cervical erosion The former term for *cervical ectopy*.

cervical incompetence Abnormal weakness of the *cervix* that can result in recurrent *miscarriages*. An incompetent cervix may gradually widen under the weight of the fetus from about the 12th week of pregnancy onwards, or may suddenly open during the second trimester. The condition is detected by an internal examination or by *ultrasound scanning*.

Treatment is with a suture (stitch) applied like a purse string around the cervix during the 4th month of pregnancy. The suture is left in position until the pregnancy is at or near full term and is then cut to allow the mother to deliver the baby normally.

cervical intraepithelial neoplasia Also known as CIN (and formerly called cervical dysplasia), abnormalities in the surface cells of the cervix that may become cancerous. There are three grades of CIN, mild (CIN1), moderate (CIN2), and severe (CIN3), based on the severity of the changes seen in cells obtained from a *cervical smear test*. In mild CIN, abnormal cells may return to a normal state without treatment; severe CIN, left untreated, may progress to cervical cancer (see *cervix, cancer of*).

CERVICAL ECTOPY

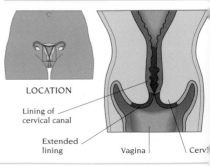

LOCATION

Lining of cervical canal

Extended lining

Vagina

Cerv

The cause of CIN is not known but risk factors include smoking, unprotected sex at an early age or with many partners, and exposure to *human papillomavirus*. Treatment depends on the severity of the condition. Mild CIN may not require treatment because the cells may return to normal, although regular monitoring is necessary. Persistent mild CIN and moderate or severe CIN are treated by destroying or removing the abnormal tissue, either by *cone biopsy* or a method called large loop excision of the transformation zone (LLETZ), which involves using a heated wire loop, passed through the vagina, to remove the abnormal tissue.

cervical mucus method A form of contraception based on identifying periods for abstinence from intercourse according to the changes in the mucus secreted by a woman's *cervix* (see *contraception, natural methods of*).

cervical osteoarthritis A degenerative disorder, also known as cervical spondylosis, that affects the joints between the cervical *vertebrae* (bones in the neck). Cervical osteoarthritis mainly affects middle-aged and elderly people, but occasionally the degeneration begins earlier due to an injury.

Symptoms of cervical osteoarthritis may include pain and stiffness in the neck, pain in the arms and shoulders, numbness and tingling in the hands, and a weak grip. Other symptoms such as dizziness, unsteadiness, and double vision when turning the head may also occur. Rarely, pressure on the spinal cord can cause weakness or paralysis in the legs and loss of bladder control.

Treatments include *heat treatment* and *analgesics*. *Physiotherapy* may improve neck posture and movement. Pressure on the spinal cord may be relieved by surgery (see *decompression, spinal canal*).

cervical rib A *congenital* abnormality in which the lowest of the seven cervical *vertebrae* (neck bones) has overdeveloped to form an extra *rib* parallel to and above the first normal rib. Symptoms may occur if the rib begins to press on the lower *brachial plexus* (the group of nerves passing from the spinal cord into the arm), causing pain, numbness, and pins-and-needles in the forearm and hand. Exercises to

strengthen the shoulder muscles and improve posture may bring relief. Severe or persistent symptoms may require surgery to remove the rib.

cervical smear test A test to detect *cervical intraepithelial neoplasia* (abnormal changes in the cells of the *cervix*) that could develop into cervical cancer (see *cervix, cancer of*). A smear test also detects some infections of the cervix, such as *human papillomavirus*, some types of which cause genital warts. A smear test is routinely carried out every three years for women aged 25–49 and every five years for women aged 50–64.

A sample of cells may be taken from the surface of the cervix using a spatula and examined under a microscope. A newer and more efficient method, known as liquid-based cytology, involves collecting the cell sample using a fine brush; the cells are then transferred from the brush into a liquid and sent for analysis. If the cells appear normal, nothing further needs to be done. If cells show abnormalities, further smears or investigations may be required.

cervical spondylosis An alternative name for *cervical osteoarthritis*.

cervicitis Inflammation of the *cervix*, usually due to an infection, such as *gonorrhoea, chlamydial infections*, genital herpes (see *herpes, genital*), or genital warts (see *warts, genital*). Cervical infection may follow injury to the cervix during childbirth or surgery. The acute form of cervicitis often does not produce symptoms, although there may be a discharge from the inflamed cervix. The chronic form may produce a vaginal discharge, irregular bleeding from the vagina, and pain low in the abdomen. Untreated cervicitis can spread to cause *endometritis, salpingitis*, or *pelvic inflammatory disease*, which may result in infertility or an increased likelihood of *ectopic pregnancy*. If cervicitis is present in the mother, her baby may be infected during delivery, resulting in *neonatal ophthalmia* or, less commonly, *pneumonia* due to chlamydial infection.

Treatment is with *antibiotics* or with *antiviral drugs*. If symptoms persist, the inflamed area of cervix may be cauterized by *electrocoagulation, cryotherapy*, or *laser treatment*.

cervix A small, cylindrical organ comprising the lower part and neck of the *uterus* and separating the body and cavity of the uterus from the *vagina*. The fibrous and smooth muscle tissue of the cervix creates a form of sphincter, which can stretch during pregnancy and childbirth.

The cervical canal runs through the cervix and allows the passage of blood during *menstruation* and of sperm from the vagina into the uterus; it also forms part of the birth canal during childbirth. After puberty, mucus is secreted from the glandular cells in the canal to assist sperm entry into the upper cervix.

CERVIX

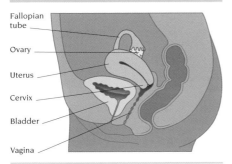

Fallopian tube
Ovary
Uterus
Cervix
Bladder
Vagina

cervix, cancer of One of the most common cancers affecting women worldwide. Cancer of the *cervix* has well-defined precancerous stages (see *cervical intraepithelial neoplasia*) that can be detected by a *cervical smear test*, allowing, in many cases, early treatment and a complete cure. Untreated, cancer of the cervix may spread to the organs in the *pelvis*.

There are two main types of cervical cancer: the squamous type is the most common and is associated with the *human papillomavirus*, acquired during sexual intercourse. Factors that predispose to this type of cancer are smoking, starting to have sex at an early age, and having many sexual partners. The second, rarer, type of cervical cancer, adenocarcinoma, sometimes occurs in women who have never had sexual intercourse. Its causes are unclear.

Symptoms do not develop until the condition is advanced, when there is vaginal bleeding or a bloodstained discharge at unexpected times, and pain if the cancer has spread within the pelvis.

Following an abnormal smear test result, *colposcopy* or a *cone biopsy* may be carried out to diagnose the condition. Early cancer may be treated by surgery to remove or destroy the abnormal tissue. In more advanced cases affecting the pelvic organs, *radiotherapy* and *chemotherapy* may be given. Radical surgery, in which the bladder, vagina, cervix, uterus, and rectum are removed, may be recommended in certain cases.

A vaccine against human papillomavirus is being developed that will provide protection against strains of the virus associated with cervical cancer.

cervix, disorders of The *cervix* is susceptible to injuries, infections, tumours, and other conditions. Minor injury to the cervix may occur during childbirth, particularly if labour is prolonged. Persistent damage to muscle fibres as a result of injury may lead to *cervical incompetence*. *Cervical ectopy* is a condition in which mucus-secreting cells form on the outside of the cervix.

The most common cervical infections are sexually transmitted, such as *gonorrhoea*, *chlamydial infections*, and *trichomoniasis*. Viral infections of the cervix include those due to the *human papillomavirus* and the herpes simplex virus (see *warts, genital; herpes, genital*).

Polyps are noncancerous growths on the cervix. Cancerous growths (see *cervix, cancer of*) are preceded by changes in the surface cells (*cervical intraepithelial neoplasia*), which can be detected by a *cervical smear test*.

cestodes The scientific name for tapeworms (see *tapeworm infestation*).

cetirizine An *antihistamine drug* used to relieve the symptoms of conditions such as allergic *rhinitis* (hay fever) and *urticaria*.

cetrimide An *antiseptic* used in preparations for cleansing the skin.

Chagas' disease An infectious parasitic disease found only in parts of South and Central America that is spread by insects commonly called cone-nosed or assassin bugs. The *parasites* live in the bloodstream and can affect the heart, intestines, and nervous system. Symptoms include swelling of the lymph nodes

C

and fever. Long-term complications include damage to the heart. The drug nifurtimox kills the parasites in the blood but has unpleasant side effects.

chalazion A round, painless swelling in the upper or lower eyelid caused by obstruction of one of the meibomian glands that lubricate the edge of the eyelids. Chalazions are also known as meibomian cysts. They are particularly common in people suffering from *acne, rosacea*, or seborrhoeic *dermatitis*. If the cyst becomes infected the eyelid becomes more swollen, red, and painful. A large swelling putting pressure on the *cornea* at the front of the eye can cause blurred vision. About a third of chalazions disappear without treatment, but large cysts may need to be removed surgically.

chancre, hard An *ulcer*, usually on the genitals, that develops during the first stage of *syphilis*.

chancroid A sexually transmitted disease, found mainly in the tropics, characterized by painful *ulcers* on the genitals and enlarged lymph nodes in the groin. The disorder is caused by the bacterium *HAEMOPHILUS DUCREYI*. Prompt treatment with *antibiotic drugs* is usually effective.

chapped skin Sore, cracked, rough skin, usually on the hands, face, and lips. It is caused by the lack, or removal, of the natural oils that keep skin supple. It tends to occur in cold weather, when oil-secreting glands produce less oil, or after repeated washing or wetting. Treatment is with a lanolin-based cream.

charcoal A form of carbon used in medicine mainly as an adsorbent agent in the emergency treatment of some types of poisoning and drug overdose.

Charcot–Marie–Tooth disease An inherited muscle-wasting disease of the legs (see *peroneal muscular atrophy*).

Charcot's joint A joint that is repeatedly damaged by injuries that have gone unnoticed because of loss of sensation in the joint (see *neuropathic joint*).

cheilitis Inflammation, cracking, and dryness of the lips that may be caused by ill-fitting dentures, a local infection, allergy to cosmetics, excessive sunbathing, or deficiency of riboflavin (vitamin B_2).

chelating agents Chemicals used in the treatment of metal poisoning that act by combining with metals such as lead, arsenic, and mercury to form less poisonous substances. *Penicillamine* is a commonly used chelating agent.

chemotherapy The term that usually describes the use of drugs to treat *cancer* but which may also describe the use of *antibiotics* to treat infectious diseases. Chemotherapy works by destroying bacteria or cancer cells or by preventing them from multiplying. Cancer chemotherapy drugs may also have effects on normal tissue such as bone marrow, the intestinal lining, the hair follicles, the ovaries and testes, and the mouth, sometimes causing severe side effects.

chenodeoxycholic acid A chemical in *bile* that reduces the amount of *cholesterol* released by the *liver* into the bile.

chest The upper part of the trunk. Known technically as the *thorax*, the chest extends from the base of the neck down to the *diaphragm*.

chest compression Also called cardiac compression massage (see *cardiopulmonary resuscitation*).

chest pain Pain in the chest, which is often without serious cause, but which may be a symptom of an underlying disorder requiring urgent treatment. The pain may be in the chest wall or in an organ within the chest. The most common causes of pain in the chest wall are a strained muscle or an injury, such as a broken rib. A sharp pain that travels to the front of the chest may be due to pressure on a nerve root attached to the spinal cord as a result of, for example, *osteoarthritis* of the *vertebrae*. Pain in the side of the chest may be due to *pleurodynia*. The viral infection *herpes zoster* (shingles) may cause severe pain along the course of a nerve in the chest wall. In *Tietze's syndrome*, inflammation at the junctions of the rib cartilages causes pain on the front of the chest wall.

Pain within the chest may be caused by *pleurisy*, as a result of *bronchitis, pneumonia*, or, rarely, *pulmonary embolism*. Cancerous tumours of the lung (see *lung cancer; mesothelioma*) may cause pain as they grow and press on the *pleura* and ribs. *Gastro-oesophageal reflux disease* may lead to heartburn, a burning pain behind the sternum.

C

The common heart disorder *angina pectoris* causes pain in the centre of the chest that may spread outwards to the throat, jaw, or arms. *Myocardial infarction* (heart attack) and acute *pericarditis* both also produce severe pain in the centre of the chest. *Mitral valve prolapse* may cause sharp chest pain, usually on the left side. Chest pain may also be a result of *anxiety* and emotional stress (see *hyperventilation*; *panic attack*).

chest thrust A first aid technique to unblock the airway in cases of *choking*, when abdominal thrusts would be dangerous (such as in infants) or impossible (such as in pregnant women). In a chest thrust, the first-aider places a fist in the other hand, and, pressing against the victim's lower breastbone, thrusts the chest wall inwards up to five times. The pressure simulates the coughing reflex and may expel the obstruction.

CHEST X-RAY

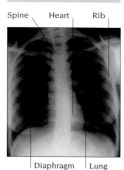

Spine | Heart | Rib

Diaphragm | Lung

chest X-ray One of the most frequently performed medical tests, usually carried out to examine the heart or lungs to confirm diagnoses of heart disorders and lung diseases. (See also *X-rays*.)

Cheyne–Stokes respiration An abnormal pattern of breathing in which the rate and depth of respiration varies. Cheyne-Stokes respiration is characterized by repeated cycles, lasting a few minutes, of deep, rapid breathing that becomes slower and shallower and then stops for 10–20 seconds. The pattern may be due to malfunction of the part of the brain that controls breathing (as occurs in some cases of *stroke* and *head injury*). It may also occur as a result of *heart failure* or in healthy people at high altitudes, especially during sleep.

chickenpox A common, mild infectious disease (also called varicella) occurring in childhood and characterized by a rash and slight fever. In adults, chickenpox is rare but usually more severe. An attack gives lifelong immunity, but the virus remains dormant in nerves and may reappear later in life to cause *herpes zoster* (shingles). The cause of chickenpox is the varicella-zoster virus, which is spread in airborne droplets. A widespread rash develops 2–3 weeks after infection, consisting of clusters of small, red, itchy spots that become fluid-filled blisters within a few hours. After several days the blisters dry out to form scabs. Scratching the blisters can lead to secondary infection and scarring. *Paracetamol* helps reduce fever and *calamine* lotion may be used to relieve itching. In severe cases, *aciclovir* (an antiviral drug) may be prescribed.

chigoe A painful, itchy, pea-sized swelling caused by a sand flea that lives in sandy soil in Africa and tropical America. The flea penetrates the skin of the feet and lays eggs. Chigoe fleas should be removed with a sterile needle, and the wounds treated with an antiseptic.

chilblain An itchy, purple-red swelling, usually on a toe or finger, caused by excessive constriction of small blood vessels below the surface of the skin in cold weather. Chilblains are most common in the young and the elderly, and women are more susceptible to them. They generally heal without treatment

child abuse The maltreatment of children. Child abuse may take the form of physical injury, sexual abuse, emotional mistreatment, and/or neglect; it occurs at all levels of society. Being deprived or ill-treated in childhood may predispose people to repeat the pattern of abuse with their own children. Children who are abused or at risk of abuse may be placed in care while the health and social services decide on the best course of action.

childbed fever See *puerperal fever*.

childbirth The process by which an infant leaves the *uterus* and enters the outside world. Childbirth (*labour*) normally takes place between 38 and 42 weeks of pregnancy and occurs in three stages.

The onset of the first stage of labour is marked by regular contractions which become progressively more painful, and occur at shorter intervals. The *cervix* becomes thinned and softened and then

CHILDBIRTH

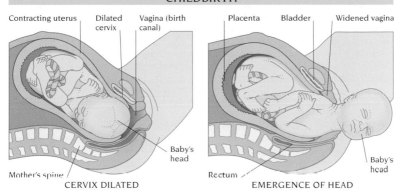

Contracting uterus | Dilated cervix | Vagina (birth canal)

Baby's head

Mother's spine

CERVIX DILATED

Placenta | Bladder | Widened vagina

Baby's head

Rectum

EMERGENCE OF HEAD

C

begins to dilate with each contraction. During this time, there may be a "show", the mucous plug that blocks the cervical canal during pregnancy is expelled as a bloody discharge. "Breaking of the waters", the rupture of the *amniotic sac*, may occur as a slow trickle of fluid or a sudden gush. The cervix is fully dilated when the opening has widened to about 10 cm in diameter. This may take 12 hours or more for a first baby, but only a few hours for subsequent babies.

In the second stage of labour, the woman feels the urge to push with each strong contraction. As the baby's head descends into the *vagina*, it rotates to face the mother's back. The *perineum* is stretched thin at this stage, and an *episiotomy* may be performed to prevent it from tearing. Once the baby's head is delivered, the rest of the body follows with the next contractions. After delivery, the *umbilical cord* is clamped and cut.

In the third stage of labour, the delivery of the placenta takes place.

The various forms of pain relief available during normal labour and delivery include opioid *analgesic drugs*, *epidural anaesthesia*, and *pudendal block*.

childbirth, complications of Difficulties and problems occurring after the onset of *labour*. Some complications are potentially life-threatening, especially if they impair the baby's oxygen supply (see *fetal distress*). Premature labour may occur, with the delivery of a small, immature baby (see *prematurity*). Pre-

mature rupture of the *amniotic sac* can lead to infection in the *uterus*, requiring prompt delivery of the baby and treatment with *antibiotic drugs*.

Slow progress in the first stage of a normal labour due to inadequate contractions of the uterus is usually treated with intravenous infusions of synthetic *oxytocin*. If the mother cannot push strongly enough, or contractions are ineffective in the second stage of labour, the baby may be delivered by *forceps delivery*, *vacuum extraction*, or *caesarean section*. Rarely, a woman has *eclampsia* during labour, requiring treatment with *anticonvulsant drugs* and oxygen, and *induction of labour* or caesarean section.

Bleeding before labour (*antepartum haemorrhage*) or during labour may be due to premature separation of the *placenta* from the wall of the uterus or, less commonly, to a condition called *placenta praevia*, in which the placenta lies over the opening of the *cervix*. Blood loss after the delivery (*postpartum haemorrhage*) is usually due to failure of the uterus to contract after delivery, or to retention of part of the placenta. If the baby lies in the breech position (see *breech delivery*), caesarean section may be necessary. Multiple pregnancies (see *pregnancy, multiple*) have an increased risk of premature labour and problems during delivery. If the mother's pelvis is too small in proportion to her baby's head, delivery by caesarean section is necessary.

C

childbirth, natural The use of relaxation and other techniques to help cope with pain and minimize the use of drugs and medical intervention during childbirth.

child development The acquisition of physical, mental, and social skills in children. Although there is wide variation in individual rates of progress, most children develop certain skills within predictable age ranges. For example, most infants start to walk at 12–18 months. Capability for new skills is linked to the maturity of the child's nervous system. Individual rates of maturity are determined genetically and modified by environmental factors in the *uterus* and after birth. Development is assessed in early childhood by looking at abilities in four main areas: locomotion; hearing and speech; vision and fine movement; and social behaviour and play. (See also *developmental delay*.)

child guidance A multidisciplinary diagnosis and advice team service for children suffering from emotional or behavioural problems (see *behavioural problems in children*). Indications of problems include poor performance at school, disruptive or withdrawn behaviour, and *drug abuse*.

Child guidance professionals include psychiatrists, psychologists, and psychiatric social workers. For young children, *play therapy* may be used for diagnosis. Older children may be offered *counselling*, *psychotherapy*, or *group therapy*. *Family therapy* may be used in cases where there are difficulties between the child and one or both parents.

chill A shivering attack accompanied by chattering teeth, pale skin, goose pimples, and feeling cold. Chill frequently precedes a fever. Repeated or severe shivering suggests serious illness.

Chinese medicine Traditional Chinese medicine is generally based on the theory that a universal life-force, called chi, manifests itself in the body as two complementary qualities that are known as *yin and yang*. According to this belief, vigorous yang and restraining yin must be in balance, and the chi must flow evenly for good health. Treatments for illness aim to restore the yin-yang balance and normalize the flow of chi using techniques such as Chinese *herbal medicine*, *acupressure*, *acupuncture*, and *t'ai chi*.

chiropody The examination, diagnosis, treatment, and prevention of diseases and malfunctions of the foot and its related structures.

chiropractic A complementary treatment for a range of disorders, including *back pain*, based on manipulation of the spine.

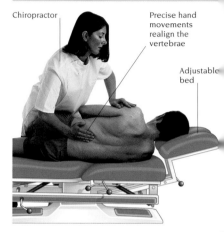

CHIROPRACTIC

Chiropractor

Precise hand movements realign the vertebrae

Adjustable bed

chlamydial infections Infectious diseases caused by chlamydiae, a group of microorganisms. Two main species of chlamydiae cause disease in humans.

The first, CHLAMYDIA TRACHOMATIS, has several strains. In men, it is a major cause of *nongonococcal urethritis*, which may cause a discharge from the penis. In women, the infection is usually symptomless, but without treatment it can lead to *pelvic inflammatory disease*, which in turn may result in *ectopic pregnancy*, *miscarriage*, or infertility. A baby born to a woman with chlamydial infection may acquire an acute eye condition called neonatal *ophthalmia*. In parts of Africa and Asia, certain strains of CHLAMYDIA TRACHOMATIS cause *trachoma*, a serious eye disease.

A second species of chlamydiae, CHLAMYDIA PSITTACI, mainly affects birds but may spread to people who have contact with pigeons, parrots, or poultry, causing a type of pneumonia called *psittacosis*.

Treatment for chlamydial infections is with *antibiotic drugs*.

C

chloasma A condition, also called melasma, in which blotches of pale brown pigmentation appear on the forehead, cheeks, and nose. The pigmentation is aggravated by sunlight. Chloasma sometimes develops during pregnancy. More rarely, it is associated with the menopause or use of *oral contraceptives*. The condition usually fades but may recur.

chlorambucil An *anticancer drug* used to treat some types of cancer, for example *Hodgkin's disease*.

chloramphenicol An *antibiotic* commonly used in the form of drops to treat superficial eye infections. It is also used to treat life-threatening infections when the causative organism is unknown. Rarely, tablets or injections are associated with aplastic *anaemia*.

chlorate poisoning The toxic effects of chemicals present in some defoliant weedkillers. Ingesting chlorates can cause kidney and liver damage, corrosion of the intestine, and methaemoglobinaemia (a chemical change in *haemoglobin* in the blood). Small doses of chlorates can prove fatal. Symptoms of poisoning include ulceration in the mouth, abdominal pain, and diarrhoea.

chlordiazepoxide A *benzodiazepine drug* mainly used to treat *anxiety*.

chlorhexidine A type of disinfectant mainly used to cleanse the skin before surgery or before taking a blood sample.

chlorine A poisonous, yellowish-green gas with powerful bleaching and disinfecting properties. Inhaling even small amounts is highly irritating to the lungs; large amounts are rapidly fatal.

chloroform A colourless liquid producing a vapour that was formerly used as a general anaesthetic (see *anaesthesia, general*). Chloroform is associated with liver damage and heart problems, and safer drugs are now used instead.

chloroquine A drug used mainly in the prevention and treatment of *malaria*. It is also a *disease-modifying antirheumatic drug* used to treat systemic *lupus erythematosus* and *rheumatoid arthritis*. Possible side effects include nausea, headache, diarrhoea, rashes, and abdominal pain. Long-term use may damage the retina.

chlorphenamine An *antihistamine drug* used to treat allergies such as allergic *rhinitis* (hay fever), allergic *conjunctivitis*, *urticaria*, and *angioedema*. It is also found in some *cold remedies*.

chlorpheniramine An alternative name for *chlorphenamine*.

chlorpromazine A widely prescribed *antipsychotic* drug used to relieve symptoms of major psychotic illnesses such as *schizophrenia* and *mania*. The drug reduces delusional and hallucinatory experiences and may have an effect on irritability and overactivity. It is also used as an antiemetic. Chlorpromazine may cause photosensitivity of the skin and, in some cases, *parkinsonism*, slow reactions, and blurred vision.

chlorpropamide A drug that is used to treat *diabetes mellitus* (see *hypoglycaemics, oral*).

choanal atresia A *congenital* defect of the *nose* in which one or both of the nasal cavities are not fully developed.

choking Partial or complete inability to breathe due to an obstruction of the airways. Choking is often due to food or drink entering the *trachea* and bronchi instead of passing from the *pharynx* into the *oesophagus*. Coughing normally dislodges the food or drink. An obstruction that partially blocks the airway and cannot be dislodged by coughing is more serious. If the airway is completely blocked, total suffocation will result if the blockage is not removed. If an obstruction cannot be cleared by first aid techniques, such as the *Heimlich manoeuvre* or removed manually, an emergency *tracheostomy* may be performed to restore the airway before removal of the obstruction with instruments.

cholangiocarcinoma A cancerous tumour in one of the *bile ducts*, which causes jaundice and weight loss.

cholangiography A procedure that uses a *contrast medium* to make *bile ducts* visible on *X-rays*. Cholangiography is used to look for biliary stones or to diagnose narrowing or tumours of the bile ducts.

cholangitis Inflammation of the common bile duct (see *biliary system*). There are two types: acute ascending cholangitis and sclerosing cholangitis. Acute ascending cholangitis is usually due to bacterial

C

infection of the duct and its bile, generally as a result of blockage of the duct by, for example, a gallstone (see bile *duct obstruction*). The infection spreads up the duct and may affect the liver. The main symptoms are recurrent bouts of jaundice, abdominal pain, chills, and fever. Mild attacks are treated with *antibiotics* and a high intake of fluids. In severe, life-threatening attacks, which may be accompanied by *septicaemia* and *kidney failure*, the infected material may be drained from the bile duct by surgery or *endoscopy*.

Sclerosing cholangitis is a rare condition in which all the bile ducts within and outside the liver become narrowed. The condition causes *cholestasis*, chronic jaundice, and itching of the skin. The liver is progressively damaged. *Colestyramine* may relieve itching. The only other treatment available is a *liver transplant*.

chole- A prefix that means relating to the *bile* or the *biliary system*.

cholecalciferol An alternative name for *colecalciferol*, also known as vitamin D_3 (see *vitamin D*).

cholecystectomy Surgery to remove the *gallbladder*, usually to deal with *gallstones*. Cholecystectomy is also used in acute *cholecystitis* and as an emergency treatment for perforation of the gallbladder or *empyema*. The procedure is carried out using conventional surgery or, more commonly, by *minimally invasive surgery* using a *laparoscope*.

cholecystitis Acute or chronic inflammation of the *gallbladder*, causing severe abdominal pain. Acute cholecystitis is usually caused by a *gallstone* obstructing the outlet from the gallbladder. The trapped bile causes irritation of the gallbladder walls and may become infected by bacteria. The main symptom is severe constant pain in the right side of the abdomen under the ribs, accompanied by fever and, occasionally, *jaundice*. Treatment is usually with *analgesic drugs*, *antibiotic drugs*, and an intravenous infusion of nutrients and fluids. In some cases, complications develop, which may include *peritonitis*, if the gallbladder bursts, and *empyema*. Both require urgent surgical treatment.

Repeated mild attacks of acute cholecystitis can lead to a chronic form, in which the gallbladder shrinks, its walls thicken, and it ceases to store bile. Symptoms (indigestion, pains in the upper abdomen, nausea, and belching) may be aggravated by eating fatty food. *Cholecystectomy* is the usual treatment.

cholecystography An X-ray procedure that uses a *contrast medium* to examine the *gallbladder* and common *bile duct*, usually to detect *gallstones*. Cholecystography has largely been replaced by *ultrasound scanning* of the gallbladder.

cholecystokinin A *gastrointestinal hormone* produced in the *duodenum* in response to the ingestion of fats and other food substances. It stimulates the release of bile from the *gallbladder* and digestive enzymes from the *pancreas*, thus facilitating the digestive process.

cholera An infection of the small intestine by the bacterium VIBRIO CHOLERAE causing profuse watery diarrhoea, which can lead to dehydration and death. Infection is acquired by ingesting contaminated food or water. Outbreaks of cholera occur regularly in northeast India, but worldwide the disease is controlled by sanitation. Treatment is with water containing salts and sugar (see *rehydration therapy*) and, in severe cases, intravenous infusion. *Antibiotic drugs* can shorten the period of diarrhoea and infectiousness. With adequate rehydration, affected people usually make a full recovery from the infection. Oral cholera vaccination is available for travellers to endemic areas.

cholestasis Stagnation of *bile* in the small *bile ducts* within the liver, leading to *jaundice* and liver disease. The obstruction to the flow of bile may be intrahepatic (within the liver) or extrahepatic (in the bile ducts outside the liver). Intrahepatic cholestasis may occur as a result of viral hepatitis (see *hepatitis, viral*) or as a side effect of a number of drugs. The flow of bile improves gradually as the inflammation from the hepatitis resolves or the drug is discontinued. The bile ducts outside the liver can become obstructed by, for example, gallstones or tumours (see *bile duct obstruction*); rarely, the ducts are absent from birth (see *biliary atresia*). Bile duct obstruction and biliary atresia are often treated surgically.

cholesteatoma A rare but serious condition in which skin cells proliferate and grow inwards from the ear canal into the middle ear. Cholesteatoma usually occurs as a result of long-standing *otitis media* together with a defect in the eardrum (see *eardrum, perforated*). Left untreated, it may damage the small bones in the middle ear and other structures. Cholesteatoma needs to be removed surgically through the eardrum or by *mastoidectomy*.

cholesterol A fat-like substance that is an important constituent of body cells and is also involved in the formation of hormones and bile salts. Cholesterol in the blood is made by the liver from foods, especially saturated fats, although a small amount is absorbed directly from cholesterol-rich foods such as eggs. High blood cholesterol levels increase the risk of *atherosclerosis*, and with it the risk of *coronary artery disease* or *stroke*. In general cholesterol transported in the blood in the form of low-density lipoproteins (LDLs) or very low-density lipoproteins (VLDLs) is a risk factor for these conditions, while cholesterol in the form of high-density lipoproteins (HDLs) seems to protect against arterial disease. Blood cholesterol levels are influenced by diet, weight, heredity, and metabolic diseases such as *diabetes mellitus*, and can be measured by blood tests. Levels below 5.0 mmol/L are acceptable; higher levels may require further tests. Dietary changes (including reducing saturated fat intake and eating oily fish) and exercise can lower cholesterol; drugs such as *simvastatin* achieve a greater reduction.

cholestyramine An alternative spelling for *colestyramine*.

chondritis Inflammation of a *cartilage*, usually caused by pressure, stress, or injury. Costochondritis is inflammation affecting the cartilage between the ribs and the sternum (breastbone).

chondro- A prefix denoting a relationship to *cartilage*, as in chondrocyte, a cell that produces cartilage.

chondroma A noncancerous tumour composed of *cartilage*, affecting the bones. Chondromas most often occur in the hands and feet (see *chondromatosis*).

chondromalacia patellae A painful disorder of the knee in which the cartilage behind the patella (kneecap) is damaged. Adolescents are most commonly affected. The condition may result from knee injuries or sporting activities in which the knee is bent for long periods. This action weakens the inner part of the quadriceps muscle (at the front of the thigh) causing the patella to tilt when the knee is straightened and rub against the lower end of the *femur*. The cartilage that covers both bones becomes roughened, causing pain and tenderness. Treatment is with *analgesic drugs* and exercises to strengthen the thigh muscles. Rarely, surgery may be needed.

chondromatosis A condition in which multiple noncancerous tumours, called *chondromas*, arise in the bones, most commonly the bones of the hands and feet. The tumours consist of *cartilage* cells and usually cause no symptoms.

chondrosarcoma A cancerous growth of *cartilage* occurring within or on the surface of large bones, causing pain and swelling. Usually occurring in middle age, the tumour develops slowly from a noncancerous tumour (see *chondroma; dyschondroplasia*) or from normal bone. *Amputation* of the bone above the tumour usually results in a permanent cure.

chordee Abnormal curvature of the penis, usually downwards. Chordee mainly occurs in males with *hypospadias*, a birth defect in which the urethral opening lies on the underside of the penis. Corrective surgery is usually performed between the ages of 1 and 3 years.

chorea A condition characterized by irregular, rapid, jerky movements, usually affecting the face, limbs, and trunk. It is a feature of *Huntington's disease* and *Sydenham's chorea*, and may occur in pregnancy. Chorea may also be a side effect of certain drugs, including *oral contraceptives*; certain drugs for psychiatric disorders; and drugs for treating *Parkinson's disease*. Symptoms usually disappear when the drug is withdrawn. Underlying causes of chorea are treated with drugs that inhibit nerve pathways concerned with movement.

choreoathetosis A condition in which the jerky, uncontrolled movements characteristic of *chorea* are combined with the slower, continuous writhing move-

C

ments of *athetosis*. Choreoathetosis occurs in children with *cerebral palsy* and as a side effect of certain drugs.

choriocarcinoma A rare cancerous *tumour* that develops from *placental* tissue in the uterus, usually as a complication of a *hydatidiform mole* (a noncancerous tumour) but sometimes after a normal pregnancy or a miscarriage. Untreated, it destroys the walls of the uterus and may spread to the vagina and vulva and, eventually, to the liver, lungs, brain, and bones. Successful treatment relies on early diagnosis.

If a woman has a hydatidiform mole, she is screened regularly after treatment using *ultrasound scanning* and tests to measure blood and urine levels of the hormone human chorionic gonadotrophin (HCG). High levels of HCG are associated with choreocarcinoma. Treatment is with *anticancer drugs*.

chorion One of the two membranes that surround the *embryo*. The chorion lies outside the *amnion*, has small finger-like projections called the chorionic villi, and develops into the *placenta*.

chorionic villus sampling A method of diagnosing genetic abnormalities in a *fetus* using a small sample of tissue taken from the chorionic *villi* at edge of the *placenta*. Because the cells have the same chromosome makeup as those in the fetus, they can be used to detect genetic abnormalities. Chorionic villus sampling (CVS) is performed between the 10th and 13th weeks in women who are at a higher-than-normal risk of having a child with a chromosomal disorder, such as *Down's syndrome*, or a genetic disease, such as *thalassaemia*. *Chromosome analysis* of the villi cells takes place in the laboratory. CVS slightly increases the risk of *miscarriage*.

choroid A layer of tissue at the back of the eye, behind the *retina*. The choroid contains many blood vessels that supply nutrients and oxygen to the retinal cells and to surrounding tissues in the eye.

choroiditis Inflammation of the *choroid*. It is often caused by infections such as *toxocariasis* or *toxoplasmosis*, more rarely by *sarcoidosis*, *syphilis*, and *histoplasmosis*. It sometimes has no obvious cause. Treatment includes *corticosteroid drugs*

for the inflammation, and *antibiotic drugs* for any causative infection.

choroid plexus A network of thin-walled blood vessels in the *eye* or *brain*. The choroid plexus of the eye supplies blood to the *retina*. In the brain, the choroid plexus lines the *ventricles* and produces *cerebrospinal fluid*.

Christmas disease A rare genetic bleeding disorder in which there is deficient production of one of the proteins in blood needed for blood coagulation (see *blood clotting*). Christmas disease has similar features to *haemophilia*.

chromium A metallic element that has a vital role in the activities of several *enzymes* in the body. Chromium is required only in minute amounts (see *trace elements*). In excess, chromium is toxic and produces inflammation of the skin and, if inhaled, damages the nose and may increase the risk of lung cancer.

chromosomal abnormalities Variations from normal in the number or structure of *chromosomes* contained in a person's cells. The cause is generally a fault in the process of chromosome division, either during the formation of an egg or sperm, or during the first few divisions of a fertilized egg. Chromosomal abnormalities are classified according to whether they involve the 44 *autosomes* or the two X and Y sex chromosomes. A complete extra set of chromosomes per cell is called polyploidy and is lethal.

Autosomal abnormalities cause physical and mental defects of varying severity. Some types of autosomal abnormality, known as trisomy, consist of an extra chromosome on one of the 22 pairs of autosomes. The most common trisomy is *Down's syndrome*. Sometimes, part of a chromosome is missing, as in *cri du chat syndrome*. In *translocation*, a part of a chromosome is joined to another, causing no ill effects in the person but a risk of abnormality in his or her children.

Sex chromosome abnormalities include *Turner's syndrome*, in which a girl is born with a single X chromosome in her cells instead of two, causing physical abnormalities, defective sexual development, and infertility. A boy with one or more extra X chromosomes has *Klinefelter's syndrome*, which causes defective sexual development and infertility. The presence of an extra X chromosome in women or an extra Y chromosome in men normally has no physical effect but increases the risk of mild learning difficulties.

Chromosomal abnormalities are diagnosed by *chromosome analysis* in early pregnancy, using *amniocentesis* or *chorionic villus sampling*.

chromosome analysis Study of the *chromosomes* in body cells to discover whether a *chromosomal abnormality* is present or to establish its nature. Fetal cells for analysis can be obtained in the uterus by *amniocentesis* or *chorionic villus sampling*. If a serious abnormality such as *Down's syndrome* is identified, termination of the pregnancy and *genetic counselling* is offered. Chromosome analysis is also carried out when a baby is stillborn without an obvious cause, or is born with abnormal physical characteristics that suggest a chromosomal defect, such as *Turner's sydrome*.

Chromosome analysis in children and adults uses white blood cells taken from a blood sample. Analysis of the sex chromosomes may be carried out to establish the chromosomal sex of a child in cases where the genitals have an ambiguous appearance (see *genitalia, ambiguous*); to confirm or exclude the diagnosis of *chromosomal abnormalities*; or to investigate *infertility*.

chromosomes Thread-like structures in the nuclei of cells. Chromosomes carry inherited information in the form of genes, which govern all cell activity and function. Each chromosome contains up to several thousand genes arranged in single file along a long double filament of *DNA*. The sequence of chemical units, or bases, in the DNA provides the coded instructions for cellular activities.

All an individual's body cells (with the exception of egg or sperm cells) carry precisely the same chromosomal material copied by a process of *cell division* from the original material in the fertilized egg. Each human cell normally contains 46 chromosomes made up of 23 pairs. Half of each pair is of maternal and half of paternal origin. 22 pairs are autosomal chromosomes, which are the same in both sexes; the remaining pair is made up

of two sex chromosomes. In females, the sex chromosomes are a pair of X chromosomes. In males, one is an X chromosome and the other is a Y chromosome. One sex chromosome (an X) originates from the mother's egg and the other (an X in girls; a Y in boys) from the father's sperm.

CHROMOSOMES

Chromosome pair

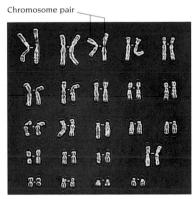

SET OF HUMAN CHROMOSOMES

chronic A term describing a disorder or set of symptoms that has persisted for a long time. A chronic illness implies a continuing disease process with little change in symptoms from day to day. (See also *acute*.)

chronic fatigue syndrome Also known as ME or myalgic encephalomyelitis, a condition causing extreme fatigue over a prolonged period, often over years.

The cause of the condition is unclear. In some cases, it develops after recovery from a viral infection or after an emotional life event such as bereavement. In other cases, there is no such preceding illness or event. The main symptom is persistent, overwhelming tiredness. Other symptoms of the syndrome vary, but commonly include impairment of short-term memory or concentration, sore throat, tender lymph nodes, muscle and joint pain, muscle fatigue, unrefreshing sleep, and headaches. The syndrome is often associated with *depression* or *anxiety*.

There is no specific test; investigations are usually aimed at excluding other

C

possible causes of the symptoms, such as *anaemia*. A physical examination, blood tests, and psychological assessment may be carried out. If no cause can be found, diagnosis is made from the symptoms. There is no known cure but commonly tried treatments include graded exercise and *cognitive-behavioural therapy*. Antidepressants may also sometimes be prescribed. Chronic fatigue syndrome is a long-term disorder, but symptoms may clear up after several years.

chronic obstructive pulmonary disease See *pulmonary disease, chronic obstructive*.

ciclosporin An *immunosuppressant drug* used following *transplant surgery*. The drug reduces the risk of tissue rejection and the need for large doses of *corticosteroid drugs*. It may need to be taken indefinitely after a transplant. It is also a *disease-modifying antirheumatic drug* and is used to treat *rheumatoid arthritis* and other *autoimmune disorders*. In addition, ciclosporin may be used in the treatment of severe *eczema* and *psoriasis*. Because ciclosporin suppresses the immune system, it increases susceptibility to infection. Swollen gums and increased hair growth are fairly common side effects. The drug may also cause kidney damage, and regular monitoring of kidney function is required.

cilia Hair-like filaments on the surface of some epithelial cells (see *epithelium*). Cilia are found particularly in the linings of the respiratory tract, where they propel dust and mucus out of the airways.

ciliary body A structure in the *eye* containing muscles that alter the shape of the lens to adjust focus. (See also *accommodation*.)

cimetidine An H_2-receptor antagonist used as an *ulcer-healing drug*. It promotes healing of gastric and duodenal ulcers (see *peptic ulcer*) and reduces symptoms of *oesophagitis*. Side effects include dizziness, fatigue, and, more rarely, erectile dysfunction and *gynaecomastia*.

CIN The abbreviation for *cervical intraepithelial neoplasia*.

cinnarizine An *antihistamine drug* used to control nausea and vomiting due to travel sickness or to reduce nausea and vertigo in inner-ear disorders, such as *labyrinthitis* and *Ménière's disease*. High doses are sometimes used to improve circulation in *peripheral vascular disease* and *Raynaud's disease*. Side effects may include drowsiness, lethargy, dry mouth, and blurred vision.

ciprofibrate A *lipid-lowering* drug that reduces levels of *cholesterol* and *triglycerides* in the blood and is a treatment for some types of *hyperlipidaemia*.

ciprofloxacin An *antibacterial drug* used mainly to treat infections of the respiratory, gastrointestinal, and urinary tracts.

circadian rhythms Any biological pattern based on a cycle approximately 24 hours long, also called a diurnal rhythm. (See also *biorhythms*.)

circulation, disorders of Conditions affecting blood flow around the body (see *arteries, disorders of; veins, disorders of*).

circulatory system The *heart* and *blood vessels*, which together maintain a continuous flow of blood throughout the body. The system provides tissues with oxygen and nutrients, and carries away waste products. The circulatory system consists of two main parts: the systemic circulation, which supplies blood to the whole body apart from the lungs; and the pulmonary circulation to the lungs. Within the systemic circulation, there is a bypass (the portal circulation), which carries nutrient-rich blood from the stomach, intestine, and other digestive organs to the liver for processing, storage, or re-entry into general circulation.

In the systemic circulation, oxygen-rich blood from the pulmonary circulation is pumped under high pressure from the left *ventricle* of the heart into the *aorta*, from where it travels through arteries and smaller arterioles to all parts of the body. Within body tissues, the arterioles branch into networks of fine blood vessels called capillaries. Oxygen and other nutrients pass from the blood through the capillaries' thin walls into body tissues; carbon dioxide and other wastes pass in the opposite direction. Deoxygenated blood is returned to the heart via venules, veins, and the *venae cavae*.

Venous blood returns to the right atrium of the heart to enter the pulmonary circulation. It is pumped from the right ventricle through the pulmonary artery to the lungs, where carbon dioxide is exchanged for oxygen. The reoxygenated blood then returns through the pulmonary veins to the heart and re-enters the systemic circulation.

CIRCULATORY SYSTEM

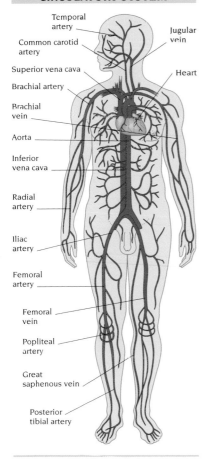

Temporal artery
Jugular vein
Common carotid artery
Superior vena cava
Heart
Brachial artery
Brachial vein
Aorta
Inferior vena cava
Radial artery
Iliac artery
Femoral artery
Femoral vein
Popliteal artery
Great saphenous vein
Posterior tibial artery

circumcision Surgical removal of the foreskin of the *penis*. Circumcision may be needed to treat *phimosis*, recurrent attacks of *balanitis*, or *paraphimosis*. It may also be performed for religious, cosmetic, or social reasons.

circumcision, female Removal of all or parts of the *clitoris*, labia majora, and labia minora (see *labia*), sometimes combined with narrowing of the entrance to

the *vagina*. Female circumcision is common in parts of Africa but has no valid medical purpose. It can cause retention of urine and injuries during sexual intercourse and childbirth.

cirrhosis A condition of the *liver* arising from long-term damage to its cells. In cirrhosis, bands of fibrosis (internal scarring) develop, leaving *nodules* of regenerating cells that are inadequately supplied with blood. Liver function is gradually impaired; the liver no longer effectively removes toxic substances from the blood (see *liver failure*). The distortion and fibrosis also lead to *portal hypertension*. The most common cause of cirrhosis is heavy *alcohol* consumption. Other causes include forms of *hepatitis* and, more rarely, disorders of the *bile ducts*, *haemochromatosis*, *Wilson's disease*, *cystic fibrosis*, and *heart failure*.

Cirrhosis may go unrecognized until symptoms such as mild *jaundice, oedema*, and vomiting of blood develop. There may be enlargement of the liver and spleen and, in men, enlargement of the breasts and loss of body hair due to an imbalance in sex hormones caused by liver failure. Complications of cirrhosis include *ascites, oesophageal varices*, and *hepatoma*. Treatment is focused on slowing the rate at which liver cells are being damaged, if possible by treating the cause. In some cases, however, the condition progresses and a *liver transplant* may be considered.

cisplatin An *anticancer drug* used to treat some cancers of the *testis* and *ovary*.

citalopram An *antipressant drug*.

CJD The abbreviation for *Creutzfeldt–Jakob disease*.

clap A slang term for *gonorrhoea*.

clarithromycin An *antibiotic drug* used to treat infections of the skin and respiratory tract.

claudication A cramp-like pain in a muscle, most often in the legs, due to inadequate blood supply. Claudication in the legs is usually caused by blockage or narrowing of arteries due to *atherosclerosis* (see *peripheral vascular disease*). A rarer cause is spinal *stenosis*. In intermittent claudication, pain is felt in the calves after walking a certain distance and is relieved by rest.

C

claustrophobia Intense fear of being in enclosed spaces, such as lifts, or of being in crowded areas. *Behaviour therapy* is the usual form of treatment.

clavicle The collarbone. The two clavicles, one on each side, form joints with the top of the sternum (breastbone) and the scapula (shoulderblade). The clavicles support the arms and transmit forces from the arms to the central skeleton.

CLAVICLE

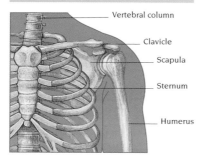

- Vertebral column
- Clavicle
- Scapula
- Sternum
- Humerus

claw-foot A deformity of the foot in which the arch of the foot is exaggerated and the tips of the toes turn under. Claw-foot may be congenital (present from birth), or it may result from damage to the nerve or blood supply to the muscles of the foot. The condition may be improved by surgery.

claw-hand A deformity, resulting from injury to the *ulnar nerve*, in which the fingers are permanently curled. Treatment of claw-hand includes repair of the damaged nerve, if possible, by the use of splints to hold the finger straight, or cutting a tendon in the wrist to allow the fingers to straighten.

claw-toe A deformity of unknown cause in which the end of one or more affected toes bends downwards so that the toe curls under. A painful *corn* may develop on the tip of the toe or on the top of the bent joint. Protective pads can relieve pressure from footwear. In severe cases, surgery may be required.

cleft lip and palate A split in the upper lip and/or palate that is present at birth. Cleft lip is a vertical, usually off-centre split in the upper lip that may be a small notch or may extend to the nose. The upper gum may also be cleft, and the nose may be crooked. The term hare lip refers only to a midline cleft lip, which is rare. Cleft palate is a gap that may extend from the back of the palate to behind the teeth and be open to the nasal cavity. Cleft palate is often accompanied by partial deafness and there may be other *birth defects*. Oral corticosteroids taken early in pregnancy may be associated with an increased risk of cleft lip and/or palate.

Surgery to repair a cleft lip may be undertaken in the first few days after birth or at about 6 months. It improves appearance; after repair, speech defects are rare. A cleft palate is usually repaired at about 6 months, but further surgery, *orthodontic* treatment, and *speech therapy* may be required.

clemastine An *antihistamine drug* used to relieve the symptoms of allergies such as *urticaria* and allergic *rhinitis* (hay fever). Clemastine can cause drowsiness.

clergyman's knee Inflammation of the *bursa* that cushions the pressure point over the tibial tubercle (the bony prominence just below the knee) caused by prolonged kneeling (see *bursitis*).

climacteric See *menopause*.

clindamycin An *antibiotic drug* with severe side effects, used only to treat serious infections that do not respond to other antibiotic drugs.

clitoridectomy An operation to remove the *clitoris* (see *circumcision, female*).

clitoris Part of the female genitalia, the clitoris is a small, sensitive, erectile organ, located just below the pubic bone, that is partly enclosed within the folds of the *labia*. The clitoris swells and becomes more sensitive during sexual stimulation.

clomifene A drug used to treat female *infertility* caused by failure to ovulate. Minor side effects may include hot flushes, nausea, headache, breast tenderness, and blurred vision. Occasionally, *ovarian cysts* develop, but these shrink when the dose is reduced. Use of the drug may result in multiple births.

clomipramine A *tricyclic antidepressant drug* used as treatment for *depression*. Side effects include dry mouth, blurred vision, and constipation.

clonazepam A *benzodiazepine drug* that is used mainly as an *anticonvulsant drug* to prevent and treat epileptic fits (see *epilepsy*). Clonazepam also prevents *petit mal* attacks in children. Side effects of the drug include drowsiness, dizziness, fatigue, and irritability.

clone An exact copy. In medicine, the term usually refers to copies of cells, genes, or organisms. Clones of cells are all descended from one original cell. In many types of cancer, cells are thought to be derived from one abnormal cell. Clones of genes are duplicates of a single gene. In research, several copies of a gene can be made to enable the gene to be studied in detail. Clones of organisms are produced by removing the nuclei from cells of a donor individual and transplanting them into the egg cells of another individual. When the eggs mature into living plants or animals, they are identical to the donor.

clonidine An *antihypertensive drug* used to reduce high blood pressure. Possible side effects include drowsiness, dizziness, dry mouth, and constipation. Abrupt withdrawal of high doses can cause a dangerous rise in blood pressure.

clonus A rapid series of abnormal *muscle* contractions that occur in response to stretching. Clonus is a sign of damage to nerve fibres that carry impulses from the motor cortex in the *cerebrum* to a particular muscle. It is also a feature of seizures in grand mal *epilepsy*.

clopidogrel An *antiplatelet drug* used to help prevent strokes or heart attacks in people at risk of these conditions, particularly those who have previously had them. Possible side effects include indigestion, abdominal pain, and diarrhoea. With prolonged use, there is also an increased risk of internal and/or external bleeding, especially in those who are also taking aspirin.

clostridium Any of a group of rod-shaped *bacteria*. Clostridia are found in soil and in the gastrointestinal tracts of humans and animals. They produce powerful toxins and are responsible for potentially life-threatening diseases such as *botulism*, *tetanus*, and *gangrene*.

clotrimazole A drug used to treat yeast and fungal infections, especially *candidiasis* (see *antifungal drugs*).

clove oil An oil distilled from the dried flower-buds of *EUGENIA CARYOPHYLLUS*, used mainly as a flavouring in pharmaceuticals. Clove oil is sometimes used as a remedy for toothache.

clubbing Thickening and broadening of the tips of the fingers and toes, usually with increased curving of the nails. It is associated with chronic lung diseases, such as *lung cancer*, *bronchiectasis*, and fibrosing *alveolitis*; with certain heart abnormalities; and, occasionally, with *Crohn's disease* and *ulcerative colitis*.

club-foot A deformity of the foot, present from birth (see *talipes*).

cluster headaches Brief but severe headaches that recur up to several times a day over a few weeks. Cluster headaches affect one side of the head or face. The cause is uncertain but they may be due to dilation of blood vessels in the brain as in *migraine*. There may also be a family history of cluster headaches.

Cluster headaches may be treated with injections of *sumatriptan* or inhalation of pure oxygen. Ergotamine is also sometimes used to treat the condition.

CNS An abbreviation for *central nervous system* (the brain and spinal cord).

CNS stimulants Drugs that increase mental alertness (see *stimulant drugs*).

coagulation, blood The main mechanism by which blood clots are formed, involving a complex series of reactions in the blood *plasma* (see *blood clotting*).

coal tar A thick, black, sticky substance distilled from coal. It is a common ingredient of ointments and medicinal shampoos prescribed for skin and scalp conditions such as *psoriasis* and some forms of *dermatitis* and *eczema*.

co-amoxiclav A *penicillin drug* containing a mixture of *amoxicillin* and clavulanic acid. Because it is a more powerful antibiotic than amoxicillin alone, co-amoxiclav is used to treat infections caused by amoxicillin-resistant strains of bacteria.

coarctation of the aorta A *congenital* heart defect of unknown cause, in which there is narrowing in a section of the aorta that supplies blood to the lower body and legs. In response, the heart has to work harder, causing *hypertension* in the upper part of the body.

COCCYX

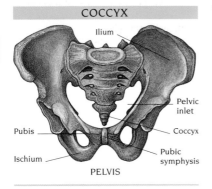

Ilium

Pelvic inlet

Pubis

Coccyx

Ischium

Pubic symphysis

PELVIS

Symptoms usually appear in early childhood and include headache, weakness after exercise, cold legs, and, rarely, breathing difficulty and swelling of the legs due to *heart failure*. Associated abnormalities include a heart *murmur*, weak or absent pulse in the groin, lack of synchronization between groin and wrist pulses, and higher blood pressure in the arms than in the legs. Diagnosis may be made by *aortography*, *MRI*, and/or *chest X-rays*. Corrective surgery is usually performed at 4–8 years of age.

cobalamin A *cobalt*-containing complex molecule, part of *vitamin B₁₂*.

cobalt A metallic element and a constituent of *vitamin B₁₂* A radioactive form of cobalt is used in *radiotherapy*.

cocaine A drug obtained from the leaves of the coca plant ERYTHROXYLON COCA, once used as a local anaesthetic (see *anaesthesia, local*) for minor surgical procedures. Cocaine affects the brain, producing euphoria and increased energy. Because of its effects, cocaine is subject to *drug abuse*. Continued use can lead to psychological dependence (see *drug dependence*), and *psychosis* if high doses are taken. Regular inhaling of the drug can damage the lining of the nose. Overdose can cause seizures and *cardiac arrest*. "Crack", a purified form of cocaine, produces a more intense reaction and has caused deaths due to adverse effects on the heart.

cocci Spherical *bacteria*, some of which are responsible for certain infections in humans (see *staphylococcal infections*; *streptococcal infections*).

coccydynia A pain in the region of the *coccyx*. Coccydynia may result from a blow to the base of the spine in a fall, from prolonged pressure due to poor posture when sitting, or the use of the *lithotomy* position during childbirth. The pain usually eases in time. Treatment may include heat, injections of a local anaesthetic, and *manipulation*.

coccyx A small triangular bone made up of four tiny bones fused together at the base of the *spine*. Together with a larger bone called the *sacrum*, it forms the back section of the *pelvis*. There is very little relative movement between the coccyx and sacrum. Later in life, they commonly become fused together.

cochlea The spiral-shaped organ situated in the labyrinth of the inner ear that transforms sound vibrations into nerve impulses for transmission to the brain, enabling *hearing*.

COCHLEA

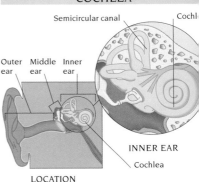

Semicircular canal

Cochl

Outer ear Middle ear Inner ear

INNER EAR

Cochlea

LOCATION

cochlear implant A device used to treat profoundly deaf people who are not helped by hearing aids. A cochlear implant consists of tiny electrodes surgically implanted in the cochlea deep in the inner ear and a receiver that is embedded in the skull just behind and above the ear. A microphone, sound processor, and transmitter are worn externally. A cochlear implant does not restore normal hearing, but it enables patterns of sound to be detected. Combined with lip-reading, it may enable speech to be understood.

co-codamol A compound *analgesic drug* containing *paracetamol* and *codeine*.

codeine An *opioid analgesic drug* derived from the *opium* poppy plant. Codeine is a useful treatment for mild to moderate pain and may be used in combination with other opioid analgesics. It is also used as a *cough remedy* and as an *antidiarrhoeal drug*. It may cause dizziness and drowsiness, especially if taken with alcohol. Taken long-term, codeine may cause constipation and be habit-forming.

cod-liver oil An oil obtained from the liver of fresh cod, which is a valuable source of *vitamin A* and *vitamin D*.

coeliac disease An uncommon condition in which the lining of the small intestine is damaged due to *hypersensitivity* to *gluten*, a protein found in wheat, rye, and some other cereals. Damage to the intestinal lining causes *malabsorption*, weight loss, and vitamin and mineral deficiencies that can lead to *anaemia* and skin problems. Faeces are bulky and foul-smelling. The disease tends to run in families and varies in severity. In babies, symptoms usually develop within six months of the introduction of gluten into the diet. The baby may become listless and irritable, develop vomiting and acute diarrhoea, and become dehydrated and seriously ill. In adults, symptoms such as tiredness, breathlessness, diarrhoea, vomiting, abdominal pain, and swelling of the legs may develop gradually over months. A chronic, distinctive rash called *dermatitis herpetiformis* may develop. Some people suffer damage to the intestinal lining but never develop symptoms.

Diagnosis is made by blood, urine, and faeces tests and *jejunal biopsies*, in which small samples of the lining of the intestine are taken for examination. Coeliac disease is treated by a lifelong gluten-free diet, which usually relieves symptoms within weeks of introduction.

co-dydramol A compound *analgesic* containing *paracetamol* and dihydrocodeine.

cognitive-behavioural therapy A method of treating psychological disorders such as *depression* based on the idea that problems arise from a person's faulty cognitions (erroneous ways of perceiving the world and oneself). In cognitive–behavioural therapy, the patient is helped to identify negative or false cognitions and then encouraged to try out new thought strategies.

coil Any of the various types of intrauterine contraceptive device (see *IUD*).

coitus Another term for *sexual intercourse*.

coitus interruptus A method of contraception (see *contraception, withdrawal method of*) in which the male partner withdraws his penis from the vagina before ejaculation occurs. Coitus interruptus is unreliable because sperm can be released before orgasm occurs, and it may cause *psychosexual dysfunction* in men and women.

colchicine A drug extracted from the autumn crocus flower used to treat acute attacks of *gout* and to reduce their frequency. Side effects include vomiting and diarrhoea.

cold, common A common viral infection that causes inflammation of the mucous membranes lining the nose and throat. Symptoms include a stuffy or runny nose, sore throat, headache, and cough. The symptoms of a common cold usually intensify over 24–48 hours, unlike those of *influenza*, which worsen rapidly over a few hours.

There are at least 200 highly contagious viruses that are known to cause the common cold. These viruses are easily transmitted in the minute airborne droplets sprayed from the coughs or sneezes of infected people. In many cases, the viruses are also spread to the nose and throat by way of hand-to-hand contact with an infected person or by way of objects that have become contaminated with the virus.

Most colds clear up within about a week. In some cases, infection spreads and causes *laryngitis*, *tracheitis*, acute *bronchitis*, *sinusitis*, or *otitis media*. In these cases, a more serious secondary bacterial infection may follow. *Antibiotic drugs* may be needed if this happens.

cold injury Localized tissue damage caused by chilling, the most serious form of which is *frostbite*. Cold injury is distinct from *hypothermia*, which refers to chilling of the whole body.

In frostbite, an area of skin and flesh becomes frozen, hard, and white as a result of exposure to very cold, dry air.

C

Sometimes there is restriction of the blood supply to the affected area. Another type of cold injury, *immersion foot*, occurs when the legs and feet are kept cold and damp for hours or days. The main risk of both conditions is that blood flow will be slowed so much that the tissues will die, leading to *gangrene*. Less serious forms of cold injury include *chilblains* and *chapped skin*.

cold remedies Preparations for the relief of symptoms of the common cold (see *cold, common*). The main ingredient is usually a mild *analgesic drug*, such as *paracetamol* or *aspirin*, which helps to relieve aches and pains. Other common ingredients include *antihistamine drugs* and *decongestant drugs* to reduce nasal congestion; *caffeine*, which acts as a mild stimulant; and *vitamin C*.

cold sore A small skin blister, usually around the mouth, commonly caused by a strain of the *herpes simplex* virus called HSV1 (herpes simplex virus type 1). The first attack of the virus, often in childhood, may be symptomless or may cause a flu-like illness with painful mouth and lip ulcers called *gingivostomatis*. The virus then lies dormant in nerve cells, but may occasionally be reactivated and cause cold sores. Reactivation may occur after exposure to hot sunshine or a cold wind, during a common cold or other infection, or in women around the time of their menstrual periods. Prolonged attacks can occur in people with reduced immunity to infection due to illness or treatment with *immunosuppressant drugs*.

In many cases, an outbreak of cold sores is preceded by tingling in the lips, followed by the formation of small blisters that enlarge, causing itching and soreness. Within a few days they burst and become encrusted. Most disappear within a week. The antiviral drug *aciclovir* in a cream may prevent cold sores if used at the first sign of tingling. Using a sunscreen may reduce the likelihood of recurrence.

colecalciferol An alternative name for vitamin D$_3$ (see *vitamin D*).

colectomy The surgical removal of part or all of the *colon*. Colectomy is used in severe cases of *diverticular disease* or to remove a cancerous tumour in the colon or a narrowed part of the intestine that is obstructing the passage of faeces. A total colectomy is carried out when *ulcerative colitis* cannot be controlled by drugs, and may be used in cases of familial *polyposis*.

In a partial colectomy, the diseased section of the colon is removed, and the ends of the severed colon are joined. A temporary *colostomy* may be required until the rejoined colon has healed. In a total colectomy, the whole of the large intestine is removed, with or without the *rectum*. If the rectum is removed, an *ileostomy* may be performed. The bowel usually functions normally after a partial colectomy. In a total colectomy, the reduced ability of the intestines to absorb water from the faeces can result in diarrhoea. *Antidiarrhoeal drugs* may therefore be required.

colestyramine A *lipid-lowering drug* used to treat some types of *hyperlipidaemia*. The drug is also used to treat diarrhoea due to excessive amounts of undigested fats in the faeces in disorders such as *Crohn's disease*.

colic A severe, spasmodic pain that occurs in waves of increasing intensity. (See also *colic, infantile*.)

colic, infantile Episodes of irritability, and excessive crying in otherwise healthy infants, thought to be due to spasm in the intestines. A baby with an attack of colic cries or screams incessantly, draws up the legs towards the stomach, and may become red in the face and pass wind. Colic tends to be worse in the evenings. The condition is distressing but harmless. Usually, it first appears at 3–4 weeks and clears up without treatment by the age of about 12 weeks.

colistin One of the *polymyxin* group of *antibiotic drugs* used in *topical* preparations for eye and ear conditions. It is only used to treat systemic infections that are resistant to other antibiotics. The drug may cause damage to the kidneys and nerve tissue.

colitis Inflammation of the *colon* causing diarrhoea, usually with blood and mucus. Other symptoms may include abdominal pain and fever. Colitis may be due to infection by various types of microorganism, such as *campylobacter* and *shigella* bacteria, viruses, or *amoebae*. A form of colitis may be provoked by *antibiotic drugs* destroying bacteria that normally live in the intestine and allowing CLOSTRIDIUM DIFFICILE, a bacterium that causes irritation, to proliferate. Colitis is a feature of *ulcerative colitis* and *Crohn's disease.*

Investigations into colitis may include examining a faecal sample, *sigmoidoscopy* or *colonoscopy, biopsy* of inflamed areas or ulcers, and a barium enema (see *barium X-ray examinations*). If the cause is an infection, antibiotics may be needed. Crohn's disease and ulcerative colitis are treated with *corticosteroid* and *immunosuppressant drugs*, and a special diet.

collagen A tough, fibrous *protein*. Collagen is the body's major structural protein, forming an important part of *tendons, bones,* and *connective tissue.*

collagen diseases See *connective tissue diseases.*

collarbone The common name for the *clavicle.*

collar, orthopaedic A soft foam or stiffened device that is worn to treat pain or instability of the neck.

Colles' fracture A break in the *radius* (one of the lower-arm bones) just above the wrist, in which the wrist and hand are displaced backwards, restricting movement and causing swelling and severe pain. The fracture is usually the result of putting out a hand to lessen the impact of a fall. The broken bones are manipulated back into position, and set in a *cast.* Healing takes up to six weeks. Hand and wrist movements usually return to normal, but there may be minor wrist deformity.

colloid A state of matter similar to a suspension (insoluble particles of a substance suspended in a liquid). Particles in a suspension are large and heavy enough to be separated from the liquid in a *centrifuge.* A colloid has smaller, lighter particles that can only be separated out of a liquid by spinning at a very high speed. In medicine, *plasma proteins* are separated from blood and used in colloid preparations to treat *shock.*

Colloid also refers to the protein-containing material in the *thyroid gland.*

colon The major part of the large *intestine.* The colon is a segmented tube, about 1.3 m long and 6.5 cm wide, that forms a large loop in the abdomen. It consists of four sections: the ascending, transverse, and descending colons, and the S-shaped sigmoid colon, which connects with the rectum. The main functions of the colon are to absorb water and mineral salts from the digested material passed on from the small intestine and to concentrate the waste material for expulsion as faeces. The colon consists of four layers: a tough outer membrane; a layer of muscles that contract and relax to move the contents along (see *peristalsis*); a submucous coat containing blood vessels that absorb water and salts; and finally an innermost layer that produces mucus to lubricate the passage of material. (See also *digestive system; intestine, disorders of.*)

colon, cancer of A *malignant* tumour of the *colon.* First symptoms of the disease include an inexplicable change in bowel movements (either constipation or diarrhoea), blood mixed in with the faeces, and pain in the lower abdomen. Sometimes, there are no symptoms until the tumour has grown big enough to cause an obstruction in the intestine (see *intestine, obstruction* of) or perforate it (see *perforation*).

A genetic basis has been found for some types of colon cancer. However, in most cases, the precise cause is unknown. Contributory factors include diet: eating a lot of meat and fatty foods and not enough fibre may increase the risk. The disease often occurs in association with other diseases of the colon, such as *ulcerative colitis* and familial *polyposis.* The chances of cure depend critically on early diagnosis. Screening for this cancer includes an *occult blood test;* if the test is positive, *sigmoidoscopy* and *colonoscopy* may be carried out. Regular screening using colonoscopy is done for those at high risk. In most cases of colon cancer, a partial *colectomy* is performed.

colon, disorders of See *intestine, disorders of.*

colon, irritable See *irritable bowel syndrome.*

colonoscopy Examination of the inside of the *colon* by means of a flexible, fibre-optic viewing instrument called a

C

colonoscope, which is introduced through the *anus* and guided along the colon. Colonoscopy is used to investigate symptoms such as bleeding from the anus and to look for disorders such as *colitis*, *polyps*, and *cancer*. Instruments may be passed through the colonoscope to take *biopsy* specimens or to remove polyps.

colon, spastic See *irritable bowel syndrome*.

colostomy An operation in which part of the *colon* is brought through an incision in the abdominal wall and formed into a *stoma*, an artificial opening through which faeces are discharged into a bag attached to the skin. A temporary colostomy may be performed at the same time as a *colectomy* to allow the colon to heal without faeces passing through it. The colostomy is closed when the rejoined colon has healed. A permanent colostomy is needed if the rectum or anus has been removed.

colostrum A thick, yellowish fluid produced by the breasts during the first few days after childbirth. Colostrum is then replaced by breast milk. Colostrum contains less fat and sugar but more minerals and protein than breast milk. It also has a high content of *lymphocytes* and *immunoglobulins*, which help to protect the baby from infection.

colour blindness See *colour vision deficiency*.

colour vision The ability to see different parts of the colour spectrum. Light perceived by the human eye consists of electromagnetic radiation (energy waves) with a spectrum of different wavelengths between about 400 and 700 nanometres. Different wavelengths produce sensations of violet, indigo, blue, green, yellow, orange, and red when they fall on the retina and stimulate nerve signals, which are processed in the brain.

As light falls on the retina, it strikes light-sensitive cells called rods and cones. The rods can detect all visible light, but only the cones can distinguish colour. There are three types of cones: red-sensitive, blue-sensitive, and green-sensitive. Each responds more strongly to a particular part of the light spectrum. Because the cones are most concentrated in a central area of the retina called the *fovea*, colour

COLOSTOMY

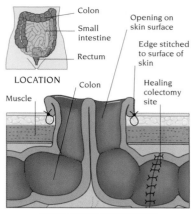

LOCATION

TEMPORARY COLOSTOMY

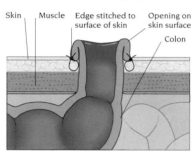

PERMANENT COLOSTOMY

vision is most accurate for objects viewed directly and is poor at the edges of vision. When light hits a cone, it causes the cone to emit an electrical signal, which passes to the brain via the *optic nerve*. Colour perception requires a minimum level of light, below which everything is seen as shades of grey. (See also *colour vision deficiency*; *eye*; *perception*; *vision*.)

colour vision deficiency Any abnormality in *colour vision* that causes difficulty distinguishing between certain colours. Total absence of colour vision (monochromatism) is rare. The most common types of colour vision deficiency are reduced discrimination of red and green. Most cases of red and green colour vision deficiency are caused by defects in the light-sensitive cells in the *retina*. These defects are usually inherited,

COLPOSCOPY

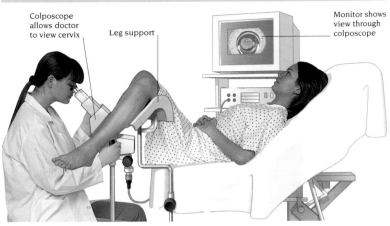

Colposcope allows doctor to view cervix

Leg support

Monitor shows view through colposcope

although occasionally defects are caused by retinal or optic nerve diseases or injury. The inherited defects tend to be sex-linked (see *genetic disorders*), which means that the majority of sufferers are male. A person with a severe green deficiency has difficulty distinguishing oranges, greens, browns, and pale reds. In severe red deficiency, all reds appear dull. A much rarer deficiency in which blue cannot be distinguished may be inherited or may be due to degeneration of the retina or optic nerve.

colposcopy Visual inspection of the *cervix* and *vagina* using a magnifying instrument called a colposcope. Colposcopy is carried out to look for the presence of areas of precancerous tissue or of early cervical cancer (see *cervical intraepithelial neoplasia; cervix, cancer of*). Colposcopy may also be used to obtain tissue biopsy samples for further tests, or to treat areas of abnormal tissue.

coma A state of *unconsciousness* and unresponsiveness to external *stimuli* (for example, pinching) or internal stimuli (such as a full bladder). Coma results from disturbance or damage to areas of the involved in conscious activity or maintenance of consciousness – in particular, parts of the *cerebrum*, upper parts of the *brainstem*, and central regions of the brain, especially the *limbic system*. There are varying depths of coma. Even

people in deep comas may show some automatic responses, such as breathing unaided and blinking. If the lower brainstem is damaged, vital functions are impaired, and artificial ventilation and maintenance of the circulation are required. With medical care, a person may be kept alive for many years in a deep coma (*persistent vegetative state*) provided the brainstem is still functioning. Complete irreversible loss of brainstem function leads to *brain death*.

combination drug A preparation containing more than one active substance.

comedo Another name for a *blackhead*.

commensal A usually harmless *bacterium* or other organism that normally lives in or on the body.

communicable disease Any disease due to a microorganism or parasite that can be transmitted from one person to another. (See also *contagious; infectious disease*.)

compartment syndrome A painful *cramp* due to compression of a group of muscles within a confined space. It may occur when muscles are enlarged due to intensive training or injury such as *shin splints*. Cramps induced by exercise usually disappear when exercise is stopped. Severe cases may require *fasciotomy* to improve blood flow and prevent development of a permanent *contracture*.

compensation neurosis A supposed psychological reaction to injury affected

C

by the prospect of financial compensation. In some cases, the condition may delay physical recovery.

complement A collection of *proteins* in *blood plasma* that helps to destroy foreign cells and is an important part of the *immune system*.

complementary medicine A group of therapies, often described as "alternative", which are now increasingly used to complement or to act as an alternative to conventional medicine. They fall into three broad categories: touch and movement (as in *acupuncture*, *massage*, and *reflexology*); medicinal (as in *naturopathy*, *homeopathy*. and *Chinese medicine*); and psychological (as in *biofeedback*, *hypnotherapy*, and *meditation*).

complex A term used in medicine to mean a group or combination of related signs and symptoms that form a syndrome (as in *Eisenmenger complex*), or a collection of substances of similar structure or function (as in *vitamin B complex*). In psychology, a complex (for example, the *Oedipus complex*) is a group of unconscious ideas and memories that have emotional importance.

compliance The degree to which patients follow medical advice.

complication A condition resulting from a preceding disorder or from its treatment.

compos mentis Latin for "of sound mind".

compress A pad of lint or linen applied under pressure to an area of skin. Cold compresses soaked in ice-cold water or wrapped around ice help to reduce pain, swelling, and bleeding under the skin after an injury (see *ice pack*). Hot compresses increase the circulation and help to bring boils to a head. A dry compress may be used to stop bleeding from a wound or may be coated with medication to help treat infection.

compression syndrome A collection of localized symptoms such as numbness, tingling, discomfort, and muscle weakness caused by pressure on a *nerve*.

compulsive behaviour See *obsessive–compulsive disorder*.

computed tomography Another name for *CT scanning*.

conception The *fertilization* of a woman's *ovum* by a man's *sperm*, followed by implantation of the resultant *blastocyst*

in the lining of the *uterus* thus starting a *pregnancy*. (See also *contraception*.)

concussion Brief *unconsciousness* due to disturbance of the electrical activity in the brain following a violent blow to the head or neck. Common symptoms following concussion include confusion, inability to remember events immediately before the injury, dizziness, blurred vision, and vomiting. If symptoms persist, or new ones develop, such as drowsiness, difficulty breathing, repeated vomiting, or visual disturbances, they could signify brain damage or an *extradural haemorrhage*. Repeated concussion can cause *punch-drunk* syndrome. (See also *head injury*.)

conditioning The formation of a specific response to a specific *stimulus*. In classical conditioning, a stimulus that consistently evokes a particular response is paired repeatedly with a second stimulus that would not normally produce the response. Eventually, the second stimulus begins to produce the response whether the first stimulus is present or not. In operant conditioning, attempts to modify behaviour are made through a system of rewards and/or punishments.

The theory that inappropriate behaviour patterns in some psychological disorders are learned through conditioning and can be modified by the same process underlies behavioural psychology (see *behaviour therapy*).

condom A barrier method of *contraception* in the form of a thin latex rubber or plastic sheath placed over the *penis* before sexual *intercourse*. Condoms also offer some degree of protection against sexually transmitted infections.

condom, female A barrier method of *contraception* in the form of a sheath inserted into the *vagina* before sexual *intercourse*. It also offers some protection against sexually transmitted infections.

conduct disorders Repetitive and persistent patterns of aggressive and/or antisocial behaviour, such as vandalism, substance abuse, and persistent lying, that occur in childhood or adolescence. (See also *behavioural problems in children*; *adolescence*.)

conductive deafness *Deafness* caused by faulty conduction of sound from the outer to the inner *ear*.

condyloma acuminatum See *warts, genital.*

cone A type of light-sensitive cell in the *retina* of the eye. Cones play a major role in *colour vision.*

cone biopsy A surgical procedure, performed under local or general anaesthesia, in which a conical or cylindrical section of the lower part of the *cervix* is removed. A cone biopsy is performed after an abnormal *cervical smear test* result if the exact precancerous or cancerous area (see *cervical intraepithelial neoplasia*) cannot be identified by *colposcopy.*

CONE BIOPSY

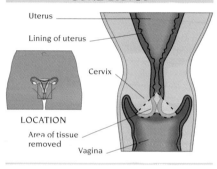

Uterus
Lining of uterus
Cervix

LOCATION
Area of tissue removed
Vagina

confabulation The use of a fictional story to make up for gaps in memory. The phenomenon occurs most commonly in chronic alcoholics suffering from *Wernicke–Korsakoff syndrome.* It may also occur with *head injuries.*

confidentiality The ethical principle that a doctor does not disclose information given in confidence by a patient.

The patient's consent is needed before a doctor supplies confidential information to an insurance company, employer, or lawyer. However, doctors must disclose information when required to by law or when faced with injuries or disorders that indicate a serious crime. Doctors are also required to notify specified infectious diseases. Treatment of young children is usually discussed with the parents, but an older child's request for confidentiality is generally respected if the doctor feels that he or she is competent enough to understand the issues involved.

confusion An acute or chronic disorganized mental state In which the abilities to

remember, think clearly, and reason are impaired. Acute confusion can arise as a symptom of *delirium,* in which brain activity is affected by fever, drugs, poisons, or injury. People with acute confusion may also have *hallucinations* and behave violently. Chronic confusion is often associated with *alcohol dependence,* long-term use of *antianxiety drugs,* and certain physically based mental disorders. Many of the conditions that cause chronic confusion (for example *dementia*) are progressive. Features include absent-mindedness, poor short-term memory, and a tendency to be repetitive. If the underlying cause of confusion can be treated, there may be marked improvement.

congenital Present at birth. Congenital abnormalities (sometimes called *birth defects*) are either inherited or result from damage or infection occurring in the *uterus* or at the time of birth.

congenital adrenal hyperplasia See *adrenal hyperplasia, congenital.*

congestion A term that usually refers to the accumulation of excess *blood, tissue fluid,* or *lymph* in part of the body. A major cause of congestion is increased blood flow to an area due to inflammation. Another cause is reduced drainage of blood from an affected area, as can occur in *heart failure,* in venous disorders such as *varicose veins,* and in *lymphatic disorders.* (See also *nasal congestion.*)

congestive heart failure See *heart failure.*

conjunctiva The transparent membrane covering the *sclera* (white of the eye) and lining the inside of the eyelids. Cells in the conjunctiva produce a fluid that lubricates the lids and the *cornea.*

conjunctivitis Inflammation of the *conjunctiva,* causing redness, discomfort, and discharge from the affected eye. There are two common types: infective conjunctivitis, caused by bacteria or viruses; and allergic conjunctivitis, which is an allergic response to substances such as cosmetics and pollen. Both types have similar symptoms but in infective conjunctivitis the discharge contains pus and may cause the eyelids to be stuck together on waking. In allergic conjunctivitis, the discharge is clear and the eyelids are often swollen.

C

Bacterial infections are treated with *antibiotic* eyedrops or ointment. Viral conjunctivitis often disappears without treatment. Allergic conjunctivitis may be relieved by eyedrops containing an *antihistamine* or a *corticosteroid drug*.

Other forms of conjunctivitis include neonatal *ophthalmia*, *keratoconjunctivitis*, and *trachoma*.

connective tissue The material that supports, binds, or separates the various structures of the body. *Tendons* and *cartilage* are made up of connective tissue, and it forms the matrix (ground substance) of *bone* and the nonmuscular structures of *arteries* and *veins*.

connective tissue diseases Types of *autoimmune disorders* that often affect blood vessels and produce secondary *connective tissue* damage. They include *rheumatoid arthritis*, systemic *lupus erythematosus*, *polyarteritis nodosa*, *scleroderma*, and *dermatomyositis*.

Conn's syndrome A disorder caused by the secretion of excessive amounts of the hormone *aldosterone* by a noncancerous tumour of one of the *adrenal glands*. (See also *aldosteronism*.)

consciousness A state of alertness in which a person is fully aware of his or her thoughts, surroundings, and intentions.

consent The legal term describing a patient's voluntary agreement to a doctor performing an operation, arranging drug treatment, or carrying out diagnostic tests. Strictly, consent is valid only if the patient has been fully informed about the purpose of the procedure, the likely outcome, and any complications and side effects. Consent cannot be given by children or by people with serious mental disorders, but a relative may give or withhold consent on their behalf. The patient's consent is also needed before a doctor supplies confidential information to an insurance company, employer, or lawyer.

constipation The infrequent or difficult passing of hard, dry *faeces*. Constipation is usually harmless. The most common cause is insufficient fibre in the diet (see *fibre, dietary*), because fibre assists the propulsion of waste matter through the *colon*. Other common causes include lack of regular bowel movements due to poor toilet-training in childhood or repeatedly ignoring the urge to move the bowels. Constipation in the elderly may be due to immobility or to weakness of the muscles of the abdomen and the pelvic floor. Self-help measures such as establishing a regular bowel routine, increasing the amount of fibre in the diet, and drinking more fluids are usually beneficial. Prolonged use of *laxative drugs* can impair the normal functioning of the colon.

Constipation is occasionally a symptom of an underlying disorder, especially if it is part of a persistent change in bowel habits after the age of 40, or if it is accompanied by blood in the faeces, pain on moving the bowels, or weight loss. Conditions that may result in constipation include *haemorrhoids*, *anal fissure*, *irritable bowel syndrome*, and narrowing of the colon in, for example, *diverticular disease* or cancer (see *colon, cancer of*).

constriction A narrowed area, or the process of narrowing.

contact dermatitis A type of *dermatitis* caused by an allergic reaction to a substance that is in contact with the skin and which would not cause a reaction in most people exposed to it. Common causes include nickel and rubber. (See also *irritant dermatitis*.)

contact lenses Very thin, shell-like, transparent discs fitted on the *cornea* of the eye to correct defective vision. Generally, contact lenses are used to correct *myopia* (shortsightedness) and *hypermetropia* (longsightedness). There are several types. Hard plastic lenses give good vision, are long-lasting and durable, inexpensive, and easy to maintain. However, they are sometimes difficult to tolerate

CONTACT LENSES

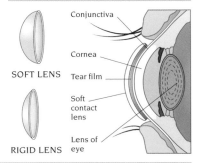

SOFT LENS

RIGID LENS

Conjunctiva

Cornea

Tear film

Soft contact lens

Lens of eye

and may fall out. Hard gas-permeable lenses are more comfortable because they allow oxygen to pass through to the eye, but are less durable. Soft lenses are the most comfortable because of their high water content. Disposable soft lenses are for single-use only; extended wear lenses are worn for up to a month.

Other types of lenses include rigid, scleral lenses that cover the whole of the front of the eye and are used to disguise disfigurement due to injury or disease; bifocal contact lenses; and toric contact lenses with an uneven surface curvature to correct astigmatism.

Hard plastic contact lenses may cause abrasion of the cornea if they are worn for too long. Soft lens wearers sometimes develop sensitivity of the eyes and lids. Other problems that may occur with any type of contact lens include infections and redness of the eye.

contact tracing A service, provided by clinics treating *sexually transmitted infections*, in which contacts of a person diagnosed as having sexually transmitted infection are traced and encouraged to be examined and treated. Contact tracing is also used in cases of infections such as *tuberculosis, meningitis,* and imported *tropical diseases.*

contagious A term used to describe a disease that can be transferred from person to person by ordinary social contact. All contagious diseases, such as the common cold or chickenpox, are *infectious.* The term contagious does not apply to the many *infectious diseases,* such as typhoid, syphilis, or AIDS, which are spread by other means.

contraception The control of fertility to prevent *pregnancy.* Methods prevent *ovulation* in the woman, stop *sperm* from meeting an *ovum* in the *fallopian tube* (preventing *fertilization*), or prevent a fertilized ovum implanting in the *uterus.*

Methods of contraception include total or periodic abstinence from *sexual intercourse* (see *contraception, natural methods of*); barrier methods (see *contraception, barrier methods of*); *coitus interruptus;* hormonal methods, including the use of *oral contraceptives,* patches, implants, and injections (see *contraceptives, injectable*), intrauterine

devices (see *IUDs*); postcoital methods (see *contraception, emergency*); or sterilization of the male (see *vasectomy*) or female (see *sterilization, female*).

contraception, barrier methods of The use of a device and/or a chemical to stop *sperm* reaching an *ovum,* preventing *fertilization* and pregnancy. Barrier methods also help prevent the sexual transmission of diseases such as *AIDS, chlamydial infections,* genital herpes (see *herpes, genital*), and viral hepatitis (see *hepatitis, viral*).

CONTRACEPTION, BARRIER

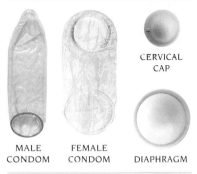

CERVICAL CAP

MALE CONDOM   FEMALE CONDOM   DIAPHRAGM

The male *condom* is one of the most widely used barrier contraceptives. Female condoms (see *condom, female*) are similar to, but larger than, male condoms.

Other female barrier methods include the diaphragm (see *diaphragm, contraceptive*), a hemispherical dome of thin rubber with a metal spring in the rim to hold it in place against the vaginal wall, blocking the entrance to the *cervix.* It is used with a *spermicide.* A cervical cap (see *cap, cervical*) is an alternative to the diaphragm.

Spermicides, in the form of aerosol foams, creams, gels, and pessaries, are placed in the vagina as close as possible to the cervix shortly before intercourse. Some spermicides should not be used with rubber barrier devices.

Mechanical and chemical means used together correctly can be highly effective in preventing conception.

contraception, emergency Measures to avoid *pregnancy* following unprotected *sexual intercourse.* There are two main methods: hormonal and physical. In the

C

first, high-dose oral *progesterone* (the "morning after" pill) should be taken in a single dose as soon as possible after unprotected sexual intercourse, preferably within 12 hours, but no later than 72 hours afterwards. In the physical method, an *IUD* is inserted by a doctor within five days of unprotected sex. Both methods are thought to work by preventing a fertilized egg from implanting in the uterus.

contraception, hormonal methods of The use by women of synthetic progestogen drugs, which are often combined with synthetic *oestrogens*, to prevent pregnancy. These drugs suppress *ovulation* and make cervical mucus thick and impenetrable to sperm. They also cause thinning of the *endometrium* (lining of the uterus), which reduces the chance of a fertilized egg implanting successfully. The best-known form of hormonal contraception is the contraceptive pill (see *oral contraceptives*). The hormones can also be given as *contraceptive implants* under the skin, as patches, by injection (see *contraceptives, injectable*), or be released by *IUDs*.

contraception, natural methods of Methods of avoiding conception based on attempts to pinpoint a woman's fertile period around the time of *ovulation*, so that sexual *intercourse* can be avoided at this time. The *calendar method* is based on the assumption that ovulation occurs around 14 days before menstruation. Because of its high failure rate, it has been largely superseded by other methods. The *temperature method* is based on the normal rise of a woman's body temperature in the second half of the menstrual cycle, after ovulation. The woman takes her temperature daily using an ovulation thermometer. Sex is considered to be only safe after there has been a sustained temperature rise for at least three days.

The *cervical mucus method* attempts to pinpoint the fertile period by observing and charting the amount and appearance of cervical mucus during the menstrual cycle. Recognized changes in the mucus occur before and often at ovulation. The *symptothermal method* combines the temperature and cervical mucus methods. Fertility devices are available that work by measuring hormone levels in the urine to predict fertile days.

contraception, withdrawal method of See *coitus interruptus*.

contraceptive Any agent that reduces the likelihood of *conception*. (See also *contraception*.)

contraceptive implant A hormonal method of *contraception* in which long-acting contraceptive drugs are inserted under the skin. An implant consists of a small rod that steadily releases a *progestogen drug* into the bloodstream.

contraceptives, injectable A hormonal method of *contraception* in which long-acting *progestogen drugs* are given by injection every 2–3 months. Injectable contraceptives are very effective but may cause menstrual disturbances, weight gain, headaches, acne, and nausea, especially during the first few months of use.

contractions, uterine Spasms of rhythmic, squeezing muscular activity affecting the walls of the *uterus* during *childbirth*. Regular contractions indicate the start of *labour* and increase in strength and frequency throughout the first stage. (See also *Braxton Hicks' contractions*.)

contracture A deformity caused by shrinkage of tissue in the skin, muscles, or tendons that may restrict movement of joints. Skin contractures commonly occur as a result of scarring following extensive burns. Other types are caused by inflammation and shrinkage of *connective tissues*. Examples are *Dupuytren's contracture* and *Volkmann's contracture*.

contraindication Factors in a patient's condition that would make it unwise to pursue a certain line of treatment.

contrast medium A substance opaque to *X-rays*, introduced into hollow or fluid-filled body parts to show them up on X-ray film. Barium is one of the most commonly used contrast media (see *barium X-ray examinations*).

controlled drug One of a number of drugs subject to restricted use because of their potential for abuse. They include *cocaine, morphine, amphetamine drugs*, and *barbiturate drugs*.

controlled trial A method of testing the effectiveness of new treatments or comparing different treatments. In a typical controlled drug trial, two comparable groups of patients suffering from the same illness are given courses of apparently identical treatment. However, only one group receives the new treatment; the second control group is given a *placebo*. Alternatively, the control group may be given an established drug that is already known to be effective. After a predetermined period, the two groups are assessed medically. Controlled trials must be conducted "blind" (the patients do not know which treatment they are receiving). In a "double-blind" trial, neither the patients nor the doctors who assess them know who is receiving which treatment.

contusion Bruising to the skin and underlying tissues from an injury.

convalescence The recovery period following an illness or surgery during which the patient regains strength before returning to normal activities.

conversion disorder A psychological disorder in which repressed emotions appear to be unconsciously converted into physical symptoms such as blindness, loss of speech, or paralysis. The condition, formerly known as hysteria, is generally treated with *psychotherapy*.

convulsion See *seizure*.

convulsion, febrile Twitching or jerking of the limbs with loss of consciousness that occurs in a child with a fever. Febrile convulsions are common, usually affecting children between the ages of 6 months and 5 years. Seizures may be prevented in susceptible children by giving *paracetamol* or *ibuprofen* at the first signs of fever. Most children who have seizures suffer no ill effects. The risk of developing *epilepsy* is very small but is increased in children with a pre-existing abnormality of the brain or nervous system, or children with a family history of epilepsy.

Cooley's anaemia See *thalassaemia*.

COPD The abbreviation for chronic obstructive pulmonary disease (see *pulmonary disease, chronic obstructive*).

copper A metallic element that is an essential part of several *enzymes*. Copper is needed by the body only in minute amounts (see *trace elements*). Copper excess may result from the rare inherited disorder *Wilson's disease*.

co-proxamol An *analgesic drug*, containing *paracetamol* and the weak *opioid* analgesic dextropropoxyphene, that has been widely used to relieve mild to moderate pain. Side effects include dizziness, drowsiness, constipation, and nausea. Co-proxamol may be habit-forming if taken over a long period. For safety reasons, it is being phased out.

cordotomy An operation to divide bundles of nerve fibres within the *spinal cord* to relieve persistent pain that has not responded to other treatment. Cordotomy is most frequently performed for pain in the lower trunk and legs, especially in people with cancer.

corn A small area of thickened skin on a toe, caused by the pressure of a tight-fitting shoe. Treatment is with a spongy ring or corn pad to ease the pressure on the corn, or the thickened skin can be removed by a chiropodist.

cornea The transparent thin-walled dome that forms the front of the eyeball. The cornea is joined at its circumference to the *sclera* (white of the eye); the black pupil and the coloured iris are visible beneath it. The main functions of the cornea are to help focus light rays on to the *retina* at the back of the eye and to protect the front of the eye. It is kept moist by tears produced by the *lacrimal gland* and the mucus-and fluid-secreting cells in the eyelids and *conjunctiva*.

CORNEA

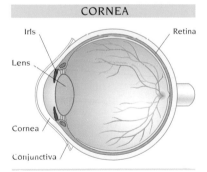

Iris — Retina
Lens
Cornea
Conjunctiva

cornea, disorders of Injuries or diseases affecting the cornea, the transparent front of the eyeball. Injuries include *corneal abrasions*, which sometimes become infected and progress to a *corneal ulcer*. Penetrating corneal injuries can cause scarring, which may lead to impairment of vision. Chemical injuries can result from contact with a corrosive

C

substance and require immediate flushing of the eye with water.

In actinic *keratopathy*, the outer layer of the cornea is damaged by ultraviolet light. In exposure keratopathy, damage is due to reduced protection by the tear film and blink reflex. The cornea can also be infected by viruses, bacteria, and fungi, the *herpes simplex* virus being especially dangerous. True inflammation of the cornea (called *keratitis*) is uncommon as the cornea contains no blood vessels.

Other disorders include: *keratomalacia* as a result of vitamin A deficiency; *keratoconjunctivitis sicca* (dry eye); corneal dystrophies such as *keratoconus*; and oedema, in which fluid builds up in the cornea and impairs vision. Rare congenital defects include microcornea (smaller cornea than normal) or megalocornea (bigger than normal) and *buphthalmos*, or "ox-eye", in which the entire eyeball is distended as a result of *glaucoma*. Degenerative conditions of the cornea such as calcium deposition, thinning, and spontaneous ulceration occur mainly in the elderly, and are more common in previously damaged eyes.

corneal abrasion A scratch or defect in the *epithelium* (outer layer) of the *cornea* caused by a small, sharp particle in the eye (see *eye, foreign body in*) or by an injury. Corneal abrasions usually heal quickly but may cause severe pain and *photophobia*. Treatment includes covering the eye with a patch, *analgesic drugs* to relieve pain, and, if the eye muscles go into spasm, eyedrops containing cycloplegic drugs (which paralyse the ciliary muscle, preventing *accommodation*). *Antibiotic* eyedrops are usually given to prevent bacterial infection, which can lead to a *corneal ulcer*.

corneal graft The surgical transplantation of donor corneal tissue to replace a damaged *cornea*. In most grafts, tissue is taken from a human *donor* after death. The success rate of corneal grafts is generally high, because the cornea has no blood vessels; this reduces access for white blood cells, which can cause *rejection* of the donor tissue.

corneal transplant See *corneal graft*.

corneal ulcer A break, erosion, or open sore in the *cornea* commonly caused by a *corneal abrasion*. It may also be due to chemical damage, or infection with *bacteria, fungi*, or *viruses* (particularly with the *herpes viruses*). Eye conditions such as *keratoconjunctivitis sicca* and eyelid deformities such as *entropion* or *ectropion* increase the risk of an ulcer.

Corneal ulcers are revealed by introducing *fluorescein* dye into the eye. Treatment depends on the underlying cause.

coronary Any structure that encircles like a crown. The term usually refers to the *coronary arteries*. It is also sometimes used as a nonmedical term for a heart attack (see *myocardial infarction*).

coronary artery Either of the two main *arteries* that supply the tissues of the heart with oxygen-rich blood. These are known as the left and right main coronary arteries and arise directly from the *aorta*. The term coronary artery is also applied to any of the arteries that branch off from the main coronary arteries, such as the left circumflex artery and the left anterior descending artery. Blockage of a coronary artery as a result of *atherosclerosis* can lead to *myocardial infarction*. (See also *coronary artery disease*.)

coronary artery bypass A major heart operation to bypass narrowed or blocked *coronary arteries* using additional blood vessels (such as a mammary artery) to improve blood flow to the heart muscle. This operation is used when symptoms of coronary artery disease have not been relieved by drugs or balloon *angioplasty* and insertion of a *stent*.

CORONARY ARTERY

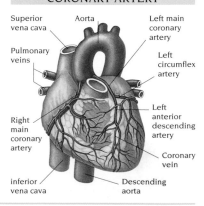

Superior vena cava
Aorta
Left main coronary artery
Pulmonary veins
Left circumflex artery
Left anterior descending artery
Right main coronary artery
Coronary vein
inferior vena cava
Descending aorta

Before surgery, sites of blockage in the arteries are identified using angiography. In some cases, *minimally invasive surgery* can be used, avoiding the need to stop the heart and use a *heart–lung machine* during the operation. The long term outlook after a bypass is good, but the grafted vessels may also eventually become blocked by *atherosclerosis*.

coronary artery disease Narrowing of the coronary arteries, which supply blood to the heart, leading to damage or malfunction of the heart. The most common heart disorders due to coronary artery disease are *angina pectoris* and *myocardial infarction* (heart attack).

The usual cause of narrowing of the arteries is *atherosclerosis*, in which fatty plaques develop on the artery linings. The vessel can become totally blocked if a blood clot forms or lodges in the narrowed area. Atherosclerosis has many interrelated causes including smoking, a high-fat diet, lack of exercise, being overweight, and raised blood cholesterol levels. Other factors include a genetic predisposition and diseases such as *diabetes mellitus* and *hypertension*.

The first symptom of coronary artery disease is frequently the chest pain of angina. Treatment is with drugs such as glyceryl trinitrate and other *nitrate drugs*, *beta-blockers*, *calcium channel blockers*, *potassium channel activators*, and *vasodilator drugs*. Aspirin to thin the blood and *statins* to lower the blood cholesterol level may be advised. Lifestyle changes, such as stopping smoking, are also vital. If drug treatment fails to relieve the symptoms or if there is extensive narrowing of the coronary arteries, blood flow may be improved by balloon *angioplasty* and insertion of a *stent* or by *coronary artery bypass* surgery.

coronary care unit A specialist ward for the care of acutely ill patients who may be suffering, or who have suffered, a *myocardial infarction* (heart attack) or another serious cardiovascular disorder.

coronary heart disease An alternative name for *coronary artery disease*.

coronary thrombosis Narrowing or blockage of one of the *coronary arteries* by a *thrombus* (blood clot), depriving a section of the heart muscle of vital oxygen. In most cases, the thrombus forms in a blood vessel already narrowed by *atherosclerosis*. Sudden blockage of a coronary artery causes an acute *myocardial infarction* (heart attack).

coroner A public officer appointed to inquire into the cause of death when it is unknown, or when it is suspected or known to result from unnatural causes. The coroner holds an inquest, sometimes before a jury.

cor pulmonale Enlargement and strain of the right side of the *heart* caused by one of a number of chronic lung diseases. Lung damage results in *pulmonary hypertension*; the resultant "back pressure" strain on the heart may eventually cause right-sided *heart failure* with *oedema*.

corpuscle Any minute body or cell, particularly red and white blood cells or certain types of *nerve* endings.

corpus luteum A small tissue mass in the *ovary* that develops from a ruptured egg *follicle* after *ovulation*. The corpus luteum secretes the female sex hormone *progesterone*, which causes the lining of the uterus to thicken in preparation for implantation of a fertilized egg. If fertilization does not occur, the corpus luteum shrinks and dies.

CORPUS LUTEUM

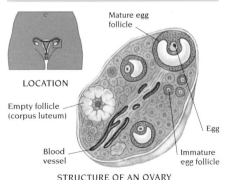

LOCATION

Mature egg follicle

Empty follicle (corpus luteum)

Blood vessel

Egg

Immature egg follicle

STRUCTURE OF AN OVARY

cortex The outer layer of certain organs, such as the brain or kidneys.

corticosteroid drugs A group of drugs that are similar to the *corticosteroid hormones* produced by the *adrenal glands*. Corticosteroids are used as hormone replacement therapy in *Addison's disease*

C

and when the *adrenal glands* or *pituitary gland* have been destroyed or removed. They are also used to treat inflammatory intestinal disorders such as *ulcerative colitis* and *Crohn's disease* and as an urgent treatment for inflammation in the artery supplying the retina in *temporal arteritis*. Other uses include treatment of *autoimmune diseases* such as systemic *lupus erythematosus* and *rheumatoid arthritis*, and treatment of *asthma*, *eczema*, and *allergic rhinitis*. Corticosteroid drugs are also used to prevent organ rejection after *transplant surgery* and in the treatment of some types of cancer, such as a *lymphoma* or *leukaemia*. Corticosteroid injections may relieve pain in disorders such as *tennis elbow* and *arthritis*.

Side effects are uncommon when corticosteroids are given as a cream or by inhaler, but tablets taken in high doses for long periods may cause *oedema*, *hypertension*, *diabetes mellitus*, *peptic ulcer*, *Cushing's syndrome*, inhibited growth in children, and, in rare cases, *cataract* or *psychosis*. High doses also impair the body's *immune system*. Long-term treatment suppresses production of corticosteroid hormones by the adrenal glands, and sudden withdrawal may lead to *adrenal failure*.

corticosteroid hormones A group of hormones produced by the *adrenal glands* that control the body's use of nutrients and the excretion of salts and water in the urine.

corticotropin An alternative name for *ACTH* (adrenocorticotrophic hormone).

cortisol Another name for *hydrocortisone*, a corticosteroid hormone produced by the *adrenal glands*.

coryza A term for the nasal symptoms of the common cold (see *cold, common*).

cosmetic dentistry Procedures to improve the appearance of the *teeth* or prevent further damage to the teeth and/or *gums*. Cosmetic dentistry procedures include fitting an *orthodontic appliance* to correct teeth that are out of alignment or where the bite is incorrect (see *malocclusion*); fitting a *crown* or veneer; *bonding* to treat chipped or stained teeth; *bleaching* of discoloured teeth; and replacing amalgam fillings with tooth-coloured fillings.

cosmetic surgery An operation performed to improve appearance rather than to cure or treat disease. Cosmetic surgery techniques include the removal of skin blemishes or *dermabrasion*; *rhinoplasty* to alter the shape or size of the nose; *face-lifts*; *mammoplasty* to reduce or enlarge the breasts; *body contour surgery* to remove excess body fat and tissue; *hair transplants*; *blepharoplasty* to remove excess skin on the eyelids; and mentoplasty to alter the size or shape of the chin. All cosmetic surgery carries the risk of side effects from the anaesthetic, as well as of complications of the procedure itself.

costalgia Pain around the chest due to damage to a *rib* or to one of the *intercostal nerves* beneath the ribs. Damage to an intercostal nerve most commonly results from of an attack of the viral infection *herpes zoster* (shingles).

cot death See *sudden infant death syndrome*.

co-trimoxazole An *antibacterial drug* containing trimethoprim and sulfa-methoxazole. Because of potentially seriously side effects, co-trimoxazole is now used to treat certain infections only when they cannot be treated with other drugs.

cough A *reflex* action that occurs as an attempt to clear the airways of mucus, sputum, a foreign body, or any other irritants or blockages. A cough is productive when it brings up mucus or sputum and unproductive, or dry, when it does not. Many coughs are due to irritation of the airways by dust, smoke (see *cough, smoker's*), or a viral infection of the upper respiratory tract (see *cold, common*; *laryngitis*; *pharyngitis*; *tracheitis*). Coughing is a feature of *bronchitis*, *asthma*, *pneumonia*, and *lung cancer*.

Over-the-counter *cough remedies* are available; but, in general, they just ease symptoms. More specific treatment is directed at the underlying disorder.

coughing up blood A symptom, medically known as haemoptysis, caused by rupture of a blood vessel in the airways, lungs, nose, or throat. The coughed-up blood may appear as bright-red or rusty-brown streaks, clots in the sputum, a pinkish froth, or, more rarely, blood alone. In all cases, medical assessment is needed. Many disorders can cause haemoptysis. The most common are infections, such as *pneumonia* or *bronchitis*; and *congestion* in and rupture of blood vessels in the lungs due to *heart failure, mitral stenosis*, or *pulmonary embolism*. A cancerous tumour can also produce haemoptysis by eroding the wall of a blood vessel.

Investigations into coughing up blood include *chest X-ray*, blood tests, and in some cases *bronchoscopy* or *CT scanning*. In some cases, no underlying cause is found. Treatment depends on the cause but stopping smoking is essential in all cases.

cough remedies Over the-counter medications for treating a *cough*. There are various preparations, but the effectiveness of most is unproven. *Expectorant* cough remedies are purported to encourage expulsion of sputum. Cough suppressants, which control the coughing reflex, include some *antihistamine drugs* and *codeine*. All cough suppressants may cause drowsiness.

cough, smoker's A recurrent *cough* in smokers. The cough is usually triggered by the accumulation of thick sputum in the airways due to inflammation caused by smoking. Giving up smoking usually stops the cough but it may take time. In general, the longer a person has been smoking, the longer it will take. Smokers with a cough should seek medical advice, particularly if their cough changes, because smoking is associated with lung *cancer* (see *tobacco-smoking*).

counselling Advice and psychological support from health professionals to help people deal with personal difficulties. Counselling is used to address problems at school, work, or in the family; provide advice on medical problems and sexual and marital problems; help people to deal with addictions; and provide support during life crises. Types of counselling include *genetic counselling*, trauma counselling, and *sex therapy*.

In most cases counselling is a one-to-one activity, but it may also be carried out in small groups. (See also *child guidance*; *family therapy*; *marriage guidance*; *psychotherapy*.)

cowpox An infection caused by the vaccinia virus, which usually affects cows.

This virus was used in the past to confer immunity against *smallpox*.

COX-2 inhibitor drugs A group of *nonsteroidal anti-inflammatory drugs* (NSAIDs) used mainly to relieve the pain and inflammation of *rheumatoid arthritis* and *osteoarthritis*. They cause less stomach irritation as a side effect than other NSAIDs, although they may still cause abdominal discomfort, which can be minimized by taking the drugs with food. However, COX-2 inhibitors are associated with an increased risk of heart disease and strokes and are therefore not generally recommended for people who have had a heart attack or stroke or who are at risk of these conditions. Examples of COX-2 inhibitors include celecoxib, etoricoxib, and lumiracoxib.

coxa vara A deformity of the *hip* in which the angle between the neck and head of the *femur* (thigh-bone) and the shaft of the femur is reduced, resulting in shortening of the leg, pain and stiffness in the hip, and a limp. The most common cause is a fracture to the neck of the femur or, during adolescence, injury to the developing part of the head of the bone. Coxa vara can also occur if the bone tissue in the neck of the femur is soft, a condition that may be *congenital* or the result of a bone disorder such as *rickets* or *Paget's disease*. Treatment may include surgery (see *osteotomy*).

coxsackievirus One of a group of *viruses* responsible for a broad range of diseases. There are two main types of coxsackievirus: A and B. The best known of the type A infections is *hand, foot, and mouth disease*, a common childhood disorder characterized by blistering of the mouth, hands, and feet. Type B viruses can cause serious illnesses such as *meningitis, pericarditis*, and *pneumonia*.

crab lice See *pubic lice*.

crack A popular term for a form of *cocaine*.

cradle cap A condition common in babies in which thick, yellow scales occur in patches over the scalp. It is a form of *seborrhoeic dermatitis*, which may also occur on the face, neck, behind the ears, and in the nappy area.

Cradle cap is harmless as long as the skin does not become infected. The condition can be treated by daily use of a

C

simple shampoo. Alternatively, warm olive oil or arachis oil may be rubbed into the baby's scalp and left on overnight in order to loosen and soften the scales, which can be washed off the next day. A mild ointment that contains an *antibiotic drug* and a *corticosteroid drug* may be prescribed if the skin becomes inflamed.

cramp A painful spasm in a *muscle* caused by excessive and prolonged contraction of the muscle fibres. Cramps often occur as a result of increased muscular activity, which causes a build-up of *lactic acid* and other chemicals in the muscles, and small areas of muscle-fibre damage. Repetitive movements, such as writing (see *cramp, writer's*) or sitting or lying in an awkward position may also cause cramp. Cramp may follow profuse sweating because loss of sodium salts disrupts muscle cell activity. Massaging or stretching the muscles involved may bring relief. *Quinine* may sometimes be given for recurrent night cramps.

Recurrent, sudden pain in a muscle that is not associated with hardness of the muscle may be caused by *peripheral vascular disease*. In this case, the condition should be investigated and treated by a doctor.

cramp, writer's Painful spasm in the muscles of the hand caused by repetitive movements, which makes writing or typing impossible.

cranial nerves Twelve pairs of *nerves* that emerge directly from the underside of the *brain*. Each of the nerves has a number as well as a name. The numbers indicate the sequence in which the nerves emerge from the brain.

The main function of some cranial nerves is to deliver sensory information from the ears, nose, and eyes to the brain. These are the *vestibulocochlear nerve* (hearing and balance), *olfactory nerve* (smell), and *optic nerve* (vision). Other cranial nerves carry impulses that move muscles of the head and neck area. These are the *oculomotor, trochlear,* and *abducent nerves* (movements of the eye), *spinal accessory nerve* (head and shoulder movements), and *hypoglossal nerve* (tongue movements).

Some cranial nerves have both sensory and motor functions. These are the *facial nerve* (facial expressions, taste, and the secretion of saliva and tears) *trigeminal nerve* (facial sensation and jaw movements) and *glossopharyngeal nerve* (taste and swallowing movements). The *vagus nerve* has branches to all the main digestive organs, the heart, and the lungs, and is a major component of the *parasympathetic nervous system*, which is concerned with maintaining the body's automatic functions.

All but two of the cranial nerve pairs connect with nuclei in the *brainstem* (the olfactory and optic nerves link directly with parts of the cerebrum). The nerves emerge through openings in the *cranium*; many then soon divide into branches.

craniopharyngioma A rare, non-hormone-secreting tumour of the *pituitary gland*. Symptoms of a craniopharyngioma may include headaches, vomiting, and defective vision. If a craniopharyngioma develops in childhood, growth may become stunted and sexual development may not occur. Craniopharyngiomas are usually removed surgically. Untreated, they may cause permanent brain damage.

CRANIAL NERVES

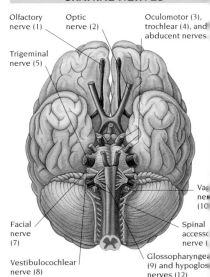

Olfactory nerve (1)
Optic nerve (2)
Oculomotor (3), trochlear (4), and abducent nerves
Trigeminal nerve (5)
Vagus nerve (10)
Facial nerve (7)
Spinal accessory nerve (11)
Vestibulocochlear nerve (8)
Glossopharyngeal (9) and hypoglossal nerves (12)

BRAIN FROM BELOW

craniosynostosis The premature closure of one or more of the joints (sutures) between the curved, flattened bones of the *skull* in infants. If all the joints are involved, the growing infant's *brain* may be compressed and there is a risk of brain damage from pressure inside the skull. If the abnormality is localized, the head may be deformed. Craniosynostosis may occur before birth and, in some cases, is associated with other *birth defects*. It may also occur in an otherwise healthy baby, or in a baby affected by a disorder such as *rickets*. If the brain is compressed, an operation may be performed to separate the fused skull bones.

craniotomy The temporary removal of a section of the skull to perform an operation on the *brain*. A craniotomy may be used in order to take a sample of tissue for analysis, remove a *tumour*, or drain an *abscess* or blood clot.

cranium The part of the *skull* around the *brain*.

C-reactive protein A protein produced in the body in response to inflammation.

cream A thick, semi-solid preparation with moisturizing properties used to apply medications to the skin.

creatinine A waste product produced by muscles and filtered from the blood by the kidneys to be excreted in *urine*.

creatinine clearance See *kidney function tests*.

crepitation A crackling sound in the lungs (heard through a *stethoscope*) caused by abnormal build-up of fluid. (See also *auscultation*.)

crepitus A grating sound or sensation caused by rough surfaces rubbing together. Crepitus may be felt or heard when the ends of a broken bone rub against each other, or when *cartilage* on the surfaces of a joint has worn away in *osteoarthritis*. Faint crepitus can be heard in the lung as a result of, for example, inflammation in *pneumonia*. Crepitus also describes the sound made when air under the skin (see *emphysema, surgical*) or gas *gangrene* is pressed.

cretinism A *congenital* condition characterized by stunted growth and failure of normal development, and, in infants, coarse facial features. Cretinism results when the *thyroid gland* fails to produce or produces insufficient amounts of the thyroid hormone *thyroxine* at birth. Replacement therapy with thyroxine is a cure, provided the condition is recognized early. (See also *hypothyroidism*.)

Creutzfeldt–Jakob disease A rare, rapidly progressive degenerative condition of the *brain*. Creutzfeldt–Jakob disease (CJD) is thought to be due to an infection with a *prion*. This is similar to the agent that causes scrapie in sheep and *bovine spongiform encephalopathy* (BSE) in cattle. One main variant of CJD largely affects middle-aged or elderly people and has no obvious cause. A second main variant, occurring in younger people, is associated with contamination during brain surgery or transplants from infected people, or treatment with human growth hormone or *gonadotrophin hormones*. A third variant, called new variant (nv) CJD, that attacks people in their teens and 20s has been identified. NvCJD causes pathological changes in the brain similar to those seen in BSE-infected cattle. It is thought to be acquired by eating infected beef. Another variant of the disease is hereditary.

Symptoms are similar for all variants. Progressive *dementia* and *myoclonus* (sudden muscular contractions) occur; muscular coordination diminishes; the intellect and personality deteriorate; and blindness may develop. As the disease progresses, speech is lost and the body becomes rigid. There is no treatment and death usually occurs within 2–3 years.

cri du chat syndrome A rare, *congenital* condition of severe *learning difficulties*, abnormal facial appearance, low birth weight, and short stature, which is characterized by a cat-like cry in infancy. The syndrome is caused by a *chromosomal abnormality*. There is no treatment. (See also *genetic counselling*.)

crisis A term for a turning point in the course of a disease (either the onset of recovery or deterioration), or for a distressing and difficult episode in life.

crisis intervention The provision of immediate advice or help by a variety of agencies such as mental health and social services departments to people with acute psychiatric or sociomedical problems.

C

critical A term used to mean seriously ill or to describe a crucial state of illness from which a patient may not recover.

Crohn's disease A chronic inflammatory disease affecting the *gastrointestinal tract*. In young people, Crohn's disease usually affects the *ileum*, causing spasms of abdominal pain, diarrhoea, loss of appetite, *anaemia*, weight loss, and *malabsorption*. In elderly people, the *rectum* is more often affected, causing rectal bleeding. In both groups, the disease may also affect the *anus*, the colon and, rarely, the mouth, *oesophagus*, stomach, and *duodenum*.

Complications include obstructions in the intestine; chronic abscesses; internal *fistulas* (abnormal passageways) between intestinal loops; and external fistulas from the intestine to the skin of the abdomen or around the anus. Complications in other parts of the body may include inflammation of the eye, severe *arthritis* in various joints, *ankylosing spondylitis*, and skin disorders (including *eczema*).

Investigatory procedures may include *sigmoidoscopy* and X-rays using barium (see *barium X-ray examinations*). *Colonoscopy* and *biopsy* may help distinguish the disease from *ulcerative colitis*.

Mesalazine and related drugs, and *corticosteroid drugs* may be prescribed. For severe cases, *azathioprine* and a high-vitamin, low-fibre diet may be beneficial. Hospital treatment may be required, and many patients need surgery at some stage.

The symptoms tend to fluctuate over many years and eventually subside in some patients. If the disease is localized, a person may remain in normal health.

crossbite A type of *malocclusion* in which some or all of the lower front teeth overlap the upper front teeth.

cross-eye A type of *strabismus* (squint) in which one or both eyes turns inwards relative to the other.

cross-matching A procedure to determine compatibility between the blood of a person requiring a *blood transfusion* and that of a *donor*. Red blood cells from one person are combined with *serum* from the other. Clumping of red blood cells indicates the presence of *antibodies*, showing the blood is not compatible.

croup A common condition in infants and young children in which narrowing and inflammation of the airways causes hoarseness, stridor (a grunting noise during breathing), and a barking cough.

Croup may be caused by a viral infection that affects the *larynx*, epiglottis (see *epiglottitis*), or *trachea*. Other causes include *diphtheria*, *allergy*, spasm caused by deficient *calcium* in the blood, and inhalation of a *foreign body*.

Humidifying the air helps make breathing easier. Nebulized or oral *corticosteroid drugs* and oxygen may be prescribed.

crowding, dental See *overcrowding, dental*.

crown, dental An artificial replacement for the crown of a *tooth* that has become decayed, discoloured, or broken. A porcelain crown is usually used on front teeth, but back teeth require the greater strength of a crown made from gold or porcelain fused to metal.

CROWN, DENTAL

Natural tooth   Peg of the original tooth   Crown

A crown may be fitted by filing the natural tooth to form a peg and cementing the crown over the top. If the tooth is badly decayed or weakened, it may be necessary to remove the entire natural crown of the tooth and then fit the artificial crown onto a post cemented in the root canal after the tooth has undergone *root-canal treatment*.

cruciate ligaments Two *ligaments* in the knee that pass over each other to form a

C

cross. The ligaments form connections between the *femur* and *tibia* inside the knee joint and prevent overbending and overstraightening at the knee.

crush syndrome Damage to a large amount of body *muscle* (usually as a result of a serious accident) causing *kidney failure*. The damaged muscles release proteins into the bloodstream, temporarily impairing kidney function. *Dialysis* is given while the kidneys recover.

crutch palsy Weakness or *paralysis* of muscles in the wrist, fingers, and thumb due to pressure on the *nerves* that supply these muscles from a crutch pressing under the arm. The condition does not occur in people who use the more common elbow crutches.

crying in infants A normal response in babies to needs or discomforts, such as hunger or thirst. Most healthy babies stop crying when their needs are attended to. In a few cases, persistent crying may be due to a physical cause such as intolerance of cow's milk or an illness (such as an ear or throat infection, or a viral fever).

cryo- A prefix meaning ice cold, used medically to indicate that a procedure uses freezing or low temperatures.

cryopreservation The preservation of living cells by freezing. The technique is used to store human eggs for *in vitro fertilization*, sperm for *artificial insemination*, or *plasma* and blood from rare blood groups.

cryosurgery The use of temperatures below freezing to destroy tissue, or the use of cold during surgery to produce *adhesion* between an instrument and body tissue. Cryosurgery causes only minimal scarring and is used to treat cancerous tumours in sites where heavy scarring can block vital openings such as in the *cervix*, the liver, and the intestines. It may be used in eye operations, for example in *cataract surgery* and treatment for *retinal detachment*. It is also commonly used for removing *warts, skin tags*, some *birthmarks*, some skin cancers, and to treat *haemorrhoids*.

cryotherapy The use of cold or freezing in treatment. (See also *cryosurgery*.)

cryococcosis A rare infection caused by inhaling the fungus CRYPTOCOCCUS NEOFORMANS found especially in soil contaminated with pigeon droppings. The most serious form the infection can take is *meningitis*. Another form of infection causes growths in the lungs, resulting in chest pain and a cough, or on the skin, causing a rash of ulcers. Most cases of cryptococcosis occur in people with reduced immunity, such as those with *AIDS*.

Cryptococcal meningitis is diagnosed from a sample of spinal fluid. A combination of *amphotericin B* and another *antifungal drug*, flucytosine, is usually prescribed. Most cases in which only the lungs are infected need no treatment.

cryptorchidism A developmental disorder of male infants in which the testes fail to descend normally into the scrotum (see *testis, undescended*).

cryptosporidiosis A type of diarrhoeal infection caused by *protozoa*, which may be spread from person to person or from domestic animals to people. The disease causes watery diarrhoea and sometimes fever and abdominal pain. It is most common in children but also occurs in male homosexuals. Treatment, apart from *rehydration therapy*, is not usually needed except for people whose *immune system* is suppressed, in whom the infection may be much more severe.

CT scanning A diagnostic technique in which the combined use of a computer and *X-rays* passed through the body at different angles produces cross-sectional images of tissues. CT (computed tomography) scanning has revolutionized the diagnosis and treatment of *tumours, abscesses*, and haemorrhages in the brain, as well as *head injuries* and *strokes*. CT scanning is also used to locate and image tumours, investigate diseases, and aid needle *biopsy* in organs of the trunk.

Newer types of CT scanners use a spiral technique: the scanner rotates around the body as the patient is moved slowly forwards on a bed, causing the X-ray beams to follow a spiral course. The computer produces 3-D images. Injected or swallowed contrast media (chemicals opaque to X-rays) may be used to make certain tissues more visible.

CT SCANNING

X-ray beam

CT scanner tilts forwards
and backwards

X-ray detector
rotates to remain
opposite X-ray
source

X-ray source
generates a beam
of X-rays and
rotates around
body

Control
panel

Direction of
rotation of
X-ray source

Motorized bed
moves forwards
after each scan

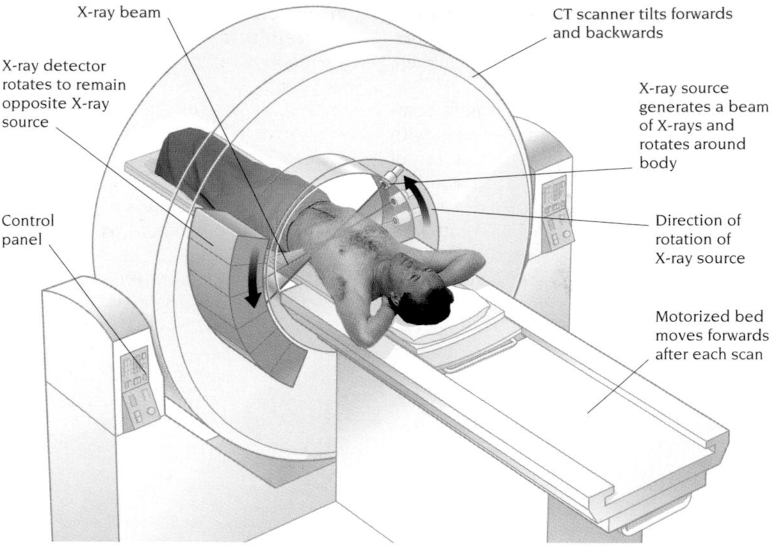

culture A growth of bacteria or other microorganisms, cells, or tissues cultivated artificially in the laboratory.

Microorganisms are collected from the site of an infection and cultured to produce adequate amounts so that tests to identy them can be performed. Cells may be cultured to diagnose disorders prenatally and for study of chromosomes (see *chromosome analysis*). Some tissues, such as skin, may be cultured to produce larger amounts for grafting.

cupping An ancient form of treatment, still used in folk healing in some countries, which draws blood to the surface by applying a small heated vessel to the skin. The inflammatory response produced is believed to help in *bronchitis*, *asthma*, and musculoskeletal pains.

curare An extract from the bark and juices of various trees that has been used for centuries by South American Indians as an arrow poison. Curare kills by causing muscle *paralysis*. Synthetic compounds related to curare are used to produce paralysis during surgery.

cure To restore to normal health after an illness. The term usually means the disappearance of a disease rather than a halt

in its progress. Medication or therapy that ends an illness may also be termed a cure.

curettage The use of a sharp-edged, spoon-shaped surgical instrument called a *curette* to scrape abnormal tissue, or tissue for analysis, from the lining of a body cavity or from the skin.

curettage, dental The scraping of the wall of a cavity or other surface with a dental *curette*. Dental curettage is one method used to remove the lining of periodontal pockets and diseased tissue from root surfaces in *periodontitis*.

curette A spoon-shaped surgical instrument for scraping away material or tissue from an organ, cavity, or surface.

Curling's ulcer A type of *stress ulcer* that occurs specifically in people who have suffered extensive skin burns.

Cushing's syndrome A hormonal disorder caused by an abnormally high level of *corticosteroid hormones* in the blood. Cushing's syndrome is characterized by a red moon-shaped face, wasting of the limbs, thickening of the trunk, and a humped upper back. Other symptoms include acne, stretch marks, bruising, weakening of the bones by *osteoporosis*, susceptibility to infection and *peptic* ulcers, and, in women, increased hairiness. Mental changes frequently occur, causing *depression, insomnia, paranoia,* or *euphoria. Hypertension, oedema,* and *diabetes mellitus* may develop. In children, growth may be suppressed.

The excess hormones are most commonly due to prolonged treatment with *corticosteroid drugs.* Such cases of Cushing's syndrome are usually mild. In other cases, high hormone levels are due to overactivity of the *adrenal glands* as a result of an *adrenal tumour,* or of a *pituitary tumour* affecting production of *ACTH* (adrenocorticotrophic hormone), which stimulates the adrenal glands.

Cushing's syndrome caused by corticosteroid drugs usually disappears if the dose is gradually reduced. A tumour of an adrenal gland is removed surgically. A pituitary tumour may be removed surgically or shrunk by irradiation and drug treatment. In both cases, surgery is followed by hormone replacement therapy.

cusp, dental A protrusion on the grinding surface of a *tooth.*

cutaneous Relating to the skin.

cutdown Creation of a small skin incision in order to gain access to a *vein* to take blood or to give intravenous fluid. This is sometimes needed when a vein cannot be identified through the skin in conditions such as shock.

cuticle The outermost layer of skin. The term commonly refers to the thin flap of skin at the base of a nail; and also to the outer layer of a hair shaft.

CVS The abbreviation for *chorionic villus sampling* and for *cardiovascular system.*

CUTICLE

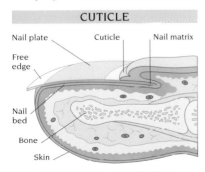

CROSS SECTION OF FINGERTIP

cyanide Any of a group of salts of hydrocyanic acid. Most are highly poisonous; inhalation or ingestion can rapidly lead to breathlessness, *paralysis,* and death.

cyanocobalamin An alternative name for *vitamin B$_{12}$.*

cyanosis A bluish coloration of the skin or mucous membranes due to too much deoxygenated *haemoglobin* in the blood. Cyanosis that is confined to the hands and feet is not serious and is usually due to slow blood flow, often as a result of exposure to cold. A blue tinge to the lips and tongue, however, could be due to a heart or lung disorder such as chronic obstructive *pulmonary disease* or *heart failure.*

cyclopenthiazide A *thiazide diuretic* drug used to reduce *oedema* associated with *heart failure* and kidney disorders, and to treat *hypertension.* Side effects include lethargy, loss of appetite, leg cramps, dizziness, rash, and erectile dysfunction.

cyclophosphamide An *anticancer drug* used in the treatment of *Hodgkin's disease* and *leukaemia.* It is also used as a *disease-modifying antirheumatic drug* to treat *rheumatoid arthritis,* and as an *immunosuppressant drug* to treat systemic *lupus erythematosus.*

cycloplegia *Paralysis* of the ciliary muscle of the eye impeding *accommodation.* Cycloplegia may be induced by cycloplegic drugs to facilitate eye examinations.

cyclosporin See *ciclosporin.*

cyclothymia A personality characteristic typified by marked changes of mood from cheerful, energetic, and sociable to gloomy, listless, and withdrawn. Mood swings may last for days or months and may follow a regular pattern.

cyproterone acetate A drug that blocks the action of *androgen hormones* and is used in the treatment of cancer of the prostate (see *prostate, cancer of*) and occasionally to reduce male sex drive. Side effects include weight gain and an increased risk of developing of blood clots.

cyst An abnormal and usually harmless lump or swelling, filled with fluid or semi-solid material. Cysts occur in body organs or tissue. Types of cysts include *sebaceous cysts, dermoid cysts, ovarian cysts, breast cysts, Baker's cysts,* and cysts that form around parasites in diseases

C

such as hydatid disease or amoebiasis. Cysts may need to be removed surgically if they disrupt the function of tissues.

cyst-/cysto- Relating to the *bladder*, as in *cystitis* (inflammation of the bladder).

cystectomy Surgical removal of the *bladder*, used for treating bladder cancer (see *bladder tumours*). It is followed by construction of an alternative channel for *urine*, usually ending in a *stoma* in the lower abdomen (see *urinary diversion*). In men, the *prostate gland* and *seminal vesicles* are also removed, usually resulting in *erectile dysfunction*. In women, the *uterus, ovaries*, and *fallopian tubes* are removed. After cystectomy an external pouch is worn for the collection of urine.

cysticercosis An infection, rare in developed countries, characterized by the presence of *cysts* in muscles and in the brain that are formed by the larval stage of the pork *tapeworm*.

cystic fibrosis A *genetic disorder*, characterized by a tendency to develop chronic lung infections and an inability to absorb fats and other nutrients from food. The main feature of cystic fibrosis (CF) is secretion of sticky mucus, which is unable to flow freely, in the nose, throat, airways, and intestines.

The course and severity of the disease vary. Typically, a child passes unformed, pale, oily, foul-smelling *faeces* and may fail to thrive. Often, growth is stunted and the child has recurrent respiratory infections. Without prompt treatment, *pneumonia, bronchitis*, and *bronchiectasis* may develop, causing lung damage. Most male sufferers and some females are infertile. CF causes excessive loss of salt in sweat, and *heatstroke* and collapse may occur in hot weather.

Prompt treatment with intensive *physiotherapy* and *antibiotics* helps to minimize lung damage from chest infections. *Pancreatin* and a diet rich in proteins and calories are given to bring about weight gain and more normal faeces. However, despite treatment, most people with CF suffer permanent lung damage and have a reduced life expectancy. Lung or heart-lung transplants have produced good results. *Amniocentesis* can determine whether or not a fetus is affected. Newborn babies may be screened for the disease (see *blood spot screening tests*). Early diagnosis and treatment improves the long-term prognosis.

cystitis Inflammation of the *bladder* lining, usually due to a bacterial infection. The main symptoms are a frequent urge to pass *urine* and burning pain on urinating. Urine may be foul-smelling or contain blood. There may be fever and chills, and lower abdominal discomfort.

Cystitis is common in women because the *urethra* is short, making it easier for bacteria to pass into the bladder. A bladder *calculus* (stone), a *bladder tumour*, or a *urethral stricture* can obstruct urine flow and increase the risk of infection. In men, cystitis is rare; it usually occurs when an obstruction, such as an enlarged prostate gland (see *prostate, enlarged*), compresses the urethra. Cystitis is children is often associated with a structural abnormality of the *ureters*, which allows *reflux* (backward flow) of urine. The use of catheters (see *catheterization, urinary*) also carries the risk of infection. Diabetics are especially susceptible to urinary tract infections.

Cystitis due to bacterial infection is treated with *antibiotic drugs*. In other cases, treatment depends on the underlying cause. It is also important to drink plenty of fluids.

cystocele A swelling in the *vagina* that is formed where the *bladder* pushes against weakened tissues in the vaginal wall. Cystocele may be associated with a prolapsed uterus (see *uterus, prolapse of*). If the urethra is pulled out of position by a cystocele, it may cause *stress incontinence* or incomplete emptying of the bladder, leading to infection of the retained urine (see *cystitis*). *Pelvic floor exercises* may relieve symptoms. Surgery may be used to lift and tighten the tissues at the front of the vagina.

cystometry A procedure used to assess *bladder* function and to detect abnormalities of the *nerves* supplying the bladder or bladder muscle. Cystometry is used to investigate urinary *incontinence* or poor bladder emptying caused by damage to bladder muscles or disrupted nerve control of these muscles.

CYSTOSCOPY

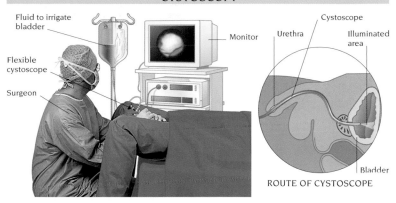

Fluid to irrigate bladder

Flexible cystoscope

Surgeon

Monitor

Cystoscope

Urethra

Illuminated area

Bladder

ROUTE OF CYSTOSCOPE

cystoscopy The examination of the *urethra* and *bladder* using a cystoscope inserted up the urethra. A cystoscope is a rigid metal or flexible fibre-optic viewing instrument, sometimes with a camera at the tip (see *endoscopy*). Cystoscopy is used to inspect the bladder for *calculi*, *bladder tumours*, and sites of bleeding and infection, and to obtain urine samples from the *ureters* to look for infection or tumour cells. *Radiopaque* dye may be injected into the ureters via the cystoscope during the X-ray procedure of retrograde pyelography (see *urography*).

Treatment, including removal of bladder tumours or calculi and insertion of *stents* (narrow tubes) into a ureter to relieve an obstruction, can all be performed via the cystoscope.

cystostomy The surgical creation of a hole in the *bladder* usually performed to drain *urine* when the introduction of a *catheter* is inadvisable or impossible.

cystourethrography, voiding An X-ray procedure for studying the *bladder* while urine is passed. Voiding cystourethrography is most commonly used in young children to detect abnormal *reflux* of urine as the bladder empties.

-cyte A suffix that denotes a *cell*. For example, a leukocyte is a white blood cell.

cyto- A prefix that means related to a *cell*, as in cytology, the study of cells.

cytokine A protein released by body cells in response to the presence of disease-causing organisms such as *viruses*.

Cytokines (which include *interferons*) bind to other cells, activating the immune response (see *immune system*).

cytology The study of individual cells. Cytology's main use in medicine is to detect abnormal cells. It is widely used to screen for cancer (as in the *cervical smear test*) or to confirm a diagnosis of cancer, and increasingly in antenatal screening for certain fetal abnormalities (using *amniocentesis* or *chorionic villus sampling* to obtain the sample of cells).

Examination of cells in a sample of fluid also helps to determine the cause of conditions such as *pleural effusion* and *ascites*. Fine-needle aspiration *biopsy* of internal organs also involves cytology.

cytomegalovirus One of the most common *herpes* viruses, which causes infected cells to take on an enlarged appearance. Cytomegalovirus (CMV) infection may cause an illness resembling *infectious mononucleosis*, but usually produces no symptoms. People who have impaired immunity are more seriously infected. A pregnant woman can transmit the virus to her unborn child; this can cause birth defects and brain damage in the child.

cytopathology The study of the microscopic appearances of *cells* in health and disease. (See also *cytology*.)

cytotoxic drugs A group of drugs that kill or damage abnormal cells; a type of *anticancer drug*. Cytotoxic drugs may also damage or kill healthy cells, especially those that are multiplying rapidly.

D

dacryocystitis Inflammation of the tear sac, usually resulting from blockage of the tear duct. The condition may occur in infants if the tear duct has not developed normally. In adults, it may follow inflammation in the nose or an injury. The cause is often unknown.

Symptoms include pain, redness, and swelling between the inner corner of the eyelids and the nose. Infection may occur and cause a discharge. The obstruction may be cleared by flushing the tear duct with saline. *Antibiotic* eye-drops or ointment are given for infection. In infants, massaging the tear sac may clear a blockage. Surgery to drain the tear sac (called dacryocystorhinostomy) is occasionally necessary.

dactylitis Inflammation of the fingers or toes, which sometimes occurs in people with *sickle cell anaemia*. More rarely, dactylitis can be caused by *tuberculosis* and *syphilis*.

danazol A drug used for treating *endometriosis*, noncancerous breast disease, and *menorrhagia*. Danazol suppresses the release of *gonadotrophin hormones*, which in turn reduces the production of the hormone oestrogen. This action usually prevents ovulation and causes irregularity or absence of menstrual periods. Possible side effects include nausea, rash, and weight gain. Pregnancy should be avoided while taking danazol.

D and C An abbreviation for dilatation and curettage, a gynaecological procedure in which the *cervix* is dilated and the *endometrium* is scraped away and a sample removed for analysis. D and C was once used to diagnose and treat disorders of the *uterus*. It has largely been replaced by hysteroscopy, an endoscopic technique for removing the endometrium (see *endometrial ablation*).

dander Minute scales that are shed from an animal's skin, hair, or feathers.

Some people are allergic to dander and develop the symptoms of allergic *rhinitis* or *asthma* if they inhale the scales.

dandruff A harmless condition in which dead skin is shed from the scalp, often producing white flakes. The usual cause is the rash seborrhoeic *dermatitis*. Frequent use of an antidandruff shampoo usually controls the dandruff.

dantrolene A *muscle-relaxant drug* used to relieve muscle spasm caused by *spinal injury*, *stroke*, or neurological disorders such as *cerebral palsy*. The drug does not cure the underlying disorder, but often improves mobility.

dantron A *laxative drug* used to treat constipation in the terminally ill who are often constipated as a side effect of opioid *analgesic drugs*. Dantron may colour the urine red.

dapsone An *antibacterial drug* used to treat *Hansen's disease* (leprosy) and *dermatitis herpetiformis*. Dapsone may cause nausea, vomiting, and, rarely, damage to the liver, red blood cells, and nerves.

daydreaming Conjuring up pleasant or exciting images or situations in one's mind during waking hours.

day surgery Surgical treatment carried out in a hospital or clinic without an overnight stay. The proportion of all operations performed on a day-surgery basis has risen substantially in recent years. Modern anaesthetics and surgical methods, such as *minimally invasive surgery*, allow a swifter recovery than in the past, and patients can usually return home within a few hours.

DDT The abbreviation for the insecticide dichlorodiphenyltrichloroethane. DDT was once widely used in the fight against diseases transmitted by insects, particularly malaria. However, because of concerns about its safety, its use is banned in most developed countries, although it is still used in some developing countries. (See also *pesticides*.)

deafness Complete or partial loss of hearing in one or both ears. There are two types of deafness: conductive deafness, which results from faulty propagation of sound from the outer to the inner ear; and sensorineural deafness, in which there is a failure in transmission of sounds to the brain.

Hearing tests can determine whether deafness is conductive or sensorineural.

The most common cause of conductive deafness in adults is earwax. Otosclerosis is a less common cause and is usually treated by an operation called stapedectomy, in which the stapes (a small bone in the middle ear) is replaced with an artificial substitute. In a child, conductive deafness usually results from otitis media or glue ear. This condition may be treated by surgery (see myringotomy). In rare cases, deafness results from a perforated eardrum (see eardrum, perforated).

Sensorineural deafness may be present from birth. This type of deafness may result from a birth injury or damage resulting from maternal infection with rubella at an early stage of pregnancy. Inner-ear damage may also occur soon after birth as the result of severe jaundice. Deafness at birth is incurable. Many children who are born deaf can learn to communicate effectively, often by using sign language. Cochlear implants may help those children born profoundly deaf to learn speech.

In later life, sensorineural deafness can be due to damage to the cochlea and/or labyrinth. It may result from prolonged exposure to loud noise, to Ménière's disease, to certain drugs, or to some viral infections. The cochlea and labyrinth also degenerate naturally with old age, resulting in presbyacusis. Sensorineural deafness due to damage to the acoustic nerve may be the result of an acoustic neuroma. Deafness may be accompanied by tinnitus and vertigo. Sometimes it can lead to depression.

People with sensorineural deafness usually need hearing-aids to increase the volume of sound reaching the inner ear. Lip-reading is invaluable for deaf people. Other aids, such as an amplifier for the earpiece of a telephone, are available. (See also ear; hearing.)

death Permanent cessation of all vital functions. The classic indicators of death are the permanent cessation of heart and lung function, and, in almost all cases, these remain the criteria by which death is certified. Brain death is the irreversible cessation of all functions of the entire brain, including the brainstem. The diagnosis of death under normal circumstances, when the individual is not on a ventilator, is based on the absence of breathing, absence of heartbeat, and on the pupils being fixed wide open and unresponsive to light.

When an individual is on a ventilator, the criteria for diagnosing brain death are based on clear evidence of irreversible damage to the brain; persistent deep coma; no attempts at breathing when the patient is taken off the ventilator; and lack of brainstem function. (See also death, sudden; mortality.)

death rate See mortality.

death, sudden Unexpected death in a person who previously seemed to be healthy. The most common cause in adults is cardiac arrest. Cardiomyopathy may cause sudden death at any age, and its presence may have been unsuspected. Sudden death may also occur as a result of stroke or in people with unsuspected myocarditis, or pneumonia. Less common causes of a sudden death include anaphylactic shock, a severe attack of asthma, and suicide.

In infants, death without warning is called sudden infant death syndrome (SIDS) or cot death. Cases of sudden death at any age must be reported to the coroner, who decides whether there should be an autopsy.

death, sudden infant See sudden infant death syndrome.

debility Generalized weakness and lack of energy. It may be due to a physical disorder (such as anaemia) or a psychological disorder (such as depression).

debridement Surgical removal of foreign material and/or dead, damaged, or infected tissue from a wound or burn in order to expose healthy tissue. Such treatment promotes the healthy healing of badly damaged skin, muscle, and other tissues in the body.

decalcification, dental The dissolving of minerals in a tooth. Dental decalcification is the first stage of tooth decay. It is caused by the bacteria in plaque acting on refined carbohydrates (mainly sugar) in food to produce acid, which leads to changes on the surface of the tooth. If the decalcification penetrates the enamel, it spreads into the dentine

D

and permits bacteria to enter the pulp. (See also *caries, dental*.)

decay, dental See *caries, dental*

decerebrate The state of being without a functioning *cerebrum*, the main controlling part of the brain. It occurs if the *brainstem* is severed, which effectively isolates the cerebrum.

deciduous teeth See *primary teeth*.

decompression sickness A hazard of divers and of others who work in or breathe compressed air or other gas mixtures. Decompression sickness is also called "the bends", and it results from gas bubbles forming in the tissues and impeding the flow of blood. At depth, divers accumulate inert gas in their tissues from the high-pressure gas mixture that they breathe (see *scuba-diving medicine*). Problems can usually be avoided by allowing the excess gas in their tissues to escape slowly into the lungs during controlled, slow ascent or release of pressure. If ascent is too rapid and pressure falls too quickly, gas can no longer be held within a tissue. Resulting bubbles may block blood vessels, causing symptoms such as skin itching and mottling and severe pain in and around the larger joints. Symptoms of nervous system impairment (such as leg weakness or visual disturbances) are particularly serious, as is a painful, tight feeling across the chest.

Divers with decompression sickness are immediately placed inside a recompression chamber. Pressure within the chamber is raised, causing the bubbles within the tissues to redissolve. Subsequently, the pressure in the chamber is slowly reduced, allowing the excess gas to escape safely via the lungs. If treated promptly, most divers with the "bends" make a full recovery. In serious, untreated cases, there may be long-term problems, such as paralysis.

decompression, spinal canal Surgery to relieve pressure on the spinal cord or a nerve root emerging from it (see *microdiscectomy*). Pressure may have various causes, including a *disc prolapse*, a tumour or abscess of the spinal cord, or a tumour, abscess or fracture of the vertebrae. Any of these conditions can cause weakness or paralysis of the limbs and loss of bladder control.

To treat major disc prolapses and tumours, a *laminectomy* (removal of the bony arches of one or more vertebrae) to expose the affected part of the cord or nerve roots may be performed. Recovery after treatment depends on the severity and duration of the pressure, the success of the surgery in relieving the pressure, and whether any damage is sustained by the nerves during the operation.

decongestant drugs Drugs that are used to relieve *nasal congestion* commonly in people with upper *respiratory tract infections*. They work by narrowing blood vessels in the membranes lining the nose. This action reduces swelling, inflammation, and the amount of mucus produced by the lining. Common drugs include ephedrine, oxymetazoline, and phenylephrine. Small amounts of these drugs are present in many over-the-counter cold remedies. Taken by mouth, decongestant drugs may cause tremor and palpitations. Adverse effects are unlikely with nose drops, but if taken for several days they become ineffective and symptoms may then recur or worsen despite continued treatment.

decubitus ulcer See *bedsores*.

deep vein thrombosis See *thrombosis, deep vein*.

DEET The commonly used abbreviation for diethyltoluamide, the active ingredient of many insect repellents. It can be applied to the skin and clothing and helps prevent bites from many types of insects, including the mosquitoes that transmit *malaria*, *dengue*, and *West Nile virus*. DEET is generally not recommended for use on children.

defaecation The expulsion of faeces from the body via the anus.

defence mechanisms Techniques used by the mind to cope with unpleasant or unwelcome emotions, impulses, experiences, or events. Repression of emotions surrounding a particular event or refusing to accept an event (denial) are both defence mechanisms.

defibrillation Administration of one or more brief electric shocks to the heart, usually via two metal plates, or paddles, placed on the chest over the heart. It is performed to return a heart's rhythm to normal in some types of *arrhythmia*

DEFIBRILLATION

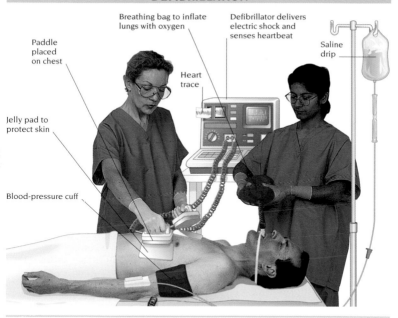

Breathing bag to inflate lungs with oxygen

Defibrillator delivers electric shock and senses heartbeat

Paddle placed on chest

Saline drip

Heart trace

Jelly pad to protect skin

Blood-pressure cuff

D

(irregular or rapid heartbeat), such as *atrial fibrillation* or *ventricular fibrillation*. Defibrillation can be carried out as an emergency procedure to treat ventricular fibrillation, which is a cause of *cardiac arrest* and most commonly occurs after a heart attack (see *myocardial infarction*). It can also be used as a planned treatment, in which case it is performed under a brief general *anaesthesia*. Breathing may be maintained artificially during the procedure.

defoliant poisoning The toxic effects of plant poisons that cause leaves to drop off. Defoliants are poisonous if swallowed. Examples of defoliants include sodium *chlorate*, potassium chlorate, phenoxy herbicides, *paraquat*, *dioxin*, hexachlorobenzene, *DDT*, and many weedkillers.

deformity Any malformation or distortion of part of the body. Deformities may be congenital (present from birth), or they may be acquired as a result of injury, disorder, or disuse. Most congenital deformities are relatively rare. Among the more common are club-foot (*talipes*) and *cleft lip and palate*. Injuries that can

cause deformity include burns, torn muscles, and broken bones. Disorders that may cause deformity include nerve problems, some deficiencies, such as *rickets*, and *Paget's disease* of the bone. Disuse of a part of the body can lead to deformity through stiffening and *contractures* of unused muscles or tendons. Many deformities can be corrected by orthopaedic techniques, *plastic surgery*, or exercise.

degeneration Physical and/or chemical changes in cells, tissues, or organs that reduce their efficiency. It is a feature of aging and may also be due to a disease process. Other known causes include injury, reduced blood supply, poisoning (by alcohol, for example), or a diet deficient in a specific vitamin. (See also *degenerative disorders*.)

degenerative disorders A term covering a range of conditions in which there is progressive impairment of the structure and function of part of the body. The definition excludes conditions due to inflammation, infection, altered immune responses, chemical or physical damage, or cancerous change.

D

The number of specialized cells or structures in the organ affected is usually reduced, and cells are replaced by *connective tissue* or scar tissue.

Degenerative nervous system disorders include *Alzheimer's disease, motor neuron disease, Huntington's disease,* and *Parkinson's disease.* Degenerative disorders of the eye include Leber's *optic atrophy* and senile *macular degeneration.* Degenerative disorders of the joints include *osteoarthritis.*

Some hardening of the arteries seems to be a feature of aging. In some people, degenerative changes in the muscle coat of arteries are unusually severe and calcium deposits may be seen on *X-rays* (as in Monckeberg's sclerosis, a type of *arteriosclerosis*). Several degenerative disorders, such as the *muscular dystrophies,* are now known to be genetic.

dehiscence The splitting open of a partly healed wound.

dehydration A condition in which a person's *water* content is at a dangerously low level. Water accounts for about 60 per cent of a man's weight and 50 per cent of a woman's. The total water (and mineral salts and other substances dissolved in the body's fluids) content must be kept within fairly narrow limits for healthy functioning of cells and tissues.

Dehydration occurs due to inadequate intake of fluids or excessive fluid loss. The latter may occur with severe or prolonged vomiting or diarrhoea or with uncontrolled *diabetes mellitus, diabetes insipidus,* and some types of *kidney failure.* Children are especially susceptible to dehydration by diarrhoea.

Severe dehydration causes extreme thirst, dry lips and tongue, an increase in heart rate and breathing rate, dizziness, confusion, lethargy, and eventual coma. The skin looks dry and loses its elasticity. Any urine passed is small in quantity and dark-coloured. If there is also salt depletion, there may also be headaches, cramps, and pallor.

For vomiting and diarrhoea, *rehydration therapy* is needed; salt and glucose rehydration mixtures are available from chemists.

In severe cases of dehydration, fluids are given intravenously. The water/salt balance is carefully monitored by blood tests and adjusted if necessary.

déjà vu French for "already seen". A sense of having already experienced an event that is happening at the moment. Frequent occurrence may sometimes be a symptom of *temporal lobe epilepsy.*

delinquency Behaviour in a young person that would be considered a crime in an adult. The term is often extended to include noncriminal behaviour such as *drug abuse,* playing truant, or running away from home. Juvenile delinquency probably results from a combination of social, psychological, and biological factors. *Child guidance* or *family therapy* may be recommended. Persistent offenders may be sent to special schools, taken into care, or made wards of court.

delirium A state of acute mental confusion, commonly brought on by physical illness. Symptoms vary according to personality, environment, and the severity of illness. They may include failure to understand events or remember what has been happening, physical restlessness, mood swings, hallucinations, and terrified panic. High fever and disturbances of body chemistry are commonly present. Children and older people are most susceptible to delirium, particularly during infection, after surgery, or when there is a pre-existing brain disturbance such as *dementia.* Drugs, poisons, and alcohol are common precipitants.

delirium tremens A state of confusion accompanied by trembling and vivid hallucinations. It usually arises in alcoholics after withdrawal or abstinence from alcohol. Early symptoms include restlessness, agitation, trembling, and sleeplessness. The person may develop a rapid heartbeat, fever, and dilation of the pupils. Sweating, confusion, hallucinations, and convulsions may also occur. Treatment consists of rehydration and sedation. Vitamin injections, particularly of thiamine (see *vitamin B complex*), may be given.

delivery The expulsion or extraction of a baby from the mother's uterus. In most cases, the baby lies lengthwise in the uterus with its head facing downwards and is delivered head first through the vaginal opening by a combination of uterine contractions and maternal effort (see *childbirth*). If the baby is lying in an abnormal position (see *breech delivery*; *malpresentation*), if uterine contractions are weak, or if the baby's head is large in relation to the size of the mother's pelvis, a *forceps delivery* or *vacuum extraction* may be required. If a vaginal delivery is impossible or dangerous to the mother or the baby, a *caesarean section* is necessary.

deltoid The triangular muscle of the shoulder region that forms the rounded flesh of the outer part of the upper arm, and passes up and over the shoulder joint. The wide end of the muscle is attached to the shoulderblade and the collarbone. The muscle fibres meet to form the apex of the triangle, which is attached to the humerus (upper-arm bone) halfway down its length. The central, strongest part of the muscle raises the arm sideways. The front and back parts of the muscle twist the arm.

DELTOID

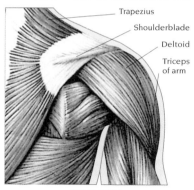

Trapezius
Shoulderblade
Deltoid
Triceps of arm

BACK VIEW

delusion A fixed, irrational idea not shared by others and not responding to reasoned argument. The idea in a paranoid delusion involves persecution or jealousy. For instance, a person may falsely believe that he or she is being poisoned (see *paranoia*). Persistent delusions are a sign of serious mental illness, most notably *schizophrenia* and *bipolar disorder*. (See also *hallucination; illusion*.)

dementia A condition characterized by a deterioration in brain function. Dementia is almost always due to *Alzheimer's disease* or to cerebrovascular disease, including strokes. Cerebrovascular disease is often due to narrowed or blocked arteries in the brain. Recurrent loss of blood supply to the brain usually results in deterioration that occurs gradually but in stages. A small proportion of cases of dementia in people younger than 65 have a underlying treatable cause such as *head injury, brain tumour, encephalitis*, or *alcohol dependence*.

The main symptoms of dementia are progressive memory loss, disorientation, and confusion. Sudden outbursts or embarrassing behaviour may be the first signs of the condition. Unpleasant personality traits may be magnified; families may have to endure accusations, unreasonable demands, or even assault. *Paranoia, depression*, and *delusions* may occur as the disease worsens. Irritability or anxiety gives way to indifference towards all feelings. Personal habits deteriorate, and speech becomes incoherent. Affected people may eventually need total nursing care.

Management of the most common Alzheimer-type illness is based on the treatment of symptoms. *Sedative drugs* may be given for restlessness or paranoia. Drugs for dementia, for example *donepezil*, can slow mental decline in some people with mild to moderate Alzheimer's disease (see *acetylcholinesterase inhibitors*), the drug memantine may be used to treat people with moderate to severe Alzheimer's disease.

De Morgan's spots Harmless red or purple raised spots in the skin, consisting of a cluster of minute blood vessels. About 2 mm across, the spots usually affect middle-aged or older people. With increasing age, the spots become more numerous but do not increase in size. They may bleed if injured. Treatment is unnecessary.

demyelination Breakdown of the fatty sheaths that surround and electrically insulate nerve fibres. The sheaths provide nutrients to the nerve fibres and are vital to the passage of electrical impulses along them. Demyelination "short-circuits" the functioning of the nerve, causing loss of sensation, coordination,

D

and power in specific areas of the body. The affected nerves may be within the *central nervous system* (CNS) or be part of the *peripheral nervous system*.

Patches of demyelination are visible on *MRI* of the brain in *multiple sclerosis*. The cause of the demyelination is not known. In many cases, demyelination attacks alternate with periods of partial or complete recovery of nerve function. In *encephalomyelitis*, there is inflammation of nerve cells within the CNS and sometimes areas of demyelination.

dendritic ulcer A type of *corneal ulcer* commonly caused by infection with *herpes simplex* virus.

dengue A tropical disease caused by a virus spread by the mosquito AEDES AEGYPTI. Symptoms include fever, headache, rash, and joint and muscle pains, which often subside after about three days. There is no specific treatment for dengue. Prevention involves protection against mosquito bites, including using insect repellents such as *DEET*.

densitometry An imaging technique that uses low-dose *X-rays* to measure bone density, as determined by the concentration of calcified material. It is used to diagnose and assess the severity of *osteoporosis*, especially in the spine and femur, and to assess its response to treatment. During the procedure, X-rays are passed through the body. A computer assesses the amount of X-rays absorbed by the body and uses this information to calculate the bone density.

density The "compactness" of a substance, defined as its mass per unit volume. In radiology, the term relates to the amount of radiation absorbed by the structure being X-rayed. Bone, which absorbs radiation well, appears white on X-ray film. A lung, which contains mostly air, absorbs little radiation and is dark on film. The same holds true in *CT scanning* and *MRI*. (See also *specific gravity*.)

dental emergencies Injuries or disorders of the teeth and gums that require immediate treatment because of severe pain and/or because delay could lead to poor healing or complications. A dislodged tooth can be reimplanted (see *reimplantation, dental*) successfully if it is done without delay. A partly dislodged tooth should be manipulated back into the socket straight away. Other dental emergencies include a broken tooth (see *fracture, dental*), severe *toothache*, which may be caused by an abscess (see *abscess, dental*), and Vincent's disease (see *gingivitis, acute ulcerative*).

dental examination An examination of the mouth, gums, and teeth by a dentist as a routine check or as part of the assessment a person complaining of a symptom. Routine examinations enable

DENSITOMETRY

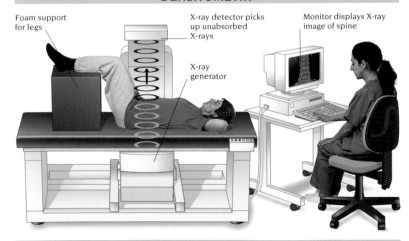

Foam support for legs

X-ray detector picks up unabsorbed X-rays

Monitor displays X-ray image of spine

X-ray generator

D

tooth decay and gum disease to be detected and treated at an early stage.

During a routine dental examination, the dentist uses a metal instrument to probe for dental cavities, chipped teeth, or fillings. *Dental X-rays* are sometimes carried out to check for problems that may not be visible. Dentists also check how well the upper and lower teeth come together. Regular examinations in children enable the monitoring of the replacement of primary teeth by permanent, or secondary, teeth. Referral for *orthodontic* treatment may be made.

dental extraction See *tooth extraction*.

dental X-ray An image of the teeth and jaws that provides information for detecting, diagnosing, and treating conditions that can threaten oral and general health. There are three types of dental *X-ray*: periapical X-ray, bite-wing X-ray, and panoramic X-ray.

Periapical X-rays are taken using X-ray film held behind the teeth. They give detailed images of whole teeth and the surrounding tissues. They show unerupted or impacted teeth, root fractures, abscesses, cysts, and tumours, and can help diagnose some skeletal diseases. Bite-wing X-rays show the crowns of the teeth and can detect areas of decay and changes in bone due to *periodontal disease*. Panoramic X-rays show all the teeth and surrounding structures on one large film. They can show unerupted or impacted teeth, cysts, jaw fractures, or tumours. The amount of radiation received from dental X-rays is extremely small. However, dental X rays should be avoided during pregnancy.

dentifrice A paste, powder, or gel used with a toothbrush to clean the teeth. It contains a mild abrasive, detergents, binding and moistening agents, thickening agents, colourings, flavourings, and sometimes *fluoride*.

dentine Hard tissue surrounding the pulp of a tooth (see *teeth*).

dentistry The science or profession concerned with the teeth and their supporting structures. Most dentists work in general dental practice; others practise in a specialized branch of dentistry.

Dentists in general practice undertake all aspects of dental care. They may refer patients to a consultant in one of the specialized branches of dentistry, such as *orthodontics, prosthetics, endodontics,* and *periodontics.* Dental hygienists carry out scaling (removal of calculi) and advise on oral hygiene methods.

dentition The arrangement, number and type of teeth in the mouth. In young children, primary dentition comprises 20 teeth (incisors, canines, and molars). These teeth are replaced between the age of 7 and 13 years by secondary (permanent) dentition. Secondary dentition

DENTITION

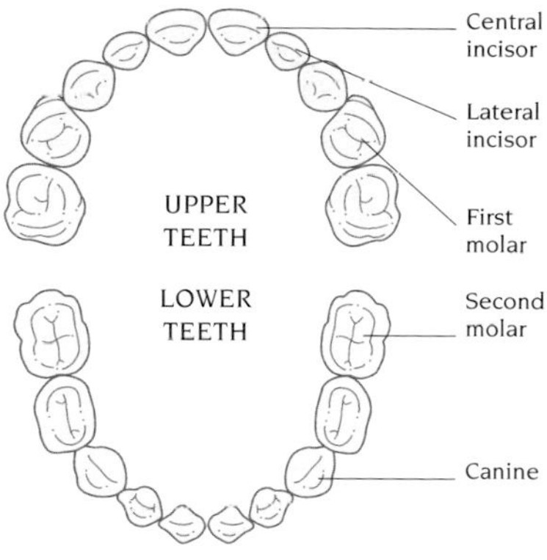

Central incisor
Lateral incisor
First molar
Second molar
Canine

UPPER TEETH
LOWER TEETH

PRIMARY TEETH

Central incisor
Lateral incisor
Canine
First molar
Third molar
Second molar
Second premolar
First premolar

UPPER TEETH
LOWER TEETH

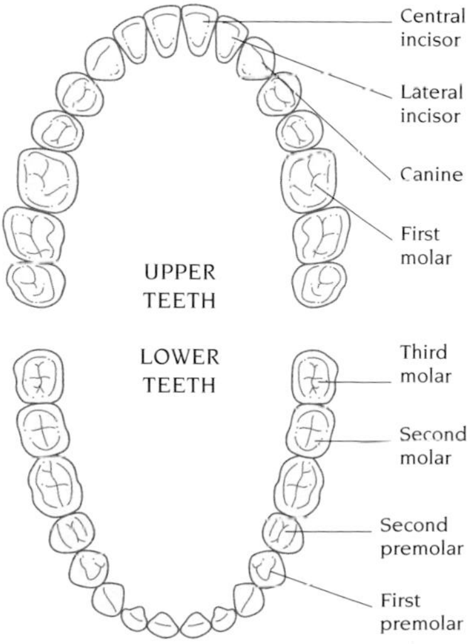

SECONDARY TEETH

D

comprises 32 teeth (incisors, canines, premolars, and molars). The third molars (wisdom teeth) may not erupt until 18–21 years of age. (See also *eruption of teeth*.)

denture An appliance that replaces missing natural teeth. It consists of a metal and/or acrylic base mounted with porcelain or acrylic teeth. The artificial teeth are matched to be similar to the original teeth. Denture baseplates, created from impressions taken from the upper and lower gums, fit the mouth accurately.

deodorant A substance that removes unpleasant odours, especially body odours.

deoxyribonucleic acid See *DNA; nucleic acids*.

dependence Psychological or physical reliance on persons or drugs. An infant is naturally dependent on parents, but, as he or she grows, dependence normally wanes. Alcohol and drugs may induce a state of physical or emotional dependence in users. A person who has a dependency may develop physical symptoms or emotional distress if deprived of the drug. (See also *alcohol dependence; drug dependence*.)

depersonalization A state of feeling unreal, in which there is a sense of detachment from self and surroundings. Depersonalization is often accompanied by *derealization*. It is rarely serious and usually comes on suddenly and may last for moments or for hours. Depersonalization most often occurs in people with *anxiety disorders*. Other causes include drugs and *temporal lobe epilepsy*.

depilatory A chemical hair remover, used topically for cosmetic reasons and to treat *hirsutism*.

depot injection An intramuscular injection of a drug that gives a slow, steady release of its active chemicals into the bloodstream. Release of the drug is slowed by the inclusion of substances such as oil or wax. The release of the active drug can be made to last for hours, days, or weeks.

A depot injection is useful for patients who may not take their medication correctly. It also prevents the necessity of giving a series of injections over a short period. Hormonal contraceptives (see *contraception, hormonal methods of*), *corticosteroid drugs*, and *antipsychotic*

drugs may be given by depot injection. Side effects may arise due to the uneven release of the drug into the bloodstream.

depression Feelings of sadness, hopelessness, and a loss of interest in life, combined with a sense of reduced emotional well-being. Symptoms vary with the severity of the depression. It may cause loss of appetite, difficulty in sleeping, tiredness, loss of interest in social activities, concentration problems, and, sometimes, anxiety. The severely depressed may have thoughts of *suicide* and feelings of worthlessness. *Hallucinations* or *delusions* may occur in extreme cases. Often, there is no single obvious cause. It may be triggered by physical illnesses (such as a viral infection), hormonal disorders (such as *hypothyroidism*), or hormonal changes after childbirth (see *postnatal depression*). Some drugs, such as *oral contraceptives*, may contribute. Inheritance may play a part. Some people become depressed in winter (see *seasonal affective disorder syndrome*). Aside from these causes, social and psychological factors may play a part.

Treatment usually includes a form of psychological treatment, such as *cognitive-behavioural therapy* or *counselling* and/or *antidepressant drugs*. Antidepressant drugs are usually effective over a period of time. ECT (electroconvulsive therapy) is infrequently used for treating severely depressed people who have not responded to other treatments. (See also *bipolar disorder*.)

derealization Feeling that the world has become unreal. It usually occurs together with *depersonalization* and may be caused by fatigue, *hallucinogenic drugs*, or disordered brain function.

dermabrasion Removal of the surface layer of the skin by high-speed sanding to improve the appearance of scars, such as from *acne*, or to remove tattoos.

dermatitis Inflammation of the skin, sometimes due to an *allergy*. Dermatitis is the same as *eczema*, and the terms can be used interchangeably.

Seborrhoeic dermatitis is a red, scaly, itchy rash that develops on the face, scalp, chest, and back. The rash often develops during times of stress and is probably caused by an excess growth of yeast on the skin. *Corticosteroid drugs* and/or drugs that kill microorganisms may help. Contact dermatitis results from a reaction to some substance that comes in contact with the skin. Common causes are detergents, nickel, certain plants, and cosmetics. It may be treated with topical corticosteroids. A patch test (see *skin tests*) may be done to identify the cause. Photodermatitis occurs in people whose skin is abnormally sensitive to light. A cluster of spots or blisters occurs on any part of the body exposed to the sun (see *photosensitivity*).

dermatitis artefacta Any self-induced skin condition. It may range from a mild scratch to extensive mutilation.

dermatitis herpetiformis A chronic skin disease in which clusters of tiny, red, intensely itchy blisters occur in a symmetrical pattern, most commonly on the back, elbows, knees, buttocks, and scalp. It usually develops in adult life and is believed to be related to *coeliac disease*.

DERMATOME

dermatology The branch of medicine concerned with the *skin* and its disorders.

dermatome An area of skin supplied with nerves by a pair of spinal nerve roots from the cervical (C2–C8), thoracic (T1–T12), lumbar (L1–L5), and sacral (S1–S5) regions. The entire body surface is an interlocking pattern of dermatomes, which is similar from one person to another. Abnormal sensation in a dermatome signifies damage to a particular nerve root, commonly due to a *disc prolapse*.

dermatome, surgical A surgical instrument for cutting varying thicknesses of skin for use in skin grafting.

dermatomyositis A rare *autoimmune disorder* in which the muscles and skin become inflamed. It causes a skin rash first on the bridge of the nose and cheeks, followed by a purple discoloration on the eyelids and sometimes a red rash on the knees, knuckles, and elbows. Muscles become weak, stiff, and painful, particularly those in the shoulders and pelvis.

Treatment is with *corticosteroid drugs* and/or *immunosuppressant drugs* and *physiotherapy*. In about 50 per cent of cases, full recovery occurs after a few years. The remainder have persistent muscle weakness. In about 20 per cent, it eventually affects the lungs and other organs and may be fatal.

dermatophyte infections A group of common fungal infections affecting the skin, hair, and nails, also known as *tinea* and, popularly, as ringworm.

dermis The inner layer of the *skin*.

dermographism Abnormal sensitivity of the skin to mechanical irritation, to the extent that firm stroking leads to the appearance of itchy weals. The condition is a form of *urticaria*. It is most common in fair-skinned people with a tendency to allergic conditions.

dermoid cyst A noncancerous tumour with a cell structure similar to that of skin. It contains hairs, sweat glands, and sebaceous glands. Dermoid cysts may also contain fragments of cartilage, bone, and even teeth. The cysts may occur in various parts of the body. Ovarian dermoid cysts account for 10 per cent of all ovarian tumours. Only rarely do they become cancerous. In the skin, dermoid cysts most commonly occur on the

D

head or neck. Surgical removal is usually recommended. (See also *teratoma*).

dermoid tumour See *dermoid cyst*.

desensitization A technique, used in *behaviour therapy* for treating *phobias*, in which the patient is gradually exposed to the cause of the fear.

desensitization, allergy See *hyposensitization*.

desferrioxamine A drug used to rid the body tissues of excess *iron* that accumulates as a result of repeated blood transfusions in anaemias, such as aplastic *anaemia* and *thalassaemia*. It is also used to treat iron poisoning and may also be used to treat excess *aluminium* in people on *dialysis*. The drug is administered by intravenous injection or subcutaneous infusion and may be given with *vitamin C* to boost excretion of the iron. Side effects may include gastrointestinal disturbances, dizziness, and skin reactions.

designer drugs A group of illegally produced chemicals that mimic the effects of specific drugs of abuse. They can cause *drug dependence* and *drug poisoning*.

There are three major groups: drugs derived from opioid *analgesic drugs* such as fentanyl; drugs similar to amphetamines, such as *ecstasy*; and variants of phencyclidine (PCP), a hallucinogenic drug. These highly potent drugs are not tested for adverse effects or for the strength of the tablets or capsules, making their use hazardous. For example, some derivatives of fentanyl are 20–2,000 times more powerful than *morphine*. Amphetamine derivatives can cause brain damage at doses only slightly higher than those required for a stimulant effect. Many designer drugs contain dangerous impurities.

desmoid tumour A growth, usually in the abdominal wall. The tumour is hard, with a well-defined edge. The tumours occur most frequently in women who have had children. They may also arise at the sites of old surgical incisions. Surgical removal is the usual treatment.

desmopressin A synthetic form of *ADH* (antidiuretic hormone) that is used to treat *diabetes insipidus* and bed-wetting (see *enuresis*).

desogestrel A *progestogen* drug used either alone or in combination with *ethinylestradiol* as an ingredient of some *oral contraceptives*. Desogestrel is reported to have a slightly higher risk of venous *thromboembolism* than older drugs. Side effects of desogestrel include menstrual irregularities, such as *amenorrhoea*, weight changes, and fluid retention. There may also be nausea, vomiting, headache, depression, and breast tenderness.

detergent poisoning The toxic effects that occur as a result of swallowing the cleaning agents in shampoos, laundry powders, and cleaning liquids.

development The process of growth and change by which an individual matures physically, mentally, emotionally, and socially. Development takes place in major phases: during the first 2 months of pregnancy (see *embryo*); to a lesser extent, during the rest of pregnancy (see *fetus*); during the first 5 years of life (see *child development*); and during *puberty* and *adolescence*.

developmental delay A term used if a baby or young child has not achieved new abilities within the normal time range. Normally, new abilities and new patterns of behaviour appear at given ages (although there is wide individual variation) and existing patterns of behaviour change and sometimes disappear (see *child development*).

Delays vary in severity and may affect the development of hand–eye coordination, walking, listening, language, speech, or social interaction. Delay may first be noticed by parents or detected during a routine developmental check.

There are many causes of developmental delay. A child who is late in most aspects of development usually has a generalized problem. This may be due to severe visual or hearing impairment, limited intellectual abilities (see *learning difficulties*), or damage to the brain before, during, or after birth. Family history and the social environment may also be associated with developmental delay.

Specific areas of delay may occur in movement and walking. Often there is no serious cause. However, specific causes may include *muscular dystrophy* and *spina bifida*. Delay in developing manipulative skills is often due to lack of adequate stimulation but may be neurological.

A lack of response to sound may be due to *deafness*. *Autism* is a rare cause of unresponsiveness to the human voice although hearing is normal. A hearing problem may cause delayed speech. Any generalized difficulty with muscle control can affect speech production; this may occur in children with cerebral palsy. Damage to, or structural defects of, the speech muscles, larynx (voice box), or mouth may also cause speech difficulties, as may any disorder affecting the speech area of the brain (see *aphasia*; *dysarthria*; *dysphonia*; *speech disorders*). Delay in bladder and bowel control have many possible causes (see *encopresis*; *enuresis*; *soiling*).

A child who shows signs of developmental delay should undergo a full assessment by a paediatrician.

developmental dysplasia of the hip (DDH) A disorder present at birth in which the head of the *femur* (thighbone) fails to fit properly into the cup-like socket in the *pelvis* to form a joint. One or occasionally both of the hips may be affected.

The cause of DDH is not known, although it is more common in girls, especially babies born by *breech delivery* or following pregnancies in which the amount of amniotic fluid was abnormally small.

If dislocation is detected in early infancy, *splints* or harnesses are applied to the thigh to manoeuvre the ball of the joint into the socket and keep it in position. These are worn for about 3 months and usually correct the problem. Progress may be monitored by *ultrasound scanning* and *X-rays*. Corrective surgery may also be required.

If treatment is delayed, there may be lifelong problems with walking. Without treatment, the dislocation often leads to shortening of the leg, limping, and early *osteoarthritis* in the joint.

deviated nasal septum See *nasal septum*.

deviation, sexual A form of sexual behaviour, most common in men, in which intercourse between adults is not the final aim. Forms of sexual deviation include *exhibitionism*, *fetishism*, and *paedophilia*.

dexamethasone A *corticosteroid drug* prescribed as a nasal spray to relieve *nasal congestion* caused by allergic *rhinitis*, as eye drops in the treatment of *iritis*, and as eardrops in the treatment of *otitis externa*. It is given in tablet form or injected to treat severe *asthma* and other inflammatory disorders in order to reduce inflammation of the brain due, for example, to *head injury*. It may be injected into an inflamed joint to relieve the symptoms of *osteoarthritis*.

The nasal spray may cause nosebleeds; eye drops may cause irritation. Prolonged use or high doses of tablets may cause adverse effects common to the corticosteroids.

dexamfetamine A central nervous system stimulant (see *amphetamine drugs*; *stimulant drugs*) sometimes used to treat *narcolepsy*. It is also used in children with *attention deficit hyperactivity disorder* for whom other treatments have not worked. Because of its stimulant properties, dexamfetamine has become a drug of abuse. With prolonged use, the stimulant effects lessen and a higher dose must be taken to produce the same effect.

DEXA scan Dual-energy X-ray absorptiometry, a technique that measures bone density by passing beams of low-dose radiation through bone. DEXA scans are used to assess the severity of *osteoporosis*. (See also *densitometry*.)

dextrocardia A rare condition, present from birth, in which the heart points to the right-hand side of the chest instead of the left. The heart may also be malformed. Sometimes, the position of the abdominal organs is also reversed. The cause of dextrocardia is unknown. Surgical treatment is only necessary if the heart is malformed.

dextromethorphan A cough suppressant available over the counter as an ingredient in *cough remedies*.

dextropropoxyphene A weak opioid *analgesic drug* that is one of the constituents of *co-proxamol*.

dextrose Another name for *glucose*.

diabetes, bronze Another name for *haemochromatosis*, a rare genetic disease in which excessive amounts of iron are deposited in tissues. It causes a bronze skin coloration, and sufferers often develop *diabetes mellitus*.

diabetes insipidus A rare condition characterized by excessive thirst and the passing of large quantities of dilute urine. It usually results from a failure of the *pituitary gland* to secrete *ADH* (antidiuretic hormone). Diseases of the pituitary gland can cause failure of ADH secretion. The condition may temporarily follow brain surgery. Treatment uses a nasal spray containing ADH. A rare form of the disease, nephrogenic diabetes insipidus, is due to the kidneys not responding to ADH; treatment is by a low-sodium diet and, paradoxically, thiazides (see *diuretic drugs*).

diabetes mellitus A disorder caused by insufficient or absent production of the hormone *insulin* by the *pancreas*, or because the tissues are resistant to the effects. Insulin is responsible for the absorption of *glucose* into cells. Lack of insulin causes high blood levels of glucose, resulting in the passage of large quantities of urine and excessive thirst. Other symptoms are weight loss, hunger, and fatigue. Urinary tract infections may also occur. *Lipid* (fat) metabolism is affected and small blood vessels degenerate. Undiagnosed diabetes can lead to blurred vision, boils, and tingling or numbness of the hands and feet.

There are two main types of diabetes mellitus, both of which tend to run in families. Type 1 (insulin-dependent) diabetes is the less common form of the disorder and usually develops in childhood or adolescence. In this type of diabetes, insulin-secreting cells in the pancreas are destroyed, and insulin production ceases. Type 2 (noninsulin-dependent) diabetes generally develops gradually, mainly in people over the age of 40. Although insulin is still produced, there is not enough for the body's needs as the tissues become relatively resistant to its effects. Symptoms may be present in only a third of people with this type of diabetes; it is often diagnosed only when complications occur. Treatment aims to keep blood glucose as normal as possible, to alleviate symptoms, and to minimize complications. It involves achieving and maintaining a normal weight, regular physical activity, dietary management, and, if necessary, treatments with *antidiabetic drugs*.

People with type 1 diabetes require regular insulin therapy. Carbohydrate intake is spread out over the day, intake of fats should be kept low, and self-monitoring of blood glucose levels is important. If the glucose/insulin balance is not maintained, *hyperglycaemia* or *hypoglycaemia* may develop. Pancreatic islet cell transplants are being researched but are not widely available. Such transplants may enable recipients to live without insulin therapy.

Treatment of type 2 diabetes usually consists of dietary measures, weight reduction, and antidiabetic drugs, often *hypoglycaemic* drugs such as sulphonylureas. Some people eventually need insulin therapy.

Complications of diabetes mellitus include *retinopathy*, peripheral neuropathy, and *nephropathy*. Ulcers on the feet are another risk. People with diabetes mellitus also have a greater risk of *atherosclerosis*, *hypertension*, other *cardiovascular disorders*, and *cataracts*.

With modern treatment and sensible self-monitoring, nearly all diabetics can look forward to a normal lifespan.

diabetic pregnancy Pregnancy in a woman with pre-existing *diabetes mellitus* or in a woman who develops diabetes during pregnancy. The latter is known as gestational diabetes. Women with established diabetes mellitus can have a normal pregnancy provided that the diabetes is controlled well. Poor control of blood glucose during the pregnancy may affect the baby's growth or increase the risk of complications during pregnancy.

Gestational diabetes is usually detected in the second half of pregnancy. The mother does not produce enough insulin to keep blood glucose levels normal. True gestational diabetes disappears with the delivery of the baby but is associated with an increased risk of developing type 2 diabetes in later life.

diagnosis The process of finding the nature of a disorder. The doctor listens to a patient's account of his or her illness and a physical examination is usually involved. Tests may be ordered after the formation of a provisional diagnosis.

dialysis A filtering technique used to remove waste products from the blood and excess fluid from the body as a treatment *for kidney failure*. The kidneys normally filter about 1,500 litres of blood daily. They maintain the fluid and *electrolyte* balance of the body and excrete wastes in the urine. Important elements, such as sodium, potassium, calcium, amino acids, glucose, and water are reabsorbed. *Urea*, excess minerals, toxins, and drugs are excreted. Dialysis is used to perform this function in people whose kidneys have been damaged due to acute kidney failure or chronic kidney failure. Without dialysis, wastes accumulate in the blood. In chronic kidney failure, patients may need to have dialysis several times a week for the rest of their lives or until they can be given a *kidney transplant*. In acute kidney failure, dialysis is carried out more intensively until the kidneys are working normally.

There are two methods of dialysis: haemodialysis and peritoneal dialysis. In both methods, excess water and wastes in the blood pass across a membrane

into a solution (dialysate), which is then discarded. Haemodialysis filters out wastes by passing blood through an artificial kidney machine. The process takes 2–6 hours. Peritoneal dialysis makes use of the *peritoneum* (the membrane that lines the abdomen) as a filter. The procedure is often carried out overnight or continuously during the day and night. Both types of dialysis carry the risk of upsetting body chemistry and fluid balance. There is also a risk of infection within the peritoneum in peritoneal dialysis.

diamorphine A synthetic, opioid *analgesic drug* similar to *morphine*; it is another name for heroin. Diamorphine is used to relieve severe pain and also to relieve distress in acute *heart failure*. It carries the risk of dependence so is prescribed with caution. The drug may also cause nausea, vomiting, and constipation. (See also *heroin abuse*.)

diaphragm, contraceptive A female barrier method of contraception in the form of a hemispherical dome of thin rubber with a metal spring in the rim. (See also *contraception, barrier methods*.)

diaphragm muscle The dome-shaped sheet of muscle that separates the chest

DIALYSIS

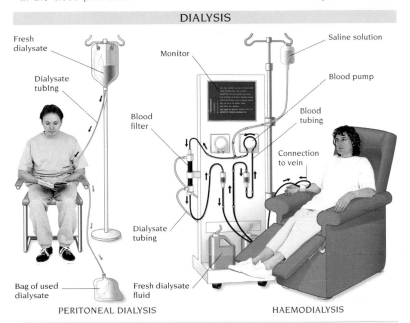

Fresh dialysate

Dialysate tubing

Monitor

Blood filter

Dialysate tubing

Bag of used dialysate

Fresh dialysate fluid

Saline solution

Blood pump

Blood tubing

Connection to vein

PERITONEAL DIALYSIS

HAEMODIALYSIS

D

from the abdomen. It is attached to the spine, ribs, and sternum (breastbone) and plays an important role in breathing. There are openings in the diaphragm for the oesophagus and major nerves and blood vessels. To inhale, the diaphragm's muscle fibres contract, pulling the whole diaphragm downwards and drawing air into the lungs. (See also *breathing*.)

diaphysis The shaft, or central portion, of a long bone, such as the *femur*. The *epiphysis* (end of the long bone) develops independently from the diaphysis, as they are initially separated by a mass of cartilage known as the epiphyseal plate. The diaphysis and epiphysis eventually fuse to form a complete bone.

DIAPHYSIS

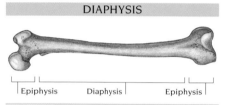

Epiphysis   Diaphysis   Epiphysis

diarrhoea Increased fluidity, frequency, or volume of bowel movements. It may be acute or chronic. Diarrhoea can be very serious in infants and elderly people because of the risk of severe, potentially fatal, *dehydration*.

Acute diarrhoea is usually a result of consuming food or water contaminated with certain bacteria or viruses (see *food poisoning*). Infective *gastroenteritis* also causes diarrhoea and may be acquired as a result of droplet infection. Other causes of acute diarrhoea include anxiety and, less commonly, *amoebiasis*, *shigellosis*, *typhoid fever* and *paratyphoid fever*, drug toxicity, *food allergy*, and *food intolerance*.

Chronic diarrhoea is generally repeated attacks of acute diarrhoea. It may be the result of an intestinal disorder such as *Crohn's disease*, *ulcerative colitis*, cancer of the colon (see *colon, cancer of*), or *irritable bowel syndrome*. Diarrhoea that recurs, persists for more than a week, or is accompanied by blood requires medical investigation.

The water and electrolytes (salts) lost during a severe attack of diarrhoea need to be replaced to prevent dehydration. Ready-prepared powders of electrolyte mixtures can be bought (see *rehydration therapy*). Antidiarrhoeal drugs, such as *diphenoxylate* and *loperamide*, should not be taken to treat attacks of diarrhoea due to infection; they may prolong it. Drugs may help if the diarrhoea is disabling or if there is abdominal pain.

Viral gastroenteritis in a child can damage the lining of the intestine, which may lead to *lactose intolerance* and further diarrhoea.

diastole The period in the heartbeat cycle when the heart muscle is at rest; it alternates with *systole*, the period of muscular contraction. (See also *cardiac cycle*.)

diastolic pressure The lowest level of *blood pressure* measured in the main arteries. Diastolic pressure is the pressure between heartbeats when the *ventricles* are relaxed and filling with blood. Systolic pressure, the highest level of blood pressure in the arteries, occurs when the ventricles contract. The normal range varies with age and between individuals, but a young adult usually has a diastolic pressure of about 80 mmHg (mm of mercury) and a systolic pressure of around 120 mmHg. A persistently high diastolic pressure occurs in most cases of *hypertension*.

diathermy The production of heat in a part of the body using high-frequency electric currents or microwaves. It can be used to increase blood flow and to reduce deep-seated pain. Diathermy can also be used to destroy tumours and diseased parts without causing bleeding. A diathermy knife is used by surgeons to coagulate bleeding vessels or to separate tissues without causing them to bleed (see *electrocoagulation*).

diathesis A predisposition towards certain disorders. For example, a bleeding diathesis is present when a *bleeding disorder* makes a person susceptible to prolonged bleeding after an injury.

diazepam One of the *benzodiazepine drugs*, used mainly for the short-term treatment of *anxiety* and *insomnia*. It is also prescribed as a *muscle-relaxant drug*, as an *anticonvulsant drug* in the emergency treatment of *epilepsy*, and to treat alcohol withdrawal symptoms. It may also be given intravenously to produce sedation in people undergoing certain procedures, such as *endoscopy.*

Diazepam may cause drowsiness, dizziness, and confusion; therefore driving and hazardous work should be avoided. Diazepam can be habit-forming.

DIC See *disseminated intravascular coagulation.*

diclofenac A *nonsteroidal anti-inflammatory drug* (NSAID) used to relieve pain and stiffness in *arthritis* and to hasten recovery following injury. Side effects may include nausea, abdominal pain, and peptic ulcer.

diet See *nutrition.*

diet and disease Several diseases are linked with diet. Diseases due to a deficiency are rare in developed countries, but many disorders are due partly to overconsumption of certain foods. A diet high in fats may contribute to *atherosclerosis* and heart disease. A high-fat diet has also been linked with cancer of the bowel (see *colon, cancer of*) and *breast cancer. Obesity* increases the risk of many other disorders, including *diabetes mellitus* and *stroke.*

Overconsumption of *alcohol* can lead to various *alcohol-related disorders.* A high salt intake predisposes a person towards *hypertension.* Some components of the diet protect against disease. For example, fibre protects against *diverticular disease*, chronic *constipation*, and *haemorrhoids.*

Some people's diets contain too few natural vitamins. Pregnant women need high intakes of *folic acid* to reduce the risk of *neural tube defects.*

Although many illnesses are commonly ascribed to *food allergy*, it is only rarely that a definite link is proved. (See also *nutritional disorders.*)

dietetics The application of nutritional science to maintain or restore health. It involves a knowledge of the composition of foods, the effects of cooking and processing, and dietary requirements, as well as psychological aspects, such as eating habits (see *nutrition*).

diethylstilbestrol A synthetic form of the female sex hormone *oestrogen.* occasionally used to treat prostate cancer (see *prostate, cancer of*) and, in postmenopausal women only, *breast cancer.* Common side effects include nausea, *oedema*, and breast enlargement (*gynaecomastia*) in men.

diethyltoluamide The chemical name of the insect repellent more commonly known as *DEET.*

differentiation The process by which the cells of the early *embryo* diversify to form the distinct tissues and organs. It also means the degree to which the microscopic appearance of cancerous tissue resembles normal tissue.

diffusion The spread of a substance in a fluid from an area of high concentration to one of lower concentration.

diflunisal A *nonsteroidal anti-inflammatory drug* (NSAID) used to relieve joint pain and stiffness in types of *arthritis.* The drug is also given for back pain, sprains, and strains. Side effects include nausea, diarrhoea, and a rash.

digestion The process by which food is broken down into smaller components that can be transported and used by the body. (See also *digestive system.*)

digestive system The group of organs responsible for *digestion.* It consists of the digestive tract (also known as the alimentary tract or canal) and various associated organs. The digestive tract consists of the *mouth, pharynx, oesophagus, stomach, intestines*, and the *anus.* The intestines are the small intestine (comprising the *duodenum, jejunum*, and *ileum*) and the large intestine (comprising the *caecum, colon*, and *rectum*). The associated organs, such as the *salivary glands, liver*, and *pancreas*, secrete digestive juices that break down food as it goes through the tract.

Food and the products of digestion are moved from the throat to the rectum by *peristalsis* (waves of muscular contractions of the intestinal wall).

Food is broken down into simpler substances before being absorbed into the bloodstream. Physical breakdown is performed by the teeth, which cut and chew, and the stomach, which churns the food. The chemical breakdown of food is performed by the action of *enzymes*, acids, and salts.

Carbohydrates are broken down into simple sugars. *Proteins* are broken down into *polypeptides, peptides*, and *amino*

D

acids. Fats are broken down into *glycerol*, glycerides, and *fatty acids*.

In the mouth, saliva lubricates food and contains enzymes that begin to break down carbohydrates. The tongue moulds food into balls (called boli) for easy swallowing. The food then passes into the pharynx. From here, it is pushed into the oesophagus and squeezed down into the stomach, where it is mixed with hydrochloric acid and pepsin. Produced by the stomach lining, these substances help breakdown proteins. When the food has been converted to a semi-liquid consistency, it passes into the duodenum where bile salts and acids (produced by the liver) help to break down fats. Digestive juices released by the pancreas into the duodenum contain enzymes that further break down food. Breakdown ends in the small intestine, carried out by enzymes produced by glands in the intestinal lining. Nutrients are absorbed in the small intestine. The residue enters the large intestine, where water is absorbed. Undigested matter is expelled via the rectum and anus as *faeces*.

DIGESTIVE SYSTEM

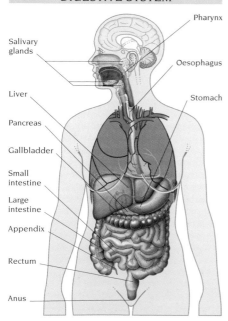

Salivary glands

Pharynx

Oesophagus

Liver

Stomach

Pancreas

Gallbladder

Small intestine

Large intestine

Appendix

Rectum

Anus

digit A division, such as a *finger* or *toe*, located at the end of a limb.

digitalis drugs A group of drugs that are extracted from plants belonging to the foxglove family. They are used to treat heart conditions, most commonly *heart failure* and *atrial fibrillation*. Those most frequently used are *digitoxin* and *digoxin*.

digital subtraction angiography See *angiography*.

digitoxin A long-acting *digitalis drug* used to treat *heart failure* and certain types of *arrhythmia*.

digoxin The most widely used of the *digitalis drugs*. It is used in the treatment of *heart failure* and certain types of *arrhythmia*, such as *atrial fibrillation*.

Blood tests may sometimes be needed to ensure the correct digoxin dose, especially in patients with kidney disease. An excessive dose may cause headache, loss of appetite, nausea, and vomiting. Digoxin occasionally disrupts the normal heartbeat, causing *heart block*.

dihydrocodeine A type of *analgesic drug*. Its side effects include nausea and vomiting.

dilatation A condition in which a body cavity, tube, or opening is enlarged or stretched due to normal physiological processes or because of disease. The term dilatation also refers to procedures for achieving such enlargement, as in dilatation and curettage.

dilatation and curettage See *D and C*.

dilation A term that is sometimes used as an alternative to *dilatation*.

dilator An instrument for stretching and enlarging a narrowed body cavity, tube, or opening.

diltiazem A *calcium channel blocker* used in the treatment of *hypertension* and *angina pectoris*. Side effects may include headache, appetite loss, nausea, constipation, and swollen ankles.

dimeticone A silicone-based substance, also known as simeticone, that is used in *barrier creams* and as an antifoaming agent in *antacid* preparations.

dioptre A unit of the power of *refraction* ("strength") of a lens; the greater the power, the stronger the lens. Lenses that cause parallel light rays to converge have a positive dioptric number and are used to correct longsightedness

D

(see *hypermetropia*). Those that cause divergence have a negative number and are used for shortsightedness (see *myopia*).

dioxin Any of a highly toxic group of chemicals. They are contaminants of some defoliant weedkillers (see *defoliant poisoning*; *Agent Orange*).

diphenhydramine An *antihistamine drug* used to treat allergic disorders such as *urticaria* and allergic *rhinitis*. It is also used for the relief of temporary sleep disturbance. Some *cough remedies* contain the drug. It can cause drowsiness, dry mouth and blurred vision.

diphenoxylate An *antidiarrhoeal drug* related to the opioid *analgesic drugs*. It lessens the contractions of the muscles in the intestinal walls, reducing the frequency of bowel movements.

diphtheria A bacterial infection that causes a sore throat, fever, and sometimes serious or fatal complications. It is caused by *CORYNEBACTERIUM DIPHTHERIAE*. During infection, the bacterium may multiply in the throat or skin. In the throat, bacterial multiplication gives rise to a membrane that may cover the tonsils and spread up over the palate or down to the larynx and trachea, causing breathing difficulties. Other symptoms are enlarged lymph nodes in the neck, increased heart rate, and fever. Sometimes, infection is confined to the skin. Life-threatening symptoms develop only in nonimmune people and are caused by a toxin released by the bacterium. A victim may collapse and die within a day of developing throat symptoms. More often the person is recovering from diphtheria when *heart failure* or paralysis of the throat or limbs develops.

Diphtheria is treated with antibiotics. An antitoxin is also given if the throat is affected. If severe breathing difficulties develop, a *tracheostomy* may be needed. Mass immunization has made diphtheria rare in developed countries. In the UK, the vaccine is given as part of routine immunization at 2, 3, and 4 months, 3–5 years, and 13–18 years of age.

diplegia *Paralysis* affecting both sides of the body (both legs and, to a lesser extent, both arms).

diplopia The medical term used to describe *double vision*.

dipsomania A form of *alcohol dependence* in which periods of excessive drinking and craving for drink alternate with periods of relative sobriety.

dipyridamole A drug that reduces the stickiness of platelets in the *blood* and thereby helps to prevent the formation of blood clots within arteries. Dipyridamole is used with *aspirin* or *warfarin* to prevent the formation of clots following *heart-valve surgery*. It may be given to people who have had a recent *myocardial infarction* or undergone a *coronary artery bypass*. Dipyridamole may also reduce the frequency of *transient ischaemic attacks*. Possible side effects include headache, flushing, and dizziness.

disability A physical or mental loss or impairment that is measurable. (See also *handicap*; *rehabilitation*.)

discharge A visible emission of fluid from an orifice or a break in the skin. A discharge may be a normal occurrence, as in some types of *vaginal discharge*, or be due to infection or inflammation.

disc, intervertebral A flat, circular, plate-like structure containing *cartilage* that lines the joints between adjacent *vertebrae* (bones) in the *spine*. Each intervertebral disc is composed of a fibrous outer layer and a soft gelatinous core. It acts as a shock absorber to cushion the vertebrae during movements of the spine. With increasing age, intervertebral discs become less supple and more susceptible to damage from injury.

DISC, INTERVERTEBRAL

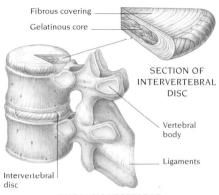

Fibrous covering

Gelatinous core

SECTION OF INTERVERTEBRAL DISC

Vertebral body

Ligaments

Intervertebral disc

THORACIC VERTEBRAE

D

disclosing agents Dyes that make the *plaque* deposits on teeth more visible so that they can be seen and removed.

discoid lupus erythematosus A form of the chronic autoimmune disorder *lupus erythematosus*.

discoloured teeth Teeth that are abnormally coloured or stained. Extrinsic stains, on the tooth's surface, are common, but are usually easily removed by polishing. They can be prevented by regular tooth cleaning. Smoking tobacco produces a brownish-black deposit. Pigment-producing bacteria can leave a visible line along the teeth, especially in children. Some dyes in foodstuffs can cause yellowing; dark brown spots may be due to areas of thinned enamel stained by foods. Some bacteria produce an orange-red stain. Stains may also follow the use of drugs containing metallic salts.

Intrinsic stains, within the tooth's substance, are permanent. Causes include death of the pulp or the removal of the pulp during *root-canal treatment* and the use of the antibiotic *tetracycline* in children. Mottling of the tooth enamel occurs if excessive amounts of fluoride are taken during development of the enamel (see *fluorosis*). *Hepatitis* during infancy may cause discoloration of the primary teeth. The teeth of children with *congenital* malformation of the *bile ducts* may be similarly affected.

Many stains can be covered or diminished with cosmetic dental procedures.

disc prolapse A common disorder of the *spine*, in which an intervertebral *disc* ruptures and part of its pulpy core protrudes. It causes painful and at times disabling pressure on a nerve root or, less commonly, on the spinal cord. The lower back is most commonly affected. A prolapsed disc may sometimes be caused by a sudden strenuous action, but it usually develops gradually as a result of degeneration of the discs with age. If the sciatic nerve root is compressed, it causes *sciatica*, which may be accompanied by numbness and tingling, and, eventually, weakness in the muscles of the leg. A prolapsed disc in the neck causes neck pain and weakness in the arm and hand.

Symptoms improve with time and analgesic drugs. However, in severe cases, surgical techniques, such as *decompression* of the spinal canal or removal of the protruding material and repair of the disc, may be necessary.

DISC PROLAPSE

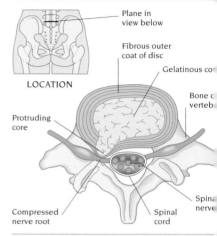

Plane in view below

Fibrous outer coat of disc

Gelatinous co

LOCATION

Bone c verteb

Protruding core

Spina nerve

Compressed nerve root

Spinal cord

disc, slipped See *disc prolapse*.

disease Illness or abnormal functioning of a body part or parts due to a specific cause, such as an infection, and identifiable by certain *symptoms* and *signs*.

disease-modifying antirheumatic drugs (DMARDs) A diverse collection of drugs that can relieve the symptoms and slow the progression of *rheumatoid arthritis* and psoriatic arthritis (a form of arthritis that sometimes occurs as a complication of *psoriasis*). DMARDs are not effective in treating osteoarthritis. The drugs, which work by directly suppressing the disease process and by modifying the immune response, may take several months to produce their full effects and are not suitable for all patients. Examples of DMARDs include *auranofin*, *azathioprine*, *chloroquine*, *ciclosporin*, *cyclophosphamide*, *gold*, hydroxychloroquine, *methotrexate*, *penicillamine*, *sodium aurothiomalate*, and *sulfasalazine*.

disinfectants Substances that kill microorganisms and thus prevent infection. The term is usually applied to strong

D

chemicals that are used to decontaminate inanimate objects, such as items of medical equipment.

dislocation, joint Complete displacement of the two bones in a joint so that they are no longer in contact, usually as a result of injury. (Displacement that leaves the bones in partial contact is called *subluxation*.) It is usually accompanied by tearing of the joint ligaments and damage to the membrane that encases the joint. Injury severe enough to cause dislocation often also causes bone to fracture. Dislocation restricts or prevents the movement of the joint; it is usually very painful. The joint looks misshapen and swells. In some cases, dislocation is followed by complications, for example, paralysis.

A dislocated joint should only be manipulated by medical personnel. First-aid treatment consists of applying a *splint* or, in the case of a dislocated shoulder, a *sling*. Sometimes, an operation is necessary to reset the bones.

disodium etidronate A drug used in the treatment of *bone disorders*. Nausea and diarrhoea are common side effects.

disopyramide An *antiarrhythmic drug* used to treat abnormally rapid heartbeat, as may occur after a *myocardial infarction* (heart attack). It reduces the force of heart muscle contraction. As a result, it may aggravate pre-existing *heart failure*. Other possible side effects include dry mouth and constipation.

disorder Any abnormality of physical or mental function.

disorientation Confusion as to time, place, or personal identity. Speech and behaviour tend to be muddled, and the person often cannot answer questions about time, date, present location, name, or address. It is usually due to a *head injury*, *intoxication*, or a chronic brain disorder, such as *dementia*. It may occasionally be due to *somatization disorder* (a psychological illness). (See also *confusion*; *delirium*.)

displacement activity The transference of feelings from one object or person to another. This is usually performed consciously to obtain emotional relief in a manner that will not cause harm to oneself or to another person.

Some psychotherapists believe that displacement is an unconscious *defence mechanism*, which prevents disturbing feelings from entering consciousness.

dissection Cutting of body tissues during surgery or for anatomical study.

disseminated intravascular coagulation (DIC) A type of *bleeding disorder* in which abnormal clotting leads to depletion of coagulation factors in the blood; the consequence may be severe spontaneous bleeding.

dissociative disorders A group of psychological illnesses in which a particular mental function becomes cut off from the mind. Types of dissociative disorder include hysterical amnesia (see *hysteria*), *fugue*, *depersonalization*, and *multiple personality*. (See also *conversion disorder*.)

distal A term describing a part of the body that is further away from another part with respect to a central point of reference, such as the trunk. For example, the fingers are distal to the arm. The opposite of distal is *proximal*.

disulfiram A drug that acts as a deterrent to drinking *alcohol*. It is prescribed for people who request help for *alcohol dependence*. Treatment is usually combined with a counselling programme. Disulfiram slows down the clearance of alcohol in the body, causing flushing, headache, nausea, dizziness, and palpitations. Symptoms may start within 10 minutes of drinking alcohol and can last for hours. Occasionally, large amounts of alcohol taken during treatment can cause unconsciousness; a person taking the drug should carry a warning card.

dithranol A drug that is used in the treatment of *psoriasis*. Dithranol is prescribed as an ointment, paste, or cream and works by slowing the rate at which skin cells multiply. This effect can be boosted by ultraviolet light treatment (see *phototherapy*). Dithranol can cause skin inflammation.

diuretic drugs Drugs that help remove excess water from the body by increasing the amount lost as *urine*. They are used in the treatment of various disorders, which include severe *premenstrual syndrome*, *hypertension*, *heart failure*, the eye condition *glaucoma*, *nephrotic syndrome*, and *cirrhosis* of the liver.

D

Types of diuretic drug differ markedly in their speed and mode of action. Thiazide diuretics cause a moderate increase in urine production. Loop diuretics are fast-acting, powerful drugs. They are often used as an emergency treatment for heart failure. Potassium-sparing diuretics are used along with thiazide and loop diuretics, both of which may cause the body to lose too much potassium. Carbonic anhydrase inhibitors block the action of the enzyme carbonic anhydrase, which affects the amount of bicarbonate ions in the blood; these drugs increase urine output moderately but are effective only for short periods of time. Osmotic diuretics are used to maintain urine output following serious injury or major surgery.

Diuretic drugs may cause chemical imbalances in the blood. Hypokalaemia (low blood levels of potassium) is usually treated with potassium supplements or potassium-sparing diuretic drugs. A diet rich in potassium may be helpful. Some diuretics raise the blood level of uric acid, increasing the risk of *gout*. Certain diuretics increase the blood glucose level, which can cause or worsen *diabetes mellitus*.

diurnal rhythms A biological pattern based on a daily cycle; also called *circadian rhythms*. (See also *biorhythms*.)

diverticula Small sacs or pouches that protrude externally from the wall of a hollow organ (such as the colon). They are thought to be caused by pressure forcing the lining of the organ though areas of weakness in the wall. Their presence in the walls of the intestines is characteristic of *diverticular disease*.

diverticular disease The presence of small protruding sacs or pouches, called diverticula, in the wall of the intestines, and the symptoms or complications caused by them. The term *diverticulosis* signifies the presence of diverticula in the intestine. *Diverticulitis* is a complication produced by inflammation in one or more diverticula.

diverticulitis Inflammation of *diverticula* in the intestine, particularly in the *colon*. It is a form of *diverticular disease* and a complication of *diverticulosis*. Diverticula may perforate and abscess-es may form in the tissue around the colon, leading to *peritonitis*. Other complications include intestinal bleeding, narrowing in the intestine, or a *fistula*.

Symptoms include fever, abdominal pain, vomiting, and rigidity of the abdomen. Intestinal haemorrhage may cause bleeding from the rectum. Diverticulitis usually subsides with bed rest and *antibiotics*. In severe cases, a liquid diet or *intravenous infusion* may be required. Surgery may be needed, in which case, the diseased section of the intestine is usually removed and the remaining sections are joined together. Some patients are given a temporary *colostomy*.

diverticulosis A form of *diverticular disease* in which there are *diverticula* present in the intestine, particularly in the *colon*. Complications of diverticulosis may include intestinal bleeding and *diverticulitis*. The cause is believed to be lack of adequate dietary fibre (see *fibre, dietary*). Diverticulosis is very rare in developing countries.

Symptoms occur in only 20 per cent of people with diverticulosis. They usually result from spasm or cramp of the intestinal muscle near diverticula. Many patients have symptoms similar to those of *irritable bowel syndrome*, such as abdominal pain, a bloated sensation, and changes in bowel habits. In severe cases, intestinal haemorrhage may produce bleeding from the rectum.

In patients with cramps, a high-fibre diet, fibre supplements, and *antispasmodic drugs* may relieve the symptoms. A high-fibre diet also reduces the incidence of complications. Bleeding from diverticula usually subsides without treatment, but surgery is an option.

diving medicine See *scuba-diving medicine*; *decompression sickness*.

dizziness A sensation of unsteadiness and light-headedness. It may be a mild, brief symptom that occurs by itself, or it may be part of a more severe, prolonged attack of *vertigo* with nausea, vomiting, sweating, or fainting.

Most attacks are harmless and are caused by a fall in the pressure of blood to the brain. This can occur when getting up quickly from a sitting or lying position (called *postural hypotension*).

Similar symptoms may result from a *transient ischaemic attack*, in which there is temporary, partial blockage in the arteries that supply the brain. Other causes include tiredness, stress, fever, *anaemia, heart block, hypoglycaemia,* and *subdural haemorrhage.*

Dizziness as part of vertigo is usually due to a disorder of the inner ear, the *acoustic nerve,* or the *brainstem.* The principal disorders of the inner ear that can cause dizziness and vertigo are *labyrinthitis* and *Ménière's disease.* Disorders of the acoustic nerve, such as *acoustic neuroma,* are rare causes of dizziness and vertigo. Brainstem disorders which can cause dizziness and vertigo include a type of *migraine, brain tumours,* and *vertebrobasilar insufficiency.* Brief episodes of mild dizziness usually clear up after taking a few deep breaths or after resting for a short time. Severe, prolonged, or recurrent dizziness should be investigated by a doctor. Treatment depends on the underlying cause.

DLE Discoid *lupus erythematosus.*

DMARDs The commonly used abbreviation for *disease-modifying antirheumatic drugs.*

DMSA scan A type of *kidney imaging* technique (see *radionuclide scanning*).

DNA The abbreviation for deoxyribonucleic acid, the principal molecule carrying genetic information in almost all organisms; the exceptions are certain viruses that use RNA. DNA is found in the *chromosomes* of cells; its double-helix structure allows the chromosomes to be copied exactly during the process of cell division. (See also *nucleic acids.*)

DNA fingerprinting See *genetic fingerprinting.*

dogs, diseases from Infectious or parasitic diseases that are acquired from contact with dogs. They may be caused by viruses, bacteria, fungi, protozoa, worms, insects, or mites living in or on a dog. Many parasites that live on dogs can be transferred to humans. The most serious disease from dogs is *rabies.* The UK is free of rabies, but travellers to countries in which rabies exists should treat any bite with suspicion. Dog bites can cause serious bleeding and shock and may become infected. *Toxocariasis* and *hydatid disease* are potentially serious diseases caused by the ingestion of worm eggs from dogs. In the tropics, walking barefoot on soil that is contaminated with dog faeces can lead to dog *hookworm infestation.*

Bites from dog *fleas* are an occasional nuisance. *Ticks* and *mites* from dogs, including a canine version of the *scabies* mite, are other common problems. The fungi that cause *tinea* infections in dogs can be caught by humans.

Some people become allergic to animal *dander* (tiny scales from fur or skin). They may, for example, have asthma or urticaria when a dog is in the house. (See also *zoonoses.*)

dominant A term used in *genetics* to describe a *gene* that shows its effects when it is present in either a single or double dose in the genotype; that is, a dominant gene has an effect whether there are one or two copies, unlike a *recessive* gene, which only has an effect when there are two copies. A dominant gene overrides an equivalent recessive gene. For example, the gene for brown eye colour is dominant, so if a child inherits a gene for brown eyes from one parent and a gene for blue eyes from the other, the child will have brown eyes. Some genetic disorders are determined by a dominant gene, for example, *Marfan's syndrome* and *Huntington's disease.* A child will have the disease if he or she inherits the gene from one or both parents.

domperidone An *antiemetic drug* used to relieve nausea and vomiting associated with some gastrointestinal disorders

DNA

Gene

Chromosome

DNA helix

D

or during treatment with certain drugs or *radiotherapy*. Adverse effects may include breast enlargement and secretion of milk from the breast.

donepezil An *acetylcholinesterase inhibitor* drug used to treat mild to moderate *Alzheimer's disease*. It slows the progression of *dementia* and loss of mental abilities. Possible side effects include nausea, vomiting, dizziness, headaches, insomnia, and difficulty in passing urine. Donepezil may also worsen the symptoms of *Parkinson's disease*.

donor A person who provides blood for transfusion, tissues or organs for transplantation, eggs, or semen for artificial insemination. The organs most frequently donated are kidneys, corneas, heart, lungs, liver, and pancreas. Certain organs can be donated during a person's lifetime; some are only used following *brain death*. All donors should be free of cancer, serious infection (such as hepatitis B), and should not carry *HIV*. Organs for transplantation must be removed within a few hours of brain death, and before or immediately after the heartbeat has stopped. In some kidney transplants, the kidney is provided by a living donor, usually a relative whose body tissues match well on the basis of *tissue-typing*.

Suitable donors may also provide bone marrow or *stem cells* for transplantation and sometimes skin for grafting. (See also *artificial insemination*; *blood donation*; *bone marrow transplant*; *organ donation*; *transplant surgery*.)

dopa-decarboxylase inhibitors Drugs used in the treatment of *Parkinson's disease*. The two main dopa-decarboxylase inhibitors, co-beneldopa and co-careldopa, are a combination of *levodopa* and benserazide and levodopa and carbidopa respectively. These drugs prevent levodopa from being activated except within the brain, which reduces the incidence of side effects such as nausea and vomiting.

dopamine A *neurotransmitter* found in the brain and around some blood vessels. It helps control body movements: a deficiency of dopamine in the *basal ganglia* (groups of nerve cells deep in the brain) causes *Parkinson's disease*.

Synthetic dopamine is injected as an emergency treatment for shock caused by a *myocardial infarction* (heart attack) or *septicaemia* (blood infection) and as a treatment for severe *heart failure*.

Doppler effect A change in the frequency with which waves (such as sound waves) from a given source reach an observer when the source is in rapid motion with respect to the observer. For example, approaching sounds appear higher in pitch (frequency) than sounds that are moving away. This is because the wavelengths of the sound from an approaching source are progressively foreshortened, whereas the wavelengths from a receding source are stretched. The Doppler effect is used in *ultrasound scanning* techniques. An emitter sends out pulses of ultrasound (inaudible high-frequency sound) of a specific frequency. When these pulses bounce off a moving object (blood flowing through a blood vessel, for example), the frequency of the echoes is changed from that of the emitted sound. A sensor detects the frequency changes and converts the data into useful information (about how fast the blood flows, for example). Doppler ultrasound techniques are also used to monitor fetal heartbeat, to detect air bubbles in *dialysis* and *heart-lung machines*, and to measure blood pressure.

dorsal Relating to the back, located on or near the back, or describing the uppermost part of a body structure when a person is lying face-down. The opposite of dorsal is *ventral*.

dose A term used to refer to the amount of a drug taken at a particular time, or to the amount of radiation an individual is exposed to during a session of *radiotherapy*. Drug dose can be expressed in terms of the weight of its active substance, the volume of liquid to be drunk, or its effects on body tissues.

The amount of radiation absorbed by body tissues during a session of radiotherapy is expressed in units called millisieverts (see *radiation units*).

dosulepin A tricyclic *antidepressant drug* used in the treatment of *depression*. The drug has a sedative action and is particularly useful in cases of depression accompanied by *anxiety* or *insomnia*. Possible adverse effects include blurred vision, dizziness, flushing, and rash.

D

dothiepin Another name for *dosulepin*.

double-blind A type of *controlled trial* that tests the effectiveness of a treatment or compares the benefits of different treatments. In double-blind trials, neither the patients nor the doctors assessing the treatments know which patients are receiving which treatment. This eliminates any expectations about which treatment will be most effective.

double vision Also known as diplopia, the seeing of two instead of one visual image of a single object. It is usually a symptom of a squint, especially of paralytic squint, in which paralysis of one or more of the eye muscles impairs eye movement. Other causes include a tumour in the eyelid or a tumour or blood clot behind the eye. Double vision can also occur in *exophthalmos*, when the eyeballs protrude because of an underlying hormonal disorder. A child with squint needs treatment to prevent *amblyopia* (lazy eye). In adults double vision needs immediate investigation.

Down's syndrome A *chromosomal abnormality* resulting in a variable degree of *learning difficulties* and a characteristic physical appearance.

People with Down's syndrome have an extra chromosome (47 instead of 46). Affected individuals have three copies of chromosome number 21 instead of two; the disorder is also called trisomy 21. In most cases, it is the result of a sperm or egg being formed with an extra *chromosome* 21. If one of these takes part in fertilization, the baby will also have the extra chromosome. This type of abnormality is more likely if the mother is aged over 35. A less common cause is a chromosomal abnormality known as a *translocation*, in which part of one parent's own chromosome number 21 has joined with another chromosome. The parent is unaffected but has a high risk of having Down's children.

Typical physical features of a person with Down's syndrome include small face and features; sloping eyes with folds of skin that cover their inner corners; large tongue; and short, broad hands. People with Down's syndrome have a greater than normal risk for certain disorders, such as a heart defect at birth (see *heart disease,*

congenital), intestinal *atresia* (a narrowing in the intestines), congenital *deafness,* and acute *leukaemia.* Down's syndrome children are especially susceptible to ear infections. A type of *Alzheimer's disease* often develops after age 40.

Down's syndrome is usually recognized soon after birth; diagnosis is confirmed by *chromosome analysis.* Screening tests during early pregnancy include *ultrasound scanning* (such as a *nuchal scan*) and blood tests to indicate fetuses likely to have the syndrome. *Chorionic villus sampling* or *amniocentesis* are then offered.

doxazosin An *antihypertensive drug* taken to reduce high blood pressure (see *hypertension*). Side effects include dizziness, headache, and nausea.

doxorubicin An *anticancer drug* given by injection, often with other anticancer drugs. It is used to treat a variety of cancers, including *leukaemias* and *lung cancer.*

doxycycline A *tetracycline drug* used in the treatment of chronic *prostatitis, pelvic inflammatory disease,* and chest infection in chronic *bronchitis.* It is also used to prevent and treat *malaria.* Taking the drug with food reduces possible side effects.

drain, surgical An appliance inserted into a body cavity or wound to release air or to permit drainage. Drains range from simple soft rubber tubes that pass from a body cavity into a dressing to wide-bore tubes that connect to a collection bag or bottle. Suction drains are thin tubes with many small holes to help collect fluid or air, which is drawn into a vacuum bottle.

dream analysis The interpretation of a person's dreams as part of *psychoanalysis* or *psychotherapy.* First developed by Sigmund Freud, it is based on the idea that repressed feelings and thoughts are revealed, in a disguised manner, in dreams.

dreaming Mental activity that happens during *sleep.* It is thought to occur only in the REM (rapid eye movement) phase of sleep, which lasts for about 20 minutes and occurs 4-5 times a night. Compared to other phases, the REM phase is active. Blood flow and brain temperature increase, and there are sudden changes in heart-rate and blood pressure.

Dreams usually closely mirror the day's preoccupations. Dreaming can be seen as a process in which the mental impressions, feelings, and ideas are sorted out. People roused during REM sleep report especially vivid dreams.

dressings Protective coverings for *wounds* that are used to control *bleeding*, absorb secretions, prevent contamination, or retain moisture.

Dressler's syndrome An uncommon disorder, also known as postinfarction syndrome, that may occur after a *myocardial infarction* (heart attack) or heart surgery. It is characterized by fever, chest pain, *pericarditis*, and *pleurisy*. Treatment is with *aspirin* or, in severe cases, with *corticosteroid drugs*.

dribbling Involuntary leakage of urine (see *incontinence, urinary*) or of saliva from the mouth (also known as drooling). Dribbling of saliva is normal in infants. In adults, it may be due to poorly fitting dentures or may be the result of facial paralysis, *dementia*, or another disorder of the nervous system, most commonly *Parkinson's disease*. Dribbling of saliva may also be caused by obstruction to swallowing.

drip See *intravenous infusion*.

drop attack A brief disturbance of the nervous system, causing a person to fall to the ground without warning. Unlike in *fainting*, the person may not lose consciousness, but injuries can occur. The causes are not fully understood, but the events may be a form of *transient ischaemic attack* (TIA) in which there is a fall in blood flow to nerve centres in the *brainstem*. Elderly men may have a drop attack while passing urine or while standing, possibly due to low blood pressure or an abrupt alteration in heart rhythm. Akinetic seizures (a rare form of *epilepsy*) are also sometimes described as drop attacks.

There is no treatment for drop attacks in elderly people. Akinetic seizures respond to *anticonvulsant drugs*.

dropsy An outmoded term for generalized *oedema* (fluid collection in body tissues). It is not a disease in itself, but a sign of disease, especially congestive *heart failure* or kidney disease.

drowning Death caused by suffocation and *hypoxia* (lack of oxygen) associated with immersion in a fluid. Most often, the person inhales liquid into the lungs;

sometimes, no liquid enters the lungs, a condition called dry drowning (see *drowning, dry*). People who are resuscitated after prolonged immersion are said to be victims of "near drowning".

Initially, automatic contraction of a muscle at the entrance to the windpipe, a mechanism called the laryngeal reflex, prevents water from entering the lungs; instead it enters the oesophagus and stomach. However, the laryngeal reflex impairs breathing and can quickly lead to hypoxia and to loss of consciousness. If the person is buoyant at this point and floats face-up, his or her chances of survival are reasonable because the laryngeal reflex begins to relax and normal breathing may resume.

An ambulance should be called and the person's medical condition assessed. If breathing and/or the pulse is absent, resuscitative measures should be started (see *artificial respiration*; *cardiopulmonary resuscitation*) and continued until an ambulance or doctor arrives. Victims can sometimes be resuscitated, despite a long period immersed in very cold water (which reduces the body's oxygen needs) and the initial appearance of being dead. In all cases of successful resuscitation, the person should be sent to a hospital.

drowning, dry A form of *drowning* in which no fluid enters the lungs. Some fatal drowning cases are "dry". Victims have a particularly strong laryngeal reflex, which diverts water into the stomach but at the same time impairs breathing.

drowsiness A state of consciousness between full wakefulness and *sleep* or *unconsciousness*. Drowsiness is medically significant if a person fails to wake after being shaken, pinched, and shouted at, or wakes but relapses into drowsiness. Abnormal drowsiness must be treated as a medical emergency. It may result from a *head injury*, high fever, *meningitis*, *uraemia* (excess urea in the blood), or *liver failure*. In a person with *diabetes mellitus*, drowsiness may be due to *hypoglycaemia* or *hyperglycaemia*. Alcohol or drugs may also produce this effect.

drug A chemical substance that alters the function of one or more organs or the process of a disease. Drugs include prescribed medicines, over-the-counter

D

remedies, and substances (such as alcohol, tobacco, and drugs of abuse) that are used for nonmedical purposes. Drugs normally have a chemical name, an officially approved generic name (see *generic drug*), and often a brand name. Those for medical use are either licensed for prescription by a doctor only or can be bought over the counter at a chemist's or supermarket.

Most drugs are artificially produced to ensure a pure preparation with a predictable potency (strength). Some are genetically engineered. A drug is classified according to its chemical make-up, the disorder it treats, or its specific effect on the body. All new drugs are tested for their efficiency and safety. In the UK, drugs are licensed by the Medicines and Healthcare Products Regulatory Agency (MHRA). A licence may be withdrawn if toxic effects are reported or if the drugs causes serious illness.

Drugs can be used to relieve physical or mental symptoms, replace a deficient natural substance, or stop the excessive production of a *hormone* or other body chemical. Some drugs are given to destroy foreign organisms, such as bacteria. Others, known as *vaccines*, stimulate the body's *immune system* to form *antibodies*.

Drugs are given by mouth or injection, or applied to the affected site by transdermal, nasal, and other routes (for example, to the lungs through an inhaler). Injected drugs act faster than oral drugs (taken by mouth) because they enter the bloodstream without passing first through the digestive system. Unabsorbed oral drugs are excreted in faeces. Drugs that have entered the bloodstream are excreted in urine.

Some drugs interact with food, alcohol, or other drugs. Most drugs can produce adverse effects; these effects may wear off as the body adapts to a drug. Adverse effects are more likely if there is a change in the absorption, breakdown, or elimination of a drug (for example, due to liver disease). Unexpected reactions sometimes occur due to a genetic disorder, an allergic reaction, or the formation of antibodies that damage tissue.

Many drugs cross the placenta; some affect growth and development of the fetus. Most drugs pass into the breast milk of a nursing mother, and some will have adverse effects on the baby.

drug abuse Use of a drug for a purpose other than that for which it is normally prescribed or recommended. Commonly abused drugs include *stimulant drugs*, such as *cocaine* and *amphetamine drugs*; central nervous system depressants, such as *alcohol* and *barbiturate drugs*; hallucinogenic drugs, such as *LSD*; and narcotics (see *opioid drugs*), such as *heroin*. Some drugs are abused in order to improve performance in sports (see *sports, drugs and*; *steroids, anabolic*).

Problems resulting from drug abuse may arise from the adverse effects of the drug, accidents that occur during intoxication, or from the habit-forming potential of many drugs, which may lead to *drug dependence*.

drug addiction Physical or psychological dependence on a drug (see *drug dependence*).

drug dependence The compulsion to continue taking a drug, either to produce the desired effects of taking it or to prevent the ill-effects that occur when it is not taken.

Drug dependence can be psychological or physical. A person is psychologically dependent if he or she feels craving or emotional distress when a drug is withdrawn. In physical dependence, the body has adapted to a drug; as a result, *withdrawal syndrome* occurs when the drug is stopped. Symptoms are relieved if the drug is taken again.

Dependence develops as a result of regular or excessive drug use, and develops most frequently with drugs that alter mood or behaviour.

Drug dependence may cause physical problems, such as lung and heart disease from smoking and liver disease from excessive *alcohol* consumption. Mental problems, such as anxiety and depression, are common during withdrawal. Dependence may also be linked with drug tolerance, in which increasingly higher doses of the substance is needed to produce the desired effect.

Complications, such as *hepatitis* or *AIDS*, contracted as a result of introducing

D

infection into the bloodstream via a dirty needle, may occur. Abusers may suffer from an overdose because of confusion about the dosage or because they take a purer, more potent preparation than they are used to.

drug interaction The effect of a *drug* when it is taken in combination with other drugs or with substances such as alcohol.

drug overdose The taking of an excessive amount of a drug, which may cause toxic effects (see *drug poisoning*).

drug poisoning Harmful effects resulting from an excessive dose of a drug. Accidental poisoning is most common in young children. In adults, it usually occurs in elderly or confused people who are unsure about their treatment and dosage requirements. Accidental poisoning may also occur in *drug abuse*. Deliberate self-poisoning is usually a cry for help (see *suicide*; *suicide, attempted*). The drugs that are most commonly taken in overdose include over-the-counter painkillers such as *paracetamol* and *antidepressant drugs*.

Anyone who has taken a drug overdose, and any child who has swallowed tablets belonging to someone else, should seek immediate medical advice. It is important to identify the drugs taken.

Treatment in hospital may involve washing out the stomach (see *lavage, gastric*). *Charcoal* may be given by mouth to reduce the absorption of the drug from the intestine into the bloodstream. To eliminate the drug, urine production may be increased by an *intravenous infusion*. Antidotes are available only for specific drugs; they include *naloxone* for *morphine* and methionine for paracetamol.

Drug poisoning may cause drowsiness and breathing difficulty, irregular heartbeat, and, rarely, cardiac arrest, seizures, and kidney and liver damage. *Antiarrhythmic drugs* are given to treat heartbeat irregularity. Seizures are treated with *anticonvulsants*. Blood tests to monitor liver function and careful monitoring of urine output are carried out if the drug is known to damage the liver or kidneys.

dry eye See *keratoconjunctivitis sicca*.

dry ice Frozen *carbon dioxide*. Dry ice is sometimes applied to the skin in *cryosurgery*: a technique used, for example, to treat *warts*.

dry socket Infection at the site of a recent tooth extraction, causing pain, bad breath, and an unpleasant taste. Dry socket occurs when a blood clot fails to form in the tooth socket after a difficult extraction, such as removal of a wisdom tooth (see *impaction, dental*). Sometimes, the clot itself becomes infected, or infection may already have been present before extraction. The inflamed socket appears dry, and exposed bone is often visible. The socket is irrigated to remove debris and may then be coated with an anti-inflammatory paste. The infection usually begins to clear up within a few days.

DSM-IV The 4th edition of the "Diagnostic and Statistical Manual of Mental Disorders", published by the American Psychiatric Association in 1994. An updated "Text Revision" version (DSM-IV-TR) was published in 2000. It classifies psychiatric illnesses and is widely accepted in other countries.

dTaP/IPV A combined vaccine that provides immunity against *diphtheria* (in a low dose), *tetanus*, *pertussis* (whooping cough), and *poliomyelitis*. It is given as a booster to children aged 3–5 years as part of the childhood *immunization* programme.

DTaP/IPV/Hib A combined vaccine that provides immunity against *diphtheria*, *tetanus*, *pertussis* (whooping cough), *poliomyelitis*, and HAEMOPHILUS INFLUENZAE type b (see *Haemophilus influenzae*). The injection is given in three doses to infants at 2, 3, and 4 months of age so that they are protected as soon as possible. Pneumococcal vaccine and/or meningitis C vaccine are given at the same time.

DTaP/IPV/Hib provides a very high level of immunity to each disease. It is less likely to cause reactions than the older vaccines. Any side effects are usually mild and occur within 12–24 hours. They include a slightly raised temperature, fretfulness, and a small lump, redness, and swelling at the injection site. Severe side effects are very rare.

Medical advice should be sought if a child has had a severe reaction to a previous dose of the vaccine or could have a severe reaction to *neomycin*, *streptomycin*, or polymyxin B (see *polymyxins*), which may be present in trace amounts in the vaccine.

DTP vaccine An injection providing immunity against *diphtheria*, *tetanus*, and *pertussis* (whooping cough). In 2004, the DTP vaccine was replaced, in the UK, by the *dTaP/IPV* and *DTaP/IPV/Hib* vaccines.

dual personality See *multiple personality*.

duct A tube or a tube-like passage leading from a gland to allow the flow of fluids, for example, the tear ducts.

dumbness See *mutism*.

dumping syndrome Symptoms due to the rapid passage of food from the stomach to the intestine. Dumping syndrome is uncommon but mainly affects people who have had a *gastrectomy*. Symptoms include sweating, fainting, and palpitations. They may occur within about 30 minutes of eating (early dumping) or after 90-120 minutes (late dumping). Some tense people may have symptoms although their stomach is intact.

duodenal ulcer A raw area in the wall of the *duodenum*, due to erosion of its inner surface lining. Duodenal ulcers and gastric ulcers (similar areas in the lining of the stomach) are also called *peptic ulcers*.

duodenitis Inflammation of the *duodenum* (first part of the small intestine), which produces vague gastrointestinal symptoms. Duodenitis is diagnosed by oesophagogastroduodenoscopy (see *gastroscopy*). examination of the upper digestive tract with a flexible viewing instrument. Treatment is similar to that for a duodenal ulcer (see *peptic ulcer*).

duodenum The first part of the small intestine. The duodenum extends from the pylorus (the muscular valve at the outlet of the stomach) to the ligament of Treitz, which marks the boundary with the jejunum (the second part of the small intestine). It is about 25 cm long and C-shaped, forming a loop around the head of the *pancreas*. Ducts from the pancreas, *liver*, and *gallbladder* feed into the duodenum through a small opening. Digestive enzymes in the pancreatic secretions and chemicals in the bile are released into it through this opening.

Dupuytren's contracture A disorder of the hand in which one or more fingers become fixed in a bent position. In about half the cases, both hands are affected. In most cases there is no apparent cause,

but the disease may in part be inherited. Men over 40 are most often affected. The tissues under the skin in the fingers or palm become thickened and shortened, causing difficulty in straightening the fingers. Surgery can correct deformity of the fingers, but in some cases there is a recurrence of the condition.

DUPUYTREN'S CONTRACTURE

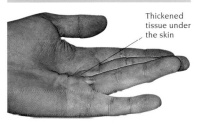
Thickened tissue under the skin

dura mater The outer of the three membranes (*meninges*) covering the brain.

dust diseases Lung disorders caused by dust particles inhaled and absorbed into the lung tissues. There they may cause *fibrosis* (formation of scar tissue) and progressive lung damage. The main symptoms are a cough and breathing difficulty. It may take at least 10 years of exposure to dusts containing coal, silica, talc, or asbestos before serious lung damage develops (see *pneumoconiosis*). Hypersensitivity to moulds on hay or grain may lead to allergic *alveolitis*. Preventive measures, such as the installation of dust extraction machinery, have reduced the incidence of dust diseases.

DVT Deep vein thrombosis (see *thrombosis, deep vein*).

dwarfism See *short stature*.

dydrogesterone A drug derived from the female sex hormone *progesterone*. It is used to treat *premenstrual syndrome* and menstrual problems (see *menstruation, disorders of*). It is also given together with an *oestrogen drug* as *hormone replacement therapy* following the menopause. Dydrogesterone is sometimes prescribed for *endometriosis* or to prevent *miscarriage*. Adverse effects include swollen ankles, weight gain, breast tenderness, and nausea.

dying, care of the Physical and psychological care with the aim of making the

D

final period of a dying person's life as free from pain, discomfort, and emotional distress as possible. Carers may include doctors, nurses, other medical professionals, counsellors, social workers, clergy, family, and friends.

Pain can be relieved by regular low doses of *analgesic drugs*. Opioid analgesics, such as *morphine*, may be given if pain is severe. Other methods of pain relief include *nerve blocks, cordotomy*, and *TENS*. Nausea and vomiting may be controlled by drugs. Constipation can be treated with *laxatives*. Breathlessness is another common problem in the dying and may be relieved by morphine.

Towards the end, the dying person may be restless and may suffer from breathing difficulty due to *heart failure* or *pneumonia*. These symptoms can be relieved by drugs and by placing the patient in a more comfortable position.

Emotional care is as important as the relief of physical symptoms. Many dying people feel angry or depressed and feelings of guilt or regret are common responses. Loving, caring support from family, friends, and others is important.

Many terminally ill people prefer to die at home. Few terminally ill patients require complicated nursing for a prolonged period. Care in a hospice may be offered. Hospices are small units that have been established specifically to care for the dying and their families.

dys- A prefix meaning abnormal, difficult, painful, or faulty, as in dysuria (pain on passing urine).

dysarthria A *speech disorder* caused by disease or damage to the physical apparatus of speech or to nerves controlling this apparatus. Affected people can formulate, select, and write out words and sentences grammatically; the problem is with vocal expression only. Dysarthria is common in many degenerative neurological conditions, such as *multiple sclerosis* and *Parkinson's disease*. Dysarthria may result from a *stroke, brain tumour*, or an isolated defect or damage to a particular nerve. Structural defects of the mouth, as occur in *cleft lip and palate*, can also cause dysarthria.

Drug or surgical treatment of the underlying disease or structural defect may improve the ability to speak clearly. *Speech therapy* is useful.

dyscalculia A disorder in which there is difficulty in solving mathematical problems. (See also *learning difficulties*.)

dyschondroplasia A rare disorder, also called multiple enchondromatosis, that is present from birth and characterized by the presence of multiple tumours of cartilaginous tissue within the bones of a limb. It is caused by a failure of normal bone development from cartilage. The bones are shortened, resulting in deformity. Rarely, a tumour may become cancerous (see *chondrosarcoma*).

dysentery An intestinal infection, causing diarrhoea (often with blood, pus, and mucus) and abdominal pain. There are two distinct forms: *shigellosis*, due to shigella bacteria; and *amoebic dysentery*, caused by the protozoan parasite ENTAMOEBA HISTOLYTICA. The main risk with dysentery is *dehydration*.

dysgraphia Problems with writing (see *learning difficulties*).

dyskinesia Abnormal muscular movements. Uncontrollable twitching, jerking, or writhing movements cannot be suppressed and may affect control of voluntary movements. The disorder may involve the whole body or be restricted to a group of muscles. Types of dyskinesia include *chorea* (jerking movements), *athetosis* (writhing), *choreoathetosis* (a combined form), *myoclonus* (muscle spasms), *tics* (repetitive fidgets), and *tremors*. Dyskinesia may result from brain damage at birth or may be a side effect of certain drugs (see *tardive dyskinesia*), which often disappears when the drug is stopped. Otherwise, dyskinesia is difficult to treat. (See also *parkinsonism*.)

dyslexia A reading disability characterized by difficulty in coping with written symbols. It is more common in males, and evidence suggests that a specific, sometimes inherited, neurological disorder underlies true dyslexia. Dyslexia is not a sign of low intelligence and therefore a dyslexic child's reading skills often lag behind other scholastic abilities. While many young children tend to reverse letters and words (for example, writing or reading p for q or was for saw), most soon correct such errors. Dyslexic children continue to confuse these symbols. Letters are transposed (as in pest for step) and spelling errors are common. These children may even be unable to read words that they can spell correctly. It is important to recognize the problem early to avoid any added frustrations.

Specific remedial teaching can help the child overcome the deficit. Avoidance of pressure from parents combined with praise for what the child can do is equally important.

dysmenorrhoea Pain or discomfort during or just before a period. Primary dysmenorrhoea is common in teenage girls and young women. It usually starts 2–3 years after *menstruation* begins but often diminishes after the age of 25. The exact cause is unknown. One possibility is excessive production of, or undue sensitivity to, *prostaglandins*, hormone-like substances that stimulate spasms in the uterus. Secondary dysmenorrhoea is due to an underlying disorder, such as *pelvic inflammatory disease* or *endometriosis*, and usually begins in adult life.

Cramp-like pain or discomfort in the lower abdomen occurs, sometimes with a dull ache in the lower back. Some women have nausea and vomiting. Mild primary dysmenorrhoea is often relieved by *analgesic drugs*. In severe cases, symptoms can usually be relieved with *oral contraceptives* or other hormonal preparations that suppress ovulation. Treatment of secondary dysmenorrhoea depends on the cause.

dyspareunia Painful sexual intercourse (see *intercourse, painful*).

dyspepsia The medical term for *indigestion*.

dysphagia The medical term for *swallowing difficulty*.

dysphasia A disturbance in the ability to select the words with which to speak and write and/or to understand speech or writing. It is caused by damage to speech and comprehension regions of the brain. (See also *aphasia*.)

dysphonia Defective production of vocal sounds in speech, as a result of disease or damage to the larynx (voice-box) or to the nerve supply to the laryngeal muscles. (See also *larynx, disorders of*; *speech disorders*.)

dysplasia Any abnormality of growth. The term applies to deformities in structures such as the skull and to abnormalities of single cells. Abnormal cell features include the size, shape, and rate of multiplication of cells.

dyspnoea The medical term for shortness of breath (see *breathing difficulty*).

dysrhythmia, cardiac A medical term meaning disturbance of heart rhythm, sometimes used as an alternative to arrhythmia (see *arrhythmia, cardiac*).

dystocia A term that means difficult or abnormal labour (see *childbirth*). Dystocia may occur, for example, if the baby is very large, or if the mother's pelvis is abnormally shaped or too small for the baby to pass through. (See also *childbirth, complications of*.)

dystonia Abnormal muscle rigidity, causing painful spasms, unusually fixed postures, or strange movements. Dystonia may affect a localized area of the body, or may be more generalized. The most common types of localized dystonia are *torticollis* (painful neck spasm) and *scoliosis* (abnormal sideways curvature of the spine). Generalized dystonia may be due to neurological disorders such as *Parkinson's disease*, or may also be a side effect of *antipsychotic drugs*.

Dystonia may be resolved with *anticholinergic drugs* or with *benzodiazepine drugs*. In some cases, *biofeedback training* may help. Injections of botulinum toxin into the affected muscles are effective in treating some types of dystonia.

dystrophy Any disorder in which the structure and normal activity of cells within a tissue have been disrupted by inadequate nutrition. The usual cause is poor circulation of blood through the tissue, but dystrophy can also be due to nerve damage or deficiency of a specific enzyme in the tissue. Examples include *muscular dystrophies* and *leukodystrophies*. Corneal dystrophies, in which cells lining the cornea are damaged, are a rare cause of blindness.

dysuria The medical term for pain, discomfort, or difficulty in passing urine (see *urination, painful*).

E

E

ear The organ of *hearing* and *balance*. It consists of three parts: the outer ear, the middle ear, and the inner ear.

The outer ear comprises the *pinna* and the ear canal. The outer part of the ear canal produces *earwax*, which traps dust and foreign bodies. The canal is closed at its inner end by the *eardrum*, which vibrates in response to changes in air pressure that make sound.

The middle ear is a cavity that conducts sound to the inner ear by means of three tiny, linked, movable bones known as *ossicles*. The first bone, the malleus, is joined to the inner surface of the eardrum. The second, the incus, is linked to the malleus and to the third bone, the stapes. The base of the stapes fills the oval window leading to the inner ear. The *eustachian tube* links the middle ear to the back of the nose.

The inner ear is an intricate series of structures deep within the skull. The front part, the *cochlea*, is a tube containing nerve fibres that detect different sound frequencies. The rear part of the inner ear contains three semicircular canals and is concerned with balance. The semicircular canals are connected to a cavity called the *vestibule* and contain hair cells bathed in fluid. Some of these cells are sensitive to gravity and acceleration; others detect direction of movement. Information from the inner ear is conducted to the brain via the *vestibulocochlear nerve*.

earache Pain in the *ear*. Earache is a common symptom, especially in childhood. The most frequent cause is acute *otitis media*, which results in severe, stabbing pain. Another common cause of earache is *otitis externa*. The pain may be accompanied by irritation and a discharge of *pus*. Intermittent earache may accompany dental problems, *tonsillitis*, throat cancer (see *pharynx, cancer of*), or pain in the jaw or neck muscles.

EAR

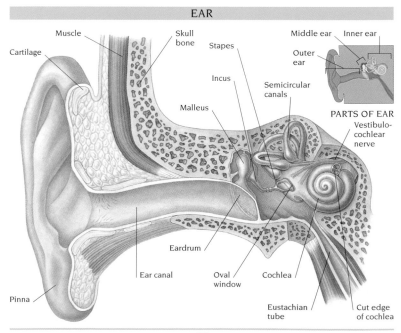

Muscle — Skull bone — Stapes — Middle ear — Inner ear
Cartilage — Outer ear
Incus — Semicircular canals
Malleus
PARTS OF EAR
Vestibulo-cochlear nerve
Eardrum
Ear canal — Oval window — Cochlea
Pinna
Eustachian tube — Cut edge of cochlea

To determine the cause of earache, the ear is inspected (see *ear, examination of*). *Analgesic drugs* may relieve the pain, and *antibiotic drugs* may be given for infection. Pus in the outer ear may be removed by suction. Pus in the middle ear may be drained by *myringotomy*.

ear, cauliflower See *cauliflower ear*.

ear, discharge from An emission of fluid from the ear, also called *otorrhoea*. It may be due to outer-ear infection (see *otitis externa*). It may also follow perforation of the eardrum (see *eardrum, perforated*), usually due to middle-ear infection (see *otitis media*). Rarely, after a *skull fracture*, *cerebrospinal fluid* or blood may be discharged.

A swab may be taken of the discharge and analysed to identify any infection. *Hearing tests* may be performed. *X-rays* of the skull are taken if there has been a *head injury* or serious middle-ear infection is suspected. Treatment usually includes *antibiotic drugs*.

ear, disorders of The *ear* is susceptible to various disorders, some of which can lead to *deafness*. In rare cases, the ear canal, *ossicles* in the middle ear, or *pinna* are absent or deformed at birth. *Rubella* in early pregnancy can damage the baby's developing ear, leading to deafness. Most cases of congenital *sensorineural deafness* are genetic.

Infection is the most common cause of ear disorders; it may occur in the ear canal, leading to *otitis externa*, or affect the middle ear, causing *otitis media*. This can lead to perforation of the eardrum (see *eardrum, perforated*). Persistent *glue ear*, often due to infection, is the most common cause of childhood hearing difficulties. Viral infection of the inner ear may cause *labyrinthitis*.

Cauliflower ear is the result of one large or several small injuries to the pinna. Perforation of the eardrum can result from poking objects into the ear or loud noise. Prolonged exposure to loud noise can cause *tinnitus* and/or deafness. Pressure changes associated with flying or scuba diving can also cause minor damage (see *barotrauma*).

Tumours of the ear are rare. *Acoustic neuroma* is a noncancerous tumour of the *acoustic nerve* that may press on

structures in the ear to cause deafness, tinnitus, and problems with balance.

In *cholesteatoma*, skin cells and debris collect in the middle ear. Obstruction of the ear canal is most often the result of *earwax*, although in small children, an object may have been pushed into the ear (see *ear, foreign body in*).

In *otosclerosis*, a hereditary condition, a bone in the middle ear becomes fixed, causing deafness. *Ménière's disease* is an uncommon condition in which deafness, *vertigo*, and tinnitus result from the accumulation of fluid in the inner ear. Deafness in many elderly people is due to *presbyacusis*, in which hair cells in the *cochlea* deteriorate.

Certain drugs, such as *aminoglycoside drugs*, can damage ear function.

eardrum The circular membrane that separates the outer *ear* from the middle ear. The eardrum vibrates in response to sound waves, conducting the sound to the inner ear through the *ossicles*.

eardrum, perforated Rupture or erosion of the *eardrum*. Perforation of the eardrum can cause brief, intense pain. There may be slight bleeding, a discharge from the ear (see *ear, discharge from*), and some reduction in hearing.

Most commonly, perforation occurs as a result of the build-up of pus in the middle ear due to acute *otitis media*. Perforation may also be associated with *cholesteatoma*. Another cause is injury, for example from insertion of an object into the ear, a loud noise, *barotrauma*, or a fracture to the base of the skull.

Diagnosis is confirmed by examination of the ear (see *ear, examination of*). *Hearing tests* may also be performed. *Analgesic drugs* may relieve any pain and *antibiotic drugs* may be prescribed to treat or prevent infection. Most perforations heal quickly. If the perforation fails to heal, *myringoplasty* may be needed.

ear, examination of The ear may be examined to investigate *earache*, discharge from the ear (see *ear, discharge from*), hearing loss, a feeling of fullness in the ear, disturbed *balance*, *tinnitus*, or swelling of lymph nodes (see *glands, swollen*) around the ear.

To view the ear canal and eardrum, an *otoscope* may be used. To obtain images

E

E

of the middle and inner ears, *X-rays*, *CT scanning*, or *MRI* may be carried out. Hearing and balance can be assessed by means of *hearing tests* or *caloric tests*. *Electronystagmography* assesses balance by watching eye movements when water is inserted into the ear.

ear, foreign body in Foreign bodies can easily enter the ear canal. Children often insert objects into their ears, and insects may crawl or fly in. Objects in the ear must be removed by a doctor. This can be done by *syringin g of the ear* or by using fine-toothed *forceps*. Insects can sometimes be floated out with olive oil or lukewarm water.

ear, nose, and throat surgery See *otorhinolaryngology*.

ear piercing Making a hole in the earlobe or another part of the external ear to accommodate an earring.

ears, pinning back of See *otoplasty*.

earwax A yellow or brown secretion, also called cerumen, produced by glands in the outer ear canal. Some people produce so much wax that it regularly obstructs the canal. Excess earwax may produce a sensation of fullness in the ear and partial *deafness*. Prolonged blockage may irritate the canal.

Wax that causes blockage or irritation may come out after being softened with oil. Otherwise, it should be removed by a doctor. This is usually done, after wax is softened, by *syringing of the ears*.

eating disorders Illnesses characterized by obsessions with weight and body image. Eating disorders are most common in young adolescent females but can affect males. In *anorexia nervosa*, patients, despite being painfully thin, perceive themselves as fat and starve themselves. Binge-eating followed by self-induced vomiting is a major feature of *bulimia*, although, in this disorder, weight may be normal. Both conditions may occur together. In morbid *obesity*, there is a constant desire to eat large quantities of food.

Ebola fever A dangerous and highly contagious viral infection that causes severe *haemorrhaging* from the skin and *mucous membranes*. Ebola fever occurs predominantly in Africa. There is no specific treatment for the disease, which is fatal in many cases.

ecchymosis The medical term for a *bruise* that is visible through the skin.

eccrine gland A type of *sweat gland*.

ECG The abbreviation for electrocardiography, a method of recording the electrical activity of the *heart* muscle. An ECG is useful for diagnosing heart disorders, many of which produce deviations from normal electrical patterns.

ECG

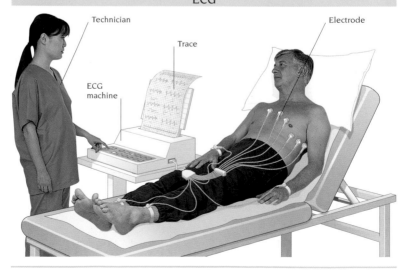

Technician

Trace

Electrode

ECG machine

Electrodes connected to a recording machine are placed on the chest, wrists, and ankles. The machine displays the electrical activity of the heart on a screen or as a printed trace. (See also *ambulatory ECG*)

echinachea A preparation of the plant *ECHINACEA ANGUSTIFOLIA*, used in *herbal medicine*. Echinachea is believed to boost the *immune system* and therefore increase the body's resistance to infection.

echocardiography A method of obtaining an image of the structure and movement of the heart with *ultrasound*. Echocardiography is a major diagnostic technique used to detect structural, and some functional, abnormalities of the heart wall, heart chambers, *heart valves*, and large *coronary arteries*. It is also used to diagnose congenital heart disease (see *heart disease, congenital*), *cardiomyopathy, aneurysms, pericarditis*, and blood clots in the heart.

A transducer (an instrument that sends out and receives sound signals) is placed on the chest. Ultrasound waves are reflected differently by each part of the heart, resulting in a complex series of echoes, which are viewed on a screen and can be recorded or the results printed out. Developments such as multiple moving transducers and computer analysis give clear anatomical pictures of the heart. Transoesophageal echocardiography is a newer, more sophisticated technique in which the transducer is placed in the oesophagus using an *endoscope*. This technique enables very detailed images to be obtained, as may be needed when planning heart-valve surgery, for example.

Doppler echocardiography measures the velocity of blood flow through the heart, allowing assessment of structural abnormalities, such as *septal defects*. Stress echocardiography can be used as an alternative to an *exercise ECG* in the assessment of *coronary artery disease*.

echolalia The compulsive repetition of what is spoken by another person. The tone and accent of the speaker are copied as well as the words. Echolalia may be a symptom of *schizophrenia* and sometimes occurs in people with a *learning disability* or autism.

eclampsia A rare, but serious condition that develops in late *pregnancy*, during *labour*, or after delivery. Eclampsia is characterized by *hypertension, proteinuria, oedema*, and the development of *seizures*; it threatens the life of both the mother and the baby. Eclampsia occurs as a complication of moderate or severe (but not mild) *pre-eclampsia*,

The warning symptoms of impending eclampsia include headaches, confusion, blurred or disturbed vision, and abdominal pain If untreated, seizures can then occur and may be followed by *coma*. Levels of blood *platelets* may fall severely, resulting in bleeding; liver and kidney function may be affected.

Careful monitoring of blood pressure and proteinuria throughout pregnancy ensures prompt treatment of impending eclampsia. Immediate delivery, often by *caesarean section*, together with *antihypertensive* and *anticonvulsant drugs* is needed. Patients may need intensive care to prevent the development of complications such as kidney failure. Blood pressure often returns to normal in the months after delivery, but it may remain high. There is a risk of recurrence in subsequent pregnancies.

econazole An *antifungal drug* used as a cream for fungal skin infections (see *athlete's foot; tinea*), and in cream or pessary form to treat vaginal *candidiasis*. Skin irritation is a rare side effect.

Ecstasy An illegal *designer drug*, related to the *amphetamine drugs*. Ecstasy has a mildly hallucinogenic effect and generates feelings of euphoria. In most people, the drug has no ill effects in the short-term, but repeated use carries a risk of liver damage. The most common side-effect is *hyperthermia*. Taking the drug causes intense thirst, and drinking large quantities of water to combat this may result in fatal damage to the body, including brain swelling.

ECT The abbreviation for electroconvulsive therapy, in which an electric current is passed through the brain to induce *seizures* in order to treat severe *depression*. It is sometimes administered under a short-lived general anaesthetic. Temporary *amnesia* is a possible side effect. ECT usually relieves depression

E

more rapidly than drug treatment and may be lifesaving in severe depression that is resistant to other treatments.

ectasia A term meaning widening, usually used to refer to a disorder of a *duct*. For example, mammary duct ectasia is abnormal widening of the ducts that carry secretions from the breast tissue to the nipple.

-ectomy A suffix that denotes surgical removal. For example, tonsillectomy is surgical removal of the tonsils.

ectoparasite A *parasite* that lives in or on its host's skin and derives nourishment from the skin or by sucking the host's blood. Various *lice*, *ticks*, *mites*, and some types of *fungi* are occasional ectoparasites of humans.

ectopic A term used to describe a body structure that occurs in an abnormal location or position, or a body function that occurs at an abnormal time.

ectopic heartbeat A contraction of the heart muscle that is out of normal timing. An ectopic *heartbeat* occurs shortly after a normal beat and is followed by a longer than usual interval before the next one.

Ectopic beats can occur in a heart that is otherwise normal and may cause no symptoms. Multiple ectopic beats can cause *palpitations*. After a *myocardial infarction*, multiple ectopic beats are a sign of damaged heart muscle. Multiple ectopic beats may lead to ventricular *fibrillation*, a rapid uncoordinated heartbeat that may be fatal.

Multiple ectopic beats that are causing palpitations, or that occur after a myocardial infarction, are often treated with an *antiarrhythmic drug*. (See also *arrhythmia, cardiac*.)

ectopic pregnancy A *pregnancy* that develops outside the *uterus*, most commonly in the *fallopian tube*, but sometimes in the *ovary* or in the abdominal cavity or *cervix*. As the pregnancy develops, it may damage surrounding tissue, causing serious bleeding, which is potentially life-threatening and requires emergency treatment.

Ectopic pregnancy is more common in women who have had previous pelvic infections (see *pelvic inflammatory disease*) and with some types of *IUD* and progestogen-only *oral contraceptives*.

Most ectopic pregnancies are discovered in the first 2 months, often before the woman realizes she is pregnant. Symptoms usually include severe pain in the lower abdomen and vaginal bleeding. Internal bleeding may cause symptoms of *shock*, such as *pallor*, sweating, and faintness.

Diagnosis is made by a transvaginal *ultrasound* examination and can be confirmed by ectopic *laparoscopy*. If the diagnosis is made early, medical treatment using the drug *methotrexate* may be considered. In most cases, surgery, usually *minimally invasive surgery*, to remove the pregnancy is carried out. If blood loss is severe, *blood transfusions* are needed. An affected fallopian tube is removed if it cannot be repaired.

ECTOPIC PREGNANCY

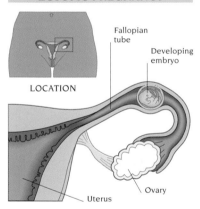

LOCATION

Fallopian tube

Developing embryo

Ovary

Uterus

ectropion Turning outwards of the *eyelid* so that the inner surface is exposed. It is most common in elderly people, in whom it usually affects the lower lid and is due to weakness of the muscle around the eye. It may also be caused by contraction of scar tissue in the skin near either lid. Ectropion often follows *facial palsy*, which causes paralysis of muscles around the eye. Even slight ectropion interferes with normal drainage of tears, which may lead to *conjunctivitis*. Surgery to tighten the lid may be needed.

eczema An inflammation of the skin, usually causing itching and sometimes scaling or blisters. There are several different types of eczema; some forms are known as *dermatitis*.

Atopic eczema is a chronic, superficial inflammation that occurs in people with an inherited tendency towards *allergy*. The condition is common in babies. An intensely itchy rash occurs, usually on the face, in the elbow creases, and behind the knees. The skin often scales, and small red pimples may appear. For mild cases, *emollients* help keep the skin soft. In severe cases, *corticosteroid* ointments may be used. *Antihistamine drugs* may reduce itching. Atopic eczema often clears up on its own as a child grows older. Severe atopic eczema occurring in adults may be treated with *immunosuppressant drugs*, such as oral *ciclosporin* or topical tacrolimus.

Nummular eczema usually occurs in adults. The cause is unknown. It produces circular, itchy, scaling patches anywhere on the skin, similar to those of *tinea* (ringworm). Topical corticosteroids may reduce the inflammation, but the disorder is often persistent.

Hand eczema is usually caused by irritant substances such as detergents, but may occur for no apparent reason. Itchy blisters develop, usually on the palms, and the skin may become scaly and cracked. Hand eczema usually improves if emollients are used and cotton gloves with rubber gloves over them are worn when coming into contact with irritants. If the eczema is severe, corticosteroids may be prescribed.

Stasis eczema occurs in people with *varicose veins*. The skin on the legs may become irritated, inflamed, and discoloured. The most important factor is swelling of the legs, which may be controlled with compression bandages or stockings. Ointments containing corticosteroids may give temporary relief.

EDD The abbreviation for expected date of delivery, the date on which a baby is due to be born. The EDD is calculated as 40 weeks from the first day of the woman's last menstrual period (see *period, menstrual*). In practice, babies are rarely born exactly on their EDD.

edentulous Without teeth.

EEG The abbreviation for electroencephalography, a method of recording the activity of the *brain*. A trace of the activity is displayed on a monitor or printed out on a moving strip of paper. In an EEG, a number of small electrodes are attached to the *scalp* and connected to

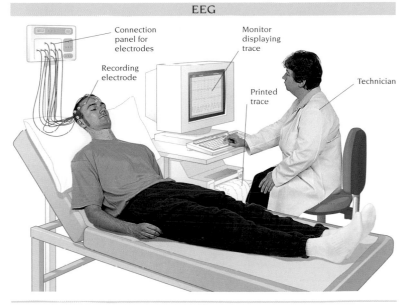

EEG

Connection panel for electrodes

Monitor displaying trace

Recording electrode

Printed trace

Technician

an instrument that records the minute electrical impulses that are produced by the brain's activity. By revealing characteristic wave patterns, an EEG can help in diagnosing different types of *epilepsy* and identifying areas in the brain where abnormal electrical activity develops.

effusion The process by which fluid escapes. The term also describes an abnormal collection of fluid, such as blood, *pus*, or *plasma*, in the tissues or a body cavity. An effusion can form as a result of inflammation or changes in pressure within blood vessels, or it can be due to changes in blood constituents, as in *nephrotic syndrome*. Effusion commonly occurs around the lung (*pleural effusion*) or heart (*pericardial effusion*) or within joints, causing swelling.

effusion, joint The accumulation of fluid in a joint space, causing swelling, limitation of movement, and usually pain and tenderness. A joint is enclosed by a capsule lined with a membrane called the *synovium*. The synovium normally secretes small amounts of fluid to lubricate the joint, but if it is damaged or inflamed (for example, by *arthritis*) it produces excessive fluid.

Pain and inflammation may be relieved by *analgesic drugs*, *nonsteroidal anti-inflammatory drugs*, and injections of *corticosteroid drugs*. Swelling usually reduces with rest, firm bandaging, ice-packs, and keeping the affected joint raised. In some cases, the fluid is drawn out with a needle and syringe.

egg See *ovum*.

ego The conscious sense of oneself, equivalent to "I". In Freudian *psychoanalytic theory*, this part of the personality maintains a balance between the primitive, unconscious instincts of the *id*, the controls of the *superego*, and the demands of the outside world.

Ehlers–Danlos syndrome An inherited disorder of *collagen*, the most important structural protein in the body. Affected individuals have abnormally stretchy, thin skin that bruises easily. Wounds are slow to heal and leave paper-thin scars, and the joints are loose and prone to recurrent dislocation. Sufferers bleed easily from the gums and digestive tract. Ehlers–Danlos syndrome is most often inherited

in an autosomal dominant pattern (see *genetic disorders*). There is no known specific treatment.

Eisenmenger complex A condition in which deoxygenated blood flows directly back into the circulation rather than through the lungs, due to an abnormal connection between the left and right sides of the heart and *pulmonary hypertension*. The resultant *hypoxia* causes *cyanosis*, fainting, and breathing difficulty. The disorder most often occurs in people with certain congenital heart defects (see *heart disease, congenital*), such as ventricular *septal defect*, that have not been corrected.

The diagnosis is confirmed by cardiac *catheterization*. Once Eisenmenger complex has developed, surgical correction of the original defect will not help. Drug treatment may control symptoms.

ejaculation Emission of *semen* from the penis at *orgasm*. Shortly before ejaculation, the muscles around the epididymides (the ducts where sperm are stored; see *epididymis*), the *prostate gland*, and the *seminal vesicles* contract rhythmically, forcing the *sperm* from the epididymides to move forwards and mix with secretions from the seminal vesicles and prostate. At ejaculation, this fluid is propelled through the *urethra* and out of the body.

Because both semen and urine leave the body by the same route, the bladder neck closes during ejaculation. This not only prevents ejaculate from going into the bladder but also stops urine from contaminating the semen (See also *reproductive system, male*.)

ejaculation, disorders of Conditions in which the normal process or timing of *ejaculation* is disrupted.

In *premature ejaculation*, emission of semen occurs before or almost immediately following penetration. Premature ejaculation is the most common sexual problem in men, and is often due to over-stimulation or anxiety about sexual performance. If the problem occurs frequently, sexual counselling and techniques for delaying ejaculation may help (see *sex therapy*).

Inhibited ejaculation is a rare condition in which erection is normal, or even prolonged, but ejaculation is abnormally delayed or fails to occur. The problem may be psychological in origin, in which case counselling may help, or it may be a complication of a disorder such as *diabetes mellitus* or *alcohol dependence*. In some cases, inhibited ejaculation occurs as a side effect of particular drugs, such as some *antihypertensive* and *antidepressant drugs*.

In retrograde ejaculation, the valve at the base of the *bladder*, which normally closes during ejaculation, stays open. As a result, ejaculate is forced back into the bladder. Retrograde ejaculation may occur as a result of a neurological disease, after surgery on the bladder or *prostatectomy*. There is no treatment, but intercourse with a full bladder can sometimes result in normal ejaculation. (See also *azoospermia; erectile dysfunction; psychosexual dysfunction; sexual problems*.)

elbow The hinge joint formed where the lower end of the *humerus* meets the upper ends of the *radius* and ulna. The elbow is stabilized by *ligaments* at the front, back, and sides. It enables the arm to be bent and straightened, and the forearm to be rotated through almost 180 degrees around its long axis without more than very slight movement of the upper arm.

Disorders of the elbow include *arthritis* and injuries to the joint and its surrounding muscles, tendons, and ligaments. Repetitive strain on the tendons of the muscles of the forearm, where they attach to the elbow, can result in an inflammation that is known as *epicondylitis*. There are two principal types of epicondylitis: *tennis elbow* and *golfer's elbow*. Alternatively, a *sprain* of the ligaments may occur. Olecranon *bursitis* develops over the tip of the elbow in response to local irritation. Strain on the joint can produce an

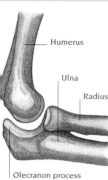

ELBOW

- Humerus
- Ulna
- Radius
- Olecranon process

effusion or traumatic *synovitis*. A fall on to the hand or on to the elbow can cause a fracture or dislocation.

elderly, care of the Appropriate care to help minimize physical and mental deterioration in the elderly. For example, failing vision and hearing are often regarded as inevitable in old age, but removal of a *cataract* or use of a *hearing-aid* can often improve quality of life. Isolation or inactivity leads to *depression* in some elderly people. Attending a day-care centre can provide social contact and introduce new interests.

Many elderly people are cared for by family members. Voluntary agencies can often provide domestic help to ease the strain on carers. Sheltered housing allows independence while providing assistance when needed. Elderly people who have *dementia* or physical disability usually require supervision in a residential care or hospital setting. (See also *geriatric medicine*.)

elective A term used to describe a procedure, usually a surgical operation, that is not urgent and can be performed at a scheduled time.

electrical injury Damage to the tissues caused by the passage of an electric current through the body and by its associated heat release. The internal tissues of the body, being moist and salty, are good conductors of electricity. Dry skin provides a high resistance to current flow, but moist skin has a low resistance and thus allows a substantial current to flow into the body. Serious injury or death from domestic voltage levels is thus more likely to occur in the presence of water.

All except the mildest electric shocks may result in unconsciousness. Alternating current (AC) is more dangerous than direct current (DC) because it causes sustained muscle contractions, which may prevent the victim from letting go of the source of the current. A current as small as 0.1 of an amp passing through the heart can cause a fatal *arrhythmia*. The same current passing through the *brainstem* may cause the heart to stop beating and breathing to cease. Larger currents, generated by high voltages, may cause charring of tissues, especially where the current enters and exits the body.

electric shock treatment See *ECT*.

electrocardiography See *ECG*.

electrocautery A technique for destroying tissue by the application of heat produced by an electric current. Electrocautery can be used to remove skin blemishes such as *warts*. (See also *cauterization*; *diathermy*; *electrocoagulation*.)

electrocoagulation The use of a high-frequency electric current to seal blood vessels by heat and thus stop bleeding. Electrocoagulation is used in surgery; the current can be delivered through a surgical knife, enabling the surgeon to make bloodless incisions. It is also used to stop nosebleeds and to destroy abnormal blood vessel formations, such as *spider naevi*, in which case the current is applied through a fine needle.

electroconvulsive therapy See *ECT*.

electroencephalography See *EEG*.

electrolysis Permanent removal of unwanted hair by introducing short-wave electric current into the hair *follicle*, which destroys the hair root.

electrolyte A substance whose molecules dissociate into its constituent *ions* when dissolved or melted.

electromyography See *EMG*.

electronystagmography A method of recording the types of *nystagmus* in order to investigate their cause. Electrical changes caused by eye movements are picked up by electrodes placed near the eyes and are recorded on a graph.

electrophoresis The movement of electrically charged particles suspended in a *colloid* solution under the influence of an electric current. The direction, distance, and rate of movement of the particles vary according to their size, shape, and electrical charge. Electrophoresis is used to analyse mixtures (to identify and quantify the proteins in blood, for example). It may be used as a diagnostic test for *multiple myeloma*, a bone marrow tumour that produces abnormally high levels of a specific *immunoglobulin* in the blood.

elephantiasis A disease that occurs in the tropics, characterized by massive swelling of the legs, arms, and *scrotum*, with thickening and darkening of the skin. Most cases of elephantiasis are due to chronic lymphatic obstruction caused by *filariasis* (a worm infestation).

ELISA test A laboratory blood test commonly used in the diagnosis of infectious diseases. ELISA stands for enzyme-linked immunosorbent assay. (See also *immunoassay*.)

elixir A clear, sweetened liquid, often containing alcohol, that forms the basis for many liquid medicines, such as *cough remedies*.

embolectomy Surgical removal of an *embolus* that has blocked an *artery* (see *embolism*). There are two methods: either an incision is made in the affected artery and the embolus is removed by suction, or it is removed by passing a *balloon catheter* into the affected vessel.

embolism Blockage of an *artery* by an *embolus*. Blood clots that have broken off from a larger clot located elsewhere in the circulation are the most common type of embolus. *Pulmonary embolism* is usually the result of a fragment breaking off from a deep vein *thrombosis* and being carried via the heart to block an artery supplying the lungs; this is a common cause of sudden death. Blood clots may form on the heart lining after a *myocardial infarction*, or in the atria in *atrial fibrillation*, and then travel to the brain, resulting in a cerebral embolism, which is an important cause of *stroke*. *Air embolism*, in which a small artery is blocked by an air bubble, is rare. Fat embolism, in which vessels are blocked by fat globules, is a possible complication of a major fracture of a limb.

Symptoms of an embolism depend on the site of the embolus. Pulmonary embolism can lead to breathlessness and chest pains. If the embolus lodges in the brain, a stroke may occur, affecting speech, vision, or movement. If an embolism blocks an artery to the leg, the limb will become painful and turn white or blue. Untreated, gangrene may develop. In serious cases of fat embolism, heart and breathing rates rise dramatically, and there is restlessness, confusion, and drowsiness.

Embolectomy (surgery to remove the blockage) may be possible. If surgery is not possible, *thrombolytic* and *anticoagulant drugs* may be given.

embolization The deliberate obstruction of a blood vessel in order to stop internal bleeding or to cut off the blood supply to a *tumour*. In the latter case, the technique can relieve pain; cause the tumour to shrivel, making surgical removal easier; or stop the tumour from spreading. Embolization can also be used to block flow through vascular abnormalities such as *haemangiomas* both in the skin and the internal organs.

A *catheter* is introduced into a blood vessel near the one to be blocked and the *embolus* that will block the vessel is released through the catheter. Emboli are made of materials such as blood-clotting agents or *silicone*.

embolus A fragment of material, usually a blood clot, that travels in the bloodstream and causes obstruction of an *artery*. An embolus is life-threatening if it blocks blood flow through a vital artery (see *embolism*).

embrocation A medication rubbed into the skin in order to relieve muscular or joint pain.

embryo The unborn child during the first 8 weeks of its development following *conception*; for the rest of the pregnancy it is known as a *fetus*.

The embryo develops from an egg that has been fertilized by a sperm (see *fertilization*). It starts as a single cell, but divides several times as it travels along the *fallopian tube* to the *uterus* to form a spherical mass of cells. About 6 days after conception, this mass becomes embedded in the uterus lining. At the site of attachment, the outer layer of cells obtains nourishment from the woman's blood; this part will later become the *placenta*. In the cell mass, a flat disc forms, consisting of layers of cells from which all the baby's tissues will form. The *amniotic sac* develops around the embryo.

Early in the 3rd week, the head of the embryo forms and the neural tube, which will later become the *brain* and *spinal cord*, forms along the embryo's back. In the 4th week, the neural tube extends towards the head, where a fold becomes visible that will eventually form the brain. Developing ears appear as pits. Rudimentary eyes form as stalks. Within the embryo, buds of tissue form that will become the lungs,

pancreas, liver, and gallbladder. A heart starts to develop in the form of a tube. Outer layers of the embryo begin to form the limb buds.

During the 5th week, the external ears become visible, pits mark the position of the nose, the jaws form, and the limb buds extend. Folds of tissue fuse to form the front wall of the chest and abdomen. The *umbilical cord* develops.

During weeks 6–8, the face becomes recognizably human, the neck forms, the limbs become jointed, and fingers and toes appear. After 8 weeks, most of the internal organs have formed and all external features are present.

EMBRYO

Cardiac bulge | Limb buds | Developing eye
Head bud
Umbilical stalk
20 DAYS | 4 WEEKS

embryology The study of the development of the *embryo* and then the *fetus* from *conception* until birth.

emergency Any condition requiring urgent medical treatment, such as *cardiac arrest*, or any procedure that must be performed immediately, such as *cardiopulmonary resuscitation*.

emergency contraception See *contraception, emergency*.

emesis The medical term for *vomiting*.

emetic A substance that causes *vomiting*, used to treat some types of poisoning and drug overdose. The most widely used emetic is *ipecacuanha*.

EMG The abbreviation for electromyogram, a recording of electrical activity in *muscle*. An EMG can help diagnose muscle disorders, such as *muscular dystrophy*, or disorders in which the nerve supply to muscle is impaired, such as *neuropathy* or *radiculopathy*.

E

Electrical activity is measured during muscle contraction and at rest; either small disc electrodes are attached to the skin over the muscle, or needle electrodes are inserted into the muscle. The impulses are displayed on a screen.

EMLA An abbreviation for eutetic mixture of local anaesthetics. This is a cream that is applied to the skin to produce local anaesthesia (see *anaesthesia, local*). EMLA is used to reduce discomfort before *intravenous* injection and *venepuncture*, particularly in children, and in skin *grafting*.

emollient A substance such as lanolin or petroleum jelly that has a soothing and softening effect when applied to the skin, eyes, or *mucous membranes*. Emollients are used in creams, ointments, nasal sprays, and suppositories.

emotional deprivation Lack of sufficient loving attention and of warm, trusting relationships during a child's early years, so that normal emotional development is inhibited. Emotional deprivation may result if *bonding* does not occur in the early months of life. Emotionally deprived children may be impulsive, crave attention, be unable to cope with frustration, and may have impaired intellectual development.

emotional problems A common term for a range of psychological difficulties, often related to *anxiety* or *depression*, which may have various causes.

empathy The ability to understand and share the thoughts and feelings of another person. In *psychoanalysis*, the therapist partly relies on empathy to establish a relationship with a patient.

emphysema A disease in which the walls of the air sacs in the lungs, known as alveoli (see *alveolus, pulmonary*), are progressively destroyed, thus reducing the area of lung available for exchange of gases. Emphysema usually develops along with chronic *bronchitis*, in a condition known as chronic obstructive pulmonary disease (see *pulmonary disease, chronic obstructive*). In almost all cases, emphysema is due to smoking. Rarely, an inherited deficiency of a chemical known as alpha$_1$-antitrypsin results in tissue damage, particularly in the lungs and liver. As the disease progresses, damage to the alveoli

causes increasing shortness of breath. Once the damage to the lungs has occurred, there is no treatment that can reverse it. Stopping smoking will reduce the rate at which the lungs deteriorate.

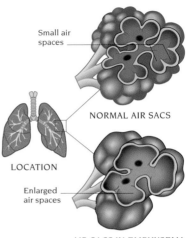

EMPHYSEMA

Small air spaces

NORMAL AIR SACS

LOCATION

Enlarged air spaces

AIR SACS IN EMPHYSEMA

emphysema, surgical The abnormal presence of air in tissues under the skin following surgery or injury.

empirical treatment Treatment given because its effectiveness has been observed in previous, similar cases rather than because there is an understanding of the nature of the disorder and the way the treatment works.

empyema An accumulation of *pus* in a body cavity or in certain organs. Empyema can occur around a lung as a rare complication of an infection such as *pneumonia* or *pleurisy*. The main symptoms are chest pain, breathlessness, and fever. Treatment is by *aspiration* (removal of the pus by suction) and the injection of *antibiotic drugs*, or by an operation to open the chest cavity and drain the pus. Empyema of the *gallbladder* may occur as a complication of *cholecystitis*, when it causes abdominal pain, fever, and *jaundice*. It is treated by surgical removal of the gallbladder.

emulsifying ointment A type of *emollient* containing emulsifying wax, white soft paraffin, and liquid paraffin that is used to smooth, soothe, and hydrate the skin in all dry or scaling conditions. Rarely, ingredients such as preservatives may result in sensitization.

enalapril An *ACE inhibitor drug* used to treat *hypertension* and *heart failure*.

enamel, dental The hard outer layer of a *tooth* that covers and protects the inner structures.

encephalitis Inflammation of the *brain*, and sometimes also the *meninges*, usually due to a viral infection. Encephalitis varies in severity from mild, in which symptoms are barely noticeable, to serious and potentially life-threatening. Mild cases can be due to glandular fever (see *infectious mononucleosis*) or may be a complication of childhood diseases such as *mumps* or *measles*. The most common cause of life-threatening encephalitis is *herpes simplex*, particularly in people with *HIV*.

Mild cases usually develop over several days and may cause only a slight fever and mild headache. In serious cases, symptoms develop rapidly and include weakness or *paralysis*, speech, memory, and hearing problems, and gradual loss of consciousness; *coma* and *seizures* may also occur. If the meninges are inflamed, other symptoms may develop, such as a stiff neck and abnormal sensitivity to light.

Diagnosis is based on results of blood tests, *CT scanning* or *MRI*, *EEG*, *lumbar puncture*, and, rarely, a brain *biopsy*. Encephalitis due to herpes simplex is treated with *intravenous infusion* of the antiviral drug *aciclovir*, but there is no known treatment for encephalitis caused by other viral infections.

encephalitis lethargica An epidemic form of *encephalitis*. There have been no major outbreaks since the 1920s, but rare sporadic cases still occur. Many people who survived the initial illness during the major epidemics developed a syndrome resembling severe *Parkinson's disease*.

encephalocele A type of *neural tube defect* that results in defects of the brain rather than of the spinal cord, as occurs in *spina bifida*.

encephalomyelitis Inflammation of the brain and spinal cord, causing damage to the nervous system. Encephalomyelitis develops as a rare complication of *measles* or, less commonly, of other viral infections such as *chickenpox*, *rubella*, or *infectious mononucleosis*. Symptoms include fever, headache, drowsiness, seizures, partial *paralysis* or loss of sensation, and, in some cases, *coma*. Diagnosis is as for *encephalitis*. There is no cure, but *corticosteroid drugs* are given to reduce inflammation and *anticonvulsant drugs* to control seizures. The disease is often fatal; those who survive may have permanent damage to the nervous system.

Myalgic encephalomyelitis is another term for *chronic fatigue syndrome*.

encephalopathy Any disorder affecting the *brain*, especially chronic degenerative conditions.

Wernicke's encephalopathy is a degenerative condition of the brain caused by a deficiency of vitamin B$_1$ (see *Wernicke–Korsakoff syndrome*). It is most common in those with chronic alcohol dependence.

Hepatic encephalopathy is caused by the effect on the brain of toxic substances (see *toxin*) that have built up in the blood as a result of *liver failure*. It may lead to impaired consciousness, memory loss, a change in personality tremors, and *seizures*.

Bovine spongiform encephalopathy, or BSE, is a disorder contracted by cattle after they are given feed containing material from sheep or cattle. The cause seems to be an infective agent known as a *prion*. Some cases of new variant *Creutzfeldt–Jakob disease* in humans have been attributed to infection with the prions responsible for BSE, probably transmitted in meat products.

Other causes of encephalopathy include *HIV* infection, *chickenpox*, and *Reye's syndrome*. Treatment of encephalopathy depends on the cause.

encopresis A type of *soiling* in which children pass normal faeces in unacceptable places after the age at which bowel control is normally achieved. The cause of encopresis is usually an underlying behavioural problem.

endarterectomy An operation to remove the lining of an *artery* affected by *atherosclerosis*, restoring normal blood flow. Endarterectomy is used to treat

E

cerebrovascular disease and peripheral vascular disease. The procedure can be performed endoscopically (see endoscopy) or by open surgery.

New lining grows in the artery within a few weeks of surgery. When narrowing is widespread, arterial reconstructive surgery may have to be performed.

endemic A term applied to a disease or disorder that is constantly present in a particular region or in a specific group of people. AIDS, for example, is endemic in central Africa. (See also epidemic).

endocarditis Inflammation of the endocardium (the membrane that lines the inside of the heart), particularly of the heart valves. Endocarditis is most often due to infection with bacteria, fungi, or other microorganisms, which may be introduced into the bloodstream during surgery or by intravenous injection with dirty needles. People whose endocardium has previously been damaged by disease are particularly vulnerable to endocarditis, as are intravenous drug users and people whose immune system is suppressed. Endocarditis is also a rare feature of some types of cancer.

Endocarditis may be either subacute or acute. In the subacute form, symptoms are general and nonspecific, although serious damage may be caused to a heart valve; the sufferer may complain of fatigue, feverishness, and vague aches and pains. On physical examination, the only evident abnormality may be a heart murmur. Acute endocarditis, which occurs less frequently, comes on suddenly, and causes severe chills, high fever, shortness of breath, and rapid or irregular heartbeat. The infection progresses quickly and may destroy the heart valves, leading to heart failure.

Endocarditis is diagnosed by physical examination and analysis of blood samples. Tests on the heart may include ECG, echocardiography, and angiography. Treatment is with high doses of antibiotic drugs, which are usually given intravenously. Heart-valve surgery may be needed to replace a damaged valve.

endocrine gland A gland that secretes hormones directly into the bloodstream rather than through a duct. Examples include the thyroid gland, pituitary gland, ovaries, testes, and adrenal glands. (See also exocrine gland.)

endocrine system The collection of glands around the body that produce hormones. These glands include the thyroid gland, pancreas, testes, ovaries, and adrenal glands. Their hormones are responsible for numerous bodily processes, including growth, metabolism, sexual development and function, and response to stress. Any increase or decrease in the production of a specific hormone interferes with the process it controls. To prevent under- or overproduction, hormone secretion from many endocrine glands is regulated by the pituitary gland, which is in turn influenced by the hypothalamus in the brain according to a feedback mechanism.

endocrinology The study of the endocrine system, including the investigation and treatment of its disorders.

endodontics The branch of dentistry concerned with the causes, prevention, diagnosis, and treatment of disease and injury affecting the nerves and pulp in teeth and periapical tissues in the gum. Common endodontic procedures are root-canal treatment and pulpotomy.

endogenous Of a disease or disorder that arises within the body rather than being caused by external factors. (See also exogenous.)

endometrial ablation A treatment for persistent menorrhagia (heavy menstrual blood loss) that involves endoscopic examination of the uterus (see endoscopy) and removal of the uterus lining, the endometrium, by diathermy or laser.

endometrial cancer See uterus, cancer of.

endometriosis A condition in which fragments of the endometrium are located in other parts of the body, usually in the pelvic cavity.

Endometriosis is most common in women aged 25–40 and may cause infertility. The cause of endometriosis is unclear. In some cases, it is thought to occur because fragments of the endometrium shed during menstruation do not leave the body but instead travel up the fallopian tubes and into the pelvic cavity, where they adhere to and grow on any pelvic organ. These displaced patches of endometrium continue to respond to hormones produced in the menstrual cycle and bleed each month. This blood cannot, however, escape and causes the formation of cysts, which may be painful and can grow to a size as large as a grapefruit.

The symptoms of endometriosis vary greatly, with abnormal or heavy menstrual bleeding being most common. There may be severe abdominal pain and/or lower back pain during menstruation. Other possible symptoms include dyspareunia (see *intercourse, painful*), diarrhoea, constipation, and pain during defaecation; in rare cases, there is bleeding from the rectum. Sometimes, endometriosis causes no symptoms.

Laparoscopy confirms the diagnosis. Drugs (including *danazol, progestogen drugs, gonadorelin* analogues, or the combined *oral contraceptive* pill) may be given to prevent menstruation. In some cases, local ablation of the endometrial deposit, using either *laser* or *electrocautery* during laparoscopy, may be needed. If the woman is not infertile, pregnancy often results in significant improvement of the condition. A *hysterectomy* may be suggested if the woman does not want children.

endometritis Inflammation of the *endometrium* that results from infection. Endometritis is a feature of *pelvic inflammatory disease*. It may also be a complication of *abortion* or childbirth, occur after insertion of an *IUD*, or be the result of a *sexually transmitted infection*, such as chlamydia. Symptoms include fever, vaginal discharge, and lower abdominal pain. Treatment includes removing any foreign body (such as an IUD or retained placental tissue) and *antibiotic drugs*.

endometrium The lining of the inside of the *uterus*. The endometrium contains numerous glands and gradually increases in thickness during the menstrual cycle (see *menstruation*) until *ovulation* occurs. The surface layers are shed during menstruation if *conception* does not take place.

endorphins A group of *protein* molecules produced in the body that relieve pain by activating *opiate* receptors in the nervous system. Endorphins have a

similar chemical structure to the pain-relieving drug *morphine*. In addition, endorphins are thought to be involved in the body's response to stress, as well as in regulating intestinal contractions, determining mood, and controlling the release of certain hormones from the *pituitary gland*. (See also *enkephalins*.)

ENDOSCOPE

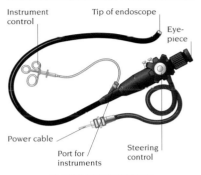

Instrument control

Tip of endoscope

Eye-piece

Power cable

Port for instruments

Steering control

FLEXIBLE ENDOSCOPE

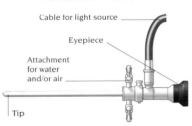

Cable for light source

Eyepiece

Attachment for water and/or air

Tip

RIGID ENDOSCOPE

endoscope A tube-like viewing instrument that is inserted into a body cavity to investigate or treat disorders. Endoscopes can be either flexible or rigid, depending on the part of the body to be examined. A flexible *fibre-optic* endoscope is a bundle of light-transmitting fibres. At the head, it has an eyepiece, steering device, and power source; at the tip, there is a light, a lens, an outlet for air or water, and sometimes a camera that transmits a picture to a screen. Side channels enable various surgical instruments to be passed down the endoscope. A rigid endoscope is a straight tube with a light attached.

endoscopy Examination of a body cavity for diagnosis or treatment by means of

E

an *endoscope*. Endoscopy makes use of both *fibre-optics* and video technology, and enables almost any hollow structure in the body to be inspected directly. The endoscope is inserted through a natural body opening, such as the mouth or vagina, or into a small incision. The operator can inspect and photograph the organ and carry out a *biopsy*. Many operations can be performed by passing surgical instruments down an endoscope. (See also *minimally invasive surgery*.)

endothelium The layer of *cells* that lines the heart, blood vessels, and lymphatic ducts (see *lymphatic system*). The cells are squamous (thin and flat), providing a smooth surface that aids the flow of blood and lymph and helps prevent the formation of blood clots. (See also *epithelium*.)

endotoxin A *poison* produced by certain *bacteria* that is not released until the bacteria die. Endotoxins that are released in infected people cause fever. They also make the *capillary* walls more permeable, causing fluid to leak into the surrounding tissue, sometimes resulting in a drop in blood pressure, a condition called endotoxic shock. (See also *enterotoxin*; *exotoxin*.)

endotracheal tube A tube that is passed into the *trachea* through the nose or mouth that enables delivery of oxygen during artificial *ventilation* or of anaesthetic gases (see *anaesthesia*) during surgery. An inflatable cuff around the lower end of the endotracheal tube

ENDOTRACHEAL TUBE

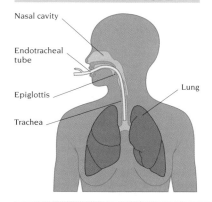

Nasal cavity

Endotracheal tube

Epiglottis

Trachea

Lung

prevents secretions or stomach contents from entering the lungs.

enema A procedure in which fluid is passed into the *rectum* through a tube inserted into the anus. An enema may be given to clear the intestine of faeces, to relieve constipation or in preparation for intestinal surgery. Enemas are also used to administer medicine, such as *corticosteroid drugs* to treat *ulcerative colitis*. A barium enema is used to diagnose disorders of the large intestine (see *barium X-ray examinations*).

energy The capacity to do work or effect a physical change. Nutritionists refer to the fuel content of a food as its energy.

There are many forms of energy, including light, sound, heat, chemical, electrical, and kinetic, and most of them play a role in the body. For instance, the *retina* converts light energy to electrical nerve impulses, making vision possible. *Muscles* use chemical energy obtained from food to produce kinetic energy, movement, and heat.

Energy is measured in units called *calories* and *joules*. Because these units are extremely small, more practical units used in *dietetics* are the kilocalorie (kcal, 1,000 calories), and kilojoule (kJ, 1,000 joules). *Carbohydrates* and *proteins* provide 4 kcal per gram (g), *fats* provide 9 kcal per g (see *metabolism*). In general, the energy liberated from the breakdown of food is stored as chemical energy in *ATP* molecules. The energy in these molecules is then available for processes that consume energy, such as muscle contraction.

energy requirements The amount of *energy* that is needed by a person for cell *metabolism*, muscular activity, and growth. This energy is provided by the breakdown of *carbohydrates*, *fats*, and *proteins* supplied by food in the diet and by stored *nutrients* in the liver, muscles, and *adipose tissue*.

Energy is needed to maintain the heartbeat, lung function, and constant body temperature. The rate at which these processes use energy is called the basal metabolic rate (BMR). Any form of movement increases energy expenditure above the BMR. A person's energy requirement increases during periods of growth and during *pregnancy* and *lactation*.

When more energy is ingested as food than is used, the surplus is stored and there is usually a gain in weight. When less energy is consumed than is spent, weight is usually lost as the stores are used up. (See also *nutrition*; *obesity*.)

engagement The descent of the head of the *fetus* into the mother's *pelvis*. In a woman's first pregnancy, engagement usually occurs by the 37th week but in subsequent pregnancies it may not occur until labour begins.

ENGAGEMENT

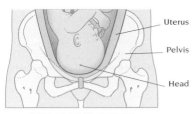

BEFORE ENGAGEMENT

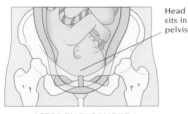

AFTER ENGAGEMENT

engorgement Overfilling of the *breasts* with *milk*. Engorgement is common a few days after childbirth. It causes the breasts and nipples to become swollen and tender, and can make *breast-feeding* difficult. The problem can be relieved by *expressing milk*.

enkephalins A group of small *protein* molecules produced in the *brain* and by nerve endings elsewhere in the body. Enkephalins have an analgesic effect and are also thought to affect mood. Enkephalins are similar to *endorphins* but have a slightly different chemical composition and are released by different nerve endings.

enophthalmos A sinking inwards of the eyeball. Enophthalmos is most often caused by fracture of the eye socket or

shrinkage of the eye due to the formation of scar tissue following injury.

enteric-coated tablet A tablet whose surface is covered with a substance that is resistant to the action of stomach juices. Enteric-coated tablets pass undissolved through the stomach into the small intestine, where the covering dissolves and the contents are absorbed. Such tablets are used either when the drug might harm the stomach lining or when the stomach juices may affect the efficacy of the drug.

enteric fever An alternative name for *typhoid fever* or *paratyphoid fever*.

enteritis Inflammation of the small intestine. The inflammation may be the result of infection, particularly *giardiasis* and *tuberculosis*, or of *Crohn's disease*. Enteritis usually causes diarrhoea. (See also *gastroenteritis*; *colitis*.)

enteritis, regional Another name for *Crohn's disease*.

enterobiasis A medical term for *threadworm* infestation of the intestines.

enterostomy An operation in which a portion of small or large intestine is joined to another part of the gastrointestinal tract or to the abdominal wall, for example in a *colostomy* or *ileostomy*.

enterotoxin A type of *toxin* released by certain *bacteria* that inflames the intestinal lining, leading to diarrhoea and vomiting. Enterotoxins cause the symptoms of staphylococcal *food poisoning* (see *staphylococcal infections*) and *cholera*. (See also *endotoxin*; *exotoxin*.)

entrapment neuropathy A condition, such as *carpal tunnel syndrome*, in which local pressure on a *nerve* causes muscle pain, numbness, and weakness in the area that the nerve supplies.

entropion A turning in of the margins of the *eyelids* so that the lashes rub against the *cornea* and the *conjunctiva*. Entropion is sometimes present from birth, especially in overweight babies. It is common in the elderly, due to weakness of the muscles around the lower eye. Entropion of the upper or lower lid may be caused by scarring, for example that due to *trachoma*.

Entropion in babies does not disturb the eye and usually disappears within a few months. In later life, entropion can

E

cause irritation, *conjunctivitis*, damage to the cornea, or problems with vision. Surgery to correct entropion can prevent such conditions.

ENT surgery See *otorhinolaryngology*.

enuresis The medical term for bed-wetting. In most cases, it occurs in children and affects boys slightly more commonly than girls. Usually, enuresis occurs as a result of slow maturation of nervous system functions concerned with bladder control. It may also result from psychological stress. In a small number of bed-wetters, there is a physical cause, such as a *urinary tract infection*.

If a child wets the bed persistently, tests, including *urinalysis*, may be performed to rule out a physical cause. For bed-wetting that is not caused by a disorder, treatment starts with training the child to pass urine regularly during the day. Getting the child to go to the toilet just before bed may be helpful. Alarm systems are available that involve the placement of humidity-sensitive pads in the child's bed. The child is woken by the alarm if urine is passed and eventually learns to wake before urinating.

environmental medicine The study of the effects on health of natural environmental factors, for example climate, altitude, sunlight, and the presence of various minerals. The study of working environments is a separate discipline (see *occupational medicine*.)

enzyme A *protein* that regulates the rate of a chemical reaction in the body. There are thousands of enzymes, each with a different chemical structure. It is this structure that determines the specific reaction regulated by an enzyme. Different enzymes occur in different tissues, reflecting their specialized functions. In order to function properly, many enzymes need an additional component, known as a coenzyme, which is often derived from a *vitamin* or *mineral*. Enzyme activity is influenced by many factors, and can be increased or inhibited by certain drugs.

Measuring enzyme levels in the blood can be useful in diagnosing certain disorders. For example, the level of heart muscle enzymes is raised following a *myocardial infarction* because the damaged heart muscle releases enzymes into the bloodstream. Many different inherited metabolic disorders, including *phenylketonuria*, *galactosaemia*, and *G6PD deficiency*, are caused by defects in, or deficiencies of, specific enzymes.

Enzymes can play a valuable role in treating certain disorders. Pancreatic enzymes may be given as digestive aids to people who have *malabsorption* related to pancreatic disease. Enzymes such as *streptokinase* and *tissue-plasminogen activator* are used to treat acute *thrombosis* and *embolism*.

eosinophil A type of leukocyte (white *blood cell*) that plays a role in the body's allergic responses and in fighting parasitic infections.

ependymoma A rare *brain tumour* of the *glioma* type that occurs most often in children.

ephedrine A drug that stimulates the release of the neurotransmitter *noradrenaline*. It is used as a *decongestant drug* to treat nasal congestion.

epicanthic fold A vertical fold of skin extending from the upper eyelid to the side of the nose. Epicanthic folds are common in Oriental people but rare in other races, except in babies, in whom they usually disappear as the nose develops. Abnormal epicanthic folds are a feature of *Down's syndrome*.

epicondyle A bony outgrowth to which *tendons* are attached (for example, at the lower end of the *humerus* bone of the upper arm where it forms part of the *elbow* joint). Overuse of muscles, leading to repeated tugging on the tendons, can cause pain and inflammation at an epicondyle (see *epicondylitis*).

epicondylitis Painful inflammation of an *epicondyle*, specifically one of the bony prominences of the *elbow* at the lower end of the humerus. It is due to overuse of forearm muscles, which causes repeated tugging on the tendons attaching to the bone. Epicondylitis affecting the prominence on the outer elbow is called *tennis elbow*. When the prominence on the inner elbow is affected it is called *golfer's elbow*.

epidemic A term applied to a disease that for most of the time is rare in a community but suddenly spreads rapidly to affect a large number of people. Epidemics of new strains of *influenza* are common. A widespread epidemic is known as a *pandemic*. (See also *endemic*.)

epidemiology The branch of medicine concerned with the occurrence and distribution of disease, including *infectious diseases* and noninfectious diseases such as cancer.

In epidemiological studies, the members of a population are counted and described in terms of such variables as race, sex, age, social class, occupation, and marital status. Then the *incidence* and *prevalence* of the disease of interest are determined. These observations may be repeated at regular intervals in order to detect changes over time. The result is a statistical record that may reveal links between particular variables and distribution of disease.

In comparative epidemiological studies, two or more groups are chosen. For example, in a study of the link between smoking and lung cancer, one group may consist of smokers and the other of nonsmokers; the proportion with cancer in each group is calculated.

epidermis The thin outermost layer of the *skin*.

epidermolysis bullosa A group of rare, inherited conditions, varying widely in severity, in which blisters appear on the skin after minor injury or occur spontaneously. The conditions can be diagnosed by a skin *biopsy*. There is no specific treatment. The outlook varies from gradual improvement in mild cases to progressive serious disease in the most severe cases.

epididymal cyst A harmless swelling, usually painless, that develops in the *epididymis*. Small cysts are common in men over 40 and need no treatment. Rarely, they become tender or enlarge and cause discomfort, in which case surgical removal may be necessary.

epididymis A long, coiled tube that runs along the back of the testis and connects the vasa efferentia (small tubes leading from the testis) to the *vas deferens* (the sperm duct leading to the urethra) Sperm cells, which are produced in the *testis*, mature as they pass slowly along the epididymis and are then stored in the *seminal vesicles* until *ejaculation* takes place.

EPIDIDYMIS

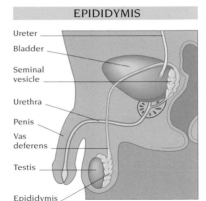

Ureter
Bladder
Seminal vesicle
Urethra
Penis
Vas deferens
Testis
Epididymis

Disorders of the epididymis include *epididymo orchitis* and *epididymal cysts* Infection or injury can block the epididymis, which, if both testes are affected, may result in *infertility*.

epididymitis See *epididymo-orchitis*.

epididymo-orchitis Acute inflammation of a *testis* along with its associated *epididymis*. Epididymo-orchitis causes severe pain and swelling at the back of the testis, and, in severe cases, swelling and redness of the *scrotum*.

The inflammation is caused by infection. Often, there is no obvious source of infection, but sometimes the cause is a bacterial *urinary tract infection* that has spread via the *vas deferens* to the epididymis. Treatment is with *antibiotic drugs*. If there is an underlying urinary tract infection, its cause will be investigated. (See also *orchitis*.)

epidural anaesthesia A method of pain relief in which a local anaesthetic (see *anaesthetic, local*) is injected into the epidural space (the space around the membranes surrounding the spinal cord) in the middle and lower back to numb the nerves that supply the chest and lower body. Epidural anaesthesia is used to relieve pain during and after surgery and during *childbirth*.

epiglottis The flap of *cartilage* lying behind the tongue and in front of the entrance to the *larynx* (voice-box). The epiglottis is usually upright to allow air to pass through the larynx and into the rest of the respiratory system. During

E

swallowing, it tilts downward to cover the entrance to the larynx, preventing food and drink from being inhaled.

epiglottitis A potentially life-threatening infection causing inflammation and swelling of the *epiglottis*. Epiglottitis is now rare due to routine *immunization* of infants against *HAEMOPHILUS INFLUENZAE*, the causative bacterium.

EPIGLOTTIS

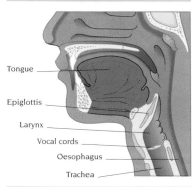

Tongue
Epiglottis
Larynx
Vocal cords
Oesophagus
Trachea

epilepsy A tendency to have recurrent *seizures*. In many people with epilepsy, the cause is unclear, although a genetic factor may be involved. In other cases, seizures may be the result of brain damage from *head injury*, birth trauma, brain infection (such as *meningitis* or *encephalitis*), *brain tumour*, *stroke*, drug intoxication, or a *metabolic disorder*.

Many people with epilepsy do not have any symptoms between seizures. Some people experience an *aura* shortly before. In some cases, a stimulus such as a flashing light triggers a seizure. Epileptic seizures may occur more frequently in times of illness or stress.

Epileptic seizures can be classified into two groups: generalized and partial. Generalized seizures cause loss of consciousness and may affect all areas of the brain. There are two types: grand mal and absence (petit mal) seizures. During a grand mal seizure, there may be an aura initially, then the body becomes stiff and consciousness is lost; breathing may be irregular or may stop briefly, then the body jerks uncontrollably. The person may be disorientated for hours

afterwards and have no memory of the event. Prolonged grand mal seizures are potentially life-threatening. Absence seizures occur mainly in children. Periods of altered consciousness last for only a few seconds and there are no abnormal movements of the body. This type of seizure may occur hundreds of times daily.

Partial seizures are caused by abnormal electrical activity in a more limited area of the brain. They may be simple or complex. In simple partial seizures, consciousness is not lost and an abnormal twitching movement, tingling sensation, or *hallucination* of smell, vision, or taste occurs, lasting several minutes. In complex partial seizures, also known as *temporal lobe epilepsy*, conscious contact with the surroundings is lost. The sufferer becomes dazed and may behave oddly. Typically, the person remembers little, if any, of the event.

Diagnosis is made from examination of the nervous system and an *EEG*. *CT scanning* or *MRI* of the brain and blood tests may also be carried out. *Anticonvulsant drugs* usually stop or reduce the frequency of seizures. Surgery may be considered if a single area of brain damage is causing the seizures. Epilepsy that develops during childhood may disappear following adolescence.

epiloia See *tuberous sclerosis*.

epinephrine An alternative name for *adrenaline*.

epiphora See *watering eye*.

epiphysis The end section of a long bone (such as the femur) separated from the *diaphysis* (shaft) by the epiphyseal plate. During childhood and adolescence, the ephiphyseal plate is made of cartilage but is gradually replaced by bone.

epiphysis, slipped See *femoral epiphysis, slipped*.

episcleritis A localized patch of *inflammation* affecting the outermost layers of the *sclera* (white of the eye) immediately

EPIPHYSIS

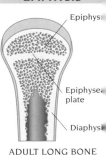

Epiphysis
Epiphyseal plate
Diaphysis

ADULT LONG BONE

underneath the *conjunctiva*. The condition usually occurs for no known reason, mainly affecting middle-aged men. In some cases, it is a complication of *rheumatoid arthritis*. The inflammation may cause a dull, aching pain and there may be *photophobia*. The disorder usually disappears by itself in a week or so but may recur. Symptoms may be relieved by using eye-drops or ointment containing a *corticosteroid drug*.

episiotomy A surgical procedure in which an incision is made in the *perineum* (the tissue between the vagina and the anus) to facilitate the delivery of a baby. After delivery, the cut tissues are stitched back together. Episiotomy is usually necessary in a *forceps delivery* and in a *breech delivery*.

epispadias A rare *congenital* abnormality in which the opening of the *urethra* is not in the *glans* (head) of the *penis*, but on its upper surface. In some cases, the penis also curves upwards. Surgery is carried out during infancy, using tissue from the *foreskin* to reconstruct the urethra. (See also *hypospadias*.)

epistaxis A medical term for *nosebleed*.

epithelium The layer of *cells* that covers the entire surface of the body and lines most of the hollow structures within it. Epithelial cells vary in shape according to their function. There are three basic shapes of cell: squamous (thin and flat), cuboidal, and columnar. Most internal organs lined with epithelium are covered with only one layer of cells, but the skin, which is subjected to more trauma, consists of many layers.

epoetin A genetically engineered preparation of the *hormone* erythropoietin, which is produced by specialized cells in the kidneys and stimulates the *bone marrow* to make red blood cells. Epoetin may be used for treating *anaemia* resulting from the lack of erythropoietin that occurs in *kidney failure*. It is also used for anaemia occurring in chronic disorders such as *rheumatoid arthritis* and itching associated with uraemia.

Epstein–Barr virus A *virus* that causes *infectious mononucleosis*; the virus is also associated with *Burkitt's lymphoma* and cancer of the nasopharynx (see *nasopharynx, cancer of*).

ERCP The abbreviation for endoscopic retrograde cholangiopancreatography, an *X-ray* procedure used for examining the *biliary system* and the pancreatic duct.

An *endoscope* is passed down the oesophagus, through the stomach, and into the *duodenum*. A *catheter* is passed through the endoscope into the common bile duct and pancreatic duct. A *contrast*

E

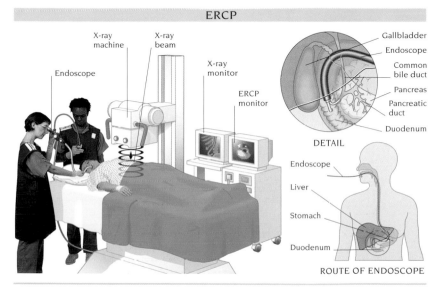

ERCP

E

medium is introduced through the catheter to make the pancreatic duct and ducts of the biliary system visible on X-rays. In some cases, it may be possible to relieve a blockage due to a gallstone during the procedure.

erectile dysfunction The inability to achieve or maintain an *erection*, also sometimes known as impotence. Erectile dysfunction may be caused by psychological factors, including concerns about performance or relationship difficulties, or by physical disorders, such as *atherosclerosis*, *diabetes mellitus*, and neurological disorders including *multiple sclerosis* and damage to the *spinal cord*. Some drugs cause erectile dysfunction as a side effect but this reverses when the drugs are stopped. Erectile dysfunction also tends to be more common with increasing age.

Treatment depends on the cause but may include *counselling* or *sex therapy* for psychological problems. The drugs *sildenafil* or *tadalafil* may be used to treat both organic and psychological erectile dysfunction. Other treatments for erectile dysfunction include self-administered injections into the penis and a surgical implant, which can produce a sustained erection.

erection The hardness, swelling, and elevation of the *penis* that occurs in response to sexual arousal or physical stimulation. The erectile tissue of the penis fills with blood as the blood vessels in it dilate. Muscles around the vessels contract and stop blood leaving the penis, so maintaining the erection.

erection, disorders of Conditions in which the normal process of *erection* of the penis is disrupted. They include total or partial failure to attain or maintain erection (see *erectile dysfunction*), persistent erection in the absence of sexual desire (see *priapism*), and curving of the penis during erection (see *chordee*).

ergocalciferol An alternative name for vitamin D$_2$ (see *vitamin D*).

ergometer A machine that measures and records the amount of physical work done and the body's response to a controlled amount of exercise. An ergometer makes continuous recordings, both during and after activity, of heart-rate and rhythm (using an *ECG*),

blood pressure, rate of breathing, and volume of oxygen taken in from the air.

ergometrine A drug given after *childbirth*, *miscarriage*, or *abortion* in order to reduce loss of blood from the *uterus*. It works by causing blood vessels in the uterine wall to contract.

ergot A product of CLAVICEPS PURPUREA, a *fungus* that grows on cereals. Ergot contains poisonous *alkaloids*, some of which have medicinal properties when taken in controlled doses. The drugs *ergotamine* and *ergometrine* are both produced from ergot.

ergotamine A drug used in the prevention and treatment of *migraine* and sometimes in the treatment of *cluster headaches*.

erosion, dental Loss of enamel from a tooth's surface due to attack by *plaque* acids or other chemicals. Erosion of the outer surfaces of the front teeth is most frequently caused by excessive intake of fruit juices and carbonate d drinks. Erosion of the inner surfaces of the molars may be a result of the regurgitation of stomach acid, as occurs in people suffering from *gastro-oesophageal reflux disease* or *bulimia*. (See also *caries, dental*.)

eroticism The character and emotive nature of sexual excitement. Sexual arousal may be stimulated by erotic thoughts, touching erogenous zones, or a variety of other sensations (such as the look and feel of certain clothes).

eruption The process of breaking out, as of a skin rash or a new tooth.

eruption of teeth The process by which developing *teeth* move upwards through the jawbone and break through the gum to project into the mouth.

Primary teeth (also known as deciduous or milk teeth) usually begin to appear at about 6 months of age. All 20 primary teeth have usually erupted by 3 years (see *teething*).

Permanent teeth (also known as secondary teeth) usually begin to appear at about 6 years of age. The first permanent molars erupt towards the back of the mouth and appear in addition to the primary teeth. The eruption of permanent teeth nearer the front of the mouth is preceded by reabsorption of the roots of the primary teeth, which become loose

ERUPTION OF TEETH

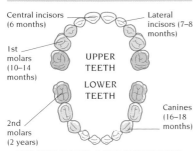

Central incisors (6 months)
Lateral incisors (7–8 months)
1st molars (10–14 months)
UPPER TEETH
LOWER TEETH
Canines (16–18 months)
2nd molars (2 years)

PRIMARY TEETH: AGES OF ERUPTION

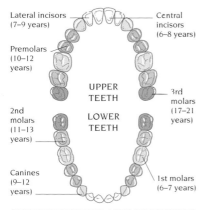

Lateral incisors (7–9 years)
Central incisors (6–8 years)
Premolars (10–12 years)
UPPER TEETH
LOWER TEETH
3rd molars (17–21 years)
2nd molars (11–13 years)
Canines (9–12 years)
1st molars (6–7 years)

PERMANENT TEETH: AGES OF ERUPTION

and detach. Eventually, permanent teeth replace all the primary ones. Wisdom teeth (the backmost, or third, molars) usually erupt between ages 17 and 21, but, in some people, they never appear.

erysipelas An infection, producing *inflammation* and blistering of the face, that is associated with a high fever and *malaise*. Caused by a *streptococcal infection*, erysipelas most often affects young children and the elderly. Treatment is with *penicillin drugs*. (See also *cellulitis*.)

erythema A term that means redness of the skin. Disorders in which skin redness is one feature include *erythema multiforme*, *erythema nodosum*, *erythema ab igne*, *lupus erythematosus*, and erythema infectiosum (also known as *fifth disease*) Erythema can have many causes, including *blushing*, *hot flushes*, *sunburn*, and inflammatory, infective, or allergic skin conditions such as *acne*, *dermatitis*, *eczema*, *erysipelas*, *rosacea*, and *urticaria*.

erythema ab igne Red, mottled skin that may also be dry and itchy, caused by exposure to strong direct heat, such as when sitting too close to a fire. The condition is most common in elderly women. Dryness and itching can often be relieved by an *emollient*. The redness fades in time but may not disappear.

erythema infectiosum See *fifth disease*.

erythema multiforme Acute *inflammation* of the skin, and sometimes of the *mucous membranes*. The disease can occur as a reaction to certain drugs, or may accompany viral infections such as *herpes simplex* or bacterial infections such as *streptococcal infections*. Other possible causes are pregnancy, *vaccination*, and *radiotherapy*. Half of all cases occur for no apparent reason.

A symmetrical rash of red, often itchy spots erupts on the limbs and sometimes on the face and the rest of the body. The spots may blister or form raised, pale-centred weals, called target lesions. Those affected may have a fever, sore throat, headache, and/or diarrhoea. In a severe form of erythema multiforme, known as *Stevens–Johnson syndrome*, the mucous membranes of the mouth, eyes, and genitals are affected and become ulcerated

Corticosteroid drugs may be given to reduce the inflammation. People with Stevens–Johnson syndrome are also given *analgesic drugs* and may need intensive care.

erythema nodosum A condition characterized by the eruption of red-purple, tender swellings on the legs.

The most common cause is a *streptococcal infection* of the throat, but the condition is also associated with other diseases, mainly *tuberculosis* and *sarcoidosis*, and may occur as a reaction to drugs, including *oral contraceptives*, *aspirin*, *penicillin drugs*, and *sulphonamide drugs*. Sometimes there is no apparent cause.

Treatment of any underlying condition clears the swellings. Bed rest, *analgesics*, and, occasionally, *corticosteroid drugs* may be necessary.

erythrasma A skin infection, caused by *CORYNEBACTERIUM*, that affects the groin, armpits, and the skin between the toes. Raised, irregularly shaped, discoloured patches appear in affected areas. Erythrasma is more common in people with *diabetes mellitus*. It usually clears up when treated with *antibiotics*.

erythrocyte Another name for a red blood cell (see *blood cells*).

erythroderma See *exfoliative dermatitis*.

erythromycin An *antibiotic drug* used to treat infections of the skin, chest, throat, and ears. Erythromycin is useful in the treatment of *pertussis* and *legionnaires' disease*. Adverse effects include nausea, diarrhoea, and an itchy rash.

eschar A *scab* on the surface of the skin formed to cover tissue damage.

Escherichia coli (E. coli) A *bacterium* normally found in the intestines which, if it enters the bladder through the urethra, is a common cause of *urinary tract infections*. Types of *E. COLI* are often the cause of traveller's diarrhoea, usually a mild illness, but some strains of the bacterium (such as strain O157) can cause serious food-borne infections that can result in *gastroenteritis* and *haemolytic-uraemic syndrome*. Attention to good food hygiene and handwashing can help to prevent the spread of food-borne *E. COLI* infections.

Esmarch's bandage A broad, rubber bandage wrapped around the elevated limb of a patient to force blood out of the blood vessels towards the heart; this creates a blood-free area, enabling surgery to be performed more easily.

esotropia An alternative term for a convergent *squint*.

ESR The abbreviation for erythrocyte sedimentation rate, which is the rate at which *erythrocytes* (red blood cells) sink to the bottom of a test tube. The ESR is increased if the level of *fibrinogen* (a type of protein) in the blood is raised. Fibrinogen is raised in response to a range of illnesses, including *inflammation*, especially when this is caused by infection or by an *autoimmune disease*. The ESR is also increased if levels of *immunoglobulins* are very high, as occurs in *multiple myeloma*. ESR is therefore useful for helping to diagnose these conditions as well as in monitoring their treatment.

estradiol The most important of the *oestrogen hormones*, essential for the healthy functioning of the female reproductive system and breast development. In synthetic form, estradiol is used to treat symptoms and complications of the *menopause* (see *hormone replacement therapy*) and to stimulate sexual development in female *hypogonadism*.

estriol One of the *oestrogen hormones*. Estriol is the predominant oestrogen produced during pregnancy. Synthetic estriol is prescribed to treat symptoms and complications of the *menopause* (see *hormone replacement therapy*) and to stimulate sexual development in female *hypogonadism*.

estrone An *oestrogen hormone*. A synthetic form is used to treat symptoms and complications of the menopause (see *hormone replacement therapy*).

ESWL Extracorporeal shock wave lithotripsy (see *lithotripsy*).

ethambutol A drug used in conjunction with other drugs to treat *tuberculosis*. Ethambutol rarely causes side effects, although it may occasionally result in *inflammation* of the *optic nerve*, leading to blurred vision.

ethanol The chemical name for the *alcohol* in alcoholic drinks.

ether A colourless liquid that produces unconsciousness when inhaled. Ether was the first general anaesthetic.

ethinylestradiol A synthetic form of the female sex hormone *estradiol*. It is most often used in *oral contraceptives*, in which it is combined with a *progestogen drug*. Less frequently, it is used in *hormone replacement therapy*.

ethosuximide An *anticonvulsant drug* used to treat absence seizures (*petit mal epilepsy*). Ethosuximide may cause nausea and vomiting and, in rare cases, affects production of blood cells in bone marrow (see *anaemia, aplastic*).

ethyl alcohol Another name for ethanol, the *alcohol* in alcoholic drinks.

ethyl chloride A colourless liquid applied to the skin as a spray to numb an area before minor surgery or to relieve muscle pain.

etidronate sodium See *disodium etidronate*.

eucalyptus oil A substance distilled from the leaves of eucalyptus trees. Because of its aromatic smell and refreshing taste, it is used as a flavouring, and – applied as a rub, inhaled as vapour, or incorporated in tablets – is also used in cough and cold remedies. There is little evidence that it has any curative properties, although it may relieve symptoms.

eunuch A man whose *testes* have been removed or destroyed so that he is sterile and lacks male hormones. A male who has been castrated before *puberty* will have broad hips, narrow shoulders, and undeveloped male secondary *sexual characteristics*.

euphoria A state of confident well-being. Euphoria is a normal reaction to personal success, but it can also be induced by drugs, including prolonged use of *corticosteroid drugs*. Euphoria with no rational cause may be a sign of *mania*, or brain damage due to *head injury*, *dementia*, *brain tumours*, or *multiple sclerosis*.

eustachian tube The passage that runs from the *middle ear* into the back of the nose, just above the soft *palate*. The tube acts as a drainage channel from the middle ear and maintains hearing by opening periodically to regulate air pressure. The lower end of the tube opens during swallowing and yawning, allowing air to flow up to the middle ear, equalizing the air pressure on both sides of the *eardrum*.

When a viral infection such as a cold causes blockage of the eustachian tube, equalization cannot occur, resulting in severe pain and temporary impairment of hearing. A person with a blocked eustachian tube who is subjected to rapid pressure changes may suffer from *barotrauma*. *Glue ear* or chronic *otitis media* may occur if the tube is blocked,

preventing adequate drainage from the middle ear. These conditions, which often result in partial hearing loss, are more common in children. This is partly because their adenoids are larger and more likely to cause a blockage if they become infected and partly because children's eustachian tubes are shorter than those of adults.

euthanasia The use of medical knowledge to end a person's life painlessly in order to relieve suffering. Euthanasia is illegal in the UK.

euthyroid The term used to describe a person whose *thyroid gland* is functioning normally, especially someone who has been successfully treated for either *hypothyroidism* or *hyperthyroidism*.

evening primrose oil An oil that is extracted from the seeds of the plant *OENOTHERA BIENNIS*, commonly known as the evening primrose. The oil contains a substance called gamolenic acid, and is believed by some to be of benefit in treating *eczema* and *premenstrual syndrome*.

EVENING PRIMROSE OIL

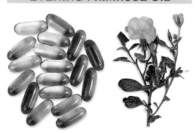

CAPSULES   EVENING PRIMROSE

eversion A turning outwards. The term is used medically to describe a type of ankle injury or deformity in which the foot is turned outwards.

evidence-based medicine Health care based on evidence, acquired through expert practice and research, that a particular test or treatment is appropriate for an individual patient.

evoked responses The tracing of electrical activity in the brain in response to a specific external stimulus. The procedure is similar to that for an *EEG*.

The technique is used to check the functioning of various sensory systems

EUSTACHIAN TUBE

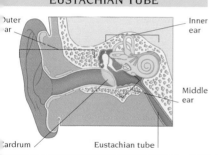

Outer ear

Inner ear

Middle ear

Eardrum   Eustachian tube

E

(such as sight, hearing, or touch). The information obtained can be used to reveal abnormalities caused by *inflammation*, pressure from a *tumour*, or other disorders, and to help confirm a diagnosis of *multiple sclerosis*.

Ewing's sarcoma A rare malignant form of *bone cancer*. It arises in a large bone, usually the *femur*, *tibia*, *humerus*, or a pelvic bone, and spreads to other areas at an early stage. The condition is most common in children aged 10–15. An affected bone is painful and tender. It may also become weakened and fracture easily. Other symptoms include weight loss, fever, and *anaemia*.

The sarcoma is diagnosed by *X-rays* and a *biopsy*. If cancer is found, the whole skeleton is examined by X-rays and *radionuclide scanning*, and the lungs viewed by *CT scanning*, to determine if, and how far, the cancer has spread. Treatment is with *radiotherapy* and *anticancer drugs*. If the cancer has not spread, the outlook is good.

examination, physical The part of a medical consultation in which the doctor looks, feels, and listens to various parts of the patient's body to assess the patient's condition or to gather information to help make a *diagnosis*.

Most examinations include *palpation*, by which the doctor examines relevant parts of the body for signs such as swelling, tenderness, or enlargement of organs. In some cases, *percussion* of the chest, or other parts of the body, may be performed by tapping with the fingers and then listening to the sound produced. *Auscultation* may be used to listen to blood flow through arteries and sounds made by the heart and lungs. The doctor may take the pulse or *blood pressure*, examine the eyes and ears, and assess the strength and coordination of the muscles.

exchange transfusion A treatment for *haemolytic disease of the newborn*, in which the infant's blood is replaced with rhesus negative donor blood (see *rhesus incompatibility*). It is used to treat dangerously high levels of *bilirubin* in the blood and the severe *anaemia* which result from the condition.

excimer laser A *laser* used to reshape the *cornea* to correct *myopia* (short

sight), *hypermetropia* (long sight), or *astigmatism* by removing very thin layers of tissue from the corneal surface (see *LASIK; PRK*).

excision Surgical cutting out of diseased tissue, such as a breast lump, from surrounding healthy tissue.

excoriation Injury to the surface of the skin or a *mucous membrane* caused by physical *abrasion*, such as scratching.

excretion Discharge of waste material from the body, including the by-products of digestion, waste products from the repair of tissues, and excess water.

The *kidneys* excrete excess nitrogen in the *urine* in the form of urea, along with excess water, salts, some acids, and most drugs. The *liver* excretes bile, which contains waste products and bile pigments formed from the breakdown of red blood cells. Some of the bile passes from the body in the *faeces*. The large *intestine* excretes undigested food, some salts, and excess water in the form of faeces. The *lungs* discharge carbon dioxide and water vapour into the air. *Sweat glands* excrete salt and water onto the skin's surface as a method of regulating body temperature.

exenteration The surgical removal of all organs and soft tissue in a body cavity, usually to arrest the growth of a *cancer*. It is sometimes used in *ophthalmology* when the eye and the contents of the eye orbit are removed.

exercise The performance of any physical activity that improves health or that is used for recreation or for the correction of physical injury or deformity (see *physiotherapy*). Different types of exercise have different effects on the body. During aerobic exercise, such as jogging or swimming, the heart and lungs work faster and more efficiently to supply the muscles' increased demand for oxygen; regular aerobic exercise improves the condition of both the cardiovascular and respiratory systems. Exercises such as weight training increase muscle strength and endurance. Activities such as yoga and pilates improve flexibility.

Regular aerobic exercise usually leads to a reduction in blood pressure. It also results in an increased amount of high-density lipoprotein (*HDL*) in the blood, which is thought to help protect against atherosclerosis and myocardial infarction. Exercise can relieve the symptoms of peripheral vascular disease and of some psychological disorders, particularly depression. Regular weightbearing exercise, such as running, increases the density of, and thereby strengthens, the bones. The bone disease osteoporosis is less common in people who have exercised throughout their adult lives.

However, vigorous exercise may cause injury and increase the risk of a heart attack in people who are out of condition. Professional sportsmen such as footballers have an increased risk of osteoarthritis in later life because of repeated minor damage to the joints. People who frequently run long distances on hard surfaces risk damage to the knee cartilage.

exercise ECG The use of electrocardiography (see ECG) to assess the function of the heart when it is put under the stress of exercise. Exercise ECG is usually carried out when coronary artery disease is suspected. It involves raising the heart rate by exercising, usually on a treadmill with an adjustable gradient or an exercise bicycle, and recording the heart's electrical activity for analysis.

exfoliation Flaking off, shedding, or peeling from a surface in scales or thin layers, as in exfoliative dermatitis.

exfoliative dermatitis A skin disorder characterized by inflammation, redness, and scaling of the skin over most of the body. Exfoliative dermatitis may be the result of an allergic response to a drug or may be due to worsening of a skin condition such as psoriasis or eczema. The condition sometimes occurs in lymphoma and leukaemia.

There is a widespread rash with severe flaking of the skin, which results in increased loss of water and protein from the surface of the body. Protein loss may cause oedema and muscle wasting. Further possible complications include heart failure and infection. The treatment and outlook depend on the cause.

exhibitionism The habit of deliberately exposing the genitalia as a deviant sexual act. This type of behaviour is almost always confined to men. Psychotherapy or behaviour therapy may help persistent offenders.

exocrine gland A gland that secretes substances through a duct on to the inner surface of an organ or the outer surface of the body. Examples include the salivary glands and sweat glands. The release of exocrine secretions can be triggered by a hormone or a neurotransmitter. (See also endocrine gland.)

exogenous Of a disease or disorder, having a cause that is external to the body, such as infection, poisoning, or injury. (See also endogenous.)

exomphalos A rare birth defect, in which a membranous sac containing part of the intestines protrudes through the navel. The condition may sometimes be diagnosed before birth by ultrasound examination. Exomphalos is treated by surgery, the success of which depends on the extent of the defect.

exophthalmos Protrusion of one or both eyeballs caused by a swelling of the soft tissue in the eye socket. It is most commonly associated with thyrotoxicosis. Other causes include an eye tumour, inflammation, or an aneurysm behind the eye. Exophthalmos may restrict eye movement and cause double vision. In severe cases, increased pressure in the socket may restrict blood supply to the optic nerve, causing blindness. The eyelids may be unable to close, and vision may become blurred due to drying of the cornea.

In exophthalmos due to thyroid disease, treatment of the thyroid disorder may relieve the exophthalmos, but, if the cause is Graves' disease, exophthalmos may persist even if thyroid function returns to normal. Early treatment of the condition usually returns vision to normal. Occasionally, surgery may be required to relieve pressure on the eyeball and optic nerve.

exostosis The most common type of benign bone tumour, in which there is an outgrowth of bone. Exostosis occurs most frequently at the end of the femur or tibia. It may be due to hereditary factors or prolonged pressure on a bone.

In most cases, exostosis produces no symptoms. Often, it is recognized only after an injury, when it appears as a hard swelling. Occasionally, the tumour presses on a nerve, causing pain or

E

weakness in the affected area. Diagnosis can be confirmed by *X-rays*. Treatment, by surgical removal, may be carried out if the tumour is causing symptoms or for cosmetic reasons.

exotoxin A poison released by certain types of *bacteria* that enters the bloodstream and causes widespread effects around the body. Exotoxins are among the most poisonous substances known. Infections by *tetanus*, *diphtheria*, and some other bacteria that release lifethreatening exotoxins can be prevented by *immunization*. Treatment of such infections usually includes administration of *antibiotic drugs* and an *antitoxin*. (See also *endotoxin*; *enterotoxin*.)

exotropia A term for a divergent *squint*.

expectorants *Cough remedies* that encourage the coughing up of sputum.

expectoration The coughing up and spitting out of sputum.

exploratory surgery Any operation that is carried out to investigate or examine part of the body to discover the extent of known disease or to establish a diagnosis. Advances in imaging techniques, such as *MRI*, have reduced the need for exploratory surgery.

exposure A term used to describe the effects on the body of being subjected to very low temperatures, or to a combination of low temperatures, wetness, and high winds. The primary danger in these conditions is *hypothermia*.

The term is also used to describe subjection to radiation or pollutants.

expressing milk A technique used by *breast-feeding* women for removing milk from the breasts. It may be needed if the woman's breasts are overfull (see *engorgement*). A woman may want to express milk so that it can be given to the baby in her absence, or so that an infant unable to feed at the breast, due to prematurity, for example, can benefit from breast milk. Milk can be expressed by hand or with a *breast pump*.

exstrophy of the bladder A rare *birth defect* in which the *bladder* is turned inside out and is open to the outside of the body through a space in the lower abdominal wall. Usually, there are also other defects, such as *epispadias* in males and failure of the pubic bones to join at the front. Surgical treatment involves reconstructing the bladder and closing the abdominal wall. If the bladder is very small, it is removed and the urine diverted (see *urinary diversion*).

extraction, dental Removal of *teeth* by a dentist. Extraction may be performed when a tooth is severely decayed or too badly broken to be repaired, or when an abscess (see *abscess, dental*) has formed. Teeth may also be removed if there is crowding or *malocclusion*, if the teeth are loose due to gum disease, or if they are preventing another tooth from erupting (see *eruption of teeth*).

For most extractions, local anaesthesia is used (see *anaesthesia, dental*). Teeth are usually extracted with dental forceps, which grasp the root of the tooth. In difficult extractions, some gum and bone may also need to be removed from around the tooth.

extradural haemorrhage Bleeding into the space between the inner surface of the skull and the external surface of the *dura mater*, the outer layer of the *meninges*. Extradural haemorrhage usually results from a blow to the side of the head that fractures the skull and ruptures an artery running over the surface of the dura mater. A *haematoma* (collection of clotted blood) forms and enlarges, causing an increase in pressure inside the skull and resulting in symptoms several hours or even days after the injury. Symptoms may include headache, drowsiness, vomiting, paralysis affecting one side of the body, and *seizures*. Untreated, extradural haemorrhage may be life-threatening.

CT scanning or *MRI* confirms the diagnosis. Surgical treatment consists of *craniotomy*, draining the blood clot, and clipping the ruptured blood vessel.

extrapyramidal system A network of *nerve* pathways that links nerve nuclei in the surface of the *cerebrum*, the *basal ganglia*, and parts of the *brainstem*. The system influences and modifies electrical impulses sent from the brain to initiate movement in skeletal muscles.

Damage or degeneration of components in the extrapyramidal system can disrupt the execution of voluntary movements and can produce involuntary tremors or jerks. Such disturbances are seen in *Hunt-*

ington's disease, Parkinson's disease, some types of *cerebral palsy*, and can also occur as a side effect of *phenothiazine drugs*.

extrovert A person whose interests are constantly directed outwards, to other people and the environment. Extroverts are active, sociable, and have many outside interests. (See also *personality*.)

exudation The discharge of fluid from *blood vessels* into surrounding tissue. In most cases, exudation is due to *inflammation*. Exudate contains cells (mainly white blood cells) and protein.

eye The organ of sight. The eye consists of structures that focus an image on to the *retina* at the back of the eye and nerve cells that convert this image into electrical impulses. These impulses are carried by the *optic nerve* to the visual cortex (an area at the back of the brain concerned with *vision*) for interpretation.

The eyes work in conjunction with each other, under the control of the brain, aligning themselves on an object so that a clear image is formed on each retina. If necessary, the eyes sharpen images by altering focus in an automatic process called *accommodation*.

The eyeballs lie within the bony *orbits*. Each eyeball is moved by six delicate muscles. The eye has a tough outer coat, the *sclera*. At the front of the sclera, the transparent *cornea* serves as the main "lens" of the eye and does most of the focusing. Behind the cornea is a chamber of watery fluid, at the back of which is the *iris* with its *pupil*, which appears black. Tiny muscles alter the size of the pupil in response to changes in light intensity to control the amount of light entering the eye. Immediately behind the iris is the *lens*, suspended by fibres from a circular muscle ring called the *ciliary body*. Contraction of the ciliary body changes the shape of the lens, enabling fine focusing. Behind the lens is the main cavity of the eye, containing a clear gel, the vitreous humour. On the inside of the back of the eye is the retina, a complex structure of nerve tissue. The retina requires a constant supply of oxygen and glucose, and a network of blood vessels, the *choroid*, surrounds it.

The eyeball is sealed off from the outside by a flexible membrane called the *conjunctiva*, which is attached to the skin at the corners of the eye and forms the inner lining of the lids. The conjunctiva contains tear- and mucus-secreting glands. They, along with an oily secretion

E

EYE

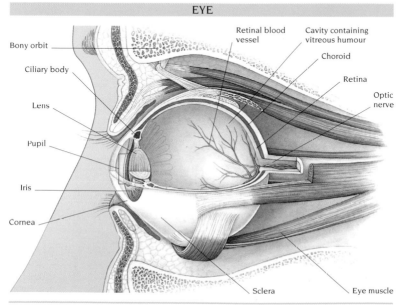

Bony orbit

Ciliary body

Lens

Pupil

Iris

Cornea

Retinal blood vessel

Cavity containing vitreous humour

Choroid

Retina

Optic nerve

Sclera

Eye muscle

E

from the meibomian glands in the lids, provide the tear film that protects the cornea and conjunctiva. The blink reflex is protective and helps to spread the tear film evenly over the cornea to enable clear vision.

eye, artificial A *prosthesis* to replace an *eye* that has been removed. It is worn for cosmetic reasons. Some movement of the artificial eye may be achieved by attaching the muscles that normally move the eye to the remaining conjunctival membrane (see *conjunctiva*) or to a plastic implant in the eye socket.

eye, disorders of Many eye disorders are minor, but some can cause loss of vision unless treated. (See also *cornea, disorders of; retinal detachment.*)

Squint is sometimes present at birth. Rarely, babies are born with *microphthalmos.* Other *congenital* disorders that affect the eye are *nystagmus, albinism,* and developmental abnormalities of the cornea and retina.

Conjunctivitis is the most common eye infection and rarely affects vision. *Trachoma* or severe bacterial conjunctivitis can impair vision. Corneal infections can lead to blurred vision or corneal *perforation* if not treated early. Endophthalmitis (infection within the eye) can occur as a result of eye injury or infection elsewhere in the body.

Narrowing, blockage or *inflammation* of the blood vessels of the *retina* may cause partial or total loss of vision.

Malignant melanoma of the *choroid* is the most common cancerous tumour of the eye. *Retinoblastoma* is a cancerous tumour of the retina that most commonly affects children.

Various *vitamin* deficiencies (particularly of vitamin A) can affect the eye and may lead to *xerophthalmia, night blindness,* or, ultimately, *keratomalacia.*

Uveitis may be caused by infection or an *autoimmune disorder* such as *ankylosing spondylitis* and *sarcoidosis.*

Macular degeneration of the retina is common in the elderly, as is *cataract.*

Glaucoma, in which the pressure inside the eyeball becomes raised, can lead to permanent loss of vision. In *retinal detachment,* the retina lifts away from the underlying layer of the eye.

Ametropia is a general term for any focusing error, such as *astigmatism, myopia,* or *hypermetropia. Presbyopia* is the progressive loss with age of the ability to focus at close range. *Amblyopia* is often due to squint.

eye-drops Medication in solution used to treat *eye disorders* or to aid in diagnosis. Examples of drugs given in this form are *antibiotic drugs, corticosteroid drugs, antihistamine drugs,* and drugs used to dilate or constrict the pupil.

eye, examination of An inspection of the structures of the *eyes,* either as part of a *vision test* or to make a diagnosis when an *eye disorder* is suspected.

An eye examination usually begins with inspection of the external appearance of the eyes, lids, and surrounding skin. A check of eye movements is usually performed and the examiner looks for *squint.* A check of the *visual acuity* in each eye using a *Snellen chart* follows. *Refraction* testing (using lenses of different strengths) may be performed to determine what glasses or contact lenses, if any, may be needed. A test of the *visual fields* may be performed, especially in suspected cases of *glaucoma* or neurological conditions. *Colour vision* may be checked because loss of colour perception is an indication of certain disorders of the *retina* or *optic nerve.* To check for abrasions or ulcers, the *conjunctiva* and *cornea* may be stained with *fluorescein.* Applanation *tonometry* is an essential test for glaucoma.

The *ophthalmoscope* is an instrument used to examine the inside of the eye, particularly the retina. The slit-lamp microscope, with its illumination and lens magnification, allows examination of the conjunctiva, cornea, front chamber of the eye, *iris,* and *lens.* For a full view of the lens and the structures behind it, the *pupil* must be widely dilated with *eye-drops.*

eye, foreign body in Any material on the surface of the *eye* or under the lid, or an object that penetrates the eyeball.

A foreign body may cause irritation, redness, increased tear production, and *blepharospasm.* In some cases, a foreign body left in the eye may cause a reaction that results in permanent loss of sight in both eyes.

Medical investigation of a foreign body in the eye may include using fluorescein eye-drops to reveal *corneal abrasions* or sites of penetration. *Ultrasound scanning* or an *X-ray* of the eye may also be performed. Local anaesthetic eye-drops may be applied and a spatula used to remove an object from the cornea. The eye may then be covered with a patch. *Antibiotic drugs* may also be prescribed.

eye injuries Serious eye injuries may be caused either by penetration of the eye by a foreign body (see *eye, foreign body in*) or by a blow to the eye.

A blow to the eye may cause tearing of the *iris* or the *sclera*, with collapse of the eyeball and possible blindness. Lesser injuries may lead to a *vitreous haemorrhage*, *hyphaema*, *retinal detachment*, or injury to the trabeculum (the channel through which fluid drains from inside the eye), which can lead to *glaucoma*. Injuries to the centre of the *cornea* impair vision by causing scarring. Damage to the lens may cause a *cataract to* form.

eyelashes, disorders of The eyelashes are arranged in two rows at the front edge of the lid and normally curve outwards. Growth in an abnormal direction may be due to injury to the lid or, more commonly, to infection. Severe *blepharitis* may destroy the roots of the lashes. *Trachoma*, an infection in which the lid is distorted by scarring, may lead to *trichiasis*. With age, the lashes become finer and fewer.

eye, lazy A popular term for *amblyopia* or a convergent *squint*.

eyelid A fold of tissue at the upper or lower edge of an eye socket. The eyelids are held in place by *ligaments* attached to the socket's bony edges. They consist of thin plates of fibrous tissue (called tarsal plates) covered by muscle and a thin layer of skin. The inner layer is covered by an extension of the *conjunctiva*. Along the edge of each lid are two rows of eyelashes. Immediately behind the eyelashes are the openings of the ducts leading from the meibomian glands, which secrete the oily part of the tear film. The lids act as protective shutters, closing as a reflex action if anything approaches the eye. They also smear the tear film across the *cornea*.

eyelid, drooping See *ptosis*.

eyelid surgery See *blepharoplasty*.

eye, painful red A common combination of eye symptoms that may be due to any of several eye *disorders*.

Uveitis is a common cause of dull, aching pain. The redness is caused by widening of blood vessels around the *iris*. Another serious cause of pain and redness in one eye is acute closed-angle *glaucoma*. Other causes include *keratitis*, usually due to a *corneal ulcer*, or a foreign body in the eye (see *eye, foreign body in*). The most common cause of redness and irritation in the eye is *conjunctivitis*.

eye-strain A common term for aching or discomfort in or around the eye. This is usually due to a headache caused by fatigue, tiredness of muscles around the eye, *sinusitis*, *blepharitis* (inflammation of the eyelids), or *conjunctivitis*.

eye teeth A common name for canine *teeth*.

eye tumours *Tumours* of the eye are rare. When eye tumours do occur, they are usually cancerous and painless.

Retinoblastoma is a cancerous tumour of the *retina* that occurs in one or both eyes and most often affects children. It may be treated by *radiotherapy, laser treatment*, or *cryosurgery*, but the eye may have to be removed to prevent spread of the tumour.

Malignant melanoma is a cancer of the *choroid*. It usually affects older people. There are no symptoms in the early stages, but it eventually causes *retinal detachment* and distortion of vision. Small tumours can be treated by laser, but the eye may need to be removed to avoid spread of the tumour.

Secondary eye tumours occur when cancer elsewhere in the body spreads to the eye. Symptoms depend on the tumour's location and growth rate. It may be controlled by radiotherapy.

Basal cell carcinoma is the most common type of tumour affecting the eyelid. It usually has a crusty central crater and a rolled edge. In the early stages, treatment may be possible by surgery, radiotherapy, or cryosurgery.

E

F

face-lift A cosmetic operation to smooth out wrinkles and lift sagging skin on an aging face. The effect is achieved by lifting the skin off the face and removing the excess. The skin is then stitched back together within the hairline. The effect may last for up to 10 years.

facet joint A type of joint found in the *spine*, formed by the bony knob (called a process) of one vertebra fitting into a hollow in the vertebra above. Facet joints allow a degree of movement between individual vertebrae, which gives the spine its flexibility.

facial nerve The 7th *cranial nerve*, which arises from structures in the *brainstem* and sends branches to the face, neck, salivary glands, and outer ear.

FACIAL NERVE

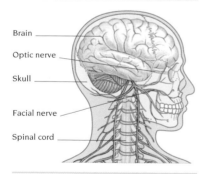

Brain

Optic nerve

Skull

Facial nerve

Spinal cord

The facial nerve performs both motor and sensory functions. It controls the muscles of the neck and of facial expression, stimulates the secretion of saliva, and conveys sensory information from the tongue and from the outer ear.

Damage to the nerve causes weakness of the facial muscles (see *facial palsy*) and, in some cases, loss of taste. Such damage is most often due to a viral infection but may also occur in *stroke*.

facial pain Pain in the face may be due to a variety of causes, of which injury is the most obvious. Facial pain is also commonly due to infection, particularly in *sinusitis* and *mumps*. Problems with the teeth and jaws are another common cause of facial pain. They include severe caries (see *caries, dental*), an abscess (see *abscess, dental*), impacted wisdom teeth (see *impaction, dental*), or partial dislocation of the jaw (see *jaw, dislocated*). Damage to a nerve that supplies the face can produce severe pain, including the knife-like pain that precedes the one-sided rash in *herpes zoster* and the intermittent shooting pain of *trigeminal neuralgia*.

A disorder elsewhere in the body may result in *referred pain* in the face. For example, in *angina*, pain may be felt in the jaw. In *migraine*, pain may occur on one side of the face. Facial pain that occurs for no apparent reason may be a symptom of *depression*.

Analgesic drugs can provide temporary relief, but severe or persistent facial pain requires medical attention.

facial palsy Weakness of the facial muscles due to inflammation of or damage to the *facial nerve*. The condition is usually temporary and affects only one side of the face.

Facial palsy is most often due to Bell's palsy, which occurs for no known reason. Less commonly, facial palsy is associated with *herpes zoster* affecting the ear and facial nerve. Facial palsy may also result from surgical damage to this nerve or compression of the nerve by a tumour.

Facial palsy usually comes on suddenly. The eyelid and corner of the mouth droop on one side of the face and there may be pain in the ear on that side. The sense of taste may be impaired or sounds may seem to be unnaturally loud.

In many cases, facial palsy clears up without treatment. Pain can be relieved by taking

FACIAL PALSY

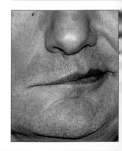

analgesic drugs, and exercising the facial muscles may aid recovery. In some cases, it may be necessary to tape the eyelid shut at bedtime in order to avoid the risk of corneal abrasion. Bell's palsy may be treated with corticosteroid drugs to reduce inflammation and speed recovery. Re-routing or grafting of nerve tissue may help people with palsies as a result of injury or a tumour.

facial spasm An uncommon disorder in which there is frequent twitching of facial muscles, which are supplied by the facial nerve. Facial spasm affects predominantly middle-aged women and is of unknown cause.

factitious disorders A group of disorders in which a patient's symptoms mimic those of a true illness but which have been invented by, and are controlled by, the patient. There is no apparent cause for a factitious disorder other than a wish for attention. The most common disorder of this type, Munchausen's syndrome, is characterized by physical symptoms. In a second form, Ganser's syndrome, there are psychological symptoms. These disorders differ from malingering, in which the person claims to be ill for a particular purpose, such as obtaining time off work.

factor V One of the blood proteins that maintains the balance between the blood clotting too easily or too slowly after an injury. About 5 per cent of the population have an inherited mutation in the gene controlling factor V production, known as factor V Leiden. They are at increased risk of deep-vein thrombosis (see thrombophilia), particularly if they are taking the oral contraceptive pill or go on long aircraft journeys.

factor VIII One of the blood proteins involved in blood clotting. People with haemophilia have a reduced level of factor VIII in their blood and, consequently, have a tendency to abnormal and prolonged bleeding when injured.

factor IX A protein in blood that plays an important role in the clotting mechanism. A deficiency of factor IX causes a rare genetic bleeding disorder known as Christmas disease.

faecal impaction A condition in which a large mass of hard faeces cannot be evacuated from the rectum. It is usually associated with long-standing constipation. Faecal impaction is most common in very young children and in the elderly, especially those who are bedridden.

The main symptoms are an intense desire to pass a bowel movement; pain in the rectum, anus, and centre of the abdomen; and, in some cases, watery faeces that are passed around the mass. Treatment is with enemas or by manual removal of the faecal mass.

faecalith A small, hard piece of impacted faeces that forms in a sac in the wall of the intestine. A faecalith is harmless unless it blocks the entrance to the sac, causing diverticulitis, or to the appendix, causing appendicitis.

faeces Waste material from the digestive tract that is expelled through the anus. Solidified in the large intestine, faeces are composed of indigestible food residue (dietary fibre), dead bacteria, dead cells from the tract lining, intestinal secretions, bile (which makes faeces brown), and water.

faeces, abnormal Faeces that differ from normal in colour, odour, consistency, or content. Abnormal faeces may indicate a disorder of the digestive system or related organ, such as the liver, but a change in the character of faeces is most often due to a change in diet.

Diarrhoea may be due simply to anxiety or may be caused by an intestinal infection (see gastroenteritis); by an intestinal disorder such as ulcerative colitis or Crohn's disease; or by irritable bowel syndrome. Loose stools may indicate malabsorption. Constipation is generally harmless but, if it develops unexpectedly, may be caused by a large-intestine disorder such as colon cancer.

Pale faeces may be caused by diarrhoea, a lack of bile in the intestine as a result of bile duct obstruction, or a disease that causes malabsorption (such as coeliac disease). Such faeces may be oily, foul-smelling, and difficult to flush away. Dark faeces may result from taking iron tablets. However, if faeces are black, there may be bleeding in the upper digestive tract.

Faeces containing excessive mucus are sometimes associated with constipation

F

or irritable bowel syndrome. *Enteritis, dysentery,* or a tumour of the intestine (see *intestine, tumours of*) may result in excess mucus, which is often accompanied by blood.

Blood in the faeces differs in appearance depending on the site of bleeding. Bleeding from the stomach or duodenum is usually passed in the form of black, tarry faeces. Blood from the colon is red and is usually passed at the same time as the faeces. Bleeding from the rectum or anus, which may be due to tumours or to *haemorrhoids*, is usually bright red. (See also *rectal bleeding.*)

faeces, blood in the See *faeces, abnormal; rectal bleeding.*

Fahrenheit scale A temperature scale in which the melting point of ice is 32° and the boiling point of water is 212°. On this scale, normal body temperature is 98.4°F, which is the equivalent of 37° Celsius (C). To convert a Fahrenheit temperature to Celsius, subtract 32 and multiply by 0.56 (or 5/9). To convert a Celsius temperature to Fahrenheit, multiply by 1.8 (or 9/5) then add 32. (See also *Celsius scale.*)

failure to thrive Failure of expected growth in an infant or toddler, usually assessed by comparing the rate at which a baby gains weight with a standardized growth chart. An undiagnosed illness such as a urinary infection may be the cause. Emotional or physical deprivation can also cause failure to thrive. A child who fails to grow at the appropriate rate needs tests to determine the cause.

fainting Temporary loss of consciousness due to reduced blood flow to the brain. Episodes of fainting are usually preceded by sweating, nausea, dizziness, and weakness, and are commonly caused by pain, stress, shock, a stuffy atmosphere, or prolonged coughing. An episode may also result from postural *hypotension*, which may occur when a person stands still for a long time or suddenly stands up. This is common in the elderly, in people with *diabetes mellitus*, and in those on *antihypertensive drugs* or *vasodilator drugs*.

In most cases, recovery from fainting occurs when normal blood flow to the

brain is restored. This restoration usually happens within minutes because the loss of consciousness results in the person falling into a lying position, which restores the flow of blood to the brain. Medical attention should be sought for prolonged *unconsciousness* or repeated attacks of fainting.

faith-healing The supposed ability of certain people to cure disease by a healing force inexplicable to science.

falciparum malaria The most severe form of *malaria*, caused by the parasitic protozoan PLASMODIUM FALCIPARUM.

fallen arches A cause of *flat-feet*. Fallen arches can develop as a result of weakness of the muscles that support the arches of the foot.

fallopian tube One of the two tubes that extend from the *uterus* to the *ovary*. The fallopian tube transports eggs and sperm and is where *fertilization* takes place.

FALLOPIAN TUBE

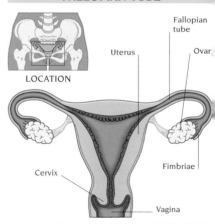

LOCATION

Uterus — Fallopian tube

Ovar

Fimbriae

Cervix

Vagina

The tube opens into the uterus at one end, and the other end, which is divided into fimbriae (finger-like projections), lies close to the ovary. The tube has muscular walls lined by cells with cilia (hair-like projections). The fimbriae take up the egg after it is expelled from the ovary. The beating cilia and muscular contractions propel the egg towards the uterus. After intercourse, sperm swim up the fallopian tube from the uterus. The lining of the tube and its secretions sustain the egg and sperm, encouraging fertilization, and nourish the egg until it reaches the uterus.

Salpingitis is inflammation of the fallopian tube, usually the result of a sexually transmitted bacterial infection, that can lead to *infertility*. An *ectopic pregnancy* (development of an embryo outside the uterus) most commonly occurs in the fallopian tube.

Fallot's tetralogy See *tetralogy of Fallot.*

fallout See *radiation hazards.*

falls in the elderly The tendency to fall increases steadily with age. Reflex actions become slower, and an elderly person who trips is frequently too slow to prevent a fall. Various medical conditions common in the elderly, including poor sight, *walking* disorders, cardiac *arrhythmias*, *hypotension*, and *Parkinson's disease*, increase the risk of falls, as does taking *sleeping drugs* or *tranquillizer drugs.*

Broken bones (see *fracture*) are a common complication of falls, especially in women. Not only do women have more falls, they are also more likely to suffer fractures because their bone strength may be reduced due to *osteoporosis*. A fall, or the fear of falling, can also have adverse psychological effects on an elderly person, who may become reluctant to leave the home.

Falls may be prevented by taking common-sense measures such as ensuring that handrails are secure, good lighting is available, suitable footwear is worn, and floor coverings and wiring are safe.

false teeth See *denture.*

familial A term applied to a characteristic or disorder that runs in families.

familial Mediterranean fever An inherited condition that affects certain Sephardic Jewish, Armenian, and Arab families. Its cause is unknown. Symptoms usually begin between the ages of 5 and 15 years, and include recurrent episodes of fever, abdominal and chestpain, and arthritis. Red skin swellings sometimes occur, and affected people may also suffer psychiatric problems. Attacks usually last from 24–48 hours but may be longer. Between attacks there are usually no symptoms. Although there is no specific treatment for familial

Mediterranean fever, known sufferers can reduce the incidence of attacks by taking *colchicine*. Death may eventually occur from *amyloidosis*, which is a complication of the condition.

family planning The deliberate limitation or spacing of births. Strategies for family planning include the different methods of *contraception*. (See also *birth control*.)

family therapy A form of psychotherapy that aims to promote greater harmony and understanding between members of a family, most often between parents and adolescent children.

famotidine An H_2 *receptor antagonist* drug that promotes healing of peptic ulcers and reduces inflammation of the oesophagus (*oesophagitis*) by suppressing acid production from the stomach. Side effects, which include headaches and dizziness, are uncommon.

Fanconi's anaemia A rare type of aplastic *anaemia* characterized by severely reduced production of all types of blood cells by the bone marrow.

Fanconi's syndrome A rare kidney disorder that occurs most commonly in childhood. Various important chemicals, such as amino acids, phosphate, calcium, and potassium, are lost in the urine, leading to failure to thrive, stunting of growth, and bone disorders such as *rickets*. Possible causes of the syndrome include several rare inherited abnormalities of body chemistry and an adverse reaction to certain drugs.

The child may resume normal growth if an underlying chemical abnormality can be corrected. Alternatively, a *kidney transplant* may be possible.

fantasy The process of imagining objects or events that are not actually occurring or present. The term also refers to the mental image. Fantasy can give the illusion that wishes have been met. In this sense, it provides satisfaction and can be a means of helping people to cope when reality becomes too unpleasant. Fantasy can also stimulate creativity. Psychoanalysts believe that some fantasies are unconscious and represent primitive instincts; these fantasies are presented to the conscious mind in symbols.

F

farmer's lung An occupational disease affecting the lungs of farm workers. Farmer's lung is a type of allergic *alveolitis*, in which affected people develop *hypersensitivity* to certain moulds that grow on hay, grain, or straw. Symptoms develop about 6 hours after exposure to dust containing fungal spores and include shortness of breath, headache, fever, and muscle aches. In acute attacks, the symptoms last for about a day. Repeated exposure to spores may lead to a chronic form of the disease, causing permanent scarring of lung tissues.

Diagnosis of farmer's lung may involve a *chest X-ray*, *pulmonary function tests*, and blood tests for a specific *antibody*. *Corticosteroid drugs* will relieve the symptoms. Further exposure to the spores of the fungus should be avoided. (See also *fibrosing alveolitis*.)

fascia Fibrous *connective tissue* that surrounds many structures in the body. One layer of the tissue, known as the superficial fascia, envelops the entire body just beneath the skin. Another layer, the deep fascia, encloses muscles, forming a sheath for individual muscles and separating them into groups; it also holds in place soft organs such as the kidneys. Thick fascia in the palm of the hand and sole of the foot have a cushioning, protective function.

fasciculation Spontaneous, irregular, and usually continual contractions of a muscle that is apparently at rest. Unlike the contractions of *fibrillation*, fasciculation is visible through the skin.

Minor fasciculation, such as that which occurs in the eyelids, is common and is no cause for concern. However, persistent fasciculation with weakness in the affected muscle indicates damage to nerve cells in the spine that control the muscle or nerve fibres that connect the spinal nerves to the muscle; *motor neuron disease* is one such disorder.

fasciitis Inflammation of a layer of *fascia* (fibrous connective tissue), causing pain and tenderness. Fasciitis is usually the result of straining or injuring the fascia surrounding a muscle; it most commonly affects the sole of the foot. Fasciitis may occur in people who suffer from *ankylosing spondylitis* (a rheumatic disorder affecting the spine) or *Reiter's syndrome* (inflammation of the urethra, conjunctivitis, and arthritis).

Treatment involves resting the affected area and protecting it from pressure. In some cases, a local injection of a *corticosteroid drug* is given. If fasciitis is part of a widespread disorder of the joints, treatment of this condition will generally improve symptoms.

fascioliasis A disease affecting the liver and bile ducts that is caused by infestation with the *liver fluke* species *FASCIOLA HEPATICA*.

fasciotomy An operation to relieve pressure on muscles by making an incision in the *fascia* (fibrous connective tissue) that surrounds them. The operation is usually performed to treat *compartment syndrome*, a painful condition in which constriction of a group of muscles causes obstruction of blood flow. Fasciotomy is also sometimes performed as a surgical emergency after an injury has resulted in muscle swelling or bleeding within a muscle compartment.

fasting Abstaining from all food and drinking only water. In temperate conditions and at moderate levels of physical activity, a person can survive on water alone for more than 2 months; however, without food or drink, death usually occurs within about 10 days.

About 6 hours after the last meal, the body starts to use glycogen (a carbohydrate stored in the liver and muscles). This continues for about 24 hours, after which the body obtains energy from stored fat and by breaking down protein in the muscles. If fasting continues, the body's *metabolism* slows down to conserve energy, and the fat and protein stores are consumed more slowly.

In the initial stages of fasting, weight loss is rapid. Later it slows down, because metabolism slows down and the body starts to conserve its salt supply, which causes water retention. In prolonged fasting, the ability to digest food may be impaired because the stomach stops secreting digestive juices. Prolonged fasting also halts production of sex hormones, causing *amenorrhoea* (absence of menstruation) in women.

fatigue See *tiredness*.

fats and oils Nutrients that provide the body with its most concentrated form of *energy*. Fats, which are also called lipids, are compounds containing chains of carbon and hydrogen with very little oxygen. Chemically, fats consist mostly of *fatty acids* combined with *glycerol*. They are divided into two main groups, saturated and unsaturated, depending on the proportion of hydrogen atoms. If the fatty acids contain the maximum possible quantity of hydrogen, the fats are saturated. If some sites on the carbon chain are unoccupied by hydrogen, they are unsaturated; when many sites are vacant, they are polyunsaturated. Monounsaturated fats are unsaturated fats with only one site that could take an extra hydrogen. Animal fats, such as those in meat and dairy products, are largely saturated, whereas vegetable fats tend to be unsaturated.

Fats are usually solid at room temperature; oils are liquid. The amount and types of fat in the diet have important implications for health. A diet containing a large amount of fat, particularly saturated fat, is linked to an increased risk of *atherosclerosis* and subsequent heart disease and stroke.

Some dietary fats, mainly triglycerides (combinations of glycerol and three fatty acids), are sources of the fat-soluble vitamins A, D, E, and K and of essential fatty acids. Triglycerides are the main form of fat stored in the body. These stores act as an energy reserve and also provide insulation and a protective layer for delicate organs. Phospholipids are structural fats found in cell membranes. Sterols, such as *cholesterol*, are found in animal and plant tissues; they have a variety of functions, often being converted into hormones or vitamins.

Dietary fats are first emulsified by bile salts before being broken down by lipase, a pancreatic enzyme. They are absorbed via the lymphatic system before entering the bloodstream.

Lipids are carried in the blood bound to protein; in this state they are known as lipoproteins. There are four classes of lipoprotein: very low-density lipoproteins (VLDLs), low-density lipoproteins (LDLs), high-density lipoproteins (HDLs), and chylomicrons. LDLs and VLDLs contain large amounts of cholesterol, which they carry through the bloodstream and deposit in tissues. HDLs pick up cholesterol and carry it back to the liver for processing and excretion. High levels of LDLs are associated with atherosclerosis, whereas HDLs have a protective effect. (See also *nutrition; omega-3 fatty acids.*)

fatty acids Organic acids, containing carbon, hydrogen, and oxygen, that are constituents of *fats and oils* There are more than 40 fatty acids, which are found in nature and which are distinguished by their constituent number of carbon and hydrogen atoms.

Certain fatty acids cannot be synthesized by the body and must be provided by the diet. These are linoleic, linolenic, and arachidonic acids, sometimes collectively termed essential fatty acids. Strictly speaking, only linoleic acid is essential, since the body can make the other two from linoleic acid obtained from food. (See also *nutrition; omega-3 fatty acids.*)

favism A disorder characterized by an extreme sensitivity to the broad bean *VICIA FABA* (fava). If an affected person eats these beans, a chemical in the bean causes rapid destruction of red blood cells, leading to a severe type of anaemia (see *anaemia, haemolytic*).

Favism is uncommon except in some areas of the Mediterranean. The disorder is caused by a sex-linked *genetic disorder*. Affected people have *G6PD deficiency*, a defect in a chemical pathway in their red cells that normally helps protect the cells from injury.

Children with a family history of favism can be screened for the disorder at an early age. If it is found, they must avoid fava beans and certain drugs, including some *antimalarial drugs* and *antibiotic drugs*, that can have a similar effect on their red blood cells.

febrile Feverish or related to *fever*, as in febrile *convulsions*.

febrile convulsion See *convulsion, febrile*.

feedback A self-regulating mechanism that controls certain body processes such as hormone and enzyme production. If, for example, levels of a hormone are too high, output of any substance that stimulates the hormone's release is inhibited; the result is reduced hormone production (negative feedback). The reverse process (positive feedback) restores the balance if the level of hormone becomes too low.

feeding, artificial The administration of nutrients other than by mouth, usually by way of a tube passed through the nose into the stomach (see *gastrostomy*) or small intestine. If long-term artificial feeding is anticipated, a tube is inserted directly into the stomach or upper small intestine using endoscopic surgery. If the gastrointestinal tract is not functioning, nutrients must be introduced into the bloodstream. This type of feeding is known as *parenteral nutrition*.

Tube feeding may be necessary for people who have gastrointestinal disorders or disorders affecting the nervous system or kidneys. Premature babies often require tube feeding if their sucking reflexes are undeveloped, as do critically ill patients due to their increased nutritional requirements. Intravenous feeding is usually given when large areas of the small intestine have been damaged or have been surgically removed.

feeding, infant A baby grows more rapidly in its first year than at any future time in its life. A good diet is essential for healthy growth and development.

During the first 6 months, most babies' nutritional requirements are met by *milk* alone, whether by *breast-feeding* or *bottle-feeding*; however, sometimes vitamin D supplements may be recommended for breast-fed babies. Both human milk and artificial milk contain carbohydrate, protein, fat, vitamins, and minerals in similar proportions. However, human milk also contains antibodies and white blood cells that protect the baby against infection. From 6 months, supplementary vitamins A, C, and D should be given to breast-fed babies. Formula milk already contains vitamin supplements.

At 1 year of age, a baby can be safely fed with full-fat cow's milk as part of a good mixed diet. Solids, initially in the form of purees, should be introduced from 6 months of age, depending on the birthweight, rate of growth, and contentment with feeding. By 7–8 months,

the baby should be eating true solids, such as chopped-up meat and vegetables. Between 1 and 5 years of age, supplementary vitamins A and D are recommended if there is any doubt that the baby is getting sufficient amounts from his or her diet.

A few babies have an intolerance to certain foods such as lactose or cow's milk protein (see *food intolerance*; *nutritional disorders*).

femoral artery A major blood vessel that supplies oxygenated blood to the leg. The femoral artery is formed in the pelvis from the iliac artery (the terminal branch of the *aorta*). It then runs from the groin, down in front of the thigh, and passes behind the knee to become the popliteal artery, which branches again to supply the lower leg.

FEMORAL ARTERY

femoral epiphysis, slipped Displacement of the upper *epiphysis* (growing end) of the *femur* (thigh bone). Such displacement is rare; it usually affects children between 11 and 13, and occurs more often in boys and obese children. The condition may also run in families. During normal growth, the epiphysis is separated from the shaft of the bone by a plate of cartilage. This is an area of relative weakness, so that a fall or other injury can cause the epiphysis to slip out of position. A limp develops, and pain is felt in the knee or groin. The leg tends to turn outwards and hip movements are restricted.

Surgery is needed to fix the epiphysis into its correct position and is usually completely successful. In some cases, the other hip may also need to be stabilized.

femoral hernia A type of *hernia* that occurs in the groin area, where the *femoral artery* and femoral vein pass from the lower abdomen to the thigh.

femoral nerve One of the main nerves of the leg. The nerve fibres making up the femoral nerve emerge from the lower spine and run down into the thigh, where they branch to supply the skin and *quadriceps muscles*.

Damage to the femoral nerve (which impairs the ability to straighten the knee) is usually caused by a slipped disc in the lumbar region of the spine (see *disc prolapse*). Damage may also result from a backward dislocation of the hip or a *neuropathy*.

femur The medical name for the thigh-bone, the longest bone in the body. The lower end hinges with the tibia (shin) to form the knee joint. The upper end is rounded into a ball (head of the femur) that fits into a socket in the pelvis to form the hip joint. The head of the femur is joined to the bone shaft by a narrow piece of bone called the neck of the femur, which is a common fracture site (see *femur, fracture of*).

At the lower end, the bone is enlarged to form two lumps (the condyles) that distribute the weight-bearing load through the knee joint. On the outer side of the upper femur is a protuberance called the greater trochanter. The shaft of the femur is surrounded by muscles which move the hip and knee joints.

femur, fracture of The symptoms, treatment, and possible complications of a fracture of the femur (thigh-bone) depend on whether the bone has broken across its neck (the short section between the top of the shaft and the ball of the hip joint) or across the shaft.

Fracture of the neck of the femur, often called a broken hip, is very common in elderly people, especially in women

with *osteoporosis*, and is usually associated with a fall. In a fracture of the neck of the femur, the broken bone ends are often considerably displaced; in such cases there is usually severe pain in the hip and groin, making standing impossible. Occasionally, the broken ends become impacted. In this case, there is less pain and walking may be possible.

Diagnosis is confirmed by X-ray. If the bone ends are displaced, an operation under general anaesthesia is necessary, either to realign the bone ends and to fasten them together, or to replace the entire head and neck of the femur with an artificial substitute (see *hip replacement*). If the bone ends are impacted the fracture may heal naturally, but surgery may still be recommended to avoid the need for bed rest.

Complications include damage to the blood supply to the head of the femur, causing it to disintegrate. *Osteoarthritis* may develop in the hip joint after fracture of the femur neck itself. However, immobility and the need for surgery in the elderly may result in complications, such as pneumonia, that are not directly related to the fracture site.

Fracture of the bone shaft usually occurs when the femur is subjected to extreme force, such as that which occurs in a traffic accident. In most cases, the bone ends are considerably displaced, causing severe pain, tenderness, and swelling.

Diagnosis is confirmed by X-ray. With a fractured femoral shaft there is often substantial blood loss from the bone. In most cases, the fracture is repaired by surgery in which the ends of the bone are realigned and fastened together with a metal pin or a more extensive fixation device. Sometimes the bone ends can be realigned by manipulation, and surgery is not necessary. After realignment, the leg is supported with a *splint* and put in *traction* to hold the bone together while it heals.

Complications include failure of the bone ends to unite or fusion of the broken ends at the wrong angle, infection of the bone (*osteomyelitis*), or damage to a nerve or artery. A fracture of the lower shaft can cause permanent stiffness of the knee.

fenbufen A *nonsteroidal anti-inflammatory drug* (NSAID) used to relieve pain and stiffness caused, for example, by *rheumatoid arthritis, osteoarthritis*, and *gout*. Fenbufen is also used to reduce pain and to help speed recovery following muscle and ligament sprains. In common with other NSAIDs, it can cause bleeding from the stomach and may also cause a rash.

fenoprofen A *nonsteroidal anti-inflammatory drug* (NSAID) that is used to relieve pain and stiffness caused, for example, by *rheumatoid arthritis, osteoarthritis*, and *gout*. Fenoprofen is also used to treat muscle and ligament sprains; it reduces pain and helps to speed recovery. In common with many NSAIDs, fenoprofen may cause irritation of the stomach.

fentanyl An *opioid* analgesic drug that is given by injection for pain relief during surgery and also to enhance general anaesthesia (see *anaesthesia, general*). Fentanyl is also used in the form of a skin patch or lozenge to control the severe chronic pain of conditions such as cancer. In common with other opioid drugs, fentanyl has side effects that include depressed breathing, constipation, nausea, and vomiting. The administration of patches may be associated with local irritation of the skin.

ferritin A complex of *iron* and protein, found mainly in the liver and spleen, which is the principal form of iron storage in the body.

ferrous fumarate A form of *iron* given in the form of an oral preparation to treat iron-deficiency *anaemia*. Ferrous fumarate can cause diarrhoea, constipation, and abdominal pain.

ferrous sulphate Another name for iron sulphate (see *iron*).

fertility The ability to produce children without undue difficulty.

A man's fertility depends on the production of normal quantities of healthy *sperm* in the testes (see *testis*), which, in turn, depends on adequate production of *gonadotrophin hormones* by the pituitary gland at the base of the brain. Fertility in males is also dependent on the ability to achieve an *erection* and to ejaculate *semen* into the vagina during *sexual intercourse*. Males become fertile at puberty and usually remain so, but to a lesser degree, well into old age.

A woman's ability to conceive depends on normal *ovulation* (the monthly production of a healthy *ovum* by one of the *ovaries*) and the ovum's unimpeded passage down a fallopian tube towards the uterus; on thinning of the mucus surrounding the mouth of the cervix to enable sperm to penetrate; and on changes in the lining of the uterus which prepare it for the implantation of a fertilized ovum. These processes are in turn dependent on normal production of gonadotrophins by the pituitary gland, and of the sex hormones *oestrogen* and *progesterone* by the ovaries. Women become fertile at puberty, and they remain so until the *menopause* around the age of 45 to 55. (See also *fertility drugs; infertility*.)

fertility drugs A group of hormonal or hormone-related drugs used to treat some types of *infertility*.

In women, fertility drugs may be given when abnormal hormone production by the pituitary gland or ovaries disrupts *ovulation* or causes mucus around the cervix to become so thick that sperm cannot penetrate it. In men, fertility drugs are less effective, but they may be used when abnormal hormone production by the pituitary gland or testes interferes with sperm production. (See also *clomifene; gonadotrophin hormones; testosterone*.)

fertilization The union of a *sperm* and an *ovum*. In natural fertilization, the sperm and ovum unite in the fallopian tube of the woman following *sexual intercourse*. A single sperm penetrates the ovum by releasing enzymes that can dissolve the outer layers of the ovum. Once inside, the sperm's nucleus fuses with that of the ovum, and its empty body shell and tail drop off. Then, the newly fertilized ovum, called a zygote, forms an outer layer that is impenetrable to other sperm. The zygote undergoes repeated cell divisions as it passes down the fallopian tube to the uterus, where it implants and will eventually grow into an embryo.

Fertilization may also occur as a result of semen being artificially introduced into the cervix (see *artificial insemination*) or may take place in a laboratory (see *in vitro fertilization*).

fetal alcohol syndrome A rare condition consisting of a combination of *congenital* defects that result from the continuous consumption of excessive amounts of *alcohol* by the mother throughout *pregnancy*. The affected baby has diminished growth, delayed mental development, a small head, a small brain, and small eyes. He or she may have a cleft palate, a small jaw, heart defects, and joint abnormalities. As a newborn, the baby sucks poorly, sleeps badly, and is irritable as a result of alcohol withdrawal. Almost one-fifth of affected babies die during the first few weeks of life; and many who survive are, to some degree, mentally and physically handicapped.

fetal circulation Blood circulation in the fetus is different from the normal circulation after birth (see *circulatory system*). The fetus neither breathes nor eats. Therefore, oxygen and nutrients are obtained and waste products such as carbon dioxide are removed via the *placenta*. Fetal blood reaches the placenta through blood vessels in the *umbilical cord*. The maternal and fetal circulations are separated by a thin membrane in the placenta, which allows the exchange of nutrients and waste products. The other fundamental difference in circulation is that most blood bypasses the lungs in the fetus through two special channels in the fetal heart. Blood passes from the right atrium of the heart to the left atrium through the foramen ovale. Another channel, known as the ductus arteriosus, allows blood to pass from the pulmonary artery to the aorta. Both channels normally close after birth. In rare cases, they fail to close, causing a congenital heart disorder (see *heart disease, congenital*).

fetal distress The physical stress experienced by a fetus during labour as a result of its not receiving enough oxygen. During a contraction, the uterus tightens and reduces the oxygen supply from the placenta to the fetus. If, in addition, there are problems, such as pressure on the umbilical cord or the mother's losing blood, there may be an inadequate amount of oxygen reaching the fetus.

Fetal distress may cause the baby's heart-rate to slow or to fail to show normal variability, which can be recorded on a cardiotocograph (see *fetal heart monitoring*). *Acidosis* (high acidity in the body), which can be detected in a sample of blood taken from the scalp, indicates that the oxygen supply to the fetus is inadequate. Signs of *meconium* in the amniotic fluid can also be an indication of fetal distress.

Fetal distress sometimes occurs as a temporary episode, but, if acidosis is severe, the distressed fetus may need to be delivered promptly by *caesarean section*, *forceps delivery*, or *vacuum extraction*. (See also *childbirth*.)

fetal heart monitoring The use of an instrument to record and/or listen to an unborn baby's heartbeat during pregnancy and labour. Monitoring is carried out at intervals throughout pregnancy if tests indicate that the placenta is not functioning normally or if the baby's growth is slow. During labour, monitoring can detect *fetal distress*, in which oxygen deprivation causes abnormality in the fetal heart-rate.

FETAL CIRCULATION

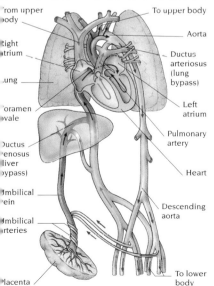

From upper body

To upper body

Aorta

Right atrium

Ductus arteriosus (lung bypass)

Lung

Left atrium

Foramen ovale

Pulmonary artery

Ductus venosus (liver bypass)

Heart

Umbilical vein

Descending aorta

Umbilical arteries

To lower body

Placenta

FETAL HEART MONITORING

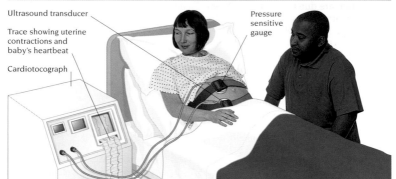

Ultrasound transducer

Trace showing uterine
contractions and
baby's heartbeat

Cardiotocograph

Pressure
sensitive
gauge

F

EXTERNAL FETAL HEART MONITORING

The simplest form of fetal heart monitoring involves the use of a special fetal stethoscope. Cardiotocography, a more sophisticated electronic version, makes a continuous paper recording of the heartbeat together with a recording of the uterine contractions. The heartbeat is picked up either externally by an *ultrasound* transducer strapped to the mother's abdomen or, as an alternative during labour, internally by an electrode attached to the baby's scalp that passes through the vagina and cervix.

fetishism Reliance on special objects in order to achieve sexual arousal. The objects need not have an obvious sexual meaning; they may include shoes, rubber or leather garments, and parts of the body, such as the feet or ears.

Fetishism usually has no obvious cause. According to psychoanalysts, the origin may be a childhood *fixation* of sexual interest upon some aspect of the mother's appearance. Treatment is necessary only if the behaviour is causing distress or persistent criminal acts.

fetoscopy A procedure for directly observing a fetus inside the uterus by means of a fetoscope, a type of *endoscope*. Fetoscopy is used to diagnose various *congenital* abnormalities before the baby is born. Because the technique carries some risks, it is performed only when other tests such as *ultrasound scanning* have detected an abnormality. By attaching additional instruments, it

is also possible to use the fetoscope to take samples of fetal blood or tissue for analysis and to correct surgically some fetal disorders. (See also *amniocentesis; chorionic villus sampling.*)

fetus The unborn child from the end of the 8th week after conception until birth. For the first 8 weeks, the unborn child is called an *embryo.*

fever Elevation above normal of body temperature. Normal body temperature is 37°C in the mouth and 0.6°C lower in the axilla (armpit). A fever may be accompanied by symptoms such as shivering, headache, sweating, thirst, faster-than-normal breathing, and a flushed face. *Confusion* or *delirium* sometimes occur, especially in the elderly; a high fever may cause seizures in a child under 5 years (see *convulsion, febrile*) or *coma.*

Most fevers are caused by a bacterial infection such as *tonsillitis* or a viral infection such as *influenza*. In these cases, proteins called pyrogens are released when the white blood cells fight the microorganisms that are responsible for the infection. Pyrogens act on the temperature controlling centre in the brain, causing it to raise the body temperature in an attempt to destroy the invading microorganisms. Fever may also occur in conditions, such as *dehydration, thyrotoxicosis, lymphoma,* and *myocardial infarction,* where infection is not present.

Drugs such as *aspirin* or other *nonsteroidal anti-inflammatory drugs,* or *paracetamol* may be given to reduce fevers that are due to infections. Otherwise, treatment is directed at the underlying cause (for example, giving *antibiotic drugs* for a bacterial infection).

feverfew The common name for the plant TANACETUM PARTHENIUM, which is used in herbal medicine to treat headache and migraine.

fibrates A group of *lipid-lowering drugs* used to treat high blood levels of *triglycerides* or *cholesterol*.

fibre, dietary Indigestible plant material in food. Dietary fibre includes certain types of polysaccharides, cellulose, hemicelluloses, gums and pectins (see *carbohydrates*), and lignin. Humans do not have the necessary enzymes to digest these substances, which pass through the digestive system virtually unchanged and cannot be used as a source of energy.

Some components of dietary fibre hold water, thereby adding bulk to the faeces and aiding bowel function. For this reason, dietary fibre can be effective in treating *constipation, diverticular disease,* and *irritable bowel syndrome*. Unrefined carbohydrate foods such as wholemeal bread, cereals, and root vegetables are rich in fibre. (See also *nutrition*.)

fibre-optics The transmission of images through bundles of thin, flexible glass or plastic threads which propagate light by total internal reflection. This means that all the light from a powerful external source travels the length of the fibre without losing its intensity. Fibre-optics have led to the development of *endoscopes*, which enable structures deep within the body to be viewed directly.

fibrillation Localized spontaneous, rapid contractions of individual muscle fibres. Unlike *fasciculation* (muscular quivering), fibrillation cannot be seen through the skin. In skeletal muscles, fibrillation is detected by an *EMG*. In heart muscle, it is detected by an *ECG*.

Fibrillation usually occurs once a nerve supplying a muscle is destroyed, which causes the affected muscle to become weak and waste away. Fibrillation of the heart muscle is caused by disruption to the spread of nerve impulses through the muscle wall of a heart chamber (see *atrial fibrillation; ventricular fibrillation*).

fibrin A substance that is produced in the blood during the process of *blood clotting*. A dissolved protein called *fibrinogen* is converted to fibrin, which forms long filaments that bind clumps of *platelets* and other blood cells into a mass which plugs the bleeding point.

fibrinogen A protein that is present in blood and which is converted into *fibrin* during the *blood clotting* process.

fibrinolysis The breakdown of *fibrin*, the principal component of any blood clot. Fibrin is a stringy protein that is formed in blood as the end product of coagulation (see *blood clotting*). Blood also contains a fibrinolytic system, which is activated in parallel with the coagulation system when a blood vessel is damaged. The fibrinolytic system prevents the formation of clots in undamaged blood vessels, thereby preventing blockage, and it dissolves a clot once a broken vessel wall has healed. *Thrombosis* (abnormal clot formation) occurs if there is a disturbance in the balance between coagulation and fibrinolytic mechanisms.

fibrinolytic drugs Another name for *thrombolytic drugs*, which are used to dissolve blood clots.

fibroadenoma A noncancerous fibrous tumour most commonly found in the breast. Fibroadenomas of the breast are painless, firm, round lumps and are usually 1–5 cm in diameter and movable. They occur most often in women under 30 and black women. Multiple tumours may develop in one or both breasts.

The lumps are removed surgically and the tissue examined to confirm diagnosis.

fibroadenosis An outdated term for the general lumpiness that is a normal feature of some women's breasts. Cyclical changes in hormone levels often lead to lumpiness, which is more obvious before a menstrual period. Lumpy breasts do not increase the risk of developing breast cancer. However, a new solitary, discrete *breast lump* should be assessed by a doctor to rule out the possibility of breast cancer.

fibrocystic disease A term used to refer either to the inherited disorder *cystic fibrosis* or the presence of general

F

lumpiness of the breasts that is a variation of normal. (See also *fibroadenosis*).

fibroid A slow-growing, noncancerous tumour of the *uterus*, consisting of smooth muscle and *connective tissue*. There may be one or more fibroids, and they may be as small as a pea or as large as a grapefruit.

Fibroids are common, appearing most often in women aged 35 to 45. The cause is thought to be related to an abnormal response to *oestrogen hormones*. *Oral contraceptives* containing oestrogen can cause fibroids to enlarge, as can *pregnancy*. Decreased oestrogen production after the *menopause* usually causes them to shrink.

In many cases, there are no symptoms. If a fibroid enlarges and projects into the cavity of the uterus, it may cause heavy or prolonged periods. A large fibroid may exert pressure on the bladder, causing frequent passing of urine, or on the bowel, causing backache or constipation. Fibroids that distort the uterine cavity may be responsible for recurrent miscarriage or infertility.

Fibroids that do not cause symptoms are often discovered during a routine pelvic examination. *Ultrasound scanning* can confirm the diagnosis. Small, symptomless fibroids usually require no treatment, but regular examinations may be needed to assess growth. Surgery is required for fibroids that cause serious symptoms. In some cases, they can be removed with a *hysteroscope* or under general *anaesthesia*, leaving the uterus intact. Sometimes, however, a *hysterectomy* is necessary.

fibroma A noncancerous tumour of the cells that make up *connective tissue*. For example, a neurofibroma is a tumour of the cells that surround nerve fibres (see *neurofibromatosis*). Treatment is necessary only if the tumour causes symptoms.

fibromyalgia Also sometimes known as fibrositis, a poorly understood condition in which there is generalized aching and stiffness of the muscles of the trunk, hips, and shoulders. Parts of the affected muscles (known as trigger points) are tender to the touch; common tender sites are the base of the skull and the muscles near the shoulderblades.

Fibromyalgia commonly develops during periods of stress and may follow a chronic course. Treatment may include heat, massage, exercise, stress reduction, and drugs such as *nonsteroidal anti-inflammatory drugs* and, sometimes, *antidepressant drugs*, which may relieve the symptoms.

fibrosarcoma A rare, cancerous tumour of the cells that make up *connective tissue*. A fibrosarcoma may develop from a noncancerous *fibroma* or may be cancerous from the start. Treatment is by surgical removal and/or *radiotherapy*.

fibrosing alveolitis Inflammation and thickening of the walls of the alveoli in the lungs (see *alveolus, pulmonary*) that results in scarring of lung tissue (see *interstitial pulmonary fibrosis*). Fibrosing alveolitis most commonly occurs in people over 60 and is more common in men.

In some cases, fibrosing alveolitis is due to an *autoimmune disorder* and may be associated with conditions such as *rheumatoid arthritis* or systemic *lupus erythematosus*. Other possible causes include radiotherapy of the organs in the chest and *anticancer drug* treatment. In many cases, however, the cause is unknown, and the condition is then known as idiopathic pulmonary fibrosis.

Symptoms of fibrosing alveolitis include shortness of breath, a persistent dry cough, and joint pains.

Treatment of the condition involves *corticosteroid drugs* combined with other *immunosuppressant drugs* to slow the progress of lung damage.

fibrosis An overgrowth of scar tissue or *connective tissue*. Fibrous tissue may be formed as an exaggerated healing response to infection, inflammation, or injury. Fibrosis can also result from a lack of oxygen in a tissue, usually due to inadequate blood flow through it (in heart muscle damaged by a *myocardial infarction*, for example). In fibrosis, specialized structures (such as kidney or muscle cells) are replaced by fibrous tissue, which causes impaired function of the organ concerned.

fibrositis See *fibromyalgia*.

fibula The outer and thinner of the two long bones of the lower leg. The fibula is much narrower than the other lower-leg bone, the *tibia* (shin), to which it runs parallel and to which it is attached at both ends by ligaments. The top end of the fibula does not reach the knee, but the lower end extends below the tibia and forms part of the *ankle joint*. The fibula is one of the most commonly broken bones. *Pott's fracture* is fracture of the fibula just above the ankle combined with dislocation of the ankle and sometimes with fracture of the tibia.

fifth disease An infectious disease that causes a widespread rash. Also known as slapped cheek disease or erythema infectiosum, fifth disease mainly affects children and is caused by a virus called parvovirus. The rash starts on the cheeks as separate, rose-red, raised spots, which subsequently converge to give the characteristic appearance. Within a few days, the rash spreads in a lacy pattern over the limbs but only sparsely on the trunk. It is often accompanied by mild fever. The rash usually clears after about 10 days. Adults, who contract the disease only rarely, may have joint pain and swelling lasting for up to 2 years. The incubation period is 7 to 14 days, and the only treatment is drugs to reduce the fever.

fight-or-flight response Arousal of the sympathetic part of the *autonomic nervous system* in response to fear but which also occurs in *anxiety disorders*. *Adrenaline* (epinephrine), *noradrenaline* (norepinephrine), and other hormones are released from the adrenal glands and nervous system, leading to a raised heart-rate, pupil dilation, and increased blood flow to the muscles. These effects make the body more efficient in either fighting or fleeing the apparent danger.

filariasis A group of tropical diseases, caused by various parasitic worms or their larvae, which are transmitted to humans by insect bites.

Some species of worm live in the lymphatic vessels. Swollen lymph nodes and recurring fever are early symptoms. Inflammation of lymph vessels results in localized *oedema*. Following repeated infections, the affected area, commonly a limb or the scrotum, becomes very enlarged and the skin becomes thick, coarse, and fissured, leading to a condition known as *elephantiasis*. The larvae

of another type of worm invade the eye, causing blindness (see *onchocerciasis*). A third type, which may sometimes be seen and felt moving beneath the skin, causes *loiasis*, characterized by irritating and sometimes painful areas of oedema called calabar swellings.

The diagnosis of filariasis is confirmed by microscopic examination of the blood. The *anthelmintic drugs* diethylcarbamazine or ivermectin most often cure the infection but may cause side effects such as fever, sickness, muscle pains, and increased itching. The use of insect repellents and protective clothing help to protect against insect bites. (See also *roundworms; insects and disease*.)

filling, dental The process of replacing a chipped or decayed area of tooth with an inactive material. Dental filling is also used to describe the restorative material itself. Amalgam, a hard-wearing mixture of silver, mercury, and other metals is generally used for back teeth. If a front tooth is chipped, a bonding technique (see *bonding, dental*) may be used, in which plastic or porcelain tooth-coloured material is attached to the surface of the tooth.

FILLING, DENTAL

film badge A device that enables hospital staff members to monitor their exposure to radiation. Film badges are worn by those people who work in X-ray and radiotherapy departments. A badge consists of a piece of photographic film in a holder worn on the clothing. The film has a fast (sensitive) emulsion on

F

one side and a slow emulsion on the other. Small doses of radiation blacken only the fast emulsion; higher doses start to blacken the slow emulsion and make the fast emulsion opaque.

finasteride A specific *enzyme* inhibitor drug that prevents *testosterone* from being converted into the more potent male hormone, dihydrotestosterone. The drug is used to treat noncancerous prostatic enlargement (see *prostate, enlarged*), improving the flow of urine. Side effects include *erectile dysfunction* and decreased libido and ejaculate volume.

finger One of the digits of the *hand*. Each finger has three phalanges (bones), which join at hinge joints moved by muscle tendons, and an artery, vein, and nerve running down each side. The entire structure is enclosed in skin with a *nail* at the tip.

Common finger injuries are *lacerations*, *fractures*, tendon ruptures, and *mallet finger*. Infections such as *paronychia* can occur, and inflamed flexor tendons may cause *trigger finger*. Congenital finger disorders include *syndactyly*, *polydactyly*, missing fingers, or a webbed appearance due to deep membrane between the fingers; other finger disorders include *rheumatoid arthritis*, *osteoarthritis*, *Raynaud's disease*, and dactylitis (swelling) due to *sickle cell anaemia*. Clubbing of the fingers is a sign of chronic lung disease or some forms of congenital heart disease. Tumours of the finger are rare but may occur in *chondromatosis*.

finger-joint replacement A surgical procedure in which one or more artificial joints made of metal, plastic, or silicone rubber are used to replace finger joints destroyed by disease, usually *rheumatoid arthritis* or *osteoarthritis*. The procedure is usually successful in relieving arthritic pain and enabling the patient to use his or her hands again, but it rarely restores normal movement.

fingerprint An impression left on a surface by the pattern of fine curved ridges on the skin of the fingertips. The ridges occur in four patterns: loops, arches, whorls, and compounds (combinations of the other three). No two people, not even identical twins, have the same fingerprints. (See also *genetic fingerprinting*.)

first aid The immediate treatment of any injury or sudden illness before professional medical care can be provided. Most first aid consists of treating minor injuries and *burns*, and *fractures*.

The aims of first-aid treatment in an emergency are to preserve life, to protect the individual from further harm, to provide reassurance, to make the victim comfortable, to arrange for medical help, and to find out as much as possible about the circumstances of the accident or injury. Various techniques can be used to achieve these aims. For example, the *recovery position* helps to maintain an open airway in an unconscious person who is breathing; *artificial respiration* is necessary if a person is not breathing. *Cardiopulmonary resuscitation* is essential if a person is not breathing and has no heartbeat. Heavy bleeding can lead to *shock* but can be controlled by applying pressure at appropriate *pressure points*.

fish oil A product occurring naturally in some species of oily fish such as mackerel. Fish-oil preparations, which are rich in omega-3 fatty acids, are used as *lipid-lowering drugs*.

fistula An abnormal passage from an internal organ to the body surface or between two organs. Fistulas may be present from birth or may be acquired as a result of tissue damage. Congenital types include *tracheoesophageal fistulas*, branchial fistulas (see *branchial disorders*), and thyroglossal fistulas (see *thyroglossal disorders*). Acquired fistulas may result from injury, infection, or cancer. Fistulas between the intestine and the skin may occur in *Crohn's disease*. Some types of *arteriovenous fistula* (between an artery and a vein) are surgically constructed to provide ready access to the circulation in people who are having *dialysis*. Some types of fistula close spontaneously but most need to be treated surgically.

fit See *seizure*.

fitness The capacity for performing physical activities without exhaustion. Fitness depends on strength, flexibility, and endurance. Because cardiovascular fitness is the precondition for all other forms of fitness, regular aerobic exercise (see *aerobics*), which makes the body's use of oxygen more efficient, is the basis of any fitness programme. Specific activities, such as weight training or yoga, can help develop strength and flexibility when included in a programme (see *exercise*). When the body is fit, the maximum work capacity and endurance are increased. A fit person has a better chance of avoiding *coronary artery disease* and preventing the effects of age and chronic disease.

fitness testing A series of exercises designed to determine an individual's level of *fitness*, primarily cardiovascular fitness and muscle performance. Fitness testing is often carried out before a person starts an exercise programme to evaluate its safety and suitability or to monitor progress thereafter.

A physical examination is usually performed, including measurement of body fat, height, and weight. Blood and urine tests may be done, including an analysis of blood *cholesterol*. The performance of the heart is measured by taking the pulse before, during, and after aerobic exercise. Another test involves measuring a person's overall performance in a standard exercise. (See also *aerobics; exercise*.)

fixation In *psychoanalytic theory*, the process by which an individual becomes or remains emotionally attached to real or imagined objects or events during early childhood. If the fixations are powerful, resulting from traumatic events, they can lead to immature and inappropriate behaviour. Regression to these events is regarded by some analysts as the basis of certain emotional disorders.

Fixation also describes the alignment and stabilization of fractured bones. Fixation may be external, as with a plaster cast, or internal, using pins, plates, or nails introduced surgically.

flail chest A type of chest injury that usually results from a traffic accident or from violence. In flail chest, several adjacent ribs are broken in more than one place, producing a piece of chest wall that moves in the opposite way to normal as the victim breathes. The injury may lead to *respiratory failure* and *shock*.

flat-feet A condition, usually affecting both feet, in which the arch is absent and the sole rests flat on the ground. The arches form gradually as supportive ligaments and muscles in the soles develop and are not usually fully formed until about age 6. In some people, the ligaments are lax or the muscles are weak and the feet remain flat. Less commonly, the arches do not form because of a hereditary defect in bone structure. Flat-feet can be acquired in adult life because of fallen arches, sometimes as the result of a rapid increase in weight. Weakening of the supporting muscles and ligaments may occur in neurological or muscular diseases such as *poliomyelitis*.

In most cases, flat-feet are painless and require no treatment, although in some cases the feet may ache on walking or standing. Arch supports can be worn in the shoes for comfort.

flatulence Abdominal discomfort or fullness that is relieved by passing wind through the anus or belching. Flatulence is a feature of many gastrointestinal conditions, such as *irritable bowel syndrome* and *gallbladder* disorders.

flatus Gas, commonly known as "wind", which is passed through the anus. Gas is formed in the large intestine by the action of bacteria on carbohydrates and amino acids in food. Large amounts of gas may cause abdominal discomfort (see *flatulence*), which may be relieved by the passage of wind or by defaecation.

flatworm Any species of worm that has a flattened shape. Two types of flatworm are parasites of humans: cestodes (*tapeworms*) and trematodes (flukes, schistosomes; see *liver fluke; schistosomiasis*).

flea bites See *insect bites*.

flecainide An *antiarrhythmic drug* used in the treatment of *tachycardia, atrial fibrillation*, and *arrhythmias* associated with conditions such as Wolff–Parkinson-White syndrome (a congenital abnormality of heart-rhythm). It is given, as tablets or injection, to people resistant to or intolerant of other treatment; and treatment is always initiated in hospital. Side effects may include dizziness, visual disturbances, and worsening, or a new type of, arrhythmia. Rarely, nausea, vomiting, urticaria, vertigo, and jaundice occur.

flies See *insects and disease*.

floaters Fragments perceived to be floating in the field of vision. Floaters move rapidly with eye movement but drift slightly when the eyes are still.

They do not usually affect vision. Most floaters are shadows cast on the retina by microscopic structures in the *vitreous humour* (the jelly-like substance behind the lens). The sudden appearance of a cloud of dark floaters, especially when accompanied by light flashes, suggests *retinal tear* or *retinal detachment*. A large red floater that obscures vision is usually due to a *vitreous haemorrhage*.

flooding A technique used in *behaviour therapy* for treating *phobias*.

floppy infant A description of a baby whose muscles lack normal tension or tone (see *hypotonia in infants*).

floppy valve syndrome See *mitral valve prolapse*.

flossing, dental The removal of plaque (see *plaque, dental*) and food particles from around the teeth and gums by using soft nylon or silk thread or tape. Dental floss may be waxed or unwaxed. Flossing should be carried out as an adjunct to toothbrushing.

FLOSSING, DENTAL

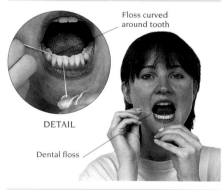

Floss curved around tooth

DETAIL

Dental floss

flu See *influenza*.

flucloxacillin A *penicillin drug* usually used to treat *staphylococcal infections*.

fluconazole An *antifungal drug* used to treat *candidiasis*, a fungal infection commonly affecting the vagina or mouth. It may cause nausea and diarrhoea.

fluctuant A term used to describe the movement within a swelling when it is examined by touch. It is a sign that the swelling contains fluid. The term is often used to describe an abscess.

fluid retention Excessive accumulation of fluid in body tissues. Mild fluid retention is common with *premenstrual syndrome* but disappears with the onset of menstruation. However, more severe fluid retention may be associated with an underlying heart, liver, or kidney disorder (see *ascites*; *nephrotic syndrome*; *oedema*). *Diuretic drugs* may be used to treat the condition.

fluke A type of flattened worm, also known as a trematode, that may infest humans or animals. The two main diseases caused by flukes are *liver fluke* infestation, which occurs worldwide, and *schistosomiasis*, a debilitating tropical disease.

fluorescein A harmless orange dye used in *ophthalmology* as an aid to the diagnosis of certain eye disorders.

fluoridation The addition of *fluoride* to the water supply as a means of reducing the incidence of dental *caries*.

fluoride A mineral that helps to prevent dental *caries* by strengthening tooth enamel (see *teeth*), making it more resistant to acid attacks. Fluoride may also reduce the acid-producing ability of microorganisms in *plaque*. In the UK, fluoride is added to the water supply in some areas; it can also be applied directly to the teeth as part of dental treatment or used in the form of mouthwashes or toothpastes. Ingestion of excess fluoride during tooth formation can lead to *fluorosis*.

fluorosis Mottling of the tooth enamel caused by ingestion of excess *fluoride* as the *teeth* are formed. In severe cases, the enamel develops brown stains. Such cases occur mostly where the fluoride level in water is far greater than the recommended level or when additional fluoride supplements are taken.

fluorouracil An *anticancer drug* used in the treatment of cancers of the breast, bladder, ovaries, and intestine.

fluoxetine A type of *antidepressant drug*.

flurazepam A type of *benzodiazepine drug* used as a sleeping drug to treat *insomnia*. The drug's effects may persist the following day; and prolonged use may result in dependence.

flurbiprofen A *nonsteroidal anti-inflammatory drug* used particularly to ease the symptoms of musculoskeletal disorders such as *rheumatoid arthritis*.

flush Reddening of the face, and sometimes the neck, caused by dilation of the blood vessels near the skin surface. Flushing may occur during *fever* or as a result of embarrassment. *Hot flushes* are common at the *menopause*.

foam, contraceptive See *spermicides*.

foetus An alternative spelling for *fetus*.

folic acid A *vitamin* that is essential for the production of red *blood cells* by the *bone marrow*. Folic acid is contained in a variety of foods, particularly liver and raw vegetables; adequate amounts are usually included in a normal diet but it is destroyed by prolonged cooking.

During pregnancy, folic acid is important for fetal growth and in the development of the nervous system and formation of blood cells. To help prevent *neural tube defects* (such as *spina bifida*), women who are planning a pregnancy should take the recommended dose of folic acid supplement before conceiving and then during the first 12 weeks of pregnancy. If there is a family history of neural tube defects, a higher dose of folic acid supplement is recommended.

Folic acid deficiency is a cause of megaloblastic *anaemia*, which produces symptoms such as headaches, fatigue, and pallor. Deficiency can occur during any serious illness or can be the result of a nutritionally poor diet.

folie à deux A French term that is used to describe the unusual occurrence of two people sharing the same psychotic illness (see *psychosis*). Commonly, the two are closely related and share one or more paranoid *delusions*. If the sufferers are separated, one of them almost always quickly loses the symptoms, which have been imposed by the dominant, and genuinely psychotic, partner.

folk medicine Any form of medical treatment that is based on popular tradition, such as the charming of warts or the use of copper bracelets to treat rheumatism.

follicle A small cavity in the body. For example, a *hair* follicle is a pit on the skin surface from which hair grows.

follicle-stimulating hormone A *gonadotrophin hormone* that is produced and secreted by the pituitary gland and acts on the ovary or testes.

folliculitis Inflammation of one or more hair follicles as a result of a *staphylococcal infection*. Folliculitis can occur almost anywhere on the skin but commonly affects the neck, thighs, buttocks, or armpits, causing a *boil*; it may also affect the bearded area of the face, producing pustules (see *sycosis barbae*). Treatment is with *antibiotic drugs*.

fomites Inanimate objects, such as bed linen, clothing, books, or a telephone receiver, that are not harmful in themselves but may be capable of harbouring harmful microorganisms or parasites and thus convey an infection from one person to another. Fomites mainly transmit respiratory infections, such as influenza. The singular form of the word is fomes.

fontanelle One of the two membrane-covered spaces between the bones of a baby's skull. At birth, the skull bones are not yet fully fused, and two soft areas can be felt through the scalp. These are the anterior fontanelle, which is diamond-shaped and usually closes up by age 18 months, and the posterior fontanelle, which is triangular and closes up within the first 2 months. It is normal for the fontanelles to become tense and bulge out when a baby cries. Persistent tension at other times may indicate an abnormality, particularly *hydrocephalus* (the accumulation of fluid in the skull). A sunken fontanelle may be a sign of *dehydration*. If a fontanelle is abnormally large, or takes a long time to close, the cause may be a brain abnormality or a disorder, such as *rickets*, affecting the skull bones. Early closure of the fontanelles results in a deformity called *craniosynostosis*.

Occasionally, a third fontanelle is present between the other two; this occurs in *Down's syndrome*.

food additives Any substance added to food for the purposes of preservation or

FONTANELLE

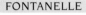

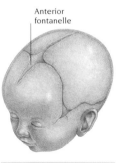

Anterior fontanelle

F

to improve its acceptability in terms of taste, colour, or consistency.

Preservatives, such as sodium nitrate, are added to food to control the growth of bacteria, moulds, and yeasts. Other additives, such as antioxidants, improve the keeping quality of food by preventing undesirable changes (they stop rancidity in foods containing fat, for example). Additives that improve texture include emulsifiers, stabilizers, thickeners, and gelling agents. Appearance and taste are improved by the use of colourings, flavourings, sweeteners, and flavour enhancers. *Artificial sweeteners*, such as aspartame, may be used instead of sugar, especially in products for diabetics or slimmers.

Certain additives may produce an allergic reaction in some people, and some are thought to be a factor in behavioural problems in children.

food allergy An inappropriate or exaggerated reaction of the *immune system* to a food. Sensitivity to cow's milk protein is a fairly common food allergy in young children. Other foods most commonly implicated in food allergy are nuts, wheat, fish, shellfish, and eggs. Food allergy is more common in people who suffer from other forms of *allergy* or *hypersensitivity*, such as *asthma*, allergic *rhinitis*, and *eczema*.

Immediate reactions, occurring within an hour or sometimes minutes of eating the trigger food, include lip swelling, tingling in the mouth or throat, vomiting, abdominal distension, abnormally loud bowel sounds, and diarrhoea. Some serious allergies can cause *anaphylactic shock*, requiring immediate self-injection with *adrenaline* (epinephrine). The only effective treatment for food allergy is avoidance of the offending food. (See also *food intolerance*.)

food-borne infection Any infectious illness caused by eating food contaminated with viruses, bacteria, worms, or other organisms. There are two mechanisms by which food can become infected. First, many animals that are kept or caught for food may harbour disease organisms in their tissues or organs; and, if meat or milk from such an animal is eaten without being thor-

oughly cooked or pasteurized, the organisms may cause illness in their human host. In the UK, the only common infection of this type is *food poisoning*. Second, food may be contaminated with organisms spread from an infected person or animal, usually by flies moving from faeces to food.

Immunization is available against certain food- and *water-borne infections* such as *typhoid fever*.

food fad A like or dislike of a particular food or foods that is taken to extremes. A food fad may lead to undue reliance on, or avoidance of, a particular foodstuff. Fads are common in toddlers, adolescents, and in people who are under stress. When a food fad becomes obsessive or persistent, it may indicate a serious eating disorder. (See also *anorexia nervosa*; *bulimia*.)

food intolerance An adverse reaction to a food or food ingredient that occurs each time the substance is eaten, that is not due to a psychological cause or to *food poisoning*, and that does not involve the *immune system*.

Food intolerance is often of unknown cause. Certain foods may be poorly tolerated due to impaired digestion and absorption associated with disorders of the pancreas or biliary system. Some people have a genetic deficiency of a specific *enzyme*, such as *lactase*, which is required to digest the sugar in milk.

food poisoning A term used for any gastrointestinal illness of sudden onset that is suspected of being caused by eating contaminated food. Most cases of food poisoning are due to contamination of food by bacteria or viruses.

The bacteria commonly responsible for food poisoning belong to the groups *SALMONELLA*, *CAMPYLOBACTER*, and *E. COLI*, certain strains of which are able to multiply rapidly in the intestines to cause widespread inflammation. Food poisoning may also be caused by *LISTERIA* (see *listeriosis*). *Botulism* is an uncommon, life-threatening form of food poisoning caused by a bacterial toxin.

The viruses that most commonly cause food poisoning are astravirus, rotavirus, and Norwalk virus (which affects shellfish). This can occur when raw or partly cooked foods have been in contact with water that is contaminated by human excrement.

Non-infective causes include poisonous mushrooms and toadstools (see *mushroom poisoning*) and fresh fruit and vegetables contaminated with high doses of insecticide.

The onset of symptoms depends on the cause of poisoning. Symptoms usually develop within 30 minutes in cases of chemical poisoning, between 1 and 12 hours in cases of bacterial toxins, and between 12 and 48 hours with most bacterial and viral infections. Symptoms usually include nausea and vomiting, diarrhoea, stomach pain, and, in severe cases, *shock* and collapse. Botulism affects the nervous system, causing visual disturbances, difficulty with speech, paralysis, and vomiting.

The diagnosis of bacterial food poisoning can usually be confirmed from examination of a sample of faeces. Chemical poisoning can often be diagnosed from a description of what the person has eaten, and from analysis of a sample of the suspect food.

Mild cases can be treated at home. Lost fluids should be replaced by intake of plenty of clear fluids (see *rehydration therapy*). In severe cases, hospital treatment may be necessary. Except for botulism, and some cases of mushroom poisoning, most food poisoning is not serious, and recovery generally occurs within 3 days. However, some strains of *E. COLI* can seriously damage red blood cells and cause *kidney failure*. (See also *cholera*; *dysentery*; *typhoid fever*.)

foot The foot has two vital functions: to support the weight of the body in standing or walking and to act as a lever to propel the body forwards.

The largest bone of the foot, the heelbone (see *calcaneus*), is jointed with the ankle bone (the talus). In front of the talus and calcaneus are the tarsal bones, which are jointed the five metatarsals. The phalanges are the bones of the toes; the big toe has two phalanges; all the other toes have three.

Tendons passing around the ankle connect the muscles that act on the foot bones. The main blood vessels and

nerves pass in front of and behind the inside of the ankle to supply the foot. The undersurface of the normal foot forms an arch supported by ligaments and muscles. Fascia (fibrous tissue) and fat form the sole of the foot, which is covered by a layer of tough skin.

Injuries to the foot commonly result in *fracture* of the metatarsals and phalanges. Congenital foot abnormalities are fairly common and include club-foot (see *talipes*), and *claw-foot*. A *bunion* is a common deformity in which a thickened *bursa* (fluid-filled pad) lies over the joint at the base of the big toe. *Corns* are small areas of thickened skin and are usually a result of tight fitting shoes. Verrucas (see *plantar warts*) develop on the soles of the feet. *Athlete's foot* is a fungal infection that mainly affects the skin in between the toes. *Gout* often affects the joint at the base of the big toe. An ingrowing toenail (see *toenail, ingrowing*) commonly occurs on the big toe and may result in inflammation and infection of the surrounding tissues (see *paronychia*). *Foot-drop* is the inability to raise the foot properly when walking and is the result of a nerve problem.

FOOT

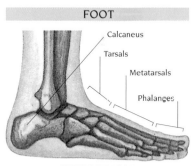

Calcaneus
Tarsals
Metatarsals
Phalanges

BONES OF FOOT

foot-drop A condition in which the foot cannot be raised properly and hangs limp from the ankle. *Neuritis* affecting the nerves that supply muscles that move the foot is a common cause and may be due to *diabetes mellitus*, *multiple sclerosis*, or a *neuropathy*. Weakness in the foot muscles can also result from pressure on a nerve (due to a *disc*

F

prolapse or a tumour) as it leaves the spinal cord. Treatment is of the underlying cause, but in many people the weakness persists. A lightweight plastic *caliper splint* can be used to keep the foot in place when walking.

foramen A natural opening in a bone or other body structure, usually to allow the passage of nerves or blood vessels. For example, the foramen magnum is a hole in the base of the *cranium* through which the *spinal cord* passes.

forceps A tweezer-like instrument used for handling tissues or equipment during surgical procedures. Various types of forceps are designed for specific purposes. (See also *forceps, obstetric.*)

forceps delivery The use of forceps (see *forceps, obstetric*) to ease out the baby's head during a difficult birth (see *childbirth*). Forceps delivery is used if the mother is unable to push out her baby unaided, or if the baby is showing signs of *fetal distress*. Forceps are also used to control the head once the body has been delivered in *breech delivery* to prevent too rapid a birth.

FORCEPS DELIVERY

Forceps   Fetus   Umbilical   Uterus
                    cord

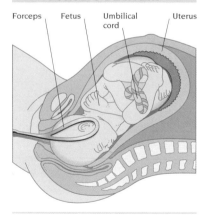

An *episiotomy* (making of a cut in the perineum) is usually needed for a forceps delivery. Recovery and care for mother and child is usually the same as after a vaginal delivery.

forceps, obstetric Surgical instruments that are used in *forceps delivery* to deliver the head of a baby in a difficult labour. Obstetric forceps consist of two blades that can be locked together and that cup the baby's head.

foreign body An object that is present in an organ or passage of the body but which should not be there. Common sites for foreign bodies include the airways (see *choking*), ear (see *ear, foreign body in*), eye (see *eye, foreign body in*), rectum, and vagina.

forensic medicine The branch of medicine concerned with the law, especially criminal law. The forensic pathologist is a doctor who specializes in the examination of bodies when circumstances suggest death was unnatural. Forensic pathologists may also examine victims of alleged sexual assault. Forensic scientists use laboratory methods to study body fluids (such as blood and semen) found on or near the victim and compare them with those from suspects. They are also trained in ballistics and the identification of fibres from clothing. In addition, forensic scientists may advise on *blood groups* and *genetic fingerprinting* in legal investigations.

foreskin The popular name for the prepuce, the loose fold of skin that covers the glans of the *penis* when it is flaccid and which retracts during erection. At birth, the foreskin is attached to the glans and is not retractable. It then separates over the first 3 to 4 years of life. The foreskin may be removed (see *circumcision*) for religious, cosmetic, medical, or social reasons.

In *phimosis*, the foreskin remains persistently tight after the age of 5, causing difficulty in passing urine and ballooning of the foreskin. There may also be recurrent *balanitis* (infection of the glans). In *paraphimosis*, the foreskin becomes stuck in the retracted position, causing painful swelling of the glans that needs emergency treatment.

forgetfulness The inability to remember (see *memory*).

formaldehyde A colourless, pungent, irritant gas. In medicine, a solution of formaldehyde and a small amount of alcohol in water, a preparation known as formalin, is used to preserve tissue specimens or to harden them before they are stained and examined.

formication An unpleasant sensation, as if ants were crawling over the skin. This may occur following abuse of certain drugs, such as alcohol or morphine.

formula, chemical A way of expressing the constituents of a chemical in symbols and numbers. Water, for example, has the formula H_2O, indicating that each molecule is composed of 2 atoms of hydrogen (H_2) and 1 of oxygen (O).

formulary A book of formulae. The term formulary is commonly used to refer to a publication that lists drug preparations and their components and effects. The contents of a formulary can be decided by a group of medical professionals working together to ensure similar patterns of drug usage.

fovea An area of the *retina* in the eye that has the highest concentration of light-sensitive cells. It is responsible for detailed vision. (See also *colour vision*.)

fracture A break in a bone, usually across its width. There are two main types: closed (simple) or open (compound) fractures. In a closed fracture, the broken bone ends remain beneath the skin and little surrounding tissue is damaged; in an open fracture, one or both bone ends project through the skin. If the bone ends are not aligned, the fracture is termed "displaced". Fractures can be further divided according to the pattern of the break, for example, transverse or spiral fractures of long bones. In a greenstick fracture, the break is not through the full width of the bone. This type of fracture occurs only in children because their bones are more pliable. In an avulsion fracture, a small piece of bone is pulled off by a tendon.

Most fractures are the result of a fall, but in *osteoporosis* the bone is weakened, and fractures such as compression fractures of the vertebrae are common.

Common sites of fracture include the hand, wrist (see *Colles' fracture*), *ankle joint*, *clavicle*, and the neck of the femur (see *femur, fracture of*). There is usually swelling and tenderness at the fracture site. The pain is often severe and is usually made worse by movement.

X-rays can confirm a fracture. Because bone begins to heal soon after it has broken, the first aim of treatment is to ensure that the bone ends are aligned. Displaced bone ends are manoeuvred back into position, under general anaesthetic, by manipulation either through the skin or through an incision. The bone is then immobilized. In some cases the ends of the bone may be fixed with metal pins or plates.

Most fractures heal without any problems. Healing is sometimes delayed because the blood supply to the affected bone is inadequate (as a result of damaged blood vessels) or because the bone ends are not close enough together. If the fracture fails to unite, internal fixation or a *bone graft* may be needed. Osteomyelitis is a possible complication of open fractures. (See also *Monteggia's fracture; pelvis, Pott's fracture; rib, fracture of; skull, fracture of.*)

FRACTURE

TRANSVERSE
FRACTURE

SPIRAL
FRACTURE

GREENSTICK
FRACTURE

COMMINUTED
FRACTURE

COMPRESSION
FRACTURE

AVULSION
FRACTURE

fracture, dental A break in a tooth (see *teeth*) most commonly caused by falling onto a hard surface or by being hit in the mouth with a hard object. Fractures may involve the crown or the root of a tooth, or both. Fractures of the enamel can usually be repaired by bonding (see *bonding, dental*); in some cases, a replacement crown may be fitted (see *crown, dental*). Fractures of the root may be treated by splinting (see *splinting,*

F

dental), *root-canal treatment*, or removing the tooth (see *extraction, dental*).

fragile X syndrome An inherited defect of the *X chromosome* that causes learning difficulties. The disorder occurs within families according to an X-linked recessive pattern of inheritance (see *genetic disorders*). Although mainly males are affected, women can become carriers of the genetic defect. In addition to having learning difficulties, affected males tend to be tall and physically strong, with large testes, a prominent nose and jaw, increased ear length, and are prone to epileptic seizures. About a third of female carriers show some intellectual impairment. The condition cannot be treated.

freckle A tiny patch of *pigmentation* that occurs on sun-exposed skin. Freckles tend to become more numerous with continued exposure to sunlight. A tendency to freckling is inherited and occurs most often in fair and red-haired people.

free-floating anxiety Vague apprehension or tension, often associated with *generalized anxiety disorder*.

free radicals Molecules that bind to and destroy body cells. Free radicals can derive from external sources such as smoke, sunlight, and food, but they are mostly produced in the body following chemical reactions.

frequency See *urination, frequent*.

Freudian slip A slip of the tongue or a minor error of action that could be what the person really wanted to say or do.

Freudian theory A discipline developed by Sigmund Freud (1856–1939) that formed the basis of *psychoanalysis*. Freud believed that feelings, thoughts, and behaviour are controlled by unconscious wishes and conflicts originating in childhood. Problems occur when the desires are not fulfilled or conflicts remain unresolved into adulthood. The essence of his theory concerns early psychological development, particularly sexual development. He also identified three components of personality: the *id*, the *ego*, and the *superego*. (See also *psychoanalytic theory*; *psychotherapy*.)

friar's balsam A name for tincture of benzoin. Friar's balsam is used with hot water as a *steam inhalation* to relieve nasal congestion, acute rhinitis, sinusitis, and to loosen coughs.

Friedreich's ataxia A very rare inherited disease in which degeneration of nerve fibres in the spinal cord causes loss of coordinated movement and balance. Once symptoms have developed, the disease becomes progressively more severe. Treatment can help with the symptoms but cannot alter the course of the disease.

frigidity Lack of desire for or inability to become aroused during sexual stimulation (see *sexual desire, inhibited*). (See also *orgasm, lack of*.)

frontal A term referring to the front part of an organ (for example, the frontal lobe of the *brain*).

frostbite Damage to tissues caused by extremely cold temperatures. Frostbite can affect any part of the body, but the extremities (the nose, ears, fingers, and toes) are most susceptible. The first symptoms of frostbite are a pins-and-needles sensation, followed by complete numbness. The skin appears white, cold, and hard and then becomes red and swollen. If damage is restricted to the skin and immediately underlying tissues, recovery may be complete. If blood vessels are affected, *gangrene* may follow. In such cases, amputation of the affected part may be necessary.

frottage A sexual *deviation* in which an individual rubs against another person in order to achieve sexual arousal.

frozen section A method of preparing a *biopsy* specimen that provides a rapid indication of whether or not a tissue, such as a *breast lump*, is cancerous. Frozen section can be undertaken during an operation so that the results can be used to determine the appropriate surgical treatment.

frozen shoulder Stiffness and pain in the *shoulder* that makes normal movement of the joint impossible. In severe cases, the shoulder may be completely rigid, and pain may be intense.

Frozen shoulder is caused by inflammation and thickening of the lining of the joint capsule. In some cases, it occurs following a minor injury to the shoulder or a *stroke*. The condition is more common in middle-aged people and those with *diabetes mellitus*.

Moderate symptoms of frozen shoulder can be eased by exercise, physiotherapy, by taking *analgesic drugs* and *non-steroidal anti-inflammatory drugs*, and by applying *ice-packs*. In severe cases, injections of *corticosteroid drugs* into the joint may be used. Manipulation of the joint under a general anaesthetic can restore mobility, but this treatment carries the risk of increasing pain in the joint initially. Recovery is often slow but the shoulder is usually back to normal and pain free within 2 years.

frusemide An alternative name for *furosemide*, a *diuretic drug*.

frustration A deep feeling of discontent and tension because of unresolved problems, unfulfilled needs, or because the path to a goal is blocked. In some people, frustration may lead to *regression*, *aggression*, or *depression*.

FSH An abbreviation for *follicle-stimulating hormone*, a *gonadotrophin hormone* produced by the pituitary gland.

fugue An episode of altered consciousness in which a person apparently purposelessly wanders away from home or work and, in some cases, adopts a new identity. When the fugue ends, the person has no recollection of what has occurred. Fugues are uncommon, and causes include *dissociative disorders*, *temporal lobe epilepsy*, *depression*, *head injury*, and *dementia*. (See also *amnesia*.)

fulminant A term used to describe a disorder that develops and progresses suddenly and with great severity. A virulent infection, a severe form of *arthritis*, or a cancer that has spread rapidly is usually described as being fulminant.

fumes See *pollution*.

functional disorders A term for any illness in which there is no evidence of organic disturbance even though physical performance is impaired.

fundus The part of a hollow body organ, such as the stomach, that is farthest away from its opening. An optic fundus is the appearance of the retina when viewed through an ophthalmoscope.

fungal infections Diseases that are caused by the multiplication and spread of *fungi*. Some fungi are harmlessly pre-

sent all the time in areas of the body such as the mouth, skin, intestines, and vagina. However, they are prevented from multiplying by competition from bacteria. Other fungi are dealt with by the body's *immune system*.

Fungal infections are therefore more common and serious in people taking long-term *antibiotic drugs* (which destroy the bacterial competition) and in those whose immune systems are suppressed by *immunosuppressant drugs*, *corticosteroid drugs*, or by a disorder such as *AIDS*. Such serious fungal infections are described as *opportunistic infections*. Some fungal infections are more common in people with *diabetes mellitus*.

Fungal infections can be classified into superficial (affecting skin, hair, nails, inside of the mouth, and genital organs); subcutaneous (beneath the skin); and deep (affecting internal organs).

The main superficial infections are *tinea* (including ringworm and athlete's foot) and *candidiasis* (thrush), both of which are common. Subcutaneous infections, which are rare, include *sporotrichosis* and *mycetoma*. Deep infections are uncommon but can be serious and include *aspergillosis*, *histoplasmosis*, *cryptococcosis*, and *blastomycosis*. The fungal spores enter the body by inhalation.

Treatment of fungal infections is with *antifungal drugs*, either used topically on the infected area or given by mouth for generalized infections.

fungi Simple parasitic life-forms that include mushrooms, toadstools, yeasts, and moulds. Disease-causing fungi can be divided into two groups: filamentous fungi and yeasts. Filamentous fungi are made up of branching threads known as hyphae, which form a network called a mycelium. Mushrooms and toadstools are the reproductive structures (known as fruiting bodies) of a filamentous fungus that has spread in dead matter or soil. Yeasts are single-celled organisms.

Most fungi are either harmless or beneficial to human health, but some can cause illness and disease. The fruiting bodies of some fungi contain toxins that can cause poisoning if eaten (see *mushroom poisoning*). Certain fungi infect food crops and produce toxins

FUNGI

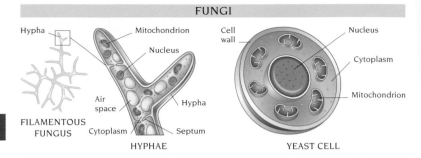

Hypha

Mitochondrion

Nucleus

Air space

Hypha

FILAMENTOUS FUNGUS

Cytoplasm

Septum

HYPHAE

Cell wall

Nucleus

Cytoplasm

Mitochondrion

YEAST CELL

that can cause food poisoning. The best known of these is a fungus that infects cereals and produces *ergot*, a toxin that constricts blood vessels; and another that grows on peanuts and produces *aflatoxin*, a poison and *carcinogen*. The inhaled spores of some fungi can cause allergic *alveolitis*, a persistent allergic reaction in the lungs. Fungal spores are sometimes responsible for other allergic disorders such as allergic *rhinitis* and *asthma*. Some fungi are able to invade and form colonies in the lungs, in the skin, or sometimes in various different tissues throughout the body, leading to conditions that range from mild irritation to severe, even fatal, widespread infection (see *fungal infections*) and illness. (See also *candidiasis*.)

fungicidal A term describing the ability to kill fungi (see *antifungal drugs*).

funny-bone A popular term for the small area at the back of the *elbow* where the ulnar nerve passes over a prominence of the humerus (upper-arm bone). A blow to the nerve causes acute pain, numbness, and a tingling sensation in the forearm and hand.

furosemide A *diuretic drug* used to treat *oedema* and *heart failure*. When given by injection, it has a rapid effect.

furuncle Another name for a *boil*.

fusidic acid A type of *antibiotic drug* used to treat bacterial infections that are resistant to *penicillin drugs*. Fusidic acid is commonly used in preparations applied to the skin, eye, and ear.

G

G6PD deficiency An *X-linked disorder* that affects the chemistry of red blood cells, making them prone to damage by infectious illness or certain drugs or foods. Red blood cells are missing G6PD (the *enzyme* glucose 6 phosphate dehydrogenase). The disorder most often affects southern European and black men. Women are unaffected but can carry the abnormal gene.

Some *antimalarial drugs* and *antibiotics* can precipitate destruction of red cells in affected people. In one form of G6PD deficiency called *favism*, affected people are sensitive to a chemical in broad beans, which they must avoid eating. After taking a precipitating drug or food, or during an infectious illness, a person with G6PD deficiency develops the symptoms (see *anaemia, haemolytic*).

G6PD deficiency is diagnosed with a blood test. There is no particular treatment but symptoms caused by a drug or food can be relieved by avoiding it.

GABA The abbreviation for gamma-aminobutyric acid, a *neurotransmitter*. GABA controls the flow of nerve impulses by blocking the release of other neurotransmitters (e.g. *noradrenaline* and *dopamine*) that stimulate nerve activity. GABA activity is increased by *benzodiazepine drugs* and *anticonvulsants*.

gabapentin An *anticonvulsant drug* used either alone or with other anticonvulsants to treat some types of *epilepsy*. Common side effects include dizziness, unsteadiness, and fatigue.

galactorrhoea Spontaneous, persistent production of milk by a woman who is not pregnant or lactating (see *lactation*), or, very rarely, by a man.

Lactation is initiated by a rise in the level of *prolactin*, a hormone produced by the *pituitary gland*. Galactorrhoea is caused by excessive secretion of prolactin due to a *pituitary tumour* or other endocrine disease, such as *hypothyroidism*. Some *antipsychotic drugs* may also cause excessive secretion. Treatment with *bromocriptine* suppresses prolactin production, but the underlying cause may also need treatment.

galactosaemia A rare, inherited condition in which the body is unable to convert the sugar galactose into *glucose* due to the absence of a liver enzyme. It causes no symptoms at birth, but *jaundice*, diarrhoea, and vomiting soon develop and the baby fails to gain weight. Untreated, the condition results in liver disease, *cataract*, and *learning difficulties*. The diagnosis is confirmed by urine and blood tests. The major source of galactose is the milk sugar lactose. Lactose-free milk must be used throughout life.

gallbladder A small, pear-shaped sac situated under the liver that stores *bile*. Bile, produced by the liver, passes into the gallbladder via the hepatic and cystic ducts. It is released into the intestine via the common *bile duct*.

GALLBLADDER

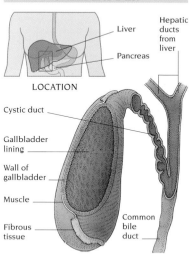

LOCATION

Liver
Hepatic ducts from liver
Pancreas
Cystic duct
Gallbladder lining
Wall of gallbladder
Muscle
Fibrous tissue
Common bile duct

gallbladder cancer A rare *cancer* of unknown cause that occurs mainly in the elderly. The cancer may cause *jaundice* and tenderness in the abdomen, but it is sometimes symptomless. It is usually diagnosed by *ultrasound scanning*.

Treatment is by surgical removal of the tumour, but the cancer has often spread to the liver by the time it is detected, making the outlook poor.

gallbladder, disorders of The principal *gallbladder* disorder is *gallstones*, which are common and often symptomless. Attempts by the gallbladder to expel the stones can cause *biliary colic*. If a gallstone becomes stuck in the gallbladder outlet, acute *cholecystitis* may develop. Occasionally, this leads to a painful condition called *empyema* of the gallbladder. If a gallbladder is empty when a stone obstructs its outlet, it may fill with mucus, resulting in a *mucocele*. *Gallbladder cancer* is rare.

gallium A metallic element whose radioactive form is used in *radionuclide scanning* to detect areas of inflammation such as those that occur in cancers, *abscesses*, *osteomyelitis*, and *sarcoidosis*.

gallstones Lumps of solid matter found in the *gallbladder*, or in the *bile ducts*. Gallstones are composed mainly of *cholesterol* and bile pigments from the breakdown of red blood cells. They develop when there is a disturbance in the chemical composition of *bile*.

Gallstones are rare in childhood and become increasingly common with age. Women are affected more than men. Risk factors include a high-fat diet and being overweight.

Most gallstones cause no symptoms. When symptoms do occur, they often begin when a stone gets stuck in the duct leading from the gallbladder, causing *biliary colic* and nausea. Gallstones may cause indigestion and *flatulence*. Possible complications are *cholecystitis*, *pancreatitis*, and *bile duct obstruction*.

Diagnosis is usually by *ultrasound scanning*. Stones that are not causing symptoms are usually left alone. In other cases, the gallbladder and stones may be removed by *cholecystectomy*, which can often be done by *laparoscopy*. Ultrasonic shock waves (see *lithotripsy*) are sometimes used to shatter stones; the fragments pass into the bowel and are excreted in the faeces. Drugs such as *ursodeoxycholic acid* may be used to dissolve stones but long-term treatment may be needed.

gambling, pathological Chronic inability to resist impulses to gamble, resulting in personal or social problems.

gamete A sex cell, which is either the *sperm* of the male or the *ovum* (egg cell) of the female.

gamete intrafallopian transfer (GIFT) A technique for assisting *conception* (see *infertility*), which can only be used if a woman has normal *fallopian tubes*. In GIFT, eggs are removed from an *ovary* during *laparoscopy* and mixed with sperm in the laboratory before both are introduced into a fallopian tube. A fertilized egg may then become implanted in the *uterus*.

gamma-globulin A substance prepared from human blood that contains *antibodies* against most common infections. (See *immunoglobulin injections*.)

gamolenic acid An essential *fatty acid* found in *evening primrose oil* and starflower oil (borage oil).

ganciclovir An *antiviral drug* that is used to treat serious *cytomegalovirus* infection in people with an impaired or suppressed immune system as a result of AIDS or following organ transplantation. Side effects include nausea, diarrhoea, abdominal pain, weakness, and bone marrow suppression.

ganglion A group of nerve cells that have a common function; for example, the *basal ganglia* in the brain are concerned with the control of muscular movements.

The term is also used to describe a fluid-filled swelling associated with the sheath of a *tendon*.

gangrene Death of tissue, usually as a result of loss of blood supply. Gangrene may affect a small area of skin or a substantial portion of a limb. Pain is felt in the dying tissues, but once dead they become numb. The affected tissue turns black. There are two types of gangrene: dry and wet. In dry gangrene, there is usually no infection, and the tissue dies because it has no blood supply. Dry gangrene does not spread, and it may be caused by *arteriosclerosis*, *diabetes mellitus*, *thrombosis*, frostbite, or an *embolism*. Wet gangrene develops when dry gangrene or a wound becomes infected by *bacteria*. The gangrene spreads and gives off an unpleasant smell. There may be redness, swelling, and oozing pus around the blackened area. A virulent type called gas gangrene is caused by a bacterium that destroys muscles and produces a foul-smelling gas.

Treatment of dry gangrene consists of attempting to improve the circulation to the affected area before the tissues die. *Antibiotic drugs* can prevent wet gangrene from setting in. *Amputation* of the affected part and the surrounding tissue is necessary.

Ganser's syndrome A rare *factitious disorder* in which a person seeks, consciously or unconsciously, to mislead others about his or her mental state and may simulate symptoms of *psychosis*.

Gardnerella vaginalis A *bacterium* that is often found in the vaginal discharge of women with *bacterial vaginosis*.

gargle A liquid preparation to wash and freshen the mouth and throat. Some gargles contain *antiseptics* or local *anaesthetics* to relieve sore throats.

gas-and-air A mixture of *nitrous oxide* and *oxygen* that is used mainly used for temporary emergency pain relief.

gastrectomy Removal of the *stomach* (total gastrectomy) or, more commonly, part of the stomach (partial gastrectomy). Total gastrectomy is used to treat some *stomach cancers*. Partial gastrectomy used to be a treatment for *peptic ulcers* but has largely been replaced by drug treatment.

Possible postoperative complications are fullness and discomfort after meals; regurgitation of bile, which may lead to *gastritis, oesophagitis*, and vomiting of bile; diarrhoea; and *dumping syndrome*. Other complications include *malabsorption*, which may lead to *anaemia* or *osteoporosis*. After total gastrectomy, patients cannot absorb vitamin B_{12} and are given it in the form of injections for the rest of their lives.

gastric erosion A break in the surface layer of the membrane lining the *stomach*. A break deeper than this layer is called a gastric ulcer (see *peptic ulcer*). Gastric erosions occur in some cases of *gastritis*. Many erosions result from ingestion of *alcohol, iron* tablets, *corticosteroid drugs*, or *nonsteroidal*

anti-inflammatory drugs (NSAIDs) such as *aspirin* and *ibuprofen*. The physical stress of serious illness, such as *kidney failure*, major head injury, or *burns* may bring on an erosion. Often there are no symptoms, but erosions may bleed, causing *vomiting of blood* or blood in the faeces. Persistent loss of blood may lead to *anaemia*. Gastric erosions are diagnosed by *gastroscopy*. They usually heal in a few days when they are treated with *antacid drugs* and *ulcer-healing drugs*.

gastric ulcer See *peptic ulcer*.

G

gastrin A *hormone* produced by cells in the *stomach* lining. Gastrin causes the stomach to produce more acid and helps to propel food through the digestive tract. (See also *gastrointestinal hormones*.)

gastritis *Inflammation* of the *stomach* lining. This may be *acute* or *chronic*. Acute gastritis may be caused by irritation of the stomach lining by drugs, usually *aspirin, ibuprofen*, or other *nonsteroidal anti-inflammatory drugs* (NSAIDs), or by *alcohol*. Severe physical stress, such as *burns* or *liver failure*, can also cause gastritis. Chronic gastritis is due to infection with the HELICOBACTER PYLORI bacterium in the majority of cases. It can also be caused by prolonged irritation of the stomach by alcohol, tobacco smoking, or *bile*; by an *autoimmune disorder* that damages the stomach lining (see *anaemia, megaloblastic*); or by degeneration of the lining with age.

Symptoms include discomfort in the upper abdomen, nausea, and vomiting. In acute gastritis, the faeces may be blackened by blood lost from the stomach; in chronic gastritis, slow blood loss may lead to anaemia (see *anaemia, iron-deficiency*). Diagnosis may be made with *gastroscopy*, during which a *biopsy* of the stomach lining may be carried out. Specific tests for HELICOBACTER PYLORI may also be performed. Treatment is usually with *ulcer-healing drugs*. These may be combined with antibiotics if HELICOBACTER PYLORI is the cause.

gastroenteritis *Inflammation* of the *stomach* and intestines, usually causing sudden upsets that last for 2 or 3 days. *Dysentery, typhoid fever, cholera, food poisoning*, and *travellers' diarrhoea* are

G

all forms of gastroenteritis. The illness may be caused by any of a variety of *bacteria*, bacterial *toxins*, *viruses*, and other organisms in food or water.

Appetite loss, nausea, vomiting, cramps, and diarrhoea are the usual symptoms. Symptom onset and severity depend on the cause; symptoms may be mild or so severe that *dehydration*, *shock*, and collapse occur. Mild cases usually require rest and *rehydration therapy* only. For severe illness, treatment in hospital may be necessary, with fluids given by *intravenous infusion*. *Antibiotic drugs* may be given for some bacterial infections, but others need no specific treatment.

gastroenterology The study of the *digestive system* and the diseases and disorders affecting it.

gastroenterostomy Surgery to create a connection between the *stomach* and the *jejunum*, sometimes combined with partial *gastrectomy*. The operation was formerly performed to treat duodenal ulcer (see *peptic ulcer*) but is now rare.

gastrointestinal hormones A group of *hormones* released from specialized cells in the *stomach*, *pancreas*, and intestine that control various functions of the digestive organs. *Gastrin*, *secretin*, and *cholecystokinin* are the best known of these hormones.

gastrointestinal tract The part of the *digestive system* consisting of the *mouth*, *oesophagus*, *stomach*, and *intestine*.

gastro-oesophageal reflux disease (GORD) Also sometimes known as acid reflux, GORD is regurgitation of acidic fluid from the stomach into the oesophagus due to inefficiency of the muscular valve at the lower end of the oesophagus. GORD may inflame the oesophagus, resulting in *heartburn* due to *oesophagitis*. It may occur in pregnancy and often affects overweight people.

gastroscopy Examination of the *stomach* using a type of *endoscope* inserted through the mouth. Although the term specifies examination of the stomach, the *oesophagus* and *duodenum* are also inspected during the procedure, which is more correctly known as OGD (see *oesophagogastroduodenoscopy*). Gastroscopy, in which the patient is usually sedated, is used to investigate symptoms such as bleeding from the upper gastrointestinal tract and disorders of the oesophagus, stomach, or duodenum.

Attachments to the instrument enable a *biopsy* to be taken and treatments such as *laser treatment* to be carried out. A gastroscope may also be used to ease the passage of a gastric feeding tube through the skin (see *gastrostomy*).

gastrostomy An opening in the *stomach* made surgically, usually connecting the stomach to the outside so that a feeding tube can be passed into the stomach or small intestine. Gastrostomy may be performed on people who cannot eat properly due to oesophageal cancer (see *oesophagus, cancer of*) or who are unable to chew and swallow due to a *stroke*. (See also *feeding, artificial*.)

Gaucher's disease A *genetic disorder* in which the lack of the *enzyme* gluco-

GASTROSCOPY

Monitor
Endoscope
Endoscope
Mouth guard
Site of intravenous sedation
Oesophagus
Stomach

ROUTE OF ENDOSCOPE

cerebrosidase leads to accumulation of a fatty substance, glucosylceramide, in the liver, spleen, bone marrow, and, sometimes, in the brain. It is treated by regular injections of the missing enzyme.

gauze An absorbent, open-weave fabric, usually made of cotton. Sterilized gauze is often used as a *dressing* for wounds.

gavage The process of feeding liquids through a *nasogastric tube*. (See *feeding, artificial*.) Gavage can also refer to *hyperalimentation*.

gemfibrozil A drug that lowers the level of fats in the blood. Gemfibrozil is usually given to people with *hyperlipidaemia* after dietary measures have failed to reduce blood fat. Gemfibrozil may cause nausea and diarrhoea, and should not be taken by people with kidney or liver disease.

gender identity The inner feeling of maleness or femaleness. Gender identity is not necessarily the same as biological sex. It is fixed within the first 2–3 years of life and is reinforced during puberty; once established, it cannot usually be changed. Gender identity problems, such as *transsexualism*, occur when a person has persistent feelings of discomfort about his or her sexual identity.

gene A unit of the material of *heredity*. A gene corresponds to a particular area of *DNA* within a *chromosome*. There are about 30,000 different genes arranged on the 23 pairs of chromosomes. These genes control the development and functioning of organs and body systems, providing an "instruction manual" for an individual's growth, survival, reproduction, and possibly also for aging and death. Genes also play a part, together with environmental factors, in determining a person's intelligence, personality, and behaviour.

Genes fulfil these functions by directing the manufacture of *proteins*. Many proteins have a structural or catalytic role in the body. Others switch genes "on" or "off". The genes that make these regulatory proteins are called control genes. The activities of control genes determine the specialization of cells; within any cell some genes are active and others idle, according to its particular function. If the control genes are disrupted, cells lose

their specialist abilities and multiply out of control; this is the probable mechanism by which cancers form (see *carcinogenesis; oncogenes*).

Each of a person's body cells contains an identical set of genes because all the cells are derived, by a process of division, from a single fertilized egg, and with each division the genes are copied to each offspring cell (see *mitosis; meiosis*). Occasionally, a fault occurs in the copying process, leading to a *mutation*. The gene at any particular location on a chromosome can exist in any of various forms, called *alleles*. If the effects of an allele mask those of the allele at the same location on its partner chromosome, it is called *dominant*. The masked allele is *recessive*. (See also *genetic code; inheritance*.)

generalized anxiety disorder A psychiatric illness characterized by chronic and persistent apprehension and tension that has no particular focus. There may also be physical symptoms such as trembling, sweating, lightheadedness, and irritability. The condition can be treated with *psychotherapy* or with drugs such as *beta blockers, sedatives* or *tranquillizers* that relieve symptoms but do not treat the underlying condition. (See *anxiety; anxiety disorders*.)

general paralysis of the insane An outdated term used to describe the stage of mental and physical deterioration that occurs in untreated or unsuccessfully treated *syphilis*.

general practice The term used in the UK to describe the provision of personal medical care outside a hospital setting. The term is now more commonly known as primary care.

generic drug A medicinal drug marketed under its official medical name (its generic name) rather than under a patented brand name.

gene therapy A technique used for the treatment of certain *genetic disorders*, such as cystic fibrosis, and certain types of *cancer*. In gene therapy, copies of a normal *gene* are inserted, using *genetic engineering* techniques, into the *DNA* of cells to counter the effects of a faulty gene or to produce substances that help fight cancer.

G

genetic code The inherited instructions, contained in *genes*, that specify the activities of cells and thereby the development and functioning of the whole body. Each gene in a *chromosome* contains the coded instructions for a cell to make a particular *protein*, which may have a specific structural or catalytic function in the body.

The DNA that makes up genes consists of two long intertwined strands, each consisting of a sequence of four different chemicals called nucleotide bases. These four bases are adenine, thymine, cytosine, and guanine (often abbreviated to A, T, C, and G). The sequence of these bases along the DNA strands makes up the genetic code.

genetic counselling Medical guidance offered to prospective parents based on an assessment of the probability that a future child would be affected by a *genetic disorder*. This assessment is made from individual and family medical histories and, in some cases, the results of tests such as *chromosome analysis* and *genetic probes*. Genetic counselling enables people to make informed decisions about parenthood, which may involve the use of techniques such as selective termination of pregnancy or *in vitro fertilization* to optimize the chances of having a healthy child.

genetic disorders Any disorder caused, wholly or partly, by one or more faults in a person's *DNA*. Genetic disorders may be *congenital* or may become apparent later in life. Many of them are *familial*. However, a child may be born with a genetic disorder when there is no previous family history.

A genetic disorder can occur in two ways: one or both parents have a defect in their own genetic material which is then inherited, or a *mutation* occurs during the formation of the *egg* or *sperm* cell.

Genetic disorders fall into three broad categories: *chromosomal abnormalities*, unifactorial defects, and multifactorial defects. In the first, a child is born with an abnormal number of whole *chromosomes* (as in *Down's syndrome*), or extra or missing bits of chromosomes.

Unifactorial disorders are rare, and are caused by a single defective gene or pair of genes. They may be sex-linked (with the defective gene carried on one of the sex chromosomes) or autosomal (with the defective gene carried on one of the other 44 chromosomes). X-linked recessive disorders are the most common type of sex-linked disorder. In these conditions, the defective gene is on the X chromosome. Women have two X chromosomes in their cells; men have only one, inherited from their mothers. When a woman inherits one defective gene, its effect is masked by the normal gene on her other X chromosome and she has no outward abnormality. She is still capable of passing the gene onto her children, and is called a carrier. Carrier females transmit the defective gene on average to half their sons, who are affected, and to half their daughters, who become carriers in turn. When a male inherits the defective gene from his mother, there is no normal gene on a second X chromosome to mask it, and he displays the abnormality. Affected males therefore far outnumber affected females. They pass the defective gene to none of their sons but to all of their daughters, who become carriers. *Haemophilia* is a disorder of this type. Unifactorial disorders of autosomal chromosomes affect males and females equally. Examples of such disorders include *cystic fibrosis*, *sickle cell anaemia*, and *thalassaemia*.

Multifactorial disorders are inherited but the pattern of inheritance is complicated. Often such disorders are influenced not only by genes but also by lifestyle and environmental factors, as in some cases of *asthma* and *schizophrenia*.

genetic engineering A branch of genetics concerned with the alteration of the genetic material of an organism to produce a desired change in the organism's characteristics. Genetic engineering has been used to mass-produce a variety of substances that are useful in medicine. A gene responsible for making a useful protein is identified and inserted into another cell (most often a bacterium or a yeast) that reproduces rapidly to form a colony of cells containing the gene. This colony produces the protein in large amounts. Some human hormones (notably *insulin* and *growth hormone*) and proteins such as *factor VIII* (used to treat *haemophilia*) are made in this way. Vaccines against infectious diseases and some drugs can also be produced by genetic engineering.

genetic fingerprinting A technique that can be used to demonstrate relationships between people (for example in *paternity testing*) or in forensic investigations to identify a criminal suspect. *DNA* contains a *genetic code* that is unique to each individual (except for identical twins). DNA can be extracted from a sample of a person's body fluids, such as blood and semen, and analysed to reveal differences in the code: the "genetic fingerprint".

genetic probe A specific fragment of *DNA* that is used in laboratory tests to determine whether particular genetic defects are present in an individual's *DNA*. Genetic probes are used in antenatal diagnosis of *genetic disorders*, and in investigating whether people with a family history of a genetic disorder carry the defective gene themselves. Genetic probes are also sometimes used for the rapid identification of infectious microorganisms.

genetics The study of *inheritance*, the chemical basis by which characteristics are determined, and the causes of the similarities and differences among individuals of a species or between different species. Branches of human genetics include population genetics, which studies the relative frequency of various *genes* in different races; molecular genetics, which is concerned with the structure, function, and copying of *DNA*; and clinical genetics, which is concerned with the study and prevention of *genetic disorders*.

genital herpes See *herpes, genital.*

genitalia The reproductive organs, especially those that are external. The male genitalia include the *penis, testes* (in the *scrotum*), *prostate gland, seminal vesicles*, and associated ducts, such as the *epididymis* and *vas deferens*. The female genitalia include the *ovaries, fallopian tubes, uterus, vagina, clitoris, vulva*, and *Bartholin's glands.*

genitalia, ambiguous A group of conditions in which the external sex organs are not clearly male or female, or in which they appear to be those of the opposite chromosomal sex. This may result from an abnormality of the *sex chromosomes* or a *hormonal disorder* (see *hermaphroditism; sex determination; adrenal hyperplasia, congenital*).

genital ulcer An eroded area of skin on the *genitalia*. The most common cause is a *sexually transmitted infection*, particularly *syphilis* and genital herpes (see *herpes, genital*). *Chancroid* and *granuloma inguinale* are tropical bacterial infections that cause genital ulcers. *Lymphogranuloma venereum* is a viral infection producing genital blisters. *Behçet's syndrome* is a rare condition that causes tender, recurrent ulcers in the mouth and on the genitals. Cancer of the penis or vulva may first appear as a painless ulcer with raised edges.

genital warts See *warts, genital.*

genito-urinary medicine The branch of medicine concerned with *sexually transmitted infections.*

genome, human The complete set of human genetic material. The human genome consists of 23 *chromosomes*, which, together, contain about 30,000 genes. All body cells contain two sets of the 23 chromosomes, one set inherited from the father and the other from the mother. An international research programme, the Human Genome Project, was launched in 1990 with the aim of identifying all the human genes. The project was completed in 2003.

gentamicin An *antibacterial drug* given by injection to treat serious infections such as *meningitis* and *septicaemia*. Gentamicin can damage the kidneys or inner ear if the dosage is not carefully controlled. The drug is also used in eye and ear drops but is unlikely to cause serious side effects with this use.

genu valgum The medical term for *knock-knee.*

genu varum See *bowleg.*

geriatric medicine The medical specialty concerned with care of the elderly. Elderly people require specialist medical treatment because they respond differently from younger people to illness and its treatment. Physical and mental decline due to *aging* can mean that illnesses are more severe in older

G

people. Because the liver becomes less efficient with age, drug dosages for elderly people need to be carefully controlled to avoid dangerous side effects. Geriatricians (also known as care-of-the-elderly physicians) also help older people to cope with everyday life following illness or injury. (See also *rehabilitation*.)

germ The popular term used to describe any microorganisms that cause disease, such as *viruses* and *bacteria*. (See also *germ cell*.)

German measles The common name for the viral infection *rubella*.

germ cell An embryonic *cell* with the potential to develop into a *spermatozoon* or *ovum*, which, on maturity, are called *gametes*. The term also describes a gamete or any cell that is undergoing gametogenesis (the process by which gametes are formed).

germ cell tumour A growth comprised of immature *sperm* cells in the male *testis* or of immature *ova* in the female *ovary*. A *seminoma* is one type of germ cell tumour (see *testis, cancer of*).

gerontology The study of *aging*. (See also *geriatric medicine*.)

Gestalt theory A school of *psychology* that emphasizes viewing things as a whole rather than breaking them down into collections of stimuli and responses. Gestalt therapy aims to increase self-awareness by looking at all aspects of an individual in his or her environment.

gestation The period of about 9 months from *conception* to birth, during which the infant develops in the *uterus*. (See also *embryo*; *fetus*; *pregnancy*.)

gestational diabetes *Diabetes* that develops for the first time during pregnancy, usually clearing up after delivery. (See *diabetic pregnancy*.)

gestodene A *progestogen drug* used with the oestrogen drug *ethinylestradiol* in low-strength combined *oral contraceptives*. Gestodene is reported to have a slightly higher risk of venous *thromboembolism* than older drugs.

giant cell arteritis An alternative name for *temporal arteritis*.

giardiasis An infection of the small intestine caused by the *protozoan* parasite *GIARDIA LAMBLIA*. Giardiasis is spread by eating or drinking food or water that is contaminated or by way of direct contact with someone who is infected.

Most of those infected do not have symptoms. If, however, symptoms do occur, they begin 1–3 days after infection and include diarrhoea and wind. The faeces of those infected tend to be highly foul-smelling, greasy, and float. Abdominal discomfort, cramps, and swelling, loss of appetite, and nausea may also occur. In some cases, giardiasis becomes *chronic*.

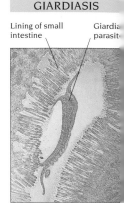

GIARDIASIS

Lining of small intestine · Giardia parasite

GIARDIA LAMBLIA

Infection is diagnosed from examination of a faecal sample or by a *jejunal biopsy*. Acute giardiasis usually clears up without treatment, but the drug *metronidazole* quickly relieves symptoms and prevents the spread of infection.

giddiness See *dizziness*.

GIFT See *gamete intrafallopian transfer*.

gigantism Excessive growth (especially in height), resulting from overproduction of *growth hormone* during childhood or adolescence by a tumour of the pituitary gland (see *pituitary tumours*). Untreated, the tumour may compress other hormone-producing cells in the pituitary gland, causing symptoms of hormone deficiency (see *hypopituitarism*). The condition may be treated with drugs such as *bromocriptine* that block the release of growth hormone, or by surgery or *radiotherapy* to remove or destroy the tumour. (See also *acromegaly*.)

Gilbert's disease A common inherited condition that affects the way in which *bilirubin* is processed by the *liver*. Usually there are no symptoms, but *jaundice* may be brought on by an unrelated illness. Sufferers are otherwise healthy. No treatment is necessary.

Gilles de la Tourette's syndrome A rare, inherited neurological disorder. It starts in childhood with repetitive grimaces and tics. Involuntary barks, grunts, or other noises may appear as the disease progresses. In some cases, the sufferer has episodes of issuing foul language. The syndrome is more common in males. It is usually of lifelong duration, but *antipsychotic drugs* can help in some cases.

gingiva The Latin name for the *gums.*

gingival hyperplasia See *hyperplasia, gingival.*

gingivectomy The surgical removal of part of the *gum* margin. Gingivectomy may be used to treat severe cases of gingival *hyperplasia* or to remove pockets of infected gum in advanced cases of *periodontitis.*

gingivitis Inflammation of the *gums.* Gingivitis is a reversible stage of gum disease and is usually the result of a build-up of *plaque* around the base of the teeth. *Toxins* produced by bacteria in the plaque irritate the gums, causing them to become infected, swollen, tender, and red-purple in colour. Gingivitis can also result from injury to the gums, usually through rough toothbrushing or flossing. Pregnant women and people with *diabetes mellitus* are especially susceptible.

Good *oral hygiene* is the main means of preventing and treating gingivitis. Untreated, it may damage gum tissue, which may lead to chronic *periodontitis.* Acute ulcerative gingivitis may develop in people with chronic gingivitis, especially those with lowered resistance to infection (see *gingivitis, acute ulcerative*).

gingivitis, acute ulcerative Painful infection and ulceration of the *gums* due to abnormal growth of bacteria that usually exist harmlessly in small numbers in gum crevices. Predisposing factors include poor *oral hygiene*, smoking, throat infections, and emotional stress. In many cases the disorder is preceded by *gingivitis* or *periodontitis.* The condition is uncommon, primarily affecting people aged 15–35.

The gums become sore and bleed at the slightest pressure. Crater-like ulcers develop on the gum tips between teeth, and there may be a foul taste in the mouth, bad breath, and swollen lymph nodes. Sometimes, the infection spreads

to the lips and cheek lining (see *noma*). A *hydrogen peroxide* mouthwash can relieve the inflammation. *Scaling* is then performed to remove plaque. The antibacterial drug *metronidazole* may be given to control infection.

gingivostomatitis Widespread inflammation of the mouth and gums, most often due to a viral infection, particularly *herpes simplex.* The condition can also be due to a bacterial infection or an adverse reaction to a prescribed drug. (See also *cold sore.*)

ginkgo An extract from the maidenhair tree *GINKGO BILOBA*, claimed to be helpful in circulatory disorders, reduced circulation in the brain, senility, depression, and premenstrual syndrome. Possible side effects are spasms and cramps.

GINKGO

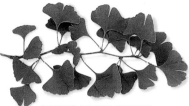

GINKGO BILOBA LEAVES

gland A group of specialized *cells* that manufacture and release chemical substances, such as *hormones* and *enzymes*, into the body. There are two main types of glands: endocrine and exocrine. *Endocrine glands* do not have ducts and release their secretions directly into the bloodstream; examples include the pituitary, thyroid, and adrenal glands. *Exocrine glands* have ducts and release their secretions either on to the surface of the skin (sebaceous glands) or into a hollow structure such as the mouth or digestive tract (salivary glands).

Lymph nodes are sometimes referred to as glands, particularly when they are enlarged (see *glands, swollen*). Strictly speaking, this is incorrect usage because lymph nodes do not secrete chemical substances.

glanders An infection of horses caused by the bacterium *PSEUDOMONAS MALLEI.* In rare cases, it is transmitted to humans,

G

causing symptoms including fever and general aches and pains. Ulcers may develop where bacteria entered the skin; if bacteria enters the lungs, *pneumonia* may occur. In severe cases, *septicaemia* may follow. Treatment is with *antibiotics*.

glands, swollen Enlargement of the *lymph nodes* as a result of inflammation and/or proliferation of white blood cells within them. Swollen lymph nodes are a common symptom, especially in children, and are usually caused by a minor infection or an allergic reaction (see *allergy*). Rarer causes include *Hodgkin's disease* and other forms of *lymphoma*.

glandular fever See *mononucleosis, infectious*.

glans The head of the *penis*.

glasses Optical devices that use lenses to correct focusing errors in the eyes to achieve clear vision. Lenses are made of glass or plastic, and the shape and thickness are chosen during a *vision test*. Convex lenses are needed for *hypermetropia* (longsightedness), and concave lenses for *myopia* (shortsightedness). Glasses for *astigmatism* use "cylindrical" lenses that are fixed in the frame at the specific angle necessary to compensate for the uneven curvature of the person's *cornea*; if required, such lenses can also be convex or concave to additionally correct for hypermetropia or myopia. Tinted lenses protect the eyes from sunlight. (See also *bifocal*; *contact lenses*)

glass eye See *eye, artificial*.

glass test A test for *meningitis* that involves pressing a clear glass against a rash. If the rash remains visible, it may be a form of *purpura*, which sometimes occurs in meningitis.

GLASS TEST

Rash visible through glass

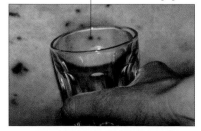

glaucoma A condition in which the pressure of the fluid in the eye is abnormally high, causing the compression and obstruction of the small blood vessels that nourish the *retina*. This may result in nerve fibre destruction and gradual loss of vision.

The most common form of glaucoma is chronic simple (open-angle) glaucoma, which rarely occurs before age 40 and often causes no symptoms until visual loss is advanced. It is caused by a gradual blockage of the outflow of *aqueous humour* over a period of years, causing a slow rise in pressure. The condition tends to run in families.

In acute (closed-angle) glaucoma, there is a sudden obstruction to the outflow of aqueous humour from the eye and the pressure rises suddenly. This causes a severe, dull pain in and above the eye, fogginess of vision, and the perception of haloes around lights at night. Nausea and vomiting may occur, and the eye may be red with a dilated pupil.

Congenital glaucoma is due to an abnormality in the drainage angles of the eyes before birth. Glaucoma can also be caused by eye injury or a serious eye disease such as *uveitis* or lens *dislocation*.

Applanation *tonometry* is used to check for glaucoma by measuring the pressure within the eye. An *ophthalmoscope* may show depression of the head of the optic nerve due to the increase in pressure. Visual field testing will be needed to assess whether vision has already been damaged, because longstanding or severe glaucoma can result in loss of peripheral vision (see *tunnel vision*). Early detection is important, before there are any symptoms, and people with a family history of glaucoma should have regular eye tests and tonometry.

Prompt treatment is essential to prevent permanent loss of vision. Chronic simple glaucoma can usually be controlled with eye-drops (e.g. *timolol*) or tablets that reduce pressure in the eye. Treatment needs to be continued for life. If drugs are ineffective, surgery may be needed to unblock the drainage channel or create an artificial channel (see *trabeculectomy*). Acute glaucoma requires emergency drug treatment, often in hospital. Surgery, usually laser *iridotomy*, may be necessary to prevent a further attack.

glibenclamide An oral hypoglycaemic drug (see *hypoglycaemics, oral*) used to treat type 2 *diabetes mellitus.*

gliclazide An oral hypoglycaemic drug (see *hypoglycaemics, oral*) used to treat type 2 *diabetes mellitus* in conjunction with dieting. Side effects are usually mild.

glioblastoma multiforme A fast-growing and highly cancerous type of primary *brain tumour.* Glioblastoma multiforme is a type of *glioma* that often develops in the *cerebrum.* The cause is unknown. Treatment may include surgery, *radiotherapy,* and/or *chemotherapy.*

glioma A type of *brain tumour* arising from the supporting connective tissue, (glial cells), in the brain. Types of glioma include *astrocytoma, glioblastoma multiforme, ependymoma, medulloblastoma,* and *oligodendroglioma.* Symptoms, diagnosis, and treatment are as for other types of brain tumour.

glipizide An oral hypoglycaemic drug (see *hypoglycaemics, oral*) used to treat type 2 *diabetes mellitus.* Side effects are usually mild and infrequent, but dizziness and drowsiness may occur. Rarely, glipizide can cause an abnormal reaction of the skin to sunlight and can reduce blood sodium levels.

globulin Any of a group of proteins that are insoluble in water but soluble in dilute salt solutions. There are a number of globulins in the blood, including *immunoglobulins* (also called antibodies).

globus hystericus A condition in which there is an uncomfortable feeling of a "lump in the throat". This lump is felt to interfere with swallowing and breathing, although there is no physical basis for the condition. In severe cases, *hyperventilation* and symptoms of a *panic attack* ensue. In most cases, the condition occurs most commonly in people who are anxious or depressed. Treatment is by reassurance, breath-control training, or *psychotherapy.*

glomerulonephritis Inflammation of the glomeruli (see *glomerulus*), affecting both kidneys. Damage to the glomeruli hampers the removal of waste products, salt, and water from the bloodstream, which may cause serious complications.

Some types of glomerulonephritis are caused by immune complexes (components of the *immune system* produced in response to infection) becoming trapped in the glomeruli. The condition occurs in some *autoimmune disorders.* Infectious diseases such as *malaria* and *schistosomiasis* are important causes of glomerulonephritis in tropical countries.

Mild glomerulonephritis may produce no symptoms. Some sufferers experience a dull ache over the kidneys. The urine may become bloodstained. Loss of protein into the urine may cause *oedema* (see *nephrotic syndrome*). *Hypertension* is a potentially serious complication. Long-term glomerulonephritis is a common cause of chronic *kidney failure.*

Diagnosis involves *kidney function tests, urinalysis,* and *kidney biopsy.* Treatment depends on the cause and severity of the disease. Children with nephrotic syndrome usually respond to *corticosteroid drugs.* In adults, kidney failure can sometimes be prevented or delayed by drug treatment and dietary control to reduce the work of the kidneys.

glomerulosclerosis Scarring caused by damage to the glomeruli (see *glomerulus*). Mild glomerulosclerosis occurs normally with age. Glomerulosclerosis may occur in some severe types of *glomerulonephritis.* It is also sometimes associated with *diabetes mellitus, hypertension, AIDS,* or intravenous *drug abuse.*

glomerulus A filtering unit of the *kidney* that consists of a cluster of capillaries

GLOMERULUS

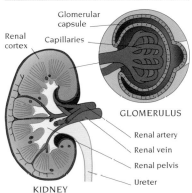

Glomerular capsule

Renal cortex

Capillaries

GLOMERULUS

Renal artery

Renal vein

Renal pelvis

Ureter

KIDNEY

G

enclosed in a capsule and supplied with blood from the renal artery. Each glomerulus is a part of a larger filtering unit called a *nephron*. Filtered blood eventually leaves the kidney via the renal vein. (See also *glomerulonephritis*.)

glomus tumour A small, bluish swelling in the skin, usually on a finger or toe near or under the nail, which is tender to touch and more painful if the limb is hot or cold. The cause is overgrowth of the nerve structures that normally control blood flow and temperature in the skin. The tumours are harmless but are surgically removed.

glossectomy Removal of all or part of the *tongue*. Glossectomy may be performed to treat *tongue cancer*.

glossitis *Inflammation* of the *tongue*. The tongue feels sore and swollen and looks red and smooth; adjacent parts of the mouth may also be inflamed.

Glossitis occurs in various forms of *anaemia* and in *vitamin B* deficiency. Other causes include infection of the mouth (especially by *herpes simplex*), irritation by dentures, and excessive use of alcohol, tobacco, or spices. Treatment is for the underlying cause. Rinsing of the mouth with a salt solution and good *oral hygiene* may help.

glossolalia Speaking in an imaginary language that has no actual meaning or syntax. (See also *neologism*.)

glossopharyngeal nerve The 9th *cranial nerve*. This nerve performs both sensory and motor functions. It conveys sensations, especially taste, from the back of the *tongue*, regulates secretion of saliva by the *parotid gland*, and controls movement of the throat muscles.

glottis The part of the *larynx* that consists of the *vocal cords* and the slit-like opening between them.

glucagon A *hormone* that stimulates the breakdown of stored *glycogen* into *glucose* and is released by the *pancreas* when the blood level of glucose is low.

Glucagon is used as an injected drug in the emergency treatment of people with *diabetes mellitus* who are unconscious as a result of low blood glucose. Nausea and vomiting are occasional adverse effects.

glucocorticoids *Hormones* produced by the cortex of the *adrenal glands* that affect carbohydrate metabolism by increasing the blood sugar level and are also involved in the body's response to physical stress. The main glucocorticoid is *hydrocortisone*.

glucosamine A molecule that occurs naturally as a component of various substances in the body, including *collagen*. Glucosamine is also sold as a food supplement and may be recommended to relieve symptoms of *arthritis*.

glucose A simple *sugar* that is naturally present in fruits and is a product of the digestion of *starch* and sucrose. It is the chief source of energy for the body and is carried to all tissues in the blood. The term "blood sugar" refers to glucose in the bloodstream.

The level of glucose in the blood is normally kept fairly constant by the actions of various *hormones*, notably *insulin*, *glucagon*, *adrenaline*, *corticosteroid hormones*, and *growth hormone*. An abnormally high blood glucose level (known as *hyperglycaemia*) may cause glucose to be lost into the urine. An abnormally low blood glucose level is called *hypoglycaemia*.

glue ear Accumulation of fluid in the cavity of the *middle ear*, causing impaired hearing. Persistent glue ear is most common in children. It is often accompanied by enlarged *adenoids* and frequently occurs with viral respiratory tract infections, such as the common *cold*. Usually both ears are affected. The lining of the middle ear becomes overactive, producing large amounts of sticky fluid, and the *eustachian tube* becomes blocked so that the fluid cannot drain away. The accumulated fluid interferes with the movement of the delicate bones of the middle ear.

Glue ear is sometimes first detected by *hearing tests*. Examination with an *otoscope* can confirm the diagnosis. In mild cases, the condition often clears up without specific treatment. If the condition persists, it may be necessary to insert *grommets*, which allow air into the middle ear and encourage fluid to drain. *Adenoidectomy* may also be required.

glue-sniffing See *solvent abuse.*

glutaraldehyde A *topical* preparation for the treatment of *warts*, particularly *plantar warts.* Glutaraldehyde may cause a rash or irritation and may stain the skin brown.

gluten A combination of gliadins and glutenins (types of proteins) formed when certain cereal flours (notably wheat flour) are mixed with water. Sensitivity to gluten causes *coeliac disease.*

gluten enteropathy See *coeliac disease.*

gluten intolerance See *coeliac disease.*

gluteus maximus The large, powerful *muscle* in each of the buttocks that gives them their rounded shape. The gluteus maximus is responsible for moving the thigh sideways and backwards.

glycerol A colourless syrupy liquid that has a sweet taste. Glycerol is prepared from *fats and oils*; it is an essential constituent of *triglycerides* (simple fats).

In rectal *suppositories*, glycerol relieves *constipation* by softening hard *faeces*. Glycerol is used in moisturizing creams. It is also used in eardrops to soften earwax and in *cough remedies* to help soothe a dry, irritating cough.

glyceryl trinitrate A *vasodilator drug* used to treat and prevent symptoms of *angina pectoris.* Possible side effects include headaches, dizziness, and flushing. A topical preparation is available to treat *anal fissures.* Additional side effects of this preparation include anal irritation and rectal bleeding.

glycogen The main form of *carbohydrate* stored in the body, found mainly in the liver and muscles. When there is too much glucose in the blood, the excess is converted to glycogen by the action of *insulin* and *corticosteroid hormones.* When the blood glucose level is low, glycogen is converted back to glucose (a process regulated by *adrenaline* and *glucagon*) and released into the bloodstream.

glycosuria The presence of *glucose* in the urine. Glycosuria results from failure of the *kidneys* to reabsorb glucose back into the bloodstream after the blood has been filtered. This may be due to *hyperglycaemia*, as in *diabetes mellitus*, or may occur if the kidney tubules have been damaged. However, glycosuria is usually only significant if

accompanied by a high blood glucose level. Glycosuria often occurs during pregnancy when the blood glucose level is normal. Glycosuria is diagnosed by *urinalysis.* Treatment depends on the cause.

glycosylated haemoglobin A form of *haemoglobin* that is bound to the sugar glucose. In most people, 4–7 per cent of haemoglobin is glycosylated. In people with *diabetes mellitus*, the level of glycosylated haemoglobin may be raised if treatment has not kept the blood glucose level within the normal range. Glycosylated haemoglobin levels indicate blood glucose levels over the preceding 3 months. However, in people with abnormal haemoglobin, such as those with *sickle cell anaemia*, glycosylated haemoglobin cannot be used to monitor blood glucose levels.

goitre Enlargement of the *thyroid gland*, visible as a swelling on the neck. The thyroid gland may enlarge (without any disturbance of its function) at *puberty*, during pregnancy, or as a result of taking *oral contraceptives.* In many parts of the world the main cause of a goitre is lack of *iodine* in the diet. A condition called toxic goitre develops in *Graves' disease* and in other forms of *hyperthyroidism* that lead to *thyrotoxicosis.* A goitre is also a feature of different types of *thyroiditis.* Other causes include a tumour or nodule in the gland and, in rare cases, *thyroid cancer.*

A goitre can range in size from a barely noticeable lump to a large swelling, depending on the cause. Large swellings

GOITRE

Swelling due to enlarged thyroid gland (goitre)

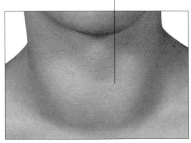

may press on the *oesophagus* or *trachea*, making swallowing or breathing difficult.

A goitre not caused by disease may eventually disappear. Goitre due to iodine deficiency can be treated by dietary measures. When a goitre is the result of disease, treatment is for the underlying disorder. Large goitres can be treated surgically (see *thyroidectomy*).

gold A *disease-modifying antirheumatic drug* used to treat active progressive *rheumatoid arthritis* and, occasionally, arthritis arising as a complication of *psoriasis*. It is given either as regular injections or orally (see *auranofin*). A common adverse effect is *dermatitis*. Gold may cause loss of appetite, nausea, and diarrhoea. It may also damage the kidneys, liver, and bone marrow, and therefore regular monitoring with blood tests is necessary for people taking the drug.

golfer's elbow A painful condition caused by inflammation of the *epicondyle* (bony prominence) on the inner *elbow*, at the site of attachment of some forearm muscles. Golfer's elbow is caused by overuse of these muscles, which bend the wrist and fingers. Activities such as using a screwdriver or playing golf with a faulty grip can cause the condition. Treatment consists of resting the elbow, applying ice-packs, and taking *analgesic drugs* to relieve pain. If the pain is severe or persistent, injection of a *corticosteroid drug* into the area may help.

gonadorelin The hormone released by the *hypothalamus* that stimulates the pituitary gland to secrete the *gonadotrophin hormones* follicle-stimulating hormone (FSH) and luteinizing hormone (LH).

Gonadorelin can be given by injection and is used to investigate suspected disease of the hypothalamus and also to stimulate the *ovaries* in the treatment of infertility. Synthesized gonadorelins (known as gonadorelin analogues) are used to treat *endometriosis* and hormone-dependent cancers, including *breast cancer* and *prostate cancer*.

gonadotrophin hormones *Hormones* that stimulate cell activity in the *ovaries* and *testes*. Gonadotrophins are essential for fertility. The two most important

gonadotrophins are follicle-stimulating hormone (FSH) and luteinizing hormone (LH), which are secreted by the *pituitary gland*. Another gonadotrophin, HCG (see *gonadotrophin, human chorionic*), is produced by the placenta during pregnancy. Certain gonadotrophins are used as drugs in the treatment of *infertility*.

gonadotrophin, human chorionic A *hormone* produced by the *placenta* in early *pregnancy*. Human chorionic gonadotrophin (HCG) stimulates the *ovaries* to produce *oestrogen* and *progesterone*, which are needed for a healthy pregnancy. HCG is excreted in the urine, and its presence in urine is the basis of pregnancy tests on urine samples.

gonads The sex glands – the *testes* in men and the *ovaries* in women.

gonorrhoea One of the most common *sexually transmitted infections*. Gonorrhoea, caused by the bacterium NEISSERIA GONORRHOEAE, is most often transmitted during sexual activity, including oral and anal sex. An infected woman may also transmit the disease to her baby during childbirth.

Gonorrhoea has an incubation period of 2–10 days. In men, symptoms include a discharge from the *urethra* and pain on passing urine. Many infected women have no symptoms; if symptoms are present, they usually consist of vaginal discharge or a burning sensation on passing urine. Infection acquired by anal sex can cause gonococcal *proctitis*. Oral sex with an infected person may lead to gonococcal *pharyngitis*. A baby exposed to infection during its birth may acquire the eye infection gonococcal *ophthalmia*.

Untreated gonorrhoea may spread to other parts of the body. In men, it may cause *prostatitis* or *epididymo-orchitis*, affecting fertility. In women, untreated gonorrhoea results in *pelvic inflammatory disease*, causing damage to the *fallopian tubes*. This increases the risk of *ectopic pregnancy* and may lead to *infertility*. Gonococcal bacteria in the bloodstream may result in *septicaemia* or *septic arthritis*.

Tests are performed on a sample of discharge or on swabs taken from the urethra, *cervix*, or *rectum* in order to confirm the diagnosis. Gonorrhoea is treated with *antibiotic drugs*.

Goodpasture's syndrome A rare *autoimmune disorder* causing *inflammation* of the glomeruli in the kidney (see *glomerulus*) and the alveoli in the lungs, and *anaemia*. It is a serious disease; unless treated early it may lead to life-threatening bleeding into the lungs and progressive *kidney failure*. The disease is most common in young men, but can develop at any age and in women. Sometimes, it responds to treatment with *immunosuppressant drugs* and *plasmapheresis*. People who have severe or repeated attacks require *dialysis* and, eventually, a *kidney transplant*.

GORD The abbreviation for *gastro-oesophageal reflux disease*.

goserelin A synthetic drug chemically related to the hypothalmic hormone *gonadorelin*. Goserelin is used to treat *breast cancer* and *prostate cancer*, *fibroids*, *infertility*, and *endometriosis*. Adverse effects include loss of bone density after prolonged application.

gout A common *metabolic disorder* that causes attacks of *arthritis*, usually in a single joint (most commonly the base of the big toe). Gout is due to high levels of uric acid in the blood (see *hyperuricaemia*), the arthritis is due to the deposition of uric acid crystals in joint tissue. The affected joint is red, swollen, and tender. Attacks last a few days and often recur. They are sometimes accompanied by fever. Gout may be associated with kidney stones (see *calculus, urinary tract*), and affects 10 times more men than women. In men, it occurs any time after *puberty*; in women it usually occurs after the *menopause*. The condition tends to run in families.

GOUT

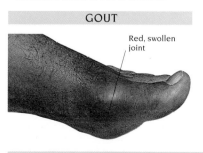

Red, swollen joint

The diagnosis is confirmed by tests on blood or fluid from the affected joint to measure uric acid levels. Pain and inflammation can usually be controlled by *nonsteroidal anti-inflammatory drugs* or *colchicine*. If these are ineffective, a *corticosteroid* may be injected into the joint. Long-term treatment with drugs such as *allopurinol* can stop or reduce the frequency of attacks.

grafting The process of transplanting healthy tissue from one part of the body to another (autografting), from one person to another (allografting), or from an animal to a person (xenografting).

Grafting is used to repair or replace diseased, damaged, or defective tissues or organs. The most common operations of this type are *skin graft, bone graft, stem cell* or *bone marrow transplant, corneal graft, kidney transplant, heart transplant, liver transplant, heart–lung transplant, heart-valve surgery*, and *microsurgery* on blood vessels and nerves.

With autografting, the grafted tissue is usually assimilated well into the surrounding tissue at the new site. The general risks of tissue rejection following other forms of grafting are discussed in *transplant surgery*.

graft-versus-host disease A complication of a *bone marrow transplant* in which *immune system* cells in the transplanted marrow attack the recipient's tissues. Graft-versus-host (GVH) disease may occur soon after transplantation or appear some months later. The first sign is usually a skin rash. This may be followed by diarrhoea, abdominal pain, *jaundice*, *inflammation* of the eyes and mouth, and breathlessness. GVH disease does not occur with *stem cell* transplants.

GVH disease can usually be prevented by administration of *immunosuppressant drugs*. If the disease develops, it can be treated with *corticosteroid drugs* and immunosuppressant drugs such as *ciclosporin* In some cases, however, it can be difficult to control.

Gram's stain An *iodine*-based stain that is used to differentiate between types of *bacterium*.

grand mal A type of epileptic seizure (see *epilepsy*) in which the sufferer falls unconscious and has generalized jerky

G

G

muscle contractions. The seizure may last for a few minutes; the person may have no recall of it on awakening.

granulation tissue A mass of red, moist, granular tissue that develops on the surface of an ulcer or open *wound* during the process of *healing*.

granulocyte A type of white *blood cell*.

granuloma An aggregation of cells of a type associated with chronic *inflammation*. They usually occur as a reaction to certain infections, such as *tuberculosis*, or a foreign body, such as a suture, but they may develop for unknown reasons in conditions such as *sarcoidosis*.

A pyogenic granuloma is an excess of granulation tissue developing at the site of an injury to the skin or mucous membrane. (See also *granuloma annulare*; *granuloma inguinale*.)

granuloma annulare A harmless skin condition characterized by a circular, raised area of skin, which spreads outwards to form a ring. The disorder occurs most commonly in children, usually on the hands. The cause is unknown. No treatment is necessary. In most cases, the affected skin heals completely over a period of several months or years.

granuloma inguinale A *sexually transmitted infection* that causes ulceration of the genitals. The infection is caused by *CALYMMATOBACTERIUM GRANULOMATIS*, also known as Donovan's bodies. Granuloma inguinale is common in parts of the tropics but is rare in developed countries. The antibiotics *tetracycline* or *erythromycin* are effective treatments.

Graves' disease An *autoimmune disorder* that is characterized by toxic *goitre* (an overactive and enlarged thyroid gland), excessive production of thyroid hormones leading to *thyrotoxicosis*, and *exophthalmos*.

gravida The medical term for a pregnant woman. The term gravida is often combined with a prefix to indicate the total number of pregnancies a woman has undergone (including the present one). For example, a primigravida is a woman who is pregnant for the first time.

gray An SI unit of radiation dosage (see *radiation unit*).

greenstick fracture A type of *fracture* that occurs when a long bone in the arm

or the leg bends and cracks on one side only. This type of fracture occurs only in children, whose bones are still growing and flexible.

grey matter Regions of the *central nervous system* consisting principally of closely packed and interconnected *nerve* cell bodies and their branching dendrites, rather than their filamentous *axons*, which make up the *white matter*. Grey matter is mostly found in the outer layers of the *cerebrum* (the main mass of the *brain* and the region responsible for advanced mental functions) and deeper regions of the brain, such as the basal ganglia. Grey matter also makes up the inner core of the *spinal cord*.

GREY MATTER

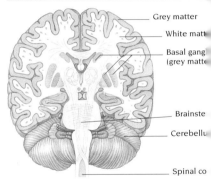

Grey matter

White matter

Basal ganglia (grey matter)

Brainstem

Cerebellum

Spinal cord

SECTION THROUGH BRAIN

grief An intensely painful emotion, usually caused by loss of a loved one. (See *bereavement*.)

grip The ability of the *hand* to hold objects firmly. The hand is well adapted for gripping, with an opposable thumb (one that is able to touch each of the fingers), specialized skin on the palm and fingers to provide adhesion, and a complex system of muscles, tendons, joints, and nerves that enables precise movements of the *digits*.

Gripping ability can be reduced by any condition that causes muscular weakness or impairment of sensation in the palms or fingers (e.g. a *stroke* or *nerve injury*) or by disorders that affect the bones or joints of the hand or wrist, such as *arthritis* or a *fracture*.

gripe Severe abdominal pain (see *colic*).

griseofulvin A drug given orally to treat some *fungal infections*. Griseofulvin is particularly useful for infections affecting the scalp, beard, palms, soles of the feet, and nails. Common side effects are headache, dry mouth, abdominal pain, and *photosensitivity*. Long-term treatment with the drug may cause liver or bone marrow damage.

groin The hollow between the lower abdomen and top of the thigh.

groin, lump in the A swelling in the *groin*, most commonly due to enlargement of a lymph node as a result of an infection (see *glands, swollen*). Another common cause is a *hernia*. Rarely, in men, an undescended testis may be the cause (see *testis, undescended*). Treatment depends on the cause.

groin strain Pain and tenderness in the *groin* as a result of overstretching of a muscle, typically while running or playing sports. The *muscles* commonly affected are the adductors and the rectus femoris. Groin strain is usually treated with *physiotherapy*, but recovery may be slow.

grommet A small tube that may be inserted through an incision in the *eardrum* during surgery to treat *glue ear*, usually in children. The grommet equalizes the pressure on both sides of the eardrum, permitting mucus to drain down the *eustachian tube* into the back of the throat. The tubes are usually allowed to fall out on their own as the hole in the eardrum closes, 6–12 months after insertion.

group therapy Any treatment of psychological problems in which a group of patients meets regularly with a therapist. Interaction among group members is considered therapeutic. Group therapy may be useful for people with personality problems and for sufferers from *alcohol dependence*, *drug dependence*, *anxiety disorders*, and *eating disorders*.

growing pains Vague aches and pains that occur in the limbs of children. The pains are usually felt at night and most often affect the calves of children aged between 6–12. The cause of growing pains is unknown, but they do not seem to be related to the process of growth itself. Growing pains are of no medical significance and require no treatment. Limb pain that occurs in the morning, causes a limp, or prevents normal use of the limb is not due to growing pains and should be assessed by a doctor.

growth Abnormal proliferation of cells in a localized area (see *tumour*). Also, an increase in size, usually as a result of increasing age (see *growth, childhood*).

growth, childhood The increase in height and weight as a child develops. The period of most rapid growth occurs before birth. After birth, although growth is still rapid in the first few years of life, especially in the first year, the rate of growth steadily decreases. *Puberty* marks another major period of growth, which continues until adult height and weight are reached, usually at about age 16–17 in girls and 19–21 in boys.

Body shape changes during childhood because different areas grow at different rates. For example, at birth, the head is already about three quarters of its adult size, it grows to almost full size during the first year. Thereafter, it becomes proportionately smaller because the body grows at a much faster rate.

Growth can be influenced by *heredity* and by environmental factors such as nutrition and general health. *Hormones* also play an important role, particularly *growth hormone*, *thyroid hormones*, and, at puberty, the *sex hormones*.

GROMMET

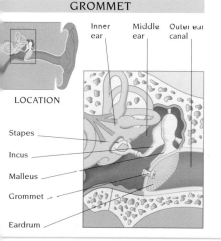

Inner ear   Middle ear   Outer ear canal

LOCATION

Stapes

Incus

Malleus

Grommet

Eardrum

A chronic illness, such as *cystic fibrosis*, may retard growth. Even a minor illness can slow growth briefly, although the growth rate usually catches up when the child recovers. In some cases, slow growth may be the only sign that a child is ill or malnourished, in which case it is known as *failure to thrive*. However, *short stature* does not necessarily indicate poor health. Abnormally rapid growth is rare. Usually, it is a familial trait, but it may occasionally indicate an underlying disorder, such as a pituitary gland tumour causing *gigantism*. (See also *age*; *child development*.)

growth factor Any of various chemicals involved in stimulating new cell growth and maintenance. Some growth factors, such as vascular endothelial growth factor, which stimulates the formation of new blood vessels, are important in the growth and spread of cancers.

growth hormone A substance that is produced by the *pituitary gland* and which stimulates normal body growth and development. Growth hormone stimulates the production of protein in muscle cells and the release of energy from the breakdown of fats. Oversecretion of growth hormone results in *gigantism* if it occurs before puberty or *acromegaly* if it occurs after.

Synthetic growth hormone given by injection may be used to treat *short stature* when the cause is a pituitary disorder or a genetic disorder.

GTN The abbreviation for *glyceryl trinitrate*.

Guillain–Barré syndrome A rare condition affecting the peripheral nerves (see *peripheral nervous system*) that causes weakness, usually in the limbs. The cause is believed to be an allergic reaction to an infection, usually viral; the nerves are damaged by *antibodies* produced by the body to eliminate the infection. In most cases, the disease develops 2 or 3 weeks after the onset of infection. Weakness, often accompanied by numbness and tingling, usually starts in the legs and spreads to the arms. The weakness may become progressively worse, resulting in *paralysis*. The muscles of the face and those controlling speech, swallowing, and breathing may also be affected.

Diagnosis of Guillain–Barré syndrome is confirmed by electrical tests to measure how fast nerve impulses are being conducted, or by a *lumbar puncture*. Most people recover fully with only supportive treatment. However, in severe cases, treatment with *plasmapheresis* or *immunoglobulin* may be given. Mechanical *ventilation* may be needed to aid breathing if the respiratory muscles and *diaphragm* are severely affected. Some people are left with permanent weakness in affected areas and/or suffer from further attacks of the disease.

guilt A painful feeling that arises from the awareness of having broken a moral code. Guilt is self-inflicted, unlike shame, which depends on how other people view the transgression. Some psychoanalysts view guilt as a result of the prohibitions of the *superego* instilled by parental authority in early life. Others see guilt as a conditioned response to actions that in the past have led to punishment. Feeling guilty for no reason or for an imagined crime is one of the main symptoms of psychotic *depression*.

Guinea worm disease A tropical disease caused by a female parasitic worm more than 1 m long. Infection is the result of drinking water containing the water flea cyclops, which harbours larvae of the worm. The larvae pass through the intestine and mature in body tissues. After about a year, the adult female worm, now pregnant, approaches the skin surface and creates an inflamed blister that bursts, exposing the end of the worm. *Urticaria*, nausea, and diarrhoea often develop while the blister is forming. The disease occurs in Africa, South America, the Caribbean, Middle East, and India.

The traditional remedy is to wind the worm from the skin on to a small stick. Once the worm is out, the condition usually clears up. The drugs *tiabendazole* and niridazole are given to reduce inflammation, *antibiotics* are given to control secondary infection, and the patient is immunized against *tetanus*.

Gulf War syndrome A term that has been used to describe a wide range of debilitating symptoms first reported by

Gulf War veterans. Common symptoms include headaches, chronic fatigue, limb pains, difficulty concentrating, and memory problems. Exposure to chemicals, intensive vaccination programmes, and combat stress have all been implicated as possible causes of the syndrome.

gullet Common name for the *oesophagus*.

gum The soft tissue surrounding the *teeth* that protects underlying structures and keeps the teeth in position in the jaw.

Healthy gums are pink or brown and firm. Careful *oral hygiene* helps prevent gum disease. *Gingivitis* may occur if *plaque* is allowed to collect around the base of the teeth. Untreated gingivitis may lead to chronic *periodontitis*. Bleeding gums are nearly always a symptom of gingivitis; rarely, they are due to *leukaemia* or *scurvy*. Gingival *hyperplasia* occurs most often as a side effect of treatment with *phenytoin*.

gumboil See *abscess, dental*

gumma A soft tumour that may develop in the late stages of untreated *syphilis*. These tumours are very uncommon in developed countries.

gut A common name for the *intestine*.

Guthrie test A blood test performed routinely on a heel-prick blood sample taken from newborn babies to check for the inherited disorder *phenylketonuria* Newborn screening programmes have progressed since the introduction of the Guthrie test and the blood sample is now also tested for several other conditions (see *blood spot screening tests*).

gynaecology The medical speciality concerned with the female *reproductive tract*. Gynaecology deals with *contraception*, the investigation and treatment of menstrual problems (see *menstruation, disorders of*), *sexual problems*, *infertility*, problems relating to the *menopause*, and disorders such as uterine *fibroids* and *ovarian cysts*. Gynaecology also covers disorders of early pregnancy, such as recurrent *miscarriage*.

gynaecomastia Enlargement of one or both *breasts* in the male, due, in some cases, to an excess of the female sex hormone *oestrogen* in the blood.

Mild, temporary gynaecomastia can occur at birth as a result of maternal hormones, and it is common at *puberty*.

Gynaecomastia developing in later life may be due to chronic liver diseases such as *cirrhosis*. Hormone secreting tumours such as pituitary or testicular tumours may also be a cause.

Adult gynaecomastia, which sometimes occurs in only one breast, can also occur when synthetic hormones and some drugs, such as *digoxin*, *spironolactone*, and *cimetidine*, change the balance of sex hormones. Rarely, a discrete lump that develops on one breast may be due to a male breast cancer.

Investigation may involve *blood tests*. If cancer is suspected, a *biopsy* will be performed. Treatment depends on the cause. If a drug is responsible, an alternative will be prescribed if possible. If there is no underlying disease, swelling usually subsides without treatment. Cosmetic surgery may be considered in severe cases (see *mammoplasty*).

G

GUTHRIE TEST

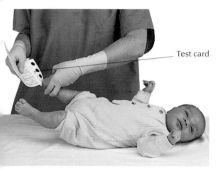

Test card

COLLECTING SAMPLE FOR
GUTHRIE TEST

H

H₂-receptor antagonists A common abbreviation for histamine₂-receptor antagonists, a group of *ulcer-healing drugs*. (See also *cimetidine; ranitidine; famotidine*.)

H5N1 virus A virus that causes a virulent strain of *avian influenza*.

habituation The process of becoming accustomed to an experience. In general, the more a person is exposed to a stimulus, the less he or she is affected by it. People can become habituated to certain drugs and develop a reduced response to their effects (see *tolerance*).

haem A compound that contains iron and which combines with globin to form *haemoglobin*.

haem- A prefix indicating *blood*.

haemangioblastoma A rare type of brain tumour consisting of blood-vessel cells. Haemangioblastomas develop slowly as cysts, often in the cerebellum, and are mostly noncancerous. Symptoms include headache, vomiting, *nystagmus* and, if the tumour is in the cerebellum, *ataxia*. Most can be removed surgically.

haemangioma A birthmark caused by abnormal distribution of blood vessels. Types of haemangioma include *port-wine stains*, *stork marks*, and *strawberry naevi*. They generally disappear without leaving a scar by the age of 5–7 years.

Haemangiomas do not usually require treatment. However, a haemangioma that bleeds persistently or that looks unsightly may need to be removed, by *laser treatment*, *cryosurgery*, *radiotherapy*, *embolization*, or *plastic surgery*.

haemarthrosis Bleeding into a *joint*, causing the capsule that encloses the joint to swell, and resulting in pain and stiffness. Haemarthrosis is usually the result of severe injury to a joint. Less common causes are *bleeding disorders*, such as *haemophilia*, and overuse of *anticoagulant drugs*.

Ice-packs may reduce swelling and pain. Fluid may be withdrawn for pain relief and for diagnosis. Haemophiliacs are given *factor VIII* to promote blood clotting. Resting the joint in an elevated position can prevent further bleeding.

Repeated haemarthrosis may damage joint surfaces, causing *osteoarthritis*.

haematemesis The medical term for *vomiting blood*.

haematology The study of *blood* and its formation, as well as the investigation and treatment of disorders that affect the blood and the *bone marrow*.

haematoma A localized collection of *blood* (usually clotted) that is caused by bleeding from a ruptured blood vessel. Haematomas can occur almost anywhere in the body and vary from a minor to a potentially fatal condition.

Less serious types of haematoma include haematomas under the nails or in the tissues of the outer ear (*cauliflower ear*). Most haematomas disappear without treatment in a few days, but if they are painful they may be drained. More serious types include extradural and subdural haematomas, which press on the brain (see *extradural haemorrhage*; *subdural haemorrhage*).

haematoma auris The medical term for *cauliflower ear*.

haematuria Blood in the *urine*, which may or may not be visible to the naked eye. In small amounts, it may give the urine a smoky appearance.

Almost any *urinary tract* disorder can cause haematuria. *Urinary tract infection* is a common cause; *prostatitis* may be a cause in men. *Cysts*, *kidney tumours*, *bladder tumours*, stones (see *calculus, urinary tract*), and *glomerulonephritis* may cause haematuria. *Bleeding disorders* may also cause the condition.

Blood that is not visible to the naked eye may be detected by a dipstick *urine test* or microscopic examination. *CT scanning, ultrasound scanning*, or intravenous *urography* can help determine the cause. If bladder disease is suspected, *cystoscopy* is performed.

haemochromatosis An inherited disease in which too much dietary iron is absorbed. Excess iron gradually accumulates in the liver, pancreas, heart, testes, and other organs. Men are more frequently affected because women regularly lose iron in menstrual blood.

Loss of sex drive and a reduction in the size of the testes are often the first signs. Excess iron over a period of time causes liver enlargement and *cirrhosis*, and can lead to *diabetes mellitus*, bronzed skin coloration, cardiac *arrhythmia*, and, eventually, *liver failure* and *liver cancer*.

Diagnosis is based on *blood tests* and a *liver biopsy*. Treatment is by regular venesection. (See also *haemosiderosis*.)

haemodialysis One of the two means of *dialysis* used to treat *kidney failure*.

haemoglobin The oxygen-carrying pigment that is present in red *blood cells*. Haemoglobin molecules, which are produced by *bone marrow*, are made up of four protein chains (two alpha- and two betaglobin) and four haem (a red pigment that contains iron).

HAEMOGLOBIN

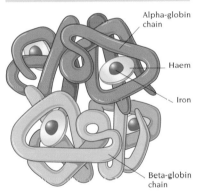

Alpha-globin chain

Haem

Iron

Beta-globin chain

STRUCTURE OF HAEMOGLOBIN

Oxygen from the lungs enters red blood cells in the bloodstream. The oxygen then combines chemically with the haem within the haemoglobin to form oxyhaemoglobin, which gives blood in the *arteries* its distinctive bright red colour and is carried around the body. In areas that need oxygen, the oxyhaemoglobin releases its oxygen and reverts to haemoglobin, giving blood in the *veins* its darker colour.

Some defects in haemoglobin production result from a *genetic disorder*; such defects are subdivided into errors of haem production, known as *porphyrias*, and those of globin production, known as *haemoglobinopathies*. Other defects, such as some types of *anaemia*, have a nongenetic cause.

haemoglobinopathy A term used to describe the *genetic disorders* in which there is a fault in the production of the globin chains of *haemoglobin*. Examples of haemoglobinopathies include *sickle cell anaemia* and the *thalassaemias*.

haemoglobinuria The presence in the urine of *haemoglobin*. Haemoglobin is mainly contained in red blood cells, but a small amount is free in the blood plasma. Excessive breakdown of red blood cells, which may be due to heavy exercise, cold weather, falciparum *malaria*, or haemolytic *anaemia*, increases the concentration of free haemoglobin in the plasma. The excess haemoglobin is excreted in the urine.

haemolysis The destruction of red *blood cells*. Haemolysis is the normal process by which old red blood cells are destroyed, mainly in the *spleen*. *Bilirubin*, a waste product of haemolysis, is excreted into the *bile* by the liver. Abnormal haemolysis, in which red blood cells are destroyed prematurely, may cause anaemia and jaundice (see *anaemia, haemolytic*).

haemolytic anaemia See *anaemia, haemolytic*.

haemolytic disease of the newborn Excessive *haemolysis* (destruction of red blood cells) in the fetus and newborn by *antibodies* produced by the mother. Haemolytic disease of the newborn is most often caused by *rhesus incompatibility*. This occurs when a mother with Rh-negative type blood, who has previously been exposed to Rh-positive blood through birth, miscarriage, abortion, or amniocentesis, is pregnant with a baby that has Rh-positive blood. Haemolytic disease has become uncommon since the introduction of routine preventive treatment for Rh-negative women during pregnancy (see *anti-D (Rh_0) immunoglobulin*).

In mild cases of haemolytic disease, the newborn baby becomes slightly jaundiced during the first 24 hours of life

H

H

(due to excess bilirubin in the blood) and slightly anaemic. In more severe cases, the level of *bilirubin* in the blood may increase to a dangerous level, causing a risk of *kernicterus* (a type of brain damage). Severely affected babies have marked anaemia while still in the uterus. They become swollen (*hydrops fetalis*) and are often stillborn.

In mild cases, no treatment is necessary. In other cases, the aim is to deliver the baby before the anaemia becomes severe, usually by *induction of labour* at 35–39 weeks' gestation. If the baby is too young to be delivered safely, fetal blood transfusions may be necessary. After birth, *phototherapy* (light treatment that converts bilirubin in the skin into a water-soluble form that is more easily excreted from the body) can help to reduce *jaundice*. An exchange blood transfusion may be needed.

haemolytic–uraemic syndrome A rare disease in which red *blood cells* are destroyed prematurely and the *kidneys* are damaged, causing acute *kidney failure*. *Thrombocytopenia* can also occur. Haemolytic–uraemic syndrome most commonly affects young children and may be triggered by a serious bacterial or viral infection. Symptoms include weakness, lethargy, and a reduction in the volume of urine. *Seizures* may occur.

Blood and urine tests can determine the degree of kidney damage. *Dialysis* may be needed until the kidneys have recovered. Most patients recover normal kidney function.

haemophilia An inherited *bleeding disorder* caused by deficiency of a blood protein, *factor VIII*, which is essential for blood clotting. Haemophiliacs suffer recurrent bleeding, usually into their joints, which may occur spontaneously or after injury. The lack of factor VIII is due to a defective gene, which shows a pattern of *sex-linked inheritance*; haemophilia affects males in most cases.

Episodes of bleeding are painful and, unless treated promptly, can lead to joint deformity. Injury, and even minor operations such as tooth extraction, may lead to profuse bleeding. Internal bleeding can lead to blood in the urine or extensive bruises.

Haemophilia is diagnosed by *blood-clotting tests*, and by *amniocentesis* or *chorionic villus sampling* in a fetus. Bleeding can be prevented or controlled by infusions of factor VIII concentrates.

Haemophilus influenzae A bacterium that causes various infectious diseases in humans. There are several types of HAEMOPHILUS INFLUENZAE; type b (Hib) causes infections such as *meningitis*, *epiglottitis*, *septicaemia*, and *pneumonia*. Infants are routinely immunized against HAEMOPHILUS INFLUENZAE type b as part of the childhood immunization schedule (see *Hib vaccine*).

haemoptysis The medical term for *coughing up blood*.

haemorrhage The medical term for *bleeding*. (See also *haematoma*.)

haemorrhoidectomy The surgical removal of *haemorrhoids*. The procedure is used to treat large, prolapsing, or bleeding haemorrhoids.

haemorrhoids Swollen veins in the lining of the *anus*. Sometimes these veins protrude outside the anal canal, in which case they are called prolapsing haemorrhoids. Straining repeatedly to pass hard faeces is one of the main causes of haemorrhoids. Haemorrhoids are also common during pregnancy and just after childbirth.

Rectal bleeding and discomfort on defaecation are the most common features. Prolapsing haemorrhoids often produce a mucous discharge and itching around the anus. A complication of prolapse is *thrombosis* and *strangulation*; this can cause extreme pain.

Diagnosis is usually by *proctoscopy*. Mild cases are controlled by drinking lots of fluids, eating a high-fibre diet, and establishing regular toilet habits. Rectal suppositories and creams containing *corticosteroid drugs* and local *anaesthetics* reduce pain and swelling. More troublesome haemorrhoids may be treated by *sclerotherapy*, *cryosurgery*, or by banding, in which a band is tied around the haemorrhoid, causing it to wither and drop off. A *haemorrhoidectomy* is generally required for prolapsing haemorrhoids.

haemosiderosis A general increase in *iron* stores in the body. Haemosiderosis may occur after repeated blood transfusions or, more rarely, as a result of excessive intake of iron.

haemospermia The medical term for blood in the semen (see *semen, blood in the*).

haemostasis The arrest of *bleeding*. There are three main natural mechanisms by which bleeding is stopped after injury. First, small blood vessels constrict. Second, small *blood cells* called platelets aggregate and plug the bleeding points. Third, the plasma coagulates, forming filaments of a substance called *fibrin*, which help to seal the damaged blood vessel (see *blood clotting*). Defects in any of these mechanisms can cause a *bleeding disorder*.

haemostatic drugs A group of drugs used to treat bleeding disorders and to control bleeding. Haemostatic preparations that help blood clotting are given to people who have deficiencies of natural clotting factors. For example, *factor VIII* is used to treat haemophilia. Drugs that prevent the breakdown of fibrin in clots, such as *tranexamic acid*, can also improve haemostasis.

haemothorax A collection of blood in the pleural cavity (see *pleura*). Haemothorax is most commonly caused by chest injury, but it may arise spontaneously in people with defects of blood coagulation or as a result of cancer. Symptoms include pain in the affected side of the chest and upper abdomen, and breathlessness. If extensive, there may be partial lung collapse. Blood in the pleural cavity is withdrawn through a needle.

hair A thread-like structure composed of dead cells containing *keratin*, a fibrous protein. The root of each hair is embedded in a tiny pit in the dermis layer of the *skin* called a hair *follicle*. Each shaft of hair consists of a spongy semihollow core (the medulla), a surrounding layer of long, thin fibres (the cortex) and, on the outside, several layers of overlapping cells (the cuticle). While a hair is growing, the root is enclosed by tissue called a bulb, which supplies the hair with keratin. Once the hair has stopped growing, the bulb retracts from the root and the hair eventually falls out.

Hair is involved in the regulation of body temperature (known as thermo-

regulation). If the body is too cold, arrector pili muscles in the skin contract, pulling the hairs upright to form goose pimples. Erect hairs trap an insulating layer of air next to the skin.

HAIR

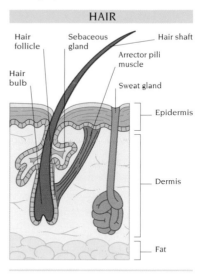

Brittle hair may be due to excessive styling, *hypothyroidism*, or severe vitamin or mineral deficiency. Very dry hair can be caused by malnutrition. Ingrown hairs occur when the free-growing end of the hair penetrates the skin near the follicle, which may cause inflammation. (See also *hirsutism*; *hypertrichosis*.)

hairball A ball of hair in the stomach, found in people who nervously suck or chew their hair (see *bezoar*).

hairiness, excessive See *hirsutism*; *hypertrichosis*.

hair removal Hair is usually removed from the body for cosmetic reasons. It may also be shaved from around an incision site before surgery. Temporary methods include shaving, waxing, *depilatory* creams, and waxing; *electrolysis* is the only permanent method of removal.

hair transplant A cosmetic operation in which hairy sections of scalp are removed and transplanted to hairless areas to treat *alopecia* (baldness). There are several different techniques.

In strip grafting, a strip of skin and hair is taken from a donor site, usually at the

HAIR TRANSPLANT

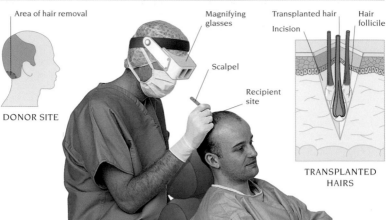

Area of hair removal

Magnifying glasses

Transplanted hair

Incision

Hair follicile

Scalpel

Recipient site

DONOR SITE

TRANSPLANTED HAIRS

STRIP GRAFTING TECHNIQUE

back of the scalp or behind the ears. The removed hairs and their follicles are then inserted into numerous incisions made in a bald area, known as the recipient site. The procedure usually takes 60–90 minutes. The patient is given a mild sedative and anaesthetic on the donor and recipient sites. The donor site heals in about 5 days. Transplanted hairs fall out shortly afterwards, but new hairs grow from the follicles 3 weeks to 3 months later.

Other transplant techniques include punch grafting, in which a punch is used to remove small areas of bald scalp, which are replaced with areas of hairy scalp; flap grafting, in which flaps of hairy skin are lifted, rotated, and stitched to replace bald areas; and male pattern baldness reduction, which involves cutting out areas of bald skin and stretching surrounding areas of hair-bearing scalp to replace them.

half-life The time taken for the activity of a substance to reduce to half its original level. The term is usually used to refer to the time taken for the level of *radiation* emitted by a radioactive substance to decay to half its original level. The concept is useful in *radiotherapy* for assessing how long material will stay radioactive in the body. Half-life is also used to refer to the length of time taken by the body to eliminate half the quantity of a drug.

halitosis The medical term for bad breath. Halitosis is usually a result of smoking, drinking alcohol, eating garlic or onions, or poor oral hygiene. Persistent bad breath not caused by any of these may be a symptom of mouth infection, *sinusitis*, or certain lung disorders, such as *bronchiectasis*.

hallucination A perception that occurs when there is no external stimulus. Auditory hallucinations (the hearing of voices) are a major symptom of *schizophrenia* but may also be caused by *bipolar disorder* and certain brain disorders. Visual hallucinations are most often found in states of *delirium* brought on by a physical illness (such as *pneumonia*) or alcohol withdrawal (*delirium tremens*). *Hallucinogenic drugs* are another common cause of visual hallucinations. Hallucinations of smell are associated with *temporal lobe epilepsy*. Those of touch and taste are rare, however, and occur mainly in people with *schizophrenia*. People subjected to *sensory deprivation* or overwhelming physical stress sometimes suffer from temporary hallucinations.

hallucinogenic drug A drug that causes *hallucination*. Hallucinogens include certain drugs of abuse, such as *LSD, marijuana, mescaline,* and *psilocybin.* Some prescription drugs, including *anticholinergic drugs* and *levodopa,* occasionally cause hallucinations.

hallux The medical name for the big *toe.*

hallux rigidus Loss of movement in the large joint at the base of the big *toe* as a result of *osteoarthritis.* The joint is usually tender and swollen. Treatment of hallux rigidus comprises resting the toe and wearing a support insert in the shoe. Surgery may be required.

hallux valgus A deformity of the big *toe* in which the joint at the base projects out from the foot, and the top of the toe turns inwards. The condition is more common in women, because it is usually associated with wearing narrow, pointed, high-heeled shoes, but it may be caused by an inherited weakness in the joint. A hallux valgus often leads to formation of a *bunion* or to *osteoarthritis* in the joint, causing pain and limiting foot movement. Severe deformity may be corrected by *osteotomy* or *arthrodesis.*

haloperidol An *antipsychotic drug* used to treat mental illnesses such as *schizophrenia* and *mania.* Haloperidol is also given to control symptoms of *Gilles de la Tourette's* syndrome and, in small doses, to treat agitation and restlessness in the elderly. Side effects include drowsiness, lethargy, weight gain, dizziness, involuntary movements (*tardive dyskinesia*), and *parkinsonism.*

halothane A colourless liquid inhaled as a vapour to induce and maintain general anaesthesia (see *anaesthesia, general*).

hamartoma A noncancerous mass, resembling a tumour, which consists of an overgrowth of tissues that are normally found in the affected part of the body. Hamartomas are common in the skin (the most common is a *haemangioma*), but they also occur in the lungs, heart, or kidneys.

hammer-toe A deformity of the *toe* (usually the second toe) in which the main joint stays bent due to a *tendon* abnormality. A painful *corn* often develops on this joint. A protective pad can ease pressure on the joint and relieve pain, but surgery may be needed if the pain is persistent.

hamstring muscles A group of *muscles* at the back of the thigh. The upper ends of the hamstring muscles are attached by *tendons* to the *pelvis;* the lower ends are attached by tendons called hamstrings to the *tibia* and *fibula.* The hamstring muscles bend the knee and swing the leg backwards from the thigh. Tearing of the hamstring muscles is common in sports. Repeated strenuous exercise may sprain the muscles (see *overuse injury*).

hand The hand is made up of the *wrist,* palm, and fingers. Movement of the hand is achieved mainly by *tendons* that attach the muscles of the forearm to the bones of the hand (the carpals, metacarpals, and phalanges) or by short muscles in the palm of the hand.

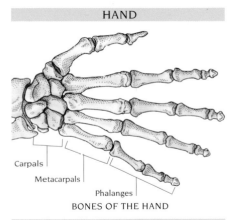

HAND

Carpals

Metacarpals

Phalanges

BONES OF THE HAND

The hands are highly susceptible to injury. *Dermatitis* is also common. The hand may be affected by *Dupuytren's contracture* or *Volkmann's contracture.* Degeneration of a tendon sheath on the upper side of the wrist may cause a harmless swelling called a *ganglion. Osteoarthritis* commonly affects the joint at the base of the thumb. *Rheumatoid arthritis* may cause deformity.

hand–arm vibration syndrome Pain and numbness in the *hand* and arm due to prolonged use of vibrating tools. Symptoms often also include blue or white coloration of the fingers and a tingling sensation in affected areas. Hand–arm vibration syndrome tends to develop slowly over years and is the result of repeated damage to blood vessels and nerves. Exposure to cold tends to aggravate the condition. There is no specific treatment, but avoiding vibrating tools is essential to prevent the disease progressing. In some cases, *calcium channel blockers* may help relieve some symptoms.

handedness Preference for using the right or left hand. Some 90 per cent of adults use the right hand for writing; two thirds prefer the right hand for most activities requiring coordination and skill. The others are either left-handed or ambidextrous (able to use both hands equally well).

Handedness is related to the division of the brain into two hemispheres, each of which controls movement and sensation on the opposite side of the body. In most right-handed people the speech centre is in the left brain hemisphere. *Inheritance* is probably the most important factor in determining handedness.

hand-foot-and-mouth disease An infectious disease, mainly affecting young children, that is caused by the *coxsackievirus*. Hand-foot-and-mouth disease may occur in small epidemics, usually in the summer. The illness is usually mild and lasts for only a few days. Symptoms include blistering of the palms, soles of the feet, and inside of the mouth, and a slight fever. There is no treatment other than mild *analgesic drugs*. The illness is not related to foot-and-mouth disease, which occurs in cattle.

handicap The extent to which a physical or mental *disability* interferes with normal functioning and causes the person to be disadvantaged.

hangnail A strip of skin torn away from the side or base of a fingernail, exposing a raw, painful area.

hangover The unpleasant effects that can be experienced after over-indulgence in *alcohol*, characterized by headache, nausea, *vertigo*, and depression. Alcohol increases production of urine, and some of the symptoms of a hangover are due to mild dehydration. (See also *alcohol intoxication*.)

Hansen's disease A chronic bacterial infection, also called leprosy, that damages nerves, mainly in the limbs and facial area, and may cause skin damage.

The disease is caused by a bacterium, MYCOBACTERIUM LEPRAE, which is spread in droplets of nasal mucus. Hansen's disease is not highly contagious, and a person is infectious only in the early stages. Prolonged close contact puts people at risk. The disease is most prevalent in Asia, Central America, South America, and Africa.

Hansen's disease has a long incubation period – about 3–5 years. There are two main types: the lepromatous type, in which damage is widespread, progressive, and severe; and the tuberculoid type, which is milder. In both types, damage is initially confined to peripheral nerves supplying the skin and muscles. Skin areas supplied by affected nerves become lighter or darker and sensation and sweating are reduced. As the disease progresses, the peripheral nerves swell and become tender. Hands, feet, and facial skin eventually become numb and muscles become paralysed, leading to deformity. Other possible features include blindness, destruction of bone, and sterility.

The presence of the causative bacteria is confirmed by a *skin biopsy*. Drug treatment may be with a combination of *dapsone*, *rifampicin*, and clofazimine, which kills most of the bacteria in a few days. Any damage that has occurred before treatment, however, is irreversible. *Plastic surgery* may be necessary to correct deformities; and nerve and tendon transplants may improve the function of damaged limbs.

hantavirus A viral infection that is transmitted to humans through the urine or faeces of infected rodents, such as rats. Symptoms range from a minor flu-like illness with headache and a sore throat to high fever, nausea and vomiting, and abnormal bleeding. Some strains of hantavirus can cause severe infections which may lead to *kidney failure*, serious lung damage, and death.

hardening of the arteries The popular term for *atherosclerosis*.

hare lip A common term for the *birth defect* in which there is a split in the upper lip due to failure of the two sides to fuse during fetal development. A hare lip is often associated with a similar failure of the two halves of the palate to join. (See also *cleft lip and palate*.)

Hashimoto's thyroiditis An *autoimmune disorder* in which the body's immune system develops *antibodies* against its own thyroid gland cells. As a result, the thyroid gland cannot produce enough *thyroid hormones*, a condition known as *hypothyroidism*. The principal symptoms of Hashimoto's thyroiditis are tiredness, muscle weakness, and weight gain, and the thyroid gland becomes enlarged.

Diagnosis is confirmed by *blood tests*. Treatment is by thyroid hormone replacement therapy, which is life-long.

hashish Another name for *marijuana*.

hay fever The popular name for a seasonal form of allergic rhinitis (see *rhinitis, allergic*).

HDL The abbreviation for *high density lipoprotein*.

headache One of the most common types of pain. A headache is only rarely a symptom of a serious underlying disorder. The pain arises from tension in the *meninges*, and in the blood vessels and muscles of the scalp.

Many headaches are simply a response to some adverse stimulus, such as hunger. Such headaches usually clear up quickly. Tension headaches, caused by tightening in the face, neck, and scalp muscles as a result of stress or poor posture, are also common, and may last for days or weeks. *Migraine* is a severe, incapacitating headache preceded or accompanied by visual and/or stomach disturbances. *Cluster headaches* cause intense pain behind one eye.

Common causes of headache include *hangover* and noisy or stuffy environments. *Food additives* may also be a cause. Some headaches are due to overuse of painkillers (see *analgesic drugs*). Other possible causes include *sinusitis*, *toothache*, *cervical osteoarthritis*, and *head injury*. Among the rare causes of headache are a *brain tumour*, *hypertension*, *temporal arteritis*, an *aneurysm*, and increased pressure within the skull.

Most headaches can be relieved by painkillers and rest. If a neurological cause is suspected, *CT scanning* or *MRI* may be performed.

head-banging The persistent, rhythmic banging of the head against a wall or hard object. Head-banging is seen in some people with severe *learning difficulties*, particularly those who lack stimulation. It also occurs in some normal toddlers, often when they are frustrated or angry; most children grow out of the behaviour.

head injury Injury to the head may occur as a result of a blow or a fall. The severity of the injury depends on whether the brain is affected. A blow may shake or bruise the brain (see *brain damage*). If the skull is broken (see *skull, fracture of*), foreign material or bone may enter the brain and lead to infection. A blow or a penetrating injury may cause swelling of the brain, or tear blood vessels, which may lead to *brain haemorrhage*.

If the head injury is mild, there may only be a slight headache. In some cases there is *concussion*. More severe head injuries may result in unconsciousness or *coma*, which may be fatal. *Amnesia* may occur. After a severe brain injury, there may be some muscular weakness or *paralysis* and loss of sensation. Symptoms such as persistent vomiting, double vision, or a deteriorating level of consciousness could suggest progressive brain damage.

Investigations may include *skull X-rays* and *CT scanning*. A blood clot inside the skull may be life-threatening and requires surgical removal; severe skull fractures may also require surgery. Recovery from concussion may take several days. There may be permanent physical or mental disability if the brain has been damaged. Recovery from a major head injury can be very slow, but there may be signs of progressive improvement for several years after the injury occurred.

head lag The backward flopping of the head that occurs when an infant is placed in a sitting position. Head lag is obvious in a newborn because the neck muscles are still weak, but by 4 months the baby can hold his or her head upright (see *child development*).

healing The process by which the body repairs bone, tissue, or organ damage caused by injury, infection, or disease.

The initial stages of healing are the same in all parts of the body. After injury, *blood clots* form in damaged tissues. White *blood cells, enzymes, histamine,* other chemicals, and *proteins* from which new cells can be made accumulate at the site of damage. Fibrous tissue is laid down within the blood clot to form a supportive structure, and any dead cells are broken down and absorbed by the white blood cells. Some tissues, such as bone and skin, are then able to regenerate by the proliferation of new cells around the damaged area. In skin injuries, the fibrous tissue shrinks as new skin forms underneath. The tissue hardens to form a scab, which falls off when new skin growth is complete. A scar may remain.

An inadequate blood supply or persistent infection prevents regeneration, and some tissues, such as nerve tissue, may be unable to regenerate. In these cases, the fibrous tissue may develop into tough scar tissue, which keeps the tissue structure intact but may impair its function.

health At its simplest, the absence of physical and mental disease. A wider concept promoted by the World Health Organization is that all people should have the opportunity to fulfil their genetic potential. This includes the ability to develop without the impediments of poor nutrition, environmental contamination, or infectious diseases. (See *diet and disease*; *health hazards*.)

health centre A building owned by a local authority and leased to general practitioners and other healthcare professionals as premises for their work.

health food A term applied to any food products thought to promote health.

health hazards Environmental factors that are known to cause, or are suspected of causing, disease. The main types of health hazard are: *infectious disease* (see *bacteria*; *fungal infections*; *insects and disease*; *viruses*; *zoonosis*); an insufficient supply, or the contamination, of food and water (see *food additives*; *food-borne infection*; *food poisoning*); work-related hazards (see *occupational disease and injury*); hazards associated with domestic and social life; tobacco-*smoking* and *alcohol*; and global environmental hazards (see *pollution*; *radiation hazards*; *sunlight, adverse effects of*).

hearing The sense that enables sound to be perceived. The *ear* transforms the sound waves it receives into nerve impulses that pass to the *brain*.

Each ear has three distinct regions: the outer, middle, and inner ear. Sound waves are channelled through the ear canal to the middle ear, from where a complex system of membranes and tiny bones conveys the vibrations to the inner ear. The vibrations are converted into nerve impulses in the *cochlea*. These impulses travel along the auditory nerve to the medulla of the brain. From there, they pass via the *thalamus* to the superior temporal gyrus, part of the cerebral cortex involved in perceiving sound. (See also *deafness*.)

hearing aids Electronic devices that improve hearing in people with certain types of *deafness*. A hearing aid consists of a tiny microphone (to pick up sounds), an amplifier (to increase their volume), and a speaker (to transmit sounds). (See also *cochlear implant*.)

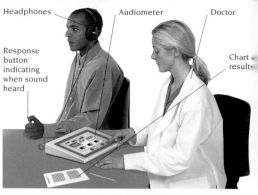

HEARING TESTS

Headphones — Audiometer — Doctor

Response button indicating when sound heard

Chart results

AUDIOMETRY

hearing loss A deterioration in the ability to perceive sound. (See also *deafness*.)

hearing tests Tests carried out to assess *hearing*. Hearing tests are performed as part of a routine assessment of *child development* and when hearing impairment is suspected. The tests are sometimes included in a general medical examination. Hearing tests may also be used to identify the cause of *tinnitus* or dizziness.

An audiometer (an electrical instrument) is used to test an individual's ability to hear sounds at different frequencies and volumes. The lowest level at which a person can hear and repeat words (the speech reception threshold) is tested, as is the ability to hear words clearly (speech discrimination). The type of hearing loss (see *deafness*) is determined by holding a tuning fork to different parts of the ear. (See also *tympanometry*.)

heart The hollow muscular pump in the centre of the chest that beats continuously and rhythmically to send *blood* to the lungs and the rest of the body. Much of the heart consists of myocardium, a special type of muscle. The heart muscle is supplied with oxygen and nutrients by two *coronary arteries*.

The internal surface of the heart is lined with a smooth membrane, called the endocardium, and the entire heart is enclosed in a tough, membranous bag, *pericardium*. Inside the heart there are four chambers. A thick central muscular wall, the septum, divides the heart cavity into right and left halves. Each half consists of an upper chamber, called an *atrium*, and a larger lower chamber, called a *ventricle*.

The right atrium receives deoxygenated blood from the entire body via two large veins called the *venae cavae*. This blood is transferred to the right ventricle and pumped to the lungs via the pulmonary artery to be oxygenated and to lose carbon dioxide. The left atrium of the heart receives oxygenated blood from the lungs (via the pulmonary veins); this blood is transferred to the left ventricle and then pumped to all tissues in the body. One-way valves at the exits from each chamber ensure that blood flows in only one direction (see *heart valves*).

As resistance to blood flow through the general circulation is much greater than resistance through the lungs, the left side of the heart must contract more forcibly than the right, and has greater muscular bulk.

heart, artificial An implantable mechanical device that takes over the action of the *heart* or assists the heart in maintaining the circulation. Problems that may occur with artificial hearts include the formation of blood clots within the mechanical device, and infection. They are therefore used as a temporary measure until a *heart transplant* can be performed.

HEART

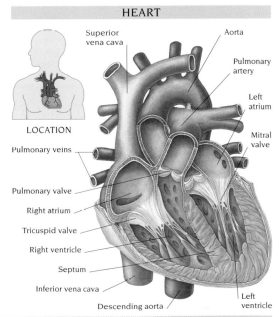

LOCATION

Superior vena cava
Aorta
Pulmonary artery
Left atrium
Mitral valve
Pulmonary veins
Pulmonary valve
Right atrium
Tricuspid valve
Right ventricle
Septum
Inferior vena cava
Descending aorta
Left ventricle

H

heart attack See *myocardial infarction*.

heartbeat A contraction of the *heart* that pumps blood to the lungs and the rest of the body. The different parts of the heart contract in a precise sequence that is brought about by electrical impulses that emanate from the *sino-atrial node* at the top of the right *atrium*. Three phases make up a cycle of one heartbeat: the diastole (resting phase), the atrial systole (atrial contraction), and the ventricular systole (ventricular contraction). The rate at which contractions occur is called the *heart-rate*. The term *pulse* refers to the character and rate of the heartbeat when it is felt at certain points around the body (at the wrist, for example).

heart block A common disorder of the *heartbeat* caused by an interruption to the passage of impulses through the heart's conducting system.

There are several grades of heart block, from a slight delay between the contractions of the atria (see *atrium*) and *ventricles* (called a prolonged P-R interval) to complete heart block, in which the atria and ventricles beat independently. Heart block may be due to *coronary artery disease, myocarditis,* overdose of a *digitalis drug,* or *rheumatic fever.*

A prolonged P-R interval causes no symptoms. In more severe heart block, the rate of ventricular contraction does not increase in response to exercise. This may cause breathlessness as a result of *heart failure,* or chest pains due to *angina pectoris.* If the ventricular beat becomes very slow, or if it stops altogether for a few seconds, loss of consciousness and *seizure* may occur due to insufficient blood reaching the brain. If the delay is prolonged, a stroke may result.

Symptomless heart block may not need treatment. Heart block that is causing symptoms is usually treated by the fitting of an artificial *pacemaker.*

heartburn A burning pain in the centre of the chest, which may travel from the tip of the breastbone to the throat. It may be caused by eating rich or spicy food, or by drinking alcohol. Recurrent heartburn is a symptom of *oesophagitis,* which is usually caused by *gastro-oesophageal reflux disease.* Heartburn is often brought on by lying down or bending forwards.

heart disease, congenital Any abnormality of the *heart* present from birth. Defects may affect the heart chambers, *valves,* or main blood vessels. Major abnormalities are *septal defects, coarctation of the aorta, transposition of the great vessels, patent ductus arteriosus, tetralogy of Fallot, hypoplastic left heart syndrome, pulmonary stenosis,* and *aortic stenosis.*

Developmental errors leading to defects arise early in the life of the *embryo.* In most cases, there is no known cause. *Rubella* in the mother is the most common known cause.

The onset and severity of symptoms depend on the defect. Some anomalies cause *cyanosis* and breathlessness but others may go undetected. Possible complications of an untreated heart defect include impaired growth, *pneumonia* as a result of mild respiratory infections, rapid tiring during exercise, and *Eisenmenger complex.*

Antenatal diagnosis, using specialized *ultrasound scanning,* is possible for most defects. After birth, any suspected defect is investigated using *chest X-rays, ECG,* or *echocardiography.*

Oxygen and various drug treatments may improve the symptoms of heart block. Some conditions, such as small septal defects or patent ductus arteriosus, may get smaller or disappear of their own accord. Other defects will require surgical correction. Narrowed heart valves can often be treated by balloon *valvuloplasty.* In other cases, *open heart surgery* or a *heart transplant* may be required.

Children with heart defects are at an increased risk of bacterial *endocarditis;* to prevent this, they are given *antibiotic drugs* before all surgical procedures including dental treatments.

heart disease, ischaemic The most common form of heart disease, in which narrowing or obstruction of the coronary arteries, usually by *atherosclerosis,* results in a reduced blood supply (see *coronary artery disease*).

heart, disorders of A wide range of disorders can disrupt the heart's action. In general, genetic factors do not play a large part in causing heart disorders, however they do contribute to the *hyperlipidaemias* that predispose a person to *atherosclerosis* and *coronary artery disease*. Structural abnormalities in the heart are among the most common birth defects (see *heart disease, congenital*).

Infections after birth may result in *endocarditis* or *myocarditis*. Tumours arising from the heart tissues are rare. They include noncancerous *myxomas* and cancerous *sarcomas*.

The heart muscle may become thin and flabby from lack of protein and calories. *Thiamine* (vitamin B_1) deficiency, common in alcoholics, causes *beriberi* with congestive *heart failure*. Alcohol poisoning over many years may cause a type of *cardiomyopathy*. *Obesity* is an important factor in heart disease, probably through its effect on other risk factors, such as *hypertension, diabetes*, and *cholesterol*.

The coronary arteries may become narrowed due to *atherosclerosis*, depriving areas of heart muscle of oxygen. The result may be *angina pectoris* or, eventually, a *myocardial infarction*.

Some drugs, such as the anticancer drug *doxorubicin*, *tricyclic antidepressants*, and even drugs used to treat heart disease, may disturb the heartbeat or damage the heart muscle.

Many common and serious heart disorders may be a complication of an underlying condition, such as cardiomyopathy or a congenital defect. Such disorders include cardiac *arrhythmia*, some cases of *heart block*, and heart failure. *Cor pulmonale* is a failure of the right side of the heart as a consequence of lung disease.

heart failure Inability of the *heart* to cope with its workload of pumping blood to the lungs and to the rest of the body. Heart failure can primarily affect the right or the left side of the heart, although it most commonly affects both sides, in which case it is known as congestive, or chronic, heart failure.

Left-sided heart failure may be caused by *hypertension*, *anaemia*, hyperthyroidism, a *heart valve* defect (such as *aortic stenosis*, *aortic incompetence*, or *mitral incompetence*), or a congenital heart defect (see *heart disease, congenital*). Other causes of left-sided heart failure include *coronary artery disease*, *myocardial infarction*, *cardiac arrhythmias*, and *cardiomyopathy*.

The left side of the heart fails to empty completely with each contraction, or has difficulty in accepting blood that has been returned from the lungs. The retained blood creates a back pressure that causes the lungs to become congested with blood. This condition leads to *pulmonary oedema*.

Right-sided heart failure most often results from *pulmonary hypertension*, which is itself caused by left-sided failure or by lung disease (such as chronic obstructive pulmonary disease (see *pulmonary disease, chronic obstructive*). Right-sided failure can also be due to a valve defect, such as *tricuspid incompetence*, or a congenital heart defect.

There is back pressure in the circulation from the heart into the venous system, causing swollen neck veins, enlargement of the liver, and *oedema*, especially of the legs and ankles. The intestines may become congested, causing discomfort.

Treatment depends on the underlying cause but may include *diuretic drugs*, *ACE inhibitor drugs*, *digitalis drugs*, and oxygen. Acute left-sided failure is an emergency and needs immediate hospital treatment.

heart imaging Techniques that provide images of heart structure. Imaging is used to detect disease or abnormalities.

A *chest X-ray*, the simplest and most widely used method of heart imaging, shows heart size and shape, and the presence of abnormal *calcification*. Pulmonary oedema and engorgement of the vessels connecting the heart and lungs are also usually detectable.

Echocardiography is useful for investigating congenital heart defects and abnormalities of the valves or heart wall. An ultrasound technique using the *Doppler effect* allows measurement of blood flow through valves. *Radionuclide scanning* and *CT scanning* provide information about the efficiency of heart function. *Angiography* may be used to show the heart chambers and to assess the condition of the coronary arteries and valves. High-quality images of the heart can be obtained by *MRI*.

heart–lung machine A machine that temporarily takes over the function of the *heart* and *lungs* to facilitate operations such as *open heart surgery*, *heart transplants*, and *heart-lung transplants*.

A heart–lung machine consists of a pump (to replace the heart's function) and an oxygenator (to replace the lung's function). The machine bypasses the heart and lungs, and the heart can be stopped.

Use of a heart–lung machine tends to damage red blood cells and to cause blood clotting. These problems can be minimized, however, by the administration of *heparin*, an anticoagulant drug, beforehand.

heart–lung transplant A procedure in which the *heart* and *lungs* of a patient are removed, and replaced with donor organs. This surgery is used to treat diseases in which the lung damage has affected the heart, or vice versa. Such diseases include *cystic fibrosis*, *fibrosing*

alveolitis, and some severe congenital heart defects (see *heart disease, congenital*). A *heart–lung machine* is used to take over the function of the patient's heart and lungs during the operation, which is no more dangerous than a *heart transplant*.

heart-rate The rate at which the *heart* contracts to pump blood around the body. Most people have a heart-rate of between 60 and 100 beats per minute at rest. This rate tends to be faster in childhood and to slow slightly with age. Very fit people may have a resting rate below 60 beats per minute.

The heart muscle responds automatically to any increase in the amount of blood returned to it from active muscles by increasing its output. During extreme exercise, heart-rate may increase to 200 contractions per minute and the output to almost 250 ml per beat.

The heart-rate is also regulated by the *autonomic nervous system*. The parts of this system concerned with heart action are a nucleus of nerve cells, called the cardiac centre, in the *brainstem*, and two sets of nerves (the parasympathetic and sympathetic).

HEART–LUNG MACHINE

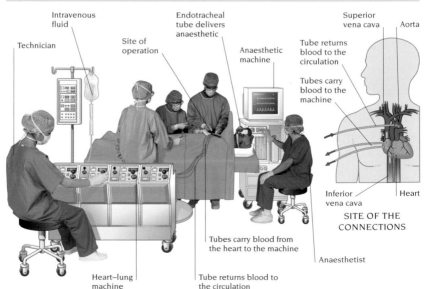

Intravenous fluid

Technician

Site of operation

Endotracheal tube delivers anaesthetic

Anaesthetic machine

Superior vena cava · Aorta

Tube returns blood to the circulation

Tubes carry blood to the machine

Inferior vena cava · Heart

SITE OF THE CONNECTIONS

Tubes carry blood from the heart to the machine

Anaesthetist

Heart–lung machine

Tube returns blood to the circulation

At rest, the parasympathetic nerves – particularly the *vagus nerve* – act on the sinoatrial node to maintain a slow heart-rate. During or in anticipation of muscular activity, this inhibition lessens and the heart-rate speeds up. Sympathetic nerves release *noradrenaline*, which further increases the heart-rate and force of contraction. Sympathetic activity can be triggered by fear or anger, low blood pressure, or a reduction of oxygen in the blood.

Release of *adrenaline* and noradrenaline by the adrenal glands also acts to increase heart-rate.

The rate and rhythm of the heart can be measured by feeling the *pulse* or by listening with a *stethoscope*; a more accurate record is provided by an *ECG*.

A resting heart-rate above 100 beats per minute is termed a *tachycardia*, and a rate below 60 beats per minute a *bradycardia*. (See also *arrhythmia, cardiac*.)

heart sounds The sounds made by the *heart* during each *heartbeat*. In each heart cycle, there are two main heart sounds that can clearly be heard through a *stethoscope*. The first is like a "lubb". It results from closure of the *tricuspid* and *mitral valves* at the exits of the atria, which occurs when the ventricles begin contracting to pump blood out of the heart. The second sound is a higher-pitched "dupp" caused by closure of the pulmonary and aortic valves at the exits of the ventricles when the ventricles finish contracting.

Abnormal heart sounds may be a sign of various disorders. For example, high-pitched sounds or "clicks" are due to the abrupt halting of valve opening, which can occur in people with certain *heart valve* defects. Heart *murmurs* are abnormal sounds caused by turbulent blood flow. These may be due to heart valve defects or congenital heart disease.

heart surgery Any operation that is performed on the *heart*. Open heart surgery allows the treatment of most types of heart defect present at birth (see *heart disease, congenital*) and various disorders of the *heart valves*. Coronary artery *bypass* is performed to treat obstruction of the coronary arteries. Narrowing of the coronary arteries can be treated by balloon *angioplasty* and insertion of a *stent*. Angioplasty balloons have also been used to open up narrowed heart valves in cases where the patient is unsuitable for open heart surgery (see *valvuloplasty*). *Heart transplant* surgery can offer hope to people with progressive, incurable heart disease.

heart transplant Replacement of a patient's damaged or diseased *heart* with a healthy heart taken from a donor at the time of death. Typically, transplant patients have advanced *coronary artery disease* or *cardiomyopathy*. During the operation, the function of the heart is taken over by a *heart–lung machine*. Most of the diseased heart is removed, but the back walls of the atria (upper chambers) are left in place. The ventricles (upper chambers) are then attached to the remaining areas of the recipient's heart. Once the immediate post-operative period is over, the outlook is good. Patients face the long-term problems associated with other forms of *transplant surgery*. (See also *heart–lung transplant*.)

HEART TRANSPLANT

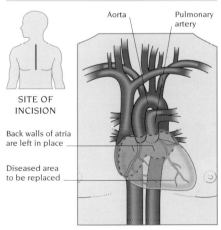

Aorta

Pulmonary artery

SITE OF INCISION

Back walls of atria are left in place

Diseased area to be replaced

heart valve A structure at the exit of a *heart* chamber that allows blood to flow out of the chamber, but prevents backwash. There are four heart valves: aortic, pulmonary, mitral, and tricuspid. Their opening and closing during each heart cycle produces *heart sounds*.

Any of the four heart valves may be affected by *stenosis* (narrowing), which causes the heart to work harder to force blood through the valve, or by incompetence or insufficiency (leakiness), which makes the valve unable to prevent backwash of blood. These defects cause characteristic heart *murmurs*.

Heart-valve defects may be present at birth (see *heart disease, congenital*), or they may be acquired later in life. The most common congenital valve defects are *aortic stenosis* and *pulmonary stenosis*. Acquired heart-valve disease is usually the result of degenerative changes or *ischaemia* affecting part of the heart and leading to aortic stenosis or *mitral incompetence*. *Rheumatic fever* can cause *mitral stenosis*, mitral incompetence, aortic valve defects, *tricuspid stenosis* and *tricuspid incompetence*. The heart valves may also be damaged by bacterial *endocarditis*.

Heart-valve disorders commonly lead to *heart failure, arrhythmias*, or symptoms resulting from reduced blood supply to body tissues.

Heart-valve defects may be diagnosed by *auscultation, chest X-ray, ECG*, or *echocardiography* and may be corrected by *heart-valve surgery*.

heart-valve surgery An operation to correct a *heart valve* defect or to remove a diseased or damaged valve. A heart valve may have to be repaired, widened, or replaced because it is either incompetent (leaky) or stenotic (narrowed). Widening of a valve may involve *valvotomy* or *valvuloplasty*. A damaged valve can be replaced by a mechanical one (fashioned from metal and plastic), a valve constructed from human tissue, a pig valve, or a valve taken from a human donor after death. A *heart–lung machine* is used during replacement.

After heart-valve surgery, symptoms such as breathlessness may take weeks to improve and require medication to be continued. Some people need long-term treatment with *anticoagulant drugs* to prevent the formation of blood clots around the new valve.

heat cramps Painful contractions in muscles that are caused by excessive salt loss as a result of profuse *sweating*.

Heat cramps are usually brought on by strenuous activity in extreme heat. The condition may occur independently, or is sometimes a symptom of *heat exhaustion* or *heatstroke*. Prevention and treatment consist of taking salt tablets or drinking weak salt solution.

heat disorders The body functions most efficiently around 37°C, and any major temperature deviation disrupts body processes. The malfunctioning or overloading of the body's mechanisms for keeping internal temperature constant may cause a heat disorder.

The mechanisms by which the body loses unwanted heat are controlled by the *hypothalamus* in the brain. When blood temperature rises, the hypothalamus sends out nerve impulses to stimulate the *sweat glands* and dilate blood vessels in the skin, which cools the body down. However, excessive sweating may result in an imbalance of salts and fluids in the body, which may lead to *heat cramps* or *heat exhaustion*. When the hypothalamus is disrupted (for example, by a *fever*), the body may overheat, leading to *heatstroke*. Excessive external heat may cause *prickly heat*.

Most heat disorders can be prevented by gradual acclimatization to hot conditions and taking salt tablets or solution. A light diet and frequent cool baths or showers may also help. Alcohol and strenuous exercise should be avoided.

heat exhaustion *Fatigue*, culminating in collapse, caused by overexposure to heat. There are three main causes of heat exhaustion: insufficient water intake, insufficient salt intake, and a deficiency in *sweat* production. In addition to fatigue, symptoms may include faintness, dizziness, nausea and vomiting, headache, and, when salt loss is heavy, *heat cramps*. The skin is usually pale and clammy, breathing is fast and shallow, and the pulse is rapid and weak. Unless it is treated, heat exhaustion may develop into *heatstroke*. Treatment of heat exhaustion involves rest, and replenishment of lost water and salt. Prevention is usually by gradual acclimatization to hot conditions.

heatstroke A life-threatening condition in which overexposure to heat coupled with a breakdown of the body's heat-regulating mechanisms cause the body to become dangerously overheated.

Heatstroke is most commonly caused by prolonged, unaccustomed exposure to the sun in a hot climate. Strenuous activity, unsuitable clothing, overeating, and drinking too much alcohol are sometimes contributory factors.

Heatstroke is often preceded by *heat exhaustion*, which consists of fatigue and profuse *sweating*. With the onset of heatstroke, the sweating diminishes and may stop entirely. The skin becomes hot and dry, breathing is shallow, and the pulse is rapid and weak. Body temperature rises dramatically and, without treatment, the victim may lose consciousness and even die.

Heatstroke can be prevented by gradual acclimatization to hot conditions (see *heat disorders*). If heatstroke develops, emergency hospital treatment is required.

heat treatment The use of heat to treat disease, aid recovery from injury, or to relieve pain. Heat treatment is useful for certain conditions, such as ligament sprains, as it stimulates blood flow and promotes healing of tissues.

Moist heat may be administered by soaking the affected area in a warm bath, or by applying a hot *compress* or *poultice*. Dry heat may be administered by a heating pad, hot-water bottle, or by a heat lamp that produces *infra-red* rays. More precise methods of administering heat to tissues deeper in the body include *ultrasound treatment* and short-wave *diathermy*.

heel The part of the *foot* below the *ankle* and behind the arch. The heel consists of the *calcaneus* (heel bone), an underlying pad of fat that acts as a cushion, and a layer of skin, which is usually thickened due to pressure from walking.

Heimlich manoeuvre A first-aid treatment for *choking*. The sole aim of the Heimlich manoeuvre is to dislodge the material that is causing the blockage by placing one fist, covered by the other, just below the victim's ribcage, and pulling sharply inwards and upwards to give an abdominal thrust.

Helicobacter pylori A bacterium that is the cause of most *peptic ulcers* as well as

a factor in *stomach cancer*. The bacterium damages the mucus layer of the stomach and duodenum, allowing gastric acid to cause ulceration. HELICOBACTER PYLORI infection may be diagnosed by testing the breath, blood, or faeces. Treatment with *antibiotics* to eradicate the infection and drugs to suppress acid production, such as *omeprazole*, has proved successful in achieving long-term recovery from peptic ulcers. After treatment, reinfection with HELICOBACTER PYLORI is rare.

heliotherapy A form of *phototherapy* involving exposure to sunlight.

helminth infestation Infection by any parasitic worm. (See *worm infestation*.)

hemianopia Loss of half of the *visual field* in each eye. Hemianopia may be "homonymous" (in which the same side of both eyes is affected) or "heteronymous" (in which the loss is in opposite sides of the eyes). Visual loss may be temporary or permanent.

Hemianopia is not due to a disorder of the eyes themselves but results from damage to the *optic nerves* or brain. Transient homonymous hemianopia in young people is usually caused by *migraine*. In older people, it occurs in *transient ischaemic attacks*. Permanent homonymous hemianopia is usually caused by a *stroke*, but it may result from brain damage by a tumour, injury, or infection. Hemianopia may also be

HEIMLICH MANOEUVRE

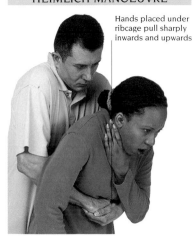

Hands placed under ribcage pull sharply inwards and upwards

caused by pressure on the optic nerve from a *pituitary tumour*.

hemiballismus Irregular, uncontrollable, flinging arm and leg movements on one side of the body, caused by disease of the *basal ganglia*. (See also *athetosis*; *chorea*.)

hemicolectomy The surgical removal of half, or a major portion, of the *colon*. (See also *colectomy*.)

hemiparesis Muscular weakness or partial *paralysis* affecting only one side of the body (see *hemiplegia*).

hemiplegia *Paralysis* or weakness on one side of the body, caused by damage or disease affecting the motor nerve tracts in the opposite side of the brain. A common cause is a *stroke*. Others include *head injury*, *brain tumour*, *brain haemorrhage*, *encephalitis*, *multiple sclerosis*, complications of *meningitis*, or a *conversion disorder*. Treatment is for the underlying cause, and is carried out in conjunction with *physiotherapy*.

Henoch–Schönlein purpura Inflammation of small blood vessels, causing leakage of blood into the skin, joints, kidneys, and intestine. The disease is most common in young children, and may occur after an infection such as a sore throat. The condition may also be due to an abnormal allergic reaction.

The main symptom is a raised purplish rash on the buttocks and backs of the limbs. The joints are swollen and often painful, and colicky abdominal pain may occur. In some cases, there is intestinal bleeding, leading to blood in the faeces. The kidneys may become inflamed, resulting in blood and protein in the urine.

The only treatment usually required is bed rest and *analgesic drugs*. Complications may arise if kidney inflammation persists. In severe cases, *corticosteroid drugs* may be given.

heparin An *anticoagulant drug* used to prevent and treat abnormal *blood clotting*. Heparin is given by injection and is used as an immediate treatment for *deep vein thrombosis* or for *pulmonary embolism*. Low molecular weight heparins, such as *tinzaparin*, which need to be injected once a day, are now widely used and can be self-administered at home.

Adverse effects of heparin include rash, aching bones, and abnormal bleeding

in different parts of the body. Long-term use may cause *osteoporosis*.

hepatectomy, partial Surgical removal of part of the *liver*. Surgery may be needed to remove a damaged area of liver following injury, or to treat noncancerous liver tumours and *hydatid disease*. Rarely, *liver cancer* is treated in this way.

hepatectomy, total Surgical removal of the *liver*. Hepatectomy is the first stage in a *liver transplant* operation.

hepatic Relating to the *liver*.

hepatitis Inflammation of the *liver*, with accompanying damage to liver cells. The condition may be acute (see *hepatitis, acute*) or chronic (see *hepatitis, chronic*) and have various causes. (See also *hepatitis A*; *hepatitis B*; *hepatitis C*; *hepatitis D*; *hepatitis E*; *hepatitis, viral*.)

hepatitis A Also called epidemic *hepatitis*, a disorder caused by the hepatitis A virus, which is transmitted in contaminated food or drink. The incubation period lasts for 15–40 days, after which nausea, fever, and *jaundice* develop. Recovery usually occurs within 3 weeks. Serious complications are rare. *Immunization* provides the best protection against hepatitis A, and may be advised for people visiting Mediterranean or developing countries. An attack can confer immunity against further infection.

hepatitis, acute Short-term inflammation of the *liver*. In some cases, acute hepatitis may progress to chronic hepatitis (see *hepatitis, chronic*), but it rarely leads to acute *liver failure*.

Acute hepatitis is fairly common. The most frequent cause is infection with a hepatitis virus (see *hepatitis, viral*), but it can be caused by other infections such as *cytomegalovirus* infection or *Legionnaires' disease*. It may also result from an overdose of *halothane* or *paracetamol* or exposure to toxic chemicals including alcohol (see *liver disease, alcoholic*). However, in some cases no cause can be identified. Symptoms range from few and mild to severe with pain, fever, and *jaundice*. Blood tests, including *liver function tests*, may be used for diagnosis. In most cases, natural recovery occurs within a few weeks. If the disorder is caused by exposure to a chemical or drug, detoxification using an *antidote* may be possible.

Intensive care may be required if the liver is badly damaged. Rarely, a *liver transplant* is the only way of saving life. In all cases, alcohol should be avoided.

hepatitis B A disorder caused by the hepatitis B virus. The virus is transmitted in blood, blood products, or other body fluids, often through sharing needles, blood transfusions, or sexual contact. The incubation period lasts for 1–6 months, then symptoms, such as headache, fever, and *jaundice*, develop suddenly. Most people recover, but hepatitis B can be fatal. *Immunization* may be advised for people at high risk of exposure to the virus, such as healthcare workers or visitors to areas where hepatitis B is prevalent.

In about 5 per cent of cases, the virus continues to cause inflammation and can still be detected in the blood 6 months after infection. People who suffer from persistent infection are at long-term risk of *liver cancer* and *cirrhosis* and may be treated with *interferon*.

hepatitis C Caused by the hepatitis C virus, this infection is often transmitted through sharing needles. Blood transfusions no longer pose a significant risk because of blood screening.

Hepatitis C has an incubation period of 6–12 months and begins as a mild illness which may go undetected. In about 3 in 4 patients, chronic hepatitis develops (see *hepatitis, chronic*), which can progress to *cirrhosis* of the liver and an increased risk of *hepatoma*.

hepatitis, chronic Long-term inflammation of the *liver*. It eventually causes scar tissue to form and leads to liver *cirrhosis* and *portal hypertension*.

Chronic hepatitis may develop following an attack of acute hepatitis (see *hepatitis, acute*). It may also occur as the result of an *autoimmune disorder*, a viral infection (see *hepatitis, viral*), a reaction to certain types of drugs or, more rarely, to a *metabolic disorder*, such as *haemochromatosis* or *Wilson's disease*.

Chronic hepatitis may cause slight tiredness or no symptoms at all. It is diagnosed by *liver biopsy*. Autoimmune hepatitis is treated with *corticosteroid drugs* and *immunosuppressants*. Viral infections often respond to *interferon*.

In the drug-induced type, withdrawal of the medication can lead to recovery. For metabolic disturbances, treatment depends on the underlying disorder.

hepatitis D An infection of the liver caused by the hepatitis D virus, which occurs only in people who already have *hepatitis B* infection. People who develop hepatitis D will usually suffer from severe chronic liver disease.

hepatitis E A type of *hepatitis*, caused by the hepatitis E virus, transmitted in contaminated food or drink. The disease is similar to *hepatitis A*.

hepatitis, viral Any type of *hepatitis* caused by a viral infection. Five viruses that attack the liver as their primary target have been identified. They cause *hepatitis A*, *hepatitis B*, *hepatitis C*, *hepatitis D*, and *hepatitis E*.

hepatoma A type of *liver cancer*.

hepatomegaly Enlargement of the *liver*, occurring as a result of any liver disorder (see *liver, disorders of*).

herbal medicine Systems of medical treatment in which various parts of different plants are used to promote health and to treat symptoms.

hereditary spherocytosis See *spherocytosis, hereditary*.

heredity The transmission of traits and disorders through genetic mechanisms. Each individual inherits a combination of *genes* via the sperm and egg cells from which he or she is derived. The interaction of the genes determines inherited characteristics, including, in some cases, disorders or susceptibility to disorders. (See also *genetic disorders*; *inheritance*.)

heritability A measure of the extent to which a disease or disorder is the result of inherited factors, as opposed to environmental influences such as diet and climate. Certain disorders (such as *haemophilia* or *cystic fibrosis*) are known to be caused entirely by hereditary factors. Others are caused by environmental factors. Between these extremes are many disorders (such as *schizophrenia*) in which both inheritance and environment probably play a part.

A rough estimate of heritability can be obtained from the known incidence of a disorder in the first-degree relatives of affected people compared with the incidence of the disorder in a population exposed to similar environmental influences. Estimates of heritability are useful in *genetic counselling*. (See also *genetic disorders*.)

hermaphroditism A *congenital* disorder in which *gonads* of both sexes are present, and the external genitalia are not clearly male or female. True hermaphroditism is extremely rare and its cause unknown. A more common condition is *pseudohermaphroditism*, in which the gonads of only one sex are present, but the external genitalia are not clearly either male or female.

hernia The protrusion of an organ or tissue through a weak area in the muscle or other tissue that normally contains it. The term is usually applied to a protrusion of the intestine through the abdominal wall. In a *hiatus hernia*, the stomach protrudes through the diaphragm and into the chest.

Abdominal hernias are usually due to a *congenital* weakness in the wall of the abdomen. The hernias may result from damage caused by lifting heavy objects, persistent coughing, or straining to defaecate, or may develop after an operation.

There are several types of hernia, and they are classified according to their location in the body. The most important are inguinal hernias, which mainly affect men; femoral hernias, which are more common in overweight women; and umbilical hernias, which occur in babies.

The first symptom of an abdominal hernia is usually a bulge in the abdominal wall. There may also be abdominal discomfort. Sometimes the protruding intestine can be pushed back into place. Severe pain occurs when the hernia bulges out and cannot be put back; surgery (see *hernia repair*) is usually necessary. If the blood supply to a twisted, trapped portion of intestine becomes impaired (a strangulated hernia), *gangrene* of the bowel may develop. A strangulated hernia requires urgent treatment. Umbilical hernias in babies can usually be left untreated as they tend to disappear naturally by age 5.

hernia repair Surgical correction of a *hernia*. Surgery is usually performed to treat a hernia of the abdominal wall that is painful or cannot be pushed back into place. A strangulated hernia requires an emergency operation. During surgery, the protruding intestine is pushed back into the abdomen and the weakened muscle wall is strengthened. Either open or *minimally invasive surgery* may be used.

herniated disc See *disc prolapse*.

herniorrhaphy Surgical correction of a *hernia*. (See *hernia repair*.)

heroin A *narcotic drug* similar to *morphine*. When used for medical purposes, it is generally known as *diamorphine*. Heroin is a white or brownish powder that can be smoked, sniffed, or dissolved in water and injected.

As well as having an analgesic effect, heroin produces sensations of warmth, calmness, drowsiness, and a loss of concern for outside events. Long-term use of the drug causes *tolerance* and psychological and physical dependence (see *drug dependence*; *heroin abuse*). Sudden withdrawal produces shivering, abdominal cramps, diarrhoea, vomiting, and restlessness.

heroin abuse Nonmedical use of heroin. Heroin addiction has many adverse effects on the user, including injection scars, skin abscesses, weight loss, impotence, and the risk of infection with *hepatitis B*, *hepatitis C*, and *HIV* through sharing needles. Death commonly occurs from accidental overdose.

herpangina A throat infection caused by *coxsackievirus*. Herpangina most commonly affects young children. The virus is usually transmitted via infected droplets coughed or sneezed into the air. Many people harbour the virus but do not

HERNIA

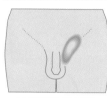

INGUINAL HERNIA

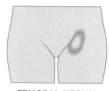

FEMORAL HERNIA

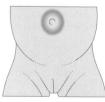

UMBILICAL HERNIA

have symptoms. Symptoms may include fever, sore throat, headache, abdominal discomfort, and muscular pains. The throat becomes red and a few small blisters appear, which enlarge and burst. Symptoms usually clear up within a week, without specific treatment

herpes Any of a variety of conditions characterized by an eruption of small, usually painful, blisters on the skin. The term usually refers to an infection with the *herpes simplex* virus. Forms of this virus are responsible for *cold sores* and genital herpes (see *herpes, genital*), among other conditions.

A closely related virus, varicella–zoster, is responsible for two other conditions in which skin blisters are a feature: *chickenpox* and *herpes zoster* (shingles).

herpes, genital A *sexually transmitted infection* caused by a form of the *herpes simplex* virus known as HSV2. After an incubation period of about a week, the virus may produce symptoms including soreness, burning, itching, and small blisters in the genital area. The blisters burst to leave small, painful ulcers, which heal in 10–21 days. The lymph nodes in the groin may become enlarged and painful, and the person may develop headache and fever. However, some infected people may not have any visible symptoms or signs.

Genital herpes cannot be cured, but treatment can reduce the severity of symptoms. *Antiviral drugs* such as *aciclovir* make the ulcers less painful and also encourage healing. Other measures include taking *analgesic drugs* and bathing with a salt solution.

Once the virus enters the body, it stays there for the rest of the person's life. Recurrent attacks may occur, usually during periods when the person is feeling run down, anxious, or depressed, before menstruation, or after sexual intercourse. The virus can be spread to others through sexual intercourse even when symptoms are absent. Recurrent attacks tend to become less frequent and less severe over time.

Genital herpes may be passed from a pregnant woman to her baby during delivery. If the virus can be detected in vaginal swabs, delivery by *caesarean section* is usually recommended.

herpes gestationis A rare skin disorder of pregnant women that produces crops of blisters on the legs and abdomen. The cause is not known.

Severe herpes gestationis is treated with *corticosteroid drugs* in tablet form and may require hospital admission. The disorder usually clears up completely after birth of the baby, but tends to recur in subsequent pregnancies.

herpes simplex A common viral infection, characterized by small, fluid-filled blisters. Herpes simplex infections are *contagious* and usually spread by direct contact. The virus has two forms, HSV1 (herpes simplex virus, type 1) and HSV2 (herpes simplex virus, type 2).

Most people are infected with HSV1 at some point in their lives, usually during childhood. The initial infection may be symptomless, or may cause a flu-like illness with multiple mouth ulcers. Thereafter, the virus remains dormant in nerve cells in the facial area. In many people, the virus is periodically reactivated, causing *cold sores*. Rarely, the virus infects the fingers, causing a painful eruption called a herpetic *whitlow*. HSV1 may produce eczema herpeticum (an extensive rash of skin blisters) in a person with a pre-existing skin disorder, such as *eczema*. Eczema herpeticum may require hospital admission. If the virus gets into an eye, it may cause *conjunctivitis* or a *corneal ulcer*. Rarely, HSV1 spreads to the brain, leading to *encephalitis*. The virus may cause a potentially fatal generalized infection in a person with an *immunodeficiency disorder* or in someone taking *immunosuppressant drugs*. HSV2 is the usual cause of sexually transmitted genital herpes (see *herpes, genital*).

Treatment of herpes simplex depends on its type, site, and severity. *Antiviral drugs, such as aciclovir*, may be helpful, particularly if used early in an infection.

herpes zoster An infection of the *nerves* supplying certain skin areas that is characterized by a painful rash. Also called shingles, herpes zoster is especially common among older people. It often affects one side of the body only. Sometimes the infection involves the face and eye and is called herpes zoster ophthalmicus.

Herpes zoster is caused by the *varicella-zoster* virus, which also causes *chickenpox*. After an attack of chickenpox, some of the viruses survive and lie dormant for many years. In some people, a decline in the efficiency of the *immune system*, especially in old age or because of disease, allows the viruses to re-emerge and cause herpes zoster. Herpes zoster is also common in people whose immune system is weakened by stress or by certain drugs, such as *corticosteroid drugs* or *anticancer drugs*.

The first indication of herpes zoster is excessive sensitivity in the skin, followed by pain. After about 5 days, the rash appears as small, raised, red spots that soon turn into blisters. These dry and develop crusts that drop off, sometimes leaving small pitted scars.

The most serious feature of herpes zoster is pain after the attack (postherpetic pain), caused by nerve damage, which may last for months or years. Herpes zoster ophthalmicus may cause a *corneal ulcer* or *uveitis*.

If treatment is begun soon after the rash appears, *antiviral drugs*, such as *aciclovir*, will reduce the severity of the symptoms and minimize nerve damage. *Analgesic drugs* may also be helpful.

heterosexuality Sexual attraction to members of the opposite sex. (See also *bisexuality*; *homosexuality*.)

heterozygote A term used to describe a person whose cells contain two different *alleles* controlling a specified inherited trait. A *homozygote* has identical alleles controlling that trait. (See also *inheritance*; *genetic disorders*.)

hiatus hernia A condition in which part of the *stomach* protrudes upwards into the chest through the opening in the *diaphragm* that is normally occupied by the *oesophagus*. The cause is unknown but it is more common in obese people and those with a long-term cough, such as smokers. In some cases, it is present at birth. Many people have no symptoms. In some people, there is *gastro-oesophageal reflux disease*. This may lead to *oesophagitis* or *heartburn*.

Antacid drugs or H_2 blockers may be given to reduce stomach acidity. In severe cases, surgery may be required.

Hib vaccine A vaccine administered routinely at 2, 3, and 4 months of age, with a booster at 12 months, to provide immunity to the bacterium *HAEMOPHILUS INFLUENZAE* type b (Hib). Before the vaccine was generally available, Hib infection was a common cause of bacterial *meningitis* and *epiglottitis* in children.

hiccup A sudden, involuntary contraction of the *diaphragm* followed by rapid closure of the *vocal cords*. Most attacks of hiccups last only a few minutes, and are not medically significant. Rarely, they may be due to a condition, such as *pneumonia* or *pancreatitis*, that causes irritation of the diaphragm or *phrenic nerves*. *Chlorpromazine*, *haloperidol*, or *diazepam* may be prescribed for frequent, prolonged attacks.

Hickman catheter A flexible plastic tube, also known as a skin-tunnelled catheter, that is passed through the chest and inserted into the subclavian vein, which leads to the heart. It is often used in people who have *leukaemia* or other cancers and need regular *chemotherapy* and blood tests. The catheter allows drugs to be injected directly into the bloodstream and blood samples to be obtained easily. The catheter is inserted under local *anaesthesia*. It can remain in position for months; the external end is plugged when not in use.

hidradenitis suppurativa Inflammation of the *sweat glands* in the armpits and groin due to a bacterial infection. Abscesses develop beneath the skin, which becomes reddened and painful and may ooze pus. The condition tends to be recurrent and can eventually cause scarring in the affected areas. *Antibiotic drugs* may help to reduce the severity of an outbreak.

high density lipoprotein One of a group of proteins that transport *lipids* in the blood. High levels of high density lipoprotein (HDL) can help protect against *atherosclerosis*. (See also *fats and oils*; *low density lipoprotein*.)

hip The *joint* between the *pelvis* and the upper end of the *femur*. The hip is a ball-and-socket joint; the smooth, rounded head of the femur fits securely into the acetabulum, a cup-like cavity in the pelvis. Tough ligaments attach the femur to the pelvis, further stabilizing the joint and providing it with the necessary strength to support the weight of the body and take the strain of leg movements. The structure of the hip allows a considerable range of leg movement.

hip, clicking A fairly common condition in adults in which a characteristic clicking is heard and felt during certain movements of the hip joint. Clicking hip is caused by a tendon slipping over the bony prominence on the outside of the *femur*, and does not indicate disease. Clicking of the hip that can be heard during examination of newborn babies indicates possible dislocation of the hip (see *developmental dysplasia of the hip*).

hip, congenital dislocation of See *developmental dysplasia of the hip*.

hip dysplasia, developmental See *developmental dysplasia of the hip*.

hippocampus A structure in the *limbic system* of the brain. The hippocampus, consisting of a band of *grey matter*, is involved with some learning processes and long-term memory storage.

Hippocratic oath A set of ethical principles derived from the writings of the Greek physician Hippocrates that is concerned with a doctor's duty to work for the good of the patient.

hip replacement A surgical procedure to replace all or part of a diseased *hip joint* with an artificial substitute. Hip replacement is most often carried out in older people whose joints are stiff and painful as a result of *osteoarthritis*. It may also be needed if *rheumatoid arthritis*

HIP REPLACEMENT

Pelvis
Pelvic socket
Area of pelvis hollowed out
Femoral component
Head of femur (thighbone) removed
Skin incision
ARTIFICIAL HIP JOINT
Shaft of femur

has spread to the hip joint or if the top end of the femur is badly fractured (see *femur, fracture of*).

Hirschsprung's disease A *congenital* disorder in which the *rectum*, and sometimes the lower part of the *colon*, lack the ganglion cells that control the intestine's rhythmic contractions. The affected area becomes narrowed and blocks the movement of faecal material.

The disease is rare and tends to run in families. It occurs about four times more often in boys. Symptoms, which include constipation and bloating, usually develop in the first few weeks of life, but may become evident in infancy or early childhood. The child usually has a poor appetite and may fail to grow properly.

A *barium X ray examination* can show the narrowed segment of the intestine. A *biopsy* may be taken. Treatment of Hirschsprung's disease involves removing the narrowed segment and rejoining the normal intestine to the anus.

hirsutism Excessive hairiness, particularly in women. The additional hair is coarse and grows in a male pattern on the face, trunk, and limbs. Hirsutism is a symptom of certain conditions, such as polycystic ovary syndrome (see *ovary, polycystic*) and congenital *adrenal hyperplasia*, in which the level of male hormones in the blood is abnormally high. Hirsutism can also be a result of taking anabolic steroids (see *steroids, anabolic*). More commonly, however, hirsutism is not a sign of any disorder; it occurs in many normal women, especially after the menopause. (See also *hypertrichosis*.)

histamine A chemical that is present in cells (mainly *mast cells*) throughout the body that is released during an allergic reaction (see *allergy*). Histamine activates two main types of receptors, H_1 and H_2. H_1 activation is responsible for the swelling and redness that occur in *inflammation*. It also narrows the airways in the lungs and causes itching. H_2 activation stimulates acid production by the stomach. These effects can be counteracted by *antihistamine drugs*.

histamine$_2$-receptor antagonists See *H_2-receptor antagonists*.

histiocytosis X A rare childhood disease in which there is an overgrowth of

H

a type of tissue cell called a histiocyte. The cause is unknown, but histiocytosis X probably results from a disturbance of the *immune system*. In the mildest form, rapid cell growth occurs in one bone only, usually the skull, a *clavicle*, a rib, or a *vertebra*, causing swelling and pain. In the most severe, and least common, form, there is a rash and enlargement of the *liver*, *spleen*, and *lymph nodes*.

histocompatibility antigens A group of proteins that have a role in the *immune system*. Certain types of histocompatibility antigens are essential for the immunological function of killer T cells (see *lymphocytes*). The *antigens* act as a guide for killer T cells to recognize and kill abnormal or foreign cells.

The main group of histocompatibility antigens is the human leukocyte antigen (HLA) system, which consists of several series of antigens. A person's tissue type (the particular set of HLAs in the body tissues) is unique, except for identical twins, who have the same set.

HLA analysis has some useful applications. Comparison of HLA types may show that two people are related, and it has been used in *paternity testing*. The HLA system is also used in *tissue-typing* to help match recipient and donor tissues before *transplant surgery*. Certain HLA types occur more frequently in people with particular diseases, such as *multiple sclerosis*, *coeliac disease*, and *ankylosing spondylitis*. HLA testing can help to confirm the presence of such diseases and identify people at risk of developing them.

histology The study of tissues, including their cellular structure and function. The main application of histology in medicine is in the diagnosis of disease.

histopathology A branch of *histology* concerned with the effects of disease on the microscopic structure of tissues.

histoplasmosis An infection caused by inhaling the spores of the fungus HISTO-PLASMA CAPSULATUM, which is found in soil contaminated with bird or bat droppings. It occurs in parts of the Americas, the Far East, and Africa.

history-taking The process by which a doctor learns from patients the symptoms of their illnesses and any previous disorders. (See also *diagnosis*.)

HIV The abbreviation for human immunodeficiency virus. HIV is a retrovirus (see *virus*) and is the cause of *AIDS*. There are two closely related viruses: HIV-1, which is the most common cause of AIDS throughout the world; and HIV-2, which is largely confined to West Africa.

HIV gains access to the body through contaminated blood transfusions, nonsterile needles, or sexual intercourse. A woman with untreated HIV infection can pass the virus to her baby during pregnancy, delivery, and through her breast milk.

In the body, the virus multiplies in white blood cells called CD4 lymphocytes, destroying them and weakening the immune system, which, impairs the body's ability to fight infection.

People with HIV infection should have regular monitoring in order to determine when specific treatments, such as *antiretroviral drugs*, are necessary.

HIV

Cross-sectioned virus — Genetic material — Outer shell of virus —

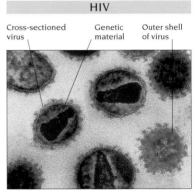

HUMAN IMMUNODEFICIENCY VIRUS

hives An alternative name for *urticaria*.

HLA The abbreviation for *human leukocyte antigen*.

HLA types See *histocompatibility antigens*.

hoarseness A rough, husky, or croaking voice. Short-lived hoarseness is often due to overuse of the voice, which strains the muscles in the *larynx*. It is also commonly caused by inflammation of the vocal cords in acute *laryngitis*. Persistent hoarseness may be due to chronic irritation of the larynx, which can be caused by smoking, excessive consumption of alcohol, chronic *bronchitis*, or constant dripping of mucus from the nasal passages. *Polyps* on the vocal cords may also cause hoarseness. In people with *hypothyroidism*, hoarseness can result from formation of tissue on the vocal cords. In young children, hoarseness may be a symptom of *croup*. Occasionally persistent hoarseness in adults has a more serious cause, such as cancer of the larynx (see *larynx, cancer of*), *thyroid cancer*, or *lung cancer*.

Resting the voice helps in strain- or laryngitis-related cases. If hoarseness persists for more than 2 weeks, a doctor should be consulted. A *laryngoscopy* may be performed to exclude a serious underlying cause.

Hodgkin's disease An uncommon, cancerous disorder in which there is a proliferation of cells in the lymphoid tissue (found mainly in the *lymph nodes* and *spleen*). Men are affected more than women. The cause is unknown.

The most common sign is the painless enlargement of lymph nodes, typically in the neck or armpits. There may be a general feeling of illness, with fever, weight loss, and night sweats. There may also be generalized itching. As the disease progresses, the *immune system* becomes increasingly impaired and life-threatening complications may result from normally trivial infections.

Diagnosis of Hodgkin's disease depends on the identification of characteristic cells in a *biopsy* of affected tissue. The extent of the disease (its *stage*) can be assessed by *chest X-ray, CT scanning* or *MRI* of the abdomen, a *bone marrow biopsy* and a *liver biopsy*. If the disease is localized to a small area, *radiotherapy* is usually curative. If the disease has spread to involve many organs, long-term treatment with *anticancer drugs* is needed. (See also *lymphoma, non-Hodgkin's*.)

hole in the heart The common name for a *septal defect*.

holistic medicine A form of therapy that treats the whole person, not just specific disease symptoms. A holistic approach is emphasized by many practitioners of *complementary medicine*.

Holter monitor A wearable device used in *ambulatory electrocardiography (ECG)* to record the heart's electrical activity

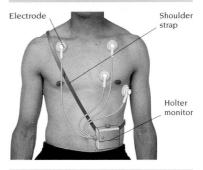

HOLTER MONITOR

Electrode

Shoulder strap

Holter monitor

continuously for 24 hours or longer. The monitor records by means of electrodes attached to the chest and allows the detection of intermittent *arrhythmias*.

homeopathy A system of *complementary medicine*. Homeopathy involves treating a condition by administering minute doses of a substance that, in larger doses, would be capable of inducing or worsening symptoms of the condition that is being treated.

homeostasis The automatic processes by which the body maintains a constant internal environment despite external changes. Homeostasis regulates conditions such as temperature and acidity by negative *feedback*. For example, when the body overheats, *sweating* is stimulated until the temperature returns to normal. Homeostasis also involves the regulation of *blood pressure* and *blood glucose* levels.

homocystinuria A rare, inherited condition caused by an *enzyme* deficiency. Homocystinuria is a type of inborn error of metabolism (see *metabolism, inborn errors of*) in which there is an abnormal presence of homocystine (an *amino acid*) in the blood and urine. Affected people are very tall, with long limbs and fingers. Some have skeletal deformities and abnormalities of the eye *lens*. The condition is incurable but may be improved by a special diet.

homosexuality Sexual attraction to people of the same sex. (See also *bisexuality*; *heterosexuality*.)

homozygote A term used to describe a person whose cells contain two identical *alleles* controlling a specified inherited trait. The cells of a *hetero-zygote* contain two different alleles controlling that trait. (See also *inheritance*; *genetic disorders*.)

hookworm infestation An infestation of the small intestine by small, round, blood-sucking worms of the *NECATOR AMERICANUS* or *ANCYLOSTOMA DUODENALE* species. Hookworm infestation occurs mainly in the tropics.

The larvae penetrate the skin of the feet or are ingested. They migrate throughout the body and mature in the small intestine. Adult worms lay eggs, which pass out in the faeces.

When larvae penetrate the skin, a red, itchy rash may develop on the feet. In light infestations, there may be no further symptoms. In heavier infestations, migration of the larvae through the lungs may produce cough and *pneumonia*; adult worms in the intestines may cause abdominal discomfort. The most important problem is iron-deficiency *anaemia* due to loss of blood.

Diagnosis is made by microscopic examination of the faeces for worm eggs. *Anthelmintic drugs* kill the worms. (See also *larva migrans*.)

hordeolum The medical name for a *stye*.

hormonal disorders Conditions caused by malfunction of an *endocrine gland*.

hormone A chemical released into the bloodstream by a gland or tissue that has a specific effect on tissues elsewhere in the body.

Many hormones are produced by *endocrine glands*. Hormones are also secreted by other organs, including the brain, kidneys, intestines, and, in pregnant women, the *placenta*. They control many body functions, including *metabolism* of cells, growth, sexual development, and the body's response to stress or illness.

hormone antagonist A drug that blocks the action of a *hormone*.

hormone replacement therapy (HRT) The use of a synthetic or natural *hormone* to treat a hormone deficiency.

Most commonly, HRT refers to the use of female hormones to relieve symptoms associated with the *menopause*, such as hot flushes and vaginal dryness. Usually, an *oestrogen drug* is taken in combination with a *progestogen*. The hormones

may be taken orally or may be released into the bloodstream from an implant, a skin patch, gel, or nasal spray. HRT for menopausal symptoms is given for short-term use around the menopause. It is no longer generally recommended for long-term relief of menopausal symptoms or for treating *osteoporosis* because HRT carries an increased risk of *breast cancer*, *thromboembolism*, and *stroke*, and may also increase the risk of *coronary artery disease*.

Minor adverse effects of HRT include nausea, breast tenderness, fluid retention, and leg cramps.

horn, cutaneous A hard, noncancerous protrusion occasionally found on the skin of elderly people and caused by an overgrowth of *keratin*.

Horner's syndrome A group of physical signs (narrowing of the eye pupil, drooping of the eyelid, and absence of *sweating*) affecting one side of the face that indicates damage to part of the sympathetic nervous system (see *autonomic nervous system*).

horseshoe kidney A *congenital* abnormality in which the two kidneys are fused at the base, forming a horseshoe shape. The joined kidneys usually function normally, but may be associated with other congenital kidney defects.

hospice A hospital or part of a hospital devoted to the care of patients who are terminally ill (see *dying, care of the*).

hot flushes Temporary reddening of the face, neck, and upper trunk that is accompanied by a sensation of heat and is often followed by *sweating*. Hot flushes are usually caused by decreased *oestrogen* production during or after the *menopause*, and they sometimes occur following removal of the ovaries (see *oophorectomy*). Hot flushes can often be alleviated by treatment with *hormone replacement therapy (HRT)*.

housemaid's knee Inflammation of the *bursa* that acts as a cushion over the kneecap. The inflammation is usually caused by prolonged kneeling but may develop after a blow to the front of the knee. (See also *bursitis*.)

HPV The abbreviation for *human papillomavirus*.

HRT See *hormone replacement therapy*.

5HT   See *serotonin agonists; serotonin antagonists.*

human chorionic gonadotrophin   See *gonadotrophin, human chorionic.*

human genome   See *genome, human.*

human leukocyte antigen (HLA)   A type of protein belonging to the group known as *histocompatibility antigens,* which play a role in the *immune system.*

human papillomavirus   A type of *virus* that is responsible for *warts* and *genital warts.* There are over 50 strains of human papillomavirus. Infection with some of these strains is thought to be a causative factor in *cervical cancer* (see *mouth cancer; pharynx, cancer of),* and anal cancer. A vaccine that protects against strains of human papillomavirus associated with cervical cancer is being developed.

humerus   The bone of the upper arm. The dome-shaped head of the bone lies at an angle to the shaft and fits into a socket in the scapula to form the shoulder joint. Below its head, the bone narrows to form a cylindrical shaft. It flattens and widens at its lower end, forming a prominence on each side called an *epicondyle.* At its base, it articulates with the *ulna* and *radius* to form the elbow.

HUMERUS

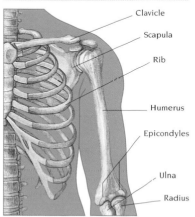

- Clavicle
- Scapula
- Rib
- Humerus
- Epicondyles
- Ulna
- Radius

humerus, fracture of   The *humerus* is most commonly fractured at its neck (the upper end of the shaft, below the head), particularly in elderly people.

Fractures of the shaft occur in adults of all ages. Fractures of the lower humerus occur most commonly in children.

An *X-ray* can show a fracture of the humerus. A fracture of the bone's neck usually requires only a *sling* to immobilize the bone; a fracture of the shaft or lower bone normally needs a plaster cast. Most fractures of the humerus heal in 6–8 weeks.

humours   Liquid or jelly-like substances in the body. The term humours usually refers to the *aqueous humour* and *vitreous humour* that occur in the *eye.*

hunchback   See *kyphosis.*

hunger   A disagreeable feeling caused by the need for food. Hunger occurs when the stomach is empty and the blood glucose level is low, often following strenuous exercise. In response to these stimuli, messages from the *hypothalamus* cause the muscular stomach wall to contract rhythmically; these contractions, if they are pronounced, produce hunger pains.

Hunger due to a low blood sugar level can also occur in *thyrotoxicosis,* and in *diabetes mellitus* when an incorrect balance between insulin and carbohydrate intake causes *hypoglycaemia.*

Huntington's disease   An uncommon disease in which degeneration of the *basal ganglia* results in *chorea* and *dementia.* Symptoms of Huntington's disease do not usually appear until age 35–50. The disease is due to a defective *gene* and is inherited in an autosomal dominant manner (see *genetic disorders*). Tests are available to identify whether a person has the defective gene.

The chorea usually affects the face, arms, and trunk, resulting in random grimaces and twitches, and clumsiness. Dementia takes the form of irritability, personality and behavioural changes, memory loss, and apathy.

At present, there is no cure for Huntington's disease, and treatment is aimed at reducing symptoms with drugs.

Hurler's syndrome   A rare, inherited condition caused by an *enzyme* defect. The syndrome is a type of inborn error of metabolism (see *metabolism, inborn errors of*) in which there is an abnormal accumulation of substances known as mucopolysaccharides in the tissues.

Affected children may appear normal at birth but, at 6–12 months of age, they develop cardiac abnormalities, umbilical *hernia*, skeletal deformities, and enlargement of the tongue, *liver*, and *spleen*. Growth is limited and mental development slows. If the condition is diagnosed in early infancy, a *stem cell* or *bone marrow transplant* may be curative.

hydatid disease A rare infestation that is caused by the larval stage of the small tapeworm ECHINOCOCCUS GRANU-LOSUS (see *tapeworm infestation*). Larvae mostly settle in the liver, lungs, or muscle, causing the development of cysts. In rare cases, the brain is affected.

The infestation is generally confined to dogs and sheep, but may be passed on to humans through accidental ingestion of worm eggs from materials contaminated with dog faeces.

The cysts grow slowly, and symptoms may not appear for some years. In many cases, there are no symptoms. Cysts in the liver may cause a tender lump or lead to *bile duct obstruction* and *jaundice*. Cysts in the lungs may press on an airway and cause inflammation; rupture of a lung cyst may cause chest pain, the coughing up of blood, and wheezing. Cysts in the brain may cause *seizures*. Ruptured cysts may rarely cause *anaphylactic shock*, which can be fatal.

Diagnosis of hydatid disease is by *CT scanning* or *MRI*. The cysts are usually drained or removed surgically.

hydatidiform mole An uncommon non-cancerous tumour that develops from placental tissue early in a pregnancy in which the embryo has failed to develop normally. The mole, which resembles a bunch of grapes, is caused by degeneration of the chorionic villi. The cause of the degeneration is unknown. In a small number of affected pregnancies, the mole develops into a *choriocarcinoma*.

Vaginal bleeding and severe morning sickness generally occur. *Ultrasound scanning* reveals the tumour. Urine and blood tests detect excessive amounts of human chorionic gonadotrophin (see *gonadotrophin, human chorionic*), which is produced by the tumour. The tumour can be removed by suction, a *D and C*, or, less commonly, a *hysterectomy*.

hydralazine An *antihypertensive drug* used principally as an emergency treatment for *hypertension*. Hydralazine may cause nausea, headache, dizziness, irregular heartbeat, loss of appetite, rash, and joint pain. Taken long term in high doses it may cause *lupus erythematosus*.

hydramnios See *polyhydramnios*.

hydrocele A soft, painless swelling in the *scrotum* caused by the space around a *testis* filling with fluid. A hydrocele may be caused by inflammation, infection, or injury to the testis; occasionally, the cause is a tumour. More often, there is no apparent cause. Hydroceles commonly occur in middle-aged men, and treatment is rarely necessary. If the swelling is uncomfortable or painful, however, the fluid may be withdrawn through a needle. Recurrent swelling may be treated by surgery.

HYDROCELE

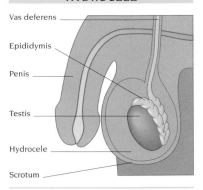

Vas deferens

Epididymis

Penis

Testis

Hydrocele

Scrotum

hydrocephalus An excessive amount of *cerebrospinal fluid*, usually under increased pressure, within the skull. The condition may be present at birth, when it is often associated with other abnormalities, such as *spina bifida*, or it may develop as a result of major *head injury*, brain *haemorrhage*, infection (such as *meningitis*), or a tumour.

With *congenital* hydrocephalus, the main feature is an enlarged head that continues to grow rapidly. Other features include rigidity of the legs, vomiting, *epilepsy*, irritability, lethargy, and the absence of normal reflex actions. If it is not treated, hydrocephalus progresses to severe brain damage, which may result in death within weeks. When the condition occurs later in life, symptoms include headache, vomiting, loss of coordination, and the deterioration of mental function.

In most cases, treatment of hydrocephalus is by draining the fluid from the brain to another part of the body, such as the abdominal cavity, where it can be absorbed.

hydrochloric acid A strong acid released by the stomach lining. This acid forms part of the stomach juices and helps to digest proteins.

hydrochlorothiazide A thiazide *diuretic drug* used in various combined preparations to treat *hypertension* and also to reduce *oedema* in people with *heart failure* or liver *cirrhosis*. Adverse effects include leg cramps, dizziness, rash, and *erectile dysfunction*. Hydrochlorothiazide may rarely cause *gout* and may aggravate *diabetes mellitus*.

hydrocortisone A *hormone* produced naturally by the *adrenal glands*. Synthetic hydrocortisone is used as a *corticosteroid drug* to treat inflammatory or allergic conditions, such as *ulcerative colitis* or *dermatitis*. Used in excess, hydrocortisone creams may thin the skin.

hydrogen peroxide An *antiseptic* solution used to treat infections of the skin or mouth and to bleach hair.

hydronephrosis A condition in which a *kidney* becomes swollen with urine as a result of an obstruction in the *urinary tract*. Many people with hydronephrosis have a *congenital* narrowing of the ureter. The obstruction of a ureter may be caused by a stone (see *calculus, urinary tract*), a *kidney tumour*, or a blood clot. Occasionally, hydronephrosis is caused by obstruction to the outflow of urine from the bladder by an enlarged prostate gland (see *prostate, enlarged*).

Acute hydronephrosis, with sudden blockage of the ureter, causes severe pain in the loin. Chronic hydronephrosis, in which the obstruction develops slowly, may cause no symptoms until total blockage results in *kidney failure*. If the blockage can be removed surgically, the kidney is likely to function normally again. Occasionally, however, a kidney is so badly damaged that it requires removal (see *nephrectomy*).

hydrophobia A popular term, now almost obsolete, for *rabies*.

hydrops An abnormal accumulation of fluid in body tissues or in a sac.

hydrops fetalis Serious swelling, or *oedema*, that occurs in a *fetus* before birth. Hydrops fetalis is often the result of *Rhesus incompatibility* (see *haemolytic disease of the newborn*).

hydrotherapy The use of exercises in water to aid recovery from injury or improve mobility.

hydroxocobalamin A long-acting synthetic preparation of *vitamin B_{12}*, given by injection.

hygiene The science and practice of preserving health. The word hygiene is commonly equated with cleanliness, but it can also refer to *public health*.

hygiene, oral See *oral hygiene*.

hygroma, cystic A *lymphangioma* that occurs around the head and neck, the armpits, or the groin and contains clear fluid. Cystic hygromas are usually present from birth and disappear naturally from the age of about 2 years.

hymen The thin membrane around the vaginal opening. The hymen has a central perforation which is usually stretched or torn by the use of tampons or during sexual intercourse for the first time.

Imperforate hymen is a rare condition in which the hymen has no perforation; at the onset of menstruation, menstrual blood collects in the *vagina*, causing lower abdominal pain. The condition is easily corrected by a minor operation.

hyoid A small, U-shaped bone situated centrally in the upper part of the neck. It is not joined to any other bone but is suspended by ligaments from the base of the skull. It provides an anchor point for the muscles of the tongue and of the upper front part of the neck.

hyoscine An *anticholinergic drug* prescribed in two distinct forms. Hyoscine butylbromide is used to relieve *irritable bowel syndrome*. Hyoscine hydrobromide is used to control *motion sickness* and to reduce nausea in *Ménière's disease*. An injection of hyoscine hydrobromide is often given as part of a *premedication* because it

H

dries secretions in the mouth and lungs. Possible adverse effects of both forms include dry mouth, blurred vision, drowsiness, and constipation.

hyper- A prefix meaning above, excessive, or greater than normal.

hyperacidity A condition in which excess acid is produced by the stomach. Hyperacidity is often confused with *gastro-oesophageal reflux disease* or *waterbrash*. It occurs in people with a duodenal ulcer (see *peptic ulcer*) or *Zollinger–Ellison syndrome*.

hyperactivity A behaviour pattern in which children are overactive and have difficulty in concentrating. The occasional occurrence of such behaviour in small children is considered normal. However, persistent hyperactivity is known as *attention deficit hyperactivity disorder (ADHD)*, which may require treatment.

hyperacusis An excessively sensitive sense of hearing. In hyperacusis, exposure to loud noises may cause pain or discomfort in the ears.

hyperaldosteronism A metabolic disorder caused by an overproduction of the hormone *aldosterone* by the *adrenal glands* (see *aldosteronism*).

hyperalimentation Administration of excessive amounts of *calories*, usually intravenously or by stomach tube (see *feeding, artificial*).

hyperbaric oxygen treatment A method of increasing the amount of *oxygen* in the tissues. This is achieved by placing a person in a special chamber and exposing him or her to oxygen at a much higher atmospheric pressure than normal. Hyperbaric oxygen treatment is used to treat poisoning from *carbon monoxide* and in cases of gas *gangrene*.

hyperbilirubinaemia A raised blood level of *bilirubin*. It may be undetectable except by a blood test, but *jaundice* occurs if the blood bilirubin rises to twice the normal level.

hypercalcaemia An abnormally high level of *calcium* in the blood, commonly caused by *hyperparathyroidism*. Cancer may also cause hypercalcaemia, either by spreading to bone or producing abnormal hormones that cause bones to release calcium. Less commonly, the condition is a result of excessive intake of *vitamin D* or of certain inflammatory disorders, such as *sarcoidosis*.

Hypercalcaemia causes nausea, vomiting, lethargy, depression, thirst, and passing urine excessively. Higher blood levels of calcium produce confusion, extreme fatigue, and muscle weakness. Without treatment, the condition can result in cardiac *arrhythmias*, *kidney failure*, *coma*, and even death. Long-standing hypercalcaemia may cause *nephrocalcinosis* or kidney stones (see *calculus, urinary tract*). Diagnosis is by blood tests. Treatment is of the underlying cause.

hypercapnia Excessive carbon dioxide in the blood caused by failure of mechanisms, such as breathing rate, that normally control the carbon dioxide levels in the blood. Hypercapnia leads to respiratory *acidosis*.

hyperemesis The medical term for excessive *vomiting*, which may cause dehydration and weight loss. When the condition occurs in pregnancy, it is known as hyperemesis gravidarum.

hyperglycaemia An abnormally high level of *glucose* in the blood that occurs in people with untreated or inadequately controlled *diabetes mellitus*. Hyperglycaemia may also occur in diabetics as a result of an infection, stress, or surgery. Features of the condition include passing large amounts of urine, thirst, *glycosuria*, and *ketosis*. If severe, hyperglycaemia may lead to confusion and *coma*, which need emergency treatment with *insulin* and *intravenous infusion* of fluids.

hypergonadism Overactivity of the gonads (*testes* or *ovaries*) that results in overproduction of *androgen hormones* or *oestrogen hormones*. Hypergonadism may be due to disorders of the gonads or a disorder of the *pituitary gland* that results in overproduction of *gonadotrophin hormones*. During childhood, the condition causes precocious sexual development and excessive growth.

hyperhidrosis Excessive *sweating*, which may be localized (affecting only the armpits, feet, palms, or face) or affect all body areas supplied by *sweat glands*. Excessive sweating may be caused by hot weather, exercise, or anxiety. In some cases it is due to an infection, *thyrotoxicosis*, *hypoglycaemia*, or a nervous system disorder. Usually, the disorder has no known cause, and begins at puberty, disappearing by the mid-20s or early 30s.

If hyperhidrosis is severe, persistent, and cannot be controlled by antiperspirants, injections of *botulinum toxin* into the skin may be used. In extreme cases, surgery may be considered to destroy the nerve centres that control sweating.

hyperkalaemia Abnormally high blood levels of *potassium*, often due to failure of the kidneys to excrete it.

hyperkeratosis Thickening of the skin's outer layer due to an increased amount of *keratin*. The most common forms of hyperkeratosis affect small, localized areas of skin and include *corns, calluses* and *warts*. A rare, inherited form affects the whole of the soles and palms. The term hyperkeratosis may also be used to describe thickening of the nails.

hyperlipidaemias *Metabolic disorders* that are characterized by high levels of *lipids* in the blood. Hyperlipidaemias may be inherited or associated with another disorder, such as *hypothyroidism, diabetes mellitus, kidney failure,* or *Cushing's syndrome*. They may also be a result of use of *corticosteroid drugs*. Hyperlipidaemias are associated with *atherosclerosis* and *coronary artery disease*.

The signs depend on the type of hyperlipidaemia and may include fatty nodules in the skin or over joints, and a white line around the rim of the *cornea*. Diagnosis depends on blood tests. Treatment aims to reduce blood lipid levels, usually by a low-fat diet and *lipid-lowering drugs*.

hypermetropia Commonly known as longsightedness, hypermetropia is an error of *refraction* that initially causes difficulty in seeing near objects and

then affects distance vision. Hypermetropia tends to run in families.

Hypermetropia is caused by the eye being too short from front to back, which results in images not being clearly focused on the *retina*. The error is present from birth, but symptoms generally do not appear until later life because the focusing power of *accommodation*, which compensates for hypermetropia, declines with age.

Glasses or *contact lenses* with convex lenses reinforce focusing power.

hypernephroma A type of *kidney cancer*, also known as renal cell carcinoma.

hyperparathyroidism Overproduction of parathyroid hormone by the *parathyroid glands* that raises the calcium level in the blood (*hypercalcaemia*) by removing calcium from bones. This may lead to bone disorders, such as *osteoporosis*. To try to normalize the high calcium level, the kidneys excrete large amounts of calcium in the urine, which can lead to the formation of kidney stones (see *calculus, urinary tract*).

Hyperparathyroidism is most often caused by a small noncancerous tumour of one or more of the parathyroid glands. It may also occur when the glands become enlarged for no known reason. It usually develops after age 40 and is twice as common in women as in men.

Hyperparathyroidism may cause depression and abdominal pain. However, often the only symptoms are those caused by kidney stones. If hypercalcaemia is severe, there may be nausea, tiredness, excessive urination, confusion, and muscle weakness.

The condition is diagnosed by *X rays* of the hands and skull and by *blood*

HYPERMETROPIA

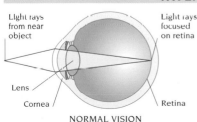

Light rays from near object

Light rays focused on retina

Lens

Cornea

Retina

NORMAL VISION

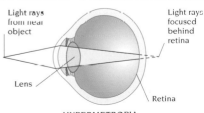

Light rays from near object

Light rays focused behind retina

Lens

Retina

HYPERMETROPIA

tests. Surgical removal of abnormal parathyroid tissue usually cures the condition. If the remaining tissue is unable to produce enough parathyroid hormone, treatment for *hypoparathyroidism* is required.

hyperplasia Enlargement of an organ or tissue due to an increase in the number of its cells. The new cells are normal, unlike those of a tumour. Hyperplasia is usually the result of hormonal stimulation. It may occur normally (such as in the enlargement of breast tissue in pregnancy) or it may indicate a disorder. (See also *hypertrophy*.)

hyperplasia, gingival Abnormal enlargement of the gums. Causes include *gingivitis*, persistent breathing through the mouth, the anticonvulsant drug *phenytoin*, and ill-fitting dentures. Surgical treatment may be needed.

hyperpyrexia A term for extremely high body temperature.

hypersensitivity Overreaction of the *immune system* to an *antigen*. There are four main types of hypersensitivity.

Type I is associated with *allergy*. After a first exposure to an antigen, *antibodies* are formed; these coat cells called mast cells in various tissues. On second exposure, the antigen and antibodies combine, causing the mast cells to disintegrate and release chemicals that cause the symptoms of *asthma*, allergic *rhinitis, urticaria, anaphylactic shock*, or other allergic illnesses.

In type II reactions, antibodies that bind to antigens on cell surfaces are formed, leading to possible destruction of the cells. Type II reactions may lead to certain *autoimmune disorders*.

In type III reactions, antibodies combine with antigens to form particles called immune complexes. These lodge in various tissues and activate further immune system responses, leading to tissue damage. This type of reaction is responsible for *serum sickness* and for the lung disease allergic *alveolitis*.

In type IV reactions, sensitized *T-lymphocytes* (a class of white *blood cell*) bind to antigens and release chemicals called lymphokines, which promote an inflammatory reaction. Type IV reactions are responsible for *contact dermatitis* and

measles rash; they may also play a part in "allergic" reactions to drugs.

Treatment of hypersensitivity depends on the type, cause, and severity. When possible, exposure to the offending antigen should be avoided.

hypersplenism An overactivity of the *spleen* resulting in, and associated with, blood disease. One of the functions of the spleen is to break down *blood cells* as they age and wear out. An overactive spleen may begin to destroy cells indiscriminately, causing a deficiency of any of the types of blood cell. In most cases, the spleen will also be enlarged. Hypersplenism may be primary, occurring for no known reason, but more commonly it is secondary to another disorder in which the spleen has become enlarged, such as *Hodgkin's disease* or *malaria*.

Hypersplenism causes *anaemia* and *thrombocytopenia*, and there may be a decrease in resistance to infection. Primary hypersplenism is treated with *splenectomy*. Treatment of secondary hypersplenism aims to control the cause.

hypertension Persistently raised *blood pressure* exceeding about 140 mmHg (systolic) and 85 mmHg (diastolic) at rest. Hypertension is very common, particularly in men, and its incidence is highest in middle-aged and elderly people.

Hypertension is usually symptomless but may cause headaches and visual disturbances when severe. It increases the risk of *stroke, coronary artery disease*, and *heart failure*, and may eventually lead to kidney damage and *retinopathy*.

In many cases, there is no obvious cause. Factors associated with hypertension include high alcohol intake, a high-salt diet, obesity, a family history of the condition, a sedentary lifestyle, a high degree of stress, and smoking.

Specific causes include various *kidney* disorders, certain disordes of the *adrenal glands, pre-eclampsia, coarctation of the aorta*, and use of certain drugs. Taking the combined *contraceptive* pill can increase the risk.

With mild to moderate hypertension, if no underlying cause is found, lifestyle changes are recommended, for example, introducing regular exercise and stopping smoking. *Biofeedback training* and relaxation techniques can help reduce blood pressure. If self-help measures have no effect, or hypertension is severe, one or a combination of *antihypertensive drugs* may be given.

hyperthermia A medical term for very high body temperature.

hyperthermia, malignant A rapid rise in body temperature to a dangerously high level, brought on by general *anaesthesia*. The condition is rare. In most cases, susceptibility is inherited; people suffering from certain muscle disorders may also be at risk. The patient's body temperature rises soon after the anaesthetic is given. Emergency treatment and intensive care are needed.

hyperthyroidism The overproduction of *thyroid hormones* by an overactive *thyroid gland*. The most common form of hyperthyroidism is *Graves' disease*, which is an *autoimmune disorder*. Less commonly, the condition is associated with the development of enlarged nodules within the thyroid gland.

The characteristic signs of hyperthyroidism include weight loss, increased appetite, increased *sweating*, intolerance to heat, a rapid *heart-rate*, and protruding eyes. In severe cases, the thyroid gland often becomes enlarged (see *goitre*) and there is physical and mental hyperactivity and muscle wasting.

The diagnosis of hyperthyroidism is confirmed by measuring the level of thyroid hormones present in the blood. The condition can be treated with drugs that inhibit the production of thyroid hormones, by radioactive *iodine* or by removal of part of the thyroid gland.

hypertonia Increased rigidity in a muscle, which may be caused by damage to its nerve supply or changes within the muscle. Hypertonia causes episodes of continuous muscle spasm. Persistent hypertonia in limb muscles following a *stroke* or *head injury* leads to *spasticity*.

hypertrichosis Growth of excessive *hair*, often in places that are not normally hairy. Hypertrichosis often occurs as a result of taking certain drugs (including *ciclosporin* and *minoxidil*). The term hypertrichosis is also used to describe hair growth in a mole. Hypertrichosis is

HYPERTRICHOSIS

Abnormal hair growth

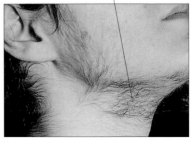

FEMALE WITH HYPERTRICHOSIS

not the same as *hirsutism*, which is due to abnormal levels of male hormones.

hypertrophy Enlargement of an organ or tissue due to an increase in the size, rather than number, of its constituent cells. For example, skeletal muscles enlarge in response to increased physical demands. (See also *hyperplasia*.)

hyperuricaemia An abnormally high level of *uric acid* in the blood. Hyperuricaemia may lead to *gout* due to the deposition of uric acid crystals in the joints; it may also cause kidney stones (see *calculus, urinary tract*) and *tophus*.

Hyperuricaemia may be caused by an inborn error of metabolism (see *metabolism, inborn errors of*), by the rapid destruction of cells in a disease such as *leukaemia*, or by medication that reduces the excretion of uric acid by the kidneys, such as *diuretic drugs*. Large amounts of *purine* in the diet may also cause hyperuricaemia.

Drugs such as *allopurinol* or *sulfinpyrazone* are prescribed for the duration of the patient's life. Purine-rich foods should be avoided.

hyperventilation Abnormally deep or rapid breathing that is usually caused by *anxiety*. Hyperventilation may also occur as a result of uncontrolled *diabetes mellitus*, oxygen deficiency, *kidney failure*, and some lung disorders.

Hyperventilation causes an abnormal loss of carbon dioxide from the blood, which can lead to an increase in blood alkalinity. Symptoms include numbness of the extremities, faintness, *tetany*, and a sensation of not being able to take a full breath. Breathing into a paper bag may help to reduce the symptoms in people with anxiety.

hyphaema Blood in the front chamber of the *eye*, usually caused by an injury that ruptures a small blood vessel in the *iris* or *ciliary body*. Initially, there may be blurred vision, but the blood usually disappears completely within a few days and vision is restored.

hypnosis A trance-like state of altered awareness characterized by extreme suggestibility. Some psychoanalysts induce a hypnotic state as a means of helping patients remember and come to terms with disturbing events. More often, hypnosis is used to help patients to relax. It may be useful in people suffering from *anxiety*, *panic attacks*, or *phobias*, or in those wishing to correct addictive habits.

hypnotherapy The use of *hypnosis* as part of a psychological therapy.

hypnotic drugs Drugs that induce sleep (see *sleeping drugs*).

hypo- A prefix meaning under, below, or less than normal.

hypoaldosteronism A rare deficiency of the hormone *aldosterone*, which is produced by the *adrenal glands*. The condition may be caused by damage or disease affecting the adrenal glands. It may produce weakness, and is treated by the drug fludrocortisone.

hypocalcaemia An abnormally low level of *calcium* in the blood. The most common cause is *vitamin D* deficiency. Rarer causes include chronic *kidney failure* and *hypoparathyroidism*. In mild cases, hypocalcaemia is symptomless; in severe cases, it leads to *tetany*. It may also result in bone softening, causing *rickets* in children and *osteomalacia* in adults.

hypochondriasis A person's unrealistic belief that he or she is suffering from a serious illness, despite medical reassurance. Hypochondriacs worry constantly about their health and interpret any symptom, however trivial, as evidence of disease.

Hypochondriasis may be a complication of other psychological disorders, including *phobia*, *obsessive–compulsive disorder*, *generalized anxiety disorder*, and brain diseases such as *dementia*.

Other factors include social stresses and personality type. Where possible, treatment is of the underlying mental disorder. Hypochondriasis without an underlying cause is difficult to treat.

hypochondrium The region on each side of the upper abdomen, situated below the lower ribs.

hypoglossal nerve The 12th *cranial nerve*, which controls tongue movement.

hypoglycaemia An abnormally low level of *glucose* in the blood. Almost all cases of hypoglycaemia occur in people with *diabetes mellitus*, in whom the *pancreas* fails to produce enough *insulin*, resulting in an abnormally high level of glucose. To lower the blood glucose level, *hypoglycaemic drugs* or insulin are given. Too high a dose of either can reduce the blood glucose to too low a level. Hypoglycaemia can also occur if a diabetic person misses a meal or takes strenuous exercise. Rarely, the condition can result from drinking too much alcohol or from an insulin-producing pancreatic tumour.

The main symptoms include *sweating*, hunger, dizziness, trembling, headache, *palpitations*, confusion, and sometimes double vision. Behaviour is often irrational and aggressive. *Coma* may occur in severe cases. Hypoglycaemia may also be the cause of seizures and jittery behaviour in newborns.

Sugar should be eaten at the first sign of a diabetic attack. An injection of either glucose solution or the hormone glucagon may be given in an emergency.

hypoglycaemics, oral A group of *antidiabetic drugs* that are used to lower blood glucose. Too high a dose may provoke the onset of *hypoglycaemia*.

hypogonadism Underactivity of the *testes* or *ovaries*. Hypogonadism may be caused by disorders of the gonads or a disorder of the *pituitary gland* that causes deficient production of *gonadotrophin hormones*. In men, hypogonadism causes the symptoms and signs of *androgen hormone* deficiency; in women, it causes those of *oestrogen* deficiency.

hypohidrosis Reduced activity of the *sweat glands*. Hypohidrosis is a feature of hypohidrotic ectodermal dysplasia, a rare, inherited, incurable condition that is characterized by reduced sweating and is accompanied by dry, wrinkled skin, sparse hair, small, brittle nails, and conical teeth. Other causes of hypohidrosis include *exfoliative dermatitis* and some *anticholinergic drugs*.

hypokalaemia A deficiency of *potassium* in the blood. Hypokalaemia is usually caused by excess fluid loss due, for example, to severe diarrhoea, but which may be the result of treatment with *diuretic drugs*.

hypomania A mild degree of *mania*.

hypoparathyroidism Insufficient production of *parathyroid hormone* by the *parathyroid glands*. A deficiency of this hormone results in low levels of *calcium* in the blood (*hypocalcaemia*).

The most common cause of hypoparathyroidism is damage to the parathyroid glands during surgery. Occasionally, the parathyroid glands are absent from birth, or they may cease to function for no apparent reason.

A low blood calcium level may cause *tetany*. Occasionally, *seizures* similar to those of an epileptic attack may occur.

The condition is diagnosed by *blood tests*. To relieve an attack of tetany, calcium may be injected slowly into a vein. To maintain the blood calcium at a normal level, a lifelong course of calcium and *vitamin D* tablets is necessary.

hypophysectomy The surgical removal or destruction (by means of a radioactive implant) of the *pituitary gland*. This may be performed to remove *pituitary tumours* or to treat some cancers of the breast, *ovary*, or *prostate gland*, the growth of which is stimulated by hormones secreted by the pituitary gland.

hypopituitarism Underactivity of the *pituitary gland*, resulting in inadequate production of one or more pituitary *hormones*. The effects depend on which hormones are affected. Possible causes are a *pituitary tumour*, an abnormality affecting the *hypothalamus*, or injury to the pituitary gland. Hypopituitarism may also follow surgery or *radiotherapy* of the pituitary gland. Treatment involves replacing the deficient hormones.

hypoplasia The failure of an organ or a body tissue to develop fully and to reach its normal adult size.

hypoplasia, enamel A defect in tooth enamel (see *enamel, dental*), usually due to *amelogenesis imperfecta*. It may also be caused by vitamin deficiency, injury, or infection of a primary tooth that interferes with enamel maturation.

hypoplastic left-heart syndrome A very serious form of congenital heart disease (see *heart disease, congenital*). The baby is born with a poorly formed left *ventricle*, often associated with other heart defects. The aorta is malformed and blood can reach it only via a duct (the ductus arteriosus) that links the aorta to the pulmonary artery.

At birth, the baby may seem healthy. However, within a day or two the ductus arteriosus naturally closes off and the baby collapses, becoming pale and breathless. In most cases, hypoplastic left-heart syndrome cannot be treated surgically, and most affected babies die within a week. A few infants have been treated with heart transplants.

hyposensitization A preventive treatment of *allergy* to specific substances, such as grass pollens and insect venom. Hyposensitization involves giving gradually increasing doses of the allergen so that the *immune system* becomes less sensitive to that substance. The treatment may need to be repeated annually for a few years. Increasing concerns about the risk of *anaphylactic shock*, which may be life-threatening, have severely restricted the use of hyposensitization.

hypospadias A *congenital* defect of the *penis*, in which the opening of the *urethra* is on the underside of the *glans* or shaft. In some cases, the penis curves downwards, a condition that is known as called *chordee*. Hypospadias can usually be corrected by surgery.

hypotension The medical term for low *blood pressure*. In its most common form, known as postural hypotension, symptoms occur after abruptly standing or sitting up. Normally, blood pressure increases slightly with changes in posture; in people with postural hypotension, this normal increase fails to occur. Postural hypotension may be a side effect of *antidepressant drugs* or *antihypertensive drugs*. It may also occur in people with *diabetes mellitus*. Acute hypotension is a feature of *shock*, and may be caused by serious injury or a disease such as *myocardial infarction* or *adrenal failure*. Treatment depends on the cause. In the absence of serious disease, low blood pressure is associated with decreased risk from *cardiovascular disorders* and *stroke*. Symptomless hypotension does not require treatment.

hypothalamus A region of the *brain*, roughly the size of a cherry, situated behind the eyes and the thalamus.

The hypothalamus controls the sympathetic nervous system (part of the *autonomic nervous system*). In response to sudden alarm or excitement, signals are sent from higher regions of the brain to the hypothalamus, initiating sympathetic nervous system activity. This causes a faster *heartbeat*, widening of the pupils, an increase in breathing rate and blood flow to muscles.

Other nerve cells in the hypothalamus are concerned with the control of body temperature, thirst, and appetite for food. The hypothalamus is also involved in regulating sleep, motivating sexual behaviour, and determining mood and emotions. It indirectly controls many *endocrine glands* through its influence on the *pituitary gland*.

Disorders of the hypothalamus are usually due to an *intracerebral haemorrhage* or a *pituitary tumour*. They have diverse effects, ranging from hormonal disorders to disturbances in temperature regulation, and increased or decreased need for food and sleep.

hypothermia A fall in body temperature to below 35°C. Most cases occur in sick, elderly people exposed to low temperatures. The body loses its sensitivity to cold as it ages, becoming less able to reverse a fall in temperature. Babies also have an increased risk of hypothermia because they lose heat rapidly and cannot easily reverse a fall in temperature.

A person suffering from hypothermia is usually pale and listless. The *heart-rate* is slow, the body is cold, and the victim is often drowsy and confused. In severe hypothermia, breathing becomes slow and shallow, the muscles are stiff, the victim may become unconscious, and the heart may stop beating.

Hypothermia is a medical emergency and requires hospital admission. In most cases, it can be prevented by self-help measures, such as dressing warmly and keeping moving in cold weather.

hypothermia, surgical The deliberate reduction of body temperature to prolong the period for which the vital organs can safely be deprived of their normal blood supply during *open heart surgery*. Cold reduces the rate of metabolism in tissues and thus increases their tolerance to lack of oxygen. Cooling may be achieved by continuously instilling cold saline at about 4°C into the open chest cavity.

hypothyroidism The underproduction of *thyroid hormones* by an underactive *thyroid gland*. Most cases are caused by an *autoimmune disorder* such as *Hashimoto's thyroiditis*. Hypothyroidism may also result from removal of part of the thyroid gland to treat hyperthyroidism. In rare cases, babies are born with an underactive thyroid gland (congenital hypothyroidism).

In adults, symptoms include tiredness, lethargy, muscle weakness, cramps, a slow heart-rate, dry skin, hair loss, a deep and husky voice, and weight gain. A syndrome called *myxoedema*, in which the skin and other tissues thicken, may develop. Enlargement of the thyroid gland may also occur (see *goitre*). Babies with congenital hypothyroidism may have feeding difficulties, constipation, jaundice (see *jaundice, neonatal*), and excessive sleepiness. If the condition is not diagnosed and treated early, it may retard mental development in childhood.

Hypothyroidism is diagnosed by measuring the level of thyroid hormones in the blood. Babies are screened for the condition shortly after birth (see *blood spot screening tests*). In all cases, treatment consists of replacement therapy with the thyroid hormone *thyroxine*, usually for life.

hypotonia Abnormal *muscle* slackness. Normally, a muscle that is not being used has a certain inbuilt tension, but in a number of disorders affecting the nervous system (such as *Huntington's disease*) this natural tension is reduced.

hypotonia in infants Excessive limpness in infants, also known as floppy infant syndrome. Hypotonic babies cannot hold their limbs up against gravity and so tend to lie flat with their arms and legs splayed.

Hypotonia may be caused by *Down's syndrome* or *hypothyroidism* and may be an early feature of *cerebral palsy*. It occurs in disorders of the spinal cord, such as *Werdnig–Hoffman disease*, and in some children who have *muscular dystrophy*.

hypovitaminosis Any condition that results from insufficiency of one or more *vitamins*. Hypovitaminosis may be due to an inadequate dietary intake or a digestive disorder that causes *malabsorption*.

hypovolaemia An abnormally low volume of blood in the circulation, usually following blood loss due to injury, internal bleeding, or surgery. It may also be due to loss of fluid from *diarrhoea* and *vomiting*. Untreated, it can lead to *shock*.

hypoxia An inadequate supply of *oxygen* to the tissues. Temporary hypoxia may result from strenuous exercise. More serious causes include impaired breathing (see *respiratory failure*), *ischaemia*, and severe *anaemia*. A rare cause is *carbon monoxide* poisoning. Severe, prolonged hypoxia may lead to tissue death.

Hypoxia in muscles forces the muscle cells to produce energy *anaerobically*, which can lead to cramps. Hypoxia in heart muscle may cause *angina pectoris*. Hypoxia of the brain causes confusion, dizziness, and incoordination, causing unconsciousness and death if persistent.

Hypoxia can be assessed by using an *oximeter* to measure the oxygen concentration of blood in the tissues. Severe hypoxia may require *oxygen therapy* or artificial *ventilation*.

hysterectomy Surgical removal of the *uterus*. It is performed in order to treat *fibroids*, and cancer of the uterus (see *uterus, cancer of*) or cervix (see *cervix, cancer of*). It may also be performed to relieve heavy menstrual bleeding or *endometriosis*, and to remove a prolapsed uterus (see *uterus, prolapse of*).

The most common type is a total hysterectomy, in which the uterus and cervix are removed. Occasionally, the fallopian tubes and ovaries are removed as well. For cervical cancer, a radical hysterectomy is performed, in which the uterus, cervix and pelvic lymph nodes

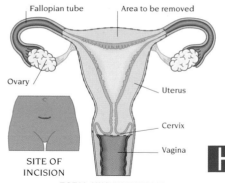

HYSTERECTOMY

Fallopian tube — Area to be removed

Ovary

Uterus

Cervix

Vagina

SITE OF INCISION

TOTAL HYSTERECTOMY

are removed. Hysterectomy may be performed through the vagina or through an incision in the abdomen.

hysteria An old-fashioned term encompassing a wide range of physical or mental symptoms attributed to mental stress. Symptoms formerly grouped under this term are now included in the more specific diagnostic categories of *conversion disorder*; *somatization disorder*; *dissociative disorders*; and *factitious disorders*. The term is still used loosely to describe irrational behaviour.

hysterosalpingography An *X-ray* procedure in which a dye (*radiopaque contrast medium*) is introduced into the cavity of the *uterus* via the *cervix* to make the uterus and *fallopian tubes* visible on X-rays. Hysterosalpingography is used to investigate *infertility*.

hysteroscopy A technique that uses a hysteroscope (see *endoscope*) to diagnose disorders, such as uterine *polyps*, inside the *uterus* and *fallopian tubes*. Hysteroscopy can be performed under local *anaesthesia*. Minor surgery, such as the removal of *fibroids*, may also be carried out through the hysteroscope.

I

iatrogenic A term meaning "physician-produced". It can be applied to any medical condition, disease, or adverse event resulting from medical treatment.

IBS See *irritable bowel syndrome*.

ibuprofen A *nonsteroidal anti-inflammatory drug* (NSAID) used as a painkiller to treat conditions such as headache, menstrual pain, and injury to soft tissues (such as muscles and ligaments). The drug's anti-inflammatory effect helps to reduce the joint pain and stiffness that occurs in types of *arthritis*. Side effects may include abdominal pain due to inflammation of the stomach lining, nausea, heartburn, and diarrhoea. Ibuprofen should not be used by people who have had a previous reaction to it (for example, *asthma*, *rhinitis*, or rash) or to any other NSAID, including aspirin. Ibuprofen should also not be used by people who have, or have ever had, a peptic ulcer.

ice-packs The means of applying ice to the skin (in a towel or other material) in order to relieve pain, stem bleeding, or reduce inflammation. Cold causes the blood vessels to contract, reducing blood flow. Ice-packs are used to relieve pain in a variety of disorders, including severe *headache*. They are used on sports injuries to minimize swelling and bruising, and they also help to stop bleeding from small vessels, as in a nosebleed.

ichthyosis A rare, inherited condition in which the skin is dry, thickened, scaly, and darker than normal due to abnormal production of *keratin*. It usually appears at or shortly after birth and improves during childhood. Commonly affected areas are the thighs, arms, and backs of the hands. Lubricants, emulsifying ointments, and bath oils are helpful. Ichthyosis may also be treated with the retinoid drug *acitretin*.

icterus A term for *jaundice*.

ICSI See *intracytoplasmic sperm injection*.

id One of the three parts of the personality (together with the *ego* and *superego*) described by Sigmund Freud. The id is the primitive, unconscious energy store from which come the instincts for food, love, sex, and other basic needs. The id seeks simply to gain pleasure and avoid pain. (See also *psychoanalytic theory*.)

idiopathic Of unknown cause. For example, epilepsy with no apparent cause is called idiopathic epilepsy.

idiopathic thrombocytopenic purpura (ITP) An *autoimmune disorder* in which *platelets* are destroyed, leading to bleeding beneath the skin (see *purpura*).

ileostomy An operation in which the *ileum* is cut and the end brought through the abdominal wall and formed into an artificial opening called a stoma. Waste is discharged from the remaining ileum into a disposable bag (stoma bag) or drained into a pouch made from the end of the ileum and situated beneath the skin (a procedure called a continent ileostomy). In the latter, faeces draining into the pouch are emptied regularly through a catheter. An ileostomy can be permanent or temporary.

Permanent ileostomy is usually performed on people with severe, uncontrolled *ulcerative colitis*. Temporary ileostomy is sometimes done at the time of partial *colectomy* (removal of part of the colon) to allow the colon to heal before waste material passes through it. It may also be done as an emergency treatment for an obstruction in the intestine. The stoma is created from a loop of the intestine that is brought to the surface. (This is later reversed by a second operation.)

During convalescence, patients are given counselling and taught the practical aspects of stoma care or drainage of continent ileostomies. Full recovery from the operation takes about 6 weeks.

ileum The final, longest, and narrowest section of the small intestine. It is joined at its upper end to the *jejunum* and at its lower end to the large intestine (comprising the caecum, colon, and rectum). The function of the ileum is to absorb nutrients from food that has been digested in the stomach and the first two sections of the small intestine (the *duodenum* and the jejunum).

Occasionally the ileum becomes obstructed, for example by pushing through a weakness in the abdominal wall (see *hernia*) or by becoming caught up with scar tissue following abdominal surgery (see *adhesion*). Other disorders of the ileum include *Meckel's diverticulum* and diseases in which absorption of nutrients is impaired, such as *Crohn's disease*, *coeliac disease*, tropical *sprue*, and *lymphoma*.

ILEUM

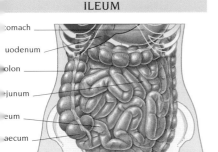

stomach
duodenum
colon
jejunum
ileum
caecum
rectum

ileus, paralytic A failure, usually temporary, of the normal contractility of the muscles of the intestine. Paralytic ileus commonly follows abdominal surgery and may also be induced by severe abdominal injury, *peritonitis*, internal bleeding, acute *pancreatitis*, or interference with the blood or nerve supply to the intestine. Symptoms include a swollen abdomen, vomiting, and failure to pass faeces. The condition is treated by resting the intestine. A tube passed through the nose or mouth into the stomach or intestine removes accumulated fluids and keeps the stomach empty. Body fluid levels are maintained by *intravenous infusion* (drip).

ilium The largest of the hip-bones that form part of the *pelvis*.

illness Perception by a person that he or she is not well. Illness is a subjective sensation; it may have physical or psychological causes. The term is also used to mean disease or disorder.

illusion A distorted sensation based on misinterpretation of a real stimulus (for example, a pen is seen as a dagger). It is differs from a *hallucination*, in which a perception occurs without any stimulus. Usually, illusions are brief and can be understood when explained. They may be due to tiredness or anxiety, to drugs, or to forms of brain damage. *Delirium tremens* is a classic inducer of illusions.

imaging techniques Techniques that produce images of structures within the body. The most commonly used and simplest techniques are *X-rays* (to view dense structures such as bone) and contrast X-rays, in which a medium, such as barium, that is opaque to X-rays is introduced into the body. Contrast X-ray techniques include *barium X-ray examinations* (used to examine the gastrointestinal tract); *cholecystography* (used to visualize the gallbladder and common bile duct); *bronchography* (to view the airways connecting the windpipe to the lungs); *angiography* and *venography* (to provide images of the blood vessels), *intravenous urography* (to visualize the kidneys and urinary tract); and *ERCP* (by which the pancreatic duct and biliary system are examined).

Many X-ray imaging techniques have been superseded by newer procedures. These include *ultrasound scanning*, *MRI* (magnetic resonance imaging), *PET scanning*, and *radionuclide scanning*. However, X-rays are used in *CT scanning*. Some of these techniques use computers to process the raw imaging data and produce the actual image. Others can produce images without a computer, although one may be used to enhance the image.

imipramine A tricyclic *antidepressant drug* most commonly used as a long-term treatment for *depression*. Possible adverse effects include excessive sweating, blurred vision, dizziness, dry mouth, constipation, nausea, and, in older men, difficulty passing urine.

immersion foot A type of *cold injury*, also called trench foot, occurring when the feet are wet and cold for a long time. Initially, the feet turn pale and have no detectable pulse; later, they become red, swollen, and painful. If the condition is ignored, muscle weakness, skin ulcers, or *gangrene* may develop.

immobility Reduced physical activity, for example, through disease, injury, or following major surgery. Immobility is particularly harmful in the elderly because it causes muscle wasting and progressive loss of function.

Total immobility can produce complications including *bedsores*, *pneumonia*, or *contractures*. A common complication of partial immobility is *oedema* (fluid retention), which causes swelling of the legs. Rarely, sluggish blood flow encourages formation of a *thrombus* (abnormal blood clot) in a leg vein. Regular *physiotherapy* and adequate nursing care are important for any person who is totally immobile.

immobilization An orthopaedic term for techniques used to prevent movement of joints or displacement of fractured bones so that the bones can unite properly (see *fracture*).

immune response The body's defensive reaction to microorganisms, cancer cells, transplanted tissue, and other substances or materials that are recognized as antigenic or "foreign". The response consists of the production of cells called *lymphocytes*, substances called *antibodies*, or *immunoglobulins*, and other substances and cells that act to destroy the antigenic material. (See also *immune system*.)

immune system A collection of cells and proteins that works to protect the body from harmful microorganisms, such as *bacteria*, *viruses*, and *fungi*. It also plays a role in the control of *cancer* and is responsible for the phenomena of *allergy*, *hypersensitivity*, and rejection after *transplant surgery*.

The term innate immunity is given to the protection that we are born with, such as the skin and the mucous membranes that line the mouth, nose, throat, intestines, and vagina. It also includes *antibodies*, or *immunoglobulins* (protective proteins), that have been passed to the child from the mother. If microorganisms penetrate these defences, they encounter "cell-devouring" white blood cells called phagocytes, and other types of white cells, such as natural cell-killing (cytotoxic) cells. Microorganisms may also meet naturally produced substances (such as *interferon*) or a group of blood proteins called the complement system, which act to destroy the invading microorganisms.

The second part of the immune system, adaptive immunity, comes into play when the body encounters organisms that overcome the innate defences. The adaptive immune system responds specifically to each type of invading organism, and retains a memory of the invader so that defences can be rallied instantly in the future.

The adaptive immune system first must recognize part of an invading organism or tumour cell as an antigen (a protein that is foreign to the body). One of two types of response – humoral or cellular – is then mounted against the antigen.

Humoral immunity is important in the defence against bacteria. After a complex recognition process, certain B-*lymphocytes* multiply and produce vast numbers of antibodies that bind to antigens. The organisms bearing the antigens are then engulfed by phagocytes. Binding of antibody and antigen may activate the complement system, which increases the efficiency of the phagocytes.

Cellular immunity is particularly important in the defence against viruses, some types of parasites that hide within cells, and, possibly, cancer cells. It involves two types of T-lymphocyte: helper cells, which play a role in the recognition of antigens and activate the killer cells (the second type of T-lymphocyte), which destroy the cells that have been invaded.

Disorders of the immune system include immunodeficiency disorders and *allergy*, in which the immune system has an inappropriate response to usually innocuous antigens such as pollen.

In certain circumstances, such as after tissue transplants, *immunosuppressant drugs* are used to suppress the immune system and thus prevent rejection of the donor tissue as a foreign organism.

immunity A state of protection against disease through the activities of the *immune system*. Innate immunity is present from birth; acquired (adaptive) immunity develops either through exposure to invading microorganisms or through *immunization*.

immunization The process of inducing *immunity* as a preventive measure against *infectious diseases.* Immunization may be active or passive. In the passive form, *antibodies* are injected into the blood to provide immediate but short-lived protection against specific *bacteria, viruses,* or *toxins.* Active immunization, also called vaccination, primes the body to make its own antibodies and confers longer-lasting immunity.

Routine childhood immunization programmes exist for diseases such as diphtheria, tetanus, pertussis, *Haemophilus influenzae* type b (Hib) infection, and *poliomyelitis;* measles, mumps, and rubella (see *MMR vaccination);* meningitis C, and *pneumococcus.* Additional immunizations before foreign travel may also be necessary (see *travel immunization).*

Most immunizations are given by injection, and usually have no after effects. However, some vaccines cause pain and swelling at the injection site and may produce a slight fever or flu-like symptoms. Some may produce a mild form of the disease. Very rarely, severe reactions occur due, for example, to an allergy to one of the vaccine's components.

People with *immunodeficiency disorders,* widespread cancer, or those taking high-dose *corticosteroid drugs* should not be given live vaccines and should discuss their condition with their doctor before starting a vaccination programme. Those who have had a severe reaction to a vaccine should consult their doctor before having a vaccination of the same type. Some vaccines should not be given to young children or during pregnancy.

immunoassay A group of laboratory techniques, which include ELISA (enzyme-linked immunosorbent assay) and radioimmunoassay, that are used in the diagnosis of infectious diseases and *allergies,* and in the measurement of *hormone* levels in the blood.

immunodeficiency disorders Disorders in which there is a failure of the *immune system's* defences to fight infection and tumours. They may be due to an inherited or a *congenital* defect or may be the result of acquired disease. The result is persistent or recurrent infection, including with organisms that would not ordinarily cause disease, and an undue susceptibility to certain forms of *cancer.* The infections in people with immunodeficiency disorders are sometimes called *opportunistic infections;* examples include *pneumocystic pneumonia, fungal infections,* and widespread *herpes simplex* infections.

Congenital or inherited deficiencies can occur in either of the two prongs of the adaptive immune system: humoral or cellular. Deficiencies of the humoral system include hypogammaglobulinaemia and agammaglobulinaemia. The former may cause few or no symptoms, depending on the severity of the deficiency, but agammaglobulinaemia can be fatal if not treated with *immunoglobulin.* Congenital deficiencies of T *lymphocytes* may lead to problems such as persistent and widespread *candidiasis* (thrush). A combined deficiency of both humoral and cellular components of the immune system, called severe combined immunodeficiency (SCID), is usually fatal in the 1st year of life unless treatment can be given by *stem cell* transplant or *bone marrow transplant.*

Acquired immunodeficiency may be due either to disease processes (such as infection with *HIV,* which leads to *AIDS)* or damage to the immune system as a result of its suppression by drugs. Severe malnutrition and many cancers can also cause immunodeficiency. Mild immunodeficiency arises through a natural decline in immune defences with age.

immunoglobulin A type of protein found in blood and tissue fluids, also known as an *antibody.* Such proteins are produced by B-lymphocytes (a type of white blood cell), and their function is to bind to substances in the body that are recognized as foreign *antigens.* This binding is crucial for the destruction of antigen-bearing microorganisms. Immunoglobulins also play a key role in *allergies* and *hypersensitivity* reactions.

Immunoglobulin G (IgG) is the major class of immunoglobulin of the five in the blood (IgA, IgD, IgE, IgG, and IgM). Its molecule consists of two parts: one binds to an antigen; the other binds to other cells, which then engulf the microorganisms bearing the antigen.

Immunoglobulins can be extracted from the blood of people who have recovered from certain infectious diseases and used for passive *immunization*.

immunoglobulin injection Administration of *immunoglobulin* preparations (*antibodies*) to prevent or treat infectious diseases. Such preparations, also known as immune globulin or gammaglobulin, work by passing on antibodies obtained from the blood of people who have previously been exposed to these diseases.

The main use of these injections is to prevent infectious diseases, such as chickenpox, in people exposed to infection who are not already immune or are at special risk (during cancer treatment, for example). They are also given regularly for *immunodeficiency disorders*. Side effects include rash, fever, and pain and tenderness at the injection site.

immunology The discipline concerned with the *immune system*. Immunologists study the immune system's functioning and investigate and treat its disorders, including *allergies*, *autoimmune disorders*, and *immunodeficiency disorders* such as *AIDS*. Immunologists are also concerned with finding ways in which the immune system can be stimulated to provide immunity. In addition, they play a role in *transplant surgery*, looking preoperatively for a good match between recipient and donor organ, and suppressing the recipient's immune system after transplantation to minimize the chances of organ rejection.

immunostimulant drugs A group of drugs that increase the efficiency of the body's *immune system*. Immunostimulant drugs include *vaccines*, *interferon* and aldesleukin (interleukin-2). Interferon is used to treat persistent viral infections, such as hepatitis C, and some types of *multiple sclerosis*. Aldesleukin is used in the treatment of some types of *cancer*.

immunosuppressant drugs A group of drugs that reduce the activity of the *immune system*. They include *azathioprine*, *ciclosporin*, *cyclophosphamide*, *methotrexate*, and *prednisolone*. Immunosuppressants are given to prevent rejection after *transplant surgery* and to slow the progress of *autoimmune disorders* such as *rheumatoid arthritis* and systemic *lupus erythematosus*.

The drugs work by suppressing the production and activity of white blood cells called *lymphocytes*. Side effects vary, but all the drugs increase the risk of infection and of the development of certain *cancers*.

immunotherapy Stimulation of the *immune system* as a treatment for *cancer*. The term is also used to describe *hyposensitization* treatment for *allergy*. One type of immunotherapy used in the treatment of cancer uses *immunostimulant drugs*. More recently, monoclonal antibodies (see *antibody, monoclonal*) directed against tumours have been produced artificially by *genetic engineering*. *Interferon* or chemical poisons can be linked to these antibodies to increase their ability to destroy tumour cells without damaging normal cells.

impaction, dental Failure of a tooth to emerge completely from the gum. It may occur because of *overcrowding* or when a tooth grows in the wrong direction.

Impacted wisdom teeth are common, and, if symptomless, may not need to be removed. In some cases, however, symptoms necessitate their removal.

impedance audiometry A *hearing test* used to investigate the middle ear in cases of conductive *deafness*.

imperforate Without an opening. The term is used to describe a body structure, such as the *hymen* or anus (see *anus, imperforate*), in which a normal perforation is lacking.

impetigo A highly contagious skin infection, common in children, that usually occurs around the nose and mouth. It is caused by bacteria (usually staphylococci) entering areas of broken skin. The skin reddens and small, fluid-filled blisters appear. The blisters tend to burst, leaving moist, weeping areas that dry to leave honey-coloured crusts. In severe cases, there may be swelling

IMPETIGO

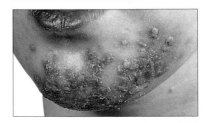

of the *lymph nodes* in the face or neck and fever.

Topical *antibiotic drugs* can be used, but if the condition is widespread oral antibiotics are usually given. To prevent spread of the infection, towels, flannels, and pillowcases should not be shared. Children should not go to school or mix with others until they have been treated.

implant Any material, either natural or artificial, inserted into the body for medical or cosmetic purposes. For example, artificial joints can replace diseased structures and breast implants can improve appearance. Implants are also used to maintain proper functioning of an internal organ, treat certain disorders, or deliver drugs or hormones.

implantation, egg Attachment of a fertilized *ovum* (egg) to the wall of the *uterus*. It occurs about 6 days after *fertilization*, when the blastocyst (early embryo) comes into contact with the wall of the uterus. As the cells of the developing *embryo* continue to divide, the outer cell layer penetrates the lining of the uterus to obtain oxygen and nutrients from the mother's blood; later, this layer develops into the *placenta*. The embryo usually implants in the upper part of the uterus; if it implants low down near the cervix, *placenta praevia* may develop. Rarely, implantation occurs outside the uterus, possibly in a fallopian tube, resulting in an *ectopic pregnancy*.

implant, dental A post, surgically embedded in the jaw for the attachment of a dental prosthesis (an artificial tooth). Titanium or synthetic materials may be used. A dental implant is fitted under local *anaesthesia*. A hole is drilled in the jaw and a post inserted. Several months later, an attachment that protrudes from the gum is screwed into the post; a few weeks after that, the prosthesis is fitted.

impotence The inability to achieve or maintain an erection, now more commonly known as *erectile dysfunction*.

impression, dental A mould taken of the *teeth*, *gums*, and *palate*. A quick-setting material, such as alginate, is placed in a mould over the teeth. The mould is removed, and plaster of Paris is poured into it to obtain a model of the area. This model is then used as a base on which to build a *denture*, *bridge*, or dental *inlay* or *crown*. Dental impressions are also used in *orthodontics* to study the position of the teeth and to make *orthodontic appliances* to correct irregularities.

incest Sexual intercourse between close relatives, such as with a parent, a son or daughter, a brother or sister, an uncle or aunt, a nephew or niece, or a grandparent or grandchild. It is illegal or taboo in most societies and against the teaching of many religions.

incidence One of the two principal measures (the other is *prevalence*) of how common a disease is in a defined population. The incidence of a disease is the number of new cases that occur during a given period (for example, 17 new cases per 100,000 people per year).

incision A cut made into the tissues of the body by a scalpel (surgical knife). Most incisions are made to gain access to tissue inside the body, usually to repair or remove a diseased organ. An incision may also be made to allow pus to drain from an *abscess* or boil.

incisional hernia A type of *hernia* in which the intestine bulges through a scarred area of the abdominal wall because the muscle has been weakened by a previous surgical *incision*.

incisor One of the eight front teeth (four each in upper and lower jaws) used for cutting through solid food (see *teeth*).

incontinence, faecal Inability to retain *faeces* in the *rectum* until a movement appropriate to expel them. A common cause is *faecal impaction*, which often results from long-standing *constipation*. The rectum becomes overfull, causing faecal fluid and small pieces of faeces to be passed involuntarily around the

IMPLANT, DENTAL

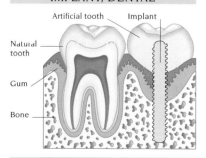

Artificial tooth   Implant

Natural tooth

Gum

Bone

impacted mass of faeces. Temporary loss of continence may also occur in severe *diarrhoea*. Other causes include injury to the anal muscles (as may occur during childbirth), *paraplegia*, and *dementia*.

If the underlying cause of faecal impaction is constipation, recurrence may be prevented by a high-fibre diet. Suppositories containing *glycerol* or *laxative drugs* may be given. Faecal incontinence in people with dementia or a nerve disorder may be avoided by regular use of *enemas* or *suppositories* to empty the rectum.

incontinence, urinary Involuntary passing of *urine*, often due to injury or disease of the *urinary tract*. Damage to or disorders of the nervous system are also common causes. There are several types of incontinence. Stress incontinence refers to the involuntary escape of urine when a person coughs, picks up a heavy package, or moves excessively. It is common in women, particularly after childbirth, when the urethral sphincter muscles are stretched. In urge incontinence, also known as irritable bladder, an urgent desire to pass urine is accompanied by inability to control the bladder as it contracts. Once urination starts, it cannot be stopped. Total incontinence is a complete lack of bladder control due to an absence of sphincter activity, which may be associated with spinal cord damage. Overflow incontinence occurs in long-term *urinary retention*, often because of an obstruction such as an enlarged *prostate gland*. The bladder is always full, leading to constant dribbling of urine.

Incontinence may also be due to urinary tract disorders (including infections, bladder stones, or tumours) or *prolapse* of the uterus or vagina. Incontinence due to lack of control by the brain commonly occurs in the young (see *enuresis*) or elderly and those with learning difficulties.

If weak pelvic muscles are causing stress incontinence, *pelvic floor exercises* may help. Sometimes, surgery may be needed to tighten the pelvic muscles or correct a prolapse. *Anticholinergic drugs* may be used to relax the bladder muscle if irritable bladder is the cause.

If normal bladder function cannot be restored, incontinence pants can be worn; men can wear a penile sheath leading into a tube connected to a urine bag. Some people can avoid incontinence by self-catheterization (see *catheterization, urinary*). Permanent catheterization is necessary in some cases.

incoordination Loss of the ability to produce smooth, muscular movements, leading to clumsiness and unsteady balance. Incoordination can also mean the failure of a group of organs to work together successfully. (See also *ataxia*.)

incubation period The time during which an *infectious disease* develops, from the point when the infecting organism enters the body until symptoms appear. Different infections have characteristic incubation periods; for example, the incubation period is 14–21 days for chickenpox and 7–14 days for measles. The incubation period for cholera may be as short as several hours.

incubator A transparent plastic cot in which oxygen, temperature, and humidity are controlled in order to provide premature or sick infants with ideal conditions for survival. Incubators have portholes to allow handling of the baby and smaller holes through which monitoring cables and intravenous and respiratory tubing can pass.

incus One of the three tiny, linked bones (*ossicles*) in the middle *ear*. The incus (the Latin name for anvil) is so-called because of its shape.

Indian medicine Traditional Indian, or Ayurvedic, medicine was originally based largely on herbal treatment, although simple surgical techniques were also used. Indian medicine later developed into a scientifically based system with a wide range of surgical techniques (such as operations for cataracts and kidney stones) along with the herbal tradition.

indigestion A common term (known medically as dyspepsia) covering a variety of symptoms brought on by eating, including *heartburn*, *abdominal pain*, *nausea*, and *flatulence*. Discomfort in the upper abdomen is often caused by eating too much, too quickly, or by eating very rich, spicy, or fatty foods. Persistent or recurrent indigestion may be due to a *peptic ulcer*, *gallstones*, *oesophagitis*, or, rarely, *stomach cancer*. *Antacid drugs* help relieve symptoms, but they can mask an underlying cause that needs medical attention. They should not be taken for longer than 2 weeks without medical advice.

indometacin A *nonsteroidal anti-inflammatory drug* (NSAID) used to relieve pain, stiffness, and inflammation in disorders such as *osteoarthritis*, *rheumatoid arthritis*, and *tendinitis*. It is also prescribed to relieve pain caused by injury to soft tissues, such as muscles and ligaments. Side effects include abdominal pain, nausea, heartburn, headache, dizziness, and increased risk of *peptic ulcer* and gastrointestinal bleeding.

induction of labour Use of artificial means to initiate childbirth when the health of the mother or baby would be at risk if pregnancy continued. The most common reason for inducing labour is that the pregnancy has continued past the estimated delivery date, which increases the chance of complications during childbirth. Other reasons for induction are *pre-eclampsia*, *Rhesus incompatibility*, or *intrauterine growth retardation*. Different methods of induction are used, depending on the stage of labour: a *prostaglandin* pessary may be inserted into the vagina to encourage the cervix to open; if the cervix is already open, the membranes containing the fetus may be ruptured; or the hormone *oxytocin* may be given intravenously to stimulate uterine contractions.

industrial diseases See *occupational disease and injury*.

infant A term usually applied to a baby up to the age of 12 months.

infantile spasms A rare type of recurrent seizure, also called progressive myoclonic encephalopathy or salaam attacks, that affects babies. The condition is a form of *epilepsy* and occurs most commonly from 4–9 months of age. Spasms may occur hundreds of times a day, each lasting a few seconds. These seizures are usually a sign of brain damage; affected babies usually have severe *developmental delay*.

infant mortality The number of infants who die during the 1st year of life per 1,000 live births, usually expressed as per year. About 2 in 3 of all infant deaths occur during the neonatal period (the 1st month of life). Most of those who die are very premature (born before the 30th week of pregnancy) or have severe birth defects. Cot death (*sudden infant death syndrome*) is a major cause of infant mortality.

infarction Death of an area of tissue due to *ischaemia* (lack of blood supply). Common examples include *myocardial infarction*, which is also known as heart attack, and pulmonary infarction, which is lung damage caused by a *pulmonary embolism* – a blood clot that has moved into a vessel in the lung and is obstructing the flow of blood. (See also *necrosis*.)

INDUCTION OF LABOUR

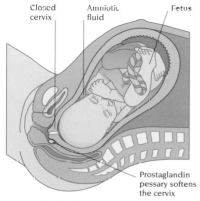

Closed cervix | Amniotic fluid | Fetus

Prostaglandin pessary softens the cervix

PROSTAGLANDIN PESSARY

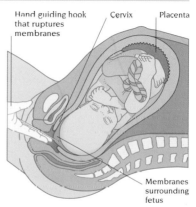

Hand guiding hook that ruptures membranes | Cervix | Placenta

Membranes surrounding fetus

RUPTURE OF MEMBRANES

INFECTION

infection The establishment in the body of disease-causing microorganisms (such as *bacteria*, *viruses*, or *fungi*). The organisms reproduce and cause disease by direct damage to cells or by releasing toxins. This normally provokes the immune system into responding, which accounts for many common symptoms. Infection can be localized within a particular area or tissue, as in a boil, or be systemic (spread throughout the body), as in *influenza*. Weakness, aching joints, and fever are symptoms of infectious disease. Localized infection may result from the spread of organisms through wounds, or during surgery and is generally associated with pain, redness, swelling, formation of a pus-filled abscess at the site of infection, and a rise in temperature.

Many minor infections are dealt with by the immune system and need no specific treatment. Severe systemic infections may need treatment with drugs such as *antibacterials* or *antivirals*. A localized infection that has produced pus may be drained surgically.

infection, congenital Infection acquired in the uterus or during birth. Many microorganisms can pass from the mother, by way of the placenta, into the circulation of the growing fetus. Particularly serious infections acquired in the uterus are *rubella*, *syphilis*, *toxoplasmosis*, and *cytomegalovirus*; all these infections may cause *intrauterine growth retardation*. Rubella that occurs in early pregnancy may cause *deafness*, congenital *heart disease*, and eye disorders. Some infections in later pregnancy, particularly with a *herpes* virus, may also damage the fetus severely. A woman with *HIV* risks passing on the virus to her baby during pregnancy; the risk can be reduced by use of *antiretroviral drugs* during pregnancy.

Infections acquired during birth are almost always the result of microorganisms in the mother's vaginal secretions or uterine fluid. Premature rupture of the membranes is associated with increased risk of infection, particularly *streptococcal*. Conditions that can be acquired during delivery include herpes, *chlamydial infections*, and *gonorrhoea*.

Treatment of the baby depends on the type of infection. Some birth defects caused by infection (such as certain types of heart defect) can be treated; others (such as congenital deafness) are usually not treatable.

infectious disease Any illness caused by a specific microorganism. The most important disease-causing organisms are *viruses*, *bacteria*, including rickettsiae, chlamydiae, and mycoplasmas, and *fungi*. Others are *protozoa* and *worms*.

In developed countries, infectious diseases are generally less of a threat than in the past because of better methods to control the spread of disease organisms (such as better sanitation and water purification); effective drugs; *immunization*; and better general health and nutrition.

For most infectious diseases, there is a time gap between the entry of the microorganisms into the body and the first appearance of symptoms. This incubation period, during which an infected person is likely to pass the microorganism to others, may be a few hours, a few days, or, in some cases, months.

Antibiotics and other antimicrobial drugs are the mainstay of treatment for bacterial infection. For viral infection, however, drug treatment is usually restricted to severe infections.

infectious mononucleosis See *mononucleosis, infectious*.

inferiority complex A neurotic state of mind that develops because of repeated hurts or failures in the past. Inferiority complex arises from a conflict between the positive wish to be recognized as someone worthwhile and the haunting fear of frustration and failure. Attempts to compensate for the sense of worthlessness may take the form of aggression and violence, or an overzealous involvement in activities. (See also *superiority complex*.)

infertility The inability to produce offspring, which may result from a problem in either the male or the female reproductive system, or, in many cases, from a combination of problems in both.

The main cause of male infertility is a lack of healthy sperm. In *azoospermia*, there are no sperm in the ejaculate; in *oligospermia*, there is an abnormally low number of sperm in the ejaculate.

In some cases, sperm are produced but are malformed or short-lived. The underlying cause of these problems may be blockage of the spermatic tubes or damage to the spermatic ducts, usually due to a *sexually transmitted infection*. Abnormal development of the testes due to an endocrine disorder (see *hypogonadism*) or damage to the testes by *orchitis* may also cause defective sperm. Smoking, toxins, or various drugs can lower the sperm count. Other causes are disorders affecting ejaculation (see *ejaculation, disorders of*). Rarely, male infertility is due to a chromosomal abnormality, such as *Klinefelter's syndrome*, or a genetic disease, such as *cystic fibrosis*.

The most common cause of female infertility is failure to ovulate. Other causes are blocked, damaged or absent *fallopian tubes*; disorders of the uterus, such as *fibroids* and *endometriosis*; problems with *fertilization*, or implantation in the uterus (see *implantation, egg*). Infertility also occurs if the woman's cervical mucus provides antibodies that kill or immobilize her partner's sperm. Rarely, a chromosomal abnormality, such as *Turner's syndrome*, is the cause of a woman's infertility.

Investigations to discover the cause of a woman's infertility may include blood and urine tests, to check that ovulation is occurring, and *laparoscopy* to determine whether or not an abnormality is present. The initial investigation for male infertility is *seminal fluid analysis*.

There are various possible treatments for male infertility, depending on the cause. In azoospermia due to blockage of the spermatic tubes or damage to the spermatic ducts, it may be possible to take sperm directly from the testis or epididymis. The sperm sample may then be used for *intracytoplasmic sperm injection* (ICSI) in conjunction with *in vitro fertilization* (IVF). In some cases of male infertility due to a hormonal imbalance, drugs such as *clomifene* or *gonadotrophin hormone* therapy may prove useful. If no sperm at all are produced by the testis, the only options are adoption of children or *artificial insemination* by a donor.

Failure of the woman to ovulate requires ovarian stimulation with a drug such as clomifene, either with or without a gonadotrophin hormone. *Microsurgery* can sometimes repair damage to the fallopian tubes. If surgery is unsuccessful, in vitro fertilization (IVF) is the only option. Uterine abnormalities or disorders, such as fibroids, may require treatment. In some cases, provided the woman has normal fallopian tubes, *gamete intrafallopian transfer* (GIFT) or *zygote intrafallopian transfer* (ZIFT) may be carried out.

infestation The presence of animal parasites (such as mites, ticks, or lice) in the skin or hair, or of worms (such as tapeworms) inside the body.

infibulation A form of female circumcision in which the labia majora (the outer lips surrounding the vagina) are removed and the entrance to the vagina narrowed (see *circumcision, female*).

infiltrate Build-up of substances or cells within a tissue that are either not normally found in it or are usually present only in smaller amounts. Infiltrate may refer to a drug (such as a local anaesthetic) that has been injected into a tissue, or to the build-up of a substance within an organ (for example, fat in the liver caused by excessive alcohol consumption). Radiologists use the term to refer to the presence of abnormalities, most commonly on a *chest X-ray*, due to conditions such as infection.

inflammation Redness, swelling, heat, and pain in a tissue due to injury or infection. When body tissues become damaged, *mast cells* release the chemical *histamine* and other substances. Histamine increases the flow of blood to the damaged tissue and also makes the blood capillaries more leaky; fluid then oozes out and into the tissues, causing localized swelling. Pain is caused by the stimulation of nerve endings by the inflammatory chemicals.

Inflammation is usually accompanied by a local increase in the number of white blood cells. These cells help to destroy any invading microorganisms and are involved in repairing the damaged tissue. Inappropriate inflammation (as in *rheumatoid arthritis* and some other *autoimmune disorders*) may be suppressed by *corticosteroid drugs* or by *nonsteroidal anti-inflammatory drugs*.

INFLAMMATION

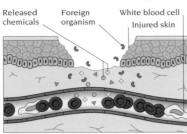

Released chemicals | Foreign organism | White blood cell / Injured skin

INJURED TISSUE

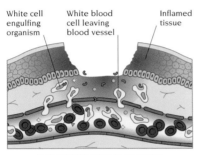

White cell engulfing organism | White blood cell leaving blood vessel | Inflamed tissue

RESULTING INFLAMMATION

inflammatory bowel disease A collective term for chronic disorders affecting the small and/or large intestine that cause abdominal pain, bleeding, and diarrhoea. *Crohn's disease* and *ulcerative colitis* are the most common types of inflammatory bowel disease.

influenza A viral infection of the respiratory tract (air passages), typically causing fever, headache, muscle ache, and weakness. Popularly known as "flu", it is spread by infected droplets from coughs or sneezes. Influenza usually occurs in small outbreaks or every few years in epidemics. There are three main types of influenza virus: A, B, and C. A person who has had an attack caused by the type C virus acquires *antibodies* that provide immunity against type C for life. Infection with a strain of type A or B virus produces immunity to that particular strain. However, type A and B viruses are capable of altering to produce new strains: type A has been the cause of *pandemics* in the last century. Occasionally, another strain of influenza virus that

primarily affects birds may also affect humans, such as *avian influenza*.

Types A and B produce classic flu symptoms; type C causes a mild illness that is indistinguishable from a common cold. The illness usually clears up completely within 7–10 days. Rarely, flu takes a severe form, causing acute *pneumonia* that may be fatal within a day or two even in healthy young adults. Type B infections in children sometimes mimic *appendicitis*, and they have been implicated in *Reye's syndrome*. In the elderly and those with lung or heart disease, influenza may be followed by a bacterial infection such as *bronchitis* or pneumonia.

Analgesic drugs help to relieve aches and pains and reduce fever. The drugs *oseltamivir*, *zanamivir*, and *amantadine* may be used for the prevention and/or treatment of influenza in certain cases. *Antibiotic drugs* may be used to combat secondary bacterial infection.

Flu vaccines, containing killed strains of the types A and B virus currently in circulation, are available but have only a 60–70 per cent success rate. Immunity is short-lived, and vaccination must be repeated annually. Influenza vaccination is advised for those over 65 and for people with chronic respiratory disease, chronic heart disease, chronic kidney disease, chronic liver disease, immunosuppression (which may be due to disease or medication), or *diabetes mellitus*. Vaccination is also recommended for people in long-stay residential care, and for health-care workers who have regular contact with vulnerable groups. The human influenza vaccines do not protect against avian influenza.

infra-red A term denoting the part of the electromagnetic spectrum immediately beyond the red end of the visible light spectrum. Directed onto the skin, infra-red radiation heats the skin and the tissues immediately below it. An infra-red lamp is one means of giving *heat treatment*.

infusion, intravenous See *intravenous infusion*.

ingestion The act of taking any substance (for example, food, drink, or medications) into the body through the mouth. The term also refers to the process by which certain cells (for example, some white blood cells) surround and then engulf small particles.

ingrowing toenail See *toenail, ingrowing*.

inguinal Relating to the groin (the area between the abdomen and thigh), as in *inguinal hernia*.

inguinal hernia A type of *hernia* in which part of the intestine protrudes through the abdominal wall in the groin. It can be direct, in which there is a localized weakness in the abdominal wall, or, in men, indirect, in which the intestine protrudes through the inguinal canal, the passage through which the testes descend into the scrotum.

inhalation The act of taking in breath (see *breathing*). An inhalation is also a substance, in the form of a gas, vapour, powder, or aerosol, to be breathed in.

inhaler A device used for administering a drug in powder or vapour form, used mainly in the treatment of various respiratory disorders, including *asthma* and chronic *bronchitis*. Metered-dose inhalers deliver a precise dose when the inhaler is pressed. Drugs taken by inhalation include *bronchodilators* and *corticosteroids*.

INHALER

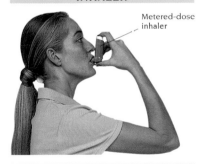

Metered-dose inhaler

inheritance The transmission of characteristics and disorders from parents to their children through the influence of *genes*. Genes are the units of *DNA* (deoxyribonucleic acid) that are contained in a person's cells; DNA controls all growth and functioning of the body. Half of a person's genes come from the mother, half from the father.

Genes are organized into *chromosomes* in the cell nucleus. Genes controlling most characteristics come in pairs, one from the father, the other from the mother. Everyone has 22 pairs of chromosomes (called autosomes) bearing these paired genes, in addition to two sex chromosomes. Females have two X chromosomes; males have an X and a Y chromosome.

Most physical characteristics, many disorders, and some mental abilities and aspects of personality are inherited. The inheritance of normal traits and disorders can be divided into those controlled by a single pair of genes on the autosomal chromosomes (unifactorial inheritance, such as eye colour); those controlled by genes on the sex chromosomes (sex linked inheritance, such as haemophilia); and those controlled by the combination of many genes (multifactorial inheritance, such as height).

Either of the pair of genes controlling a trait may take any of several forms, known as *alleles*. For example, the genes controlling eye colour exist as two main alleles, coding for blue and brown eye colour. The brown allele is dominant over blue in that it "masks" the blue allele, which is called recessive to the brown allele. Only one of the pair of genes controlling a trait is passed to a child from each parent. For example, someone with the brown/blue combination for eye colour has a 50 per cent chance of passing on the blue gene, and a 50 per cent chance of passing on the brown gene, to any child. This factor is combined with the gene coming from the other parent, according to dominant or recessive relationships, to determine the child's eye colour. Certain genetic disorders are also inherited in a unifactorial manner (for example, *cystic fibrosis* and *achondroplasia*).

Sex-linked inheritance depends on the two sex chromosomes, X and Y. The most obvious example is gender. Male gender is determined by genes on the Y chromosome, which is present only in males. Any faults in a male's genes on the X chromosome tend to be expressed outwardly because such a fault cannot be masked by the presence of a normal gene on a second X chromosome (as it can in females). Faults in the genes of the X chromosome include those responsible for colour vision deficiency, haemophilia,

I

and other sex-linked inherited disorders, which almost exclusively affect males.

Multifactorial inheritance, along with the effects of environment, may play a part in causing certain disorders, such as *diabetes mellitus* and *neural tube defects.*

inhibition The process of preventing any mental or physical activity. Inhibition in the brain and spinal cord is carried out by certain *neurons*, which damp down the action of other nerve cells to keep the brain's activity in balance. In *psychoanalysis*, inhibition refers to the unconscious restraint of instinctual impulses.

injection Introduction of a substance into the body from a syringe via a needle. Injections may be intravenous (into a vein), intramuscular (into a muscle), intradermal (into the skin), intra-articular (into a joint), or subcutaneous (under the skin).

injury Harm to any part of the body. It may arise from many causes, including physical influences (for example, force, heat, cold, electricity, vibration, and radiation), chemical causes (for example, poisons), bites, or oxygen deprivation.

ink-blot test An outdated psychological test in which the subject was asked to interpret the appearance of a number of ink blots. The most widely used example was the *Rorschach test.*

inlay, dental A filling of porcelain or gold used to restore a badly decayed tooth. An inlay may be needed for the back teeth or to protect a weakened tooth.

inoculation The act of introducing a small quantity of a foreign substance into the body, usually by injection, for the purpose of stimulating the *immune system* to produce *antibodies* (protective proteins) against the substance. Inoculation is usually done to protect against future infection by particular bacteria or viruses (see *immunization*).

inoperable A term applied to any condition that cannot be alleviated or cured by surgery, particularly cancers.

inorganic A term used to refer to any of the large group of substances that do not contain carbon and to a few simple carbon compounds (for example, *carbon dioxide* and *carbon monoxide*). Examples of inorganic substances include table salt (sodium chloride) and bicarbonate of soda (sodium bicarbonate).

inpatient treatment Care or therapy in hospital following admission.

inquest An official inquiry by a *coroner* into a death that is of unknown cause or is suspected of being unnatural.

insanity A term for serious mental disorder. The term has no technical meaning.

insect bites Puncture wounds inflicted by bloodsucking insects such as gnats, mosquitoes, fleas, and lice. Most bites cause only temporary pain or itching, but some people have severe skin reactions. In the tropics and subtropics, insect bites are potentially more serious because certain biting species can transmit disease (see *insects and disease*).

All insect bites provoke a skin reaction to substances in the insect's saliva or faeces, which may be deposited at or near the site of the bite. Reactions vary from red pimples to painful swellings or an intensely itching rash; some insects, such as bees and wasps, have stings (see *insect stings*) that can produce fatal allergies. (See also *lice*; *spider bites*; *mites and disease*; *ticks and disease*.)

insects and disease Relatively few insect species cause disease directly in humans. Some parasitize humans, living under the skin or on the body surface (see *lice*; *chigoe*; *myiasis*). The most troublesome insects are flies and biting insects. Flies can carry disease organisms from human or animal excrement via their feet or legs and contaminate food or wounds.

A number of serious diseases are spread by biting insects. These include *malaria* and *filariasis* (transmitted by mosquitoes), *sleeping sickness* (tsetse flies), *leishmaniasis* (sandflies), epidemic *typhus* (lice), and *plague* (rat fleas). Mosquitoes, sandflies, and ticks can also spread illnesses such as *yellow fever*, *dengue*, *Lyme disease*, and some types of viral *encephalitis*. Organisms picked up when an insect ingests blood from an infected animal or person are able to survive or multiply in the insect. Later, the organisms are either injected into a new human host via the insect's saliva or deposited in the faeces at or near the site of the bite.

Most insect-borne diseases are confined to the tropics and subtropics, although tick-borne Lyme disease occurs in some parts of the UK. The avoidance of insect-borne disease is largely a matter of keeping flies off food, discouraging insect bites by the use of suitable clothing and insect repellents (such as *DEET*), and, in parts of the world where malaria is present, the use of mosquito nets and screens, *pesticides*, and antimalarial tablets.

insect stings Reactions produced by the sting of insects such as bees and wasps. Venom injected by the insect contains inflammatory substances that cause local pain, redness, and swelling for about 48 hours. Any sting in the mouth or throat is dangerous because the swelling may obstruct breathing. About 1 person in 200 is allergic to insect venom, and a severe allergic reaction can occur, leading to *anaphylactic shock*. A procedure known as *hyposensitization* is occasionally used for such people.

If the symptoms of anaphylactic shock develop, it is essential to seek emergency medical treatment. Any person who is hypersensitive to bee or wasp venom should carry an emergency kit for self injection of *adrenaline* (epinephrine).

insecurity Lack of self-confidence and uncertainty about one's abilities, aims, and relationships with others. A feeling of insecurity may be a feature of *anxiety* and other neurotic mental disorders.

insight Being aware of one's own mental state. In a general sense, this means knowing one's own strengths, weaknesses, and abilities. The term also has the specific psychiatric meaning of knowing that one's symptoms are an illness. Loss of insight may be a feature of psychotic and neurotic disorders.

in situ A Latin term meaning "in place". The phrase "carcinoma in situ" is used to describe tissue (particularly of the skin or cervix) that is cancerous only in its surface cells.

insomnia Difficulty in falling asleep or in staying asleep. About 1 in 3 adults suffer from insomnia at some time in their lives. The most common cause is worry, but other causes include physical symptoms such as a cough or itching or conditions such as *restless legs*. Environmental and lifestyle factors or misuse of *sleeping drugs* are also common causes. Insomnia can also be a symptom of

a psychiatric illness, such as *anxiety* and/or *depression*. Withdrawal symptoms from *antidepressants*, *antianxiety drugs*, sleeping drugs, and some illicit drugs (see *drug abuse*), may cause insomnia.

instinct An innate primitive urge. The need for warmth, food, love, and sex are all forms of instinct, but the instinct for survival is probably the most powerful.

institutionalization Loss of personal independence that stems from living for long periods under a rigid regime, such as in a prison or other large institution. Apathy, obeying orders unquestioningly, accepting a standard routine, and loss of interests are the main features.

insulin A hormone produced by the *pancreas* that regulates *glucose* levels in the blood. It is normally produced in response to raised glucose levels following a meal and promotes glucose absorption into the *liver* and muscle cells (where it is converted into energy). Insulin thus prevents a build-up of glucose and ensures that tissues have sufficient amounts of glucose. Failure of insulin production results in *diabetes mellitus*. An *insulinoma* is a rare tumour that causes excessive production of insulin and consequent attacks of *hypoglycaemia*.

Insulin replacement, self-administered by injection or though an infusion pump (see *pump, insulin*) is used in the treatment of diabetes mellitus. Inhaled insulin is also available and may be used by some adults with type 1 or type 2 diabetes. Insulin cannot be taken orally because it is destroyed by stomach acid. Preparations of insulin are commonly produced by genetic engineering and closely mimic human insulin. Animal-derived insulin is also available but its use is declining. Insulin treatment prevents excessively high glucose levels in the blood (*hyperglycaemia*) and *ketosis* (a build-up of certain acids in the blood), which in severe cases may cause coma.

Too high a dose of insulin will cause hypoglycaemia, which can be relieved by consuming food or a sugary drink. Severe hypoglycaemia may cause coma, for which emergency treatment with an injection of glucose or *glucagon* (a hormone that opposes the effects of insulin) is necessary.

insulinoma A rare noncancerous tumour of the insulin-producing cells of the *pancreas*. Abnormal quantities of insulin are produced with the result that the amount of glucose in the blood can fall to dangerously low levels (*hypoglycaemia*) and, unless sugar is given immediately, can cause *coma* and death. Once diagnosed, a drug (diazoxide) is given to prevent hypoglycaemia until the tumour is removed.

intelligence The ability to understand concepts and to reason them out. Intelligence can also be considered as having three separate forms: abstract (understanding ideas and symbols); practical (aptitude in dealing with practical problems such as repairing machinery); and social (coping reasonably and wisely with human relationships). Intelligence is partly inherited and partly influenced by external factors such as environment and physical health.

Intelligence is formally evaluated with *intelligence tests*, which test a range of mental abilities and express the result as an intelligence quotient (IQ). The tests are designed so that a person of average mental ability has an IQ of around 100. Extremes of intelligence occur in *learning difficulties* (defined by a low IQ) and in the gifted (defined by an IQ of over 140).

intelligence tests Tests designed to provide an estimate of a person's mental abilities. The most widely used are Wechsler tests of which there are two basic types: the Wechsler Adult Intelligence Scale (WAIS) and the Wechsler Intelligence Scale for Children (WISC). Each is divided into verbal (concerned with language skills) and performance sections, including measures of constructional ability and visual-spatial and perceptual ability (interpretation of shapes). Other tests include the Stanford-Binet test, which is used mainly as a measure of scholastic ability.

In most intelligence tests, scoring is based on mental age (MA) in relation to chronological age (CA). The intelligence quotient (IQ) is MA divided by CA, multiplied by 100. The tests are devised to ensure that 3 in 4 people have an IQ between 80 and 120. They are standardized so that the score indicates the same relative ability at different age levels.

Intelligence tests may be used to assess school or job aptitude. However, they have been criticized for their alleged bias regarding gender and race.

intensive care Constant close monitoring and treatment of seriously ill patients that enables treatment to be tailored to the patient's condition on an hour-by-hour basis. Intensive care units (ICUs), sometimes known as intensive treatment units (ITUs), contain electronic equipment to monitor vital functions such as blood pressure and heart-rate and rhythm. Frequently, patients in these units require mechanical ventilation, in which a machine takes over or assists with breathing. Urine output, fluid balance, and blood chemistry are recorded regularly. Fluids are given intravenously. If nutrients are required, they are supplied to the stomach through a tube. There is a high ratio of specially trained nursing and medical staff to patients. (See also *coronary care unit*.)

inter- A prefix that means between, as in *intercostal* (between the ribs). (See also *intra-*.)

intercostal The medical term for between the *ribs*, as in the intercostal muscles, thin sheets of muscle between each rib.

intercourse, painful Pain during *sexual intercourse*, known medically as dyspareunia, which can affect both men and women. Pain may be superficial (around the external genitals) or deep (within the pelvis).

In men, superficial pain may be due to anatomical abnormalities such as *chordee* (bowed erection) or *phimosis* (tight foreskin). *Prostatitis* may cause a widespread pelvic ache, a burning sensation in the penis, or pain on ejaculation.

Scarring (after childbirth, for example) and lack of vaginal lubrication, especially after the *menopause*, may cause painful intercourse in women. *Psychosexual dysfunction* may also cause pain during intercourse. *Vaginismus*, a condition in which the muscles of the vagina go into spasm, is usually psychological in origin. Deep pain is frequently caused by pelvic disorders (such as *fibroids*, *endometriosis*, *ectopic pregnancy*, or *pelvic*

INTENSIVE CARE

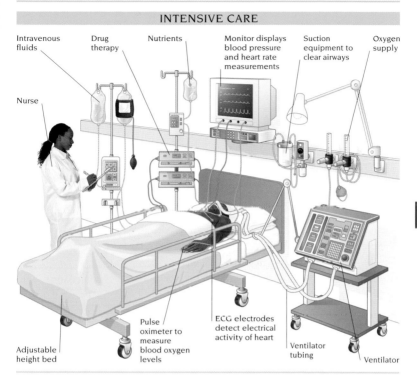

Intravenous fluids

Drug therapy

Nutrients

Monitor displays blood pressure and heart rate measurements

Suction equipment to clear airways

Oxygen supply

Nurse

Adjustable height bed

Pulse oximeter to measure blood oxygen levels

ECG electrodes detect electrical activity of heart

Ventilator tubing

Ventilator

inflammatory disease due to sexually transmitted infections), disorders of the ovary (such as *ovarian cysts*), and disorders of the *cervix*. Other causes are *cystitis* and *urinary tract infections*.

Treatment is directed at the underlying cause of the pain. If the discomfort is psychological in origin, special counselling may be needed (see *sex therapy*).

interferon A protein produced naturally by body cells in response to viral infections and other stimuli. It inhibits viral multiplication and increases the activity of natural killer cells (a type of *lymphocyte* that forms part of the body's *immune system*). It is also produced artificially for use in treatment of a number of disorders. There are three main types: interferon alfa is used in the treatment of certain *lymphomas*, malignant melanoma (see *melanoma, malignant*), a type of *leukaemia*, and chronic *hepatitis* B and C. Interferon beta is used in the treatment of relapsing *multiple sclerosis*.

Interferon gamma is used to reduce the risk of serious infections in some types of *immunodeficiency*. Adverse reactions include fever, headaches, lethargy, depression, and dizziness.

intermittent claudication A cramping pain in the legs due to inadequate blood supply (see *claudication*).

intersex A group of abnormalities in which the affected person has ambiguous genitalia (abnormal external sex organs) or external genitalia that have the opposite appearance to the chromosomal sex of the individual (see *sex determination*).

interstitial Referring to gaps (interstices) between cells, tissues, or other body structures. For example, *tissue fluid* between body cells is known as interstitial fluid. (See also *interstitial radiotherapy*.)

interstitial pulmonary fibrosis Scarring of lung tissue mainly involving the alveoli. There are a number of causes, including occupational exposure to dusts and *fibrosing alveolitis*, which is an *autoimmune disorder*.

interstitial radiotherapy Treatment of a cancerous tumour by inserting radioactive material into the growth or into neighbouring tissue. Using this method, which is a form of brachytherapy, radiation can be targeted at the diseased area.

Radioactive material (usually artificial radioisotopes) contained in wires, small tubes, or seeds is then implanted into or near the diseased tissue under general *anaesthesia*. The material is left in place for variable amounts of time depending on the radioactive substance and the tumour being treated. (See also *intracavitary therapy*; *radiotherapy*.)

intertrigo Inflammation of the skin due to two surfaces rubbing together. Intertrigo is most common in obese people. The affected skin is red and moist and may have an odour, often with a fungal infection such as *candidiasis*; there may also be scales or blisters. The condition worsens with sweating. Treatment consists of weight reduction and keeping the affected areas clean and dry. A cream containing a *corticosteroid* and/or *antifungal drug* is used if candidiasis is present.

intervertebral disc See *disc, intervertebral*.

intestinal imaging See *barium X-ray examinations*.

intestinal lipodystrophy See *Whipple's disease*.

intestine The major part of the digestive tract (see *digestive system*), extending from the exit of the stomach to the anus. It forms a long tube divided into two main sections: the small and large intestines.

The small intestine is about 6.5 m in length and has three sections: the *duodenum*, the *jejunum* and the *ileum*. Partially digested food from the stomach is forced along the intestine by *peristalsis*.

The small intestine is concerned with the digestion and absorption of food. Digestive enzymes and bile are added to the partly digested food in the duodenum via the bile and pancreatic ducts (see *biliary system*). Glands within the walls of each section of the small intestine produce mucus and other enzymes, which help to break down the food. Blood vessels in the intestinal walls absorb nutrients and carry them to the liver for distribution to the rest of the body.

The large intestine is about 1.5 m long. The main section, the *colon*, is divided into an ascending, a transverse, a descending, and a pelvic portion (the sigmoid colon). The *appendix* hangs from a pouch (the *caecum*) between the small intestine and the colon. The final section before the *anus* is the *rectum*.

Unabsorbed material leaves the small intestine as liquid and fibre. As this material passes through the large intestine, water, vitamins, and mineral salts are absorbed into the bloodstream, leaving faeces made up of undigested food residue, fat, various secretions, and bacteria. The faeces are compressed and pass into the rectum for evacuation.

intestine, cancer of A malignant tumour in the intestine. Both the small and large intestine may develop carcinoid tumours (leading to *carcinoid syndrome*) and *lymphomas*. Cancer of the small intestine is rare, but cancer of the large intestine is one of the most common of all cancers (see *colon, cancer of*; *rectum, cancer of*).

intestine, disorders of The intestine is subject to various structural abnormalities and to the effects of many infective organisms and parasites; it may also be affected by tumours and other disorders.

Structural abnormalities may be present from birth (congenital) or may develop later. They cause blockage of the intestine (see *intestine, obstruction of*) and include *atresia*, *stenosis*, and *volvulus*. In newborns, meconium (fetal intestinal contents) may block the intestine.

Generalized inflammation of the intestine may result from viral or bacterial infections or from noninfectious causes, as in *ulcerative colitis* and *Crohn's disease*. *Gastroenteritis* is the term commonly applied to inflammation of the stomach and intestines. Infection encompasses *food poisoning, traveller's diarrhoea, typhoid fever, cholera, amoebiasis*, and *giardiasis*. Intestinal worm infestations include *roundworms* and *tapeworms*. Sometimes inflammation is localized, such as in *appendicitis* and *diverticular disease*.

Tumours of the small intestine are rare, but noncancerous growths, *lymphomas*, and carcinoid tumours (causing *carcinoid syndrome*) occur. Tumours of the large intestine are common (see *colon, cancer of; rectum, cancer of*). Some forms of familial *polyposis* may progress to cancer.

Impaired blood supply (*ischaemia*) to the intestine may occur as a result of partial or complete obstruction of the arteries in the abdominal wall (from diseases such as *atherosclerosis*) or from the blood vessels being compressed or trapped, as in *intussusception* or *hernias*. Loss of blood supply may cause *gangrene*.

Other disorders that affect the intestine include *peptic ulcers, diverticulosis, malabsorption, coeliac disease*, and *irritable bowel syndrome*.

intestine, obstruction of A partial or complete blockage of the small or large intestine. Causes include a strangulated *hernia*; stenosis (narrowing) of the intestine, often due to cancer in the intestine; intestinal *atresia; adhesions; volvulus*; and *intussusception*. Intestinal obstruction also occurs in diseases that affect the intestinal wall, such as *Crohn's disease*. In less common cases, internal blockage of the intestinal canal is caused by impacted food, *faecal impaction, gallstones*, or an object that has been accidentally swallowed.

A blockage in the small intestine usually causes intermittent cramp-like pain in the centre of the abdomen with increasingly frequent bouts of vomiting and failure to pass wind or faeces. An obstruction in the large intestine causes pain, distension of the abdomen, and failure to pass wind or faeces.

Treatments involve emptying the stomach via a *nasogastric tube* and replacing lost fluids through an intravenous drip. In some cases, this will be sufficient to correct the problem. However, in many cases, surgery to deal with the cause of the blockage is necessary.

intestine, tumours of Cancerous or noncancerous growths in the intestine. Cancerous tumours commonly affect the large intestine (see *colon, cancer of; rectum, cancer of*); the small intestine is only rarely affected. *Lymphomas* and carcinoid tumours (leading to *carcinoid syndrome*) may sometimes develop in the intestine; noncancerous tumours include *polyps* in the colon, and

adenomas, leiomyomas, lipomas, and *angiomas* in the small intestine.

intoxication A general term for a condition resulting from *poisoning*. It customarily refers to the effects of excessive drinking (see *alcohol intoxication*), but also includes *drug poisoning*, poisoning from the accumulation of the by-products of *metabolism* in the body, or the effects of industrial poisons.

intra- A prefix that means within, as in the term intramuscular (within a muscle). (See also *inter-*.)

intracavitary therapy Treatment of a cancerous tumour in a body cavity or the cavity of a hollow organ by placing a radioactive implant or anticancer drugs within the cavity. Intracavitary *radiotherapy* with a radioactive implant is a form of brachytherapy that is mainly used to treat cancers of the uterus and cervix (see *uterus, cancer of; cervix, cancer of*). If implants (usually in the form of artificial radioisotopes embedded in wires or small tubes) are used, they are left there for a period of time.

INTRACAVITARY THERAPY

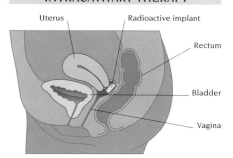

INTRACAVITARY RADIOTHERAPY

Intracavitary therapy may be used to treat a malignant effusion (a collection of fluid that contains cancerous cells). A needle, sometimes with a *catheter* attached, is passed through the wall of the abdomen or the chest into the abdominal cavity or pleural cavity (the space around the lungs). As much of the fluid as possible is withdrawn from the cavity before anticancer drugs are injected directly into it. (See also *interstitial radiotherapy*.)

intracerebral haemorrhage Bleeding into the brain from a ruptured blood vessel. It is one of the three principal mechanisms by which a stroke can occur. It mainly affects middle-aged or elderly people and is usually due to *atherosclerosis*. Untreated *hypertension* increases the risk of intracerebral haemorrhage.

The ruptured artery is usually in the *cerebrum*. The escaped blood seeps out, damaging brain tissue. The symptoms are sudden headache, weakness, and confusion, and often loss of consciousness. Speech loss, facial paralysis, or one-sided weakness may develop, depending on the area affected. Surgery is usually impossible; treatment is aimed at life-support and the reduction of blood pressure. Large haemorrhages are usually fatal. For the survivor of an intracerebral haemorrhage, rehabilitation and outlook are as for any type of stroke.

intracytoplasmic sperm injection (ICSI) A treatment for male *infertility* in which a single sperm, collected from a sample of semen or directly from the testis or epididymis, is injected into an *ovum* in vitro (see *in vitro fertilization*) to fertilize it. The fertilized ovum is then placed in the uterus.

intractable A term to describe any condition that does not respond to treatment.

intradermal A medical term meaning into or within the upper layers of the skin. An intradermal injection is made into the skin; whereas a *subcutaneous injection* is made under it.

intramuscular A medical term meaning within a muscle, as in an intramuscular injection, in which a drug is injected deep within a muscle.

intraocular pressure The pressure within the eye that helps to maintain the shape of the eyeball, due to the balance between the rate of production and removal of aqueous *humour*. Aqueous humour is continually produced from the *ciliary body* and exits from the drainage angle (a network of tissue between the iris and cornea). If drainage is impeded, intraocular pressure builds up (a condition known as *glaucoma*). If the ciliary body is damaged (as a result of prolonged inflammation), less fluid is produced and the eye becomes soft.

intrauterine contraceptive device See *IUD*.

intrauterine growth retardation Poor growth in a fetus, usually resulting from a failure of the *placenta* to provide adequate nutrients (often related to *pre-eclampsia*) or sometimes from a fetal defect. Severe maternal disease, such as chronic *kidney failure*, can reduce fetal growth. Fetal problems such as an intrauterine infection or *genetic disorder* can also impair growth. Smoking during pregnancy may reduce fetal growth and birth weight.

Intrauterine growth retardation may be suspected on *antenatal* examination; *ultrasound scanning* may be performed to assess the problem. The underlying cause is treated, if possible. If the baby's growth is slowing, *induction of labour* or a *caesarean section* may be necessary. Most babies whose growth was retarded in the uterus gain weight rapidly after delivery. However, if an intrauterine infection or genetic disorder was the cause, poor growth may continue.

intravenous A term meaning within a vein, as in intravenous infusion (slow introduction of a substance into a vein) and intravenous injection (rapid introduction of a substance into a vein).

intravenous infusion The slow introduction, over hours or days, of fluid into the bloodstream through a cannula (thin plastic tube) inserted into a vein. Commonly known as a drip, an intravenous injection is used to give blood (see *blood transfusion*) or, more commonly, fluids and essential salts. Other uses include providing nutrients to people unable to digest food (see *feeding, artificial*) and the administration of certain drugs.

intravenous urography An X-ray procedure, commonly called IVU, used to give a clear image of the *urinary tract*. The procedure involves intravenous infusion of a *contrast medium* into the arm. The medium is carried in the blood to the urinary system, where it passes through the kidneys, ureters, and bladder to be excreted in the urine. X-rays taken at intervals show outlines of the urinary system. IVU detects abnormalities such as tumours and obstructions, and signs of kidney disease.

INTRAVENOUS UROGRAPHY

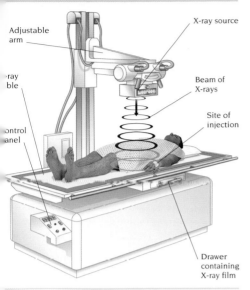

Adjustable arm

X-ray source

X-ray table

Beam of X-rays

Site of injection

Control panel

Drawer containing X-ray film

intrinsic factor A chemical produced by the stomach lining that is necessary for the absorption of vitamin B_{12}.

introitus A general term for the entrance to a body cavity or space, most commonly used for the vagina.

introvert A person more concerned with his or her inner world. Introverts prefer to work alone, are shy, quiet, and withdrawn when under stress. (See also *extrovert; personality*.)

intubation Most commonly, the process of passing an *endotracheal tube* (breathing tube) into the trachea (windpipe). Endotracheal intubation is carried out if mechanical *ventilation* is needed to deliver oxygen to the lungs. The tube is passed through the mouth or nose and down the throat.

The term intubation is also used to refer to the placement of a gastric or intestinal tube in the stomach for purposes of suction or the giving of nutrients (see *feeding, artificial*).

intussusception A condition in which part of the intestine telescopes in on itself, forming a tube within a tube, usually resulting in intestinal obstruction (see *intestine, obstruction of*). The condition usually affects the last part of the small intestine, where it joins the large intestine. In some cases there is an association with a recent infection. In other cases, it may start at the site of a *polyp* or *Meckel's diverticulum*.

Intussusception occurs most commonly in children under the age of 2. An affected child usually develops severe abdominal colic; vomiting is common, and blood and mucus are often found in the faeces. In severe cases, the blood supply to the intestine becomes blocked and *gangrene*, followed by *peritonitis* or *perforation*, may result. In some cases, an *enema* can be used to force the abnormal area of bowel back into a normal position. In other cases, surgery may be necessary to reposition the bowel.

invasive Tending to spread throughout body tissues; the term is usually applied to cancerous tumours or harmful microorganisms. In an invasive medical procedure, body tissues are penetrated by an instrument. (See also *minimally invasive surgery; noninvasive*.)

inverted nipple An indrawing of the *nipple*, which can be longstanding or may develop in later life as a result of changes in the breast. Causes include normal changes associated with aging or, in some cases, an underlying cancer.

in vitro The performance of biological processes in a laboratory rather than within the body. The term in vitro literally means "in glass".

INTUSSUSCEPTION

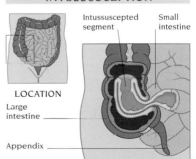

Intussuscepted segment

Small intestine

LOCATION

Large intestine

Appendix

in vitro fertilization (IVF) A method of treating *infertility* in which an egg (*ovum*) is surgically removed from the ovary and fertilized outside the body.

The woman is given a course of *fertility drugs* to stimulate release of eggs from the ovary. This is followed by *ultrasound scanning* to check the eggs, which are collected by *laparoscopy* immediately before ovulation. They are then mixed with sperm in the laboratory. Two, or sometimes more, fertilized eggs are replaced into the uterus. If they become safely implanted in the uterine wall, the pregnancy usually continues normally.

More than 1 in 4 couples who undergo in vitro fertilization eventually achieve pregnancy, although several attempts may be necessary. Modifications of the technique, such as *intracytoplasmic sperm injection (ICSI)*, *gamete intrafallopian transfer (GIFT)*, and *zygote intrafallopian transfer (ZIFT)*, are generally more effective than the original method.

in vivo Biological processes occurring within the body. (See also *in vitro.*)

involuntary movements Uncontrolled movements of the body. These movements occur spontaneously and may be slow and writhing (see *athetosis*); rapid, jerky, and random (see *chorea*); or predictable, stereotyped, and affecting one part of the body, usually the face (see *tic*). They may be a feature of a disease (for example, *Huntington's disease*) or a side effect of certain drugs used to treat psychiatric conditions.

iodine An element essential for formation of the *thyroid hormones*, triiodothyronine (T3) and thyroxine (T4), which control the rate of *metabolism* (internal chemistry) and growth and development. Dietary shortage may lead to goitre or *hypothyroidism*. Deficiency in the newborn can, if left untreated, lead to *cretinism*. Shortages are very rare in developed countries due to bread and table salt being fortified with iodide or iodate.

Radioactive iodine is sometimes used to reduce thyroid gland activity in thyrotoxicosis and in the treatment of thyroid cancer. Iodine compounds are used as antiseptics, in radiopaque contrast media in some X-ray procedures (see *imaging techniques*), and in some cough remedies.

ion A particle that carries an electrical charge; positive ions are called cations and negative ions are called anions. Many vital body processes, such as the transmission of nerve impulses, depend on the movement of ions across cell membranes. Sodium is the principal cation in the fluid that bathes all cells (extracellular fluid). It affects the flow of water into and out of cells (see *osmosis*), thereby influencing the concentration of body fluids.

The acidity of blood and other body fluids depends on the level of hydrogen cations, which are produced by metabolic processes. To prevent the fluids from becoming too acidic, hydrogen cations are neutralized by bicarbonate anions in the extracellular fluid and blood, and by phosphate anions inside cells (see *acid–base balance*).

ionizer A device that produces *ions* (electrically charged particles). Ionizers that produce negative ions can be used to neutralize positive ions in the atmosphere. Some people believe that use of an ionizer reduces symptoms, such as headaches and fatigue, that may result from a build-up of positive ions generated by electrical machines.

ipecacuanha A drug (also called ipecac) used to induce vomiting in the treatment of types of *poisoning*.

ipratropium bromide A *bronchodilator drug* used to treat breathing difficulties.

IQ The abbreviation for intelligence quotient (see *intelligence tests*).

iridectomy A procedure performed on the eye to remove part of the *iris*. The most common type of iridectomy, known as a "peripheral iridectomy", is usually performed to treat acute *glaucoma*. A small opening is made, surgically or with a laser, near the outer edge of the iris to form a channel through which *aqueous humour* can drain.

iridocyclitis Inflammation of the *iris* and *ciliary body*. Iridocyclitis is more usually known as anterior *uveitis*. (See also *eye, disorders of.*)

iridotomy A surgical procedure performed on the eye, in which an incision is made in the *iris* using a knife or a laser. Laser iridotomy may be performed to treat acute *glaucoma*. (See also *iridectomy.*)

iris The coloured part of the eye, made up of a loose framework of transparent *collagen* and muscle fibres, that lies behind the cornea and in front of the lens. It is connected at its outer edge to the ciliary body and has a central aperture, the *pupil*, through which light enters the eye and falls on the retina. The iris constantly contracts and dilates to alter the size of the pupil, which controls the amount of light that passes through the pupil.

IRIS

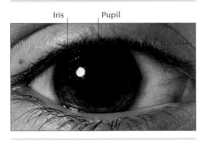

Iris   Pupil

iritis An inflammation of the *iris*, now often termed anterior *uveitis*.

iron A mineral essential for the formation of certain *enzymes*, *haemoglobin* (the oxygen-carrying pigment in red blood cells), and *myoglobin* (the oxygen carrying pigment in muscle cells). It is found in foods such as liver, cereals, fish, green leafy vegetables, nuts, and beans. During pregnancy, supplements may be needed. Iron deficiency leading to anaemia (see *anaemia, iron deficiency*) is usually caused by abnormal blood loss, such as from a *peptic ulcer* or heavy periods, but may also be due to diet.

Iron supplements may cause nausea, abdominal pain, constipation, or diarrhoea and may colour the faeces black. Excessive iron in the tissues is a feature of *haemochromatosis*, which results in organ damage, commonly *cirrhosis*.

iron-deficiency anaemia See *anaemia, iron-deficiency*.

iron lung A large machine formerly used to maintain breathing, especially in people paralysed by *poliomyelitis*. The iron lung has been replaced by more efficient means of maintaining breathing (see *ventilation*).

irradiation See *radiation hazards*; *radiotherapy*.

irradiation of food The treatment of food with ionizing *radiation* to kill bacteria, moulds, insects, and other parasites. It improves the keeping qualities of food and is a means of controlling some types of *food poisoning*. It does not destroy bacterial toxins, however, and may destroy *vitamins*. Irradiation does not render food radioactive.

irrigation, wound Cleansing of a deep wound by repeatedly washing it out with a medicated solution or sterile saline.

irritable bladder Intermittent, uncontrolled contractions of the muscles in the *bladder* wall that may cause urge incontinence (see *incontinence, urinary*). It can occur temporarily if there is a urinary tract infection (see *cystitis*); a catheter present within the bladder; a bladder stone (see *calculus, urinary tract*); or an obstruction to the outflow of urine by an enlarged *prostate gland*. In some cases, symptoms may be relieved by *antispasmodic drugs*; other treatment is directed at any underlying cause. Bladder training may also be used.

irritable bowel syndrome (IBS) A combination of intermittent abdominal pain and constipation, diarrhoea, or bouts of each, that occurs in the absence of other diagnosed disease. IBS affects about 10–20 per cent of adults; it is twice as common in women as in men, usually beginning in early or middle adulthood. It is usually recurrent throughout life but is unlikely to lead to complications.

Symptoms include cramp-like pain in the abdomen, abdominal distension, often on the left side, transient relief of pain by bowel movement or passing wind, sense of incomplete evacuation of the bowels, and excessive wind. Anxiety and stress tend to exacerbate the condition.

If constipation is the main problem, a high-fibre diet or bulk-forming agents, such as *bran* or *methylcellulose*, may be helpful. Short courses of *antidiarrhoeal drugs* may be given for persistent diarrhoea. *Antispasmodic drugs* may be prescribed to relieve muscular spasm. *Hypnosis, psychotherapy*, and *counselling* have proved effective in some cases.

ischaemia Insufficient blood supply to a specific organ or tissue. It is usually caused by disease of the blood vessels, such as *atherosclerosis*, but may also result from injury, constriction of a vessel due to spasm of the muscles in the vessel wall, or inadequate blood flow due to inefficient pumping of the heart. Symptoms depend on the area affected.

Treatment may include *vasodilator drugs* to widen the blood vessels or, in more severe cases, an *angioplasty* and insertion of a *stent* or a *bypass operation*.

ischium One of the bones that form the lower part of the *pelvis*.

isolation Nursing procedures (also called barrier nursing) designed to prevent a patient from infecting others or from being infected. The patient is usually isolated in a single room.

Complete isolation is used if a patient has a contagious disease, such as *Lassa fever*, that can be transmitted to others by direct contact and airborne germs. In this case, all bedding, equipment and clothing are either sterilized or incinerated after use. Partial isolation is carried out if the disease is transmitted in a more limited way (by droplet spread, as in *tuberculosis*, for example).

Reverse isolation, also called reverse barrier nursing, is used to protect a patient whose resistance to infection is severely lowered by a disease or treatment such as *chemotherapy*. The air supply to the room is filtered. All staff and visitors wear caps, gowns, masks, and gloves. Occasionally, long-term reverse isolation is needed for patients with severe combined immunodeficiency (see *immunodeficiency disorders*).

isometric A system of *exercise* without body movement in which muscles build up strength by working against resistance, provided by either a fixed object or an opposing set of muscles. (See also *isotonic*.)

isoniazid An *antibacterial drug* used to treat *tuberculosis*. Isoniazid is given in combination with other antituberculous drugs, usually for at least 6 months.

isoprenaline A drug used to stimulate the heart in cases of severe shock. It is used only in hospitals, mainly in intensive care units.

isosorbide A long-acting *nitrate drug* that acts as a vasodilator drug. Isosorbide is used to reduce the severity and frequency of *angina pectoris*. This drug

is also given to treat severe *heart failure*. Adverse effects include headache, hot flushes, and dizziness.

isotonic A system of *exercise*, such as weight lifting, in which muscle tension is kept constant as the body works against its own, or an external, weight. The term also describes fluids, such as intravenous fluids or drinks, with the same osmotic pressure (see *osmosis*) as the blood. (See also *isometric*.)

isotope scanning See *radionuclide scanning*.

isotretinoin A drug derived from *vitamin A* used in the treatment of severe *acne*. It works by reducing the formation of sebum (natural skin oils) and keratin (a tough protein that is the major component of the outer layer of skin).

Side effects include itching, dryness and flaking of the skin, and cracking of the lips; depression may also be exacerbated. Isotretinoin may damage a developing fetus and therefore before starting treatment a woman is given a pregnancy test to ensure she is not pregnant. She should then avoid getting pregnant while taking the drug and for at least one month after stopping it.

ispaghula A bulk-forming *laxative drug* used to treat *constipation*, *diverticular disease*, and *irritable bowel syndrome*. As ispaghula travels through the intestine, it absorbs water from surrounding blood vessels, thereby softening and increasing the volume of the faeces. Ispaghula is also used in people with chronic, watery *diarrhoea* and in patients who have had a *colostomy* or an *ileostomy* to control the consistency of faeces.

Adverse effects include flatulence, abdominal distension, and discomfort.

itching An intense irritation or tickling sensation in the skin. Generalized itching may result from excessive bathing, which removes the skin's natural oils and may leave the skin excessively dry. Some people experience general itching after taking certain drugs. Many elderly people suffer from dry, itchy skin, especially on their backs. Itching commonly occurs during pregnancy.

Many skin conditions, including *chickenpox*, *urticaria* (nettle rash), and *eczema*, produce an itchy rash. Generalized skin itchiness can be a result of *diabetes mellitus, kidney failure, jaundice,* and *thyroid* disorders.

Pruritus ani (itching around the anal region) occurs with *haemorrhoids* and *anal fissure. Threadworm infestation* is the most likely cause of anal itching in children. Pruritus vulvae (itching of the external genitalia in women) may be due to *candidiasis,* hormonal changes, or to use of spermicides or vaginal ointments and deodorants. *Insect bites, lice,* and *scabies* infestations cause intense itching. Specific treatment for itching depends on the underlying cause. Cooling lotions, such as *calamine,* relieve irritation; emollients reduce dryness.

-itis A suffix meaning "inflammation of". Virtually every organ or tissue in the body can suffer inflammation, so "itis" is by far the most common word ending in medicine. Examples of its use are bronchitis (inflammation of the bronchi) and hepatitis (inflammation of the liver).

itraconazole A type of *antifungal drug.*

IUCD An abbreviation for intrauterine contraceptive device (see *IUD*).

IUD An abbreviation for intrauterine contraceptive device. An IUD, which is also known as an IUCD or coil, is a mechanical device that is inserted into the uterus for purposes of *contraception.* Most IUDs are plastic devices with either copper or silver incorporated to improve their effectiveness. One type of IUD releases small amounts of *progestogen hormone* and is sometimes known as an intrauterine system (see *IUS*). IUDs are believed to act by inhibiting the implantation of a fertilized egg in the wall of the uterus (see *implantation, egg*).

An IUD is inserted through the vagina and cervix into the uterine cavity. Once in position, an IUD provides immediate and highly effective protection. Most IUDs have a plastic string attached to make removal easier and also to indicate its presence when in place. IUDs may be left in place for up to 10 years, depending on the type. Most IUDs can also be used as emergency contraception; the exception is the type of IUD that releases progestogen (the IUS).

IUDs are not usually recommended for women with *fibroids* or an irregular uterine cavity. If menstrual flow is heavy or if there is a history or increased risk of *pelvic inflammatory disease* (PID), a progestogen IUD may be recommended.

Rarely, pregnancy can occur, although IUDs seldom cause problems and can be removed. Nonprogestogen IUDs can increase the risk of PID in certain groups, such as women with multiple partners. A rare complication of IUD use is perforation of the uterus, which most commonly occurs at the time of insertion.

IUS An abbreviation for intrauterine system. The IUS is a mechanical contraceptive device that resembles an *IUD* but also contains the *progestogen hormone* levonorgestrel. Like the IUD, the device is fitted inside the uterus, where the hormone is released slowly and continuously for up to 5 years. The IUS prevents pregnancy by affecting the uterine lining and thickening the cervical mucus. It may be recommended for contraceptive use instead of a nonprogestogen IUD for women with a history or increased risk of *pelvic inflammatory disease* (PID) The IUS is not suitable for emergency contraception.

In addition to its contraceptive effect, the IUS may make menstrual periods lighter and less painful and so may be used as treatment for heavy periods (see *menorrhagia*). It may also sometimes be used to deliver progestogen as part of *hormone replacement therapy (HRT).*

IVF See *in vitro fertilization.*

IVU The abbreviation for *intravenous urography* (an X-ray imaging technique for visualizing the urinary tract).

IUD

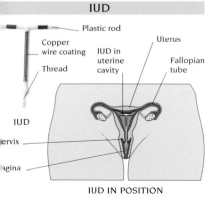

Plastic rod
Copper wire coating
Thread
IUD in uterine cavity
Uterus
Fallopian tube
IUD
ervix
agina

IUD IN POSITION

J

Jakob–Creutzfeldt disease See *Creutz-feldt–Jakob disease*.

jaundice Yellowing of the skin and the whites of the eyes, caused by an accumulation of *bilirubin* in the blood. Jaundice is the chief sign of many disorders of the *liver* and *biliary system*. Many babies develop jaundice soon after birth (see *jaundice, neonatal*).

Bilirubin is formed from *haemoglobin* when old red cells are broken down, mainly by the *spleen*. It is absorbed by the liver, where it is made soluble in water and excreted in *bile*.

There are three main types of jaundice: haemolytic, hepatocellular, and obstructive. In haemolytic jaundice, too much bilirubin is produced for the liver to process. This is caused by excessive *haemolysis* of red cells, which can have many causes (see *anaemia, haemolytic*).

In hepatocellular jaundice, bilirubin accumulates because its transfer from liver cells into the bile is prevented, usually due to acute hepatitis (see *hepatitis, acute*) or *liver failure*.

In obstructive jaundice, also known as cholestatic jaundice, bile cannot leave the liver because of *bile duct obstruction*. Obstructive jaundice can also occur if the bile ducts are not present (as in *biliary atresia*) or if they have been destroyed by disease. *Cholestasis* then occurs and bilirubin is forced back into the blood. For all types of jaundice, treatment is for the underlying cause.

jaundice, neonatal Yellowing of the skin and whites of the eyes in newborn babies, due to accumulation of *bilirubin* in the blood. It usually results from the *liver* being immature and unable to excrete bilirubin efficiently. This form of jaundice is usually harmless and disappears within a week. Rarely, severe or persistent neonatal jaundice is caused by *haemolytic disease of the newborn*, *G6PD deficiency*, hepatitis, hypothyroidism, *biliary atresia*, or infection.

Jaundiced babies usually require extra fluids and may be treated with *phototherapy*. Exchange transfusion (see *blood transfusion*) may be needed in severe cases. If severe neonatal jaundice is not treated promptly, *kernicterus* may occur.

jaw The mobile bone of the face, also known as the mandible. The term sometimes includes the *maxilla*. The mandible bears the lower teeth on its upper surface and is connected to the base of the skull at the *temporomandibular joints*. Muscles attached to the jaw allow movements needed in chewing, biting, and side-to-side and downward movement.

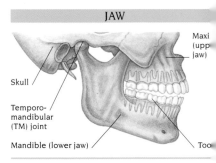

JAW

Skull

Maxi
(upp
jaw)

Temporo-mandibular
(TM) joint

Mandible (lower jaw)

Too

jaw, dislocated Displacement of the lower *jaw* from one or both *temporomandibular joints*. A dislocated jaw is usually due either to a blow or to yawning. There is pain in front of the ear on the affected side or sides, and the jaw projects forwards. The mouth cannot be fully closed, making eating and speaking difficult. Dislocation tends to recur. Surgery may be carried out to stabilize the joint but is often unsuccessful.

jaw, fractured A fracture of the *jaw*, most often caused by a direct blow. A minor fracture may cause tenderness, pain on biting, and stiffness. In more severe injuries, teeth may be loosened or damaged, jaw movement may be severely limited, and there may be loss of feeling in the lower lip. Minor fractures are normally left to heal on their own. For severe fractures with displacement of the bones, surgical treatment is necessary. To allow healing, the jaw is immobilized, usually by wiring the upper and lower teeth together. The wires are removed after about 6 weeks.

jealousy, morbid Preoccupation with the potential sexual infidelity of one's partner. The sufferer, most often a man, becomes convinced that his partner is having an affair. Morbid jealousy is usually caused by a *personality disorder*, *depression*, or *paranoia*, but may also occur in those suffering from *alcohol dependence* or organic brain syndrome (see *brain syndrome, organic*).

jejunal biopsy A diagnostic test in which a small piece of tissue is removed from the lining of the *jejunum* for microscopic examination. It is especially useful in the diagnosis of *Crohn's disease*, *coeliac disease*, *lymphoma*, and other causes of *malabsorption*. The biopsy is taken using an *endoscope* passed down the throat into the small intestine, via the stomach.

jejunum The middle, coiled section of the small *intestine*, joining the *duodenum* to the *ileum*. The jejunum's function is the digestion of food and absorption of nutrients. It may be affected by *coeliac disease*, *Crohn's disease*, and *lymphoma*.

jellyfish stings Stings from jellyfish, which belong to a group of marine animals called coelenterates or cnidarians. Stinging capsules discharge when jellyfish tentacles are touched. Usually, the sting causes only a mildly painful or itchy rash, but some jellyfish and Portuguese men-of-war (other members of the same group) can cause a severe sting. Rarely, venom may cause vomiting, sweating, breathing difficulties, and collapse. Dangerous species live mainly in tropical waters. *Antivenoms* may be available.

jet-lag Fatigue and interruption of the sleep-wake cycle caused by disturbance of normal body *biorhythms* as a result of flying across different time zones. Jet-lag provokes daytime sleepiness and *insomnia* at night. Other symptoms include reduced physical and mental activity, and poor memory. Jet-lag tends to be worse after an eastward flight (which shortens the traveller's day) than after a westward one.

jigger An alternative name for a *chigoe* or sand flea.

jogger's nipple Soreness of the nipple caused by clothing rubbing against it,

usually during sports such as jogging or long-distance running. Both men and women can be affected. Prevention is by applying petroleum jelly to the nipple before prolonged running.

joint The junction between two or more bones. Many joints are highly mobile, while others are fixed or allow only a small amount of movement.

Joints in the skull are fixed joints firmly secured by fibrous tissue. The bone surfaces of mobile joints are coated with smooth *cartilage* to reduce friction. The joint is sealed within a tough fibrous capsule lined with synovial membrane (see *synovium*), which produces a lubricating fluid. Each joint is surrounded by strong *ligaments* that support it and prevent excessive movement. Movement is controlled by muscles that are attached to bone by *tendons* on either side of the joint. Most mobile joints have at least

JOINT

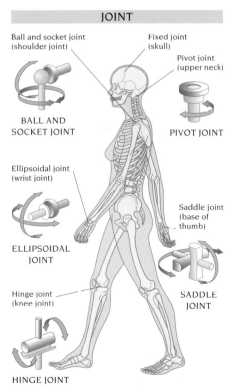

Ball and socket joint (shoulder joint)

Fixed joint (skull)

Pivot joint (upper neck)

BALL AND SOCKET JOINT

PIVOT JOINT

Ellipsoidal joint (wrist joint)

Saddle joint (base of thumb)

ELLIPSOIDAL JOINT

Hinge joint (knee joint)

SADDLE JOINT

HINGE JOINT

one *bursa* nearby, which cushions a pressure point.

There are several types of mobile joint. The hinge joint is the simplest, allowing bending and straightening, as in the fingers. The knee and elbow joints are modified hinge joints that allow some rotation as well. Pivot joints, such as the joint between the 1st and 2nd vertebrae (see *vertebra*), allow rotation only. Ellipsoidal joints, such as the wrist, allow all types of movement except pivotal. Ball-and-socket joints include the hip and shoulder joints. These allow the widest range of movement (backwards or forwards, sideways, and rotation).

Common joint injuries include sprains, damage to the cartilage, torn ligaments, and tearing of the joint capsule. Joint *dislocation* is usually caused by injury but is occasionally *congenital*. A less severe injury may cause *subluxation* (partial dislocation). Rarely, the bone ends are fractured, which may cause bleeding into the joint (*haemarthrosis*) or *effusion* (build-up of fluid in a joint) due to *synovitis* (inflammation of the joint lining). Joints are commonly affected by *arthritis*. *Bursitis* may occur as a result of local irritation or strain.

joint replacement See *arthroplasty*.

joule The international unit of *energy*, work, and heat. Approximately 4,200 joules (symbol J) or 4.2 kilojoules (kJ) equal 1 kilocalorie (kcal); 1 kJ is equal to about 0.24 kcal. (See also *calorie*.)

jugular vein One of three veins on each side of the neck that return deoxygenated blood from the head to the heart. The internal jugular, the largest of the three (internal, external, and anterior), arises at the base of the skull, travels down the neck alongside the carotid arteries, and passes behind the *clavicle*, where it joins the subclavian vein (the large vein that drains blood from the arms).

Jungian theory Ideas put forward by the Swiss psychiatrist Carl Gustav Jung (1875–1961). Jung theorized that certain ideas (called archetypes) inherited from experiences in a person's distant past were present in his or her unconscious and controlled the way he or she viewed the world. Jung called these shared ideas the "collective unconscious". He believed that each individual also had a "personal unconscious", containing experiences from his or her life, but he regarded the collective unconscious as superior. Therapy was aimed at putting people in touch with this source of ideas, particularly through dream interpretation. Jung's approach was also based on his theory of personality, which postulated two basic types: the extrovert and the introvert. One of these types dominates a person's consciousness and the other must be brought into consciousness and reconciled with its opposite for the person to become a whole individual.

juvenile arthritis See *juvenile chronic arthritis*.

juvenile chronic arthritis A rare form of *arthritis* affecting children. Juvenile chronic arthritis occurs more often in girls, and usually develops between 2 and 4 years of age or around puberty. There are three main types. *Still's disease* (systemic onset juvenile arthritis) starts with fever, rash, enlarged lymph nodes, abdominal pain, and weight loss. These symptoms last for a period of several weeks. Joint pain, swelling, and stiffness may develop after several months. Polyarticular juvenile arthritis causes pain, swelling, and stiffness in many joints. Pauciarticular juvenile arthritis affects four joints or fewer.

Possible complications include short stature, *anaemia*, *pleurisy*, *pericarditis*, and enlargement of the *liver* and *spleen*. *Uveitis* may develop, which, if untreated, may damage vision. Rarely, *amyloidosis* may occur or *kidney failure* may develop.

Diagnosis is based on the symptoms, together with the results of X-rays and *blood tests*, and is only made if the condition lasts for longer than 3 months.

Treatment may include *disease-modifying antirheumatic drugs*, such as gold, methotrexate, and azathioprine, *corticosteroid drugs*, *nonsteroidal anti-inflammatory drugs*, or *aspirin*. Splints may be worn to rest inflamed joints and to reduce the risk of deformities. *Physiotherapy* reduces the risk of muscle wasting and deformities.

The arthritis usually clears up after several years. However, in some children, the condition remains active into adult life.

K

kala-azar A form of *leishmaniasis* that is spread by insects. Kala-azar occurs in parts of Africa, India, the Mediterranean, and South America.

kaolin An *aluminium* compound used as an ingredient in some *antidiarrhoeal drugs*. Kaolin is taken orally and increases the bulk of faeces.

Kaposi's sarcoma A cancerous tumour arising from blood vessels, usually in the skin. Kaposi's sarcoma usually only occurs in those people who have *AIDS* or a weakened immune system and is associated with infection with a specific herpes virus. The tumours, which consist of pinkish brown raised areas or flat patches, can spread rapidly. They usually start on the feet and ankles, spread up the legs, and then appear on the hands and arms.

KAPOSI'S SARCOMA

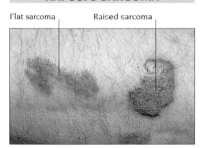

Flat sarcoma   Raised sarcoma

Tumours can also affect the gastrointestinal and respiratory tracts, where they may cause severe internal bleeding. Skin lesions may be treated with *radiotherapy*. *Anticancer drugs* may be used for wide spread skin disease or internal lesions.

karyotype The characteristics of *chromosomes*, in terms of number, size, and structure, in an individual or a species. The term "karyotype" is also applied to a diagram of chromosome pairs arranged in their assigned numerical order.

Kawasaki disease A rare acute illness of unknown cause that most commonly affects children under 2. The disease is characterized by fever lasting 1–2 weeks, *conjunctivitis*, dryness and cracking of the lips, swollen *lymph nodes* in the neck, reddening of the palms and soles, and a generalized rash. By the end of the 2nd week of illness, the skin at the tips of the fingers and toes peels and other symptoms subside. The heart muscle and *coronary arteries* are affected in about 1 in 5 cases. High dose *gammaglobulin* and *aspirin* may be given to prevent associated heart complications. Most children recover completely.

keloid A raised, hard, irregularly shaped, itchy scar on the skin due to a defective healing process in which too much *collagen* is produced, usually after a skin injury. Keloids can develop anywhere on the body, but the breastbone and shoulder are common sites. Black people are affected more than whites. After several months, most keloids flatten and cease to itch. Injection of *corticosteroid drugs* into the keloid may reduce itchiness more quickly and cause some shrinkage.

keratin A fibrous *protein* that is the main constituent of the tough outermost layer of the *skin*, *nails*, and *hair*.

keratitis Inflammation of the *cornea*. It often takes the form of a *corneal ulcer* and may result from injury, contact with chemicals, or an infection. Symptoms of keratitis include pain and excessive watering of the eye, blurring of vision, and *photophobia*. Noninfective keratitis is treated by covering the affected eye. Drugs such as *antibiotics* may be given to treat infective keratitis.

keratoacanthoma A type of harmless skin nodule that commonly occurs in elderly people, most often on the face or arm. The cause is unknown, but many years of exposure to strong sunlight or long-term use of *immunosuppressant drugs* may be factors. Initially, the nodule resembles a small wart, but it grows to 1–2cm across in about 8 weeks. Although the nodule usually disappears gradually after this, surgical removal is often recommended to prevent scarring.

keratoconjunctivitis Inflammation of the *cornea* associated with *conjunctivitis*.

The most common form, epidemic keratoconjunctivitis, is caused by a virus and is highly infectious. The conjunctivitis is often severe and may destroy the surface of the *conjunctiva*. Tiny opaque spots develop in the cornea that may interfere with vision and persist for months. There is no specific treatment, but corneal spots may be minimized by using eyedrops containing *corticosteroid drugs*.

keratoconjunctivitis sicca Persistent dryness of the *cornea* and *conjunctiva* caused by deficiency in tear production. The condition is associated with *autoimmune disorders* such as *rheumatoid arthritis*, *Sjögren's syndrome*, and systemic *lupus erythematosus*. Prolonged dryness may lead to blurred vision, itching, grittiness, and, in severe cases, the formation of a *corneal ulcer*. The most effective treatment is frequent use of artificial tears (see *tears, artificial*).

keratoconus An inherited disorder of the eye in which the *cornea* becomes gradually thinned and conical. The condition affects both eyes and usually develops around puberty, giving rise to increasing *myopia* and progressive distortion of vision that cannot be fully corrected by glasses. Hard contact lenses improve vision in the early stages, but when vision has seriously deteriorated and contact lenses are no longer helpful it generally becomes necessary to perform a *corneal graft*.

keratolytic drugs Drugs that loosen and remove the tough outer layer of skin. Keratolytic drugs, which include *urea* and *salicylic acid* preparations, are used to treat skin and scalp disorders, such as *warts, acne, dandruff*, and *psoriasis*.

keratomalacia A progressive disease of the *eye*, caused by severe *vitamin A* deficiency, in which the *cornea* becomes opaque and ulcerated. Perforation of the cornea is common, often leading to loss of the eye through infection. The condition usually occurs only in severely malnourished children and is a common cause of blindness in developing countries. In the early stages, the damage can be reversed by treatment with large doses of vitamin A but, if untreated, blindness is usually inevitable.

keratopathy A general term used to describe a variety of disorders of the *cornea*. Actinic keratopathy is a painful condition in which the outer layer of the cornea is damaged by *ultraviolet light*. Exposure keratopathy is corneal damage due to loss of the protection afforded by the tear film and blink reflex. It may occur in conditions in which the eyelids inadequately cover the cornea, including severe *exophthalmos*, *facial palsy*, and *ectropion*.

keratoplasty See *corneal graft*.

keratosis A *skin* growth caused by an overproduction of *keratin*. Keratoses occur mainly in elderly people. Seborrhoeic keratoses are harmless growths that occur mainly on the trunk. The growths range in appearance from flat, dark-brown patches to small, wart-like protrusions. They do not need treating unless they are unsightly. Solar keratoses are small, wart-like, red or flesh-coloured growths that appear on exposed parts of the body as a result of overexposure to the sun over many years. Rarely, they may develop into skin cancer, usually *squamous cell carcinoma*, and must be surgically removed.

keratosis pilaris A common condition in which patches of rough skin appear on the upper arms, thighs, and buttocks. The openings of the hair follicles become enlarged by plugs of *keratin*, and hair growth may be distorted. The condition occurs most commonly in adolescents and obese people. It is not serious and usually clears up on its

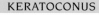

KERATOCONUS

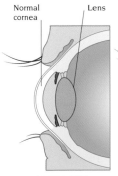

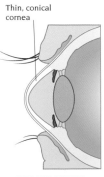

Normal cornea   Lens   Thin, conical cornea

NORMAL EYE   KERATOCONUS

own. In severe cases, applying a mixture of *salicylic acid* and soft paraffin and scrubbing with a loofah may help.

keratotomy, radial A now uncommon procedure in which radiating incisions are made in the *cornea* (up to, but not through, its innermost layer) to reduce *myopia*. Radial keratotomy has been largely replaced by laser procedures, such as *LASIK*, which carry less risk of permanent damage to the eye.

kerion A red, boggy, pustular swelling that develops as a reaction to a fungal infection, usually scalp ringworm (see *tinea*). The inflammation gradually subsides over 6–8 weeks, but, if severe, may leave a scar and permanent hair loss in the affected area. Oral *antifungal drugs* need to be taken for several weeks.

kernicterus A rare disorder in which newborn, especially premature, infants suffer brain damage because of severe jaundice (see *jaundice, neonatal*).

ketamine A general *anaesthetic*, given by injection. It is mainly given to children undergoing painful procedures, such as *bone marrow biopsy*. Ketamine is often abused for its stimulant effect.

ketoacidosis A combination of *acidosis* and *ketosis*.

ketoconazole An *antifungal drug* used to treat *fungal infections* of the gut, skin, and fingernails, and *candidiasis* (thrush) of the mouth or vagina. It is also used as a shampoo to treat dandruff. Adverse effects include nausea and rash.

ketone Any of a group of chemicals related to acetone, which is found in solvents such as nail polish remover. Certain ketones are produced during the *metabolism* of fats. Excessive amounts build up in the body in *ketosis*.

ketoprofen A type of *nonsteroidal anti-inflammatory drug* (NSAID) prescribed as an *analgesic drug* for injuries to soft tissues, such as muscles and ligaments. Ketoprofen also reduces joint pain and stiffness in arthritic conditions. It may cause abdominal pain, nausea, indigestion, and increased risk of *peptic ulcer*.

ketosis A potentially serious condition in which excessive amounts of chemicals called *ketones* accumulate in the body. Ketones are normal products of fat *metabolism* but are produced in ex-

cess when *glucose* is not available for the body to use as an energy source, for example in starvation or inadequately controlled *diabetes mellitus*. Symptoms include sweet, "fruity"-smelling breath, loss of appetite, nausea, and abdominal pain. If the condition is not treated, it may result in confusion, unconsciousness, and death. Treatment is the same as for diabetes unless the cause is fasting or starvation, in which case a nutritious diet is usually effective.

keyhole surgery Another name for *minimally invasive surgery*.

kidney Either of the two organs that filter the blood and excrete waste products and excess water as *urine*. The kidneys are situated at the back of the abdominal cavity, on either side of the spine. Each kidney is surrounded by a fibrous capsule and is made up of an outer cortex and an inner medulla.

The cortex contains specialized capillaries called glomeruli, which, together

KIDNEY

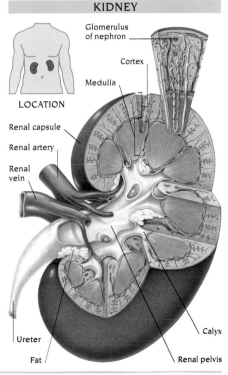

Glomerulus of nephron

Cortex

Medulla

LOCATION

Renal capsule

Renal artery

Renal vein

Ureter

Fat

Calyx

Renal pelvis

with a series of tubules, make up the *nephrons*, the filtering units of the kidney. The nephrons filter blood under pressure and then selectively reabsorb water and certain other substances back into the blood. Urine is formed from substances that are not reabsorbed. The urine is conducted through tubules to the renal pelvis (the central collecting area of the kidney) and then through tubes called ureters to the bladder.

The kidneys also regulate the body's fluid balance. To do this, the kidneys excrete excess water, and when water is lost from the body (for example as a result of sweating), they conserve it (see *ADH*). In addition, the kidneys control the body's *acid–base balance* by adjusting urine acidity. The kidneys are also involved in hormonal regulation of red *blood cell* production and *blood pressure*.

kidney biopsy A procedure in which a small sample of *kidney* tissue is removed and examined under a microscope. Kidney *biopsy* is performed to investigate and diagnose serious kidney disorders, such as *glomerulonephritis*, *proteinuria*, *nephrotic syndrome*, and acute *kidney failure*, or to assess the kidneys' response to treatment. There are two basic techniques: percutaneous needle biopsy, in which a hollow needle is passed through the skin into the kidney under local *anaesthesia*; and open surgery under general anaesthesia.

kidney cancer A cancerous tumour of the *kidney*. Most kidney cancers originate in the kidney itself, but in rare cases cancer spreads to the kidney from another organ. There are three main types of kidney cancer. The most common, renal cell carcinoma, usually occurs in people over 40. Nephroblastoma (also called *Wilms' tumour*) is a fast-growing tumour that mainly affects children under 5. Transitional cell carcinoma arises from cells lining the renal pelvis; it is more common in smokers or those who have taken *analgesic drugs* for a long time.

Symptoms of kidney cancer vary. It is often symptomless in the early stages, although later there may be blood in the urine. All types require surgical removal of the kidney and sometimes also of the ureter. For nephroblastoma, surgery is followed by treatment with *anticancer drugs*. Kidney cancer is likely to be fatal if it has spread to other organs before treatment is started.

kidney cyst A fluid-filled sac in the *kidney*. Most kidney cysts are noncancerous. Cysts commonly develop in people over 50 and may occur singly or multiply in one or both kidneys. Most cysts occur for no known reason and do not usually produce symptoms unless they become large enough to cause pain in the lower back due to pressure. However, large numbers of cysts in the kidneys may be associated with polycystic kidney disease (see *kidney, polycystic*), which often leads to *kidney failure*. Treatment of simple cysts is not usually necessary, but *aspiration* (withdrawal of fluid) or surgical removal may be carried out if a cyst is painful or recurs.

kidney disorders The *kidneys* are susceptible to a wide range of disorders. However, since only one normal kidney is needed for good health, disease is rarely life-threatening unless it affects both kidneys and is at an advanced stage.

Congenital abnormalities, such as *horseshoe kidney*, are fairly common and usually harmless. Serious inherited disorders include polycystic kidney disease (see *kidney, polycystic*), *Fanconi's syndrome*, and *renal tubular acidosis*.

Blood vessels in the kidneys can be damaged by *shock, haemolytic–uraemic syndrome, polyarteritis nodosa, diabetes mellitus*, and systemic *lupus erythematosus*. The filtering units may be inflamed (see *glomerulonephritis*). Allergic reactions to drugs, prolonged treatment with *analgesic drugs*, and some *antibiotics* can damage kidney tubules. Noncancerous kidney *tumours* are rare, as is *kidney cancer*. Metabolic disorders, such as *hyperuricaemia*, may cause kidney stones (see *calculus, urinary tract*). Infection of the kidney is called *pyelonephritis*. *Hydronephrosis* is caused by urinary tract obstruction. In *crush syndrome*, kidney function is disrupted by proteins released into the blood from damaged muscle. *Hypertension* can be a cause and an effect of kidney damage. Other effects of serious damage include *nephrotic syndrome* and *kidney failure*.

kidney failure A reduction in the function of the *kidneys*. Kidney failure can be *acute* or *chronic*. In acute kidney failure, kidney function often returns to normal once the underlying cause has been discovered and treated; in chronic kidney failure, function is usually irreversibly lost. Causes of acute kidney failure include a severe reduction in blood flow to the kidneys, as occurs in *shock*; an obstruction to urine flow, for example due to a *bladder tumour*; or certain rapidly developing types of kidney disease, such as *glomerulonephritis*. Chronic kidney failure can result from a disease that causes progressive damage to the kidneys, such as *hypertension, diabetes mellitus*, longstanding obstruction to urine flow, and excessive use of *analgesic drugs*.

The most obvious symptom of acute kidney failure is usually oliguria (reduced volume of urine). This leads to a build-up of urea and other waste products in the blood and tissues, which may cause drowsiness, nausea, and breathlessness. Symptoms of chronic kidney failure develop more gradually and may include malaise, nausea, loss of appetite, and weakness.

If acute kidney failure is due to sudden reduction in blood flow, blood volume and pressure can be brought back to normal by saline *intravenous infusion* or *blood transfusion*. Surgery may be needed to remove an obstruction in the urinary tract. Acute kidney disease may be treated with *corticosteroid drugs*. Treatment may also involve *diuretic drugs* and temporary *dialysis* (artificial purification of the blood). A high-carbohydrate, low-protein diet with controlled fluid and salt intake is important for both types of kidney failure. Chronic kidney failure may progress over months or years towards end-stage kidney failure, which is life-threatening. At this stage, long-term dialysis or a *kidney transplant* is the only effective treatment. In both acute and chronic kidney failure, good control of hypertension and diabetes is essential.

kidney function tests Tests performed to investigate *kidney disorders*. *Urinalysis* is a simple test in which a urine sample is examined under a microscope for blood cells, pus cells, and casts (cells and mucous material that accumulate in the tubules of the kidneys and pass into the urine). Urine may be tested for substances, such as proteins, that leak into the urine when the kidneys are damaged. Kidney function can be assessed by measuring the concentration in the blood of substances, such as *urea* and *creatinine*, that the kidneys normally excrete. Kidney function may also be assessed by *kidney imaging* techniques.

kidney imaging Techniques for visualizing the *kidneys*, usually performed for diagnosis. *Ultrasound scanning* can be used to identify kidney enlargement, a *cyst* or tumour, and the site of any blockage. Conventional *X-rays* show the outline of the kidneys and most kidney stones. *Intravenous urography* shows the internal anatomy of the kidney and *ureters*. *Angiography* is used to image blood circulation through the kidneys. *CT scanning* and *MRI* provide detailed cross-sectional images and can show abscesses or tumours. Two types of *radionuclide scanning* are used for the kidneys: DMSA and DTPA/MAG3 scanning. A DMSA scan gives information about the size, shape, and position of the kidneys. A DTPA/MAG3 scan provides information about blood flow to the kidneys and kidney function.

kidney, polycystic An inherited disorder in which both *kidneys* are affected by numerous *cysts* that gradually enlarge until most of the normal kidney tissue is destroyed. Polycystic kidney disease is distinguished from multiple simple *kidney cysts*, which occur commonly with age. There are two types of polycystic disease. The most common usually becomes apparent in middle age, producing abdominal swelling, pain, and blood in the urine. As the disease progresses, *hypertension* and *kidney failure* may result. The rare type causes enlargement of the kidneys and kidney failure in infants and young children. There is no effective treatment for preserving kidney function in either type, but symptoms of kidney

K

failure can be treated by *dialysis* and *kidney transplant*.

kidney stone See *calculus, urinary tract*.

kidney transplant An operation in which a person with chronic *kidney failure* receives a healthy kidney, either from a living donor or a cadaver. One donor kidney is sufficient to maintain the health of the recipient. The new kidney is placed in the pelvis through an incision in the abdomen and carefully positioned so that it can be connected easily to a nearby vein and artery and to the bladder. The diseased kidneys are left in place. The transplant avoids the need for *dialysis* and often allows a return to normal lifestyle. Kidney transplantation is more straightforward and common than the transplantation of any other major organ.

kidney tumours Growths in the *kidney*. Kidney tumours may be cancerous (see *kidney cancer*) or noncancerous. Noncancerous ones, such as *fibromas*, *lipomas*, and *leiomyomas*, are often symptomless, although a *haemangioma* (composed of a collection of blood vessels) may grow very large and cause blood to appear in the urine. Treatment is usually not needed for noncancerous tumours unless they are large or painful, in which case they may be surgically removed.

kilocalorie The unit of energy equal to 1,000 *calories*, abbreviated to kcal. In dietetics, a kilocalorie is sometimes referred to simply as a Calorie (or C).

kilojoule The unit of energy equal to 1,000 *joules*, abbreviated to kJ. One kcal (see *kilocalorie*) equals 4.2 kJ.

kiss of life A commonly used name for *artificial respiration*.

kleptomania A recurring inability to resist impulses to steal, often without any desire for the stolen objects. The condition is usually a sign of an immature personality. It is sometimes associated with *depression*, and may also result from *dementia* or some forms of *brain damage*.

Klinefelter's syndrome A *chromosomal abnormality* in which a male has one, or occasionally more, extra X chromosomes in his cells, giving a complement of XXY instead of XY. The risk of a baby having the condition increases with maternal age. Features of the syndrome vary in severity and may

KIDNEY TRANSPLANT

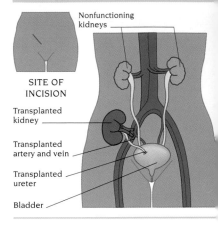

Nonfunctioning kidneys

SITE OF INCISION

Transplanted kidney

Transplanted artery and vein

Transplanted ureter

Bladder

not become apparent until puberty, when *gynaecomastia* (breast enlargement) occurs and the *testes* remain small. Affected males are usually infertile (see *infertility*). They tend to be tall and thin with a female body shape and absence of body hair. Incidence of *learning difficulties* is higher in people with Klinefelter's syndrome than in the general population. There is no cure for the disorder, but hormonal treatment can induce secondary *sexual characteristics*, and *mastectomy* may be used to treat gynaecomastia.

Klumpke's paralysis *Paralysis* of the lower arm, with wasting of the small muscles in the hand, and numbness of the fingers (excluding the thumb) and of the inside of the forearm. Klumpke's paralysis is caused by injury to the 1st thoracic nerve (one of the *spinal nerves*) in the *brachial plexus*, which is usually the result of *dislocation* of the shoulder.

knee The hinge *joint* between the *femur* (thighbone) and *tibia* (shin). The *patella* (kneecap) lies across the front of the joint. Two protective discs of cartilage called menisci (see *meniscus*) cover the surfaces of the femur and tibia to reduce friction. *Bursas* (fluid-filled sacs) are present above and below the patella and behind the knee. External *ligaments* on each side of the joint provide support. *Cruciate ligaments* within the joint prevent overstraightening and overben-

K

KNEE

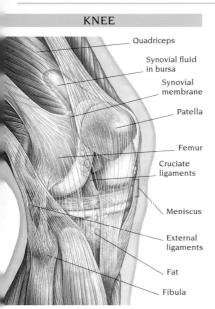

Quadriceps

Synovial fluid in bursa

Synovial membrane

Patella

Femur

Cruciate ligaments

Meniscus

External ligaments

Fat

Fibula

ding of the knee. The *quadriceps muscles* on the front of the thigh straighten the knee; the *hamstring muscles* at the back of the thigh bend it.

Knee injuries are common. They include ligament sprains, torn meniscus, *dislocation* of the patella, and *fracture* of any of the bones in the joint. *Chondromalacia patellae* is common in adolescents.

kneecap See *patella*.

knee-joint replacement Surgery to replace a diseased *knee* joint with an artificial substitute, usually a metal or plastic implant. Knee-joint replacement is most commonly carried out in older people whose knees are severely affected by *osteoarthritis* or *rheumatoid arthritis*.

knock-knee Inward curving of the legs so that the knees touch, causing the feet to be kept further apart. Knock knee is common in toddlers and may be part of normal development. In adults or children, it may be caused by a disease such as *rickets* that softens the bones; *osteoarthritis* or *rheumatoid arthritis* of the knee; or a leg *fracture* that has not healed correctly. In children, the condition usually disappears by age 10. Knock-knee that persists, or is caused

by a disorder, may require *osteotomy*, in which the *tibia* (shin) is cut and re-aligned to straighten the leg. In adults, *knee-joint replacement* may be needed.

knuckle The name for a *finger* joint.

koilonychia A condition in which the *nails* are dry, brittle, and thin, eventually becoming spoon-shaped. It may be caused by injury to the nail, and may also be associated with iron-deficiency *anaemia* or *lichen planus*.

Koplik's spots Tiny, grey-white spots that appear in the mouth during the incubation period of *measles*.

Korsakoff's psychosis See *Wernicke–Korsakoff syndrome*.

kraurosis vulvae See *vulvitis*.

kuru A rare, fatal infection of the brain that affects some inhabitants of New Guinea. The disease is caused by a *prion*, which has a long incubation period and is spread by cannibalism. Symptoms include progressive difficulty in controlling movements and *dementia*.

kwashiorkor A severe form of *malnutrition* in young children that occurs principally in poor rural areas in the tropics. Affected children have stunted growth and a puffy appearance due to *oedema*. The liver often enlarges, *dehydration* may develop, and the child loses resistance to infection, which may have fatal consequences. The more advanced stages are marked by *jaundice*, drowsiness, and a fall in body temperature. Initially, the child is frequently fed with small amounts of milk, and vitamin and mineral tablets. A nutritious diet is then gradually introduced. Most treated children recover, but those less than 2 years old may suffer from permanently stunted growth.

kyphoscoliosis A combination of *kyphosis* and *scoliosis*.

kyphosis Excessive outward curvature of the *spine*. Kyphosis usually affects the spine at the top of the back, resulting in a hump or pronounced rounding of the back. The condition may be caused by any of a variety of *spine disorders*. In some cases, a *congenital* abnormality may be the cause. Treatment, which is rarely successful, is of the underlying disorder. When combined with a curvature of the spine to one side (*scoliosis*), the condition is known as kyphoscoliosis.

K

labetalol A *beta-blocker drug* that is used to treat *hypertension* and *angina pectoris*. Possible adverse effects include indigestion, nausea, and, in rare cases, *depression,* temporary *erectile dysfunction,* and liver damage.

labia The folds of skin of the *vulva* that protect the vaginal and urethral openings. There are two pairs of labia. The outer pair, the labia majora, are fleshy folds that bear hair and contain sweat glands. They cover the smaller, hairless inner folds, the labia minora, which meet to form the hood of the *clitoris*.

labile A term meaning unstable or likely to undergo change.

labour See *childbirth*.

labyrinth The collective term for the convoluted structures of the inner *ear*. The first part of the labyrinth is the *cochlea*, which contains the mechanism of *hearing*. Situated behind the cochlea are two sacs (the saccule and the utricle) and three fluid-filled semicircular canals, all of which are concerned with *balance*.

labyrinthitis Inflammation of the *labyrinth*. The condition is almost always caused by bacterial or viral infection. Viral labyrinthitis may develop during illnesses such as influenza. Bacterial labyrinthitis is commonly a complication of *otitis media*. The main symptom is *vertigo*, sometimes with nausea, vomiting, *nystagmus*, *tinnitus*, and hearing loss. Viral labyrinthitis clears up on its own, but symptoms are relieved by *antihistamine drugs*. Immediate treatment with *antibiotic drugs* is needed for bacterial labyrinthitis, otherwise permanent *deafness* or *meningitis* may result.

laceration A torn, irregular *wound*.

lacrimal apparatus The system that produces and drains *tears*. The lacrimal apparatus of the eye includes the main and accessory lacrimal glands and the nasolacrimal drainage duct. The main

LACRIMAL APPARATUS

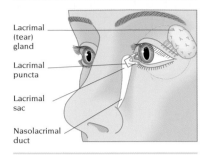

Lacrimal (tear) gland

Lacrimal puncta

Lacrimal sac

Nasolacrimal duct

gland lies just within the upper and outer margin of the eye orbit and drains on to the *conjunctiva*. It secretes tears during crying and when the eye is irritated. The accessory gland lies within the conjunctiva, and maintains the normal tear film, secreting it directly onto the conjunctiva. Tears drain through the lacrimal puncta, tiny openings towards the inner ends of the upper and lower eyelids. The puncta are connected by narrow tubes to the lacrimal sac, which lies within the lacrimal bone on the side of the nose. Leading from the sac is the nasolacrimal duct, which opens inside the nose.

lactase deficiency A condition in which there is an absence of lactase, an *enzyme* that breaks down *lactose* (milk sugar), in the cells of the small intestine. Lactase deficiency results in a reduced ability to digest lactose, also known as *lactose intolerance*. The condition may be permanent, or may occur temporarily after gastroenteritis, particularly in young children. Symptoms include abdominal cramps, bloating, *flatulence*, and *diarrhoea*, all of which are caused by the laxative effect of the undigested sugar in the intestines. Treatment is with a lactose-free diet.

lactation The production and secretion of breast milk (see *breast-feeding*).

lactic acid A weak acid that is produced when body cells break down *glucose* by *anaerobic* metabolism in order to produce energy. Lactic acid is produced by muscles during vigorous exercise and is one of the factors that contribute to *cramp*. The acid is also produced in body tissues when they receive insufficient oxygen due to impairment of their blood supply in a heart attack (see *myocardial infarction; shock*).

lactobacillus A type of rod-shaped *bacteria* found in fermented plant and dairy products. Some types of lactobacilli colonize the human intestine and the vagina, where they prevent the overmultiplication of harmful bacteria.

lactose One of the sugars present in milk; a disaccharide *carbohydrate*.

lactose intolerance The inability to digest *lactose* (see *lactase deficiency*).

lactulose A *laxative drug* that is used to treat *constipation*.

lambliasis Another name for *giardiasis*.

laminectomy Surgical removal of part or all of one or more laminae (the bony arches on each *vertebra*) to expose the spinal cord. Laminectomy is performed as the first stage of spinal canal decompression (see *decompression, spinal canal*).

lamivudine A *reverse transcriptase inhibitor* drug used in the treatment of *HIV* infection. Often, when the treatment is started, three drugs are used: two reverse transcriptase inhibitors and a third drug from another class, such as a *protease inhibitor* or a non-nucleoside reverse transcriptase inhibitor. Lamivudine may also be used to treat longstanding *hepatitis B* infections. Nausea, vomiting, and diarrhoea are the most common side effects.

lamotrigine An *anticonvulsant drug* used either alone or in combination with other anticonvulsants in the treatment of *epilepsy*. It can cause a number of minor side effects, such as nausea, headache, and blurred vision. Rarely, serious skin reactions may occur, particularly in children. In addition, there may be flu-like symptoms, bruising, sore throat, and facial swelling, which should be reported to a doctor promptly.

lance To incise using a *lancet* or a surgical *scalpel*.

lancet A small, pointed, double-edged knife used to open and drain lesions, such as boils and abscesses.

language disorders Problems affecting the ability to communicate and/or comprehend the spoken and/or written word (see *speech; speech disorders*).

lanolin A mixture of purified water and a yellow, oily substance obtained from sheep's wool. Lanolin is used as an *emollient* in the treatment of dry skin and mild *dermatitis*. Occasionally, it may cause an allergic reaction.

lansoprazole A drug used to treat disorders caused by excess stomach acid, such as *peptic ulcer* and *gastro-oesophageal reflux disease*. Side effects of lansoprazole include abdominal pain, diarrhoea, constipation, headache, and dizziness.

lanugo hair Fine, soft, downy hair that covers a *fetus*. Lanugo hair first appears in the 4th or 5th month of gestation and usually disappears by the 9th month. It can still be seen in some premature babies. Lanugo hair sometimes reappears in adults who have cancer. It may also occur in those with *anorexia nervosa* or be a side effect of certain drugs, especially *ciclosporin*.

laparoscopy Examination of the interior of the abdomen using a laparoscope, which is a type of *endoscope*. Laparoscopy is widely used in *gynaecology*. Surgical procedures such as *appendicectomy* and *cholecystectomy* are now often performed laparoscopically (see *minimally invasive surgery*).

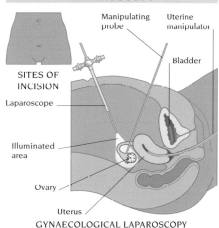

LAPAROSCOPY

Manipulating probe

Uterine manipulator

Bladder

SITES OF INCISION

Laparoscope

Illuminated area

Ovary

Uterus

GYNAECOLOGICAL LAPAROSCOPY

laparotomy Any operation in which the abdomen is opened either for diagnostic purposes or for surgical treatment.

larva migrans Infections characterized by the presence of the larval (immature) forms of certain worms in the body. *Visceral* larva migrans (*toxocariasis*) is caused by a type of worm that normally parasitizes dogs. *Cutaneous* larva migrans (creeping eruption) is caused by a form of *hookworm infestation*; the larvae penetrate the skin and move around, leaving intensely itchy red lines sometimes accompanied by blistering. Both types of larva migrans can be treated with *anthelmintic drugs*.

laryngeal nerve One of a pair of *nerves* that carry instructions from the *brain* to the *larynx* and send sensations from the larynx to the brain.

laryngectomy Surgical removal of all or part of the *larynx* to treat advanced cancer (see *larynx, cancer of*). After the operation, many patients learn to speak using their *oesophagus*. There are also mechanical devices available that are designed to help generate speech.

laryngitis Inflammation of the *larynx*. Laryngitis may be acute, lasting only a few days, or chronic, persisting for a long period. Acute laryngitis is usually caused by a viral infection, such as a cold, but can also be due to an *allergy*. Chronic laryngitis may be caused by overuse of the voice; violent coughing; irritation from tobacco smoke, alcohol, or fumes; or damage during surgery. *Hoarseness* is the most common symptom and may progress to loss of voice. There may also be throat pain or discomfort and a dry, irritating cough. Laryngitis due to a viral infection is often accompanied by fever and a general feeling of illness. If *sputum* (phlegm) is coughed up, or if hoarseness persists for more than 2 weeks, medical advice should be sought.

laryngoscopy Examination of the *larynx* using a mirror held against the back of the palate (indirect laryngoscopy), or a rigid or flexible viewing tube called a laryngoscope (direct laryngoscopy).

laryngotracheobronchitis Inflammation of the *larynx*, *trachea*, and *bronchi*, caused by a viral or a bacterial infection. The disorder is usually mild, but can be life-threatening. It is a common cause of *croup* in young children.

larynx The organ in the throat that is responsible for voice production, commonly called the voice-box. The larynx lies between the *pharynx* and the *trachea*. It consists of areas of *cartilage*, the largest of which is the thyroid cartilage that projects to form the Adam's apple. Below it are the cricoid cartilage and the two pyramid-shaped arytenoid cartilages.

Inside the larynx are two fibrous sheets of tissue, the *vocal cords*, which vibrate to produce vocal sounds when air from the lungs passes through them. These vibrations are modified by the tongue, mouth, and lips to produce *speech*.

Attached to the top of the thyroid cartilage is the *epiglottis*, a leaf-shaped flap of cartilage that drops over the larynx to prevent food from entering the trachea when swallowing.

LARYNX

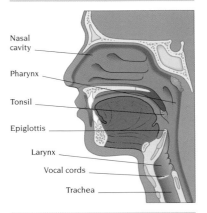

Nasal cavity

Pharynx

Tonsil

Epiglottis

Larynx

Vocal cords

Trachea

larynx, cancer of A cancerous tumour of the *larynx*. The exact causes of this cancer are not known, but smoking and high alcohol consumption may be associated factors. *Hoarseness* is the main symptom, particularly when the tumour originates on the *vocal cords*. At an advanced stage, symptoms may include difficulty in breathing and swallowing, and coughing up blood.

If *laryngoscopy* reveals a tumour on the larynx, a *biopsy* is carried out. If the tumour is small, *radiotherapy* or *laser treatment* may be used. For unresponsive and large tumours, partial or total *laryngectomy* may be considered.

larynx, disorders of Laryngeal disorders (those affecting the *larynx*) usually cause *hoarseness* as they interfere with the functioning of the *vocal cords*. In adults, the most common laryngeal disorder is *laryngitis*. In children, *croup* is common up to the age of 4. Much rarer is *epiglottitis*, a life-threatening disorder in young children. Rarely, a baby is born with a soft, limp larynx, a condition called laryngomalacia, which causes noisy breathing during feeding; the larynx usually attains normal firmness by the age of 2.

Various kinds of tumour may develop on the vocal cords. The most common is a *polyp* (a noncancerous swelling caused by smoking, an infection such as influenza, or straining the voice). Warts and small noncancerous growths called *singer's nodes* can also occur on the vocal cords. The larynx may also be affected by cancerous tumours (see *larynx, cancer of*).

laser A device that produces a concentrated beam of light radiation; "laser" is an acronym for "light amplification by stimulated emission of radiation". (See *laser treatment*.)

laser treatment Use of a *laser* beam in a variety of medical procedures. High-intensity laser beams cut through tissue and cause blood clotting. They can be used in surgery and to destroy abnormal blood vessels. Lasers are frequently used in *ophthalmology* to treat eye disorders, in *gynaecology* (for example, to unblock *fallopian tubes*), and to remove *birthmarks* and tattoos.

LASIK The abbreviation for laser-assisted in-situ keratomileusis, a type of eye surgery in which a *laser* is used to reshape the *cornea* to correct refractive errors (see *refraction*) such as shortsightedness (see *myopia*) and *astigmatism*.

Lassa fever A dangerous infectious disease caused by a virus carried by rodents. Lassa fever is largely confined to West Africa. The illness starts with fever, headache, muscular aches, and a sore throat. Later, severe diarrhoea and vomiting develop. In extreme cases, the disease can be fatal. Treatment includes injections of the drug *ribavirin*.

lassitude A term describing a feeling of *tiredness*, weakness, or exhaustion.

lateral Relating to, or situated on, one side. "Bilateral" means "on both sides".

latissimus dorsi A large, flat, triangular *muscle* in the back; contracting it moves the arm downwards and backwards.

laudanum A solution of *opium*, formerly used as a sedative and painkiller and in in the treatment of diarrhoea.

laughing gas The popular name for *nitrous oxide*.

Laurence–Biedl–Moon syndrome A rare inherited disorder characterized by increasing *obesity*, retinitis pigmentosa that may lead to blindness, *learning difficulties*, polydactyly, and hypogonadism. (See also *genetic disorders*.)

lavage, gastric Washing out the stomach with water, usually to remove toxins.

laxative drugs A group of drugs used to treat *constipation*. There are various types. Bulk-forming laxatives increase the volume and softness of faeces and make them easier to pass. Stimulant laxatives stimulate the intestinal wall to contract and speed up the elimination of faeces. Lubricant laxatives soften and facilitate the passage of faeces. Osmotic laxatives increase the water content and volume of the faeces. If used in excess, laxative drugs may cause diarrhoea, abdominal cramps, and flatulence, and may impair normal bowel function.

lazy eye An ambiguous name for the visual defect that commonly results from squint (see *amblyopia*).

LASER TREATMENT

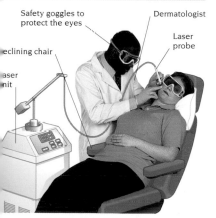

Safety goggles to protect the eyes

Dermatologist

Laser probe

Reclining chair

Laser unit

LASER SKIN TREATMENT

LDL See *low density lipoprotein*.

lead poisoning Damage to the *brain*, *nerves*, red *blood cells*, and digestive system, caused by inhaling lead fumes or swallowing lead salts. Acute poisoning, which occurs when a large amount of lead is taken into the body over a short period of time, is sometimes fatal.

Symptoms include severe, colicky abdominal pain, diarrhoea, and vomiting. There may also be *anaemia*, loss of appetite, and a blue, black, or grey line along the gum margins. Lead poisoning may be confirmed by blood and urine tests. *Chelating agents*, such as *penicillamine*, may be prescribed.

learning The process by which knowledge or abilities are acquired, or behaviour is modified. Various theories about learning have been proposed. Behavioural theories emphasize the role of *conditioning*, and cognitive theories are based on the concept that learning occurs through the building of abstract "cognitive" models, using mental capacities such as intelligence, memory, insight, and understanding.

learning difficulties Problems with *learning*, which result from a range of mental and physical problems. Learning difficulties may be either general or specific. In general learning difficulties, all aspects of mental and physical functioning may be affected. Depending on the severity of the problem, a child with general learning difficulties may need to be educated in a special school. Specific learning difficulties include *dyslexia*, dyscalculia (the inability to solve mathematical problems), and dysgraphia (writing disorders). Causes of learning difficulties include *deafness*, *speech disorders*, and disorders of *vision*, as well as genetic and chromosomal problems.

learning disability A *learning difficulty*.

leech A type of bloodsucking worm with a flattened body and a sucker at each end. Leeches of various types inhabit tropical areas. They bite painlessly, introducing their saliva into the wound before sucking blood. Leech saliva contains an anticlotting substance called hirudin, which may cause the wound to bleed for hours. Leeches are sometimes used in medicine to drain a *haematoma* from a wound.

leg, broken See *femur, fracture of*; *fibula*; *tibia*.

legionnaires' disease A form of *pneumonia* that is caused by LEGIONELLA PNEUMOPHILA, a bacterium that breeds in warm, moist conditions. The source of infection is often an air-conditioning system in a large, public building.

The first symptoms include headache, muscular and abdominal pain, diarrhoea, and a dry cough. Over the next few days, pneumonia develops, resulting in a high fever, shaking chills, coughing up of thick *sputum* (phlegm), drowsiness, and sometimes *delirium*. Treatment is with the antibiotic drug *erythromycin*.

leg, shortening of Shortening of the leg is usually caused by faulty healing of a fractured *femur* (thigh-bone) or *tibia* (shin). Other causes are an abnormality present from birth, surgery on the leg, or muscle weakness associated with *poliomyelitis* or another neurological disorder.

leg ulcer An open sore on the leg that fails to heal, usually resulting from poor blood circulation to or from the area. There are various types of ulcer. Venous ulcers (also referred to as varicose or stasis ulcers) occur mainly on the ankles and lower legs and are caused by valve failure in veins; they usually appear in conjunction with *varicose veins*. Bedsores (decubitus ulcers) develop on pressure spots on the legs due to a combination of poor circulation, pressure, and immobility over a long period. Leg ulcers can also be due to *peripheral vascular disease* and *diabetes mellitus*. In the tropics, some infections can cause *tropical ulcers*.

leiomyoma A noncancerous tumour of smooth *muscle*. Leiomyomas, also called *fibroids*, usually occur in the *uterus*. More rarely, they develop in the walls of blood vessels in the skin, forming tender lumps. Leiomyomas may require surgical removal if they cause symptoms.

leishmaniasis Any of a variety of diseases caused by single-celled *parasites* called leishmania. These parasites are harboured by dogs and rodents and are transmitted by the bites of sandflies. The most serious form of leishmaniasis is called kala-azar or visceral leishmaniasis. This disease is prevalent in some parts of Asia, Africa, and South America, and also occurs in some Mediterranean countries. In addition, there are several types of cutaneous leishmaniasis, some of which are prevalent in the Middle East, North Africa, and in the Mediterranean. Kala-azar causes persistent fever, enlargement of the *spleen, anaemia,* and, later, darkening of the skin. The illness may develop any time up to 2 years after infection, and, if untreated, may be fatal. The cutaneous forms have the appearance of a persistent ulcer at the site of the sandfly bite.

All varieties of leishmaniasis can be treated with drugs, such as sodium stibogluconate, given by intramuscular or intravenous injection.

lens The internal optical component of the *eye* responsible for focusing; also called the crystalline lens. It is situated behind the *iris* and is suspended on delicate fibres from the *ciliary body*. The lens is elastic, transparent, and slightly less convex on the front surface than on the back. Changing its curvature alters the focus so that near or distant objects can be seen sharply (see *accommodation*). Opacification of the lens is called *cataract.* (See also lens *dislocation.*)

LENS

Lens

Retina

Cornea

Iris

Ciliary body

lens dislocation Displacement of the crystalline *lens* from its normal position in the eye. Lens dislocation is almost always caused by an injury that ruptures the fibres connecting the lens to the *ciliary body.* In *Marfan's syndrome,* these fibres are particularly weak and lens dislocation is common.

A dislocated lens may produce severe visual distortion or double vision, and sometimes causes a form of *glaucoma* if drainage of fluid from the front of the eye is affected. If glaucoma is severe, the lens may need to be removed. (See also *aphakia.*)

lens implant A plastic *prosthesis* used to replace the removed opaque *lens* in *cataract surgery.*

lentigo A flat, brown area of skin similar to a freckle. Lentigines (the plural of lentigo) are usually harmless and need no treatment. However, any areas of raised, darker brown skin within a lentigo need investigation, as such areas could develop into malignant melanomas (see *melanoma, malignant*).

leprosy See *Hansen's disease.*

leptin A *protein* that has a role in the regulation of fat storage by the body.

leptospirosis A rare disease caused by a type of *spirochaete* bacterium that is harboured by rodents and excreted in their urine. It is also known as Weil's disease. Symptoms include fever, chills, headache, severe muscle aches, and a skin rash. Kidney and liver damage are also common. *Antibiotic drugs* are effective treatment but kidney and liver function may recover only slowly. The nervous system may also be affected, often producing signs of *meningitis.*

lesion An all-encompassing term for any abnormality of structure or function in any part of the body. The term may refer to a wound, infection, tumour, abscess, or chemical abnormality.

lethargy A feeling of *tiredness,* drowsiness, or lack of energy.

leukaemia Any of several types of cancer in which there is a disorganized proliferation of white *blood cells* within the bone marrow. Organs such as the liver, spleen, lymph nodes, or brain may cease to function properly if they become infiltrated by abnormal cells.

Leukaemias are classified into *acute* and *chronic* types (acute types generally develop faster than chronic leukaemia). They are also classified according to the type of white cell that is proliferating abnormally. If the abnormal cells are *lymphocytes* or lymphoblasts (precursors of lymphocytes), the leukaemia is called lymphocytic or lymphoblastic leukaemia. If abnormal cells are derived from other types of white cell or their precursors, the disease is called myeloid, myeloblastic, hairy cell, or granulocytic leukaemia. (See also *leukaemia, acute*; *leukaemia, chronic lymphocytic*; *leukaemia, chronic myeloid*.)

leukaemia, acute A type of *leukaemia* in which excessive numbers of immature white blood cells called blasts are produced in the bone marrow. If untreated, acute leukaemia can be fatal within a few weeks or months. The abnormal cells may be of two types: lymphoblasts (immature *lymphocytes*) in acute lymphoblastic leukaemia, and myeloblasts (immature forms of other types of white cell) in acute myeloblastic leukaemia.

Exposure to certain chemicals (such as benzene and some *anticancer drugs*) or high levels of radiation may be a cause in some cases. Inherited factors may also play a part; there is increased incidence in people with certain genetic disorders (such as *Fanconi's anaemia*) and chromosomal abnormalities (such as *Down's syndrome*). People with blood disorders such as chronic myeloid leukaemia (see *leukaemia, chronic myeloid*) and primary *polycythaemia* are at increased risk, as their bone marrow is already abnormal.

The symptoms and signs of acute leukaemia include bleeding gums, easy bruising, headache, bone pain, enlarged lymph nodes, and symptoms of *anaemia*, such as *tiredness*, pallor, and breathlessness on exertion. There may also be repeated infections. The diagnosis is based on blood tests and a *bone marrow biopsy*. Treatment includes transfusions of blood and platelets, the use of *anticancer drugs*, and possibly *radiotherapy*. A *stem cell* or *bone marrow transplant* may also be required. The outlook depends on the type of leukaemia and the age of the patient. *Chemotherapy* has increased success rates and 6 in 10 children with the disease can now be cured, although treatment is less likely to be completely successful in adults.

leukaemia, chronic lymphocytic A type of *leukaemia* caused by prolifera-

tion of abnormal *lymphocytes*. Although it is incurable, the disease is not always fatal. The cause is unknown.

Symptoms develop slowly, often over many years. As well as symptoms and signs common to acute forms of leukaemia (see *leukaemia, acute*), there may be enlargement of the *liver, lymph nodes,* and *spleen,* persistent raised temperature, and night sweats. Diagnosis is by blood tests and a *bone marrow biopsy*. In many mild cases, no treatment is needed. To treat severe cases, *anticancer drugs* and monoclonal antibodies (see *antibody, monoclonal*) are given, sometimes with *radiotherapy*.

leukaemia, chronic myeloid A rare type of *leukaemia*, also called chronic granulocytic leukaemia, which is caused by the overproduction of granulocytes, neutrophils, or polymorphonuclear leukocytes (see *blood cells*). The cause is unknown. This type of leukaemia usually has three phases: a chronic phase, an accelerated phase, and an acute phase. During the chronic phase, symptoms are usually mild and may include slight tiredness and weight loss. During the accelerated phase, symptoms are more marked and may include noticeable tiredness, weight loss, and abdominal pain. During the acute phase, symptoms are those of the acute form of leukaemia (see *leukaemia, acute*).

The diagnosis of chronic myeloid leukaemia is made from blood tests and a *bone marrow biopsy*. Treatment includes a *stem cell* or *bone marrow transplant*, *anticancer drugs*, and possibly *blood transfusion*.

leukocyte Any type of white *blood cell*.

leukodystrophies A rare group of inherited childhood diseases in which the *myelin* sheaths that form a protective covering around many nerves are destroyed. These diseases cause severely disabling conditions, such as impaired speech, *blindness, deafness,* and *paralysis,* and are always fatal.

leukoplakia Raised white patches on the *mucous membranes* of the *mouth* or *vulva,* caused by tissue thickening. It is most common in the elderly and is increasingly found in people with *AIDS*. Leukoplakia in the mouth, which most commonly occurs on the tongue, is usually due to tobacco-smoking or to rubbing by a rough tooth or denture. It is not known what causes the condition to develop on the vulva.

The patches are usually harmless, although occasionally they result in a cancerous change in the affected tissue. If the condition persists, the patches are removed under local *anaesthesia* and tissue is examined microscopically for signs of malignant change. (See also *mouth cancer*; *vulva, cancer of.*)

leukorrhoea See *vaginal discharge*.

leukotriene receptor antagonists A group of *antiallergy drugs*, such as *montelukast* and *zafirlukast*, used to prevent symptoms of mild to moderate *asthma*. The drugs work by blocking the effects of leukotrienes – naturally occurring substances released in the lungs during an allergic reaction.

Because they are not *bronchodilator drugs* and will not relieve an existing attack, they are usually used with bronchodilators and inhaled *corticosteroids* to reduce the frequency of attacks.

Side effects include gastrointestinal disturbances and headache. Skin and hypersensitivity reactions may also occur.

levamisole An *anthelmintic drug* given by mouth in a single dose to eliminate *roundworm* infestation. Side effects of levamisole are rare but can include mild nausea or vomiting.

levodopa A drug used to treat *Parkinson's disease*. Side effects include nausea, vomiting, nervousness, and agitation.

levonorgestrel A *progestogen drug* used in some *oral contraceptives*.

levothyroxine A synthetic version of the *thyroid hormone* thyroxine, used to treat *hypothyroidism*. Side effects, such as rapid heartbeat and tremor, may occur if the initial dose is too high.

LH The abbreviation for *luteinizing hormone*.

LH-RH The abbreviation for *luteinizing hormone-releasing hormone*.

libido Sexual desire. Loss of libido is a symptom of many physical illnesses and of *depression*, *drug abuse*, and *alcohol* abuse. (See also *sexual desire, inhibited*.)

lice Small, wingless insects that feed on human blood. There are three species:

PEDICULUS HUMANUS CAPITIS (the head louse), *PEDICULUS HUMANUS CORPORIS* (the body louse), and *PHTHIRUS PUBIS* (the crab, or pubic, louse). All have flattened bodies and measure up to 3 mm across.

Head lice live on the scalp and their bite causes intense itching. They are spread by direct contact. Their tiny eggs (nits) attach to hairs close to the scalp. Body lice live and lay eggs on clothing next to the skin. They can transmit epidemic *typhus* and *relapsing fever*. Crab lice live in pubic hair or, more rarely, in armpits, beards, or eyelashes; they are usually transmitted during sexual contact (see *pubic lice*). Various preparations can be applied to kill lice and eggs.

lichenification Thickening and hardening of the *skin* caused by repeated scratching, often to relieve the intense itching of disorders such as *atopic eczema* or *lichen simplex*.

lichen planus A common *skin* disease of unknown cause that usually affects middle-aged people. Small, shiny, intensely itchy, pink or purple raised spots appear on the skin of the wrists, forearms, or lower legs. There is often a lacy network of white spots covering the inside lining of the cheeks. The disease is treated with topical *corticosteroid drugs*.

lichen sclerosus et atrophicus A chronic skin condition of the anogenital area. The skin is scarred and white, and the anatomy of areas such as the vaginal opening or the foreskin may become distorted. Treatment is with potent topical *corticosteroid drugs*.

lichen simplex Patches of thickened, itchy, sometimes discoloured skin, due to repeated scratching. Typical sites are the neck, wrist, elbow area, and ankles. Lichen simplex is most common in women and is often stress-related. Treatment is with oral *antihistamine drugs* and creams containing *corticosteroid drugs*, and may also involve addressing any underlying stress or anxiety.

lid lag A momentary delay in the normal downward movement of the upper eyelids that occurs when the eye looks down. Lid lag is a characteristic feature of *thyrotoxicosis*, and usually occurs in conjunction with *exophthalmos*.

lidocaine A local anaesthetic (see *anaesthesia, local*) used to numb tissues before minor surgical procedures, and as a *nerve block*. It can also be used to control heart arrhythmias.

LIGAMENT

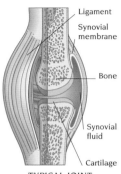

Ligament

Synovial membrane

Bone

Synovial fluid

Cartilage

TYPICAL JOINT

life expectancy The number of years a person can expect to live. Life expectancy can be estimated assuming that patterns of health and illness in a community do not change.

life support The process of keeping a person alive by artificially inflating the lungs (see *ventilation*) and, if it is needed, maintaining the heartbeat.

ligament A band of tough, fibrous, partly elastic tissue. Ligaments are important components of *joints*; they bind the bone ends together and prevent excessive movement. They also support various internal organs. Minor ligament injuries such as *sprains* are treated with ice, bandaging, and sometimes *physiotherapy*. If a ligament has been torn (ruptured), the joint is either immobilized by a *plaster cast* to allow healing or repaired surgically.

ligation The surgical process of tying off a *duct* or a blood vessel with a *ligature* in order to stop bleeding. The term is used in tubal ligation, a form of sterilization in which the fallopian tubes are tied off (see *sterilization, female*).

ligature A length of thread or other material used for *ligation*.

lightening A feeling experienced by many pregnant women when the baby's head descends into the pelvic cavity. Lightening usually occurs in the final 3 weeks of pregnancy, leaving more space in the upper abdomen and relieving pressure under the *diaphragm*.

light treatment See *phototherapy*.

lignocaine Former name for *lidocaine*.

limb, artificial An artificial leg or arm, known medically as a *prosthesis*, which is fitted to replace a limb that has been missing from birth or lost as a result of *amputation* (see *limb defects*).

limb defects Incomplete development of one or more limbs at birth. Limb defects are rare and may be inherited or form part of a *syndrome*. In a condition called *phocomelia*, hands, feet, or tiny finger- or toe-buds are attached to limb stumps or grow directly from the trunk. The drug *thalidomide*, when taken by pregnant women, is known to have caused phocomelia in fetuses.

limbic system A ring-shaped area in the centre of the *brain* consisting of a number of connected clusters of nerve

LIMBIC SYSTEM

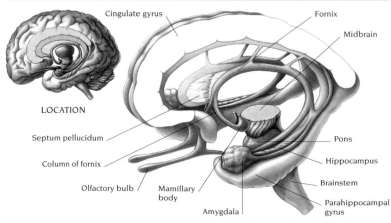

Cingulate gyrus

Fornix

Midbrain

LOCATION

Septum pellucidum

Column of fornix

Olfactory bulb

Mamillary body

Amygdala

Pons

Hippocampus

Brainstem

Parahippocampal gyrus

cells. The limbic system plays a role in influencing the *autonomic nervous system*, which automatically regulates body functions; the emotions; and the sense of smell. The system is extensive, and contains various different substructures including the *hippocampus*, the cingulate gyrus, and the amygdala.

limp An abnormal pattern of *walking* in which the movements of one leg (or of the *hip* on one side of the body) are different from those of the other. A limp in a child should always be seen within 24 hours as it may result from a hip problem that requires treatment.

linctus A bland, usually sweetened mixture taken to soothe irritation caused by an inflamed throat. A simple linctus contains no active drug, but linctuses are commonly used as a basis for cough suppressants (see *cough remedies*).

linear accelerator A device for accelerating subatomic particles, such as electrons, to a speed approaching that of light so that they have extremely high energies. A linear accelerator can also be used to generate high-energy *X-rays*. High-energy electrons or X-rays are used in *radiotherapy* to treat certain cancers.

liniment A liquid rubbed on the skin to relieve aching muscles and stiff joints. Liniments may contain rubefacients (substances that increase blood flow beneath the skin), or certain drugs, such as *nonsteroidal anti-inflammatory drugs*.

liothyronine A *thyroid hormone* used as replacement therapy in *hypothyroidism*. Liothyronine acts more quickly than *levothyroxine* and is cleared from the body more rapidly.

lip One of two fleshy folds around the entrance to the mouth. The main substructure of the lips is a ring of muscle that helps to produce speech. Smaller muscles at the corners of the lips are responsible for facial expression. Disorders of the lips include *chapped skin*, *cheilitis*, *cold sores*, and *lip cancer*.

lip cancer A *malignant* tumour, usually on the lower *lip*. Lip cancer is largely confined to older people, particularly those who have been exposed to a lot of sunlight and those who have smoked cigarettes or a pipe. The first symptom is a white patch that develops on the lip

and soon becomes scaly and cracked with a yellow crust. The affected area grows and eventually becomes ulcerated. In some cases, the cancer spreads to the *lymph nodes* in the jaw and neck. Lip cancer (usually a *squamous cell carcinoma*) is diagnosed by *biopsy*. Treatment is surgical removal, *radiotherapy*, or a combination of both.

lipectomy, suction A type of *body contour surgery* in which excess fat is sucked out through a small skin incision.

lipid disorders *Metabolic disorders* that result in abnormal amounts of *lipids* (fats) in the body. The most common lipid disorders are the *hyperlipidaemias*, which are characterized by high levels of lipids in the blood and can cause *atherosclerosis* and *pancreatitis*. There are also some very rare lipid disorders due solely to heredity, such as *Tay–Sachs disease*.

lipid-lowering drugs A group of drugs used to treat *hyperlipidaemia*. These drugs help to prevent, or slow the progression of, *atherosclerosis* and *coronary artery disease*. The most commonly used types are *statins* and *fibrates*.

lipids A general term for *fats and oils*. Lipids include triglycerides (simple fats), phospholipids (important constituents of cell membranes and nerve tissue), and sterols, such as *cholesterol*.

lipoma A common noncancerous tumour of fatty tissue. Lipomas are slow-growing, soft swellings that may occur anywhere on the body, most commonly on the thigh, trunk, or shoulder. They are painless and harmless, but may be surgically removed for cosmetic reasons.

lipoprotein Particles comprising a fatty core and protein outer layer (apolipoprotein) that allow the transport of fats in the bloodstream. Genetic variations in the structure of apolipoproteins and lipoproteins play an important part in determining susceptibility to *cardiovascular disorders* and *Alzheimer's disease*.

liposarcoma A rare cancer of fatty tissue that most commonly develops during late middle age. Liposarcomas produce firm swellings, usually in the abdomen or the thigh. The tumours can generally be removed by surgery but tend to recur.

liposuction The popular term for suction lipectomy (see *lipectomy, suction*).

L

lip-reading A way of understanding speech by interpreting movements of the mouth and tongue. Lip-reading is often used by people who are deaf.

liquid paraffin A lubricant *laxative drug* obtained from petroleum. It can cause anal irritation, and prolonged use may impair the absorption of vitamins from the intestine into the blood.

lisinopril An *ACE inhibitor drug* commonly used to treat *hypertension*.

lisp A common *speech disorder* caused by protrusion of the tongue between the teeth so that the "s" sound is replaced by "th". Sometimes the cause is a cleft palate (see *cleft lip and palate*). In most children, there is no physical defect and lisping disappears by the age of about 4.

listeriosis An infection that is common in animals and may also affect humans. It is caused by the bacterium LISTERIA MONOCYTOGENES, which is widespread in the environment, especially in soil. Possible sources of human infection include soft cheese, ready-prepared coleslaw and salads, and improperly cooked meat.

In most adults, the only symptoms are fever and aching muscles. There may also be sore throat, *conjunctivitis*, diarrhoea, and abdominal pain. *Pneumonia*, *septicaemia*, and *meningitis* may develop in severe cases. However, listeriosis can be life-threatening, particularly in elderly people, those with reduced immunity, and newborn babies. In pregnant women, infection may cause a miscarriage.

The condition is diagnosed by *blood tests* and analysis of other body fluids, such as urine. Treatment is with *antibiotic drugs*.

lithium A drug used in the long-term treatment of *mania* and *bipolar disorder*. High levels of lithium in the blood may cause vomiting, diarrhoea, blurred vision, tremor, drowsiness, rash, and, in rare cases, kidney damage. Regular tests are needed to monitor the level of lithium in the blood.

lithotomy Surgical removal of a *calculus* (stone) from part of the *urinary tract*. The procedure is only performed for large stones; smaller stones are usually crushed and removed using *cystoscopy*, or pulverized ultrasonically by *lithotripsy*.

lithotomy position Position in which a patient lies on his or her back with the hips and knees bent and the legs wide apart. Once used for *lithotomy*, the position is still used for *pelvic examinations* and some types of pelvic surgery.

lithotripsy The process of using shock waves or ultrasonic waves to break up *calculi* (stones) inside the kidneys, upper *ureters*, and *gallbladder* for excretion. There are two different procedures: extracorporeal shock-wave lithotripsy (ESWL), performed to break up small stones, and percutaneous lithotripsy, performed on larger stones. ESWL uses a machine called a *lithotripter*, which produces external shock waves. In percutaneous lithotripsy, a nephroscope (an instrument for viewing the kidney) is inserted into the kidney and an ultrasonic probe is directed through the nephroscope to destroy the stone. *Ureteric colic* (severe spasmodic pain in the side, occurring if the ureter is obstructed by small fragments of stone) may occur after ESWL. People treated for *gallstones* may need drug treatment to aid the final elimination of stone residues.

lithotripter The machine used in extracorporeal shock-wave *lithotripsy* (ESWL) to disintegrate small *calculi* (stones).

livedo reticularis A net-like, purple or blue mottling of the skin, usually on the lower legs, caused by the enlargement of blood vessels beneath the skin. It is more common in people with *vasculitis* and those who suffer from excessive sensitivity to cold. The condition is harmless, and tends to be worse in cold weather.

liver The largest organ of the body, this roughly wedge-shaped, red-brown structure lies in the upper right abdominal cavity, directly below the *diaphragm*. The liver is divided into two main lobes, each consisting of many lobules. These lobules are surrounded by branches of the hepatic artery, which supplies the liver with oxygenated blood, and the portal vein, which supplies nutrient-rich blood. Deoxygenated blood from the liver drains into the hepatic veins. A network of ducts carries *bile* from the liver to the *gallbladder* and the small intestine.

The liver plays a vital role in the body because it produces and processes a wide range of chemical substances. The

LITHOTRIPSY

Lead apron
Control unit
X-ray receiver
Monitors
X-ray beam to locate kidney stones
Water- or gel-filled cushion
Shock waves
Shock-wave generator
X-ray source

EXTRACORPOREAL LITHOTRIPSY

L

substances produced include important proteins for blood *plasma*, such as *albumin*. The liver also produces *cholesterol* and special proteins that help the blood to carry fats around the body. In addition, liver cells secrete *bile*, which removes waste products from the liver and aids

LIVER

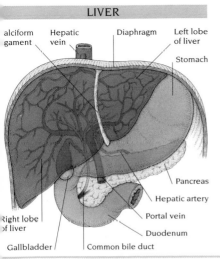

alciform gament
Hepatic vein
Diaphragm
Left lobe of liver
Stomach
Pancreas
Hepatic artery
Portal vein
Right lobe of liver
Duodenum
Gallbladder
Common bile duct

the breakdown and absorption of fats in the small intestine (see *biliary system*).

Another major function is the processing of nutrients for use by cells. The liver also stores excess *glucose* as glyco gen. In addition, it controls the blood level of *amino acids* (the building blocks of proteins). If the level of amino acids is too high, the liver converts the excess into glucose, proteins, other amino acids, or *urea* (for excretion).

Finally, the liver helps to clear the blood of drugs and poisons. These substances are broken down and excreted in the bile.

liver abscess A localized collection of *pus* in the *liver*. The most common cause is an intestinal infection. Bacteria may spread from areas inflamed by *diverticulitis* or *appendicitis*, and amoebae may invade the liver as a result of *amoebiasis* The symptoms are high fever, pain in the upper right abdomen, and (especially in elderly people) mental confusion. *Ultrasound scanning* usually reveals the abscess. It can sometimes be treated by *aspiration*, but often surgery is needed.

liver biopsy A diagnostic test in which a small sample of tissue is removed from the liver, usually under local *anaesthesia*. The main function of this test is to diagnose liver diseases. (See also *biopsy*.)

liver cancer A cancerous tumour in the *liver*. It may be primary (originating within the liver) or secondary (having spread from elsewhere, often the stomach, pancreas, or large intestine). There are two main types of primary tumour: a hepatoma, which develops in the liver cells, and a *cholangiocarcinoma*, which arises from cells lining the bile ducts.

The most common symptoms of any liver cancer are loss of appetite, weight loss, lethargy, and sometimes pain in the upper right abdomen. The later stages of the disease are marked by *jaundice* and *ascites* (excess fluid in the abdomen). Tumours are often detected by *ultrasound scanning*, and diagnosis may be confirmed by *liver biopsy*. A hepatoma can sometimes be cured by complete removal. In other cases, *anticancer drugs* can help to slow the progress of the disease. It is usually not possible to cure secondary liver cancer, but anticancer drugs or, in some cases, removal of a solitary *metastasis* may be advised.

liver, cirrhosis of See *cirrhosis*.

liver disease, alcoholic Damage to the *liver* caused by excessive *alcohol* consumption. The longer consumption goes on, the more severe the damage. The initial effect is the formation of fat globules between liver cells, a condition called fatty liver. This is followed by alcoholic *hepatitis*, and damage then progresses to *cirrhosis*. Alcohol-related liver disease increases the risk of developing *liver cancer*. *Liver function tests* show a characteristic pattern of abnormalities, and *liver biopsy* may be needed to assess the severity of damage. There is no particular treatment, but abstinence from alcohol prevents further damage. Treatment for *alcohol dependence* may be required.

liver, disorders of The *liver* is a common site of disease. The most significant liver conditions include alcohol-related disorders (see *liver disease, alcoholic*), *hepatitis*, and *liver cancer*. Disorders can also result from infection. Certain viruses cause hepatitis (see *hepatitis, viral*). Bacteria may spread up the biliary system to the liver, causing *cholangitis* or

liver abscess. Parasitic diseases affecting the liver include *schistosomiasis*, *liver fluke*, and *hydatid disease*. Certain *metabolic disorders*, such as *haemochromatosis* and *Wilson's disease*, may involve the liver. Other types of liver disorder include *Budd–Chiari syndrome*, in which the veins draining the liver become blocked. Occasionally, defects of liver structure are present at birth. Such defects principally affect the bile ducts; one example is *biliary atresia*, in which the bile ducts are absent. Because the liver breaks down drugs and toxins, damage to liver cells can also be caused through overdose or drug allergy. (See also *jaundice*; *liver failure*; *portal hypertension*.)

liver failure Severe impairment of *liver* function that develops suddenly or at the final stages of a chronic liver disease. Because the liver breaks down toxins in the blood, liver failure causes the levels of the toxins to rise, affecting the functioning of other organs, particularly the brain.

Liver failure may be acute or chronic. Symptoms of acute liver failure develop rapidly and include impaired memory, agitation, and confusion, followed by drowsiness. The functioning of other organs may become impaired, and the condition may lead to *coma* and death. Features of chronic liver failure develop much more gradually and include *jaundice*, itching, easy bruising and bleeding, a swollen abdomen due to accumulated fluid, red palms and, in males, *gynaecomastia* (enlarged breasts) and shrunken testes. Chronic liver failure may suddenly deteriorate into acute liver failure.

Acute liver failure requires urgent hospital care. Although no treatment can repair damage that has already occurred in acute and chronic liver failure, certain measures, such as prescribing *diuretic drugs* to reduce abdominal swelling, may be taken to reduce the severity of symptoms. Consumption of alcohol should cease in all cases. The prognoses for sufferers of chronic liver failure vary depending on the cause, but some people survive for many years. For acute liver failure, a *liver transplant* is necessary to increase the chances of survival.

liver fluke Any of various species of flukes (flatworms) that infest the *bile ducts* in the *liver*. The only significant fluke in the UK is FASCIOLA HEPATICA, which causes the disease fascioliasis.

Fascioliasis has two stages. During the first stage, young flukes migrate through the liver, causing it to become tender and enlarged; other symptoms include fever and night sweats. In the second stage, adult worms occupy the bile ducts. Their presence may lead to *cholangitis* and bile duct obstruction, which can cause *jaundice*. Treatment with an *anthelmintic drug* may be effective.

liver function tests Tests of blood chemistry that can detect changes in the way the *liver* is making new substances and breaking down and/or excreting old ones. The tests can also show whether liver cells are healthy or being damaged.

liver imaging Techniques that produce images of the *liver, gallbladder, bile ducts*, and blood vessels supplying the liver, to aid the detection of disease. *Ultrasound scanning, CT scanning*, and *MRI* are commonly used. *Radionuclide scanning* may reveal cysts and tumours and show bile excretion. *X–ray* techniques include *cholangiography, cholecystography*, and *ERCP* (endoscopic retrograde cholangiopancreatography). In these procedures, a *contrast medium*, which is opaque to X-rays, is introduced to show abnormalities in the *biliary system*. *Angiography* reveals the blood vessels in the liver.

liver transplant Replacement of a diseased *liver* with a healthy liver removed from a donor. Liver transplants are most successful in the treatment of advanced *liver cirrhosis* in people with chronic active *hepatitis* or primary *biliary cirrhosis*. People who have primary liver cancer are rarely considered for transplantation because there is a high risk that the tumour will recur.

During this procedure, the liver, *gallbladder*, and portions of the connected blood and *bile* vessels are removed. The donor organs and vessels are connected to the recipient's vessels. After the transplant, the recipient is monitored in an *intensive care* unit for a few days and remains in hospital for up to 4 weeks.

living will An advance directive, signed by an adult of sound mind, that gives instructions about what types of medical treatment the person does or does not want to receive if he or she becomes incapable of giving or refusing consent.

lobe One of the clearly defined parts into which certain organs, such as the brain, liver, and lungs, are divided. The term may also be used to describe any projecting, flat, pendulous part of the body, such as the earlobe.

lobectomy An operation performed to cut out a *lobe* in the liver (see *hepatectomy, partial*), lung (see *lobectomy, lung*), or thyroid gland (see *thyroidectomy*).

lobectomy, lung An operation to cut out one of the *lobes* of a *lung*, usually to remove a cancerous tumour.

lobotomy, prefrontal Cutting of some of the fibres linking the frontal lobes to the rest of the brain. This operation was formerly used to treat severe psychiatric disorders; it is very rarely performed now.

lochia The discharge, after childbirth, of blood and fragments of uterine lining from the area where the *placenta* was attached. The discharge is bright red for the first 3 or 4 days and then becomes paler. The amount of lochia decreases as the placental site heals, and discharge usually ceases within 6 weeks.

locked knee A temporary inability to move the *knee* joint. A locked knee may be caused by a torn cartilage or by *loose bodies* in the joint.

lockjaw A painful spasm of the jaw muscles that makes it difficult or impossible to open the mouth. Lockjaw is the most common symptom of *tetanus*.

LIVER TRANSPLANT

Bile duct
Transplanted liver
Recipient's aorta
SITE OF INCISION
Transplanted gallbladder
Donor's blood vessels
Recipient's blood vessels

locomotor Relating to movement of the extremities, as in locomotor *ataxia*.

lofepramine A *tricyclic antidepressant* drug that is used in the long-term treatment of *depression*.

loiasis A form of the tropical parasitic disease *filariasis*, caused by infestation with the worm LOA LOA. The worms travel beneath the skin, producing itchy areas of inflammation known as Calabar swellings, and can sometimes be seen moving across the front of the eye. Loiasis is treated with a course of diethylcarbamazine.

loin The part of the back on each side of the spine between the lowest pair of ribs and the top of the pelvis.

longsightedness See *hypermetropia*.

loose bodies Fragments of *bone*, *cartilage*, or capsule linings within a *joint*. Loose bodies may occur whenever there is damage to a *joint*, as in injury, *osteoarthritis*, or *osteochondritis dissecans*. The fragments can cause a joint to lock, resulting in severe pain. Gentle manipulation may be required to unlock the joint. If locking occurs frequently, the loose bodies may be removed during *arthroscopy* or by surgery.

loperamide An *antidiarrhoeal drug*. Loperamide occasionally produces a rash. Other rare adverse effects are fever, abdominal cramps, and bloating.

loratadine An *antihistamine drug*.

lorazepam A *benzodiazepine* drug used in the treatment of *insomnia* and *anxiety*.

lordosis Inward curvature of the *spine*. This curvature is normally present to a minor degree in the lower back, but lordosis can become exaggerated by poor posture or by *kyphosis* higher in the back. Pronounced lordosis is usually permanent and can lead to *disc prolapse* or *osteoarthritis* of the spine.

losartan An *angiotensin II antagonist* drug used to treat *hypertension* (high blood pressure). Side effects are usually mild; they include dizziness and fatigue.

lotion A liquid drug preparation applied to the skin. Some examples of drugs prepared as a lotion include *calamine* and *betamethasone*, which are used to treat skin inflammation.

Lou Gehrig's disease The most common type of *motor neuron disease*; also known as amyotrophic lateral sclerosis.

low density lipoprotein One of a group of proteins that are combined with *lipids* in the *plasma*. Low density lipoproteins (LDLs) are involved in the transport of *cholesterol* in the bloodstream. An excess of LDLs (see *hyperlipidaemias*) is associated with *atherosclerosis*. (See also *high density lipoprotein*.)

LSD Abbreviation of lysergic acid diethylamide: a synthetic *hallucinogenic drug*, derived from *ergot*, that is used illegally as a recreational drug. LSD sometimes produces panic and physical side effects such as nausea and dizziness.

Ludwig's angina A rare bacterial infection of the floor of the mouth. The condition spreads to the throat, causing life-threatening swelling. It requires immediate treatment with *antibiotic drugs*.

lumbago A general term for low *back pain*. Lumbago may be due to an intervertebral *disc prolapse*. It may also arise if *synovium* is trapped between the surfaces of a small intervertebral joint, or if there is momentary partial dislocation of an intervertebral joint with straining of ligaments. However, in many cases no cause is found. Treatment is with *analgesic drugs* and gentle physical activity. (See also *lumbosacral spasm*.)

lumbar Relating to the part of the back between the lowest ribs and the top of the pelvis. The lumbar region of the *spine* consists of the five lumbar *vertebrae*.

lumbar puncture A procedure in which a hollow needle is inserted into the lower

LUMBAR PUNCTURE

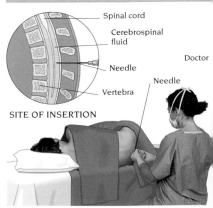

Spinal cord
Cerebrospinal fluid
Doctor
Needle
Needle
Vertebra

SITE OF INSERTION

part of the spinal canal to withdraw *cerebrospinal fluid* or to inject drugs or other substances. Lumbar puncture is usually carried out to collect a sample of cerebrospinal fluid in order to diagnose and investigate disorders of the brain and spinal cord (such as *meningitis* and *subarachnoid haemorrhage*). The procedure takes about 15 minutes and is carried out under local *anaesthesia*.

lumbosacral spasm Excessive tightening of the muscles that surround and support the lower region of the *spine*, causing *back pain*. Treatment of lumbosacral spasm may include *analgesic drugs*.

lumen The space within a tubular organ, such as the intestine.

lumpectomy A surgical treatment for breast cancer in which only the cancerous tissue is removed. (See also *mastectomy*; *quadrantectomy*.)

lunacy An outdated term for serious mental disorder.

lung One of the two main organs of the *respiratory system*. The lungs supply the body with the oxygen needed for *aerobic* metabolism and eliminate the waste product carbon dioxide. Air is delivered to the lungs via the *trachea* (windpipe); this branches into two main bronchi (air passages), with one *bronchus* supplying each lung. The main bronchi divide again into smaller bronchi and then into bronchioles, which lead to air passages that open out into grape-like air sacs called alveoli (see *alveolus, pulmonary*). Oxygen and carbon dioxide diffuse into or out of the blood through the thin walls of the alveoli. Each lung is enclosed in a double membrane called the *pleura*; the two layers of the pleura secrete a lubricating fluid that enables the lungs to move freely as they expand and contract during breathing. (See also *respiration*.)

lung cancer The most common form of *cancer* in the UK. Tobacco-*smoking* is the main cause. Passive smoking (the inhalation of tobacco smoke by non-smokers) and environmental pollution (for example, with radioactive minerals or asbestos) are also risk factors.

The first and most common symptom is a cough. Other symptoms include coughing up blood, shortness of breath, and chest pain. Lung cancer can spread to other parts of the body, especially the liver, brain, and bones. In most cases, the cancer is revealed in a *chest X-ray*. To confirm the diagnosis, tissue must be examined microscopically for the presence of cancerous cells (see *cytology*). If lung cancer is diagnosed at an early stage, *pneumonectomy* (removal of the lung) or *lobectomy* (removal of part of the lung) may be possible. *Anticancer drugs* and *radiotherapy* may also be used.

lung, collapse of See *atelectasis*; *pneumothorax*.

lung disease, chronic obstructive See *pulmonary disease, chronic obstructive*.

lung, disorders of The most common *lung* disorders are infections. These diseases include *pneumonia*, *tracheitis*, and *croup*. *Bronchitis* and *bronchiolitis*, which are inflammatory disorders affecting the airways within the lungs, can be complications of colds or *influenza*. The disorder

L

LUNG

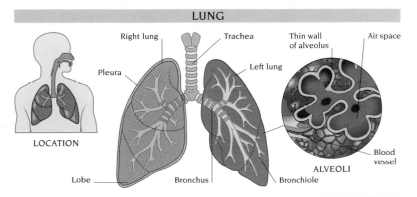

Right lung
Trachea
Thin wall of alveolus
Air space

Pleura
Left lung

LOCATION

Lobe
Bronchus
Bronchiole

ALVEOLI

Blood vessel

bronchiectasis may occur as a complication of severe bacterial pneumonia or *cystic fibrosis*. The lungs can also be affected by allergic disorders. The most important of these is *asthma*. Another such disorder is allergic *alveolitis*, which is usually a reaction to dust of plant or animal origin. Irritation of the airways, usually by tobacco-*smoking*, can cause diseases characterized by damage to lung tissue and narrowing of the airways (see *pulmonary disease, chronic obstructive*). The lungs can also be affected by cancerous tumours; *lung cancer* is one of the most common cancers. Noncancerous lung tumours are uncommon.

Injury to a lung, usually resulting from penetration of the chest wall, can cause the lung to collapse (see *pneumothorax*; *haemothorax*). Damage to the interior of the lungs can be caused by inhalation of toxic substances (see *asbestosis*; *silicosis*). Blood supply to the lungs may be reduced by *pulmonary embolism*.

Lung disorders can be investigated in various ways, such as *chest X-ray, bronchoscopy*, and *pulmonary function tests*.

lung function tests See *pulmonary function tests*.

lung imaging Techniques that provide images of the *lungs* to aid in the diagnosis of disease. Most *lung disorders* can be detected by *chest X-ray*. *CT scanning* and *MRI* play an important role in detecting the presence and spread of *lung tumours*. *Ultrasound scanning* is sometimes used to reveal pleural *effusion*. *Radioisotope scanning* is used to detect evidence of pulmonary embolism.

lung tumours Growths in the lungs. These tumours may be either cancerous (see *lung cancer*) or noncancerous.

Cancerous lung tumours are usually associated with tobacco-*smoking*. Noncancerous tumours occur less frequently than cancers. The most common form of noncancerous tumour is a bronchial *adenoma*, which arises in the lining of a *bronchus*. Adenomas often cause bronchial obstruction; affected people may also cough up blood. Treatment involves surgical removal of the tumour. Other rare noncancerous tumours include *fibromas* (which consist of fibrous tissue) and *lipomas* (which consist of fatty tis-

sue). No treatment is necessary unless the tumours are causing problems.

lupus erythematosus An *autoimmune disorder* that causes inflammation of *connective tissue*. The most common type, discoid lupus erythematosus (DLE), only affects exposed areas of the skin. The more serious form, systemic lupus erythematosus (SLE), affects many body systems, including the skin.

In both varieties of lupus erythematosus, the symptoms periodically subside and recur with varying severity. In DLE, the rash starts as one or more red, circular, thickened areas of skin that later scar. These patches may occur on the face, behind the ears, and on the scalp. Treatment is usually with topical *corticosteroid drugs*. SLE causes a variety of symptoms. A characteristic red, blotchy, butterfly-shaped rash may appear over the cheeks and the bridge of the nose; other symptoms include fatigue, fever, loss of appetite, nausea, joint pain, and weight loss. There may also be *anaemia*, neurological or psychiatric problems, *kidney failure, pleurisy, arthritis*, and *pericarditis*. Diagnosis is made by *blood tests* and sometimes a *skin biopsy*.

Sufferers of mild forms of SLE may have near normal health for many years; treatment with *corticosteroid drugs* and *immunosuppressant drugs* can improve life expectancy. Other treatments are available to treat specific features of the disease. However, SLE is still a potentially fatal disorder.

lupus pernio *Sarcoidosis* affecting the skin, in which purple, chilblain-like swellings appear on the nose, cheeks, or ears.

lupus vulgaris A rare form of *tuberculosis* affecting the skin, especially on the head and neck. Painless, clear, red-brown nodules appear and ulcerate; the ulcers eventually heal, leaving deep scars.

luteinizing hormone Also known as LH, a *gonadotrophin hormone* produced by the *pituitary gland*.

luteinizing hormone-releasing hormone A naturally occurring *hormone*, also known as LH-RH, that is released by the *hypothalamus* in the brain. This hormone is also prepared synthetically as a drug. Natural LH-RH stimulates the release of *gonadotrophin hormones* from the *pituitary gland*. Gonadotrophin hormones control the production of *oestrogen hormones* and *androgen hormones*. Synthetic LH-RH, also known as synthetic *gonadorelin*, is used to treat delayed puberty, and to treat infertility in women. LH-RH may cause headache, nausea, hot flushes, vaginal dryness, and irregular periods.

Lyme disease A disease caused by the bacterium BORRELIA BURGDORFERI, which is transmitted by the bite of a tick that usually lives on deer. At the site of the bite, a red dot may appear and gradually expand into an area up to 5 mm across. Symptoms including fever, headache, and muscle pain usually develop, followed by joint inflammation, which typically affects the knees and other large joints.

Symptoms may vary in severity and occur in cycles lasting a week or so. If the disease is not treated, complications including *meningitis*, *facial palsy*, and an abnormal heartbeat (see *arrhythmia, cardiac*) may develop. The most serious long-term complication is *arthritis*. The disease can be treated with *antibiotic drugs*. Treatment is most effective when given soon after the initial infection.

lymph A watery or milky body fluid containing *lymphocytes*, proteins, and fats. Lymph accumulates outside the blood vessels in the intercellular spaces of body tissues, and is collected by the vessels of the *lymphatic system*. This system filters the fluid and eventually returns it to the bloodstream. Lymph plays an important role in the *immune system* as well as in absorbing fats from the intestine.

lymphadenitis A medical term for inflammation of the *lymph nodes*, which is a common cause of *lymphadenopathy* (see *glands, swollen*).

lymphadenopathy The medical term for swollen *lymph nodes* (see *glands, swollen*).

lymphangiography A diagnostic procedure that involves injecting a *contrast medium* into lymph vessels (see *lymphatic system*) so that these vessels and lymph nodes, and any abnormalities, can be seen on *X-ray* film. Lymphangiography has largely been superseded by *CT scanning* and *MRI*.

lymphangioma A rare, noncancerous tumour of the skin or tongue consisting of a mass of abnormal lymph vessels.

lymphangitis Inflammation of the lymphatic vessels (see *lymphatic system*) due to the spread of *bacteria* (commonly streptococci) from an infected wound. The inflammation causes tender red streaks to appear on the skin overlying the lymphatic vessels. These red streaks extend from the infection site towards the nearest *lymph nodes*. The affected nodes become swollen and tender, and there is usually fever and a general feeling of illness. Lymphangitis requires urgent treatment with *antibiotic drugs*.

lymphatic system A system of vessels (lymphatic vessels) that drains *lymph* from tissues all over the body back into the bloodstream. The lymphatic system is part of the *immune system* and has a major function in defending the body against infection and cancer. This system also plays a part in the absorption of fats from the intestine.

All body tissues are bathed in lymph, a watery fluid derived from the bloodstream. Much of this fluid is

L

LYMPHATIC SYSTEM

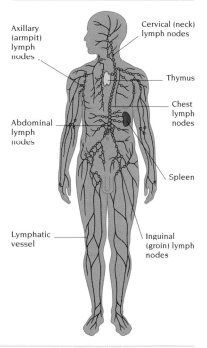

Axillary (armpit) lymph nodes

Cervical (neck) lymph nodes

Thymus

Chest lymph nodes

Abdominal lymph nodes

Spleen

Lymphatic vessel

Inguinal (groin) lymph nodes

returned to the bloodstream through the walls of the capillaries (see *circulatory system*), but the remainder is transported to the heart through the lymphatic system.

Lymph is moved along the lymphatic vessels during physical activity, as muscle contractions compress the vessels; valves inside the vessels ensure that the lymph flows in the correct direction. Situated on the lymphatic vessels are *lymph nodes*, through which the lymph passes. These nodes filter the lymph and trap infectious microorganisms or other foreign bodies. The nodes contain many *lymphocytes*, white blood cells that can neutralize or destroy invading bacteria and viruses. The lymphatic system also includes the *spleen* and the *thymus*, which produce lymphocytes.

lymph gland A popular name for a *lymph node*. (See also *lymphatic system*.)

lymph node A small organ lying along the course of a lymphatic vessel (see *lymphatic system*); commonly but incorrectly called a lymph gland. Lymph nodes vary considerably in size, from microscopic to about 2.5 cm in diameter.

A lymph node consists of a thin, fibrous outer capsule and an inner mass of lymphoid tissue. Penetrating the capsule

LYMPH NODE

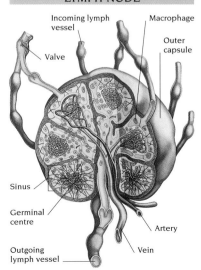

Incoming lymph vessel
Macrophage
Outer capsule
Valve
Sinus
Germinal centre
Artery
Vein
Outgoing lymph vessel

are several small lymphatic vessels (which carry lymph into the node). Each node contains sinuses (spaces), in which the lymph is filtered. The flow of the lymph slows as it moves through narrow channels in the sinuses; this reduction in flow allows macrophages (white blood cells that engulf and destroy foreign and dead material) time to filter microorganisms from the lymph. Germinal centres in the lymph node release white blood cells called *lymphocytes*, which also help to fight infection. A single, larger vessel carries lymph out of the node.

lymphocyte Any one of a group of white *blood cells* that are of crucial importance to the *immune system*. There are two principal types of lymphocyte: B- and T-lymphocytes. B-lymphocytes produce *immunoglobulins* or *antibodies*, which attach themselves to *antigens* (proteins) on the surfaces of bacteria. This starts a process leading to the destruction of the bacteria. The T-lymphocytes comprise three main groups of cells: killer (cytotoxic) cells, helper cells, and suppressor cells. The killer T-lymphocytes attach to abnormal cells (for example, tumour cells, cells that have been invaded by viruses, and those in transplanted tissue) and release chemicals called lymphokines, which help to destroy the abnormal cells. Helper T-cells enhance the activities of the killer T-cells and the B-cells, and also control other aspects of the immune response. Suppressor T-cells act to "switch off" the immune response. Some lymphocytes do not participate directly in immune responses, but serve as a memory bank for antigens that have been encountered.

lymphoedema An abnormal accumulation of *lymph* in the tissues, which occurs when the normal drainage of lymph is disrupted (see *lymphatic system*). There are various causes. In the tropical disease *filariasis*, lymphatic vessels may be blocked by parasitic worms. Cancer can lead to lymphoedema if vessels become blocked by deposits of cancer cells. Surgical removal of *lymph nodes* under the arm or in the groin, or *radiotherapy* to an area containing lymph nodes, may also result in lymphoedema. Rarely, the condition is due to a *congenital* abnormality of the lymphatic vessels known as Milroy's disease. In addition, the disorder may occur for no known cause.

Lymphoedema may develop in the arm following a radical mastectomy. Otherwise, it usually causes swelling of the legs, to an incapacitating degree in some people. There is no known cure. Treatment consists of taking *diuretic drugs*, massage, wearing an elastic bandage or compression sleeve, and special exercises; these measures may bring about some improvement.

lymphogranuloma venereum A sexually transmitted disease caused by a *chlamydial infection*; it is most common in tropical areas. The first sign of this condition may be a small genital blister that heals in a few days. There may also be fever, headache, muscle and joint pains, and a rash. The *lymph nodes*, particularly in the groin, become painfully enlarged and inflamed. *Abscesses* may form, and persistent *ulcers* may develop, on the skin over the affected glands. Treatment is with *antibiotic drugs*.

lymphoma Any of a group of cancers in which the cells of lymphoid tissue (found principally in the *lymph nodes* and the *spleen*) multiply unchecked. Lymphomas fall into two categories. If certain characteristic abnormal cells (Reed–Sternberg cells) are present, the disease is called Hodgkin's disease. All other forms are known as non-Hodgkin's lymphoma. (See *Burkitt's lymphoma*; *Hodgkin's disease*; *lymphoma, non-Hodgkin's*.)

lymphoma, non-Hodgkin's Any cancer of lymphoid tissue (found mainly in the *lymph nodes* and *spleen*) other than *Hodgkin's disease*. In most cases there is no known cause. Occasionally, the disease is associated with suppression of the *immune system*, particularly after an organ transplant. One type of non-Hodgkin's lymphoma, known as *Burkitt's lymphoma*, is thought to be caused by the *Epstein–Barr virus*.

There is usually painless swelling of *lymph nodes* in the neck, armpit, or groin. The *liver* and *spleen* may enlarge, and lymphoid tissue in the abdomen may be affected. Many other organs may become involved, leading to diverse symptoms ranging from headache to skin ulceration. Unless it is controlled, the disease (often marked by fever) progressively impairs the immune system, leading to death from infections or an uncontrolled spread of cancer. Diagnosis is based on a *biopsy*, usually taken from a lymph node. *Chest X-ray, CT scanning, MRI, lumbar puncture, bone marrow biopsy,* and *lymphangiography* of the abdomen may be needed to assess the extent of the disease.

If the lymphoma is confined to a single group of lymph nodes, treatment consists of *radiotherapy*. More often, the disease is more extensive, and in such cases *anticancer drugs* and *monoclonal antibodies* (see *antibody, monoclonal*) are given. A *stem cell* or *bone marrow transplant*, together with drug treatment and/or radiotherapy, may be performed on some people.

lysergide see *LSD*.

lysis A medical term for breaking down or destruction, usually applied to the destruction of cells by disintegration of their outer membrane. A common example is *haemolysis*, the breakdown of red blood cells. Lysis may be caused by chemical action, such as that of an *enzyme*, or by physical action, such as that of heat or cold. The term lysis is also occasionally used to refer to a sudden recovery from a fever.

lysozyme An *enzyme* found in tears, saliva, sweat, nasal secretions, breast milk, and many tissues. It destroys bacteria by disrupting their cell walls.

M

macro- A prefix meaning large, as in macrophage (a large cell in the *immune system*) or *macroglossia*.

macrobiotics A dietary system in which foods with a balance of *yin and yang* are eaten. Foods are classified as yin or yang depending on factors such as their colour, texture, and taste.

macroglossia Abnormal enlargement of the tongue. Macroglossia is a feature of *Down's syndrome, hypothyroidism,* and *acromegaly*. It is also caused by some tumours of the tongue, such as a *haemangioma* or a *lymphangioma*.

macrolide drugs A class of *antibiotic drugs* used to treat a wide range of infections including those of the ear, nose, throat, respiratory and gastrointestinal tracts, and skin. Common macrolides include *azithromycin* and *erythromycin*.

macrophage A cell in the *immune system*. Macrophages are large *phagocytes*, which can engulf and destroy microorganisms and other foreign particles. They are found in most body tissues.

macula The area of the eye's *retina* responsible for seeing fine detail. The macula surrounds the *fovea*, which contains the highest density of visual cells.

MACULA

Retina Fovea

Lens

Macula

Iris

Cornea

Optic
nerve

macular degeneration A progressive, painless disorder affecting the *macula*. The result is a roughly central, circular area of blindness that increases in size until it is large enough to obscure two or three words at reading distance. Macular degeneration does not cause total blindness as vision is retained around the edges of the visual fields. This condition is a common disorder in elderly people.

Of the two types of macular degeneration that may occur, one type may be remedied by *laser treatment*. There is no treatment for the other form, although the affected person may benefit from aids such as magnifying instruments.

macule A spot that is level with the skin's surface and discernible only by difference in colour or texture.

mad cow disease The commonly used name for *bovine spongiform encephalopathy* (BSE).

magnesium An element essential in the diet for the formation of bones and teeth, muscle contraction, nerve impulse transmission, and activation of many *enzymes*. Dietary sources include cereals, nuts, soya beans, milk, and fish.

magnesium sulphate A magnesium compound used as a *laxative drug* and an *anticonvulsant drug*.

magnesium trisilicate A magnesium compound used in *antacid drugs*.

magnetic resonance imaging See *MRI*.

malabsorption Impaired absorption of nutrients by the lining of the small intestine. Malabsorption may be caused by many conditions, including *lactase deficiency, cystic fibrosis*, chronic *pancreatitis, coeliac disease, Crohn's disease, amyloidosis, giardiasis, Whipple's disease,* and *lymphoma*. The removal of some of the small intestine, and certain operations on the stomach, may also result in malabsorption.

Common symptoms are diarrhoea and weight loss; and in severe cases, there may also be malnutrition (see *nutritional disorders*), *vitamin* deficiency, *mineral* deficiency, or *anaemia*. Diagnosis may be made by tests on faeces, *blood tests, barium X-ray examination* and *jejunal biopsy*. In most cases, dietary modifications or supplements are successful in treating the disorder. In severe cases, intravenous infusion of nutrients is needed (see *feeding, artificial*).

maladjustment Failure to adapt to a change in one's environment, resulting in inability to cope with work or social activities. Maladjustment can occur as a reaction to stressful situations, such as divorce or moving house. There may be feelings of *depression* or *anxiety*, or *behavioural problems in children* and in adolescents. Maladjustment usually disappears when a person is removed from the stressful situation or adapts to it.

malaise A vague feeling of being unwell.

malalignment Positioning of *teeth* in the *jaw* so that they do not form a smooth arch shape when viewed from above or below (see *malocclusion*).

Malalignment may also refer to a *fracture* in which the bone ends are not in a straight line.

malar flush A high colour over the cheekbones, with a bluish tinge caused by reduced oxygen concentration in the blood. Malar flush is considered to be a sign of *mitral stenosis*, which often follows *rheumatic fever*. However, malar flush is not always present in mitral stenosis, and many people with this colouring do not have heart disease.

malaria A serious disease caused by parasitic *protozoa* called plasmodia. The infection is spread by the bite of anopheles mosquitoes and is prevalent throughout the tropics. Malaria causes severe fever, and, in some cases, fatal complications affecting the kidneys, liver, brain, and blood.

There are four species of plasmodia that cause malaria: *PLASMODIUM FALCIPARUM, PLASMODIUM VIVAX, PLASMODIUM OVALE*, and *PLASMODIUM MALARIAE*. When a mosquito carrying any of these species bites a human, the plasmodia enter the bloodstream. They invade the liver and red blood cells, where they multiply. The red cells then rupture, releasing the new parasites. Some of them infect new red cells, and the others develop into forms that can infect more mosquitoes. Falciparum malaria infects more red cells than the other species and therefore causes a more

serious infection. Most cases of this form occur in Africa.

Symptoms of malaria include fever, shaking, and chills. There may also be severe headache, general malaise, and vomiting. The fever often develops in cycles, occurring every other day (in vivax and ovale infections) or every third day (in malariae infections).

Falciparum malaria can be fatal within days. Infected red cells become sticky and block blood vessels in vital organs. The *spleen* becomes enlarged and the *brain* may be affected, leading to *coma* and convulsions. Destruction of blood cells causes haemolytic anaemia (see *anaemia, haemolytic*). Kidney failure and jaundice often occur.

A diagnosis is made by examining a blood sample under a microscope to view the parasites. *Chloroquine* is the usual treatment for species other than falciparum. Falciparum malaria is treated with *quinine, proguanil* and atovaquone, or artemether and lumefantrine. People with vivax or ovale malaria must also take the drug *primaquine*. In severe cases, blood transfusions may be needed.

Preventive antimalarial drugs should be taken by all visitors to malarial countries. Doctors should be consulted for up-to-date advice on the choice and dosages of drugs to be taken. Avoiding mosquito bites by wearing suitable clothing and using insect repellents (such as *DEET*) and mosquito nets is also important in helping prevent malaria.

malathion An antiparasitic drug, which is used to treat skin or hair infestations such as *lice* and *scabies*.

malformation A deformity, particularly one resulting from faulty development.

malignant A condition that tends to become progressively worse and to result in death. The term is primarily used to refer to a cancerous *tumour* that spreads from its original location to form secondary tumours in other parts of the body.

malignant melanoma See *melanoma, malignant*.

malingering The deliberate simulation of symptoms for a purpose, such as taking time off work or obtaining compensation. Malingering is different from *factitious disorders* and *hypochondriasis*, in which

M

symptoms are not under the individual's voluntary control.

mallet finger Injury to the tendon or bone in a fingertip that forces the tip into a bent position. A common sports injury, it occurs when a ball strikes a finger.

Treatment is with a splint or with temporary insertion of wire through the bones to hold the finger straight. The injury heals within 2–3 months.

mallet toe See *claw-toe*.

malleus One of the three tiny bones (known collectively as the auditory ossicles) that are situated in the middle ear. The malleus, together with the *incus* and the *stapes*, transmits sound vibrations from the eardrum to the inner ear.

Mallory–Weiss syndrome A tear at the lower end of the *oesophagus*, causing vomiting of blood. The syndrome is commonly caused by retching and vomiting after drinking excessive amounts of alcohol. Less often, violent coughing, a severe asthma attack, or epileptic convulsions may be the cause.

An *endoscope* is passed down the oesophagus to confirm the diagnosis. The tear generally heals within 10 days and no special treatment is usually required. However, a *blood transfusion* may sometimes be necessary.

malnutrition See *nutritional disorders*.

malocclusion An abnormal relationship between the upper and lower sets of *teeth* when they are closed, affecting the bite (see *occlusion*) or appearance.

Malocclusion usually develops during childhood. It is inherited, or is caused by thumb-sucking or a mismatch between the teeth and jaws – for example, the combination of large teeth and a small mouth (see *overcrowding, dental*).

Orthodontic appliances (braces) may be used to move teeth into the proper position, and if there is dental overcrowding, some teeth may be extracted. *Orthognathic surgery* is used to treat severe recession or protrusion of the lower jaw. Treatment is best carried out in childhood or adolescence.

malpresentation A condition in which a baby is not in the usual head-first position for *childbirth*. Malpresentation includes breech presentation (the baby's bottom appears first), face presentation, and shoulder presentation (in which the baby is lying across the uterus). Breech presentations are the most common. A breech baby may be born by *breech delivery* or *caesarean section*. A shoulder presentation baby usually requires a caesarean section.

malta fever Older term for *brucellosis*.

mammary gland See *breast*.

mammography An X-ray procedure for examination of the *breast*. The

MAMMOGRAPHY

X-ray machine

Compressed breast

Plastic cover

X-ray beam

DETAIL

Plastic cover

Mammography technician

X-ray plate

breast is gently flattened between an X-ray plate and a plastic cover so that as much tissue as possible can be imaged. The procedure is used to investigate *breast lumps*, and to screen for *breast cancer*, because it allows the detection of breast tumours too small to be found during a physical examination (see *breast self-examination*). In the UK, all women aged 50–70 are offered routine mammography every 3 years. Such screening has improved the detection of early breast cancer and has led to a reduction in the number of deaths from the disease.

mammoplasty A cosmetic operation to make large or pendulous breasts smaller (breast reduction), to enlarge small breasts (breast enlargement), or to reconstruct a breast following surgery for *breast cancer*.

In breast reduction, unwanted tissue is removed and the breast is raised to correct drooping. Breast enlargement involves the insertion of an implant under the skin. Breast reconstruction may be carried out at the same time as a *mastectomy*. The normal contours of the breast are restored by the insertion of an implant. Possible complications of mammoplasty include leakage from an implant, hardening of the surrounding breast tissue, scarring, and infection.

mandible The lower *jaw*.

mania A mental disorder characterized by episodes of overactivity, elation, or irritability. Mania usually occurs as part of *bipolar disorder*.

Symptoms may include extravagant spending, repeatedly starting new tasks; sleeping less; increased appetite for food, alcohol, sex, and exercise; outbursts of inappropriate anger, laughter, or sudden socializing; and delusions of grandeur. If symptoms are mild, the condition is called hypomania.

Severe mania usually needs treatment in hospital with *antipsychotic drugs*. Relapses may be prevented by taking *lithium* or *carbamazepine*.

manic-depressive illness An alternative term for *bipolar disorder*.

manipulation A therapeutic technique involving the skilful use of the hands to move a part of the body, joint, or muscle to treat certain disorders. Manipulation is important in *orthopaedics*, *physiotherapy*, *osteopathy*, and *chiropractic*.

Manipulation may be used to treat deformity and stiffness caused by bone and joint disorders, to realign bones in a displaced *fracture*, to reposition a joint after a *dislocation*, or to stretch a *contracture*.

mannitol An osmotic *diuretic drug* used to treat *oedema* of the brain and *glaucoma*.

manometry The measuring of pressure (of either a liquid or a gas) by means of an instrument called a manometer. Manometry is used to measure blood pressure using an instrument called a *sphygmomanometer*.

mantoux test A skin test for tuberculosis (see *tuberculin tests*).

manubrium The uppermost part of the *sternum* (breastbone).

MAOI An abbreviation for *monoamine oxidase inhibitor* drugs.

marasmus A severe form of protein and calorie malnutrition that usually occurs in famine or semi-starvation conditions. Marasmus is common in young children in developing countries. The disorder causes stunted growth, emaciation, and loose folds of skin on the limbs and buttocks due to loss of muscle and fat. Other signs include sparse, brittle hair; diarrhoea; and dehydration.

Treatment includes keeping the child warm and giving a high-energy, protein-rich diet. Persistent marasmus can cause mental handicap and impaired growth. (See also *kwashiorkor*.)

marble bone disease See *osteopetrosis*.

march fracture A break in one of the *metatarsal bones* (the long bones in the foot) that is caused by running or walking for long distances on a hard surface. The fracture results in pain, tenderness, and swelling. However, it may not show on X-rays until callus (new bone) starts to form. Treatment for a march fracture is rest and, occasionally, immobilization in a plaster cast. (See also *stress fracture*.)

Marfan's syndrome A rare *genetic disorder* of *connective tissue* (material that holds body structures together) that results in skeletal, heart, and eye abnormalities. Features of Marfan's

M

syndrome usually appear after age 10. Affected people are very tall and thin, with long, spidery fingers and weak ligaments and tendons. The chest and spine are often deformed and the lens of the eye may be dislocated. The heart or *aorta* is often abnormal.

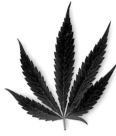

MARIJUANA LEAF

marijuana The flowering tops and dried leaves of the Indian hemp plant *CANNABIS SATIVA*, containing the active ingredient THC (tetra-hydrocannabinol). The leaves are usually smoked but can be drunk as tea or eaten in food. Physical effects of marijuana include dry mouth, mild reddening of the eyes, slight clumsiness, and an increased appetite. The main subjective feelings are usually of calmness and wellbeing, but depression occurs occasionally.

Large doses may cause panic, fear of death, and illusions. In rare cases, true *psychosis* occurs, with paranoid delusions, confusion, and other symptoms, which usually disappear within a few days. Marijuana use has also been linked with an increased risk of *schizophrenia*. Regular use of marijuana may lead to a more permanent state of apathy and loss of concern (a condition that is known as amotivational syndrome).

marriage guidance See *relationship counselling*.

marrow, bone See *bone marrow*.

marsupialization A type of surgical procedure that is used to drain some types of *abscess* or *cyst* and to prevent the formation of further abscesses. Marsupialization is used to treat certain types of cysts affecting the *pancreas* and *liver*, and cysts affecting the *Bartholin's glands* at the entrance to the vagina.

masculinization See *virilization*.

masochism A chronic desire to be physically, mentally, or emotionally abused. The term masochism is used to refer to the achievement of sexual excitement by means of one's own suffering through activities such as bondage, flagellation, and verbal abuse. (See also *sadism*; *sadomasochism*.)

massage Rubbing and kneading areas of the body, usually with the hands. Massage increases the blood flow and relaxes muscles; it may be used to relieve muscle spasm, treat muscle injury, and reduce *oedema*. Although massage is most effective when carried out by someone else, self-massage can also alleviate pain caused by muscle tension.

mastalgia The medical term for pain in the breast.

mast cell A type of cell that plays an important part in *allergy*. In an allergic response, mast cells release *histamine*.

mastectomy The surgical removal of all of the *breast*, usually performed to treat *breast cancer*. Mastectomy may be used for extensive breast cancer or for multiple cancerous tumours. For smaller cancers, *lumpectomy* or *quadrantectomy* may be appropriate.

A mastectomy involves the removal of all of the breast tissue and usually some or all of the *lymph nodes* in the armpit. Cells from the lymph nodes are examined to determine whether cancerous cells may have spread. The

MASTECTOMY

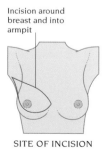

Incision around breast and into armpit

SITE OF INCISION

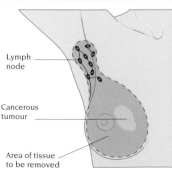

Lymph node

Cancerous tumour

Area of tissue to be removed

operation is performed under general *anaesthesia* and usually requires a stay in hospital of several days. *Plastic surgery* to reconstruct the breast may be carried out at the same time as the mastectomy or at a later time (see *mammoplasty*).

Treatment with *radiotherapy* may be given after surgery, especially if the cancer has spread to lymph nodes. It usually starts a month after surgery and is continued for 3–6 weeks. Drug treatment with *tamoxifen* or *chemotherapy* may also be given.

mastication The process of chewing food. The canines and incisors (front teeth) shear the food. The tongue then pushes it between the upper and lower premolars and molars (back teeth) to be ground by movements of the lower jaw. *Saliva* is mixed with the food to help break it down for swallowing.

mastitis Inflammation of breast tissue, usually caused by bacterial infection and sometimes by hormonal changes. Mastitis usually occurs when bacteria enter the nipple during *breast-feeding*. It can also be caused by changes in levels of *sex hormones* in the body – for example, at the onset of puberty.

Mastitis results in pain, tenderness, and swelling in one or both breasts. Bacterial mastitis during breast-feeding also causes redness and *engorgement* and may result in a *breast abscess*.

Mastitis caused by infection is treated with *antibiotic drugs* and *analgesic drugs*, and by *expressing milk* to relieve engorgement. Mastitis caused by hormone changes usually clears up in a few weeks without treatment.

mastocytosis An unusual condition in which itchy, irregular, yellow or orange-brown swellings occur on the skin, most commonly on the trunk. Mastocytosis may also affect body organs, including the liver, spleen, and intestine, and it may cause symptoms such as diarrhoea, vomiting, and fainting. Very rarely, the condition leads to *anaphylactic shock*, which can be fatal. The condition usually begins in the first year of life and clears up by adolescence. *Antihistamine drugs* may be helpful in relieving symptoms of mastocytosis.

mastoid bone The lower part of the temporal bone in the *skull*. It has a projection, known as the mastoid process, which can be felt behind the ear. The mastoid bone is honeycombed with air cells. These are connected to a cavity called the mastoid antrum, which leads into the middle ear. Infections of the middle ear (see *otitis media*) occasionally spread through the mastoid bone to cause acute *mastoiditis*.

mastoiditis Inflammation of the *mastoid bone* in the skull. The disease is caused by infection spreading from the middle ear (see *otitis media*) to the air cells in the mastoid bone through a cavity called the mastoid antrum.

Mastoiditis causes earache and severe pain, swelling, and tenderness behind the ear. There is usually also fever, a creamy discharge from the ear, progressive hearing loss, and displacement of the outer ear. If the infection spreads, it may lead to *meningitis*, a *brain abscess*, blood clotting in veins within the brain, or *facial palsy*.

Treatment is with *antibiotic drugs*. If the infection persists, an operation known as a mastoidectomy may be carried out to remove the infected air cells.

masturbation Sexual self-stimulation, usually to *orgasm*. Massaging the *penis* or the *clitoris* with the hand is the usual method of masturbation.

maternal mortality The death of a woman during *pregnancy*, or within 42 days of *childbirth*, *miscarriage*, or an induced *abortion*, from any pregnancy-related cause. Maternal mortality rate describes the number of such deaths per year per set number of pregnancies. Maternal deaths may occur as a direct result of complications of pregnancy, or indirectly due to a medical condition worsened by pregnancy. Major direct causes include *embolism*, *antepartum haemorrhage*, *postpartum haemorrhage*, *hypertension*, *eclampsia*, and *puerperal sepsis*. Indirect causes include heart disease, *epilepsy*, and some cancers.

Maternal mortality is lowest for second pregnancies. It rises with age, being greatest for women over 40.

maxilla One of a pair of bones that together form the centre of the face, the upper jaw, and the roof of the mouth. Each maxilla contains a large air-filled cavity (called the maxillary sinus) which is connected to the nasal cavity.

McArdle's disease A rare *genetic disorder* characterized by muscle stiffness and painful cramps that increase during exertion and afterwards. The cause is a deficiency of an *enzyme* in muscle cells that stimulates breakdown of the carbohydrate *glycogen* into the simple sugar glucose. The result is a build-up of glycogen and low levels of glucose in the muscles. Damage to the muscles occurs, causing myoglobinuria (muscle-cell pigment in the urine), which may lead to *kidney failure*. There is no treatment, but symptoms may be relieved by eating glucose or fructose before exercise.

MDMA The hallucinogenic substance methylenedioxymethamfetamine, which has the street name *Ecstasy*.

ME The abbreviation for myalgic encephalomyelitis (see *chronic fatigue syndrome*).

measles A potentially dangerous viral illness that causes fever and a characteristic rash. Measles mainly affects children, but can occur at any age. The virus is spread primarily by airborne droplets of nasal secretions. It can be transmitted during the *incubation period* (8–14 days after infection) and up to 7 days after symptoms appear.

The illness starts with a fever, runny nose, sore eyes, cough, and a general feeling of being unwell. After 3–4 days, a red rash appears, usually starting on the head and neck and spreading to cover the body. The spots sometimes join to produce large red blotches, and the *lymph nodes* may be enlarged. After 3 days, the rash starts to fade and the symptoms subside.

The most common complications are ear and chest infections, which usually occur 2–3 days after the rash appears. Diarrhoea, vomiting, and abdominal pain also occur. Febrile convulsions (see *convulsion, febrile*) are also common, but these are not usually serious. *Encephalitis* occurs in about 1 in 1,000 cases, causing headache, drowsiness, and vomiting. Seizures and *coma* may follow, sometimes leading to *brain damage* or even death. In very rare cases, a progressive brain disorder known as subacute sclerosing panencephalitis develops years later. If measles occurs during pregnancy, the fetus dies in about a fifth of cases. However, there is no evidence that measles causes birth defects.

There is no specific treatment for measles. Plenty of fluids and *paracetamol* are given for fever, and *antibiotic drugs* may be given to treat bacterial infections that occur as complications.

To help prevent measles, immunization with the *MMR vaccination* is recommended at around 13 months of age. This produces immunity in about 90 per cent of cases, with a booster shot given before school or nursery school entry.

meatus A canal or passageway through part of the body. The term usually refers to the external auditory meatus, the canal in the outer *ear* that leads from the outside to the eardrum.

mebendazole An *anthelmintic drug* used to treat *worm infestations* of the intestine. Possible adverse effects include abdominal pain and diarrhoea.

mebeverine An *antispasmodic drug* used to treat *irritable bowel syndrome*.

Meckel's diverticulum A common problem, present at birth, in which a small, hollow, wide-mouthed sac protrudes from the *ileum*. Symptoms only occur when the diverticulum becomes infected, obstructed, or ulcerated. The most common symptom is painless bleeding, which may be sudden and severe, making immediate *blood transfusion* necessary. Inflammation may cause symptoms very similar to those of acute *appendicitis*. Meckel's diverticulum occasionally causes *intussusception* or *volvulus* of the small intestine. Diagnosis of Meckel's diverticulum may be made by using technetium *radionuclide scanning*. If complications occur, they are treated by surgical removal of the diverticulum.

meconium The thick, sticky, greenish-black faeces passed by infants in the first day or two after birth. It consists of *bile*, mucus, and shed intestinal cells.

Occasionally, the fetus passes meconium into the *amniotic fluid* in the uterus. This is more common in babies who experience *fetal distress* during labour or who are over 40 weeks' gestation. Meconium in the amniotic fluid may be inhaled when the baby starts to breathe, sometimes blocking the airways and damaging the lungs.

In some babies with *cystic fibrosis*, the meconium is so thick and sticky that it blocks the intestine (see *intestine, obstruction of*).

medial A medical term that means "situated towards the midline of the body". Less commonly, the term refers to the middle layer of a body structure.

median nerve One of the main nerves of the arm. It is a branch of the *brachial plexus* and runs down the arm from the shoulder into the hand. The median nerve controls the muscles that carry out bending movements of the wrist, fingers, and thumb, and that rotate the forearm palm-inwards. The nerve also conveys sensations from the thumb and first three fingers, and from the region of the palm at their base.

Damage to the nerve may result from injury to the shoulder, a *Colles' fracture* just above the wrist, or pressure on the nerve where it passes through the wrist (*carpal tunnel syndrome*). Symptoms of damage include numbness and weakness in areas controlled by the nerve.

mediastinoscopy Investigation of the *mediastinum* by means of an *endoscope* inserted through an incision in the neck.

Mediastinoscopy is used mainly to perform a *biopsy* of a *lymph node*. The sample is removed by tiny blades on the endoscope.

mediastinum The membranous partition between the lungs and the other structures within the chest cavity. These structures include the *heart* and associated blood vessels, *trachea*, *oesophagus*, *thymus* gland, *lymph nodes*, lymphatic vessels, and nerves.

medication Any substance prescribed to treat disease. (See also *drug*; *medicine*.)

medicine The study of human diseases, their causes, frequency, treatment, and prevention. The term is also applied to a substance prescribed to treat illness.

medicolegal Relating to aspects of medicine and law that overlap. Among the matters on which medicolegal experts advise are the laws concerning damages for injuries due to medical negligence or malpractice, evidence concerning the extent of injury in a civil action, the use of paternity tests, the mental competence of people who have drawn up wills, and restrictions on the mentally ill.

Medicolegal issues also include an individual's right to die (see *brain death*; *euthanasia*; *living will*); the necessity for informed *consent* to any surgical procedure; the legal aspects of *artificial insemination*, *in vitro fertilization*, *sterilization*, and *surrogacy*, and a patient's right to *confidentiality* concerning his or her illness. (For the medical aspects of criminal law, see *forensic medicine*.)

meditation Concentrating on an object, a word, or an idea with the aim of inducing an altered state of consciousness.

At its deepest level, meditation can resemble a trance. More commonly, it is a calming therapy and can be a way of reducing stress levels and treating stress-related disorders. A common form of meditation practised in the west is transcendental meditation (TM).

medroxyprogesterone A *progestogen drug* used to treat *endometriosis* and uterine cancer (see *uterus, cancer of*). It is also sometimes used in *hormone replacement therapy*. Medroxyprogesterone can also be used as a contraceptive, administered by injection at 3-monthly intervals (see *contraception, hormonal methods of*). Possible adverse effects include weight gain, swollen ankles, and breast tenderness.

medulla The innermost part of an organ or other body structure; for example, the adrenal medulla is the central region of an *adrenal gland*. The term "medulla" is also sometimes used to refer to the *medulla oblongata*.

medulla oblongata Also known as the *medulla*, the lowest part of the *brain-*

M

MEDULLA OBLONGATA

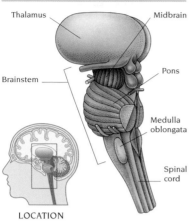

Thalamus

Midbrain

Brainstem

Pons

Medulla oblongata

Spinal cord

LOCATION

stem. The medulla oblongata lies in the skull just above the spinal cord.

medulloblastoma A type of cancerous *brain tumour* that occurs mainly in children. The tumour usually arises from the *cerebellum*, which is concerned with posture, balance, and coordination. It grows rapidly and may spread to other parts of the brain and to the *spinal cord*. A morning headache, repeated vomiting, and a clumsy gait develop. There are also frequent falls. The tumour is diagnosed by *CT scanning* or *MRI* and often responds to *radiotherapy*. Surgery and *anticancer drugs* may also be needed.

mefenamic acid A *nonsteroidal anti-inflammatory drug* used to relieve pain and inflammation. Possible adverse effects are typical for this group of drugs.

mefloquine A drug used to prevent *malaria* in parts of the world where the parasite that causes it is resistant to *chloroquine*. Side effects include nausea, vomiting, and diarrhoea. Rarely, there may be *panic attacks*, *hallucinations*, and *psychosis*.

mega- A prefix meaning very large, as in *megacolon*, a condition in which the colon is greatly enlarged. The prefix megalo- has the same meaning.

megacolon A gross distension (enlargement) of the *colon*, usually accompanied by severe, chronic *constipation*.

In children, the main causes of megacolon are *anal fissures*, *Hirschsprung's*

disease, and psychological factors that may have arisen during toilet-training. In elderly people, causes include the long-term use of strong *laxative drugs*. People suffering from chronic *depression* or *schizophrenia* often have megacolon. Other, rarer causes include *hypothyroidism*, *spinal injury*, and drugs such as *morphine* and *codeine*.

Megacolon causes constipation and abdominal bloating. Associated loss of appetite may lead to weight loss. Diarrhoea may result if semi-liquid faeces leak around the obstructing hard faeces.

Diagnosis is made by *proctoscopy*, *barium X-ray examination*, and tests of bowel muscle function. If Hirschsprung's disease is suspected, *biopsy* of the large intestine may be performed. Impacted faeces are often removed using *enemas*. In severe cases, the faeces must be removed manually.

megaloblastic anaemia See *anaemia, megaloblastic.*

megalomania An exaggerated sense of one's own importance or ability that often occurs in *mania*. Megalomania may take the form of a *delusion* of grandeur, or of a desire to organize activities that are expensive, large in scale, and involve many people.

-megaly A suffix meaning enlargement, as in *acromegaly*, a condition in which there is enlargement of the skull, jaw, hands, and feet due to excess production of *growth hormone*.

megestrol A *progestogen drug* used to treat certain types of *breast cancer* and uterine cancer (see *uterus, cancer of*). It may be prescribed when a tumour cannot be removed by surgery, if a tumour has recurred after surgery, or when other *anticancer drugs* or *radiotherapy* prove ineffective.

Possible adverse effects of megestrol include swollen ankles, weight gain, and nausea.

meibomian cyst See *chalazion.*

Meig's syndrome A rare condition in which a tumour of an *ovary* is accompanied by *ascites* and a *pleural effusion*. The fluid usually disappears when the tumour is removed.

meiosis A type of cell division that occurs in the *ovaries* and *testes* during

M

the production of egg and sperm cells. During meiosis in humans, a cell containing 23 pairs of *chromosomes* (46 in total) divides to form four sperm or egg cells, each with 23 single chromosomes.

First, the chromosomes are duplicated to produce four copies of each chromosome (92 in total). Matching pairs of chromosomes line up and exchange genetic material. The cell then divides twice to form four daughter cells, with each taking one copy of each chromosome. Egg and sperm cells therefore have only half the usual chromosome content of a body cell, so that each parent contributes half of the child's genetic material. The exchange between chromosomes means that each daughter cell has a unique genetic make-up. (See also *mitosis*.)

melaena Black, tarry *faeces* caused by bleeding, usually in the upper gastrointestinal tract. The blood is blackened by the action of secretions during digestion. Melaena is usually caused by a *peptic ulcer* but may indicate cancer.

melancholia Former term for *depression*.

melanin The brown or black pigment that gives skin, hair, and the iris of the eyes their colouring. Melanin is produced by cells called *melanocytes*.

Exposure to sunlight increases the production of melanin, which protects the skin from the harmful effects of ultraviolet rays and causes the skin to darken. Localized overproduction of melanin in the skin can result in a pigmented spot, most commonly a *freckle* or mole (see *naevus*).

melanocyte A specialized skin cell that produces the pigment *melanin*.

melanoma, juvenile A raised, reddish-brown skin blemish which sometimes appears on the face or legs in early childhood (see *naevus*). Although they are usually harmless, an unsightly growth, or one suspected of being skin cancer, can be removed surgically.

melanoma, malignant The most serious of the three types of skin cancer, the other two being *basal cell carcinoma* and *squamous cell carcinoma*. Malignant melanoma is a tumour of melanocytes, the cells that produce *melanin*, and is due to

long-term exposure to strong sunlight. There are an increasing number of new cases and deaths in the UK each year from this skin cancer.

MELANOMA, MALIGNANT

Irregular edge · · · · · · · · · · · · · · Crusted surface

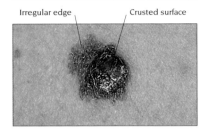

Tumours usually develop on exposed skin but may occur anywhere on the body. A melanoma usually grows from an existing mole, which may enlarge, become lumpy, bleed or crust over, change colour, develop an irregular edge, turn into a scab, or become itchy. Occasionally, a melanoma develops in normal skin. The tumour often spreads to other parts of the body. Diagnosis is by a *skin biopsy* and the melanoma is removed surgically. *Radiotherapy* or *anticancer drugs* may also be necessary.

melanosis coli Black or brown discoloration of the colon lining, associated with chronic *constipation* and prolonged use of certain *laxative drugs*, such as senna, rhubarb, and cascara.

The discoloration is most common in elderly people and is usually symptomless, clearing up when the laxatives are stopped. Rarely, it is associated with colon cancer (see *colon, cancer of*).

melasma See *chloasma*.

melatonin A *hormone* secreted by the *pineal gland* that is thought to play a part in controlling daily body rhythms.

melphalan An *anticancer drug* used to treat *multiple myeloma* as well as certain types of *breast cancer* and ovarian cancer (see *ovary, cancer of*).

Possible adverse effects include nausea, vomiting, sore throat, loss of appetite, aplastic *anaemia*, abnormal bleeding, and increased susceptibility to infection.

membrane A layer of tissue that covers or lines a body surface or forms a barrier.

M

memory The ability to remember. Memory is usually thought of as having three stages: registration, storage, and recall. In registration, information is perceived, understood, and stored in short-term memory. Unless they are constantly repeated, the contents of short-term memory are lost in minutes. In retention, important information is transferred into long-term memory and stored. Recall involves bringing information into the conscious mind at will.

Many factors determine how well something is remembered, including its familiarity and how much attention has been paid to it.

It is not known where in the brain the memory process takes place. However, the temporal lobe and *limbic system* may be involved. The mechanisms for storing memory are also unknown.

Most memory disturbances are due to failure at the retention or recall stage (see *amnesia*). In some cases, the problem occurs at the registration stage. Some people with *temporal lobe epilepsy* have uncontrollable flashbacks of distant past events. The most common memory disorder is the normal difficulty in recall that develops with age. More severe loss of memory may be an early symptom of *dementia*.

memory, loss of See *amnesia*.

menarche The onset of *menstruation*. Menarche usually occurs around age 13, 2 or 3 years after *puberty* starts.

Ménière's disease An inner *ear* disorder characterized by recurrent *vertigo*, *deafness*, and *tinnitus*. The cause is a build-up of fluid in the *labyrinth*. The fluid build-up may damage the labyrinth and sometimes the adjacent *cochlea*.

The disease is uncommon before the age of 40. There is a sudden attack of vertigo, lasting from a few minutes to several hours. This is usually accompanied by nausea, vomiting, *nystagmus*, and deafness, tinnitus, and a feeling of pressure or pain in the affected ear.

Diagnosis is usually made with audiometry (see *hearing tests*) or other hearing tests, and a *caloric test*. Treatment with certain *antihistamine drugs*, such as *cinnarizine*, or with *betahistine* usually relieves the symptoms, although *prochlorperazine* may also be given, under the tongue, rectally, or by injection, for severe attacks. Ménière's disease can also be treated by surgery to the inner ear if symptoms are not controlled by drugs. If deafness eventually becomes total, the other symptoms usually disappear.

meninges The three membranes that cover and protect the *brain* and the *spinal cord*. The outer membrane, the dura mater, is tough and fibrous; it lines the inside of the skull and forms a loose sheath around the spinal cord. The middle membrane, the arachnoid mater, is elastic and web-like. The inner membrane, the pia mater, lies directly next to the brain. It is separated from the arachnoid mater by the subarachnoid space, which contains *cerebrospinal fluid*.

MENINGES

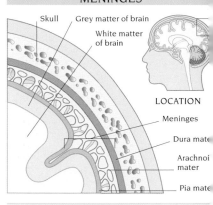

Skull
Grey matter of brain
White matter of brain

LOCATION

Meninges

Dura mater

Arachnoid mater

Pia mater

meningioma A rare, noncancerous tumour of the *meninges* of the brain that arises from the arachnoid mater (middle layer) and usually becomes attached to the dura mater (outer layer). The tumour slowly expands and may become very large before any symptoms appear. Symptoms can include headache, vomiting, and impaired mental function. There may also be speech loss or visual disturbance. If the tumour invades the skull bone, there may be thickening and bulging of the skull.

Meningiomas can be detected by *X-ray* or *CT scanning*, and *MRI* of the skull, and can often be completely

M

removed by surgery. Otherwise, treatment is by *radiotherapy*.

meningitis Inflammation of the *meninges* (membranes covering the *brain* and *spinal cord*), usually due to infection. Viral meningitis tends to occur in epidemics in the winter; it is relatively mild. Bacterial meningitis is life-threatening. It is mainly caused by HAEMOPHILUS INFLUENZAE, STREPTOCOCCUS PNEUMONIAE *(pneumococcus)*, and MENINGOCOCCUS type B and C bacteria.

The infection usually reaches the meninges via the bloodstream from an infection elsewhere in the body. Less commonly, it passes through skull cavities from an infected ear or *sinus*, or from the air following a *skull fracture*.

The main symptoms are fever, severe headache, nausea and vomiting, dislike of light, and a stiff neck. In viral meningitis, the symptoms are mild and may resemble influenza. In bacterial meningitis, the main symptoms may develop over only a few hours, followed by drowsiness and, occasionally, loss of consciousness. In about half the cases of meningococcal meningitis, there is also a rash under the skin that does not fade with pressure (see *glass test*). The rash starts as pin-prick spots that can join to give a bruise-like appearance.

To make a diagnosis, a *lumbar puncture* is performed. Viral meningitis needs no treatment and usually clears up within a week or two with no after-effects. Bacterial meningitis is a medical emergency. It is treated with intravenous *antibiotic drugs*. With prompt treatment, a full recovery is usually made. However, brain damage may occur in some cases.

Vaccines are now given to protect children against three of the major types of bacterial meningitis: those caused by the HAEMOPHILUS INFLUENZAE bacterium, the MENINGOCOCCUS type C bacterium, and pneumococcus (see *immunization*). For other types of bacterial meningitis, antibiotic drugs are given as a protective measure to people who have come into contact with the infection. Immunization against some forms of meningitis is advised for Muslim pilgrims travelling to Saudi Arabia and for people visiting Nepal and some parts of sub-Saharan Africa.

meningocele A protrusion of the spinal cord *meninges* under the skin that is caused by a congenital defect in the spine (see *spina bifida*).

meningomyelocele Another name for *myelocele* (see *spina bifida*).

meniscectomy A surgical procedure in which all or part of a damaged *meniscus* (cartilage disc) is removed from a joint, almost always from the knee. Meniscectomy may be carried out when damage to the meniscus causes the knee to lock or to give way repeatedly. The procedure cures these symptoms and reduces the likelihood of premature *osteoarthritis* in the joint.

Arthroscopy may be carried out to confirm and locate the damage, and the damaged area removed by instruments passed through the arthroscope.

Alternatively, the meniscus may be removed through an incision at the side of the *patella* (kneecap).

In either case, there may be an increased risk of osteoarthritis in later life, but this is less than if the damaged meniscus had been left in place.

meniscus A crescent-shaped disc of cartilaginous tissue found in several joints. The *knee* joint has two menisci, and the *wrist* joints, and the *temporomandibular joints* of the jaw, have one each. The menisci are held in position by *ligaments* and help to reduce friction during joint movement.

menopause The cessation of *menstruation*, which usually occurs between the ages of 45 and 55. The term is usually used to refer to a period of physical and psychological changes that occur as a result of reduced *oestrogen* production.

Symptoms of menopause include *hot flushes* and night sweats; vaginal dryness caused by thinning of the vaginal skin; and a decrease in vaginal secretions. The vagina shrinks and loses elasticity, and becomes prone to minor infections. Vaginal dryness may also make sexual intercourse more difficult and painful (see *vaginitis*). The neck of the bladder and urethra undergo similar changes, which can result in a feeling of needing to urinate frequently.

Psychological symptoms, such as poor concentration, tearfulness, loss of

M

interest in sex, and depression, are also often attributed to the menopause.

Changes in *metabolism* occur during the menopause but may not cause symptoms until later. Bones become thinner, and *osteoporosis* may develop. There is also an increased level of fats in the blood, which may cause an increase in *atherosclerosis* and a higher incidence of *coronary artery disease* and *stroke*.

Hormone replacement therapy (HRT) may relieve menopausal symptoms, but is now generally recommended only for short-term use around the menopause.

menorrhagia Excessive loss of blood during *menstruation*. Menorrhagia may be caused by an imbalance of *oestrogen hormones* and *progesterone hormone*, which control menstruation. The imbalance causes an excessive build-up of *endometrium* (lining of the uterus). Disorders that affect the uterus, such as *fibroids*, *polyps*, or a *pelvic infection*, can also cause menorrhagia.

Treatment may include *nonsteroidal anti-inflammatory drugs*, drugs that affect blood clotting, hormones, or the fitting of an *IUD* (intrauterine device) that releases small amounts of *progestogen* (see *IUS*). Menorrhagia may also be treated by *endometrial ablation*.

menotrophin A *gonadotrophin hormone* given as a drug to stimulate cell activity in the *ovaries* and *testes*. It is used as a treatment for certain types of male and female *infertility*, as it prepares the ovary for ovulation and may help stimulate sperm production. It is used along with human chorionic gonadotrophin (see *gonadotrophin, human chorionic*).

In women, menotrophin may cause multiple pregnancy, abdominal pain, bloating, and weight gain. In men, it may cause enlargement of the breasts.

menstruation The periodic shedding of *endometrium*, accompanied by bleeding, that occurs in women who are not pregnant. It usually begins at *puberty* and continues until the *menopause*.

Menstruation occurs at the end of the menstrual cycle, which usually lasts for 28 days (the normal range is 21–35 days). At the beginning of the cycle, a hormone from the *pituitary gland* stimulates an egg *follicle* in an *ovary* to mature. The follicle secretes *oestrogen hormones*, which make the endometrium thicken.

Ovulation (release of an egg from the follicle) usually occurs in the middle of the menstrual cycle. The empty follicle also produces *progesterone hormone*, which makes the endometrium become swollen and thick with retained fluid. This enables a fertilized egg to implant in the endometrium. If pregnancy fails to occur, the production of oestrogens and progesterone diminishes. The endometrium is then shed about 14 days after ovulation. Uterine contractions force the menstrual discharge to be expelled into the vagina, accompanied by bleeding, which may last for 1–8 days.

menstruation, disorders of An abnormality in the monthly cycle of menstrual bleeding. Menstrual disorders may be a sign of a problem in the pelvic area, such as *fibroids, endometriosis*, or *pelvic inflammatory disease*, but the cause is often unknown.

Dysmenorrhoea (painful periods) is the most common type of menstrual disorder. Other types of menstrual disorder are *amenorrhoea* (absence of menstruation), polymenorrhoea (too frequent menstruation), oligomenorrhoea (infrequent periods or scanty blood loss), and *menorrhagia* (excessive bleeding).

Some women have extreme variations in the length of menstrual cycles or menstrual periods, or in the amount of blood lost (see *menstruation, irregular*).

menstruation, irregular A variation in the normal pattern of *menstruation*. Irregular menstruation can include variations in the interval between periods, in the duration of menstrual bleeding, or in the amount of blood that is lost.

The most common cause of irregular menstruation is a disturbed balance of *oestrogen hormones* and *progesterone hormone*. Other causes include *stress*, travel, a change in the method of *contraception*, unsuspected pregnancy, or early *miscarriage*.

Menstruation is often irregular for the first few years, and for several years before the *menopause*.

mental age A measurement of the intellectual development of a person, with regard to the normal age at which that

M

level of achievement is attained. For example, a 13 year-old child with *learning difficulties* may have a mental age of 5.

mental handicap Impaired intellectual development, also known as general *learning difficulties* or disability.

Mental Health Act The Mental Health Act (1983) details the rights of patients with *mental illness* and the grounds for detaining mentally ill people against their will. It also outlines forms of legal guardianship for such patients.

When a person is endangering his or her own or other people's health or safety (for example, threatening harm or suicide) because of a recognized mental illness, he or she may be compulsorily taken into hospital to be given treatment. If a person breaks the law because of a mental disorder, the courts may remand him or her to hospital.

mental illness A general term that describes any form of psychiatric disorder.

mental retardation See *learning difficulties*.

menthol An alcohol prepared from mint oils. Menthol is an ingredient of several over-the-counter inhalation preparations used to treat a blocked or stuffy nose.

meprobamate An *antianxiety drug* occasionally used in the treatment of *anxiety* and *stress*. It also acts as a muscle relaxant. Prolonged use may cause dependence.

meptazinol A weak opioid *analgesic drug* used for the short-term relief of moderate to severe pain, such as after surgery and during childbirth. Possible adverse effects include nausea, vomiting, and dizziness.

mercaptopurine An *anticancer drug* used to treat certain types of *leukaemia*. Adverse effects include nausea, mouth ulcers, and appetite loss. Rarely, it may cause liver damage, *anaemia*, and abnormal bleeding.

mercury The only metal that is liquid at room temperature. Mercury is used in amalgam fillings for teeth (see *amalgam, dental*).

mercury poisoning Toxic effects of mercury on the body. The most common cause of mercury poisoning is breathing in vapour given off by liquid mercury, usually as a result of industrial exposure. Swallowing a small amount of liquid mercury is unlikely to lead to poisoning. Mercury compounds may cause poisoning by absorption through the intestines (causing nausea, vomiting, diarrhoea, and abdominal pain) or the skin (causing severe inflammation).

After entering the body, mercury accumulates in organs, principally the brain and kidneys. Mercury deposits in the brain cause tiredness, incoordination, excitability, tremors, and numbness in the limbs. In severe cases, there may be impaired vision and *dementia*. Deposits of mercury in the kidneys may lead to *kidney failure*.

Treatment may involve *chelating agents*, which help the body to excrete the mercury quickly; haemodialysis (see *dialysis*); and induced vomiting or pumping out the stomach, if mercury has been swallowed within the previous few hours.

mesalazine A drug used to treat *ulcerative colitis* and Crohn's disease. Adverse effects of mesalazine include nausea, diarrhoea, abdominal pain, and headache.

mescaline A *hallucinogenic drug* obtained from the Mexican peyote cactus.

mesenteric lymphadenitis An acute abdominal disorder, mainly affecting children, in which *lymph nodes* in the *mesentery* become inflamed. The main symptoms of pain and tenderness in the abdomen may mimic appendicitis. There may also be mild fever. Mesenteric lymphadenitis usually clears up rapidly, needing only *analgesic drugs* to reduce pain and fever.

mesentery A membrane that attaches organs to the abdominal wall. The term

MESENTERY

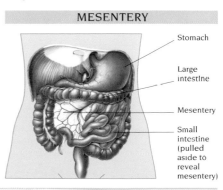

Stomach

Large intestine

Mesentery

Small intestine (pulled aside to reveal mesentery)

is used particularly to refer to the membranous fold that encloses the small intestine, attaching it to the back of the abdominal wall. The mesentery contains the blood vessels, nerves, and lymphatic vessels for the intestines.

mesothelioma A cancerous tumour of the *pleura*. Exposure to asbestos dust is a risk factor (see *asbestos-related diseases*). Symptoms, which do not always occur, include cough, chest pain, and breathing difficulty, especially if a *pleural effusion* develops. Diagnosis is made with a *chest X-ray* followed by pleural *biopsy* or examination of a fluid sample from any effusion. If the tumour is small, surgery is often successful. There is no effective treatment for large tumours, although *radiotherapy* may alleviate symptoms.

mesothelium A type of *epithelium* covering the *peritoneum*, the *pleura*, and the *pericardium*.

mesterolone An *androgen hormone* (male sex hormone) used as replacement therapy in *hypogonadism* because testosterone cannot be given orally. Side effects can include prostate problems, headache, and depression.

mestranol An *oestrogen drug* used in some *oral contraceptives*.

metabolic disorders A group of disorders in which some aspect of body chemistry is disturbed. Some metabolic disorders result from an inherited malfunction or deficiency of an *enzyme* (see *metabolism, inborn errors of*). Others result from under- or overproduction of a hormone that controls metabolic activity, such as occurs in *diabetes mellitus* and *hypothyroidism*.

metabolism A collective term for all the chemical processes that take place in the body. It is divided into catabolism (breaking down of complex substances into simpler ones) and anabolism (building up of complex substances from simpler ones). Usually, catabolism releases energy, while anabolism uses it.

The energy needed to keep the body functioning at rest is called the basal metabolic rate (BMR). It is measured in joules (or kilocalories) per square metre of body surface per hour. The BMR increases in response to factors such as stress, fear, exertion, and illness, and is controlled principally by various hormones, such as *thyroxine*, *adrenaline* (epinephrine), and *insulin*. (See also *metabolism, inborn errors of*; *metabolic disorders*.)

metabolism, inborn errors of Inherited defects of body chemistry. Inborn errors of metabolism are caused by single *gene* defects, which lead to abnormal functioning of an *enzyme*.

Some of these gene defects are harmless, but others are severe enough to result in death or physical or mental handicap. Examples include *Tay–Sachs disease, phenylketonuria, Hurler's syndrome*, and Lesch–Nyhan syndrome. Collectively, inborn errors of metabolism affect around 1 child in 5,000.

Symptoms are usually present at or soon after birth. They may include unexplained illness or failure to thrive, developmental delay, floppiness, persistent vomiting, or *seizures*.

Routine tests are performed on newborn babies for some genetic disorders, such as phenylketonuria.

Treatment is not needed for some inborn errors of metabolism. For others, avoidance of a specific environmental factor may be sufficient. In some cases, the missing enzyme or the protein that it produces can be manufactured using *genetic engineering* techniques, or a vitamin supplement can help compensate for the defective enzyme. If the enzyme is made in blood cells, a *stem cell* or *bone marrow transplant* may provide a cure.

People with a child or a close relative who is affected may benefit from *genetic counselling* before planning a pregnancy.

metabolite Any substance involved in a metabolic reaction (a biochemical reaction in the body). The term metabolite is sometimes used to refer only to the products of a metabolic reaction. (See also *metabolism*.)

metacarpal bone One of five long, cylindrical bones within the hand. The bones run from the wrist to the base of each digit, with the heads of the bones forming the knuckles.

metaplasia A change in tissue resulting from the transformation of one type of cell into another. Usually harmless, but occasionally precancerous, metaplasia can affect the lining of various organs, such as the bronchi (airways) and bladder. Metaplasia of the cervix, which occurs in *cervical ectopy*, can be detected by a *cervical smear test*.

metastasis A secondary cancerous tumour (one that has spread from a primary *cancer* to another part of the body). The term also applies to the process by which such spread occurs. Metastases can spread through the lymphatic system, in the bloodstream, or across a body cavity.

metatarsal bone One of five long, cylindrical bones within the foot. The bones make up the central skeleton of the foot and are held in an arch by the surrounding *ligaments*.

metatarsalgia Pain in the foot. Causes include fracture of a *metatarsal bone*, *flat-feet*, or *neuroma* of a nerve in the foot.

metatarsophalangeal joint The joint between each *metatarsal bone* and its adjoining toe bone (see *phalanges*). The metatarsophalangeal joint at the base of the big toe is commonly affected by *gout* and by *hallux rigidus*.

metformin An oral hypoglycaemic drug (see *hypoglycaemics, oral*) that lowers blood glucose levels and is used to treat type 2 *diabetes mellitus*. Possible adverse effects include loss of appetite, a metallic taste in the mouth, nausea, vomiting, and diarrhoea.

methadone A synthetic opioid *analgesic drug* that resembles morphine. Methadone is used under supervision to relieve withdrawal symptoms in people undergoing a heroin or morphine detoxification programme. Side effects may include nausea, vomiting, constipation, dizziness, and dry mouth.

methane A colourless, odourless, highly inflammable gas that occurs naturally in oil wells and coal mines. Methane is also produced by the decomposition of organic matter; it is one of the gases present in intestinal gas (see *flatus*).

methanol A poisonous type of *alcohol* that is used as a solvent or paint remover and in some types of antifreeze. Methanol poisoning usually occurs as a result of drinking it as a substitute for ordinary alcohol. Symptoms of poisoning include headache, dizziness, nausea, vomiting, and unconsciousness. Damage may also occur to the *retina* and the *optic nerve*, causing blurred vision. Repeated or large doses of methanol may result in permanent blindness.

methicillin-resistant staphylococcus aureus See *MRSA*.

methotrexate An *anticancer drug* and *disease-modifying antirheumatic drug*. It is used to treat *lymphoma* (cancer of the lymph nodes), some forms of *leukaemia*, and cancers of the uterus, breast, ovary, lung, bladder, and testis. Methotrexate slows the progression of disease in some inflammatory conditions and may be used to treat some cases of *rheumatoid arthritis* and severe *psoriasis*. Possible adverse effects include nausea, vomiting, diarrhoea, mouth ulcers, *anaemia*, increased susceptibility to infection, liver damage, and abnormal bleeding.

methyl alcohol An alternative name for *methanol*.

methylcellulose A bulk-forming *laxative drug* used to treat *constipation*, *irritable bowel syndrome*, and *diverticular disease*. Methylcellulose increases the firmness of faeces in chronic watery *diarrhoea* and regulates their consistency in people who have a *colostomy* or *ileostomy*. It is also given as eyedrops to relieve dry eyes. As methylcellulose causes a feeling of fullness, it is sometimes used to help treat *obesity*.

methyldopa An *antihypertensive drug*. Adverse effects include drowsiness, depression, and nasal congestion.

methylenedioxymethamfetamine See *Ecstasy*.

methylphenidate A central nervous system *stimulant drug* used, under specialist supervision, to treat *attention deficit hyperactivity disorder (ADHD)* in children. Possible adverse effects include loss of appetite, tremors, sleeplessness, and rashes.

methylprednisolone A *corticosteroid drug* used to treat severe *asthma*, skin inflammation, *inflammatory bowel disease*, and certain types of *arthritis*. Adverse effects are the same as for other *corticosteroid drugs*.

M

methysergide A drug used to prevent *migraine* and *cluster headaches*. Methysergide is usually given only under hospital supervision, when other treatments have been ineffective.

Adverse effects of this drug can include dizziness, drowsiness, and nausea. Long-term treatment may cause chest pain, *kidney failure*, or leg cramps.

metoclopramide An *antiemetic drug*. It is used to prevent and treat nausea and vomiting, including that associated with migraine or caused by anticancer drugs, radiotherapy, or anaesthetic drugs. Metoclopramide may be given with a premedication to reduce the risk of inhaling vomit when under an anaesthetic. Adverse effects can include dry mouth, sedation, or diarrhoea. Large doses may cause uncontrollable movements of the face, mouth, and tongue.

metolazone A *diuretic drug* that is used to treat *hypertension*. Metolazone is also given to reduce *oedema* in people with *heart failure*, kidney disorders, or *cirrhosis* of the liver. Adverse effects can include weakness, lethargy, and dizziness.

metoprolol A cardioselective *beta-blocker drug* that is used to treat *angina pectoris* and *hypertension* and to relieve symptoms of *hyperthyroidism*. It is also given after a *myocardial infarction* to reduce the risk of further damage to the heart. Adverse effects of metoprolol include lethargy, cold hands and feet, nightmares, and rash.

metronidazole An *antibiotic drug* used to treat infections caused by *anaerobic* bacteria, such as a dental *abscess* and *peritonitis*. Metronidazole is also used to treat protozoan infections, such as *trichomoniasis* and *amoebiasis*. Adverse effects include nausea and vomiting, loss of appetite, abdominal pain, and dark-coloured urine. Alcohol should be avoided during treatment.

mexiletine An *antiarrhythmic drug* used to treat certain heart-rhythm disorders, usually after a *myocardial infarction*. Possible adverse effects include nausea, vomiting, dizziness, and tremor.

mianserin An *antidepressant drug* used to treat severe *depression*, especially that accompanied by *anxiety* or *insom-*nia. Mianserin usually takes several weeks to become fully effective. Possible adverse effects include dry mouth, blurred vision, constipation, dizziness, and drowsiness. Rarely, prolonged use may reduce blood cell production; regular *blood counts* are therefore carried out during treatment.

miconazole An *antifungal drug* used to treat *tinea* skin infections, such as *athlete's foot*, vaginal *candidiasis* (thrush), and fungal infections of internal organs. Miconazole in the form of a cream or vaginal suppository may, in rare cases, cause a burning sensation or a rash.

micro- A prefix meaning small, as in *microorganisms* (tiny organisms).

microangiopathy Any disease or disorder of the small blood vessels. It may be a feature of conditions such as *diabetes mellitus*, *septicaemia*, *eclampsia*, *glomerulonephritis*, and advanced *cancer*. When microangiopathy occurs with these conditions, the small blood vessels become distorted, and red blood cells are damaged. This causes microangiopathic haemolytic anaemia (see *anaemia, haemolytic*)

microbe A popular term for a microorganism, particularly a harmful type that causes disease.

microbiology The study of microorganisms, particularly those that are pathogenic (disease-causing).

microcephaly An abnormally small head, usually associated with *learning difficulties*. Microcephaly may occur if the brain is damaged before or during birth, or if there is injury or disease in early infancy.

microdiscectomy Surgery to relieve pressure on the spinal cord, or a nerve root emerging from it, that is caused by protrusion of the soft core of an intervertebral disc (see *disc prolapse*). The procedure is performed under general *anaesthesia* and involves removing the protruding tissue via a small incision in the outer coat of the disc.

microorganism A tiny, single-celled living organism. Most microorganisms are too small to be seen by the naked eye.

microphthalmos A rare congenital disorder of the *eye*. Affected children are born with an abnormally small eye on one or both sides.

microscope An instrument for producing a magnified image of a small object. Microscopes are used to examine the structure and chemical composition of cells and tissues, and to investigate microorganisms and diseased tissues. In the operating theatre, microscopes are used in *microsurgery*.

Compound microscopes are the most widely used type. They have two lens systems (the objective and the eyepiece), mounted at opposite ends of a tube called the body tube. There is a stage to hold the specimen, a light source, and an optical condenser which concentrates the light. The maximum magnification is about 1,500 times.

Phase-contrast and interference microscopes are modified light microscopes that allow unstained transparent specimens to be seen. They are used for examining living cells and tissues.

Fluorescence microscopes use ultraviolet light to study specimens stained with fluorescent dyes.

Electron microscopes give much higher magnifications than light microscopes by using a beam of electrons instead of light. There are two main types: transmission electron microscopes (TEMs) and scanning electron microscopes (SEMs). TEMs can magnify up to about 5,000,000 times, enabling tiny viruses and molecules to be seen. SEMs have a lower maximum magnification (100,000 times), but produce three-dimensional images. This makes them useful for studying surface structures of cells and tissues.

microsurgery Surgery in which the surgeon views the operation site via a special binocular microscope with pedal-operated magnification, focusing, and movement. The technique of microsurgery is used for surgery involving minute, delicate, or not easily accessible tissues. Examples include surgery on the eye or the inside of the ear.

micturition A term for passing urine.

midazolam A *benzodiazepine drug* used as *premedication*. Adverse effects include confusion, drowsiness, and dizziness.

midbrain The top part of the *brainstem*, situated above the pons. The midbrain is also called the mesencephalon.

middle ear See *ear*.

middle-ear effusion, persistent See *glue ear*.

middle-ear infection See *otitis media*.

mid-life crisis A popular phrase to describe the feelings of distress that affect some people in early middle age after they realize that they are no longer young. Counselling and support are usually effective in helping people to come to terms with the changes of age.

midwifery The profession that is concerned with assisting women in pregnancy and childbirth.

mifepristone A *sex hormone* drug that is used together with a *prostaglandin drug* to induce medical termination of a pregnancy (see *abortion, induced*). Possible adverse effects include malaise, faintness, nausea, rash, and, rarely, uterine bleeding.

migraine A severe headache, typically lasting 4–72 hours, accompanied by

M

MICRODISCECTOMY

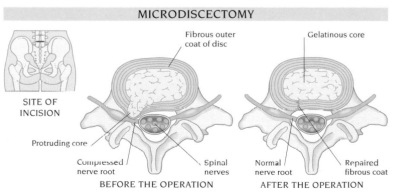

Fibrous outer coat of disc

Gelatinous core

SITE OF INCISION

Protruding core

Compressed nerve root

Spinal nerves

Normal nerve root

Repaired fibrous coat

BEFORE THE OPERATION

AFTER THE OPERATION

visual disturbances and/or nausea and vomiting. Migraine attacks may be isolated or may recur at varying intervals.

There is no single cause of migraine, although it tends to run in families. Stress-related, food-related, or sensory-related factors may trigger an attack. *Menstruation* and *oral contraceptives* may also trigger migraine.

There are two types: migraine with aura (an impression of flashing lights and/or numbness and tingling), and migraine without aura. In migraine without aura, there is a slowly worsening headache, often on one side of the head, with nausea and sometimes vomiting.

In migraine with aura, there may be visual disturbances for up to an hour, followed by a severe one-sided headache, nausea, vomiting and light-sensitivity. Other temporary neurological symptoms, such as weakness in one half of the body, may occur.

Diagnosis is usually made from the history and a physical examination. Treatment for an attack is an *analgesic drug* such as *aspirin* or *paracetamol*, plus an *antiemetic drug*, if needed. If this is not effective, treatment with *serotonin agonists* such as *sumatriptan* may be prescribed. *Ergotamine* may prevent an attack if taken before the headache begins, but is now rarely used. Sleeping in a darkened room may hasten recovery.

For frequent attacks, preventive treatment may be needed. Keeping a diary can help pinpoint trigger factors, and prophylactic drugs may be prescribed. (See also *cluster headaches*.)

milia Tiny, harmless, hard, white spots that usually occur in clusters around the nose and on the upper cheeks in newborn babies and also in young adults.

milk A nutrient fluid produced by the mammary glands of mammals.

milk–alkali syndrome A rare type of *hypercalcaemia* accompanied by *alkalosis* and *kidney failure*. The syndrome is due to excessive, long-term intake of calcium-containing *antacid drugs* and milk. It is most common in people with a *peptic ulcer* and associated kidney disorders. Symptoms include weakness, muscle pains, irritability, and

apathy. Treatment is to reduce milk and antacid intake.

milk of magnesia A magnesium preparation used as an *antacid* and *laxative drug*.

milk teeth See *primary teeth*.

Minamata disease The name given to a severe form of *mercury poisoning* that occurred in the mid-1950s, in people who had eaten polluted fish from Minamata Bay, Japan. Many people suffered severe nerve damage and some died.

mineralization, dental The deposition of calcium crystals and other mineral salts in developing teeth. (See *calcification, dental*.)

mineralocorticoid The term used to describe a *corticosteroid hormone* that controls the amount of salts that are excreted in urine.

minerals In nutrition, chemical elements that are essential in the diet. At least 20 minerals, including potassium, sodium, and calcium, are vital for health. Some, such as iron and zinc, are needed in only tiny amounts (see *trace elements*).

mineral supplements Dietary supplements containing one or more minerals in tablet or liquid form. Some mineral supplements may be harmful in excess. *Iron* is the most commonly taken mineral supplement and is used to treat iron-deficiency *anaemia*. It may also be given to pregnant or breast-feeding women. (See also individual mineral entries.)

minilaparotomy A procedure for female sterilization (see *sterilization, female*).

minimal access surgery See *minimally invasive surgery*

minimal brain dysfunction A hypothetical condition thought to account for behavioural and other problems in children for which no physical cause is found. It may be a cause of some *learning difficulties*, difficulty in concentrating, impulsiveness, and *hyperactivity*.

minimally invasive surgery Surgery using an *endoscope* passed into the body through a small incision. Further small openings may be made for surgical instruments or instruments may be passed down the endoscope so that the operation can be performed without a long surgical incision. Minimally invasive surgery may be used for

MINIMALLY INVASIVE SURGERY

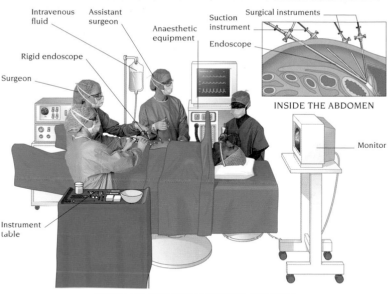

MINIMALLY INVASIVE ABDOMINAL SURGERY

M

many operations in the abdomen (see *laparoscopy*), including *appendicectomy*, *cholecystectomy*, *hernia repair*, and many *gynaecological* procedures. Knee operations (see *arthroscopy*) are also often performed by minimally invasive surgery.

minipill An *oral contraceptive* containing a *progestogen drug*. The minipill is also known as the *progestogen-only pill (POP)*.

minocycline A tetracycline *antibiotic drug* used to treat *acne*, respiratory-tract infections, and some genitourinary infections.

minoxidil A *vasodilator drug* used to treat severe *hypertension* when other drugs have been ineffective. Prolonged use can stimulate hair growth, and so it is used in lotion form as a treatment for male-pattern baldness (see *alopecia*).

miosis Constriction of the pupil of the *eye*. Miosis may be caused by drugs such as *pilocarpine* or *opium*, by a disease affecting the *autonomic nervous system*, or by bright light. A degree of miosis is normal in older people.

miotic drugs Drugs used in the treatment of *glaucoma* to reduce pressure in the eye. Used *topically*, miotic drugs cause the pupil to contract, which opens up the drainage channels and drains fluid from the front of the eye. Side effects include headache, particularly over the eye, and blurred vision. Common miotics include carbachol and *pilocarpine*. (See also *mydriatic drugs*.)

miscarriage Loss of the fetus before the 24th week of pregnancy or viability (the ability to survive outside the uterus without artificial support). The majority of miscarriages occur in the first 12 weeks of pregnancy, and may be mistaken for a late menstrual period. Miscarriages are classified into three types. In a threatened miscarriage the fetus remains alive in the uterus. In an inevitable miscarriage the fetus dies and is expelled from the uterus. In a missed miscarriage the fetus dies but remains in the uterus.

Miscarriages may occur because of *chromosomal abnormalities*, *genetic disorders*, or developmental defects in the fetus. Problems in the mother that may cause miscarriage include severe illness, placental failure, an *autoimmune disorder*, *cervical incompetence*, a defect in the uterus, or large uterine *fibroids*. However, in many cases no cause is found.

The symptoms of miscarriage are heavy bleeding with cramping. Slight blood loss with severe pain may be a symptom of either a threatened miscarriage or *ectopic pregnancy*.

A *pelvic examination*, urine test, and *ultrasound scanning* may be performed to assess the pregnancy. If all of the contents of the uterus have been expelled, no further treatment may be necessary. Otherwise, medication or a *D and C* may be required. A missed miscarriage requires medication to induce a miscarriage, a D and C, or *induction of labour*, depending on the duration of the pregnancy. Rhesus-negative women are given *anti-D(Rh$_o$) immunoglobulin* to prevent complications related to *rhesus incompatibility* in future pregnancies.

misoprostol A synthetic *prostaglandin drug* that may be used to induce a medical abortion. Misoprostol is also used to prevent and treat peptic ulcers associated with the use of *nonsteroidal anti-inflammatory drugs* (NSAIDs) because it inhibits gastric secretion; for this reason it is combined with an NSAID in some preparations.

mites and disease Mites are small animals, usually less than 1.2 mm, with eight legs. Many species have piercing and blood-sucking mouthparts.

Species causing disorders include the *scabies* mite, which burrows in human skin causing intense itching; the housedust mite, which can cause *asthma* when inhaled in dust; and chiggers (American harvest mites), which are found in thick grass and cause an itchy rash when they bite. Mites in grain or fruit may cause skin irritation, sometimes known as grocers' or bakers' itch. Certain mites transmit diseases, particularly scrub *typhus* and rickettsial *pox*.

mitochondria Small *organelles* that are found inside *cells*, in which cell *respiration* takes place. The mitochondrial wall consists of two membranes, and the inner one is highly folded to provide a surface for the respiration reactions. Cells that use a lot of energy, such as muscle cells, contain many mitochondria.

mitochondrial DNA Mitochondria have their own *DNA*. In human mitochondria, the DNA is a double-helical circle that codes for 13 proteins. Mitochondria have a distinctive genetic code, and their genomes are not changed by *meiosis* during reproduction, making the DNA useful in genetic studies.

The significance of mitochondria having their own DNA is that diseases can be inherited via abnormalities of mitochondrial DNA, and inheritance of the DNA is maternal, directly from the egg.

mitosis A type of cell division in which the *chromosomes* within the nucleus of a cell are exactly duplicated into each of two daughter cells.

Before cell division, the chromosomes duplicate themselves and coil up with the two copies joined together. The doubled chromosomes line up in the centre of the cell and are pulled apart to opposite ends of the cell, which then divides. Each daughter cell therefore has the same chromosome content as the original cell. (See also *meiosis*.)

mitral incompetence Failure of the *mitral valve* of the *heart* to close properly, allowing blood to leak back into the left atrium (upper chamber) when pumped out of the left ventricle (lower chamber). The disorder, which is also known as mitral regurgitation, may occur in conjunction with *mitral stenosis*.

Symptoms include increasing breathlessness and fatigue, sometimes with *palpitations*. Later, the ankles may swell.

Diagnosis may be made by hearing a characteristic heart *murmur*, and from chest *X-rays*, *ECG*, and *echocardiography*. Cardiac *catheterization* may also be performed. Treatment may include *diuretic drugs*, *vasodilator drugs*, and *anticoagulant drugs*. If symptoms are disabling, *heart-valve surgery* may be considered. Before dental or other surgery, patients with mitral incompetence are given *antibiotic drugs* to prevent *endocarditis*.

mitral stenosis Narrowing of the opening of the *mitral valve* in the *heart*. The left atrium (upper chamber) has to work harder to force blood through the narrowed valve. Mitral stenosis is more common in women and may be accompanied by *mitral incompetence*. Stenosis is usually due to damage to the valve caused by *rheumatic fever*.

The main symptom is breathlessness on exertion. As mitral stenosis worsens, breathing difficulty eventually occurs when at rest. Other signs include *palpitations*, *atrial fibrillation*, and flushed cheeks. There may also be coughing up of blood and fatigue.

A diagnosis is made from the patient's history, listening to heart sounds, and by investigations such as an *ECG*, *chest X-rays*, *echocardiography*, and cardiac *catheterization*. Drug treatment is broadly the same as for mitral incompetence.

If symptoms persist, balloon *valvuloplasty* may be carried out to stretch the valve. Alternatively, *heart-valve surgery* may be performed to replace the valve.

mitral valve A valve in the left side of the *heart*. The mitral valve is made up of two flaps, which allows one-way blood flow from the left *atrium* into the left *ventricle*.

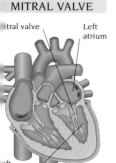

MITRAL VALVE

tral valve

Left atrium

eft entricle

STRUCTURE OF HEART

mitral valve prolapse A common, slight deformity of the *mitral valve*, in the left side of the *heart*, that can produce a degree of *mitral incompetence*. The prolapse is most common in women and causes a heart murmur. It may be inherited, but the cause is often unknown.

Usually, there are no symptoms, and treatment is not needed. Occasionally, the condition may produce chest pain, *arrhythmia*, or, rarely, *heart failure*. Often, no treatment is required for mitral valve prolapse, but some people may be treated with *beta-blocker drugs*, *diuretic drugs*, *antiarrhythmic drugs*, or, rarely, *heart-valve surgery*.

mittelschmerz Lower abdominal pain that some women have at the time of *ovulation*. The pain is usually one-sided and lasts only a few hours. It may be accompanied by slight vaginal blood loss. In cases of severe mittelschmerz, *oral contraceptives* may be prescribed to suppress ovulation.

MMR vaccination Administration of a combined *vaccine* that gives protection against *measles*, *mumps*, and *rubella*. The vaccination is offered to all children at around 13 months of age, with a booster shot at 3–5 years. Vaccination is postponed if a child is feverish, and it is not given to children with untreated cancer or *allergies* to *aminoglycoside* antibiotic drugs such as *neomycin*.

Mild fever, rash, and malaise may occur after vaccination. In 1 per cent of cases, mild, noninfectious swelling of the *parotid glands* develops 3–4 weeks after vaccination. There is no evidence for a link between MMR and bowel disease or *autism*.

mobilization The process of making a part of the body capable of movement. Mobilization refers to treatment that is designed to increase mobility in a part of the body recovering from injury or affected by disease.

Surgeons use the term to refer to the freeing of an organ or structure from surrounding *connective tissue* and fibrous adhesions (bands of tissue joining normally unconnected parts of the body).

moclobemide An *antidepressant drug* used to treat severe resistant depression and *social phobia*. Moclobemide is a reversible *monoamine oxidase inhibitor* and is less likely than other MAOIs to cause high blood pressure. But, as with all MAOIs, dietary restrictions still apply.

molar See *teeth*.

molar pregnancy A pregnancy in which a tumour develops from the placental tissue and the embryo does not develop normally. A molar pregnancy may be noncancerous (a *hydatidiform mole*) or may invade the wall of the uterus (an invasive mole). A molar pregnancy that becomes cancerous is called a *choriocarcinoma*.

If the dead embryo and placenta are not expelled from the uterus after

M

a *miscarriage*, the dead tissue is called a carneous mole.

mole A type of pigmented *naevus*. (See also *molar pregnancy*.)

molecule The smallest complete unit of a substance that can exist independently and still retain the characteristic properties of that substance. Almost all molecules consist of two or more atoms that are bonded together. Molecules that consist of only one atom are known as monatomic molecules.

molluscum contagiosum A harmless viral infection characterized by shiny, pearly white papules (tiny lumps) on the skin surface. Each papule has a central depression, and produces a cheesy fluid when it is squeezed. A crust forms before healing occurs.

MOLLUSCUM CONTAGIOSUM

Pearly white papule

The papules often appear on the genitals, the inside of the thighs, or the face. Children are more commonly affected than adults. The infection is transmitted by direct skin contact or during sexual intercourse; it usually clears up within a few months, but may last for up to 18 months.

Mongolian blue spot A blue-black pigmented spot found on the lower back and buttocks at birth. The spots are a type of *naevus* and are caused by a concentration of melanocytes (pigment-producing cells). Mongolian blue spots are commonly found in black or Asian children, and they usually disappear by the age of 3–4 years.

moniliasis See *candidiasis*.

monitor To maintain a constant watch on the condition of a patient. Also, any device used to carry out monitoring.

monoamine oxidase inhibitors Also known as MAOIs, one of the main types of *antidepressant drug*. They work by preventing the breakdown of certain *neurotransmitters* by the *enzyme* monoamine oxidase. The increased levels of neurotransmitters that result are associated with improved mood. Common drugs include *phenelzine* and isocarboxazid. All MAOIs interact with certain other drugs and foods such as cheese and red wine; but *moclobemide* is known as a reversible MAOI, which makes the adverse reactions less likely to occur.

monoarthritis Inflammation of a single joint, causing pain and stiffness. Common causes of monoarthritis include *osteoarthritis, gout*, and infection.

monoclonal antibody See *antibody, monoclonal*.

monocyte One of the main types of white blood cell. Monocytes are *phagocytes*, and play an important role in the *immune system*.

mononucleosis, infectious An acute viral infection characterized by a high temperature, sore throat, and swollen *lymph nodes*, particularly in the neck.

Commonly called glandular fever, it is caused by the *Epstein–Barr virus* and is most common during adolescence or early adulthood. One common mode of transmission is thought to be kissing.

In the body, the virus multiplies in the *lymphocytes* (also called mononuclear cells), which develop an atypical appearance. The first symptoms are a fever and headache, followed by swollen lymph nodes and a severe sore throat. Rarely, enlargement of the tonsils may obstruct breathing. Mild inflammation of the liver may occur, leading to *jaundice*.

Diagnosis is often made from the symptoms and a blood test. Recovery usually takes 4–6 weeks, with rest the only treatment needed. In rare cases, *corticosteroid drugs* are given to reduce severe inflammation, particularly if breathing is obstructed. For 2–3 months after recovery, patients often feel depressed, lack energy, and have daytime sleepiness.

monorchism The presence of only one *testis*. The most probable causes are surgery (see *orchidectomy*) and *congenital* absence of the testis.

monosodium glutamate A *food additive* that is used as a flavour enhancer and seasoning. Monosodium glutamate (MSG) is the sodium salt of an *amino acid*. A short-lived illness involving pain in the neck and chest, *palpitations*, feeling hot, and a headache may occur in some people after eating food to which large amounts of MSG have been added.

mons pubis The rounded swelling over the front of the *pubic bone*. The mons pubis, which becomes covered with hair at puberty, is formed by a pad of fatty tissue under the skin.

Monteggia's fracture Fracture of the *ulna* just below the elbow, with dislocation of the *radius* from the elbow joint.

montelukast A specific *leukotriene receptor antagonist drug* that is used in the management of asthma. It is not used to treat acute attacks.

mood disorders Disorders in which the emotions are affected: *mania*, *depression*, and *bipolar disorder*.

moon face Rounded facial appearance that is a feature of *Cushing's syndrome*.

morbid anatomy Also called pathological anatomy, the study of the structural changes that occur in body tissues as a result of disease, especially the changes visible to the naked eye.

morbidity The state or condition of being diseased. In medical statistics, the morbidity ratio is the proportion of diseased people to healthy people in a particular community.

morbilli Another name for *measles*.

morning-after pill See *contraception, emergency*.

morning sickness See *vomiting in pregnancy*.

morphine An opioid *analgesic drug* derived from the opium poppy. Morphine is given to relieve severe pain caused by *myocardial infarction*, major surgery, serious injury, and *cancer*.

Morphine blocks the transmission of pain signals at sites called opiate receptors in the *brain* and *spinal cord*. The drug also induces a sense of well-being or euphoria. Side effects include drowsiness, dizziness, constipation, nausea, vomiting, and confusion. Long-term use of morphine may lead to *drug dependence*, with severe flu-like symptoms when the drug is withdrawn (see *withdrawal syndrome*).

morphoea A condition in which one or more hard, flat patches develop on the skin. It is a type of *scleroderma* but is confined to the skin. Although harmless, the condition can be disfiguring.

mortality The death rate, which is the number of deaths per 100,000 (or 10,000 or 1,000) of the population per year. Mortality is often calculated for specific groups. For example, *infant mortality* measures the deaths of live-born infants during the 1st year of life.

Standardized mortality allows comparison of the death rate in, for example, an occupational or socioeconomic group with that for the entire population. (See also life *expectancy*; *maternal mortality*.)

morula A stage in the development of an *embryo* after *fertilization*. The fertilized egg divides repeatedly as it travels down the *fallopian tube*. When it forms a ball of cells, it is called a morula.

mosaicism The presence of two or more groups of cells containing different genetic material within one person.

Some people with syndromes caused by *chromosomal abnormalities* (such as *Down's syndrome* and *Turner's syndrome*) have mosaicism. Depending on the proportion of abnormal cells and the type of abnormality, they range from looking physically normal to having features typical of the syndrome.

mosquito bites Mosquitoes are flying insects found throughout the world. The females bite humans or animals to obtain blood, which they need to produce eggs. The males do not bite. A doctor should be consulted if there is a severe skin reaction to a mosquito bite.

As well as being irritating, mosquito bites can also transmit diseases. The main disease-transmitting mosquitoes belong to three groups: ANOPHELES (which transmits *malaria*), AEDES (which carries *yellow fever*), and CULEX (which transmits *filariasis*).

Preventive measures should be taken in any area where mosquitoes are rampant. The most effective measures are wearing clothes that cover the arms and legs, placing mosquito screens over windows, and using insect

M

repellents (such as *DEET*) or slow-burning coils that release insecticidal smoke. Mosquito nets should be placed over beds. (See also *insect bites; insects and disease.*)

motion sickness A condition that some people experience during road, sea, or air travel. Symptoms range from uneasiness and headache to distress, excessive sweating and salivation, pallor, nausea, and vomiting.

Motion sickness is caused by the effect of repetitive movement on the organ of balance in the inner *ear*. Factors such as anxiety, a fume-laden atmosphere, or the sight of food may make the condition worse. So, too, can focusing on nearby objects; sufferers should look at a point on the horizon.

Motion sickness may be prevented or controlled by *antiemetic drugs* or by acupressure bands worn on the wrist.

motor A term used to describe anything that brings about movement, such as a *muscle* or a *nerve*.

motor neuron disease A group of disorders in which there is degeneration of the *nerves* in the *central nervous system* that control muscular activity. This causes weakness and wasting of the muscles. The cause is unknown.

The most common type of motor neuron disease is amyotrophic lateral sclerosis (ALS or Lou Gehrig's disease). It usually affects people over the age of 50 and is more common in men. Some cases run in families. Usually, symptoms start with weakness in the hands and arms or legs, and muscle wasting. There may be irregular muscle contractions, and muscle cramps or stiffness. All four extremities are soon affected.

Progressive muscular atrophy and progressive bulbar palsy both start with patterns of muscle weakness different from ALS but usually develop into ALS.

There are two types of motor neuron disease that first appear in childhood or adolescence. In most cases, these conditions are inherited. *Werdnig–Hoffman disease* affects infants at birth or soon afterwards. In almost all cases, progressive muscle weakness leads to death within several years. Chronic spinal muscular atrophy begins in childhood or adolescence, causing progressive weakness but not always serious disability.

There are no specific tests for motor neuron disease. Diagnosis is based on careful clinical examination by a neurologist. Tests including *EMG*, muscle *biopsy, blood tests, myelography, CT scanning*, or *MRI* may be performed.

The disease typically goes on to affect the muscles involved in breathing and swallowing, leading to death within 2–4 years. However, about 10 per cent of sufferers survive for 10 years.

Nerve degeneration cannot be slowed down, but *physiotherapy* and the use of various aids may help to reduce disability. The drug riluzole is used to extend life (or the time until mechanical *ventilation* is required).

mould Any of a large group of *fungi* that exist as many-celled, filamentous colonies. Some moulds are the source of *antibiotic drugs*. Others can cause diseases such as *aspergillosis*.

mountain sickness An illness that can affect people who have ascended rapidly to heights above 2,400m–3,000m. Mountain sickness is caused by the reduced atmospheric pressure and oxygen levels that occur at high altitude.

mouth The oral cavity, which breaks food down for swallowing (see *mastication*) and is used in breathing. In addition, it helps to convert sound vibrations from the *larynx* into speech.

mouth cancer Forms of cancerous tumour that affect the lips, tongue, and oral cavity. Lip cancer and tongue cancer are the most common types.

Predisposing causes of mouth cancer are poor *oral hygiene*, drinking alcoholic spirits, tobacco-*smoking*, chewing tobacco, and inhaling snuff. Irritation from ill-fitting dentures or jagged teeth are other factors. Men are affected twice as often as women; most cases occur in men over the age of 40.

Mouth cancer usually begins with a whitish patch, called *leukoplakia*, or a small lump. These may cause a burning sensation, but are usually painless. As the tumour grows, it may develop into an *ulcer* or a deep fissure, which may bleed and erode surrounding tissue.

Diagnosis is based on a *biopsy*. Treatment consists of surgery, *radiotherapy*, or both. Extensive surgery may cause facial disfigurement and problems with eating and speaking, which may require reconstructive surgery. Radiotherapy sometimes damages the salivary glands (see *mouth, dry*).

When mouth cancer is detected and treated early, the outlook is good.

mouth, dry The result of inadequate production of saliva. Dry mouth is usually a temporary condition caused by fear, infection of a *salivary gland*, or the action of *anticholinergic drugs*.

Rarely, permanent dry mouth may occur as part of *Sjögren's syndrome* or from *radiotherapy* to treat mouth cancer. Dryness usually causes difficulty in swallowing and speaking, interference with taste, and tooth decay (see *caries, dental*). It may be relieved by spraying the inside of the mouth with artificial saliva.

mouth-to-mouth resuscitation See *artificial respiration*.

mouth ulcer An open sore caused by a break in the *mucous membrane* lining the mouth. The ulcers are white, grey, or yellow spots with an inflamed border. The most common types are aphthous ulcers (see *ulcer, aphthous*) and ulcers caused by the *herpes simplex* virus. A mouth ulcer may be an early stage of *mouth cancer* and may need to be investigated with a *biopsy* if it fails to heal within a month.

mouthwash A solution for rinsing the mouth. Many only leave the mouth feeling fresh and remove loose food debris from the teeth. Some, such as those containing *hydrogen peroxide*, can help to clean the teeth if the gums are too tender for proper toothbrushing, as in some types of *gingivitis*. Those containing *chlorhexidine* are effective against plaque when routine dental hygiene is impossible. *Fluoride* mouthwashes help to prevent tooth decay (see *caries, dental*), and a mouthwash of warm salt water can help to ease painful inflammation caused by tooth disorders. Antiseptic mouthwashes intended to combat *halitosis* are usually ineffective because they do not treat the cause of the problem.

movement Bodily movements include skeletal movements and movements of soft tissues and body organs. All movement is brought about by the actions of muscles and may be voluntary, involuntary, or a *reflex* action.

All voluntary skeletal movements are initiated in the part of the cerebrum (main mass of the *brain*) called the motor cortex. Signals are sent down the *spinal cord* along nerve fibres, and from there along separate nerve fibres to the appropriate muscles. Control relies on information supplied by sensory nerve *receptors*, in the muscles and elsewhere, that record the position of the different parts of the body and the amount of contraction in each muscle. This information is integrated in specific regions of the brain (including the *cerebellum* and *basal ganglia*) that control the coordination, initiation, and cessation of movement.

Skeletal movements can also occur as simple reflexes in response to certain sensory warning signals; the movement is automatic and less controlled, involving far fewer nerve connections.

Some body movements do not involve the skeleton. For example, eye and tongue movements are brought about by contractions of muscles that are attached to soft tissues. These movements may be voluntary or reflex.

Movements of the internal organs are involuntary; they include the *heartbeat* and *peristalsis*.

moxibustion A form of alternative therapy, often used in conjunction with *acupuncture*, in which a cone of wormwood leaves (moxa) or certain other plant materials is burned just above the skin for the purpose of relieving internal pain.

moxisylyte A *vasodilator drug* used in the treatment of *Raynaud's disease*. Side effects include nausea, diarrhoea, hot flushes, headache, and dizziness.

MRI The abbreviation for magnetic resonance imaging. MRI is a diagnostic technique that produces cross-sectional or three-dimensional images of organs and other body structures

The patient lies inside a scanner surrounded by a large, powerful magnet.

M

A receiving magnet is then placed around the part of the body to be investigated. If large areas, such as the abdomen, are to be imaged, the receiving magnet is fitted inside the scanner; for a smaller area, such as a joint, a magnet may be placed around the part to be scanned. The scanner generates a strong magnetic field, which causes the atoms in the body to line up parallel to each other. Short pulses of radio waves from a radiofrequency source briefly knock the atoms out of alignment. As the atoms realign they emit tiny signals, which are detected by the receiving magnet. Information about these signals is passed to a computer, which builds up an image based on the signals' strength and location. MRI images can be enhanced by use of a *contrast medium* to highlight particular body structures, such as tumours and blood vessels.

Images from MRI are similar to those produced by *CT scanning* but give greater contrast between normal and abnormal tissues. MRI is useful in studying the brain and spinal cord, the internal structure of the eye and ear, the internal organs, and blood flow. A type of MRI called functional MRI (fMRI) can reveal areas of neural activity in the brain.

There are no known risks or side effects. The technique does not use ionizing radiation and can be performed repeatedly, but the scanner may interfere with the functioning of pacemakers, hearing aids, and other electrical devices.

MRSA The abbreviation for methicillin-resistant *STAPHYLOCOCCUS AUREUS*, a bacterium resistant to methicillin and many other *antibiotic drugs*. MRSA is commonly known as the "hospital superbug" because most cases are contracted in hospital, and infection is difficult to treat and can sometimes be fatal.

MS The abbreviation for the disorder *multiple sclerosis*.

MSG The abbreviation for the food additive *monosodium glutamate*.

MSU The abbreviation for midstream specimen of urine: a specimen of urine to be examined for the presence of microorganisms. The initial part of the stream is not collected, in order to avoid bacterial contamination of the specimen from the skin or the lining of the lower urinary tract.

mucocele A swollen sac or cavity within the body that is filled with *mucus* secreted by its inner lining.

mucolytic drugs Drugs that make sputum (phlegm) less sticky and easier to cough up. An example is carbocisteine.

MRI

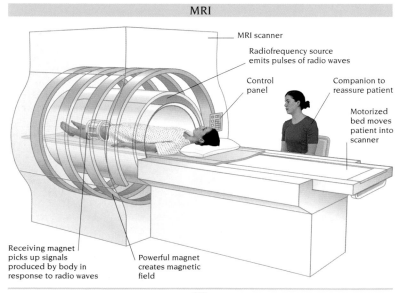

MRI scanner

Radiofrequency source emits pulses of radio waves

Control panel

Companion to reassure patient

Motorized bed moves patient into scanner

Receiving magnet picks up signals produced by body in response to radio waves

Powerful magnet creates magnetic field

mucopolysaccharidosis A group of rare inherited metabolic disorders (see *metabolism, inborn errors of*) of which *Hurler's syndrome* is the best known. All mucopolysaccharidoses are *genetic disorders* in which there is an abnormality of a specific *enzyme*. This leads to the accumulation within body cells of substances called mucopolysaccharides.

Features may include abnormalities of the skeleton and/or the central nervous system, with *learning difficulties* and, in some cases, a characteristic facial appearance. There may also be clouding of the *cornea*, liver enlargement, and joint stiffness. No specific treatment is available. However, a *stem cell* or *bone marrow transplant* may successfully be used to treat Hurler's syndrome.

Mild forms of mucopolysaccharidoses allow a child to have a relatively normal life. More severe types usually cause death during childhood or adolescence.

mucosa A term for *mucous membrane*.

mucous membrane The soft, pink, skin-like layer that lines many of the cavities and tubes in the body, including the *respiratory tract* and the *digestive tract*. Mucous membranes contain millions of cells called goblet cells, which secrete a fluid containing *mucus*.

mucoviscidosis See *cystic fibrosis*.

mucus The thick, slimy fluid secreted by *mucous membranes*. Mucus moistens, lubricates, and protects parts of the body lined by mucous membranes, such as the digestive and respiratory tracts.

mucus method of contraception See *contraception, natural methods of*.

multiple myeloma Also called myelomatosis, multiple myeloma is a rare, cancerous condition in which plasma cells in the *bone marrow* proliferate uncontrollably and function incorrectly. It occurs in middle- to old age.

Plasma cells are a type of B-*lymphocyte* that produce *immunoglobulins*, which help protect against infection. In multiple myeloma, the proliferating plasma cells produce excessive amounts of one type of immunoglobulin, while production of other types is impaired. This makes infection more likely.

Proliferation of the abnormal cells causes pain and destroys bone tissue. Affected *vertebrae* may collapse and compress nerves, causing numbness or *paralysis*. Blood calcium levels increase as bone is destroyed, as may the level of one or more immunoglobulins. These changes in the blood may damage the kidneys, leading to *kidney failure*. There may also be *anaemia* and a tendency for abnormal bleeding.

The disease is diagnosed by a *bone marrow biopsy*, by *blood tests* or *urinalysis*, and by *X-rays*. Treatment includes the use of *anticancer drugs*, *stem cell* transplantation, *radiotherapy*, and supportive measures, including *blood transfusions*, *antibiotic drugs*, and *analgesic drugs*.

multiple personality A rare disorder in which a person has two or more distinct personalities, each of which dominates at different times. The personalities are usually very different from each other.

multiple pregnancy See *pregnancy, multiple*.

multiple sclerosis A progressive disease of the central *nervous system* in which patches of *myelin* in the brain and spinal cord are destroyed. Multiple sclerosis (or MS) is an *autoimmune disorder*, in which the immune system attacks the myelin sheath that covers some nerves in the brain and spinal cord. Affected nerves cannot conduct nerve impulses, so functions such as movement and sensation may be lost. Any area of the body can be affected. Symptoms range from numbness and tingling to *paralysis* and *incontinence*.

Attacks of symptoms are followed by a variable period of remission, in which dramatic improvements may be made.

Women are more likely to develop MS than men, and there may be a genetic factor, as the disease sometimes runs in families. There may also be an environmental factor, as MS is more common in temperate zones than in the tropics.

Symptoms usually develop early in adulthood. Spinal cord damage may cause tingling, numbness, weakness in the extremities, *spasticity*, paralysis, and incontinence. Damage to white matter (myelinated nerves) in the brain may cause fatigue, *vertigo*, clumsiness, muscle

M

weakness, slurred speech, blurred vision, numbness, weakness, or facial pain.

Attacks may last several months. After a variable remission period, a relapse occurs, which may be precipitated by injury, infection, or stress. Some people have mild relapses and long periods of remission, with few permanent effects. Some people become gradually more disabled from the first attack. A few suffer gross disability within the first year.

There is no single diagnostic test, but *MRI* may show damage to white matter in the brain. *Evoked response* tests on the eyes and analysis of cerebrospinal fluid also provide strong evidence.

There is no specific treatment. Some people claim that dietary modifications such as fish oils are beneficial. In some cases, *interferon* beta can extend the time between attacks and reduce the rate of decline.

multivitamins Over-the-counter preparations, containing a combination of vitamins, that are used as a dietary supplement. (See *vitamin supplements*.)

mumps An acute viral illness, mainly of childhood. The main symptom is inflammation and swelling of one or both of the *parotid glands* situated inside the angle of the jaw. One attack of mumps confers lifelong immunity. Since routine *MMR vaccination*, epidemics of mumps no longer occur.

The mumps virus is spread in airborne droplets. The *incubation period* is 2–3 weeks; an affected person is infectious for about a week before and up to 2 weeks after symptoms appear.

Infected children often have no symptoms, or they may feel slightly unwell and have some discomfort around the parotid glands. In more serious cases, there is pain around the glands and chewing becomes difficult; one or both glands then become swollen, painful, and tender. A fever and headache may develop. The swelling subsides within a week to 10 days. When only one gland is affected, the second often swells as the first gland's swelling subsides. Complications of mumps include viral *meningitis*, *pancreatitis*, and *epididymo-orchitis*.

Diagnosis is usually made from the symptoms. There is no specific treatment.

Munchausen's syndrome A chronic *factitious disorder* in which the sufferer complains of physical symptoms that are pretended or self-induced in order to play the role of patient. Most afflicted people are repeatedly hospitalized.

The usual complaints are abdominal pain, bleeding, neurological symptoms, rashes, and fever. Sufferers typically invent dramatic histories and behave disruptively in hospital. Many have detailed medical knowledge and scars from self-injury or previous treatment. In Munchausen's syndrome by proxy, parents cause factitious disorders in their children.

Treatment consists of protecting sufferers from unnecessary operations and drug treatments.

mupirocin A topical *antibacterial* cream or ointment used to treat skin infections such as *impetigo*.

murmur A sound caused by turbulent blood flow through the *heart*, as heard through a *stethoscope*.

Heart murmurs are regarded as an indication of possible abnormality in the blood flow. Apart from "innocent" murmurs, the most common cause of extra blood turbulence is a disorder of the *heart valves*. Murmurs can also be caused by some types of congenital heart disease (see *heart disease, congenital*) or by rarer conditions such as a *myxoma* in a heart chamber.

muscle A structure composed of bundles of specialized cells capable of contraction and relaxation to create movement. There are three types of muscle: skeletal, smooth, and cardiac.

The skeletal muscles are the most prominent in the body (see *muscular system*). They are called voluntary muscles because they are under conscious control. Skeletal muscles are composed of groups of muscle fibres arranged in bundles called fascicles. A fibre is made up of longitudinal units called myofibrils, the working units of which are filaments of actin and myosin (two proteins that control contraction). A state of partial contraction is constantly maintained – this is muscle tone.

Smooth muscle is concerned with the movements of internal organs. It is not

M

MUSCLE

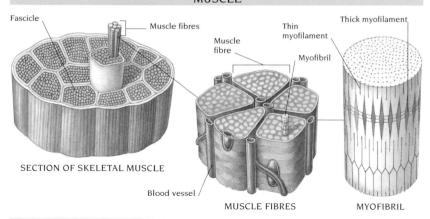

Fascicle — Muscle fibres — Thin myofilament — Thick myofilament

Muscle fibre — Myofibril

SECTION OF SKELETAL MUSCLE

Blood vessel

MUSCLE FIBRES

MYOFIBRIL

under conscious control; for this reason, it is also called involuntary muscle. Smooth muscle is made up of long, spindle-shaped cells, and contracts with the same sliding action of actin and myosin as skeletal muscle. This type of muscle is stimulated by the *autonomic nervous system*; it also responds to *hormones* and to levels of chemicals in fluid around the muscle.

Cardiac muscle (also called myocardium) is found only in the *heart*. It is able to contract rhythmically about 100,000 times a day, and has a similar structure to that of skeletal muscle. Contraction is stimulated by the autonomic nervous system, by hormones, and by the stretching of muscle fibres.

The most common muscle disorders are injury and lack of blood supply to a muscle. Rare disorders include *muscular dystrophy* and *myasthenia gravis*.

muscle-relaxant drugs A group of drugs used to relieve muscle spasm and *spasticity*. Muscle-relaxant drugs are used mainly in the treatment of nervous system disorders such as *multiple sclerosis* and painful muscular conditions such as *torticollis*. They are occasionally used to relieve muscle rigidity caused by injury. Some types are used to cause temporary paralysis during surgery under general *anaesthesia*.

Except for *dantrolene*, muscle-relaxant drugs partly block nerve signals that stimulate muscle contraction. Dantrolene interferes with the chemical activity in muscle cells needed for contraction. The drugs may cause muscle weakness and drowsiness. In rare cases, dantrolene causes liver damage.

muscle spasm Sudden and involuntary contraction of a muscle. Muscle spasm is a normal reaction to pain and inflammation around a joint. Common causes are muscle *strain*, *disc prolapse*, and stress. Usually, the cause of the spasm is treated. *Muscle-relaxant drugs* may also be needed. (See also *spasticity*.)

muscular dystrophy A group of rare inherited muscle disorders which cause slow, progressive wasting away of muscle fibres. This degeneration may lead to disability and death.

The most common and severe form of muscular dystrophy is Duchenne muscular dystrophy. This is caused by a recessive gene carried on the X chromosome (see *sex-linked inheritance*). Boys only have one X chromosome, so if they inherit a copy of the defective gene from their mother they develop the disorder. Girls (with two X chromosomes) are not affected but become carriers of the defective gene. Affected boys walk with a waddle, find climbing difficult, and may have curvature of the spine. The disorder progresses rapidly; the ability to walk is lost by the age of 12, and few boys survive beyond the teenage years.

M

Becker's muscular dystrophy starts later in childhood and progresses more slowly. Myotonic dystrophy affects the muscles of the hands, face, neck, and feet, and causes *learning difficulties*. Limb-girdle muscular dystrophy mainly affects muscles in the hips and shoulders, and facioscapulo-humeral muscular dystrophy affects muscles in the upper arms, shoulder girdle, and face. In this last form, severe disability is rare.

A diagnosis for Duchenne muscular dystrophy can be made with gene testing before symptoms develop. Once muscle weakness develops other tests become useful, including measurement of muscle *enzymes* and an *EMG*.

There is no cure, and *physiotherapy* is the main treatment. Remaining as active as possible keeps healthy muscles in good condition. Surgery to the heel *tendons* may assist walking in some cases. The long-term outlook depends on the particular form.

Families in which a child or adult has developed any form of muscular dystrophy should receive *genetic counselling*.

muscular system The muscles of the body that are attached to the *skeleton*. These muscles are responsible for voluntary movement, and also support and stabilize the skeleton. In most cases, a muscle attaches to a bone (usually by means of a *tendon*) and crosses over a joint to attach to another bone. Muscles

MUSCULAR SYSTEM

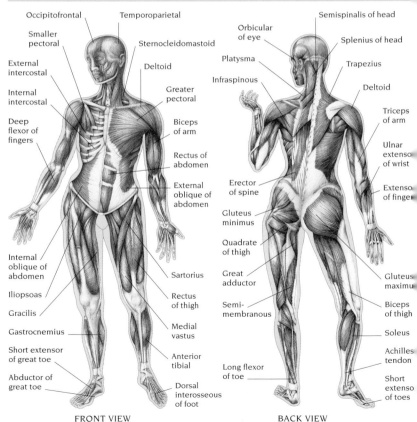

FRONT VIEW   BACK VIEW

can produce movement by contracting and shortening to pull on the bone to which they are attached. They can only pull, not push, and are therefore arranged so that the pull of one muscle or group of muscles is opposed to another, enabling a movement to be reversed. Although most actions of the skeletal muscles are under conscious control, *reflex* movements of certain muscles occur in response to stimuli.

There are more than 600 muscles in the body, classified according to the type of movement they produce. An extensor opens out a joint, a flexor closes it; an adductor draws a part of the body inwards, an abductor moves it outwards; a levator raises it, a depressor lowers it; and constrictor or sphincter muscles surround and close orifices.

musculoskeletal Relating to muscle and/or bone. The musculoskeletal system is the skeleton and the muscles attached to it.

mushroom poisoning There are many species of poisonous mushrooms and toadstools in the UK, but many of them have an unpleasant taste and are therefore unlikely to be eaten in sufficient amounts to cause problems.

Most fatal cases of mushroom poisoning in the UK are caused by AMANITA PHALLOIDES (death cap). This mushroom can be confused with the edible field mushroom, although it has white gills instead of pink-brown ones.

The death cap and some related species, such as AMANITA VIROSA (destroying angel), contain poisons called amanitins, which attack cells in the liver, kidneys, and small intestine. Symptoms such as severe abdominal pain, vomiting, and diarrhoea usually develop 8–14 hours after eating the mushrooms. Later, there may be liver enlargement and *jaundice*, which may lead to death from *liver failure*. There is no antidote, and treatment consists of supportive measures only. For those people who survive, recovery usually occurs after about a week.

AMANITA MUSCARIA (fly agaric) has a red cap flecked with white. Symptoms of poisoning appear within 20 minutes to 2 hours, and may include drowsiness, visual disturbances, *delirium*, muscle tremors, and nausea and vomiting. Treatment of this type of poisoning (and of other types with rapidly developing symptoms) is with gastric lavage (see *lavage, gastric*) and activated charcoal. Recovery usually occurs within 24 hours.

"Magic" mushrooms contain the hallucinogen *psilocybin*. These mushrooms may also cause high fever in children. The effects usually last for 4–6 hours.

mutagen Any agent that increases the rate of *mutation* in cells. The main mutagens are ionizing *radiation* (see *radiation hazards*), some chemicals, and certain illnesses.

mutation A change in a cell's *DNA*. Many mutations are harmless; however some are harmful, giving rise to *cancers*, *birth defects*, and hereditary diseases. Very rarely, a mutation may be beneficial.

A mutation results from a fault in the replication of DNA when a cell divides. A daughter cell inherits some faulty DNA, and the fault is copied each time the new cell divides, creating a cell population containing the altered DNA

Some mutations occur by chance. Any agent that makes mutations more likely is called a *mutagen*.

There are several types of mutation. Point mutations affect only one *gene* and may lead to the production of defective *enzymes* or other proteins. In other mutations, *chromosomes* (or parts of them) are deleted, added, or rearranged. This type may produce greater disruptive effects than point mutations.

If a mutated cell is a somatic (body) cell, it can, at worst, multiply to form a group of abnormal cells. These cells often die out, are destroyed by the body's *immune system*, or have only a minor effect. Sometimes, however, they may become a *tumour*.

A mutation in a *germ cell* (immature egg or sperm) may be passed on to a child, who then has the mutation in all of his or her cells. This may cause an obvious birth defect or an abnormality in body chemistry. The mutation may also be passed on to the child's descendants. *Genetic disorders* (such as *haemophilia* and *achondroplasia*) stem from point mutations that occurred in the germ cell of a parent,

M

grandparent, or more distant ancestor. *Chromosomal abnormalities* (such as *Down's syndrome*) are generally due to mutations in the formation of parental eggs or sperm.

mutism Refusal or inability to speak. Mutism may occur as a symptom of profound congenital *deafness*, severe *bipolar disorder*, catatonic *schizophrenia*, or a rare form of *conversion disorder*. The term may also apply to a religious vow of silence.

Elective mutism is a rare childhood disorder (usually starting before age 5), in which the child can speak properly but refuses to do so most of the time.

Akinetic mutism describes a state of passivity caused by some brain tumours or by *hydrocephalus*. People with akinetic mutism are incontinent, require feeding, and respond at most with a whispered "yes" or "no".

myalgia Medical term for *muscle* pain.

myalgic encephalomyelitis Also known as ME (see *chronic fatigue syndrome*).

myasthenia gravis A rare disorder in which the muscles become weak and tire easily. The muscles of the eyes, face, throat, and limbs are most commonly affected.

Myasthenia gravis is an *autoimmune disorder*. In many cases, abnormalities in the thymus gland are present, and in some cases a *thymoma* is found. Women are affected more often than men.

The disease is extremely variable in its effects. In most cases, it causes drooping eyelids, double vision, a blank facial expression, and a weak, hoarse, nasal voice that is hesitant and becomes slurred during extended conversation. The arm and leg muscles may also be affected. In severe cases, the respiratory muscles may become weakened, causing breathing difficulty.

Diagnosis of the condition is often made by injecting the drug edrophonium into a vein. This temporarily restores power to the weak muscles. *Blood tests* and *EMG* are also sometimes used. *CT scanning* or *MRI* may also be performed to look for a thymoma.

Treatment with drugs that facilitate transmission of nerve impulses often restores the patient's condition to near normal. In some cases, the condition often improves, and is sometimes cured by thymectomy (removal of the thymus gland). Regular exchanges of the patient's *plasma* for fresh plasma may be carried out in severe cases. *Corticosteroid drugs* may be given. In a minority of patients, *paralysis* of the throat and respiratory muscles may lead to death.

mycetoma An uncommon tropical infection affecting skin and bone and caused by *fungi* or by actinomycetes (bacteria that form long chain-like colonies). It usually occurs on one limb, producing a hard swelling and a discharge of pus. Infections caused by actinomycetes are treated with *antibiotic drugs*. Surgical removal of diseased tissue may be necessary for a fungal infection.

mycology The study of *fungi*.

mycoplasma Any of a group of *bacteria* that are the smallest types capable of free existence. Mycoplasmas are about the same size as *viruses* but, unlike viruses, they are capable of reproducing outside living cells. One species, MYCOPLASMA PNEUMONIAE, causes primary atypical *pneumonia*.

mycosis Any disease caused by a fungus. (See *fungi*; *fungal infections*.)

mycosis fungoides A rare type of *lymphoma* that primarily affects the skin of the buttocks, back, or shoulders. The cause of mycosis fungoides is unknown. In its mildest form, it produces a non-itchy, red, scaly rash, which may spread slowly or remain unaltered for many years. In more severe forms, thickened patches of skin, *ulcers*, and enlarged *lymph nodes* may develop.

The diagnosis is confirmed with a *skin biopsy*. Treatment may include *PUVA*, *radiotherapy*, nitrogen mustard, *anticancer drugs*, and *corticosteroid drugs*.

mydriasis Dilation (widening) of the pupil of the eye. It occurs in the dark, if a person is emotionally aroused, after the use of certain eye-drops (such as those containing *atropine*), and after consumption of alcohol.

mydriatic drugs A group of drugs used to treat *uveitis* and to dilate the pupil during examination of the inside of the eye and for surgery. Mydriatics work by relaxing the circular muscles of the *iris*, causing the pupil to dilate. Common mydriatic drugs include *tropicamide*, cyclopentolate, homatropine, and *phenylephrine*. (See also *cycloplegia; miotic drugs*.)

myectomy Surgical removal of part or all of a muscle. Myectomy may be performed to treat severely injured and infected muscles or to remove a fibroid in an operation called a *myomectomy*.

myel- A prefix that denotes a relationship to bone marrow (as in *multiple myeloma*) or to the spinal cord (as in *myelitis*). The prefix myelo- has the same meaning.

myelin The fatty material made of *lipid* (fat) and protein that forms a protective sheath around some nerve fibres and increases the efficiency of nerve impulse transmission. (See also *demyelination*.)

MYELIN

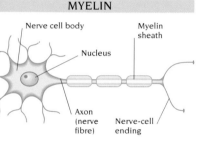

NERVE CELL

myelitis Inflammation of the spinal cord, often caused by a viral infection. In transverse myelitis, the spinal cord becomes inflamed around the middle of the back. Common symptoms are back pain and gradual *paralysis* of the legs, which, in some cases, becomes permanent.

myelocele Another name for *myelomeningocele* (see *neural tube defect*).

myelofibrosis An alternative term for *myelosclerosis*.

myelography *X-ray* examination of the spinal cord, nerves, and other tissues within the spinal canal after injection of a contrast medium (a substance that is opaque to X-rays).

The procedure has now been replaced by *CT scanning* and *MRI*.

myeloma, multiple See *multiple myeloma*.

myelomatosis See *multiple myeloma*.

myelomeningocele A protrusion of the *spinal cord* and its *meninges* (protective membranes) under the skin due to a congenital defect (see *neural tube defect*).

myelopathy Any disease or disorder of the *spinal cord*.

myelosclerosis An increase of fibrous tissue within the *bone marrow* (also known as myelofibrosis), in which the marrow's ability to produce blood cells is impaired. Myelosclerosis may be primary (occurring with no obvious cause) or secondary (resulting from another bone marrow disease).

The main symptoms of myelosclerosis are those of *anaemia*. Enlargement of the *spleen*, night sweats, loss of appetite, and weight loss also commonly occur. In secondary myelosclerosis, the underlying disease may cause other symptoms.

Treatment of primary myelosclerosis includes *blood transfusions* to relieve symptoms. A few patients may develop acute *leukaemia*. Treatment of secondary myelosclerosis depends on the underlying cause.

myiasis An infestation by fly larvae, which is primarily restricted to tropical areas. In Africa, the tumbu fly lays eggs on wet clothing left outside; the larvae hatch and penetrate the skin to cause boil-like swellings. Other flies may lay eggs in open wounds, on the skin, or in the ears or nose. Sometimes, larvae penetrate deeply into the tissues. Intestinal infestation can occur after eating contaminated food. Preventive measures include keeping flies away from food, covering open wounds, and ironing clothes that have been dried outdoors.

Myiasis of the skin is treated by placing drops of oil over the swelling. The larva comes to the surface, where it can be removed with a needle. In deeper tissues, surgery may be needed. Intestinal myiasis is treated with a *laxative*.

myo- A prefix denoting a relationship to muscle (as in *myocarditis*).

myocardial infarction Sudden death of part of the *heart* muscle due to a blockage in the blood supply to the heart. The disorder is popularly known as a heart attack. It is usually

M

M

characterized by severe, unremitting chest pain. Myocardial infarction is the most common cause of death in developed countries.

Men are more likely to have a heart attack than women, and smokers are at greater risk. Other risk factors include a family history of the condition, increased age, unhealthy diet, obesity, and disorders such as *hypertension* and *diabetes mellitus. Atherosclerosis* of the coronary arteries is usually a factor.

Symptoms include sudden pain in the centre of the chest, breathlessness, feeling restless, clammy skin, nausea and/or vomiting, or loss of consciousness. Myocardial infarction may cause immediate *heart failure* or *arrhythmias.*

Diagnosis is made from the patient's history and tests including *ECG* and measurement of *enzymes* released into the blood from damaged heart muscle. Further tests such as cardiac catheterization (see *catheterization, cardiac*) may be done to determine the extent of damage to the heart muscle.

A myocardial infarction is a medical emergency. Initial treatment may include *aspirin, thrombolytic drugs, analgesic drugs,* and *oxygen therapy. ACE inhibitor drugs,* intravenous *infusion* of fluids, *antiarrhythmic drugs,* and *beta-blocker drugs* may also be given. Electrical *defibrillation* may be used to control severe arrhythmias. Emergency *angioplasty* may sometimes be necessary.

After recovery, preventive measures such as taking more exercise, losing weight, stopping smoking, and dietary changes are recommended. *Statin* drugs are usually given to lower blood *cholesterol;* ACE inhibitors, aspirin, or *beta-blocker drugs* are given to reduce the risk of further attacks.

myocarditis Inflammation of the *heart* muscle, usually due to infection by the coxsackievirus. Myocarditis is a characteristic feature of *rheumatic fever.*

There are often no symptoms. Rarely, there may be a serious disturbance of the heartbeat, breathlessness, chest pain, and *heart failure.* In severe cases, death may result from *cardiac arrest.*

Myocarditis may be suspected from the patient's history and from a physical examination. An *ECG* will show characteristic abnormalities of the heartbeat. Diagnosis also involves *echocardiography* and *blood tests.*

There is no specific treatment. Bed rest is usually recommended and *corticosteroid drugs* may be prescribed.

myoclonus Rapid and uncontrollable jerking or spasm of one or more muscles either at rest or during movement. Myoclonus may be associated with a muscular or nervous disorder. It also occurs in healthy people, such as when the limbs twitch before sleep.

myofascial pain syndrome See *temporomandibular joint syndrome.*

myoglobin An oxygen-carrying pigment that is present in muscles. It consists of a combination of iron and protein. Myoglobin stores oxygen, releasing it when it is needed by the muscles. The presence of myoglobin in the urine is known as myoglobinuria. Slight myoglobinuria may occur during prolonged exercise. Severe myoglobinuria is usually caused by the release of myoglobin from a large area of damaged muscle, and may cause *kidney failure.*

myoma A noncancerous muscle *tumour.*

myomectomy Surgical removal of a *myoma.* The term is also used to describe the surgical removal of *fibroids* from the uterus.

myopathy A disease of *muscle* that is not caused by disease of the nervous system. A myopathy may be an inherited disorder, such as *muscular dystrophy;* it may also be caused by chemical poisoning, a chronic disorder of the *immune system,* or a *metabolic disorder.*

myopia An error of *refraction* in which objects seen in the distance appear blurred. Commonly called shortsightedness, myopia is caused by the eye being too long from front to back. As a result, images of distant objects are focused in front of the retina.

Myopia, which tends to be inherited, usually appears around puberty and increases until the early 20s. If it starts in early childhood it may become very severe. The condition is detected during

MYOPIA

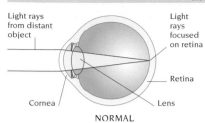

Light rays from distant object

Light rays focused on retina

Retina

Cornea

Lens

NORMAL

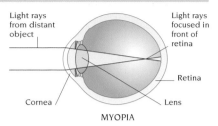

Light rays from distant object

Light rays focused in front of retina

Retina

Cornea

Lens

MYOPIA

a *vision test*. Treatment is with concave *glasses* (or *contact lenses*) or by *photo-refractive keratectomy*.

myosin A major protein component of *muscle* fibres. Together with *actin*, it provides the mechanism for muscles to contract. The myosin molecules slide along the actin filaments to make the muscle fibres shorter.

myositis Inflammation of *muscle* tissue, causing pain, tenderness, and weakness. Types of myositis include *myositis ossificans* (in which damaged muscle is replaced by bone), *polymyositis*, and *dermatomyositis*.

myositis ossificans A *congenital* or acquired condition in which bone is deposited in muscles. The congenital form is rare. The first symptoms are painful swellings in the muscles, which gradually harden and extend until the affected child is encased in a rigid sheet. There is no treatment, and death results.

The acquired form may develop after a bony injury, especially around the elbow; it causes severe pain and a swelling, which hardens. Treatment with *diathermy*, coupled with gentle, active movements, may be helpful.

myotomy A surgical procedure that involves cutting into a *muscle*.

myotonia Inability of a *muscle* to relax after the need for contraction has passed. It is a feature of myotonic dystrophy, a form of *muscular dystrophy*.

myringitis Inflammation of the eardrum. Myringitis occurs in *otitis media*.

myringoplasty Surgical closure of a perforation (hole) in the eardrum (see *eardrum, perforated*) by means of a tissue graft (see *grafting*).

myringotomy A surgical opening made through the eardrum to allow drainage of the middle-ear cavity. It is usually performed to treat persistent *glue ear* in children. A *grommet* may be inserted into the eardrum at the same time.

myxoedema A condition in which there is thickening and coarsening of the skin and other body tissues (most noticeably in the face). Myxoedema is usually due to *hypothyroidism*; in such cases, the condition is commonly accompanied by weight gain, hair loss, sensitivity to cold, and mental dullness. The term "myxoedema" is sometimes used for adult hypothyroidism.

myxoma A noncancerous, jelly-like tumour composed of soft mucous material and loose fibrous strands. Myxomas usually occur singly, and may sometimes grow very large. They may develop under the skin, in the abdomen, in the bones, or, very rarely, inside the cavities of the heart. In this case, thrombi (blood clots) may form, and the flow of blood through the heart may be obstructed. Myxomas can usually be successfully removed by surgery.

M

N

nadolol A *beta-blocker* drug used in the treatment of *hypertension* (high blood pressure), *angina pectoris* (chest pain due to impaired blood supply to heart muscle), certain types of *arrhythmia* (irregularity of the heartbeat), and to control symptoms of *hyperthyroidism* (overactivity of the thyroid gland). Possible adverse effects are typical of other beta-blocker drugs.

naevus A type of skin blemish of which there are two main groups: pigmented naevi are caused by abnormality or overactivity of melanocytes (skin cells that produce the pigment *melanin*); vascular naevi are caused by an abnormal collection of blood vessels.

The most common types of pigmented naevi are *freckles*, *lentigos*, and *café au lait spots*: flat brown areas that may occur where the skin is exposed to the sun. Another common type is a mole, sometimes called a melanocytic naevus. In rare cases, moles become cancerous (see *melanoma, malignant*). Juvenile melanomas (see *melanoma, juvenile*) are red-brown naevi that occur in childhood. Blue naevi are common in young girls. Most black and Asian infants are born with blue-black spots on their lower backs (see *Mongolian blue spot*).

Port-wine stains and strawberry marks (see *haemangioma* and *spider naevi*) are examples of vascular naevi.

Most naevi are harmless. However, if a naevus suddenly appears, grows, bleeds, or changes colour, medical advice should be sought immediately to exclude the possibility of *skin cancer*.

nail A hard, curved plate on the fingers and toes composed of *keratin* (a tough protein). Nails grow from an area called the nail bed. At the base of each nail a half-moon shape, the lunula, is crossed by a flap of skin called the cuticle. The surrounding skin is known as the nail

fold. A fingernail takes about 6 months to grow from base to tip; toenails take twice as long.

The nails are susceptible to damage through injury, or by bacterial or fungal infections, especially *tinea* and *candidiasis*. Sometimes they become abnormally thick and curved: a condition known as *onychogryphosis*. Nail abnormalities may be a sign of skin disease, such as *alopecia* areata, *psoriasis*, and *lichen planus*, or of more generalized disease, for example iron-deficiency *anaemia*. Unusual nail colour may indicate disease.

Treatment of nail infections can be difficult. Creams and lotions may not penetrate sufficiently; oral medication may take months to be effective.

NAIL

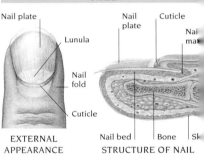

EXTERNAL APPEARANCE

STRUCTURE OF NAIL

nail-biting A common habit in children during their early years at school. Most children grow out of it, although nail-biting sometimes continues as a nervous habit in adolescents and adults.

Various preparations with an unpleasant taste can be painted on the nails as a preventive measure.

nalidixic acid An antibiotic drug used to treat and/or to prevent *urinary tract infection*. Possible adverse effects include nausea, vomiting, increased sensitivity to sunlight, blurred vision, drowsiness, and dizziness.

naloxone A drug that blocks the action of *opioid drugs*. Naloxone reverses the breathing difficulty caused by high doses of opioid drugs given during surgery. The drug is also given to newborn babies who are affected by opioid drugs used to relieve the mother's pain during labour.

Possible adverse effects include nausea, vomiting, and tremors.

nandrolone An anabolic steroid (see *steroids, anabolic*) used to treat certain types of *anaemia*.

Possible side effects include swollen ankles and *jaundice*. Nandrolone may cause difficulty in passing urine in men, and irregular menstruation and abnormal hair growth in women.

nappy rash Common skin inflammation in babies that is caused by irritant substances in urine or faeces. Occasionally, the inflammation is severe. Ointments containing mild *corticosteroid drugs* may be prescribed to suppress inflammation.

naproxen A *nonsteroidal anti-inflammatory drug* (NSAID). Naproxen is used to relieve joint pain and stiffness in *arthritis*; it is also prescribed to hasten recovery following injury to soft tissues, such as muscles or ligaments.

Possible adverse effects include nausea, abdominal pain, *peptic ulcer*, and *kidney failure*.

narcissism Intense self-love. A narcissistic personality disorder is characterized by an exaggerated sense of self-importance, constant need for attention or praise, inability to cope with criticism or defeat, and poor relationships with other people.

narcolepsy A sleep disorder characterized by chronic daytime sleepiness with recurrent episodes of sleep occurring throughout the day. Attacks may last from a few seconds to more than an hour. *Cataplexy* (sudden loss of muscle tone without loss of consciousness) occurs in about three quarters of cases. Other symptoms may include *sleep paralysis* and hallucinations. In narcolepsy, the REM (rapid eye movement) state of sleep is entered into abnormally rapidly.

Narcolepsy is often inherited. Treatment usually involves regular naps, along with *stimulant drugs* to control drowsiness, and *antidepressant drugs* to suppress cataplexy.

narcosis A state of stupor, usually caused by a drug (see *opioid drugs*) or some other chemical. Narcosis resembles sleep but, unlike someone who is sleeping, a person in narcosis cannot be roused completely.

narcotic drugs See *analgesic drugs*; *opioid*.

nasal congestion Partial blockage of the nasal passage caused by swelling of the *mucous membrane* that lines the nose. Nasal congestion is sometimes accompanied by the accumulation of thick nasal mucus.

Nasal congestion is a symptom of the common *cold* and of hay fever (see *rhinitis, allergic*); it may also be caused by certain drugs. The swelling may become persistent in disorders such as chronic *sinusitis* or *nasal polyps*.

Steam inhalation can help to loosen the mucus. This involves placing the head over a basin of hot water, possibly with the addition of aromatic oils such as menthol or eucalyptus, and inhaling the steam for several minutes. *Decongestant drugs* in the form of drops and sprays should be used for only a few days. Longer term, nasal *corticosteroid drugs*, *sodium cromoglicate*, and topical *antihistamine drugs* may control symptoms. Persistent nasal congestion should be investigated by a doctor.

nasal discharge The emission of fluid from the *nose*. Nasal discharge is commonly caused by inflammation of the mucous membrane lining the nose and is often accompanied by *nasal congestion*.

A discharge of mucus may indicate allergic *rhinitis*, a cold, or an infection that has spread from the sinuses (see *sinusitis*). A persistent runny discharge may be an early indication of a tumour (see *nasopharynx, cancer of*).

Bleeding from the nose (see *nosebleed*) is usually caused by injury or a foreign body in the nose. A discharge of cerebrospinal fluid from the nose may follow a fracture at the base of the skull.

nasal obstruction Blockage of the nasal passage on one or both sides of the *nose*.

The most common cause of nasal obstruction is inflammation of the mucous membrane lining the passage (see *nasal congestion*). Other causes include deviation of the *nasal septum*, nasal *polyps*, a *haematoma* (a collection of clotted blood) usually caused by injury, and, rarely, a cancerous tumour. In children, enlargement of the *adenoids* is the most common cause of nasal obstruction.

N

nasal polyp A growth in the lining of the *nose*, usually attached by a small stalk. Most nasal polyps are noncancerous, but they may need to be removed if they cause *nasal obstruction*.

nasal septum The dividing partition inside the *nose*. The nasal septum consists of cartilage at the front and bone at the rear, both of which are covered by *mucous membrane*.

Disorders include a deviated septum (twisting of the septum to one side), which may be present from birth or caused by injury. Surgery may be needed if breathing is obstructed.

Injury may also cause a *haematoma* (a collection of clotted blood) to form between the cartilage of the septum and the wall of one nasal cavity. A haematoma may obstruct breathing and may become infected, causing an *abscess* that could require surgical drainage.

Rarely, a hole may be eroded in the nasal septum by *tuberculosis, syphilis, Wegener's granulomatosis*, or as a result of sniffing *cocaine*.

nasogastric tube A narrow plastic tube that is passed through the nose, down the oesophagus, and into the stomach. Nasogastric tubes are commonly used to suck or drain digestive juices from the stomach when the intestine is blocked (as in *pyloric stenosis*) or is not working properly (as may occur after an abdominal operation). A nasogastric tube is also used to give liquid nourishment to patients who cannot eat (see *feeding, artificial*), to obtain specimens of stomach secretions for examination, and to wash out the stomach after a drug overdose or after swallowing a poison (see *lavage, gastric*).

nasolacrimal duct A channel that drains tears into the nose. The nasolacrimal duct forms part of the *lacrimal apparatus*.

nasopharynx The passage connecting the nasal cavity behind the *nose* to the top of the throat behind the soft *palate*. The nasopharynx is part of the respiratory tract and forms the upper section of the *pharynx*. During swallowing, the nasopharynx is sealed off by the soft palate pressing against the back of the throat, preventing food from entering. It contains the lower openings of the *eustachian tubes* (passages connecting

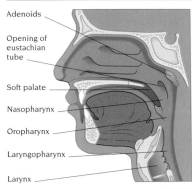

NASOPHARYNX

Adenoids
Opening of eustachian tube
Soft palate
Nasopharynx
Oropharynx
Laryngopharynx
Larynx

the back of the nose to the middle ear) and, in children, the *adenoids*, which can enlarge to block the nasopharynx, forcing the child to breathe through the mouth.

nasopharynx, cancer of A cancerous tumour of the *nasopharynx* that usually spreads to the nasal cavity, sinuses, base of the skull, and lymph nodes in the neck.

Cancer of the nasopharynx is rare in the West but common in the Far East. Most common at age 40–50, it affects twice as many men as women. One cause is believed to be the *Epstein–Barr virus*.

Common first signs are recurrent nosebleeds, a runny nose, and voice change. Loss of sense of smell, double vision, deafness, paralysis of one side of the face, and severe pain may develop.

Diagnosis is through a *biopsy, MRI* scans, and *X-rays*. Treatment is usually with *radiotherapy*, but surgery may also be performed. If treated early, the outlook can be good.

natural childbirth See *childbirth, natural*.

naturopathy A form of *alternative medicine* based on the principle that disease is a result of the accumulation of waste products and toxins in the body, and that symptoms reflect the attempts of the body to rid itself of these substances. Practitioners of naturopathy believe that health is maintained by avoiding anything artificial or unnatural in the diet or in the environment.

nausea The sensation of needing to vomit. Although nausea may occur without *vomiting*, the causes are the same.

navel A popular term for the *umbilicus*, the depression in the abdomen that marks the point at which the umbilical cord was attached to the fetus.

nebulizer An aerosol device used to administer a drug in the form of a fine mist for inhalation through a face mask or mouthpiece. Nebulizers are used to administer *bronchodilator drugs*, especially in the emergency treatment of *asthma*.

neck The part of the body that supports the head and serves as a passageway between the head and brain and the body.

The neck contains many important structures: the *spinal cord* (which carries nerve impulses to and from the brain); *trachea* (windpipe), *larynx* (voice box); *oesophagus*; *thyroid* and *parathyroid glands*; *lymph nodes*; and several major blood vessels. The upper seven vertebrae of the spine are in the neck; a complex system of muscles is connected to these vertebrae, the clavicles (collarbones), the upper ribs, and lower jaw.

Neck disorders include *torticollis* (wry neck) in which the head is twisted to one side. *Fractures* and *dislocations* of vertebrae in the neck and *whiplash injury* can injure the spinal cord causing paralysis or even death (see *spinal injury*). Any condition causing swelling in the neck may interfere with breathing or swallowing.

Degeneration of the joints between the neck vertebrae may occur due to *cervical osteoarthritis*, causing similar symptoms to those of *disc prolapse*. In *ankylosing spondylitis*, fusion of the vertebrae may result in permanent neck rigidity. *Cervical rib* is a rare congenital defect in which there is a small extra rib in the neck.

Neck pain of unknown origin is very common. As long as neurological symptoms (such as loss of sensation or muscle power) are absent, the condition is unlikely to be serious and usually disappears within a few weeks.

neck dissection, radical A surgical procedure for the removal of cancerous *lymph nodes* in the neck. The operation is commonly part of the treatment of cancer of the tongue, tonsils, or other structures in the mouth and throat.

neck rigidity Marked stiffness of the neck caused by spasm of the muscles in the neck and spine. Neck rigidity is an important clinical sign of *meningitis* (inflammation of the membranes covering the brain and spinal cord). Severe neck rigidity may cause the head to arch backwards, especially in babies.

necrolysis, toxic epidermal A severe, blistering rash in which the surface layers of the skin peel off, exposing large areas of red raw skin over the body. The condition carries a risk of widespread infection and loss of body fluid and salts.

The most common cause of toxic epidermal necrolysis is an adverse reaction to a *drug*, particularly a barbiturate, sulphonamide, or penicillin. The condition usually clears up when the drug is discontinued. Intravenous fluid replacement is sometimes necessary.

necrophilia A rare sexual perversion in which orgasm is achieved by means of sexual acts with dead bodies.

necropsy A little used alternative medical term for an *autopsy* (postmortem examination of a body).

necrosis The death of tissue cells. Necrosis can occur as a result of *ischaemia* (inadequate blood supply), which may lead to *gangrene*; infection, such as *tuberculosis*; or damage by extreme heat or cold, noxious chemicals, or excessive exposure to X-rays or other radiation.

In necrosis due to tuberculosis, the dead tissue is soft, dry, and cheese-like. Fatty tissue beneath the skin that has died as a result of damage or infection develops into tough scar tissue that may form a firm nodule.

necrotizing fasciitis A rare, serious infection of tissues beneath the skin by a type of streptococcal bacterium. Necrotizing fasciitis is most likely to occur as a complication following surgery. The initial symptoms are inflammation and blistering of the skin. The infection spreads very rapidly, and the bacteria release enzymes and toxins that can cause extensive destruction of deeper tissues and damage internal organs. Urgent treatment with *antibiotic drugs* and removal of all infected tissue are essential. The infection is life-threatening.

needle aspiration See *biopsy*.

needle exchange A health scheme that enables intravenous drug abusers to exchange used hypodermic needles for

N

new, sterile ones. The scheme is aimed at reducing the risks of infections, such as *HIV* and *hepatitis*, transmitted by the sharing of contaminated needles.

needlestick injury Accidental puncture of the skin by a contaminated hypodermic needle. Hospital staff are most likely to be at risk. Needlestick injuries carry the risk of serious infections, such as *HIV* and *hepatitis*, and need immediate attention. The wound should be cleaned thoroughly. If there is a significant risk of infection, preventive medication will be given. Blood tests will be carried out to determine whether infection has actually been transmitted.

nefopam An *analgesic drug* used to relieve moderate pain caused, for example, by injury, surgery, or cancer. Possible adverse effects include nausea, nervousness, dry mouth, and difficulty sleeping.

Nelson's syndrome A rare disorder of the *endocrine system* that causes increased skin pigmentation. Nelson's syndrome results from enlargement of the *pituitary gland*, which can follow removal of the *adrenal glands* (a treatment for *Cushing's syndrome*).

Nelson's syndrome is treated by *hypophysectomy* (removal or destruction of the pituitary gland).

nematodes The scientific name for a group of cylindrically shaped worms (*roundworms*), some of which can be parasites of humans.

neologism The act of making up new words that have a special meaning for the inventor. The term also refers to the invented words themselves. Persistent neologism can be a feature of speech in people with *schizophrenia*.

neomycin An *antibiotic drug* used to treat ear, eye, and skin infections, often in combination with other drugs. Neomycin is sometimes given to prevent infection of the intestine prior to surgery. Possible adverse effects include rash and itching.

neonate A newly born infant, under the age of 1 month (see *newborn*).

neonatology The branch of *paediatrics* concerned with the care of *newborn* infants and the treatment of disorders during the first few weeks of life.

neoplasia A medical term for *tumour* formation. The term neoplasia does not necessarily imply that the new growth is *cancerous*; neoplasia also results in tumours that are *noncancerous*.

neoplasm A medical term for a *tumour* (any new abnormal growth). Neoplasms may be *cancerous* or *noncancerous*.

neostigmine A drug that is used to treat *myasthenia gravis* (a rare autoimmune disorder that causes muscle weakness). Neostigmine increases the activity of *acetylcholine*, a *neurotransmitter* that stimulates the contraction of muscles.

Possible adverse effects of neostigmine include nausea and vomiting, increased salivation, abdominal cramps, diarrhoea, blurred vision, muscle cramps, sweating, and twitching.

nephrectomy Surgical removal of one or both of the *kidneys*.

One of the most common reasons for nephrectomy is to remove a cancerous tumour (see *kidney cancer*). A kidney may also be removed if it is not functioning normally due to injury, infection, or the presence of stones (see *calculus, urinary tract*), or if it is causing severe *hypertension* (high blood pressure).

On removal of a single kidney the remaining kidney takes over the workload. If both kidneys are removed, the patient requires *dialysis* or a *kidney transplant*.

nephritis Inflammation of one or both *kidneys*. Nephritis may be caused by an infection (see *pyelonephritis*), abnormal responses of the *immune system* (see *glomerulonephritis*), or metabolic disorders, such as gout.

nephroblastoma See *kidney cancer*.

nephrocalcinosis Deposits of calcium within the tissue of one or both *kidneys*. Nephrocalcinosis is not the same as kidney stones (see *calculus, urinary tract*), in which calcium particles develop inside the drainage channels of the kidney.

Nephrocalcinosis may occur in any condition in which the level of calcium in the blood is raised. It may also occur as a result of taking excessive amounts of certain *antacid drugs* or *vitamin D*. Treatment is of the underlying cause to prevent further calcification.

nephrolithotomy The surgical removal of a *calculus* (stone) from the *kidney*.

Nephrolithotomy may be performed through an abdominal incision, or via a puncture incision in the back. Large calculi may need to be broken up before removal. Other methods of removal are *pyelolithotomy* and *lithotripsy*.

nephrology The medical speciality concerned with the normal functioning of the *kidneys* and with the causes, diagnosis, and treatment of kidney disease.

Methods of investigating the kidneys include kidney *biopsy*, *kidney function tests*, and *kidney imaging* techniques such as *ultrasound scanning* and *intravenous urography*. Treatment of kidney disorders may involve drugs and surgery and, in advanced cases, *dialysis* or a *kidney transplant*.

nephron The microscopic unit of the kidney that consists of a glomerulus (a filtering funnel made up of a cluster of capillaries) and a tubule. There are about 1 million nephrons in each kidney. The nephrons filter waste products from the blood and modify the amount of salt and water excreted in urine, according to the body's needs. This process involves filtration of blood in the glomerulus followed by further processing as the filtrate flows through the various parts of the tubule – the proximal convoluted tubule, loop of Henle, and the distal convoluted tubule.

nephropathy A term for any disease of or damage to the *kidneys*.

Obstructive nephropathy refers to kidney damage caused by a urinary tract *calculus* (stone), a tumour, scar tissue, or pressure from an organ that is blocking the flow of urine and creating back pressure within the kidney.

Reflux nephropathy refers to kidney damage caused by backflow of urine from the bladder towards the kidney. It is caused by failure of the valve mechanism at the lower end of the ureter.

Toxic nephropathy refers to damage caused by various poisons or minerals.

nephrosclerosis Hardening of the arterioles and arteries of the *kidney*.

nephrosis See *nephrotic syndrome*.

nephrostomy The introduction of a small tube into the *kidney* to drain urine to the abdominal surface, bypassing the ureter and bladder. Nephrostomy is sometimes performed after an operation on the ureter or kidney–ureter junction.

nephrotic syndrome A collection of symptoms and signs resulting from damage to the glomeruli (filtering units of the *kidney*), causing severe *proteinuria* (loss of protein from the bloodstream into the urine). The syndrome may be a result of *diabetes mellitus*, *amyloidosis* (accumulation in tissues of an abnormal protein called amyloid), *glomerulonephritis*, severe *hypertension*, reactions to poisons, and adverse reactions to drugs.

The main symptom of nephrotic syndrome is swelling of the legs and face due to *oedema* (build-up of fluid). Also, fluid may collect in the chest cavity, resulting in *pleural effusion*, or in the abdomen, causing *ascites*. Diarrhoea, lethargy, and *anorexia* may additionally occur.

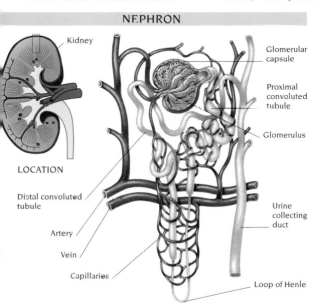

NEPHRON

Kidney

Glomerular capsule

Proximal convoluted tubule

Glomerulus

LOCATION

Distal convoluted tubule

Urine collecting duct

Artery

Vein

Capillaries

Loop of Henle

Treatment is of the underlying condition. A low-sodium diet may be recommended, and *diuretic drugs* may be given to reduce oedema. If the concentration of protein in the blood is very low, protein may need to be given intravenously.

nerve A bundle of nerve fibres which travel to a common location. Nerve fibres, known as axons, are the filamentous projections of many individual *neurons* (nerve cells).

NERVE

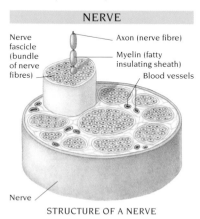

Nerve fascicle (bundle of nerve fibres)

Axon (nerve fibre)

Myelin (fatty insulating sheath)

Blood vessels

Nerve

STRUCTURE OF A NERVE

The most obvious nerves in the body are the peripheral nerves, which extend from the *central nervous system* (consisting of the *brain* and *spinal cord*). Of these, 12 pairs of *cranial nerves* link directly to the brain, and 31 pairs of *spinal nerves* join the spinal cord. In the shoulder and hip regions, the spinal nerves join to form plexuses, from which branch the main nerves to the limbs. Most nerves divide at numerous points to send branches to all parts of the body, particularly to the sense organs, the skin, skeletal muscles, internal organs, and glands.

Nerve fibres may have a sensory function, carrying information from a receptor or sense organ towards the central nervous system (CNS), or they may have a motor function, carrying instructions from the CNS to a muscle or a gland. The messages are carried by electrical impulses propagated along the fibres. Some nerves carry only sensory or motor fibres, but most carry both.

Nerve function is sensitive to cold, pressure, and injury (see *nerve injury*). The peripheral nerves can be damaged by a wide variety of disorders, including infection, inflammation, and metabolic disorders (see *neuropathy*).

nerve block The injection of a local anaesthetic around a nerve to produce loss of sensation in a part of the body supplied by that nerve. For example, the palm of the hand may be anaesthetized by giving injections at sites up the arm, blocking the ulnar and median nerves.

A nerve may be blocked as it leaves the spinal cord. This occurs in *epidural anaesthesia*, used mainly in childbirth, and in *spinal anaesthesia*, used mainly for surgery of the lower abdomen and limbs. In a caudal block an anaesthetic is injected around nerves leaving the lowest part of the spinal cord. It produces anaesthesia in the buttock and genital areas, and is occasionally used in childbirth. A pudendal nerve block involves the injection of an anaesthetic into nerves passing under the pelvis into the floor of the vagina. This type of nerve block is sometimes used in a *forceps delivery*. (See also *anaesthesia, local.*)

nerve conduction studies Tests carried out to assess the extent of nerve damage caused by disorders of the peripheral nervous system (see *neuropathy*). In the test, an electrical stimulus is applied to a nerve, and the speed at which the nerve responds to the stimulus and transmits a signal is recorded.

NERVE CONDUCTION STUDIES

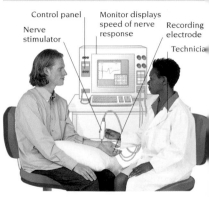

Control panel

Nerve stimulator

Monitor displays speed of nerve response

Recording electrode

Technicia

nerve injury Damage or severance of conducting fibres within a *nerve* as a result of trauma, causing loss of skin sensation and muscle power. (See *neuropathy* for nerve damage from causes other than injury.)

If a peripheral nerve (a nerve outside the brain or spinal cord) is only partially severed, the cut fibres may be able to regenerate. Provided the severed ends are still aligned, new fibres can grow across the cut to rejoin the connection, restoring function. If a nerve is totally severed, the individual fibres cannot regenerate successfully and there is no recovery of function. Nerve tracts within the brain and spinal cord are structurally different from the peripheral nerves, and severed fibres in these tracts do not regenerate. For example, vision cannot be restored if the *optic nerves* are cut.

Microsurgery can sometimes be used to stitch a severed peripheral nerve into place, but recovery is rarely complete.

nerve, trapped Compression or stretching of a nerve, causing numbness, tingling, weakness, and, sometimes, pain.

Common examples of a trapped nerve include *carpal tunnel syndrome*, in which pressure on the median nerve as it passes through the wrist causes symptoms in the thumb, index, and middle fingers; a *disc prolapse*, in which pressure on the nerve root leading from the spinal cord produces symptoms in the back and legs; and *crutch palsy*, in which the radial nerve presses against the humerus (upper-arm bone), producing symptoms in the wrist and hand.

A damaged nerve may take some time to heal. In severe cases, surgical decompression to relieve pressure on the nerve may be necessary.

nervous breakdown A nontechnical term used to describe unusual behaviour (such as episodes of tearfulness or shouting and screaming) that may be part of a crisis of severe *anxiety*, *depression*, or other psychiatric illness. The condition affects the sufferer's ability to cope with everyday life.

nervous energy A nontechnical term for the increased drive and activity of individuals who are always restless, anxious, and on the go.

nervous habit A nontechnical term for a minor repetitive movement or activity. Sometimes a nervous habit consists of involuntary twitches and facial tics, such as in *Gilles de la Tourette's syndrome* and some forms of *dyskinesia*. Voluntary nervous habits, such as *nail-biting* and *thumb-sucking*, are common in young children.

All nervous habits increase during periods of tension or anxiety, and may be severe in some forms of *depression*, *anxiety disorder*, or drug withdrawal.

nervous system The body system that gathers and stores information and is in overall control of the body.

NERVOUS SYSTEM

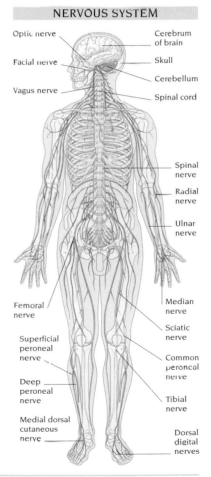

Optic nerve
Facial nerve
Vagus nerve
Cerebrum of brain
Skull
Cerebellum
Spinal cord
Spinal nerve
Radial nerve
Ulnar nerve
Median nerve
Sciatic nerve
Common peroneal nerve
Tibial nerve
Dorsal digital nerves
Femoral nerve
Superficial peroneal nerve
Deep peroneal nerve
Medial dorsal cutaneous nerve

N

N

The *brain* and *spinal cord* form the *central nervous system* (CNS), which consists of billions of interconnected *neurons* (nerve cells). Input of information to the CNS comes from the sense organs. Motor instructions are sent out to skeletal muscles, the muscles controlling speech, internal organs and glands, and the sweat glands in the skin. This information is carried along nerves that fan out from the CNS to the entire body. Each nerve is a bundle consisting of the axons (filamentous projections) of many individual neurons.

In addition to the nervous system's anatomical divisions, there are various functional divisions. Two of the most important are the *autonomic nervous system*, concerned with the automatic (unconscious) regulation of internal body functioning, and the somatic nervous system, which controls the muscles responsible for voluntary movement.

The overall function of the nervous system is to gather and analyse information about the external environment and the body's internal state, and to initiate appropriate responses, such as avoiding physical danger.

The nervous system functions largely through automatic responses to stimuli (see *reflex*), although voluntary actions can also be initiated through the activity of higher, conscious areas of the brain.

Disorders of the nervous system may result from damage to or dysfunction of its component parts (see *brain*; *spinal cord*; *neuropathy*; *nerve injury*). They may also be due to impairment of sensory, analytical, or memory functions (see *vision, disorders of*; *deafness*; *numbness*; *anosmia*; *agnosia*; *amnesia*), or of motor functions (see *aphasia*; *dysarthria*; *ataxia*).

netilmicin An *antibiotic* drug usually prescribed only to treat serious infection in hospital, when other antibiotic drugs have proved ineffective. In rare circumstances, netilmicin can damage the inner ear or the kidneys.

nettle rash A common name for *urticaria*.

neuralgia Pain caused by irritation of, or damage to, a *nerve*. The pain usually occurs in brief bouts and may be severe.

Some types of neuralgia are features of a specific disorder. *Migraine* sufferers commonly experience a form of neuralgia consisting of attacks of intense, radiating pain around the eye. Postherpetic neuralgia is a burning pain that may recur at the site of an attack of *herpes zoster* (shingles) for months or even years after the illness.

Other types of neuralgia result from disturbance of a particular nerve. In glossopharyngeal neuralgia, intense pain is felt at the back of the tongue and in the throat and ear, all of which are areas supplied by the glossopharyngeal nerve. The cause of the pain is generally unknown. The same is true of *trigeminal neuralgia*, a severe paroxysm of pain affecting one side of the face supplied by the trigeminal nerve.

Neuralgia is sometimes relieved by *analgesic drugs* (painkillers) such as paracetamol. Glossopharyngeal, trigeminal, and postherpetic neuralgia may respond to treatment with *carbamazepine* or other *anticonvulsant drugs*, or to *tricyclic antidepressant drugs*.

neural tube defect A developmental failure affecting the spinal cord or brain of the embryo. The most serious defect is *anencephaly* (total lack of a brain), which is fatal. More common is *spina bifida*, in which the vertebrae do not form a complete ring around the spinal cord. Spina bifida can occur anywhere on the spine, but it is most common in the lower back.

There are different forms of spina bifida. In spina bifida occulta, the only defect is a failure of the fusion of the bony arches behind the spinal cord, which may not cause any problems. When the bone defect is more extensive, there may be a meningocele, a protrusion of the *meninges*, or a myelomeningocele, a malformation of the spinal cord. Myelomeningocele is likely to cause severe handicap, with paralysis of the legs, loss of sensation in the lower body, *hydrocephalus*, and paralysis of the anus and bladder, causing *incontinence*. Associated problems include *cerebral palsy*, *epilepsy*, and *learning difficulties*.

Surgery is usually performed a few days after birth. In mild cases, the defect can usually be corrected, but in myelomeningocele, some handicap will remain.

NEURAL TUBE DEFECT

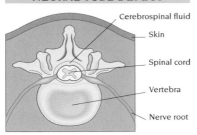

Cerebrospinal fluid
Skin
Spinal cord
Vertebra
Nerve root

NORMAL VERTEBRA

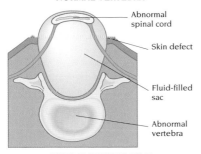

Abnormal spinal cord
Skin defect
Fluid-filled sac
Abnormal vertebra

MYELOMENINGOCELE

Genetic factors play a part in neural tube defects, which show multifactorial *inheritance*. Couples who have had an affected child or who have a family history of neural tube defects should seek *genetic counselling*. The risk of a neural tube defect occurring can be substantially reduced if a woman takes *folic acid* supplements before and during pregnancy: a woman who is planning a pregnancy should take the recommended dose of supplement before conceiving and then for the first 12 weeks of pregnancy. If there is a family history of neural tube defects, a higher dose of folic acid supplement is recommended.

Ultrasound scanning and *amniocentesis* allow accurate antenatal testing for neural tube defects.

neurapraxia A type of *nerve injury* in which the outward structure of a nerve appears intact, but some of the conducting fibres have been damaged or have degenerated and thus do not transmit signals normally.

neurasthenia An outdated term that literally means "nervous exhaustion". It was once used to describe a number of physical and mental symptoms, including loss of energy, insomnia, aches and pains, *depression*, irritability, and reduced concentration.

neuritis A term that literally means inflammation of a nerve. True nerve inflammation may be caused by infection (for example by a virus in *herpes zoster* or by a bacterium in *Hansen's disease*). The term neuritis is also often applied to nerve damage or disease from causes other than inflammation. It has become virtually synonymous with *neuropathy*.

neuroblastoma A tumour of the *adrenal glands* or the sympathetic nervous system (which is part of the *autonomic nervous system*). Most neuroblastomas develop in the adrenal glands or in the sympathetic nerves along the back wall of the abdomen. Less commonly, tumours develop in the sympathetic nerves of the chest or neck.

Neuroblastomas are the most common extracranial (outside the skull), solid tumour of childhood. Most cases develop during the first 10 years of life, especially in the first 5 years.

Common symptoms include a lump in the abdomen, tiredness, weight loss, aches and pains, paleness, and irritability. Diarrhoea, high blood pressure, and flushing of the skin sometimes occur.

The diagnosis of a neuroblastoma is from *MRI* and *CT scanning*, blood tests, urine tests, and *biopsy* of the bone marrow and any accessible tumours. Treatment consists of surgical removal of the tumour, followed by *radiotherapy*. Anticancer drugs and a *stem cell* or *bone marrow transplant* may also be required. The outlook varies because neuroblastomas range from being relatively harmless to aggressively cancerous.

neurocutaneous disorders A group of conditions characterized by abnormalities of the skin and of the nerves and/or the central nervous system.

The best known of these neurocutaneous disorders is *neurofibromatosis*, in which there are brown patches on the skin and numerous fibrous nodules on the skin and nerves. Another example is *tuberous sclerosis*, which is characterized by small skin-coloured swellings over the cheeks and nose, mental deficiency, and epilepsy.

neurodermatitis An itchy, eczema-like skin condition caused by repeated scratching. (See also *lichen simplex*.)

neuroendocrinology The study of the interactions between the *nervous system* and the *endocrine system* that control internal body functions and the body's response to the external environment.

neurofibromatosis An uncommon inherited disorder (also known as von Recklinghausen's disease) characterized by numerous neurofibromas (soft, fibrous swellings, varying significantly in size), which grow from nerves, and by *café au lait spots* (pale, coffee-coloured patches) on the skin, usually on the trunk and pelvis.

If neurofibromas occur in the central nervous system, they may cause *epilepsy* and other complications. Neurofibromatosis can lead to bone deformities. Rarely, neurofibromas become cancerous.

Surgical removal of neurofibromas is necessary only if there are complications. Anyone with this disorder, and parents of an affected child, should seek *genetic counselling* if planning a pregnancy.

neurology The medical discipline concerned with the study of the *nervous system* and its disorders (see also *neuropathology*; *neurosurgery*).

neuroma A noncancerous tumour of *nerve* tissue. In most cases, the cause is unknown; rarely, a neuroma develops as a result of damage to a nerve.

A neuroma may affect any nerve in the body. Symptoms vary, but there is often intermittent pain and sometimes weakness and numbness in the areas that are supplied by the affected nerve.

If symptoms are troublesome, the tumour may be surgically removed. (See also *acoustic neuroma*.)

neuron The term used to describe a nerve cell. A typical neuron consists of a cell body, several branching projections called dendrites, and a filamentous projection called an axon (also known as a nerve fibre). An axon branches at its end to form terminals through which electrical signals are transmitted to target cells. Most axons are coated with a layered insulating *myelin* sheath, which speeds the transmission of the signals. The myelin sheath is punctuated along its length by gaps called nodes of Ranvier, which help this process. Because the myelin sheath is nonconductive, ion exchange (depolarization) only occurs at a node, and signals leap from node to node along the axon.

The nervous system contains billions of neurons, of which there are three main types: sensory neurons, which carry

NEURON

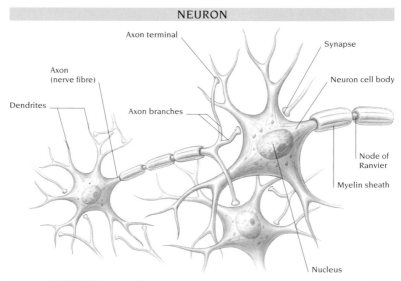

Axon terminal

Synapse

Axon (nerve fibre)

Neuron cell body

Dendrites

Axon branches

Node of Ranvier

Myelin sheath

Nucleus

signals from sense receptors into the *central nervous system* (CNS); motor neurons, which carry signals from the CNS to muscles or glands; and interneurons, which form all the complex electrical circuitry within the CNS itself.

When a neuron transmits ("fires") an electrical impulse, a chemical called a *neurotransmitter* is released from the axon terminals at *synapses* (junctions with other neurons). This neurotransmitter may make a muscle cell contract, cause an endocrine gland to release a hormone, or affect an adjacent neuron.

Different stimuli excite different types of neurons to fire. Sensory neurons, for example, may be excited by physical stimuli, such as cold or pressure. The activity of most neurons is controlled by the effects of neurotransmitters released from adjacent neurons. Certain neurotransmitters generate a sudden change in the balance of electrical potential inside and outside the cell (an "action potential"), which occurs at one point on the cell's membrane and flows at high speed along it. Others stabilize neuronal membranes, preventing an action potential. Thus, the firing pattern of a neuron depends on the balance of excitatory and inhibitory influences acting on it.

If the cell body of a neuron is damaged or degenerates, the cell dies and is never replaced. A baby starts life with the maximum number of neurons, which decreases continuously thereafter.

neuropathic joint A joint that has been damaged by inflammation and a series of injuries, which pass unnoticed due to loss of sensation in the joint resulting from *neuropathy* (nerve damage caused by disease). Neuropathic joints develop in a number of conditions, including *diabetes mellitus* and untreated *syphilis*.

When sensation to pain is lost, abnormal stress and strain on a joint do not stimulate the protective reflex spasm of the surrounding muscles; this failure of the protective reflex allows exaggerated movement that can damage the joint. *Osteoarthritis*, swelling, and deformity are features of a neuropathic joint.

An orthopaedic *brace* or *caliper splint* may be necessary to restrict any abnormal movement of the joint. Occasionally,

an *arthrodesis* (a surgical operation to fuse a joint) is performed. The nerve damage is irreversible.

neuropathology The branch of *pathology* that is concerned with the causes and effects of disorders of the *nervous system*. (See also *neurology*.)

neuropathy Disease or inflammation of, or damage to, the peripheral *nerves*, which connect the *central nervous system* (brain and spinal cord), to the muscles, glands, sense organs, and internal organs. The term neuritis is now used more or less interchangeably with neuropathy.

Most nerve cell axons (the conducting fibres that make up nerves) are insulated by a sheath of the fatty substance *myelin*. Most neuropathies arise from damage to, or irritation of, either the axons or their myelin sheaths, which may cause slowing or a complete block of the passage of electrical signals. Polyneuropathy (or polyneuritis) means damage to several nerves; mononeuropathy (or mononeuritis) indicates damage to a single nerve; neuralgia describes pain caused by irritation or inflammation of a nerve.

Some cases of neuropathy have no obvious cause. Among specific causes are *diabetes mellitus*, dietary deficiencies, excessive alcohol consumption, and metabolic upsets such as *uraemia*.

Nerves may become acutely inflamed after a viral infection, and neuropathies may also result from *autoimmune disorders*, such as *rheumatoid arthritis*. Neuropathies may occur secondarily to cancerous tumours, or with *lymphomas* and *leukaemias*. There is also a group of inherited neuropathies, the most common being *peroneal muscular atrophy*.

The symptoms of neuropathy depend on whether it affects mainly sensory nerve fibres or mainly motor nerve fibres. Damage to sensory nerve fibres may cause numbness, tingling, sensations of cold, and pain. Damage to motor fibres may cause muscle weakness and muscle wasting. Damage to autonomic nerves may lead to blurred vision, impaired or absent sweating, faintness, and disturbance of gastric, intestinal, bladder, and sexual functioning.

To determine the extent of the damage, *nerve conduction studies* are carried

N

out together with *EMG* tests, which record the electrical activity in muscles. Diagnostic tests such as *blood tests*, *MRI* scans, and nerve or muscle *biopsy* may also be required. When possible, treatment is aimed at the underlying cause. If the cell bodies of the damaged nerve cells have not been destroyed, full recovery from neuropathy is possible.

neuropsychiatry The branch of medicine dealing with the relationship between psychiatric symptoms and neurological disorder. This may include the effects of head injury and alcohol on the brain, or disorders such as brain tumours, infections, inherited illnesses, and disorders causing brain damage in childhood.

neurosis An old term for a range of psychiatric disorders excluding *psychosis*.

neurosurgery The specialty concerned with the surgical treatment of disorders of the *brain*, *spinal cord*, or other parts of the *nervous system*.

Conditions treated by neurosurgery include tumours of the brain, spinal cord, or meninges (membranes surrounding the brain and spinal cord); *brain abscess*; abnormalities of the blood vessels supplying the brain, such as an *aneurysm* (balloon-like swelling at a weak point in an artery); bleeding inside the skull (see *extradural haemorrhage*, *intracerebral haemorrhage*, and *subdural haemorrhage*); some birth defects (such as *neural tube defects* and *hydrocephalus*); certain types of *epilepsy*; and nerve damage caused by illness or accidents. Neurosurgery may also be performed to relieve *pain* that is otherwise untreatable.

neurosyphilis Infection of the brain or spinal cord that occurs in untreated syphilis many years after initial infection.

Damage to the spinal cord due to neurosyphilis may cause tabes dorsalis, characterized by poor coordination of leg movements, urinary incontinence, and pains in the abdomen and limbs. Damage to the brain may cause *dementia*, muscle weakness, and, in rare cases, total paralysis of the limbs.

neurotoxin A chemical that damages nervous tissue. The principal effects of neurotoxic nerve damage are numbness, weakness, or paralysis of the part of the body supplied by the affected nerve.

Neurotoxins are present in the venom of certain snakes (see *snake bites*), and are released by some types of bacteria (such as those that cause *tetanus* and *diphtheria*). Some chemical poisons, such as arsenic and lead, are also neurotoxic.

neurotransmitter A chemical released from a nerve ending that transmits impulses from one *neuron* (nerve cell) to another neuron, or to a muscle cell. When a nerve impulse reaches a nerve ending, neurotransmitters are released from synaptic vesicles and cross a tiny gap (synapse) to reach the target cell. Here, they cause channels in the target cell to open, letting through charged particles that stimulate an impulse in the cell. Alternatively, neurotransmitters may inhibit nerve impulses.

Scores of different chemicals fulfil this function in different parts of the *nervous system*. Many neurotransmitters act as both neurotransmitters and hormones, being released into the bloodstream to act on distant target cells.

One of the most important neurotransmitters is *acetylcholine*, which causes skeletal muscles to contract when it is released by neurons connected to the muscles. Acetylcholine is also released by neurons that control the sweat glands and the heartbeat, and transmits messages between neurons in the brain and spinal cord.

Another chemical, *noradrenaline* (norepinephrine), aids the nervous control of heartbeat, blood flow, and the body's response to stress. *Dopamine* plays an important role in parts of the brain that control movement. *Serotonin* is one of the main neurotransmitters found in parts of the brain concerned with conscious processes.

Another group of neurotransmitters is called the neuropeptides. This group includes the *endorphins*, which are used by the brain to control sensitivity to pain.

neutrophil A type of phagocyte, or white *blood cell*. They are an important part of the *immune system*, and their role is to engulf and destroy invading bacteria.

newborn An infant at birth and during the first few weeks of life (see also *prematurity*; *postmaturity*).

newborn screening tests A series of tests carried out on newborn babies to detect disorders or abnormalities so that, if necessary, treatment can be given as soon as possible. The tests include a complete physical examination to check for possible abnormalities of the heart, lungs, genitals, hips, skull, spine, hands, feet, eyes, and ears. The baby's head circumference and length are also measured. In addition, a small sample of blood is taken from the baby's heel and analysed to check for certain rare disorders (see *blood spot screening tests*). Within the first few weeks of birth, specialized hearing tests are also done to check the baby's hearing is normal.

NGU An abbreviation for *nongonococcal urethritis.*

niacin See *vitamin B complex.*

nickel A metallic element that is present in the body in minute amounts. Nickel is thought to activate certain *enzymes* (substances that promote biochemical reactions), and it may also play a part in stabilizing chromosomal material in the nuclei of cells.

Exposure to nickel may cause *dermatitis* (inflammation of the skin). *Lung cancer* has been reported in workers in nickel refineries.

niclosamide An *anthelmintic drug* used to treat *tapeworm infestation.* Niclosamide causes the tapeworm to loosen its grip on the inner wall of the intestine. The worm is then passed out of the body in the faeces.

Adverse effects include abdominal pain, lightheadedness, and itching.

nicorandil A *potassium channel activator* drug used in the prevention and long-term treatment of *angina.* Side effects, which include flushing, nausea, vomiting, and dizziness, are mainly due to nicorandil's *vasodilation* effects and usually wear off with continued treatment. Rarely, mouth ulcers and muscle pain can occur.

nicotinamide A form of niacin (see *vitamin B complex*).

nicotine A drug in tobacco which acts as a stimulant and is responsible for dependence on tobacco. After inhalation, the nicotine in tobacco smoke passes rapidly into the bloodstream. The drug acts on the nervous system until broken down by the liver and excreted in the urine.

Nicotine acts primarily on the *autonomic nervous system*, which controls involuntary body activities such as the heart rate. In habitual smokers, the drug increases the heart rate and narrows the blood vessels, the combined effect of which is to raise blood pressure. Nicotine also stimulates the *central nervous system*, thereby reducing fatigue, increasing alertness, and improving concentration.

Stopping smoking often causes withdrawal symptoms such as headaches and difficulty in concentrating. *Nicotine replacement therapy*, such as the use of nicotine skin patches and chewing gum, can be effective in aiding withdrawal from nicotine. (See also *smoking.*)

nicotine replacement therapy Preparations containing *nicotine* that are used in place of cigarettes as an aid to stopping smoking. Nicotine products are available in the form of *sublingual* tablets, chewing gum, skin patches, nasal spray, or inhaler. Side effects may include nausea, headache, palpitations, cold or flu-like symptoms, hiccups, and vivid dreaming. Nicotine replacement therapy should be used as part of a complete package of measures, including the determination to succeed.

nicotinic acid A form of niacin (see *vitamin B complex*). Nicotinic acid is prescribed as a *lipid-lowering drug* and is used together with a *statin* to treat certain types of *hyperlipidaemia.* Possible adverse effects of nicotinic acid include flushing, dizziness, nausea, palpitations, and itching.

nifedipine A *calcium channel blocker* drug used mainly to prevent and treat *angina pectoris.* Nifedipine is also often used to treat *hypertension* (high blood pressure) and disorders affecting the circulation, such as *Raynaud's disease.* Possible adverse effects include *oedema* (accumulation of fluid in tissues), flushing, headache, and dizziness.

night blindness The inability to see well in dim light. Many people with night blindness have no discernible eye disease. The condition may be an

N

inherited functional defect of the retina, an early sign of *retinitis pigmentosa*, or a result of vitamin A deficiency.

nightmare An unpleasant, vivid dream, sometimes accompanied by a sense of suffocation. Nightmares occur during REM (rapid eye movement) *sleep* in the middle and later parts of the night, and they are often clearly remembered if the dreamer awakens completely.

Nightmares are especially common in children aged between 8 and 10, and are particularly likely to occur when the child is unwell or anxious. In adults, nightmares may be a side effect of certain drugs, including *beta-blocker drugs* and *benzodiazepine* drugs. Repeated nightmares may be associated with traumatic experiences.

Nightmares should not be confused with hypnagogic *hallucinations*, which occur while falling asleep, nor with *night terror*, which occurs in NREM (nonrapid eye movement) sleep and is not remembered the next day.

night terror A disorder, occurring mainly in children, that consists of abrupt arousals from sleep in a terrified state. Night terror (also called sleep terror) usually starts between the ages of 4 and 7, gradually disappearing in early adolescence.

Episodes occur during NREM (nonrapid eye movement) *sleep*, usually half an hour to three and a half hours after falling asleep. Sufferers wake up screaming in a semiconscious state and remain frightened for some minutes. They do not recognize familiar faces or surroundings, and usually cannot be comforted. The sufferer gradually falls back to sleep and has no memory of the event the following day.

Night terror in children has no serious significance, but, in adults, is likely to be associated with an *anxiety disorder*.

nipple The small prominence at the tip of each *breast*. Women's nipples contain tiny openings through which milk can pass. The nipple and the areola, a surrounding area of dark skin, both increase in size during pregnancy. Involuntary muscle in the nipple allows it to become erect.

Structural defects of the nipple are rare. An inverted nipple is usually a harmless abnormality of development.

Nipple inversion that develops in older women is mostly due to aging, but *mammography* may be advisable to rule out the possibility of *cancer*.

Cracked nipples, common in the last months of pregnancy and during breast-feeding, may lead to infective *mastitis*. Washing, drying, and moisturizing the nipple daily can help to prevent cracking.

Papilloma of the nipple is a noncancerous swelling attached to the skin by a stalk. *Paget's disease of the nipple* appears initially as persistent eczema of the nipple and is due to a slow-growing cancer arising in a milk duct. Surgical treatment is required.

Discharge from the nipple occurs for various reasons. A clear, straw-coloured discharge may develop in early pregnancy; a milky discharge may occur after breast-feeding is over. *Galactorrhoea* (milk discharge in someone who is not pregnant or breast-feeding) may be caused by a hormone imbalance, or, rarely, a galactocele (a cyst under the areola). A discharge containing pus indicates a breast *abscess*. A blood-stained discharge may be due to a noncancerous breast disorder or cancer.

nitrate drugs A group of *vasodilator drugs* used to treat *angina pectoris* (chest pain as a result of impaired blood supply) and severe *heart failure* (reduced pumping efficiency of the heart). Two commonly used nitrate drugs are *glyceryl trinitrate* and *isosorbide*.

Possible side effects of nitrate drugs include headache, flushing, and dizziness. *Tolerance* (the need for greater amounts of a drug for it to have the same effect) may develop when the drug is taken regularly.

nitrazepam A *benzodiazepine* drug used in the short-term treatment of *insomnia*. Nitrazepam is long-acting and may cause a hangover, with drowsiness and light-headedness, the following day. Regular use can lead to reduced effectiveness.

Nitrazepam can lead to drug dependence and to withdrawal symptoms, such as nervousness and restlessness.

nitric oxide (NO) A gas that is produced both outside the body as a pollutant (for example, in car exhaust fumes), and inside the body, where it takes the form of a molecule that acts as a messenger between cells. Nitric oxide causes blood vessels to dilate, affecting the flow of oxygenated blood and regulating blood pressure. Overproduction of nitric oxide is associated with various disorders, including *toxic shock, rheumatoid arthritis,* and *diabetes mellitus;* underproduction may cause *impotence* and *angina.* The control of nitric oxide is an important element of many drug treatments.

nitrites Salts of nitrous acid (a nitrogen-containing acid). Sodium nitrite is used in meat preservation. In large amounts, nitrites can cause dizziness, nausea, and vomiting.

nitrofurantoin An *antibacterial drug* that is used in the treatment of *urinary tract infection.* Nitrofurantoin should be taken with food to reduce the risk of stomach irritation, abdominal pain, and nausea. More rarely, breathing difficulty, numbness, and jaundice occur.

nitrogen A colourless, odourless gas that makes up 78 per cent of the Earth's atmosphere. Although nitrogen gas cannot be utilized by the body, compounds of nitrogen, such as *amino acids,* are essential to life.

nitrous oxide (N$_2$O) A colourless gas, sometimes called laughing gas. Nitrous oxide is used with oxygen to provide *analgesia* (pain relief) and light anaesthesia (see *anaesthesia, general*).

Adverse effects of nitrous oxide and oxygen may include nausea and vomiting during the recovery period.

nits The eggs of lice. Both head lice and pubic lice produce eggs, which they stick to the base of hairs. Nits measure only about 0.5 mm in diameter. They are light brown when newly laid, and white when hatched. (See also *lice; pubic lice.*)

nocardiosis An infection caused by a fungus-like bacterium present in soil. The infection, acquired through inhalation, usually starts in the lung and spreads via the bloodstream to the brain and other parts of the body, such as the bones, heart, kidneys, and skin. Nocardiosis is rare except in people with *immunodeficiency disorders* or those already suffering from another serious disease.

The infection causes a pneumonia-like illness, with fever and cough. It fails to respond to short-term, antibiotic treatment, and progressive lung damage occurs. Brain abscesses may follow. Treatment is with *sulphonamide drugs,* often in conjunction with other antibacterial drugs, for example *trimethoprim.*

nocturia The disturbance of sleep at night by the need to pass *urine.*

A common cause of nocturia in men is enlargement of the prostate gland (see *prostate, enlarged*), which obstructs the normal outflow of urine and causes the *bladder* to empty incompletely. In women, a common cause is *cystitis* (inflammation of the bladder), in which irritation of the bladder wall increases its sensitivity so that smaller volumes of urine trigger a desire to urinate. Other causes of nocturia include *diabetes mellitus, heart failure* (reduced pumping efficiency), chronic *kidney failure,* and *diabetes insipidus.*

nocturnal emission Ejaculation that occurs during sleep, commonly called a 'wet dream'. Nocturnal emission is normal in male adolescents.

node A small, rounded mass of tissue. The term most commonly refers to a *lymph node,* a normal structure in the lymphatic system. (See also *nodule.*)

nodule A small lump of tissue. A nodule may protrude from the skin's surface or form deep under the skin. Nodules may be either hard or soft.

noise Any sound, particularly one that is disordered and irregular, that is unwanted or interferes with the ability to hear. (See also noise-induced hearing loss.)

noise-induced hearing loss Hearing loss caused by prolonged exposure to excessive noise or by brief exposure to intensely loud noise.

Exposure to a sudden, very loud noise, above about 120 decibels, can cause immediate and permanent damage to *hearing.* Normally, muscles in the middle *ear* respond to loud noise by altering the position of the ossicles (the chain of bones that pass vibrations to the inner ear), thus damping down the intensity of the noise. If these protective reflexes have no time to respond, the full force of the vibrations is carried to the inner ear, severely damaging the delicate hair cells in the cochlea. Occasionally, loud noises can rupture the *eardrum.*

N

NOISE-INDUCED HEARING LOSS

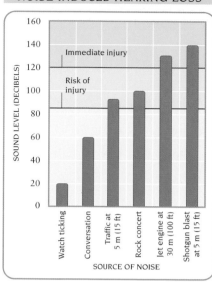

RISK OF NOISE-INDUCED HEARING LOSS

Noise damage also occurs over a period of time by prolonged exposure to lower levels of noise. Any noise above 85–90 decibels may cause damage, with gradual destruction of the hair cells of the cochlea, leading to permanent hearing loss. Prolonged exposure to loud noise causes an inability to hear certain high tones. Later, deafness extends to all high frequencies, and perception of speech is impaired. Eventually, lower tones are also affected.

Sounds at 85–90 decibels or above may cause pain and temporary deafness. Prolonged *tinnitus* (ringing or buzzing in the ears) occurring after a noise has ceased is an indication that some damage has probably occurred.

noma The death of tissue in the lips and cheeks due to bacterial infection. Also called cancrum oris, it is largely confined to young, severely malnourished children in developing countries. Noma can also occur in the last stages of *leukaemia*.

Without treatment, noma causes severe ulceration, eventual destruction of the bones around the mouth, and loss of teeth. Healing occurs naturally, but scarring may be severe.

Antibacterial drugs and improved nutrition halt the progress of the disease.

nonaccidental injury See *child abuse*.

nongonococcal urethritis Formerly known as nonspecific urethritis, inflammation of the urethra due to a cause other than gonorrhoea. Worldwide, nongonococcal urethritis is a very common type of sexually transmitted infection.

Almost 50 per cent of cases are known to be caused by CHLAMYDIA TRACHOMATIS (see *chlamydial infections*); others are caused by the virus that causes *herpes simplex*, TRICHOMONAS VAGINALIS infections (see *trichomoniasis*), or other microorganisms. In the remainder of cases, the cause remains unknown.

In men, the infection usually causes a clear or a purulent urethral discharge, often accompanied by pain or discomfort on passing urine. The equivalent condition in women, called nonspecific genital infection, may not cause symptoms unless there are complications.

Treatment may be difficult if the cause of symptoms cannot be determined. *Antibiotic drugs*, such as doxycycline and *azithromycin*, are given. Follow-up visits may be advised after treatment, and *contact tracing* is essential.

In men, *epididymitis*, *prostatitis* and *urethral stricture* (narrowing of the urethra) can occur as complications of nongonococcal urethritis. *Reiter's syndrome* (in which there is arthritis and conjunctivitis as well as urethritis) may also occur as a complication in some men.

In women, *pelvic inflammatory disease* and cysts of the *Bartholin's glands* may occur. *Ophthalmia neonatorum*, a type of conjunctivitis, sometimes develops in babies born to women with chlamydial cervicitis.

noninvasive A term used to describe any medical procedure that does not involve penetration of the skin or entry into the body through any of the natural openings. Examples include *CT scanning* and *echocardiography*. The term noninvasive is sometimes also applied to noncancerous tumours that do not spread throughout body tissues.

nonoxinol 9 A *spermicide* used in contraceptive preparations such as gels, foams, and creams.

nonspecific urethritis See *nongonococcal urethritis.*

nonsteroidal anti-inflammatory drugs
A group of drugs, also known as NSAIDs, that produce *analgesia* (pain relief) and reduce inflammation in joints and soft tissues such as muscles and ligaments. NSAIDs are among the most widely used of all drugs; common examples include *aspirin, diclofenac, diflunisal, ibuprofen, indometacin, ketoprofen, mefenamic acid, naproxen, piroxicam,* and *sulindac.* The *COX-2 inhibitor drugs,* such as *celecoxib,* are also classed as NSAIDs. The analgesic *paracetamol* is not classed as an NSAID as it has no anti-inflammatory effect.

NSAIDs are used to relieve symptoms caused by types of arthritis, such as *rheumatoid arthritis, osteoarthritis,* and *gout.* They are also used in the treatment of back pain, menstrual pain, dental pain, headaches, pain after minor surgery, and soft tissue injuries, such as sprains and strains.

The drugs reduce pain and inflammation by blocking the production of *prostaglandins* (chemicals that cause inflammation and trigger transmission of pain signals to the brain).

NSAIDs may cause a wide range of side effects, including nausea, indigestion, bleeding from the stomach and sometimes *peptic ulcer.* In general, the risk of side effects occurring is greater in the elderly. It is advisable to take the lowest effective dose of an NSAID for the shortest time possible. NSAIDs should not be used by people who have had a previous reaction to them (for example, *asthma, rhinitis,* or rash) nor by those who have or have had a peptic ulcer. Some NSAIDs have particular risks; see individual drug entries for specific risks and precautions.

NSAIDS may also interact with other drugs, such as anticoagulants, and medical advice should therefore be sought before taking an NSAID with a prescribed medication.

noradrenaline Also known as norepinephrine, a *hormone* secreted by certain nerve endings (principally those of the *sympathetic nervous system*) and by the medulla (centre) of the *adrenal glands.* Noradrenaline's primary function is to help maintain a constant blood pressure

by way of stimulating certain blood vessels to constrict (narrow) when the blood pressure falls. For this reason, it may sometimes be injected in the emergency treatment of *shock* or severe bleeding. (See also *adrenaline.*)

norepinephrine An alternative term for *noradrenaline.*

norethisterone A *progestogen drug* used primarily in some *oral contraceptives.* Norethisterone is sometimes prescribed to postpone menstruation. It is also used to treat menstrual disorders such as *menorrhagia, endometriosis,* and certain types of *breast cancer.* It is occasionally given by injection as a long-acting contraceptive. Possible side effects include swollen ankles, weight gain, depression and, rarely, jaundice.

nose The uppermost part of the respiratory tract, and the organ of *smell.* The nose is an air passage connecting the nostrils at its front to the *nasopharynx* (the upper part of the throat) at its rear. The *nasal septum,* which is made of cartilage at the front and bone at the rear, divides the passage into two chambers.

The bridge of the nose is formed from two small nasal bones and from cartilage. The roof of the nasal passage is formed by bones at the base of the skull; the walls by the maxilla (upper jaw); and the floor by the hard palate. Three conchae (thin, downward-curving plates of bone) covered with *mucous membrane* project from each wall.

Air-filled, mucous membrane-lined cavities known as paranasal sinuses open into the nasal passage. There is an opening in each wall to the nasolacrimal duct, which drains away tears. Projecting into the roof of the nasal passage are the hair-like endings of the olfactory nerves, which are responsible for the sense of smell.

A main function of the nose is to filter, warm, and moisten inhaled air before it passes into the rest of the respiratory tract. Just inside the nostrils, small hairs trap large dust particles and foreign bodies. Smaller dust particles are filtered from the air by the microscopic hairs of the conchae. The mucus on the conchae flows inwards, carrying microorganisms and other foreign bodies back towards the nasopharynx to be swallowed and destroyed in the stomach.

The nose detects smells by means of the olfactory nerve endings, which, when stimulated by inhaled vapours, transmit this information to the olfactory bulb in the brain.

The nose is susceptible to a wide range of disorders. Allergies (see *rhinitis, allergic*), infections such as colds (see *cold, common*), and small *boils* are common. Backward spread of infection from the nose occasionally causes a serious condition called *cavernous sinus thrombosis*. The nose is also particularly prone to injury (see *nosebleed; nose, broken*). Obstruction of the nose may be caused by a nasal *polyp* (a projection of swollen mucous membrane).

Noncancerous tumours of blood vessels, known as *haemangiomas*, commonly affect the nasal cavity in babies. *Basal cell carcinoma* and *squamous cell carcinoma* may occur around the nostril. The nose may also be invaded by cancers originating in the sinuses.

nosebleed Loss of blood from the mucous membrane that lines the nose. The most common causes of a nosebleed are fragile blood vessels, a blow to the nose, or the dislodging of crusts that have formed in the mucous membrane as a result of a common cold or infection. Rarely, recurrent nosebleeds are a sign of an underlying disorder, such as *hypertension* (high blood pressure), a bleeding disorder, or a tumour of the nose or paranasal sinuses.

nose, broken Fracture of the nasal bones or dislocation of the cartilage that forms the bridge of the *nose*. The fracture is usually accompanied by severe swelling of overlying soft tissue. A fractured nose is painful and remains tender for about 3 weeks after injury.

Resetting is usually carried out either before the swelling has started, or when it has subsided, usually about 10 days after the injury. Occasionally, a displaced bridge can be manipulated into position under a local anaesthetic, but, usually, a general anaesthetic is needed. A plaster splint is sometimes required during healing.

nose reshaping See *rhinoplasty*.

nosocomial A term meaning associated with hospitals. A nosocomial infection is one acquired by a patient in hospital.

notifiable diseases Medical conditions that must be reported to the local health authorities. Notification of certain potentially harmful infectious diseases enables health officers to monitor and control the spread of infection.

Examples of notifiable infectious diseases are *food poisoning*, viral *hepatitis*, *measles*, *malaria*, *tetanus*, *tuberculosis*, and *pertussis* (whooping cough).

Some categories of diseases other than infections must also be reported. These include certain *birth defects* and forms of *learning difficulties*. Cancers are registered nationally, and cancer data is now pooled in an international registry.

Certain types of *occupational disease* are also reportable; examples include *lead poisoning*, *mercury poisoning*, *cadmium poisoning*, and *anthrax*. (See also *prescribed diseases*.)

NSAID Abbreviation for *nonsteroidal anti-inflammatory drugs*.

NSU An abbreviation for nonspecific urethritis, the former term for *nongonococcal urethritis*.

nuchal scan *Ultrasound scanning* performed in early pregnancy in order to identify fetuses at high risk of *chromosomal abnormalities* such as *Down's syndrome*. The scan investigates the nuchal fold, an area of skin at the back of the neck. The amount of fluid under the nuchal fold is measured as it is an indicator of a possible chromosomal abnormality.

nuclear energy The energy released as a result of changes in the nuclei of atoms. It is also known as atomic energy and is principally released in the form of heat, light, and ionizing *radiation*.

nuclear magnetic resonance See *MRI*.

nucleic acids Substances found in all living matter that have a fundamental role in the propagation of life. Nucleic acids provide the inherited coded instructions (or "blueprint") for an organism's development.

There are two types of nucleic acid: deoxyribonucleic acid (*DNA*) and ribonucleic acid (*RNA*). In all plant and animal cells, including human cells, DNA permanently holds the coded instructions, which are translated and implemented by RNA. DNA is the main constituent of *chromosomes*, which are carried in the nucleus (central unit) of the cell.

DNA and RNA are similar in structure, both comprising long, chain-like molecules. However, DNA usually consists of two intertwined chains, whereas RNA is generally single-stranded.

The basic structure of DNA is like a rope ladder, the chains forming the two sides, with interlinking structures in between forming the rungs. The ladder is twisted into a spiral shape called a double helix.

Each DNA chain has a "backbone" consisting of a string of sugar and phosphate chemical groups. Attached to each sugar is a chemical called a base, which can be any of four types (adenine, thymine, guanine, and cytosine) and forms half a rung of the DNA ladder. The four bases can occur in any sequence along the chain. The sequence, which may be millions of individual bases long, provides the code for the cell's activities (see *genetic code*).

RNA is like a single strand of DNA, the main difference is that the base thymine is replaced by another base, uracil.

DNA controls a cell's activities by specifying and regulating the synthesis of *enzymes* and other proteins in the cell. Different *genes* (sections of DNA that code for information) regulate the production of different proteins. For a particular protein to be made, an appropriate section of DNA acts as a template for an RNA chain. This "messenger" RNA then passes out of the nucleus into the cell cytoplasm, where it is decoded to form proteins (see *genetic code*; *protein synthesis*).

When a cell undergoes mitotic (see *mitosis*) division, identical copies of its DNA must go to each of the two daughter cells. The two DNA chains separate, and two more chains are formed beside the original chains. Because only certain base pairings are possible, the new double chains are identical to the original DNA molecule. Each of a person's cells carries the same DNA replica that was present in the fertilized ovum, so the DNA message passes from one generation of cells to the next.

nucleus The central core, structure, or focal point of an object.

The nucleus of a living *cell* is a roughly spherical unit at the centre of the cell. It contains the *chromosomes* (composed mainly of *nucleic acid*), which are responsible for directing the cell's activities, and is surrounded by a membrane. The membrane has small pores through which various substances can pass between the nucleus and the cytoplasm, a thick fluid that forms the bulk of the cell. Usually, the nucleus has one nucleolus, a smaller dense region with no membrane that is concerned with protein manufacture.

NUCLEUS

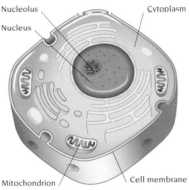

Nucleolus Cytoplasm
Nucleus
Mitochondrion Cell membrane

TYPICAL HUMAN CELL

A nerve nucleus is a group of *neurons* (nerve cells) within the brain and spinal cord that work together to perform a particular function.

The nucleus of an atom, composed of protons and neutrons, accounts for almost the total mass of the atom but only a tiny proportion of its volume. *Nuclear energy* is produced through changes in atomic nuclei.

numbness Loss of sensation in part of the body caused by interference with the passage of impulses along sensory *nerves*. Numbness may be the result of a disorder of or damage to the *nervous system* or its blood supply.

Multiple sclerosis can cause loss of sensation in any part of the body through damage to nerve pathways in the central nervous system (CNS). In a *neuropathy*, the peripheral nerves (nerves outside the CNS) are damaged. In a *stroke*, pressure on, or reduced blood supply to, nerve pathways in the brain often causes loss of feeling on one side of the body.

Severe cold causes numbness by direct action on the nerves. Numbness may also be a feature of psychological disorders, such as *anxiety, panic attack*, or a hysterical *conversion disorder*.

Treatment of numbness depends on the underlying cause.

nutrient An essential dietary factor, including carbohydrates, proteins, certain fats, vitamins, and minerals.

nutrition The scientific study of food and the processes by which it is digested and assimilated.

A good diet supplies adequate but not excessive quantities of *proteins, carbohydrates, fats, vitamins, minerals*, dietary *fibre*, and water. The daily diet should include foods from each of the four main food groups: milk and milk products; vegetables and fruits; breads and cereals; meat, eggs, and pulses. Vitamin and mineral supplements are of unproven value in most otherwise healthy people and may be harmful if excessive amounts are taken. However, specific supplements may be recommended for certain groups, such as infants and women who are pregnant or planning a pregnancy.

Personal requirements of nutrients and *energy* vary, depending on individual body size, age, sex, and lifestyle (notably, activity level). For example, an average woman requires about 2,000 kcal (8,400 kJ) daily, compared with about 2,500 kcal (10,500 kJ) for an average man. (See also *energy requirements*.)

nutritional disorders Nutritional disorders may be caused by a deficiency or excess of one or more *nutrients*, or by the presence of a *toxin* (poisonous element) in the diet.

A diet deficient in *carbohydrates* is almost inevitably also deficient in *protein*, leading to protein–calorie malnutrition. Such malnutrition is most often seen as a result of severe poverty and famine (see *kwashiorkor; marasmus*).

Inadequate intake of protein and calories may also occur in people who excessively restrict their diet to lose weight (see *anorexia nervosa*), hold mistaken beliefs about diet and health (see *food fad*), or suffer from a loss of interest in food associated with *alcohol dependence* or *drug dependence*.

Deficiency of specific nutrients is commonly associated with a disorder of the digestive system, such as *coeliac disease*, *Crohn's disease*, or pernicious anaemia (see *anaemia, megaloblastic*).

Obesity results from taking in more *energy* from the diet than is used up by the body. Nutritional disorders may also result from an excessive intake of *minerals* and *vitamins*. An excessive intake of saturated fat is thought to be a contributory factor in *coronary artery disease* and in some forms of *cancer*.

Naturally occurring toxins can interfere with the digestion, absorption, and/or utilization of nutrients, or can cause specific disorders due to their toxic effects: for example, the *ergot* fungus found on rye can cause ergotism.

nystagmus A condition in which there is involuntary movement of the eyes.

In the most common type, jerky nystagmus, the eyes repeatedly move slowly in one direction and then rapidly in the other. Less commonly, nystagmus is "pendular", with the eyes moving evenly from side to side.

Nystagmus may be congenital, in which case the cause is unknown. It also occurs in *albinism* and as a result of any very severe defect of vision present at birth, such as congenital *cataract*.

Persistent nystagmus appearing later in life usually indicates a nervous system disorder (such as *multiple sclerosis*, a *brain tumour*, or an *alcohol-related disorder*), or a disorder of the balancing mechanism in the inner ear. Adult-onset nystagmus is occasionally seen as an occupational disorder in people who work in poor light.

Electronystagmography, a method of recording eye movements, may be used to identify the type of nystagmus.

nystatin An *antifungal drug* used in the treatment of *candidiasis* (thrush). Nystatin may be safely used during pregnancy. High doses taken by mouth may cause diarrhoea, nausea, vomiting, and abdominal pain.

oat cell carcinoma A form of *lung cancer*, also known as *small cell carcinoma*.

obesity A condition of excess fat accumulation in the body. An adult with a *body mass index* (BMI) between 25 and 29.9 is classed as overweight; a BMI between 30 and 39.9 as obese; and a BMI over 40 as very obese. About 2 in 5 adults in the UK are overweight and a further 1 in 5 is obese or very obese. Childhood obesity is an increasing problem, with an estimated 1 in 6 children being overweight, obese, or very obese.

Obesity is caused by consuming more calories than are expended. A person's calorie (energy) requirements are determined by metabolic rate (see *metabolism*) and level of physical activity. Family history is sometimes a factor in becoming obese. Obesity may also be associated with some hormonal disorders, although these are not generally the cause.

Obesity increases the risk of *hypertension*, *stroke*, and type 2 *diabetes mellitus*. *Coronary artery disease* is more common in obese people, particularly in obese men under 40. Obesity in men is also associated with increased risk of cancer of the colon, rectum, and prostate, and, in women, of the breast, uterus, and cervix. Extra weight may also aggravate some existing conditions, such as *osteoarthritis*.

The first line of treatment is education in healthy eating habits and diet, plus regular exercise (see *weight reduction*). Drugs that reduce fat absorption (such as *orlistat*) or appetite suppressants (such as *sibutramine*) may be used as part of treatment in suitable patients. *Wiring of the jaws*, stapling of the stomach, and intestinal bypass operations are attempted only if obesity is seriously endangering a person's health.

obsessive-compulsive disorder A psychiatric condition in which a person is dogged by persistent ideas (obsessions) that lead to repetitive, ritualized acts (compulsions). Obsessions are commonly based on fears about security or becoming infected. In obsessional rumination, there is constant brooding over a word, phrase, or unanswerable problem. Compulsions may occur frequently enough to disrupt work and social life. The disorder is often accompanied by *depression* and *anxiety*. If severe, a person may become housebound.

The disorder usually starts in adolescence. Genetic factors, an obsessive personality, or a tendency to neurotic symptoms may contribute. Some types of brain damage, especially in *encephalitis*, can cause obsessional symptoms.

Many sufferers respond well to *behaviour therapy*, which may be combined with *antidepressant drugs*, but symptoms may recur under stress.

obstetrics The branch of medicine concerned with *pregnancy* and *antenatal care*, *childbirth*, and *postnatal care*. It is also the study of the structure and function of the female *reproductive system*. (See also *gynaecology*.)

obstructive airways disease See *pulmonary disease, chronic obstructive*.

occiput The lower back part of the head, where it merges with the neck.

occlusion Blockage of a passage, canal, opening, or vessel in the body. This may be due to disease (for example, a *pulmonary embolism*) or medically induced. Occlusion also describes eye-patching for *amblyopia*, and the relationship between the upper and lower teeth when the jaw is shut. (See also *malocclusion*.)

occult Hidden or obscure, such as occult blood in a sample of faeces.

occult blood, faecal The presence in the faeces of blood that cannot be seen by the naked eye, but can be detected by chemical tests. Such tests may be used in screening for cancer of the colon (see *colon, cancer of*) or rectum (see *rectum, cancer of*). Faecal occult blood may also be a sign of a gastrointestinal disorder such as *oesophagitis*, *gastritis*, or *stomach cancer*, cancer of the intestine (see *intestine, cancer of*); *diverticular disease*; *polyps* in the colon; *ulcerative colitis*, or irritation of the stomach or intestine by drugs such as aspirin. (See also *rectal bleeding*.)

occupational disease and injury Illnesses, disorders, or injuries that result from exposure to chemicals or dust, or are due to physical, psychological, or biological factors in the workplace.

Pneumoconiosis is *fibrosis* of the lung due to inhalation of industrial dusts, such as coal. *Asbestosis* is associated with asbestos in industry, and allergic *alveolitis* is caused by organic dusts (see *farmer's lung*).

Industrial chemicals can damage the lungs if inhaled, or other major organs if they enter the bloodstream via the lungs or skin. Examples include fumes of cadmium, beryllium, lead, and benzene. Carbon tetrachloride and vinyl chloride are causes of liver disease. Many of these compounds can cause kidney damage.

Work-related skin disorders include contact *dermatitis* and *squamous cell carcinoma*. Rare infectious diseases that are more common in certain jobs include *brucellosis* and *Q fever* (from livestock), *psittacosis* (from birds), and *leptospirosis* (from sewage). People who work with blood or blood products are at increased risk of viral hepatitis (see *hepatitis, viral*) and *AIDS*, as are healthcare professionals. The nuclear industry and some healthcare professions use measures to reduce the danger from *radiation hazards*.

Other occupational disorders include *writer's cramp*, *carpal tunnel syndrome*, *singer's nodes*, *Raynaud's phenomenon*, *deafness*, and *cataracts*.

occupational medicine A branch of medicine dealing with the effects of various occupations on health, and with an individual's capacity for particular types of work. It includes prevention of *occupational disease and injury* and the promotion of health in the working population. *Epidemiology* is used to analyse patterns of sickness absence, injury, illness, and death. Clinical techniques are used to monitor the health of a particular workforce. Assessment of psychological stress and hazards of new technology are part of the remit. Occupational health risks are reduced by dust control, appropriate waste disposal, use of safe work stations and practices, limiting exposure to harmful substances, and health screening.

occupational mortality Death due to work-related disease or injuries. Annual occupational mortality rates are usually expressed as number of deaths per million at risk.

occupational therapy Treatment comprising individually tailored programmes of activities that help people who have been disabled by illness or accident to improve their function and ability to carry out everyday tasks. Occupational therapy also involves recommending aids and changes to the home that help to increase the person's independence.

octreotide A *somatostatin analogue*, a hormone that acts on the *pituitary gland*. Given by injection, octreotide is used mainly in the treatment of *acromegaly* and hormone-secreting intestinal tumours. Octreotide is also used to prevent complications following pancreatic surgery. Side effects may include various gastrointestinal disturbances such as nausea, vomiting, abdominal pain and bloating, flatulence, and diarrhoea.

ocular Relating to or affecting the *eye* and its structures; also the eyepiece of an optical device, such as a *microscope*.

oculogyric crisis A state of gaze in which the eyes are fixed, usually upwards, for minutes or hours. The crisis may be associated with muscle spasm of the tongue, mouth, and neck, and is often triggered by stress. It may also occur following *encephalitis* and in *parkinsonism*, or may be induced by drugs, such as *phenothiazine* derivatives.

oculomotor nerve The 3rd *cranial nerve*, controlling most of the muscles that move the eye. This nerve also supplies the muscle that constricts the pupil, that which raises the upper eyelid, and the ciliary muscle, which focuses the eye. The nerve may be damaged due to a fracture to the base of the skull or a tumour. Symptoms include *ptosis*, *squint*, dilation of the pupil, inability to focus the eye, double vision, and slight protrusion of the eyeball. (See also *trochlear nerve*; *abducent nerve*.)

oedema Abnormal fluid accumulation in body tissues that may be localized (as in swelling from an injury) or generalized (as in *heart failure*). Symptoms of generalized oedema, such as swelling around the base of the spine and in the

0

ankles, occur when excess body fluid increases by more than 15 per cent. In severe cases, fluid accumulates in large body cavities, such as the peritoneal cavity of the abdomen in *ascites* or the pleural cavity of the lungs in *pleural effusion*. In *pulmonary oedema*, the air sacs of the lungs become waterlogged.

Causes include heart failure, *kidney failure*, and *nephrotic syndrome*. Often, the underlying cause of oedema cannot be treated. Treatment is focused on increasing urine output by restricting salt intake and using *diuretic drugs*.

Oedipus complex A psychoanalytic term that describes the unconscious sexual attachment of a child for the parent of the opposite sex, and the consequent jealousy of, and desire to eliminate, the parent of the same sex.

oesophageal atresia A rare *birth defect* in which the oesophagus forms into two separate, blind-ended sections during development. There is usually an abnormal channel (*tracheoesophageal fistula*) between one of the sections and the trachea. The condition may be suspected before birth if the mother had *polyhydramnios*. The infant cannot swallow, and drools and regurgitates milk continually. If there is an upper tracheoesophageal fistula, milk may be sucked into the lungs, provoking attacks of coughing and *cyanosis*. Immediate surgery is needed to join the blind ends of the oesophagus and close the fistula. If the operation is successful, the baby should develop normally. Some babies, however, do not survive.

oesophageal dilatation A procedure to stretch the *oesophagus* when it has been narrowed by disease (see *oesophageal stricture*) and swallowing is difficult. *Endoscopy* is used to locate the obstruction. The narrowed area is then stretched by passing bougies (cylindrical rods with olive-shaped tips) down the oesophagus, or by using *balloon catheters*.

oesophageal diverticulum A sac-like protrusion of part of the *oesophagus* wall in which food becomes trapped, causing irritation, difficulty swallowing, *halitosis*, and regurgitation. A diverticulum is usually removed surgically.

oesophageal spasm Uncoordinated muscle contractions in the *oesophagus*, which cause intermittent swallowing difficulties and chest or upper abdominal pain. The spasm may be caused by reflux *oesophagitis*, but often occurs for no apparent reason. Women are more commonly affected. A barium swallow (see *barium X-ray examinations*) and *endoscopy* may be used to rule out a more serious condition, such as cancer. Treatment is of the underlying cause.

oesophageal speech A technique for producing speech after surgical removal of the *larynx* (see *laryngectomy*). Air is trapped in the *oesophagus* and is gradually expelled while the tongue, palate, and lips form distinguishable sounds.

oesophageal stricture Narrowing of the *oesophagus* that may cause pain, swallowing difficulties, weight loss, and regurgitation of food. It may be due to cancer (see *oesophagus, cancer of*) or, for example, persistent reflux *oesophagitis*. Diagnosis may include a barium swallow (see *barium X-ray examinations*), *endoscopy*, and *biopsy*. Usually, the narrowed area is widened by *oesophageal dilatation*.

oesophageal varices Widened veins in the walls of the lower *oesophagus* and, sometimes, the upper part of the stomach. Varices develop as a consequence of *portal hypertension*. Blood in the portal vein, passing from the intestines to the liver, meets resistance due to liver disease. The increased blood pressure causes blood to be diverted into small veins in the walls of the oesophagus and stomach. These veins may become distended and rupture, causing vomiting of blood and black faeces. There are usually other symptoms of chronic liver disease.

To control acute bleeding, a *balloon catheter* may be passed into the oesophagus to press on the bleeding varices. The varices may be treated with an intravenous injection of *vasopressin* and/or by injection, via an *endoscope*, of a sclerosant that seals off the affected veins.

oesophagitis Inflammation of the *oesophagus*. In corrosive oesophagitis, which is caused by swallowing caustic chemicals such as cleaning fluids, there is immediate severe pain and swelling in the throat and mouth. Antidotes are of limited value, and washing out the stomach (see *lavage, gastric*) increases the damage. Treatment consists mainly of reducing pain and providing nursing care until the oesophagus heals.

Reflux oesophagitis is due to poor function of muscles in the lower oesophagus, which permits the stomach's acidic contents to rise back into the oesophagus (see *gastro-oesophageal reflux disease*). The main symptom, heartburn, may be worsened by alcohol, smoking, and obesity. Poor function of the lower oesophagus may be linked with a *hiatus hernia*. In mild cases, treatment focuses on diet and lifestyle changes; *antacid drugs* may help reduce acidity. In moderate or severe cases, H_2-*receptor antagonists* or *proton pump inhibitors*, which greatly reduce gastric acid, may be used. Surgical treatment may be necessary for a hiatus hernia.

Barrett's oesophagus, a complication of reflux oesophagitis, may lead to cancer. Severe, chronic oesophagitis can cause an *oesophageal stricture*.

oesophagogastroduodenoscopy An examination of the upper digestive tract using an *endoscope* (see *gastroscopy*).

oesophagogastroscopy Examination of the *oesophagus* and stomach using an *endoscope* (see *gastroscopy*).

oesophagoscopy *Endoscopic* examination of the *oesophagus* (see *gastroscopy*).

oesophagus The muscular tube that carries food to the stomach; a part of the digestive tract (see *digestive system*). The top end has a sphincter muscle that opens to allow the passage of food; a similar sphincter operates where the oesophagus joins the stomach. *Peristalsis* propels food and liquids down towards the stomach and intestines for digestion. (See also *swallowing*.)

oesophagus, cancer of A malignant tumour, most common in people over 50, that mainly affects the middle or lower *oesophagus* and leads to swallowing difficulties. Smoking and heavy alcohol intake are risk factors.

Symptoms progressively worsen to a point where food is immediately regurgitated and there is rapid weight loss. Regurgitated fluid spilling into the *trachea* often causes respiratory infections.

Diagnosis is with a barium swallow (see *barium X-ray examinations*) and a *biopsy*

taken during *endoscopy*. Removal of the oesophagus may be possible in some cases. *Radiotherapy* may cause regression of the cancer, relieve symptoms, and occasionally cure older patients who might not survive major surgery. Insertion of a rigid tube through the tumour, or laser treatment to burn through it, can help to relieve symptoms and improve nutrition. The overall outlook is poor, but is improved with early diagnosis.

oesophagus, disorders of Several disorders, most of which cause swallowing difficulties and/or chest pain.

Infections of the oesophagus are rare but may occur in immunosuppressed patients. The most common infections are *herpes simplex* and *candidiasis* (thrush). *Oesophagitis* is usually due to reflux of stomach contents, causing heartburn. Corrosive oesophagitis can occur as a result of swallowing caustic chemicals. Both may cause an *oesophageal stricture*.

Congenital defects include *oesophageal atresia*, which requires surgery soon after birth. Tumours of the oesophagus are quite common; about 90 per cent are cancerous (see *oesophagus, cancer of*). Injury to the oesophagus is most commonly caused by a tear or rupture due to severe vomiting and retching. (See also *swallowing difficulty*.)

OESOPHAGUS

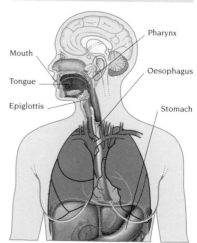

Pharynx

Mouth

Oesophagus

Tongue

Epiglottis

Stomach

oestradiol See *estradiol.*

oestriol See *estriol.*

oestrogen drugs A group of synthetically produced drugs that are used in *oral contraceptives* and to supplement or replace the body's own *oestrogen hormones.* Oestrogen drugs are often used together with *progestogen drugs.*

Oestrogens suppress the production of *gonadotrophin hormones,* which stimulate cell activity in the *ovaries.* Oestrogen drugs may be used to treat, or sometimes prevent, menopausal symptoms and disorders. Oestrogens may also be used to treat certain forms of *infertility,* female *hypogonadism,* abnormal menstrual bleeding, and prostatic cancer (see *prostate, cancer of*).

Oestrogens may cause breast tenderness and enlargement, bloating, weight gain, nausea, reduced sex drive, depression, migraine, and bleeding between periods. Side effects often subside after 2 or 3 months. The drugs can increase the risk of abnormal blood clotting (see *thrombosis, deep vein*), *breast cancer,* uterine cancer (see *uterus, cancer of*), *stroke,* and susceptibility to high blood pressure (see *hypertension*). Oestrogen drugs should not be taken in pregnancy as they may adversely affect the fetus.

oestrogen hormones A group of hormones that are essential for normal female sexual development and healthy functioning of the reproductive system. In women, they are produced mainly in the *ovaries* and also in the *placenta* in pregnancy. Small amounts are produced in the *adrenal glands* in both men and women, but oestrogens have no known specific function in men. When levels are low, oestrogen hormones can be replaced with *oestrogen drugs.*

oestrone See *estrone.*

ofloxacin A *quinolone* antibiotic used to treat skin, soft tissue, and lower *respiratory tract* and *urinary tract infections.* Ofloxacin is usually taken in tablet form to treat infections that have not responded to treatment with other drugs but is also given by intravenous infusion to treat severe *systemic* infections. Side effects may include nausea, vomiting, diarrhoea, and abdominal pain.

oils See *fats and oils.*

ointment A greasy preparation used as a vehicle to apply drugs in dry skin conditions such as *eczema* or to protect or lubricate the skin.

olanzapine An *antipsychotic drug* used for the treatment of *schizophrenia, mania,* and to prevent recurrence of *bipolar disorder.*

olecranon In the arm, the bony projection at the upper end of the *ulna* that forms the point of the elbow.

olfactory nerve The 1st *cranial nerve,* which conveys sensations of smell as nerve impulses from the nose to the brain. Each of the two olfactory nerves has receptors in the mucous membrane lining the nasal cavity. These receptors detect smells and send signals along nerve fibres, which pass through tiny holes in the roof of the nasal cavity and combine to form the olfactory bulbs. From here, nerve fibres come together to form the olfactory nerve, leading to the olfactory centre in the brain. Sense of smell may be lost or impaired due to damage to the olfactory nerves, usually as a result of head injury.

OLFACTORY NERVE

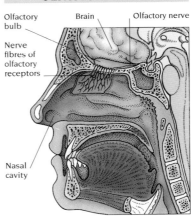

Olfactory bulb — Brain — Olfactory nerve

Nerve fibres of olfactory receptors

Nasal cavity

oligo- A prefix meaning few, scanty or little, as in *oligospermia* (too few *sperm* in the *semen*).

oligodendroglioma A rare and slow-growing type of primary *brain tumour* mainly affecting young or middle-aged adults. Surgical removal of the tumour can, in some cases, lead to a total cure.

oligohydramnios A rare condition in pregnancy in which there is insufficient *amniotic fluid* surrounding the fetus in the uterus.

oligospermia A temporary or permanent deficiency in the number of *sperm* in the *semen*. Oligospermia is a major cause of *infertility*, especially when other disorders of the sperm are also present.

Normally, there are more than 20 million sperm per millilitre of semen. A low sperm count can be due to various disorders, including *orchitis*, undescended testis (see *testis, undescended*), and, infrequently, a *varicocele* (varicose vein of the testis). Smoking, alcohol abuse, stress, and some drugs may cause temporary oligospermia. Treatment is for the underlying cause. If the cause is unknown, *gonadotrophin hormones* may be prescribed. (See also *azoospermia*.)

oliguria The production of low quantities of *urine* in proportion to the volume of fluid taken in. The condition may be caused by excessive sweating; in some cases, it is a sign of *kidney failure*.

olive oil An oil, obtained from the fruit of the olive tree *OLEA EUROPAEA*, that may be used to soften earwax or to treat *cradle cap* in babies.

-oma A suffix denoting a tumour, which may be cancerous or noncancerous, as in *lipoma* and *carcinoma*.

omega-3 fatty acids A group of *fatty acids* (constituents of fats and oils) that are vital for many body functions, including nerve function, immune system function, and fat transport. They cannot be made by the body and must be obtained from the diet. Good sources of omega-3 fatty acids include fish such as sardines, herring, mackerel, trout, and salmon, soya bean oil, and rapeseed oil. Omega-3 fatty acids are thought to help reduce blood lipid levels, blood pressure, and the risk of cardiovascular disease. They may also help brain development in children. Pregnant and breast-feeding women may be advised to have an adequate intake of omega-3 fatty acids to support development of the baby's brain. Omega-3 fatty acids are sometimes prescribed as part of treatment to lower blood lipid levels.

omentum A double fold of fatty membrane hanging in front of the intestines.

omeprazole A drug that is used to treat *peptic ulcer*, reflux *oesophagitis*, and *Zollinger-Ellison syndrome*. Adverse effects include rashes, headache, nausea, diarrhoea, and constipation.

omphalocele An alternative name for *exomphalos*.

onchocerciasis A tropical disease, also called river blindness, caused by the worm *ONCHOCERCA VOLVULUS*. The disease is a type of *filariasis* transmitted by simulium flies. The worms' dead larvae can lead to blindness if they cause an allergic reaction in or near the eyes. Treatment is with *anthelmintic drugs*.

oncogenes Genes found in every cell that control growth, repair, and replacement. Abnormalities of oncogenes are known to be a factor in the development of cancerous cells. *Mutations* in oncogenes, resulting from damage by *carcinogens*, can cause a cell to grow unrestrainedly and infiltrate and destroy normal tissues (see *cancer*). Factors known to cause cancer include ultraviolet light, radioactivity, tobacco, alcohol, asbestos, some chemicals, and certain viruses.

oncology The study of the causes, development, characteristics, and treatment of tumours, particularly cancers.

ondansetron A *serotonin antagonist* drug used to control nausea and vomiting following an operation or induced by *radiotherapy* or *anticancer drugs*. It is taken as tablets, syrup, or suppositories, or given by injection. Side effects may include constipation, headache, and hiccups.

onychogryphosis Abnormal thickening, hardening, and curving of the nails that occurs mainly in elderly people. Onychogryphosis may be associated with *fungal infection* or poor circulation.

onycholysis Separation of the nail from its bed: a feature of many skin conditions, including *psoriasis* and *dermatitis*.

oophorectomy Removal of the *ovaries*, usually to treat *ovarian cysts* or cancer (see *ovary, cancer of*). A partial oophorectomy may be performed to preserve ovarian function in women under 40. In a *hysterectomy*, both ovaries may be removed if disease has spread from the

OPERATING THEATRE

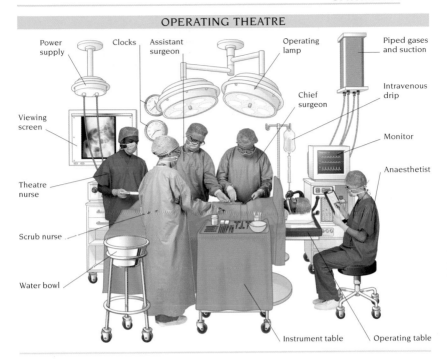

Power supply — Clocks — Assistant surgeon — Operating lamp — Piped gases and suction — Intravenous drip — Chief surgeon — Viewing screen — Monitor — Anaesthetist — Theatre nurse — Scrub nurse — Water bowl — Instrument table — Operating table

uterus, or to prevent ovarian cancer from developing in the future. The ovaries may be removed as part of the treatment for *breast cancer* if growth of the tumour depends on hormones produced by the ovary. If both ovaries are removed before the menopause, *hormone replacement therapy (HRT)* may be needed.

-opathy A suffix that denotes a disease or disorder, as in *neuropathy* (a disorder of the peripheral nerves).

open heart surgery Any operation on the *heart* in which it is stopped temporarily and its function taken over by a mechanical pump. The main forms of open heart surgery are correction of congenital heart defects (see *heart disease, congenital*), surgery for narrowed or leaky heart valves (see *heart-valve surgery*), and *coronary artery bypass* surgery. Once the pump is connected, the heart is opened, and the defects repaired. Surgical hypothermia is used to keep the heart cool and help prevent damage to the heart muscle from lack of oxygen (see *hypothermia, surgical*).

operable A term applied to a condition that is suitable for surgical treatment, such as an accessible noncancerous tumour. (See also *inoperable*.)

operating theatre A specialized hospital room in which surgical procedures are performed. The risk of infection of open wounds during surgery is reduced by a ventilation system that continually provides clean, filtered air, and walls and floors that are easily washable. Surgeons, assistants, and nurses use sterile brushes and bactericidal soaps to scrub their hands and forearms before putting on sterile gowns, masks, and gloves. The theatre is equipped with shadowless operating lights; lightboxes for viewing X-ray images; anaesthetic machines (see *anaesthesia, general*); and a *diathermy* machine, which controls bleeding. A *heart-lung machine* may also be used.

operation A surgical procedure, usually carried out with instruments but sometimes using only the hands (as in the manipulation of a simple fracture).

ophthalmia An old term for *ophthalmitis*.

O

ophthalmia neonatorum A type of *eye* inflammation and discharge (*ophthalmitis*) that occurs in newborn infants, usually as a result of infection with *gonorrhoea* or *chlamydia* at birth. The infection is treated with *antibiotic drugs*.

ophthalmitis Any inflammatory eye disorder. Types of ophthalmitis include *ophthalmia neonatorum* and sympathetic ophthalmitis: a rare condition in which a penetrating injury to one eye is followed by severe *uveitis* that can cause blindness in the other eye. Sympathetic ophthalmitis can be treated with *corticosteroid drugs*, but removal of the injured eye is sometimes necessary to save the sight of the other.

ophthalmology The study of the *eye* and the diagnosis and treatment of the disorders that affect it. Ophthalmology covers assessment of vision, prescription of glasses or contact lenses, and surgery for eye disorders, such as *cataracts* and *glaucoma*. (See also *eye, examination of*; *optician*; *optometry*; *orthoptics*.)

ophthalmoplegia Partial or total paralysis of the muscles that move the eyes. Ophthalmoplegia may be caused by disease of the muscles, such as *Graves' disease*, or by a condition that affects the brain or the nerves supplying the eye muscles, such as *stroke*, a *brain tumour*, *encephalitis*, or *multiple sclerosis*.

ophthalmoscope An instrument used to examine the inside of the *eye*.

ophthalmoscopy A noninvasive procedure in which an ophthalmologist (a doctor specializing in eye disorders) uses an opthalmoscope to examine the inside of the *eye*. The ophthalmoscope

OPHTHALMOSCOPY

Ophthalmoscope · Ophthalmologist

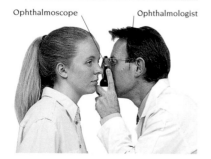

is used to direct a beam of light into the eye and examine the *retina*; the retinal blood vessels; the head of the *optic nerve*; and the *vitreous humour*.

opiate Any drug derived from, or chemically similar to, *opium*.

opioid A type of *analgesic drug* (painkiller) used to treat moderate to severe pain. Opioids, also known as narcotic drugs, may be abused for their euphoric effects; abuse may cause *tolerance* (the need for greater amounts of a drug to get the same effect), and physical and psychological *drug dependence*. Commonly used opioids include *codeine*, *diamorphine*, *morphine*, and *pethidine*.

opium A substance obtained from the unripe seed pods of the poppy plant PAPAVER SOMNIFERUM. Opium has an analgesic effect and may also cause sleepiness and euphoria. Opium and its derivatives, such as *codeine* and *diamorphine*, are known as *opioids*.

opportunistic infection Infection by organisms that rarely have serious or widespread effects in people of normal health, but which can cause serious illness or widespread infection in a person whose *immune system* is impaired. In most patients with *AIDS*, death is due to opportunistic infections, especially *pneumocystis pneumonia*. Many fungal infections, such as *candidiasis*, and some viral infections, such as *herpes simplex*, are opportunistic infections. Treatment is with appropriate antimicrobial drugs.

oppositional defiant disorder A type of behavioural disorder that usually appears in childhood or early adolescence. Typically, a child shows hostile, argumentative behaviour that includes loss of temper, defiance of rules, and swearing. To some extent such behaviour is common in adolescence, but when law-breaking or violence occur the condition is deemed to be pathological.

optic atrophy A shrinkage or wasting of the *optic nerve* fibres due to disease or injury to the optic nerve, resulting in partial or complete loss of vision. Optic atrophy may occur without prior signs of nerve disease, such as inflammation.

optic disc The area on the *retina* where nerve fibres from the eyeball join the *optic nerve*. The optic disc is also known as the blind spot due to its lack of light-sensitive cells.

optician A person who fits and sells *glasses* or *contact lenses*. An ophthalmic optician, or optometrist, also examines the eyes to test for *myopia, presbyopia, hypermetropia,* or *astigmatism.* People with suspected eye disorders are referred to a specialist called an ophthalmologist. (See also *ophthalmology; optometry.*)

optic nerve The 2nd *cranial nerve*; the nerve of *vision.* The two optic nerves each consist of about 1 million nerve fibres that transmit impulses from the *retina* to the *brain.* The optic nerves converge behind the eyes, where fibres from the inner halves of the retina cross over. Nerve fibres from the right halves of both retinas go to right side of the occipital lobes in the brain; those from the left halves go to the left side.

Disorders of the optic nerve include *optic neuritis* and *papilloedema.* The latter is caused by pressure on the nerve from disease in the *orbit* or a *brain tumour.*

optic neuritis Inflammation of the *optic nerve,* often causing sudden loss of part of the visual field. Attacks are sometimes accompanied by pain on moving the eyes. Vision usually improves within 6 weeks, but some optic nerve fibres will be damaged. Recurrent attacks usually lead to permanent loss of visual acuity.

Most cases are thought to be due to demyelination of the optic nerve fibres in *multiple sclerosis.* The condition may also result from inflammation or infection of tissues around the optic nerve. *Corticosteroid drugs* may help to restore vision, but seem to have little effect on long-term outcome. (See also *optic atrophy.*)

optometry The practice of assessing *vision* to establish whether glasses or contact lenses are needed to correct a visual defect, as carried out by an optometrist. Disorders of the eye may require treatment by an ophthalmologist. (See also *ophthalmology; optician.*)

oral Concerning the *mouth.*

oral contraceptives A group of oral drug preparations containing one or more synthetic female *sex hormones,* taken by women in a monthly cycle to prevent pregnancy. "The pill" commonly refers to the combined or the phased pill, which both contain an *oestrogen drug* and a *progestogen drug,* and the progestogen-only pill (POP), also sometimes known as the minipill. Oestrogen pills include *ethinylestradiol;* progestogens include levonorgestrel and *norethisterone.* When used correctly, the number of pregnancies among women using oral contraceptives for one year is less than 1 per cent. Actual failure rates may be four times higher.

Combined and phased pills increase oestrogen and progesterone levels. This interferes with the production of two hormones, *luteinizing hormone* (LH) and *follicle-stimulating hormone* (FSH), which in turn prevents ovulation. Most POPs work by making the lining of the cervix too thick for sperm to penetrate and also making the lining of the uterus thinner so that implantation of a fertilized ovum is less likely. A type of POP containing *desogestrel* also works by inhibiting ovulation.

Oestrogen-containing pills offer protection against uterine and ovarian cancer, *ovarian cysts, endometriosis,* and iron-deficiency *anaemia.* They also tend to make menstrual periods regular, lighter, and relatively pain-free. Possible side effects include raised blood pressure (see *hypertension*), weight changes, nausea, depression, swollen breasts, reduced sex drive, increased appetite, leg and abdominal cramps, headaches, and dizziness. There is also a risk of *thrombosis* causing a *stroke* or a *pulmonary embolism.* These pills may also aggravate heart disease or cause *gallstones, jaundice,* and, very rarely, liver cancer. All oral contraceptives can cause bleeding between periods, especially the POP. Other possible adverse effects of the POP include irregular periods, *ectopic pregnancy,* and ovarian cysts. There may be a slightly increased long-term risk of breast cancer for women taking the combined pill.

Oestrogen-based pills should generally be avoided in women with hypertension, *hyperlipidaemia, liver disease, migraine, otosclerosis, sickle cell anaemia,* or who are at increased risk of a thrombosis. They are not usually prescribed to a woman with a personal or family history of heart or circulatory disorders, or who suffers from unexplained vaginal bleeding. The POP or a low-oestrogen pill may be

O

used by women who should avoid oestrogens. Combined or phased pills may interfere with milk production and should not be taken during breast-feeding. Some drugs may impair the effectiveness of oral contraceptives. (See also *contraception*.)

oral hygiene Measures to keep the mouth and teeth clean and reduce the risk of tooth decay (see *caries, dental*), *gingivitis* and other gum disorders, and *halitosis*. Oral hygiene includes regular, thorough *toothbrushing* and flossing (see *floss, dental*) to remove *plaque*. *Disclosing agents* help to reveal build-up of plaque. Dentures are brushed on all surfaces and soaked in cleansing solution.

Professional treatment to remove *calculus* and stubborn plaque by scaling and polishing is usually carried out by a dentist or dental hygienist during a routine check-up. In *periodontal disease*, treatment may be needed more often.

oral rehydration therapy See *rehydration therapy*.

oral surgery The branch of surgery that treats deformity, injury, or disease of the teeth, jaws, and other parts of the mouth. Procedures include the extraction of impacted wisdom teeth (see *impaction, dental*) and *alveolectomy*. More complicated oral surgery includes *orthognathic surgery* to correct deformities of the jaw; repair of a broken jaw; plastic surgery to correct *cleft lip and palate*; and the removal of some noncancerous tumours from the mouth.

ORAL SYRINGE

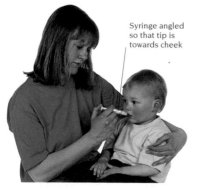

Syringe angled so that tip is towards cheek

USING AN ORAL SYRINGE

oral syringe A device used to administer liquid medicines by mouth, especially to young children. Small, accurately measured doses of the drug are drawn into the syringe via a plunger and squirted on to the inside of the cheek.

orbit The socket in the *skull* containing the eyeball, protective fat, blood vessels, muscles, and nerves. The *optic nerve* passes into the *brain* through an opening in the back of the orbit.

A severe blow to the face may fracture the orbit, but the eyeball is often undamaged as it can move back into the socket. Fractures often heal without treatment, but some cause deformity and require corrective surgery. Rarely, bacterial infection spreads from a *sinus* or the face to cause *orbital cellulitis*.

orbital cellulitis Bacterial infection of the tissues within the eye socket, or *orbit*. Infection is potentially serious as it may spread to the *brain*. Treatment is with high doses of *antibiotic drugs*.

orchidectomy The surgical removal of one or both of the *testes*. Orchidectomy may be performed for testicular cancer (see *testis, cancer of*) or gangrene due to torsion (see *testis, torsion of*), or to reduce production of *testosterone* in the treatment of cancer of the prostate gland (see *prostate, cancer of*). Removal of one testis does not affect sex drive, potency, or the ability to have children.

orchidopexy An operation to bring down an undescended testis (see *testis, undescended*) into the scrotum. Orchidopexy is usually performed in early childhood to reduce the risk of later *infertility* or testicular cancer (see *testis, cancer of*).

orchitis Inflammation of a *testis*. Orchitis may be caused by the *mumps* virus, particularly if infection occurs after puberty. Swelling and severe pain in the affected testis are accompanied by high fever. In *epididymo-orchitis*, the tube that carries sperm from the testis is also inflamed.

Treatment is with *analgesic drugs* and *ice-packs* to reduce swelling; *antibiotic drugs* may be given, but not for mumps orchitis. The condition usually begins to subside within 7 days but is occasionally followed by shrinking of the testis.

orf A skin infection occasionally transmitted to humans from sheep. Caused by a *pox* virus, orf usually produces a single persistent, fluid-filled blister on the arm or hand. Usually, no specific treatment is necessary as most cases clear up spontaneously in 3–6 weeks. However, large *lesions* may be removed surgically.

organ A collection of various *tissues* integrated into a distinct structural unit to perform specific functions. For example, the brain consists of nerve tissue and support tissue organized to receive, process, and send out information.

organ donation The agreement of a person (or his or her family) to surgical removal of one or more organs for use in *transplant surgery*. Most organs for transplantation, such as the heart, lungs, liver, and kidneys, are removed immediately after death, often in intensive care units where heart and lung function is sometimes maintained by machine after *brain death* has been certified. Compatible living donors may also be able to give a kidney (see *tissue-typing*). People can facilitate use of their organs after death by informing relatives and carrying a donor card. (See also *corneal graft; heart-lung transplant; heart transplant; heart-valve surgery; kidney transplant; liver transplant*.)

organelle One of various specialized structures contained within a body *cell*.

organic Related to a body *organ*; having organs or an organized structure; or related to *organisms* or to substances from them. In chemistry, "organic" refers to certain compounds that contain carbon. In medicine, the term indicates the presence of disease. (See also *inorganic*.)

organic brain syndrome See *brain syndrome, organic*.

organism A general term for an individual animal or plant. Microscopically small organisms, such as bacteria and viruses, are termed microorganisms.

organophosphates Highly poisonous agricultural insecticides that are harmful when absorbed through the skin, by inhalation, or by swallowing. Among the many possible symptoms are nausea, vomiting, abdominal cramps, diarrhoea, blurred vision, excessive sweating, headache, confusion, and twitching. Severe poisoning may cause breathing difficulty, palpitations, seizures, and unconsciousness. If left untreated, death may result.

Treatment may include washing out the stomach (see *lavage, gastric*) or removing soiled clothing and washing contaminated skin. Injections of *atropine* may be given, and *oxygen therapy* and/or artificial *ventilation* may be needed. With rapid treatment, people may survive doses that would otherwise have been fatal. Long term effects of organophosphates in sheep dips are thought to be responsible for debilitating illness with neural, muscular, and mental symptoms.

orgasm Intense sensations produced by a series of muscular contractions at the peak of sexual excitement. Orgasm in men usually lasts for about 3–10 seconds but can last up to a minute in women.

In men, contractions of the muscles of the inner pelvis massage seminal fluid from the *prostate gland* into the *urethra*, from which it is forcefully propelled via the urethral orifice (see *ejaculation*). Orgasm in women is associated with irregular contractions of the voluntary muscles of the walls of the *vagina* and, in some women, of the *uterus*, followed by relief of congestion in the pelvic area. Some women experience multiple orgasms if stimulation is continued. Orgasm is followed by a refractory phase during which there is no physical response to further sexual stimulation. Both men and women may experience problems with orgasm (see *ejaculation, disorders of; orgasm, lack of*).

orgasm, lack of Inability to achieve orgasm during sexual activity. It may be due to inhibited sexual desire (see *sexual desire, inhibited*) or inability to become aroused or maintain arousal (see *frigidity; erectile dysfunction*). In men, there may be a problem achieving orgasm despite normal arousal (see *ejaculation, disorders of*). The problem is common in women; some may achieve orgasm through *masturbation* but not during sexual intercourse. Sometimes it is due to pain during intercourse (see *intercourse, painful*).

For both sexes, contributory factors include problems with technique or in the relationship, unfamiliarity with sexual responses, psychological problems (such as anxiety, early sexual trauma, or inhibi-

O

tions), and fear of pregnancy. *Sex therapy, relationship counselling*, and *psychotherapy* are sometimes helpful.

orlistat An anti-obesity drug used with a slimming diet to treat severe *obesity*. Unlike *appetite suppressants*, orlistat acts on the gastrointestinal tract, preventing the digestion of fats by lipases (pancreatic *enzymes*). Instead of being absorbed, the fats pass out of the body in faeces.

Side effects are gastrointestinal and can be minimized by reducing fat intake. Flatulence and faecal urgency are common. Deficiencies of fat-soluble vitamins may develop with prolonged use.

ornithosis A disease of birds, caused by the microorganism CHLAMYDIA PSITTACI, that can cause *psittacosis* in humans.

orphan drugs Drugs that have been developed to treat rare conditions but are not manufactured generally.

orphenadrine A *muscle-relaxant drug* used to treat painful muscle spasm due to soft-tissue injury and *Parkinson's disease*. Side effects include a dry mouth and blurred vision.

ORT An abbreviation for oral hydration therapy. (See *rehydration therapy*.)

ortho- A prefix meaning normal, correct, or straight, as in *orthopaedics*, a branch of surgery concerned with correcting disorders of the bones and joints.

orthodontic appliances Fixed or removable devices, commonly known as braces, worn to correct *malocclusion*, or to reposition overcrowded or *buck teeth*. Usually fitted during childhood and adolescence, they move teeth using sustained gentle pressure. A fixed appliance has brackets attached to the teeth through which an arch wire is threaded and tightened to exert pressure. These are usually kept in place for about a year, after which time a retainer plate may be needed to hold the teeth in place until tooth and jaw growth has finished.

Removable appliances, consisting of a plastic plate with attachments that anchor over the back teeth, are used when only one or a few teeth need correcting. They apply force by springs, wire bows, screws, or rubber bands fitted to the plate.

orthodontics A branch of *dentistry* concerned with preventing and treating *malocclusion*. The procedures are usually

performed while teeth are developing and still relatively manoeuvrable, but can also be of benefit in adulthood.

An orthodontist may first make models of the teeth (see *impression, dental*) and take *X-rays* of the head and jaws. Certain teeth, often premolars, may be extracted to make room for the remaining teeth. Poorly positioned teeth are then moved by gentle pressure exerted by *orthodontic appliances*.

orthognathic surgery An operation to correct deformity of the jaw and the severe *malocclusion* that is invariably associated with it. The bones of the jaw are repositioned under general anaesthesia, and often require splinting (see *splinting, dental*) until they heal.

orthopaedics The branch of surgery concerned with disorders of the *bones* and *joints* and their associated *muscles, tendons*, and *ligaments*. Procedures include setting broken bones and applying casts; treating dislocations, slipped discs, arthritis, and back problems; treating bone tumours and birth defects of the skeleton; and repairing or replacing hip, knee, or finger joints.

orthopnoea Difficulty in breathing when lying flat. Orthopnoea is a symptom of *heart failure* and *pulmonary oedema*, and also occurs with *asthma* and chronic obstructive pulmonary disease (see *pulmonary disease, chronic obstructive*).

orthoptics Techniques used mainly in children to measure and evaluate *squint*, including eye exercises, assessment of monocular and binocular vision, and measures to combat *amblyopia*.

orthotics Use of appliances to support or correct weakened or deformed joints.

os An anatomical term for a bone; also refers to an opening in the body, as in the cervical os (entrance to the *uterus*).

oseltamivir An *antiviral drug* used to prevent or treat *influenza* A and B virus infections. To be effective, the drug should be taken within 48 hours of the onset of symptoms. Oseltamivir is not a substitute for routine influenza vaccination, and it can be taken even by those who have been vaccinated. The drug may also help protect against the most serious effects of *avian influenza*. Possible side effects are nausea, vomiting, and abdominal pain.

O

OSSICLE

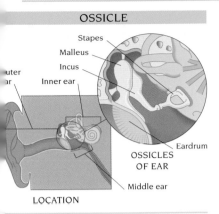

Stapes
Malleus
Incus
Inner ear
uter
ar
Eardrum
OSSICLES
OF EAR
Middle ear

LOCATION

Osgood-Schlatter disease Painful enlargement and tenderness of the tibial tuberosity (the bony prominence of the *tibia*), which occurs most commonly in boys aged 10–14. It results from excessive, repetitive pulling of the *quadriceps muscle*, due to repeated exercise. The disorder often clears up without treatment; severe pain may require *physiotherapy* or immobilization of the knee in a plaster *cast*.

osmosis The passage of a solvent from a weaker solution to a more concentrated one through a semipermeable membrane. All body cells are surrounded by such membranes, which allow water, salts, simple sugars (such as *glucose*), and *amino acids* (but not proteins) to pass through. Therefore, osmosis plays an important part in regulating the distribution of water and other substances in body tissues.

ossicle A small bone, especially any of the three tiny bones in the middle *ear* (malleus, incus, and stapes) that conduct sound from the eardrum to the inner ear.

ossification The process by which *bone* is formed, renewed, and repaired, starting in the embryo and continuing throughout life. There are three main situations in which ossification occurs: bone growth, during which new bone forms at the *epiphyses* (ends) of bones; bone renewal as part of normal regeneration; and bone repair following a *fracture*.

In newborn babies, the *diaphysis* (shaft) has begun to ossify and is composed mainly of bone, while the epiphyses are made of cartilage that gradually hardens. In children, growth plates produce new cartilage to lengthen the bones, and more bone forms at secondary ossification centres in the epiphyses. By the age of 18, the shafts, growth plates, and epiphyses have ossified and fused into continuous bone.

osteitis Inflammation of *bone*. The most common cause is infection (see *osteomyelitis*). Other causes are *Paget's disease* and *hyperparathyroidism*.

osteitis deformans An alternative term for *Paget's disease*.

osteo- A prefix denoting a relationship to bone, as in *osteoporosis*, a condition in which the bones thin and weaken.

osteoarthritis A common *joint* disease characterized by degeneration of the

OSSIFICATION

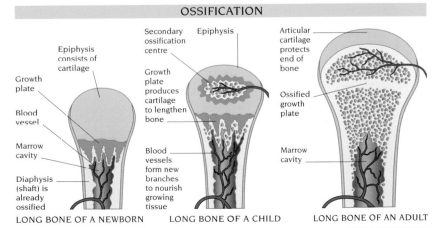

Epiphysis consists of cartilage
Growth plate
Blood vessel
Marrow cavity
Diaphysis (shaft) is already ossified

Secondary ossification centre — Epiphysis
Growth plate produces cartilage to lengthen bone
Blood vessels form new branches to nourish growing tissue

Articular cartilage protects end of bone
Ossified growth plate
Marrow cavity

LONG BONE OF A NEWBORN   LONG BONE OF A CHILD   LONG BONE OF AN ADULT cartilage that lines joints or by formation of *osteophytes*, leading to pain, stiffness, and occasionally loss of function. Osteoarthritis is due to wear and tear on joints, weight-bearing joints being the most commonly affected. Weakness and shrinkage of surrounding muscles may occur if pain prevents the joint from being used regularly. Affected joints become enlarged and distorted by osteophytes. Osteoarthritis occurs in almost all people over 60, although not all have symptoms. Factors that lead to its earlier development include excessive wear of, or injury to, a joint; congenital deformity or misalignment of bones in a joint; *obesity*; or inflammation from a disease such as *gout*. Severe osteoarthritis affects three times as many women as men.

There is no cure for osteoarthritis. Symptoms can be relieved by *nonsteroidal anti-inflammatory drugs, analgesics*, injections of *corticosteroid drugs* into affected joints, and *physiotherapy*. In overweight people, weight loss often provides relief of symptoms. Glucosamine dietary supplements may also alleviate symptoms in some people. Surgery for severe osteoarthritis includes *arthroplasty* and *arthrodesis*.

osteochondritis dissecans Degeneration of a *bone* just under a joint surface, causing fragments of bone and cartilage to become separated, which may cause the joint to lock. The condition commonly affects the knee and usually starts in adolescence. Symptoms include aching discomfort and intermittent swelling of the affected joint.

If a fragment has not completely separated from the bone, the joint may be immobilized in a plaster *cast* to allow reattachment. Loose bone or cartilage fragments in the knee are removed during *arthroscopy*. Disruption to the smoothness of the joint surface increases the risk of *osteoarthritis*.

osteochondritis juvenilis Inflammation of an *epiphysis* (growing end of bone) in children and adolescents, causing pain, tenderness, and restricted movement if the epiphysis forms part of a joint. The inflammation leads to softening of the bone, which may result in deformity. The condition may be due to

disruption of the bone's blood supply. There are several types: *Perthes' disease*; Scheuermann's disease, which affects several adjoining vertebrae; and other types that affect certain bones in the foot and wrist.

The affected bone may be immobilized in an orthopaedic *brace* or plaster cast. In Perthes' disease, surgery may be required to prevent more deformity. The bone usually regenerates within 3 years and rehardens, but deformity may be permanent and increases the risk of *osteoarthritis* in later life.

osteochondroma A noncancerous *bone* tumour, which is formed from a stalk of bone capped with cartilage, and appears as a hard round swelling near a joint. An osteochondroma develops in late childhood and early adolescence, usually from the side of a long bone near the knee or shoulder. The tumour causes problems only if it interferes with movement of tendons or the surrounding joint, in which case it may be removed surgically. Large osteochondromas can interfere with skeletal growth, causing deformity.

osteochondrosis See *osteochondritis juvenilis*.

osteodystrophy Any generalized bone defect due to *metabolic disorders*. Types of osteodystrophy include *rickets; osteomalacia; osteoporosis* due to Cushing's syndrome or excessive intake of *corticosteroid drugs*; and bone cysts and bone mass reduction associated with chronic *kidney failure* or *hyperparathyroidism*. In adults, an osteodystrophy is usually reversible if the underlying cause is treated before bone deformity occurs.

osteogenesis imperfecta A *congenital* condition characterized by abnormally brittle *bones* that are unusually susceptible to *fractures*. The condition is caused by an inherited defect in the *connective tissue* that forms the basic material of bone. Severely affected infants are born with multiple fractures and a soft skull and do not usually survive. Others have many fractures during infancy and childhood, often as a result of normal handling and activities, and it may be difficult to distinguish the condition from *child abuse*. A common sign of the condi-

O

tion is that the whites of the eyes are abnormally thin, making them appear blue. Sufferers may also be deaf due to *otosclerosis*. Very mild cases may not be detected until adolescence or later.

There is no specific treatment. Fractures are immobilized and usually heal quickly, but they may cause shortening and deformity of the limbs, resulting in abnormal, stunted growth. Skull fractures may cause brain damage or death. Parents may have *genetic counselling* to estimate the risk in future children. Severe cases can be diagnosed prenatally by *ultrasound scanning*.

osteogenic sarcoma See *osteosarcoma*.

osteoid osteoma A bone disorder in which a tiny abnormal area of bone, usually in a long bone, causes deep pain, which is typically worse at night. The condition is cured by removing the area of bone. (See also *osteoma*.)

osteoma A hard, noncancerous, usually small tumour that may occur on any *bone*. Surgical removal may be necessary if an osteoma causes symptoms by pressing on surrounding structures.

osteomalacia Softening, weakening, and demineralization of *bones* in adults due to *vitamin D* deficiency. Osteomalacia is rare in developed countries; it most commonly affects housebound, elderly, and dark-skinned people live in countries that have less sunlight than their country of origin.

Healthy bone production requires calcium and phosphorus, which cannot be absorbed from the diet without sufficient vitamin D (found in certain foods and manufactured by the skin in sunlight). Causes of osteomalacia include a diet low in vitamin D; *malabsorption* in conditions like *coeliac disease* or after intestinal surgery; or insufficient exposure to sunlight.

Osteomalacia causes bone pain, muscle weakness, and, if the blood level of calcium is very low, *tetany*. Weakened bones are vulnerable to distortion and fractures. Treatment is with a diet rich in vitamin D and increased exposure to sunlight; vitamin D supplements may also be given in some cases. Calcium supplements may be given if osteomalacia is due to malabsorption.

osteomyelitis Infection, usually by bacteria, of *bone* and *bone marrow*. It is relatively rare in developed countries but is more common in children, most often affecting the long arm and leg bones and vertebrae; in adults, it usually affects the pelvis and *vertebrae*. In acute osteomyelitis, the infection (usually STAPHYLOCOCCUS AUREUS) enters the bloodstream via a skin wound or as a result of infection elsewhere in the body. The infected bone and marrow become inflamed, and pus forms, causing fever, severe pain and tenderness in the bone, and inflammation and swelling of the skin over the affected area.

Prompt treatment over several weeks or months with high doses of *antibiotic drugs* usually cures acute osteomyelitis. If the condition fails to respond, surgery is performed to expose the bone, clean out areas of infected and dead bone, and drain the pus.

Chronic osteomyelitis may develop if acute osteomyelitis is neglected or fails to respond to treatment; after a compound *fracture*; or, occasionally, as a result of *tuberculosis* spreading from another part of the body. The condition causes constant pain in the affected bone. Complications include persistent deformity and, in children, arrest of growth in the affected bone. In the later stages of the disease, *amyloidosis* may develop. Chronic osteomyelitis requires surgical removal of all affected bone, sometimes followed by a *bone graft*; antibiotic drugs are also prescribed.

osteopathy A system of diagnosis and treatment that recognizes the role of the musculoskeletal system in the healthy functioning of the body. The basic principle of osteopathy is that all body systems operate in unison, and that disturbances in one system can alter the functions of others. The osteopath uses manipulation; rhythmic stretching, and pressure to restore joint mobility; and traditional diagnostic and therapeutic procedures to diagnose and treat dysfunction.

osteopetrosis A very rare inherited disorder in which *bones* harden and become denser. Deficiency of one of the two types of bone cell responsible for healthy bone growth results in a disruption of normal bone structure. In its mildest form, there may be no symptoms; more severe forms of osteopetrosis result in abnormally high susceptibility to *fractures*; stunted growth; deformity; and *anaemia*. Pressure on nerves may cause blindness, deafness, and facial paralysis.

Most treatments for osteopetrosis aim to reduce the severity of symptoms. Bone marrow transplants of cells from which healthy bone cells might develop are undertaken in some cases.

osteophyte An outgrowth of *bone* at the boundary of a joint. The formation of osteophytes is a characteristic feature of *osteoarthritis* that contributes to the deformity and restricted movement of affected joints.

osteoporosis Loss of bone tissue, causing the bone to become brittle and fracture easily. Bone thinning is a natural part of aging. However, women are especially vulnerable to loss of bone density after *menopause*, because their *ovaries* no longer produce *oestrogen hormones*, which help maintain bone mass.

OSTEOPOROSIS

Thinned, weakened bone

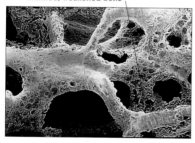

MICROSCOPIC VIEW OF BONE

Other causes include removal of the ovaries; a diet that is deficient in calcium; certain hormonal disorders; long-term treatment with *corticosteroid drugs*; and prolonged immobility. Osteoporosis is most common in heavy smokers and drinkers, and in excessively thin people.

The first sign is often a fracture, typically just above the wrist or at the top of the *femur*. One or several *vertebrae* may fracture spontaneously and cause the bones to crumble, leading to progressive height loss or pain due to compression of a spinal nerve.

Osteoporosis is confirmed using *densitometry*, such as a *DEXA scan*. Bone loss can be minimized with adequate dietary calcium and vitamin D, and regular, sustained exercise to build bones and maintain their strength. *Bisphosphonate drugs* help prevent bone loss; if bisphosphonates are not suitable, *raloxifene*, strontium ranalate (see *strontium*), or *calcitonin* may be given. *Hormone replacement therapy (HRT)* may be considered for postmenopausal women when other treatments have been ineffective or are unsuitable.

osteosarcoma A cancerous tumour of the bone that spreads rapidly to the lungs and, less commonly, to other areas. An osteosarcoma may occur in adolescents for no known reason (usually in a long bone of the arm or leg or around the knee, hip, or shoulder). In elderly people, osteosarcomas may develop in several bones as a late, rare complication of *Paget's disease*. The tumour causes pain and swelling of the affected bone if it occurs near the surface.

The condition may be treated by *radiotherapy*, but the affected bone is usually surgically removed. Sometimes it is replaced by a bone graft or artificial bone, but most often, an amputation and a prosthesis (see *limb, artificial*) are required. Anticancer drugs improve the outlook; about half of those in whom the disease is discovered early are cured.

osteosclerosis Increased *bone density*, visible on *X-rays* as an area of extreme whiteness. Localized osteosclerosis may be caused by a severe injury that compresses the bone, *osteoarthritis*, chronic *osteomyelitis*, or an *osteoma*. Osteosclerosis occurs throughout the body in the inherited bone disorder *osteopetrosis*.

osteotomy Surgery to change the alignment of, or shorten or lengthen, a *bone* by cutting it. Osteotomy is used to correct a *hallux valgus* that has caused a *bunion*; *coxa vara* (a hip deformity); or deformity due to *developmental dysplasia of the hip (DDH)*. The prodecure is also used to straighten a long bone that has healed crookedly after a *fracture*, or to shorten the uninjured leg if a fractured leg has shortened during healing (see *leg, shortening of*).

ostomy The term used to describe a surgical opening or a junction of two hollow organs (for example, *colostomy*).

otalgia The medical term for *earache*.

OTC drug See *over-the-counter drug*.

otitis externa An *ear* infection affecting the outer-ear canal. Otitis externa usually causes inflammation and swelling, discharge, and, in some people, *eczema* around the opening of the canal. The ear may be itchy and painful and blocked with pus, causing deafness.

Generalized infection of the canal, and sometimes of the pinna (external ear), may be due to a fungal or bacterial infection. The ear may also sometimes become inflamed as part of a generalized skin disorder such as atopic eczema or seborrhoeic *dermatitis*.

Often, the only treatment needed is to keep the ear clean and dry until the infection has cleared. Locally acting preparations containing *antibiotic drugs*, *antifungal drugs*, and/or *corticosteroid drugs* may be used. Oral antibiotics may be given for severe bacterial infections.

otitis media Inflammation of the middle *ear*. This condition is due to a viral or bacterial infection extending up the *eustachian tube*, which runs from the back of the nose to the middle ear. The tube may become blocked by inflammation or enlarged *adenoids*, causing fluid and pus to accumulate in the middle ear rather than draining away. Children, particularly those under 7 years, are especially susceptible to otitis media; some children have recurrent attacks.

Acute otitis media can cause sudden severe earache, a feeling of fullness in the ear, deafness, *tinnitus*, and fever. The eardrum may burst, in which case healing usually occurs within a few weeks. The condition is diagnosed by examination of the middle ear with an *otoscope*; the eardrum will appear red and possibly bulging outwards. Treatment is with *analgesic drugs*, and sometimes *antibiotic drugs*, although many childhood infections are viral.

One possible complication of otitis media is *glue ear* (chronic secretory otitis media), in which a thick fluid builds up in the ear and affects hearing. It may develop following severe or recurrent otitis media, particularly in children. Other complications include hearing impairment and a *cholesteatoma*. In rare cases, the infection responsible for otitis media spreads inwards to cause *mastoiditis*.

oto- A prefix that denotes a relationship to the *ear*, as in *otorrhoea* (discharge from the ear).

otoacoustic emission An echo emitted by the inner *ear* in response to sound. The emission is produced only by a normally functioning ear and is recorded in a test to detect impaired hearing.

otomycosis A fungal *ear* infection that causes inflammation of the ear canal and external ear (see *otitis externa*).

otoplasty Cosmetic or reconstructive surgery on the external *ear*. This procedure is usually carried out to make protruding ears lie closer to the head. Otoplasty may also be performed to construct a missing ear or to reconstruct a damaged ear.

otorhinolaryngology A surgical speciality, also known as ENT surgery, that is concerned with diseases of the *ear*, *nose*, and *throat*. ENT specialists treat *sinus* problems, *otitis media*, *glue ear*, *tonsillitis*, minor hearing loss, *otosclerosis*, *Ménière's disease*, airway problems in children, uncontrollable nosebleeds, and cancer of the *larynx* and *sinuses*.

otorrhoea A discharge of pus or other fluid from the ear (see *ear, discharge from*).

otosclerosis A disorder of the middle *ear* that causes progressive *deafness*. The condition usually develops in both ears. Otosclerosis occurs when overgrowth of bone immobilizes the *stapes* (the innermost one of the three tiny bones in the middle ear). As a result, sound vibrations are prevented from passing along the bone to the inner ear. To an affected person, sounds are muffled but can be distinguished more easily if there is background noise.

Otosclerosis frequently runs in families, and symptoms usually start to appear in early adulthood. The condition affects more women than men, and often develops during pregnancy. Hearing loss progresses slowly over 10 to 15 years and is often accompanied by *tinnitus* and, more rarely, *vertigo*. A degree of sensorineural deafness may develop,

O

OTOSCLEROSIS

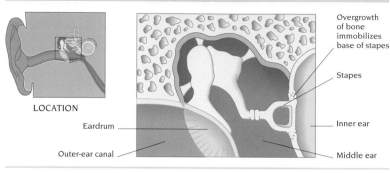

LOCATION

Overgrowth of bone immobilizes base of stapes

Stapes

Eardrum

Inner ear

Outer-ear canal

Middle ear

making high tones difficult to hear and causing the sufferer to speak loudly.

The condition is diagnosed by *hearing tests*. It can be cured by *stapedectomy*, a surgical procedure in which the stapes is replaced by a tiny piston, which moves through a hole created in the inner ear. Because the piston can move freely, it can transmit sound vibrations to the inner ear. Alternatively, a *hearing-aid* can markedly improve hearing.

otoscope An instrument, also called an auroscope, for examining the outer-ear canal and the eardrum. An otoscope illuminates and magnifies the inside of the ear. Otoscopy (examination using an otoscope) is performed to detect physical abnormalities such as inflammation or pus in the outer-ear canal (see *otitis externa*) and distortion or rupture of the eardrum.

ototoxicity Toxic damage to the structures of the inner ear. High doses of certain drugs (such as *aminoglycoside* antibiotics) may cause this type of ear damage, resulting in impaired hearing and balance.

out-of-body experience A feeling of leaving one's body and observing oneself from another dimension. Thought to be due to disturbance of brain function, it is reported by some patients after a general anaesthetic or a medical emergency.

outpatient treatment Medical care on a same-day basis in a hospital or clinic.

ovarian cyst An abnormal, fluid-filled swelling in an *ovary*. Ovarian cysts are common and, in most cases, noncancerous. The most common type, a follicular cyst, is one in which the egg-producing

follicle enlarges and fills with fluid. Cysts may also occur in the corpus luteum, a mass of tissue that forms from the follicle after *ovulation*. Other types include *dermoid cysts* and cancerous cysts (see *ovary, cancer of*).

Ovarian cysts are often symptomless, but some cause abdominal discomfort, pain during intercourse, or irregularities of menstruation such as *amenorrhoea, menorrhagia,* or *dysmenorrhoea*. Severe abdominal pain, nausea, and fever may develop if twisting or rupture of a cyst occurs. This condition requires surgery.

An ovarian cyst may be discovered during a routine *pelvic examination* and its position and size confirmed by ultrasound or *laparoscopy*. In many cases, simple ovarian cysts – thin-walled or fluid-filled cysts – resolve themselves. However, complex cysts (such as dermoid cysts) usually require surgical removal. If an ovarian cyst is particularly large, the ovary may need to be removed (see *oophorectomy*).

ovary One of a pair of almond-shaped glands situated on either side of the *uterus* immediately below the opening of the *fallopian tubes*. Each ovary contains numerous cavities called *follicles*, in which egg cells (see *ovum*) develop. The ovaries also produce the female sex hormones *oestrogen* and *progesterone*.

ovary, cancer of A malignant growth of the *ovary*. The cancer may be either primary (arising in the ovary) or secondary (due to the spread of cancer from another part of the body). Ovarian cancer can occur at any age but is most common

O

after 50 and in women who have never had children. A family history of cancer of the ovary, breast, or colon, especially in close relatives under 50, is an important risk factor. Taking the combined *oral contraceptive* pill reduces the risk.

In most cases, ovarian cancer causes no symptoms until it is widespread. The first symptoms may include vague discomfort and swelling in the abdomen; nausea and vomiting; abnormal vaginal bleeding; and *ascites*.

If ovarian cancer is suspected, a doctor will carry out a physical examination to detect any swellings in the pelvis. A *laparoscopy* will usually be done to confirm the diagnosis.

Treatment is by surgical removal of the growth or as much cancerous tissue as possible. This usually involves *salpingo-oophorectomy* and *hysterectomy* followed by *radiotherapy* and *anticancer drugs*.

ovary, disorders of Diseases and abnormalities of the ovaries can occur for various reasons. Absence of ovaries, or their failure to develop normally, is rare and is usually due to a chromosomal abnormality (see *Turner's syndrome*). Oophoritis (inflammation of an ovary) may result from infections such as *gonorrhoea* or *pelvic inflammatory disease*. *Ovarian cysts* are common and usually noncancerous. Multiple ovarian cysts, together with other characteristic features, occur in polycystic ovary syndrome (see *ovary, polycystic*). Ovarian cancer (see *ovary, cancer of*) occurs mainly in women over 50. Ovarian failure causes premature *menopause* in about 5 per cent of women.

ovary, polycystic A condition, also called Stein–Leventhal syndrome, that is characterized by oligomenorrhea or *amenorrhoea* (scanty or absent periods), *infertility*, *hirsutism* (excessive hairiness), acne, and *obesity*. Often, there are multiple *ovarian cysts*. Most women with polycystic ovaries begin menstruation at a normal age, but after a year or two periods become highly irregular and then cease.

The underlying cause of the condition is unknown but it is associated with higher than normal levels of *luteinizing hormone* (LH) and *testosterone* and with insulin resistance (in which body cells are resistant to insulin, causing excessive insulin to be produced by the pancreas to compensate).

Treatment is directed towards the symptoms and may include losing excess weight, *oral contraceptives* for menstrual irregularities and acne, *clomifene* for infertility, and *depilatories* or *electrolysis* for hirsutism.

Polycystic ovaries are often associated with high oestrogen levels in the body, which increase the risk of endometrial cancer (see *uterus, cancer of*).

overbite Overlapping of the lower front *teeth* by the upper ones. A slight degree of overbite is normal as the upper jaw is larger than the lower jaw. In *malocclusion*, overbite may be greater than normal or the lower teeth may project in front of the upper teeth.

overbreathing See *hyperventilation*.

overcrowding, dental Excessive crowding of the *teeth* so that they are unable to assume their normal positions in the jaw. Dental overcrowding is commonly inherited and may occur because the teeth are too large for the jaw or the jaw is too small to accommodate the teeth. Premature loss of primary molar (back) teeth can cause the permanent teeth beneath them to move out of position and crowd the teeth further forward.

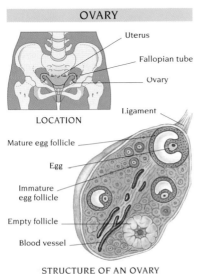

OVARY

Uterus

Fallopian tube

Ovary

Ligament

LOCATION

Mature egg follicle

Egg

Immature egg follicle

Empty follicle

Blood vessel

STRUCTURE OF AN OVARY

Overcrowded teeth may lead to *malocclusion* or may prevent certain teeth from erupting through the gum (see *impaction, dental*). They can be difficult to clean, increasing the risk of dental decay (see *caries, dental*) and *periodontal disease*.

Teeth may need to be extracted to allow room for others. Usually an *orthodontic appliance* is fitted to the remaining teeth to position them correctly.

over-the-counter (OTC) drug A drug that can be bought without a prescription at a chemist's or other store.

overuse injury Also called repetitive strain injury, a term for any injury caused by repetitive movement of part of the body. Symptoms include pain and stiffness in the affected joints and muscles.

Examples include *epicondylitis*: painful inflammation of one of the bony prominences at the elbow, caused by the pull of the attached forearm muscles during strenuous activities (see *golfer's elbow; tennis elbow*). Overuse injuries of the fingers, thumb, and wrist joints may affect assembly-line and keyboard workers, and musicians; injuries of the neck may affect violinists. Rest relieves the symptoms. A change in the technique used during the activity may prevent recurrence.

overweight See *obesity*.

ovulation The development and release of an *ovum* (egg) from a follicle within an *ovary*. During the first half of the menstrual cycle, *follicle-stimulating hormone* (FSH) causes several ova to mature in the ovary. At mid-cycle, *luteinizing hormone* (LH) causes a ripe ovum to be released. Signs of ovulation include a rise in body temperature, changes in the cervical mucus, and sometimes mild abdominal pain (see *mittelschmerz*). A yellow mass of tissue called the corpus luteum, which forms from the follicle after *ovulation*, releases progesterone during the second half of the cycle.

After its release, the ovum travels along the *fallopian tube* and, if *fertilization* does not occur, is shed during *menstruation*. Regular menstruation usually means that ovulation is occurring, except around *puberty* and approaching the *menopause*.

ovum The egg cell (female cell of reproduction). An ovum contains a nucleus suspended in cytoplasm (a gel-like substance) and is surrounded by a protective layer, the *zona pellucida*.

About 1 million immature ova are present in each *ovary* at birth, but only about 200 per ovary mature to be released at *ovulation*. A *fertilized* ovum develops into an *embryo*.

OVUM

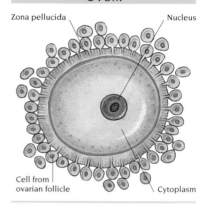

Zona pellucida — Nucleus

Cell from ovarian follicle — Cytoplasm

oxazepam A *benzodiazepine drug* used as a short-term treatment for *anxiety*. Oxazepam may cause dependence if it is taken regularly for more than 2 weeks (see *drug dependence*).

oximeter An instrument used for measuring the oxygen content of the blood.

oxprenolol A *beta-blocker drug* that is used to treat *hypertension, angina,* and cardiac *arrhythmias*. Oxprenolol may also be used to relieve symptoms of *anxiety* and control those of *hyperthyroidism*.

oxybutynin A drug that is used to treat frequent urination (see *urination, frequent*) by increasing the bladder's capacity. Common side effects include dry mouth and blurred vision.

oxygen A colourless, odourless gas that makes up 21 per cent of the Earth's atmosphere. Oxygen is essential for almost all forms of life, including humans, because it is necessary for the metabolic "burning" of foods to produce energy – a process that takes place in body cells and is known as *aerobic* metabolism.

Oxygen is absorbed through the lungs and into the blood, where it binds to the *haemoglobin* in red blood cells. As oxygen-rich blood circulates around the body, the oxygen is released from the red blood cells into the body tissues.

Additional supplies of oxygen are used to treat conditions such as severe *bronchitis* or *hypoxia*. High-pressure oxygen (see *hyperbaric oxygen treatment*) is sometimes used to treat *decompression sickness* or *carbon monoxide* poisoning. (See also *ozone*.)

oxygen concentrator An appliance used in *oxygen therapy* that separates oxygen from the air and mixes it back in at a greater concentration. This oxygen-enriched air is delivered through a tube for prolonged inhalation. The appliance is used by people who have persistent *hypoxia* due to severe *chronic obstructive pulmonary disease* (see *pulmonary disease, chronic obstructive*) (See also *hyperbaric oxygen treatment*.)

oxygen therapy The process of supplying a person with oxygen-enriched air to relieve severe *hypoxia* (inadequate oxygen in body tissues). The oxygen is usually delivered through a face-mask or a nasal cannula (a length of narrow plastic tubing with two prongs that are inserted into the nostrils). Piped oxygen is used in hospitals; oxygen in cylinders can be used at home for acute attacks of hypoxia, such as those occurring in severe asthma. Long-term therapy for people with persistent hypoxia may involve the use of an *oxygen concentrator*. (See also *hyperbaric oxygen treatment*.)

OXYGEN THERAPY

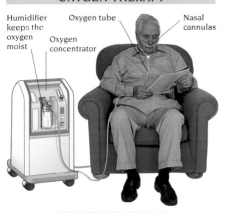

Humidifier keeps the oxygen moist

Oxygen tube

Oxygen concentrator

Nasal cannulas

HOME OXYGEN THERAPY

oxymetazoline A *decongestant drug* used in the treatment of *allergic rhinitis*, *sinusitis*, and the common *cold*.

oxytetracycline A tetracycline *antibiotic drug* that is used to treat *chlamydial infections* such as *nongonococcal urethritis*. It is also used for a variety of other infective conditions, including *bronchitis* and *pneumonia*; in addition, the drug may be used to treat severe *acne*.

Side effects may include nausea, vomiting, diarrhoea, skin rash, and increased sensitivity of the skin to sunlight. Oxytetracycline may discolour developing teeth, and is not given to children under 12 or to pregnant women.

oxytocin A *hormone* produced by the *pituitary gland*. Oxytocin causes uterine *contractions* during labour and stimulates milk flow in *breast-feeding* women.

Synthetic oxytocin is used for *induction of labour*. It is given by intravenous infusion to produce uterine contractions. It is also often given with ergotamine as a single dose after delivery to prompt placental separation and expulsion, to reduce blood flow, or to empty the uterus after a *miscarriage*. A possible adverse effect of synthetic oxytocin is abnormally strong, painful contractions. Rare side effects include nausea, vomiting, palpitations, and allergic reactions.

oxyuriasis An alternative name for enterobiasis or *threadworm infestation*.

ozena A severe and rare form of *rhinitis*, in which the mucus membrane in the nose wastes away and a thick nasal discharge dries to form crusts. Ozena often causes severe *halitosis*.

ozone A rare form of oxygen, ozone is a poisonous, faintly blue gas that is produced by the action of electrical discharges (such as lightning) on oxygen molecules. Ozone occurs naturally in the upper atmosphere, where it screens the Earth from most of the Sun's harmful ultraviolet radiation. The ozone layer is being depleted by atmospheric pollutants, allowing increasing amounts of ultraviolet radiation to reach the Earth's surface. This problem could lead to a rise in the incidence of *skin cancer* and *cataracts*, as well as having other potentially hazardous effects.

O

P

pacemaker A small device that supplies electrical impulses to the *heart* to maintain a regular *heartbeat*. A pacemaker is implanted when the *sinoatrial node* in the heart malfunctions, or when the passage of the electrical impulses that stimulate heart contractions is impaired (see *heart block*; *sick sinus syndrome*).

Pacemakers can be fixed-rate (which discharge impulses at a steady rate) or demand (which discharge only when the heart rate slows or a beat is missed). They may be external (used as a temporary measure) or internal (implanted in the chest). Some types can increase the heart rate during exercise or change an abnormal rhythm into a normal one.

PACEMAKER

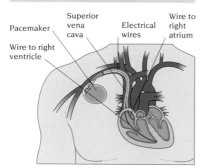

Pacemaker · Superior vena cava · Electrical wires · Wire to right atrium · Wire to right ventricle

INTERNAL PACEMAKER IN POSITION

paclitaxel An *anticancer drug* that is used to treat certain types of cancer, such as ovarian cancer (see *ovary, cancer of*) and *breast cancer*. The possible side effects of paclitaxel can include nausea, vomiting, *anaemia*, and increased susceptibility to infection.

paediatrics The branch of medicine that is concerned with the development of children, and the diagnosis, treatment, and prevention of childhood diseases.

paedophilia Sexual attraction to children. (See also child *abuse*; *incest*.)

Paget's disease A common disorder of the middle-aged and elderly, in which the formation of bone is disrupted. Affected bones become weak, thick, and deformed. Paget's disease, which is also called osteitis deformans, usually affects the pelvis, skull, collarbone, vertebrae, and long bones of the leg. The disorder may run in families and mostly affects men.

There are often no symptoms, but if symptoms do occur, the most common ones are bone pain and deformity, especially bowing of the legs. Affected bones are prone to fracture. Skull changes may lead to leontiasis (distortion of the facial bones producing a lion-like appearance) and to damage to the inner ear, sometimes causing deafness, *tinnitus*, *vertigo*, or headaches.

The disorder is diagnosed by *X-rays* and *blood tests*. Most people do not need treatment, or only need *analgesic drugs*. In more severe cases, treatment with drugs such as *calcitonin* may be prescribed or surgery may be needed.

Paget's disease of the nipple A rare type of *breast cancer* in which a tumour develops in the *nipple*. The disease resembles *eczema* and can cause itching and a burning feeling. A non-healing sore may develop. Without treatment, the tumour may spread into the breast. Diagnosis is made with a *biopsy*.

pain A localized sensation that can range from mild discomfort to an excruciating experience. Stimulation of sensory nerve endings called nociceptors in the skin leads to pain messages being sent to the brain. Some nociceptors respond only to severe stimulation, others to warning stimuli. Pain receptors are present in other structures, such as blood vessels and tendons. Pain that may be felt at a point some distance from the cause is known as *referred pain*.

Treatment for pain may include drugs, electrical stimulation (*TENS*), surgery, or therapies such as *acupuncture*. (See also *pain relief*, *endorphins*.)

painful arc syndrome A condition in which pain occurs when the arm is raised between 45 and 160 degrees from the side. The usual cause is an inflamed tendon or *bursa* around the shoulder joint being squeezed between the *scapula* and *humerus*. Treatment includes *physiotherapy* and injection of *corticosteroid drugs*.

painkillers See *analgesic drugs*.

pain relief The treatment of pain, usually with *analgesic drugs*. *Paracetamol, aspirin* and *codeine* are the most widely used drugs in this group. Pain accompanied by *inflammation* is often alleviated by *nonsteroidal anti-inflammatory drugs (NSAIDs)*. Severe pain may require treatment with *opioids*, such as *morphine*.

Other methods of pain relief include *massage, ice-packs, poultices, TENS, acupuncture*, or *hypnosis*. Surgery to destroy pain-transmitting nerves (as in a *cordotomy*) is occasionally performed when other treatments fail.

palate The roof of the mouth, which is covered with *mucous membrane* and which separates the mouth from the nasal cavity. At the front is the hard palate, a plate of bone forming part of the *maxilla*. At the rear is the soft palate, a flap of muscle and fibrous tissue that projects into the *pharynx*. (See also *cleft lip and palate*.)

palliative treatment Treatment that relieves the symptoms of a disorder but does not cure it.

pallor Abnormal paleness of the *skin* and *mucous membranes*, particularly noticeable in the face. Pallor is not always a symptom of disease. It may be due to a deficiency of the skin pigment *melanin* that may affect people who spend very little time in daylight. It is also a feature of *albinism*. In addition, pallor may be caused by constriction of small blood vessels in the skin, which may occur in response to shock, severe pain, injury, heavy blood loss, or fainting.

Disorders that cause pallor include *anaemia, pyelonephritis, kidney failure*, and *hypothyroidism*. *Lead poisoning* is a rare cause.

palpation A technique used in *physical examination*, in which parts of the body are felt with the hands.

palpitation Awareness of the *heartbeat* or a sensation of having a rapid and forceful heartbeat. Palpitations are usually felt in tense situations, or after strenuous exercise or a scare. When experienced at rest or when calm, they are usually due to *ectopic heartbeats* and are felt as fluttering or thumping in the chest. Palpitations may also be due to *cardiac arrhythmias* and *hyperthyroidism*. Recurrent palpitations, or those causing chest pain, breathlessness, or dizziness, may be investigated by a 24-hour *ECG* and *thyroid function tests*. Treatment depends on the cause.

palsy A term applied to certain forms of *paralysis*, such as *facial palsy*.

panacea A claimed remedy for all diseases. No such remedy is known.

pancreas A tapered gland that lies across the back of the abdomen, behind the stomach. The broadest part (head) is on the right-hand side. The main part (body) tapers from the head and extends horizontally. The narrowest part (tail) is on the left near the spleen.

The pancreas has a digestive and a hormonal function. It mostly consists of exocrine tissue, which secretes digestive *enzymes* into the duodenum via the pancreatic duct. Also secreted is sodium bicarbonate, which neutralizes stomach acid entering the duodenum. The pancreas also contains groups of endocrine cells called the islets of Langerhans, which secrete the hormones *insulin* and *glucagon*. These hormones regulate the levels of *glucose* in the blood.

The most common pancreatic disorder is *diabetes mellitus*.

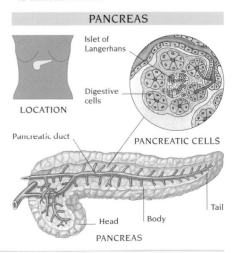

PANCREAS

LOCATION

Islet of Langerhans

Digestive cells

PANCREATIC CELLS

Pancreatic duct

Head

Body

Tail

PANCREAS

pancreas, cancer of A cancerous tumour of the exocrine tissue of the *pancreas*. The cause is unknown, but smoking and a high intake of fats or alcohol may be contributing factors. Symptoms include upper abdominal pain, loss of appetite, weight loss, and *jaundice*. There may also be indigestion, nausea, vomiting, diarrhoea, and tiredness. In many cases, symptoms do not appear until the cancer has spread to other parts of the body.

Diagnosis usually requires *ultrasound scanning*, *CT scanning* or *MRI* of the upper abdomen, or *ERCP*. In early stages, *pancreatectomy*, *radiotherapy* and *anticancer drugs* may provide a cure. In later stages, little can be done apart from provision of *palliative treatment*.

pancreatectomy Removal of all or part of the *pancreas*. Pancreatectomy may be performed to treat *pancreatitis* or localized cancer of the pancreas (see *pancreas, cancer of*). Rarely, it is performed to treat *insulinomas*. Pancreatectomy may lead to *diabetes mellitus* and *malabsorption*.

pancreatin An oral preparation of pancreatic *enzymes* required for digestion. It is used to prevent *malabsorption*, and it may be needed after *pancreatectomy* or by people with pancreatic disorders.

pancreatitis Inflammation of the *pancreas*, which may be acute or *chronic*. The main causes of acute pancreatitis are alcohol abuse and *gallstones*. Less common causes are injury, viral infections, surgery on the *biliary system*, or certain drugs. Chronic pancreatitis is usually due to alcohol abuse. Rarer causes include *hyperlipidaemias*, *haemochromatosis*, and severe acute pancreatitis. Chronic pancreatitis leads to permanent damage. Acute pancreatitis is less damaging but there may be recurrences.

Symptoms of acute pancreatitis are a sudden attack of severe upper abdominal pain, which may spread to the back, often with nausea and vomiting. Movement often makes the pain worse. The attack usually lasts about 48 hours. Chronic pancreatitis usually has the same symptoms, although the pain may last from a few hours to several days, and attacks become more frequent. If there is no pain, the principal signs may be *malabsorption* or *diabetes mellitus*.

Severe acute pancreatitis may lead to *hypotension*, *heart failure*, *kidney failure*, *respiratory failure*, *cysts*, and *ascites*. Chronic pancreatitis may also lead to the development of ascites and cysts, as well as *bile duct obstruction* and diabetes mellitus.

A diagnosis may be made by *blood tests*, abdominal *X-rays*, *ultrasound scanning*, *CT scanning*, *MRI*, or *ERCP*. Acute pancreatitis is treated with *intravenous infusion* of fluids and salts and opioid *analgesic drugs*. In some cases, the gut may be washed out with sterile fluid, or a *pancreatectomy* may be performed and any gallstones that are present removed. Treatment for the chronic form is with painkillers, *insulin*, *pancreatin*, and, in some cases, *pancreatectomy*.

pancreatography Imaging of the pancreas or its ducts using *CT scanning*, *MRI*, *ultrasound scanning*, *X-rays* (following injection of a radiopaque contrast medium into the pancreatic ducts during exploratory surgery), or with *ERCP*.

pandemic A medical term applied to a disease that occurs over a large geographical area and that affects a high proportion of the population; a widespread epidemic.

panic attack A brief period of acute *anxiety*, often dominated by an intense fear of dying or losing one's reason. Attacks are unpredictable at first, but tend to become associated with specific situations, such as a cramped lift.

Symptoms (a sense of breathing difficulty, chest pains, *palpitations*, feeling light-headed, dizziness, sweating, trembling, and faintness) begin suddenly. *Hyperventilation* often occurs, causing a *pins-and-needles* feeling, and feelings of *depersonalization* and *derealization*. The attacks end quickly.

Panic attacks are generally a feature of an *anxiety disorder*, *agoraphobia*, or other *phobias*. In some cases, such attacks are part of a *somatization disorder* or *schizophrenia*. *Behaviour therapy* and relaxation exercises may be used in treatment of this condition.

panic disorder A type of *anxiety* disorder, characterized by recurrent *panic attacks* of intense anxiety and distressing physical symptoms.

pantothenic acid One of the vitamins in the *vitamin B complex*.

papilla Any small, nipple-shaped projection from a tissue's surface, such as the mammary papilla (the breast nipple).

papilloedema Swelling of the head of the *optic nerve*, which is visible with an *ophthalmoscope*. Also called optic disc oedema, it usually indicates a dangerous rise in the pressure within the skull, sometimes caused by a *brain tumour*.

papilloma A noncancerous growth of the *epithelium* that resembles a wart and most commonly affects the skin, tongue, larynx, and urinary and digestive tracts.

pap smear See *cervical smear test*.

papule A small, solid, slightly raised area of skin. Papules are usually less than 5 mm in diameter, are raised or flat, have a smooth or warty texture, and are either pigmented or the colour of the surrounding skin.

par-/para- Prefixes that may mean beside or beyond, closely resembling or related to, or faulty or abnormal.

para-aminobenzoic acid The active ingredient of many *sunscreen* preparations. Its abbreviation is PABA.

paracentesis A procedure in which a body cavity is punctured with a needle from the outside to remove fluid for analysis, to relieve pressure from excess fluid, or to instil drugs.

paracetamol An *analgesic drug*, used to treat mild pain and to reduce fever. Paracetamol may rarely cause nausea or rash. An overdose may cause *liver damage* and can be fatal.

paraesthesia Altered sensation in the skin that occurs without a stimulus (see *pins-and-needles*).

paraffinoma A tumour-like swelling under the skin caused by prolonged exposure to paraffin. Paraffinomas may form in the lungs if paraffin is inhaled.

paraldehyde A *sedative drug* used to stop prolonged epileptic *seizures*. Paraldehyde can be administered as an *enema* or by injection into a muscle.

paralysis Complete or partial loss of controlled movement caused by the inability to contract one or more *muscles*. Paralysis may be temporary or permanent. There may also be loss of feeling in affected areas.

Paralysis of one half of the body is called *hemiplegia*; paralysis of all four limbs and the trunk is called *quadriplegia*. *Paraplegia* is paralysis of both legs and sometimes part of the trunk. Paralysis may be flaccid, causing floppiness, or spastic, causing rigidity.

Paralysis can be caused by brain disorders such as *stroke, brain tumour, brain abscess,* or *brain haemorrhage.* Some types of paralysis are caused by damage to parts of the nervous system (such as the *cerebellum* and *basal ganglia*) concerned with fine control of movement. Paralysis can also be caused by damage to or pressure on the spinal cord as a result of injury or *disc prolapse*. Diseases affecting the spinal cord (such as *multiple sclerosis* and *poliomyelitis*) and muscle disorders (such as *muscular dystrophy*) may also cause paralysis. Nerve disorders, called *neuropathies*, may cause varying degrees of paralysis.

The underlying cause is treated, if possible, and *physiotherapy* is used to prevent joints from becoming locked and to strengthen muscles and joints.

paralysis, periodic A rare, inherited condition that affects young people. Periodic paralysis is characterized by episodes of muscle weakness, which vary in frequency from daily to every few years and last from a few minutes to a few hours. In some cases, there is a drop in the *potassium* levels in the blood; in others, the levels rise. A carbohydrate-rich meal may trigger an attack. The condition often clears up without treatment by age 40.

paramedic A term for any health-care worker other than a doctor, nurse, or dentist. The term usually refers to ambulance staff who attend accidents or medical emergencies.

paranoia A condition in which the central feature is the *delusion* that people or events are especially connected to oneself. The term paranoia may also be used to describe feelings of persecution. A paranoid person builds up an elaborate set of beliefs based on the interpretation of chance remarks or events. Typical themes are persecution, jealousy (see *jealousy, morbid*), love, and grandeur.

Paranoia may be *chronic* or *acute*. Chronic paranoia may be caused by

P

brain damage, abuse of alcohol or amphetamines, *bipolar disorder*, or *schizophrenia* and is likely in those with a *personality disorder*. Acute paranoia, lasting for less than 6 months, may occur in people, such as refugees, who have experienced radical changes. In shared paranoia (see *folie à deux*), delusion develops because of a close relationship with someone else who has a delusion.

There are usually no other symptoms of mental illness apart from occasional *hallucinations*. In time, anger, suspicion, and social isolation may become severe.

If acute illness is treated early with *antipsychotic drugs*, the outlook is good. In longstanding paranoia, delusions are usually firmly entrenched, but antipsychotics may make them less prominent.

paraparesis Partial *paralysis* or weakness of both legs and sometimes part of the trunk.

paraphimosis Constriction of the *penis* behind the *glans* (head) by an extremely tight foreskin that has been pulled back, causing swelling and pain. Paraphimosis often occurs as a complication of an abnormally tight foreskin (see *phimosis*). The foreskin can often be returned manually to its normal position after application of an ice-pack. Otherwise, an injection or an operation to cut the foreskin may be necessary. *Circumcision* prevents recurrence.

paraplegia Weakness or *paralysis* of both legs and sometimes of part of the trunk, often accompanied by loss of feeling and by loss of urinary control. Paraplegia is a result of nerve damage in the *brain* or *spinal cord*.

parapsychology The branch of *psychology* dealing with experiences and events that cannot be scientifically accounted for. These include forms of extrasensory perception (ESP), such as telepathy (communication of thoughts), telekinesis (movement of objects with the mind), and precognition (being able to see into the future).

Many "paranormal" experiences can probably be explained by mental disturbances; others are probably due to coincidence, self-deception, or fraud.

paraquat A poisonous weedkiller that is available in high concentrations for agricultural use and which can be fatal if swallowed, inhaled, or absorbed through the skin. Paraquat poisoning requires urgent medical attention. The symptoms may include breathing difficulties, mouth ulcers, nosebleeds, diarrhoea, and later, respiratory and kidney failure. Treatments include eating activated charcoal or Fuller's earth. *Haemodialysis* may also be used.

parasite Any organism living in or on another living creature and deriving advantage from it, while causing the host disadvantage. The parasite obtains food from the host's blood, tissues, or diet. Parasites may spend only part of their life-cycles with the host or remain there permanently. Some parasites cause few symptoms, while others cause disease or even death.

Animal parasites of humans include *protozoa, worms, flukes, leeches, lice, ticks,* and *mites*. *Viruses* and disease-causing *fungi* and *bacteria* are also parasites.

parasitology The scientific study of *parasites*. Although viruses and many types of bacteria and fungi are parasites, their study is conducted under the title of *microbiology*.

parasuicide See *suicide, attempted*.

parasympathetic nervous system One of the two divisions of the *autonomic nervous system*.

parathion A highly poisonous agricultural *organophosphate* insecticide.

parathyroid glands Two pairs of oval, pea-sized glands that lie behind the

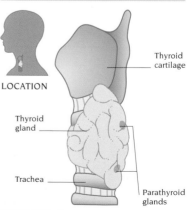

PARATHYROID GLANDS

LOCATION

Thyroid cartilage

Thyroid gland

Trachea

Parathyroid glands

thyroid gland in the neck. Some people have only one parathyroid gland or have extra glands in the neck or chest. The glands produce parathyroid *hormone*, which helps regulate the level of calcium in the blood; even small variations in calcium level can impair muscle and nerve function. Rarely, the parathyroid glands may become overactive (in a condition called *hyperparathyroidism*) or underactive (see *hypoparathyroidism*).

parathyroid tumour A growth within a *parathyroid gland*. The tumour may cause excess secretion of parathyroid hormone, leading to *hyperparathyroidism*. Cancers of the parathyroid are very rare; most parathyroid tumours are noncancerous *adenomas*. An adenoma that causes hyperparathyroidism will be surgically removed, which usually provides a complete cure.

paratyphoid fever An illness identical in most respects to *typhoid fever*, except that it is caused by SALMONELLA PARA-TYPHI and is usually less severe.

paraumbilical hernia A *hernia* occurring near the *navel*. It may occur in obese women who have had several children.

parenchyma The functional (as opposed to supporting) tissue of an organ.

parenteral A term applied to the administration of drugs or other substances by any route other than via the gastrointestinal tract (for example, by injection into a blood vessel).

parenteral nutrition Intravenous feeding (see *feeding, artificial*).

paresis Partial *paralysis* or weakness of one or more muscles.

parietal A medical term that refers to the wall of a part of the body.

parity A term that is used to indicate the number of pregnancies a woman has undergone that have resulted in the birth of a baby capable of survival.

parkinsonism Any neurological disorder characterized by a mask-like face, rigidity, and slow movements. The most common type is *Parkinson's disease*.

Parkinson's disease A neurological disorder that causes muscle tremor, stiffness, and weakness. The characteristic signs are trembling, rigid posture, slow movements, and a shuffling, unbalanced walk. The disease is caused by degeneration of, or damage to, cells in the *basal ganglia* of the brain, reducing the amount of dopamine (which is needed for control of movement). It occurs mainly in elderly people and is more common in men.

The disease usually begins as a slight tremor of one hand, arm, or leg, which is worse when the hand or limb is at rest. Later, both sides of the body are affected, causing a stiff, shuffling, walk; constant trembling of the hands, sometimes accompanied by shaking of the head; a permanent rigid stoop; and an unblinking, fixed expression. The intellect is unaffected until late in the disease.

There is no cure. Drug treatment is used to minimize symptoms in later stages. *Levodopa*, which the body converts into *dopamine*, is usually the most effective drug. It may be used in combination with benserazide or carbidopa. The effects of levodopa gradually wear off. Drugs that may be used in conjunction with it, or as substitutes for it, include *amantadine, selegiline*, pergolide, and *bromocriptine*. Surgical operations on the brain are occasionally performed. Untreated, the disease progresses over 10 to 15 years, leading to severe weakness and incapacity. About one third of sufferers eventually develop *dementia*.

paronychia An infection of the skin fold at the base or side of the *nail*. Paronychia may be acute (caused by bacteria) or chronic (usually caused by CANDIDA ALBICANS). The condition is most common in women, particularly those with poor circulation and whose work involves frequent contact with water. It also affects people with skin disease involving the nail fold. Treatment is with *antifungal drugs* or *antibiotic drugs*.

parotid glands The largest of the three pairs of *salivary glands*. The parotid glands lie above the angle of the jaw, below and in front of the ear, on each side of the face.

parotitis Inflammation of the *parotid glands*, often due to infection with the *mumps* virus.

paroxetine A *selective serotonin reuptake inhibitor* antidepressant drug. Possible side effects include nausea, indigestion, and appetite loss. It is not usually recommended for those under 18.

paroxysm A sudden attack, worsening, or recurrence of symptoms or of a disease; a *spasm* or *seizure*.

parrot fever The common name for *psittacosis*.

parturition See *childbirth*.

parvovirus A viral infection that causes a rash and joint inflammation. Many children have no symptoms, but some have a bright red rash on the cheeks, a mild fever, and sometimes mild joint inflammation. Symptoms are more severe in adults; they include a rash on the palms and soles of the feet and severe inflammation in the knee, wrist, and hand joints. A diagnosis is made from the symptoms and a *blood test*. The infection usually clears up within 2 weeks without treatment.

passive smoking Involuntary inhalation of *tobacco* smoke by people who do not smoke. Passive smoking has been shown to increase the risks of chest and ear infections in children and of tobacco-induced cancers in adults.

pasteurization The process of heating foods to destroy disease-causing *microorganisms*, and to reduce the numbers of microorganisms responsible for fermentation and putrefaction.

patch test A method of diagnosing the substances responsible for contact *dermatitis*. A selection of possible *allergens* are put on a patch and taped to the skin. A skin reaction indicates sensitivity to a particular allergen.

patella The kneecap (see *knee*).

patent A term meaning open or unobstructed (such as in *patent ductus arteriosus*). The term patent medicine is sometimes used to refer to proprietary drugs protected by a patent.

patent ductus arteriosus A defect of the *heart* in which the ductus arteriosus (a channel between the pulmonary artery and the aorta in the fetus) fails to close at birth. It affects about 60 babies per 100,000. In the fetus, blood pumped by the right side of the heart flows through the ductus arteriosus and bypasses the lungs (see *fetal circulation*). At or shortly after birth, the ductus usually closes. In some babies this closure may fail to happen, preventing normal circulation. There are usually no symptoms unless a large amount of blood is misdirected, in which case the baby fails to gain weight, becomes short of breath on exertion, and may have frequent chest infections. Eventually, *heart failure* may develop.

Diagnosis is made from hearing a heart *murmur*, from *chest X-rays*, and from an *ECG* and *echocardiography*. The drug indometacin or surgery may be used to close the duct.

paternity testing The use of blood tests to help decide whether a man is the father of a child. Blood samples are taken from the child, from the suspected father, and sometimes from the mother. The samples are tested for *blood groups*, histocompatibility antigens, and similarities in *DNA*. *Genetic fingerprinting* provides the most decisive result.

patho- A prefix denoting a relationship to disease.

pathogen Any agent, but particularly a *microorganism*, that causes disease.

pathogenesis The processes by which a disorder originates and develops.

pathognomonic A medical term applied to a symptom or sign that is characteristic of a disease or disorder and is therefore sufficient to make a diagnosis.

pathological Relating to disease or to its study (*pathology*).

pathology The study of disease – its causes, mechanisms, and effects on the body. Pathologists conduct autopsies to determine causes of death and to determine the effects that a disease or a treatment has had.

pathology, cellular Also called cytopathology, the branch of *cytology* concerned with the effects of disease on cells.

pathology, chemical Another name for clinical biochemistry, the study of abnormalities in the chemistry of body tissues in disease.

pathophysiology The study of the effects of disease on body functions.

-pathy A suffix that denotes a disease or disorder.

PCR An abbreviation for *polymerase chain reaction*.

peak-flow meter A piece of equipment that measures the maximum speed at which air can flow out of the lungs. A peak-flow meter is useful in assessing the severity of *bronchospasm*, and is most commonly used to diagnose asthma, monitor patients with asthma, and assess response to asthma treatment. The peak flow is measured by taking a deep breath and breathing out with maximum effort through the mouthpiece.

PEAK-FLOW METER

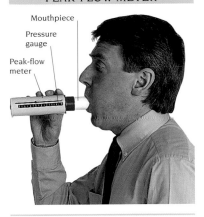

Mouthpiece

Pressure gauge

Peak-flow meter

peau d'orange A condition in which the skin has a normal colour but looks like orange peel. The skin's dimpled appearance is due to fluid retention in the nearby lymph vessels.

pectoral A medical term that means relating to the chest, as in the major and minor pectoral muscles.

pediculosis Any type of louse infestation. (See *lice; pubic lice*.)

peer review Processes by which doctors and scientists review the work of colleagues in the same field. Peer review is used to maintain standards.

pellagra A potentially fatal nutritional disorder caused by deficiency of niacin (see *vitamin B complex*) and resulting in *dermatitis*, diarrhoea, and *dementia*. It occurs primarily in poor rural communities in parts of the world, such as areas of India, where people subsist on maize. Most of the niacin in maize is unabsorbable unless the maize is treated with an alkali such as limewater. Disorders such as *carcinoid syndrome* and *inflammatory bowel disease* may also be a cause.

The first symptoms are weakness, weight loss, lethargy, depression, irritability, and inflammation and itching of skin exposed to sunlight. In acute attacks, weeping

blisters may develop on the affected skin, and the tongue becomes swollen and painful. Diagnosis is made from the patient's condition and dietary history. Daily intake of niacin and a varied diet usually bring about a cure.

pelvic examination Examination of a woman's external and internal genitalia. After examination of the external genitalia, a *speculum* is inserted into the vagina to allow a clear view of the cervix. A *cervical smear test* may be performed. The doctor inserts two fingers into the vagina and, with the other hand, feels the abdomen to evaluate the position and size of the uterus and the ovaries and to detect any tenderness or swelling.

pelvic floor exercises A programme of exercises to strengthen the muscles and tighten the ligaments at the base of the abdomen, which form the pelvic floor.

These muscles and ligaments support the uterus, vagina, bladder, urethra, and rectum. Performing the exercises may help to prevent prolapse of the uterus (see *uterus, prolapse of*) and urinary stress incontinence (see *incontinence, urinary*).

The pelvic floor muscles are those that tighten when urine flow is stopped midstream. The exercises involve stopping and starting urine flow several times by contracting and relaxing the muscles. Ideally, they should be performed for 5 minutes every hour throughout the day. They can be done standing, sitting, or lying down, by imagining that urine is being passed, contracting and holding the muscles for 10 seconds, and then slowly releasing them, repeating 5–10 times as often as possible.

pelvic infection An infection in the female reproductive system. Severe or recurrent pelvic infection is referred to as *pelvic inflammatory disease* (PID).

pelvic inflammatory disease An infection of the internal female reproductive organs. Pelvic inflammatory disease (or PID) may not have any obvious cause, but may occur as a result of a sexually transmitted infection, such as *gonorrhoea* or *chlamydia*, or after a *miscarriage*, an abortion, or *childbirth*. An *IUD* increases the risk of infection. PID may cause *infertility* or increase the risk of *ectopic pregnancy*.

P

Common symptoms include abdominal pain and tenderness, fever, and irregular menstrual periods. Pain often occurs after menstruation and may be worse during intercourse. There may also be malaise, vomiting, or backache. A diagnosis is usually made by an internal *pelvic examination*, examination of swabs to look for infection, and a *laparoscopy*. *Antibiotic drugs* and sometimes *analgesic drugs* are prescribed. An IUD may need to be removed.

pelvic pain See *abdominal pain*.

pelvimetry Assessment of the shape and dimensions of a woman's pelvis by making measurements on an *X-ray* image. Pelvimetry may be carried out to determine whether a woman is likely to have difficulty in delivering a baby vaginally. It may also be performed after a vaginal delivery has been unsuccessful, to assist in planning a future pregnancy.

pelvis The ring of bones in the lower trunk consisting of two innominate (hip) bones, which are joined to the *sacrum* at the back and the pubic *symphysis* at the front. Each hip bone consists of three fused bones: the ilium (the largest and uppermost), ischium (which bears much of the body weight when sitting), and pubis (the smallest).

In women, the pelvis is generally shallow and broad, and the pubic symphysis joint is less rigid than a man's. These differences facilitate childbirth. In men, the greater body weight needs a larger and more heavily built pelvis.

pemphigoid An uncommon chronic skin disease, mainly affecting elderly people, in which large, sometimes itchy, blisters form on the skin. Pemphigoid is thought to be an *autoimmune disorder*. Diagnosis is made with a skin *biopsy*, and treatment is usually a long-term course of *corticosteroid* or *immunosuppressant drugs*.

pemphigus A rare, serious skin disease in which *blisters* develop on the skin and in the mouth. It primarily affects people aged 40–60. The blisters usually develop in the mouth, before appearing on the skin and then rupturing to form raw areas that may become infected and later crust over. Skin that appears unaffected may also blister after gentle pressure is applied. If a large area of the body is affected, severe skin loss can lead to bacterial infection and, sometimes, death.

The diagnosis is confirmed by a skin *biopsy*. Treatment is with a long-term course of *corticosteroid drugs* and, sometimes, *immunosuppressants*. Antibiotics may also be prescribed.

penicillamine A *disease-modifying antirheumatic drug* sometimes used to treat acute, progressive *rheumatoid arthritis*. Penicillamine is also used to treat copper, mercury, lead, or arsenic poisoning; *Wilson's disease*; and primary *biliary cirrhosis*.

The possible adverse effects of penicillamine can include allergic rashes, itching, nausea, vomiting, abdominal pain, loss of taste, blood disorders, and impaired kidney function.

penicillin drugs A group of *antibiotic drugs*. Natural penicillins are derived from the mould PENICILLIUM; others are synthetic preparations. Penicillins are used to treat many infective conditions,

PELVIS

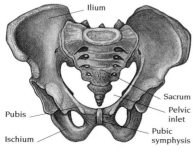

Ilium
Pubis
Ischium
Sacrum
Pelvic inlet
Pubic symphysis

MALE PELVIS

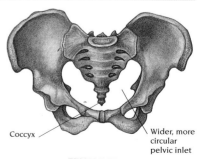

Coccyx
Wider, more circular pelvic inlet

FEMALE PELVIS

including *tonsillitis*, *bronchitis*, bacterial *endocarditis*, *syphilis*, and *pneumonia*. They are also given to prevent *rheumatic fever* from recurring. Common adverse effects of penicillins are an allergic reaction causing a rash, and diarrhoea.

penile implant A *prosthesis* inserted into the *penis* to help a man with permanent *erectile dysfunction* to achieve intercourse. The various types include a silicone splint inserted in the tissues of the upper surface of the penis, and an inflatable prosthesis that is inflated by squeezing a small bulb in the scrotum.

penile warts See *warts, genital.*

penis The male sex organ through which *urine and semen pass.* The penis consists mainly of three cylindrical bodies of erectile tissue (spongy tissue full of blood vessels) that run along its length. Two of these bodies, the corpora cavernosa, lie side by side along the upper part of the penis. The third body, the corpus spongiosum, lies centrally beneath them and expands at the end to form the *glans.* Through the centre of the corpus spongiosum runs the *urethra*, a narrow tube that carries urine and semen out of the body through an opening at the tip of the glans. Around the erectile tissue is a sheath consisting of fibrous connective tissue enclosed by skin. Over the glans, the skin forms a fold called the *foreskin.*

penis, cancer of A rare type of cancerous tumour that is more common in uncircumcised men with poor personal hygiene. Viral infection and smoking have both been shown to be additional risk factors. The tumour usually starts on the *glans* or on the foreskin as a painless, wart-like lump or a painful ulcer, and develops into a cauliflower-like mass. The growth usually spreads slowly, but in some cases it can spread to the *lymph nodes* in the groin within a few months.

Diagnosis is made by a *biopsy.* If the tumour is detected early, *radiotherapy* is usually successful. Otherwise, removal of part or all of the penis may be necessary.

pentamidine An antiprotozoal drug (see *protozoa*), administered by intravenous infusion or nebulizer to prevent and treat *pneumocystis pneumonia* in immunosuppressed people. Pentamidine is also used to treat the tropical disease *leish-*

maniasis. Side effects may include nausea and vomiting, dizziness, flushing, rash, and taste disturbances.

pentazocine An opioid *analgesic drug* used to relieve moderate or severe pain caused by injury, surgery, cancer, or childbirth. It is rarely used because of its adverse affects, which include dizziness, drowsiness, nausea, vomiting, and, rarely, hallucinations. *Drug dependence* may develop if high doses are taken for prolonged periods.

peppermint oil An oil obtained from the peppermint plant MENTHA PIPERITA. It is prescribed to relieve abdominal colic but may cause heartburn. It is also used as a flavouring in some drug preparations.

peptic ulcer A raw area that develops in the gastrointestinal tract as a result of erosion by acidic gastric juice; it most commonly occurs in the stomach or the first part of the *duodenum.*

The major cause of peptic ulcers is HELICOBACTER PYLORI bacterial infection, which can damage the lining of the stomach and duodenum, allowing the acid stomach contents to attack it. *Analgesic drugs*, alcohol, excess acid production, and smoking can also damage the stomach lining. Ulcers can also form in the *oesophagus*, when acidic juice from the stomach enters it (see *gastro-oesophageal reflux disease*), and in the duodenum.

There may be no symptoms, or there may be burning or gnawing pain in the upper abdomen. Other possible symptoms include loss of appetite, nausea, and vomiting. The ulcer may also bleed. If severe, it may result in haematemesis (vomiting of blood) and *melaena*, and is a medical emergency. Chronic bleeding may cause iron-deficiency *anaemia.* Rarely, an ulcer may perforate the wall of the digestive tract and lead to *peritonitis.*

An ulcer is usually diagnosed by an *endoscopy* of the stomach and duodenum; less commonly, a barium meal (see *barium X-ray examination*) is performed. Blood and breath tests will be carried out to see whether the person is infected with the HELICOBACTER bacterium. If this is the case, a combination of *antibiotics* and an *ulcer-healing drug* will be given. A further test may be done to check that treatment has been successful. If

P

HELICOBACTER is not detected – for example, in ulcers caused by *nonsteroidal anti-inflammatory drugs* (NSAIDs) – treatment is with *proton pump inhibitors* or *H₂-blockers*, and the NSAIDs will be stopped. Surgery is now rarely needed for peptic ulcers, except to treat complications such as bleeding or perforation. Stopping smoking and reducing alcohol consumption lessen the likelihood of recurrence.

peptide A protein fragment consisting of two or more *amino acids*. Peptides that consist of many linked amino acids are known as polypeptides; chains of polypeptides are called *proteins*. In the body, peptides occur in forms such as *hormones* and *endorphins*.

perception The interpretation of a sensation. Information is received through the five senses (taste, smell, hearing, vision, and touch) and organized into a pattern by the brain. Factors such as attitude, mood, and expectations affect the final interpretation. *Hallucinations* are false perceptions that occur in the absence of sensory stimuli.

percussion A diagnostic technique involving tapping the chest or abdomen with the fingers and listening to the sound produced to deduce the condition of the internal organs. (See also *examination, physical.*)

percutaneous A medical term meaning through the skin.

perforation A hole made in an organ or tissue by disease or injury.

peri- A prefix meaning around.

perianal haematoma A *haematoma* under the skin around the anus.

pericarditis Inflammation of the *pericardium*, which often leads to chest pain and fever. There may also be an increased amount of fluid (*effusion*) in the pericardial space, which may restrict the heart. Long-term inflammation can cause constrictive pericarditis, a condition in which the pericardium becomes scarred, thickens, and contracts, interfering with the heart's action.

Causes of pericarditis include infection; *myocardial infarction*; cancer spreading from another site; and injury to the pericardium. The disorder may accompany *rheumatoid arthritis*, systemic *lupus erythematosus*, and *kidney failure*.

Pericarditis causes pain behind the breastbone, and sometimes in the neck and shoulders. There may also be fever. Constrictive pericarditis causes *oedema* of the legs and abdomen.

Diagnosis is made from a *physical examination* and an *ECG* and *chest X-rays* or *echocardiography*. If possible, treatment is aimed at the cause. *Analgesic drugs* or *anti-inflammatory drugs* may be given. If an effusion is present, fluid may be drawn off through a needle. In constrictive pericarditis, part of the pericardium may be removed.

pericardium The membranous bag that surrounds the *heart* and the roots of the major blood vessels that emerge from it. The pericardium has two layers separated by a space called the pericardial space, which contains a small amount of fluid that lubricates the heart.

PERICARDIUM

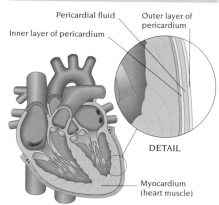

Pericardial fluid
Outer layer of pericardium
Inner layer of pericardium

DETAIL

Myocardium (heart muscle)

STRUCTURE OF HEART

perimetry A visual field test to determine the extent of peripheral vision. (See eye, *examination of.*)

perinatal Relating to the period just before or just after birth. The perinatal period is often defined as the period from the 28th week of pregnancy to the end of the 1st week after birth.

perinatology A branch of *obstetrics* and *paediatrics* concerned with the study and care of the mother and baby during pregnancy and just after birth.

perindopril An *ACE inhibitor drug* used to treat *hypertension* and *heart failure*. A combined preparation of perindopril and a *diuretic drug* may be used to improve blood pressure control. Possible side effects of perindopril include *hypotension*, a dry cough, and skin rashes.

perineum The area bounded internally by the pelvic floor (the muscles that support the pelvis) and the surrounding bony structures. Externally, the perineum is the area that lies behind the genitals and in front of the anus.

periodic fever An inherited condition causing recurrent bouts of fever. (See *familial Mediterranean fever*.)

period, menstrual See *menstruation*.

periodontal disease Any disorder of the periodontium (the tissues that surround and support the *teeth*).

periodontics The branch of *dentistry* concerned with *periodontal disease*.

periodontitis Inflammation of the periodontium (the tissues surrounding the *teeth*). There are two types: periapical and chronic. Periapical periodontitis results from neglected dental *caries* and occurs when bacteria enter the tooth pulp and spread to the root tip, sometimes causing a dental *abscess*, *granuloma*, or *cyst*. Chronic periodontitis is a result of untreated *gingivitis*, in which bacteria attack the periodontal tissues. This type is the major cause of adult tooth loss.

Periapical periodontitis may cause toothache, especially on biting. An abscess may make the tooth loose; a large dental cyst may cause swelling of the jaw. In chronic periodontitis, the signs of gingivitis are present.

Periodontitis is diagnosed by a dental examination and dental *X-rays*. Periapical periodontis is treated by draining pus and filling the tooth or by *extraction*.

Regular teeth cleaning can prevent advanced chronic periodontal disease and further destruction of the tissues. Treatment may include root planing, *scaling*, *gingivectomy*, or curettage (see *curettage, dental*). Sometimes, loose teeth can be anchored to firmer teeth by splinting (see *splinting, dental*).

period pain See *dysmenorrhoea*.

periosteum The tissue that coats all of the *bones* in the body except the joint surfaces. The periosteum contains small blood vessels and nerves, and produces new bone in the initial stages of healing following a *fracture*.

PERIOSTEUM

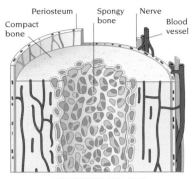

Periosteum   Spongy   Nerve
Compact bone   bone   Blood vessel

STRUCTURE OF BONE

periostitis Inflammation of the *periosteum*. The usual cause is a blow that presses directly on to bone. Symptoms include pain, tenderness, and swelling over the affected area.

peripheral nervous system All the nerves that fan out from the *central nervous system* to the muscles, skin, internal organs, and glands (see *nerve*; *cranial nerves*; *spinal nerves*).

peripheral vascular disease Narrowing of blood vessels in the legs, and sometimes in the arms, restricting blood flow and causing pain. In severe cases, *gangrene* may develop. In most affected people, peripheral vascular disease is caused by *atherosclerosis*. The greatest risk factor is *smoking*. Diseases of the peripheral vessels that are not caused by atherosclerosis include *Buerger's disease*, *Raynaud's disease*, *deep vein thrombosis*, and *varicose veins*.

The first symptom of narrowed arteries due to atherosclerosis is usually an aching feeling in the leg muscles when walking, which is relieved by resting. Pain recurs after the same amount of walking as before. Prolonged use of the arms may also cause pain. Symptoms then become worse until, eventually, pain is present even when the person is at rest and the affected limb is cold and numb.

In the final stage, there is gangrene. Sudden arterial blockage may occur, causing sudden severe pain. Movement and feeling in the limb are lost.

A diagnosis is often based on results of doppler *ultrasound* or *angiography*.

Exercise and giving up smoking are important aspects of treatment. *Arterial reconstructive surgery, bypass* surgery, or balloon *angioplasty* may be needed. *Amputation* is needed for gangrene.

peristalsis Wave-like movement caused by rhythmic contraction and relaxation of the smooth muscles in the walls of the digestive tract and the ureters. Peristalsis is responsible for the movement of food and waste products through the digestive system and for transporting urine from the kidneys to the bladder.

peritoneal dialysis See *dialysis*.

peritoneum The two-layered membrane that lines the abdominal cavity and covers and supports the abdominal organs. The peritoneum produces a lubricating fluid that allows the abdominal organs to glide smoothly over each other, and protects the organs against infection. It also absorbs fluid and acts as a natural filtering system. The peritoneum may become inflamed as a complication of an abdominal disorder (see *peritonitis*).

PERITONEUM

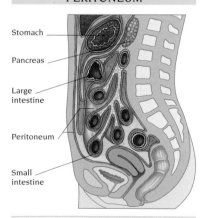

Stomach

Pancreas

Large intestine

Peritoneum

Small intestine

peritonitis Inflammation of the *peritoneum*. It is a serious, usually acute, condition. The most common cause is *perforation* of the stomach or intestine wall, which allows bacteria and digestive juices to move into the abdominal cavity. Perforation is usually the result of a *peptic ulcer, appendicitis*, or *diverticulitis*. Peritonitis may also be associated with acute *salpingitis, cholecystitis*, or *septicaemia*.

There is usually severe abdominal pain. After a few hours, the abdomen feels hard, and *peristalsis* stops (see *ileus, paralytic*). Other symptoms are fever, bloating, nausea, and vomiting.

Diagnosis is made from a *physical examination*. Surgery may be necessary to deal with the cause. If the cause is unknown, a *laparoscopy* or an exploratory *laparotomy* may be performed. *Antibiotic drugs* and *intravenous infusions* of fluid are often given. In most cases, a full recovery is made. Intestinal obstruction, caused by *adhesions*, may occur at a later stage.

peritonsillar abscess A complication of *tonsillitis*.

permanent teeth The second *teeth*, which usually start to replace the primary teeth at about the age of 6. There are 32 permanent teeth: 16 in each jaw. Each set of 16 consists of 4 incisors, 2 canines, 4 premolars and 6 molars. (See also *eruption of teeth*.)

permethrin A substance included in preparations used to treat *pubic lice* and *scabies*. Permethrin can also be used as an insecticide; sprayed on to mosquito nets and clothing, it repels mosquitoes and ticks.

pernicious anaemia A type of *anaemia* caused by a failure to absorb *vitamin* B_{12}. Deficiency leads to the production of abnormal, large red blood cells.

pernio An alternative term for *chilblain*.

peroneal muscular atrophy A rare, inherited disorder characterized by muscle wasting in the feet and calves and then in the hands and forearms. The condition, also known as Charcot–Marie–Tooth disease, is caused by degeneration of some peripheral nerves. It is more common in boys, and usually appears in late childhood or adolescence. Muscle wasting stops halfway up the arms and legs, making them look like inverted bottles; sensation may be lost. There is no treatment, but the sufferer rarely becomes totally incapacitated because the disease

P

usually progresses very slowly. Life expectancy is normal.

perphenazine A *phenothiazine*-type *antipsychotic drug* used to relieve symptoms in psychiatric disorders, such as *schizophrenia*; to sedate agitated or anxious patients; and sometimes to relieve severe nausea and vomiting.

Possible adverse effects include abnormal movements of the face and limbs, drowsiness, blurred vision, stuffy nose, and headache. Long-term use of the drug may cause *parkinsonism*.

persistent vegetative state Long-term *unconsciousness* caused by damage to areas of the brain that control higher mental functions. The eyes may open and close, and there may be random movements of the limbs, but there is no response to stimuli such as pain. Basic functions such as breathing and heartbeat are not affected. There is no treatment to reverse the situation, but, with good nursing care, survival for months or years is possible.

personality The sum of a person's traits, habits, and experiences. Temperament, intelligence, emotion, and motivation are important aspects. The development of personality seems to depend on the interaction of heredity and environment.

personality disorders A group of conditions characterized by a failure to learn from experience or to adapt appropriately to changes, resulting in distress and impairment of social functioning. Personality disorders are ways of behaving that may become especially obvious during periods of stress. They are usually first recognizable in adolescence and continue throughout life, often leading to *depression* or *anxiety*.

Specific types of personality disorders are divided into three groups but there is often overlap. The first group is characterized by eccentric behaviour. Paranoid people show suspiciousness and mistrust of others, schizoid people are cold emotionally, and schizotypal personalities have behaviour oddities similar to those of schizophrenia, but less severe.

In the second group, behaviour tends to be dramatic. Histrionic people are excitable and constantly crave stimulation, narcissists have an exaggerated sense of their own importance (see *narcissism*), and people with antisocial personality disorder fail to conform to accepted social standards of behaviour.

People in the third group show anxiety and fear. Dependent personalities lack the self-confidence to function independently. Those with compulsive personalities are rigid in their habits (see *obsessive–compulsive disorder*), and passive-aggressive people resist demands from others.

Treatment is usually *counselling, psychotherapy*, and *behaviour therapy*.

personality tests Questionnaires designed to define various personality traits or types. Tests may be designed to detect psychiatric symptoms, underlying personality traits, how outgoing or reserved a person is, and predisposition to developing neurotic illness.

perspiration The production and excretion of sweat from the *sweat glands*. Perspiration is another name for sweat.

Perthes' disease Inflammation of an *epiphysis* of the head of the *femur*. The disease is a type of *osteochondritis juvenilis*, thought to be due to disrupted blood supply to the bone. The condition is most common in boys aged 5–10, and usually affects one hip. Symptoms include pain in the thigh and groin, and a limp on the affected side. Diagnosis is made with *X-rays*. Treatment may be rest for a few weeks, followed by splinting of the hip, or surgery. The disease usually clears up by itself within 3 years, but the hip may be permanently deformed.

pertussis A highly contagious infectious disease, also called whooping cough, which mainly affects infants and young children. The main features are coughing bouts, often ending in a characteristic "whoop". The main cause is infection with BORDETELLA PERTUSSIS bacteria, which are spread in airborne droplets.

After an *incubation period* of 7–10 days, the illness starts with a mild cough, sneezing, nasal discharge, fever, and sore eyes. After a few days, the cough becomes more persistent and severe, especially at night. Whooping occurs in most cases. Sometimes the cough can cause vomiting. In infants, there is a risk of temporary *apnoea* following a coughing spasm. The illness may last for a few weeks. The possible complications include nosebleeds, *dehydration*, *pneumonia*, *pneumothorax*, *bronchiectasis*, and convulsions. If left untreated, pertussis may prove fatal.

Pertussis is usually diagnosed from the symptoms. In the early stages, *erythromycin* is often given to reduce the child's infectivity. Treatment consists of keeping the child warm, giving small, frequent meals and plenty to drink, and protecting him or her from stimuli, such as smoke, that can provoke coughing. If the child turns blue or persistently vomits after coughing, hospital admission is needed.

To protect infants, communities need to maintain a high level of immunity through *immunization*. In the UK, vaccination against pertussis is given at 2, 3, and 4 months of age, with a booster dose at 3–5 years. Possible complications include a mild fever and fretfulness. Very rarely, an infant may have a severe reaction to the vaccine, with high-pitched screaming or seizures.

perversion See *deviation, sexual*.

pes cavus See *claw-foot*.

pessary Any of a variety of devices placed in the vagina. Some types are used to correct the position of the uterus (see *uterus, prolapse of*); others are used as contraceptive devices. The term is also used to refer to a medicated vaginal suppository.

pesticides Poisonous chemicals used to eradicate pests. Different types include herbicides, insecticides, and fungicides. Pesticide poisoning, particularly in children, may result from swallowing an insecticide or a garden herbicide (see *chlorate poisoning*). Poisoning may occur in agricultural workers, often as a result of inhalation or absorption of the chemical through the skin. Exposure to pesticides can also occur indirectly, through eating pesticide-contaminated food. (See also *DDT*; *defoliant poisoning*; *organophosphates*; *paraquat*; *parathion*.)

petechiae Red or purple, flat, pinhead spots that occur in the skin or mucous membranes. Petechiae are caused by a localized *haemorrhage* from small blood vessels. They occur in *purpura* and, sometimes, bacterial *endocarditis*.

pethidine A synthetic opioid *analgesic drug* similar to, but less powerful than, *morphine*. It is used as a *premedication* and to relieve pain after operations, during childbirth, or in terminal illness. As it may cause nausea and vomiting, it is usually given with an *antiemetic drug*.

petit mal A type of seizure that occurs in *epilepsy*. Petit mal attacks occur in children and adolescents but rarely in adults. There is momentary loss of awareness, occasionally with drooping eyelids. Treatment is with an *anticonvulsant drug*.

petroleum jelly A greasy substance obtained from petroleum, also known as petrolatum or soft paraffin. The jelly is commonly used as an *ointment* base, a protective dressing, and an *emollient*.

PET scanning The abbreviation for positron emission tomography, a diagnostic technique based on the detection of positrons (a type of subatomic particle) that are emitted by radioactively labelled substances introduced into the body. PET scanning produces three-dimensional images of the metabolic and chemical activity of tissues.

Substances used in biochemical processes in the body are labelled with radioisotopes and then injected into the bloodstream. The substances are taken up in greater concentrations by tissues that are more metabolically active. The substances emit positrons, which release photons that are detected by the scanner. PET scans are used to detect brain

PET SCANNING

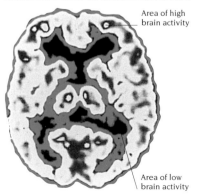

Area of high brain activity

Area of low brain activity

PET SCAN OF NORMAL BRAIN

tumours, locate epileptic activity within the brain, and examine brain function.

Peutz–Jeghers syndrome A very rare, inherited condition in which *polyps* occur in the gastrointestinal tract and small, flat, brown spots appear on the lips and in the mouth. Occasionally the polyps bleed, or cause abdominal pain or *intussusception*. Tests include *barium X-ray examination* and *endoscopy*. Bleeding polyps may be removed.

peyote A cactus plant found in northern Mexico and the southwest of the US. Its dried blossoms are used to prepare the hallucinogenic drug *mescaline*.

Peyronie's disease A disorder of the *penis* in which part of the sheath of fibrous connective tissue thickens, causing the penis to bend during erection. This commonly makes intercourse difficult and painful. Eventually, some of the penile erectile tissue may also thicken. Men over 40 are most often affected. The cause is unknown. The disease may improve without treatment. Otherwise, local injections of *corticosteroid drugs* or surgical removal of the thickened area and replacement with normal tissue may be carried out.

pH A measure of the acidity or alkalinity of a solution. The pH scale ranges from 0–14, 7 being neutral; values smaller than this are acid, values larger are alkaline. The pH of body fluids must be close to 7.4 for metabolic reactions to proceed normally (see *acid-base balance*).

phaeochromocytoma A rare tumour of cells that secrete *epinephrine* (adrenaline) and *norepinephrine* (noradrenaline). It causes increased production of these hormones, leading to *hypertension*. The tumours usually develop in the *medulla* (core) of the *adrenal glands*, and are most common in young to middle-aged adults.

Hypertension is the only sign most of the time, but pressure on the tumour, emotional upset, change in posture, or taking *beta-blocker drugs* can cause a surge of hormones. This surge brings on a sudden rise in blood pressure, *palpitations*, headache, nausea, vomiting, facial flushing, sweating, and, sometimes, a feeling of impending death.

Blood tests and *urinalysis* are used to make a diagnosis. *CT scanning*, *MRI*, and *radioisotope scanning* may be used

to locate the tumours, which are then usually removed surgically. Follow-up medical checks are required because the condition occasionally recurs.

phagocyte A cell in the *immune system* that can surround, engulf, and digest *microorganisms*, foreign particles, and cellular debris. Phagocytes are found in the blood, *spleen*, *lymph nodes*, and alveoli (small air sacs) within the lungs.

phalanges The small bones that make up the fingers, thumb, and toes. The thumb and big toe have two phalanges; all the other fingers and toes have three.

phalanx A term for any of the bones in the fingers or the toes.

phallus Any object that may symbolize the *penis*.

phantom limb The *perception* that a limb is still present after amputation.

pharmaceutical Any medicinal drug. The term is also used in relation to the manufacture and sale of drugs.

pharmacognosy The study or knowledge of the pharmacologically active ingredients of plants.

pharmacokinetics The term used to describe how the body deals with a *drug*.

pharmacology The branch of science that is concerned with the discovery and development of *drugs*; their chemical composition; their actions; their uses; and their side effects and toxicity.

pharmacopoeia Any book that lists and describes most medicinal drugs, especially an official publication, such as the British Pharmacopoeia (BP).

A pharmacopoeia describes sources, preparations, and doses of drugs. There may also be information on how drugs work and on possible adverse effects.

pharmacy The practice of preparing drugs, and making up and dispensing prescriptions. Also, a place where these activities are carried out.

pharyngeal diverticulum An alternative term for a pharyngeal pouch (see *oesophageal diverticulum*).

pharyngeal pouch See *oesophageal diverticulum*.

pharyngitis Acute or chronic inflammation of the *pharynx*, causing a sore throat. Causes of pharyngitis include viral and bacterial infections. Swallowing substances that scald, corrode, or scratch

P

the lining of the throat, and smoking, may also cause pharyngitis.

With a sore throat, there may be discomfort when swallowing, fever, earache, and swollen *lymph nodes* in the neck.

Gargling with warm salt water and taking *analgesic drugs* is usually the only treatment needed. If the sore throat is severe or prolonged a doctor may take a throat *swab* and prescribe *antibiotic drugs*.

pharynx The passage that connects the back of the mouth and nose to the *oesophagus*. The upper part, or *nasopharynx*, connects the nasal cavity to the area behind the soft *palate*. The middle part, the oropharynx, runs from the nasopharynx to below the tongue. The lower part, called the laryngopharynx, lies behind and to each side of the *larynx*.

pharynx, cancer of A cancerous tumour of the *pharynx*. Pharyngeal cancer usually develops in the *mucous membrane* lining. In the West, almost all cases of pharyngeal cancer are related to smoking and to drinking alcohol. The incidence rises with age, and the disorder is more common in men.

Cancerous tumours of the oropharynx (the middle section of the pharynx) usually cause difficulty swallowing, often with a sore throat and earache. Blood-stained sputum may be coughed up. Sometimes there is only the feeling of a lump in the throat or a visible enlarged *lymph node* in the neck. Cancer of the laryngopharynx (the lowermost part of the pharynx) initially causes a sensation of incomplete swallowing, then a muffled voice, hoarseness, and increased difficulty in swallowing. Tumours of the nasopharynx have different causes and symptoms (see *nasopharynx, cancer of*).

Diagnosis of cancer of the pharynx is made by *biopsy*, often in conjunction with *laryngoscopy, bronchoscopy*, or *oesophagoscopy*. The growth may be removed surgically or treated with *radiotherapy*. *Anticancer drugs* may also be given.

phencyclidine A drug of abuse, commonly known as angel dust or PCP.

phenelzine A monoamine oxidase inhibitor *antidepressant drug* usually given when other antidepressant drugs are ineffective. Possible side effects include dizziness, drowsiness, and rash, and,

when taken with certain foods or other drugs, a dangerous rise in blood pressure.

phenobarbital A *barbiturate drug* used mainly as an *anticonvulsant*. It is often used with *phenytoin* to treat *epilepsy*. Possible side effects include drowsiness, clumsiness, dizziness, excitement, and confusion.

phenothiazine drugs A group of drugs used to treat psychotic illnesses (see *antipsychotic drugs*) and to relieve severe nausea and vomiting (see *antiemetic drugs*). The group includes *chlorpromazine*, fluphenazine, and perphenazine.

phenoxymethylpenicillin A synthetic *penicillin drug* prescribed to treat bacterial infections including pharyngitis, tonsillitis, and tooth abscess.

Possible adverse effects include rash and nausea. A few people develop a serious allergic reaction in which there is wheezing, breathing difficulty, and swelling around the mouth and eyes.

phenylephrine A *decongestant drug* used to treat seasonal allergic *rhinitis* (hay fever) and the common *cold*. As eye-drops, it is used to dilate the pupils for eye examinations. High doses or prolonged use of nasal preparations may cause headache and blurred vision; stopping taking the drug suddenly may make nasal congestion worse.

phenylketonuria An inherited disorder in which the *enzyme* that converts the *amino acid* phenylalanine into tyrosine (another amino acid) is defective. Unless phenylalanine is excluded from the diet, it builds up in the body and causes severe learning difficulties. All newborn babies are screened for phenylketonuria (see *blood spot screening tests*; *Guthrie test*). Affected babies show few signs of abnormality, but, unless phenylalanine is avoided, they develop neurological disturbances including *epilepsy*. They may have blonde hair and blue eyes, and their urine may have a mousy odour. Many have *eczema*.

Phenylalanine is found in most protein-containing foods and in artificial sweeteners. A specially modified diet is generally recommended throughout life, (and especially during pregnancy, because high phenylalanine levels in the mother can damage the fetus).

phenytoin An *anticonvulsant* drug used to treat *epilepsy* and *trigeminal neuralgia*. Side effects include nausea, dizziness, tremor, and overgrown and tender gums.

pheromone A substance with a particular odour that, when released in minute quantities by an animal, affects the behaviour or development of other individuals of the same species.

phimosis Tightness of the foreskin, preventing it from being drawn back over the *glans* (head) of the penis. In uncircumcised babies, some degree of phimosis is normal, but it usually improves by age 3 or 4. In some boys, the condition persists and may cause the foreskin to balloon out on urination. Attempts to retract a tight foreskin may make the condition worse. Phimosis may also develop in adult men, causing painful erection that may lead to *paraphimosis*. Proper cleaning of the glans may not be possible, so *balanitis* may develop. Treatment in both adults and children is by *circumcision*.

phlebitis Inflammation of a vein. A clot often develops, in which case the condition is termed *thrombophlebitis*.

phlebography The obtaining of *X-ray* images of veins that have been injected with a *radiopaque* substance. An alternative name is *venography*.

phlebotomy Puncture of a vein to remove blood (see *venepuncture; venesection*.)

phlegm See *sputum*.

phobia A persistent, irrational fear of, and desire to avoid, a particular object or situation. A phobia is considered a psychiatric disorder when it interferes with normal social functioning. Simple phobias (specific phobias) are the most common. These may involve fear of particular animals or situations, such as enclosed spaces (*claustrophobia*). Animal phobias usually start in childhood, but others develop at any time. Treatment depends on the severity of the condition.

Agoraphobia is a more serious phobia, often causing severe impairment. It usually starts in the late teens or early 20s. Social phobia is fear of being exposed to scrutiny, such as a fear of eating or speaking in public. This disorder usually begins in late childhood or early adolescence.

Causes of phobias are unknown. Simple phobias are thought by some to be a form of *conditioning*. For example, a person with a fear of dogs may have been frightened by a dog in childhood.

Exposure to the feared object or situation causes intense *anxiety* and, in some cases, a *panic attack*. Phobias may be associated with *depression* or *obsessive–compulsive behaviour*. Treatment may be with *behaviour therapy* and sometimes *antidepressant drugs*.

phocomelia A limb defect in which the feet and/or the hands are joined to the trunk by short stumps. The condition is extremely rare, but used to occur as a side effect in the children of women who took the drug *thalidomide* in early pregnancy.

pholcodine A *cough* suppressant.

phosphates Salts that are essential in the diet. A phosphate compound called *ATP* stores energy in cells.

phosphorus An essential *mineral*, present in many foods, including cereals, dairy products, and meat. In the body, phosphorus is combined with *calcium* to form the bones and teeth.

photocoagulation Destructive heating of tissue by intense light focused to a fine point, as in *laser treatment*.

photophobia An uncomfortable sensitivity or intolerance to light. It occurs with eye disorders, such as *corneal abrasion*, and is a feature of *meningitis*.

photorefractive keratectomy A surgical treatment for *astigmatism*, *myopia*, and *hypermetropia*, in which areas of the *cornea* are shaved away by *laser*.

photosensitivity Abnormal reaction to sunlight. Photosensitivity usually causes a rash on skin exposed to sunlight. This often occurs because a photosensitizer (such as some drugs, dyes, chemicals in perfumes and soaps, and plants such as mustard) has been ingested or applied to the skin. Photosensitivity is also a feature of disorders such as systemic *lupus erythematosus*. People who are susceptible to photosensitivity reactions should avoid exposure to sunlight and photosensitizers, and use *sunscreens*.

phototherapy Treatment with light, including sunlight, *ultraviolet light*, blue light, or *lasers*. Moderate exposure to sunlight is the most basic form, and is often helpful in treating *psoriasis*.

P

447

PHOTOTHERAPY

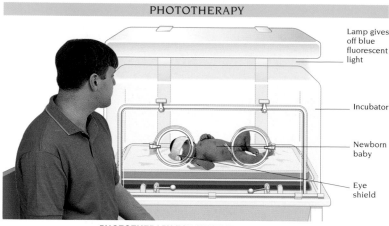

Lamp gives off blue fluorescent light

Incubator

Newborn baby

Eye shield

PHOTOTHERAPY FOR NEONATAL JAUNDICE

PUVA combines the use of long-wave ultraviolet light (UVA), with a *psoralen drug*, which sensitizes the skin to light. This is used to treat psoriasis and other skin diseases such as *vitiligo*. Psoriasis may also be treated using short-wave ultraviolet light (UVB), sometimes combined with the application of coal tar.

Visible blue light is used to treat neonatal jaundice (see *jaundice, neonatal*), which is due to high levels of the pigment *bilirubin* in the blood. In phototherapy, bilirubin is converted into a harmless substance that can be excreted. To maximize exposure, the baby is undressed and placed under lights in an incubator to keep him or her warm.

phrenic nerve One of the pair of main nerves supplying the *diaphragm*. Each phrenic nerve carries motor impulses to the diaphragm, and plays a part in controlling breathing. Injury to, or surgical cutting of, one of the nerves results in *paralysis* of half of the diaphragm.

physical examination See *examination, physical.*

physical medicine and rehabilitation A branch of medicine concerned with caring for patients who have become disabled through injury or illness.

physiology The study of body functions, including physical and chemical processes of cells, tissues, organs, and systems, and their various interactions.

physiotherapy Treatment with physical methods or agents. Physiotherapy is used to prevent or reduce joint stiffness; restore muscle strength; reduce pain; inflammation, and muscle spasm; and retrain joints and muscles after *stroke* or nerve injury. Methods include heat *treatment*, exercises, *massage*, *ice-packs*, *hydrotherapy*, and *TENS*. Physiotherapy is also used to maintain breathing in people with impaired lung function, and to prevent and treat pulmonary complications after surgery. Techniques include *breathing exercises, postural drainage*, and administration of oxygen, drugs, or moisture through a *nebulizer*.

phyto- A prefix meaning of plant origin.

phytomenadione A form of *vitamin K.*

phyto-oestrogens *Oestrogens* that occur naturally in plants.

pia mater The innermost of the three membranes of the *meninges.*

pica A craving to eat non-food substances such as earth or coal. Pica is common in early childhood and may occur during pregnancy. It may also occur in nutritional or iron-deficiency disorders, and in severe psychiatric disorders.

Pickwickian syndrome An unusual disorder characterized by extreme *obesity*, shallow breathing, and *sleep apnoea*. The cause is unclear. Symptoms usually improve with weight loss.

PID See *pelvic inflammatory disease.*

P

PINTA

pigeon toes A minor abnormality in which the leg or foot is rotated, forcing the foot and toes to point inwards. The condition is common in toddlers.

pigmentation Coloration of the skin, hair, and *iris* of the eyes by *melanin*. The more melanin present, the darker the coloration. Blood pigments can also colour skin (such as in a bruise).

There are many abnormalities of pigmentation. Patches of pale skin occur in *psoriasis, pityriasis alba, pityriasis versicolor,* and *vitiligo. Albinism* is caused by generalized melanin deficiency. *Phenylketonuria* results in a reduced melanin level, making sufferers pale-skinned and fair-haired. Areas of dark skin may be caused by disorders such as *eczema* or psoriasis, pityriasis versicolor, *chloasma,* or by some perfumes and cosmetics containing chemicals that cause *photosensitivity.* Permanent areas of deep pigmentation, such as freckles and moles (see *naevus*), are usually due to an abnormality of *melanocytes. Acanthosis nigricans* is characterized by dark patches of velvet-like, thickened skin. Blood pigments may lead to abnormal colouring. Excess of the bile pigment bilirubin in *jaundice* turns the skin yellow, and *haemochromatosis* turns the skin bronze.

piles A common name for *haemorrhoids.*

pill, contraceptive See *oral contraceptives.*

pilocarpine A drug used to treat *glaucoma.* It may initially cause blurred vision, headache, and eye irritation.

pilonidal sinus A pit in the skin, often containing hairs, in the upper part of the buttock cleft. The cause is probably hair fragments growing inwards. Although usually harmless, infection may occur, causing recurrent, painful abscesses. If a sinus is infected, a wide area around it is surgically removed. Recurrence of infection is common, and plastic surgery is sometimes required.

pimozide An *antipsychotic drug* used to treat *schizophrenia* and other psychoses and also sometimes *Gilles de la Tourette's syndrome.* It may cause sedation, dry mouth, constipation, and blurred vision. An *ECG* is recommended before and during treatment with pimozide because the

drug has been associated with abnormalities of the heart's electrical activity.

pimple A small *pustule* or *papule.*

pindolol A *beta-blocker drug* used to treat *angina pectoris* and *hypertension.* Possible side effects are typical of other beta-blocker drugs, except that pindolol is less likely to cause *bradycardia.*

pineal gland A tiny, cone-shaped structure deep within the *brain,* whose sole function appears to be the secretion of *melatonin* in response to changes in light.

PINEAL GLAND

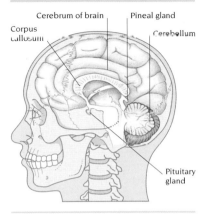

pinguecula A small, noncancerous, yellowish spot on the *conjunctiva* over the white of the eye. They are common in elderly people.

pink-eye See *conjunctivitis.*

pinna The fleshy part of the outer ear, consisting of a flap of cartilage and skin. It is also called the auricle.

pins-and-needles A tingling or prickly feeling in an area of skin that is usually associated with *numbness* and, sometimes, a burning feeling. The medical term is *paraesthesia.* Transient pins-and-needles is due to a temporary disturbance in the conduction of nerve signals from the skin. Persistent pins-and-needles may be caused by *neuropathy.*

pinta A skin infection, caused by TRE-PONEMA CARATEUM, occurring in remote areas of tropical America. A large spot, surrounded by smaller ones, appears on the face, neck, buttocks, hands, or feet. After 1–12 months it is followed by red skin patches that turn blue, then brown, and finally white. *Antibiotic drugs* clear up the infection, but the skin may be permanently disfigured.

pinworm infestation An alternative name for *threadworm infestation*.

pioglitazone An oral *hypoglycaemic drug* that is used in combination with other oral hypoglycaemics (either *metformin* or a sulphonylurea) in the treatment of type 2 *diabetes mellitus*. Side effects may include gastrointestinal disturbances, weight gain, and anaemia.

piperazine An *anthelmintic drug* used to treat *infestation* by *roundworms* and *threadworms*. Possible adverse effects include abdominal pain, nausea, vomiting, and diarrhoea.

piroxicam A *nonsteroidal anti-inflammatory drug* (NSAID) used to alleviate symptoms of *arthritis*, and to relieve pain in *bursitis*, *tendinitis*, and after minor surgery. Adverse effects may include nausea, indigestion, abdominal pain, swollen ankles, *peptic ulcer*, and liver problems.

pituitary gland Sometimes referred to as the master gland, the pituitary is the most important *endocrine gland*. It regulates and controls the activities of other endocrine glands and many body processes. It is a pea-sized structure attached by a stalk of nerve fibres to the *hypothalamus*. The anterior lobe produces *growth hormone*; *prolactin*; *ACTH*; TSH (thyroid-stimulating hormone), which stimulates

PITUITARY GLAND

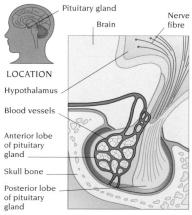

Pituitary gland
Brain
Nerve fibre

LOCATION

Hypothalamus

Blood vessels

Anterior lobe of pituitary gland

Skull bone

Posterior lobe of pituitary gland

hormone production by the *thyroid gland*; the *gonadotrophins* FSH (follicle stimulating hormone) and LH (luteinizing hormone); and melanocyte-stimulating hormone (MSH), which controls darkening of the skin. The posterior pituitary secretes *ADH* and *oxytocin*.

pituitary tumours Growths in the *pituitary gland*. Pituitary tumours are rare, and mostly noncancerous, but tumour enlargement can put pressure on the *optic nerves*, causing visual defects.

The causes of pituitary tumours are unknown. They may lead to inadequate hormone production, causing problems such as cessation of menstrual periods or reduced sperm production. They may also cause the gland to produce excess hormone. Overproduction of growth hormone causes *gigantism* or *acromegaly*; too much thyroid-stimulating hormone (TSH) can lead to *hyperthyroidism*.

Investigations include blood tests, X-rays, *MRI* of the pituitary, and usually also *vision tests*. Treatment may be by surgical removal of the tumour, *radiotherapy*, hormone replacement, or a combination of these techniques. The drug *bromocriptine* may be used; it can reduce production of hormones and shrink some tumours.

pityriasis alba A common skin condition of childhood and adolescence. Irregular, fine, scaly, pale patches appear on the face. Caused by mild *eczema*, it usually clears up with *emollients*.

pityriasis rosea A common, mild skin disorder in which a rash of flat, scaly-edged, pink spots or patches appears on the trunk and upper arms. It is not contagious and mainly affects children and young adults. Its cause is unknown. The rash lasts for 4–8 weeks, may cause itching, and usually clears up without treatment. Calamine lotion or *antihistamine drugs* may relieve any itching.

pityriasis versicolor A common skin condition in which patches of white, brown, or salmon-coloured flaking skin appear on the trunk and neck. Also known as tinea versicolor, it is caused by a fungus that exists on most people's skin. Treatment is with *antifungal drugs*.

pivmecillinam See *penicillin drugs*.

pizotifen A drug used to prevent migraine in people with frequent, disabling attacks. Adverse effects can include nausea, dizziness, drowsiness, dry mouth, and muscle pains. Prolonged use may cause weight gain.

PKU The abbreviation for *phenylketonuria*.

placebo A chemically inert substance given instead of a drug. Benefit may be gained from a placebo because the person taking it believes it will have a positive effect. As the effectiveness of any drug may be partly due to this "placebo effect", many new drugs are tested against a placebo preparation.

placenta The organ that develops in the uterus during pregnancy and that link the blood supplies of mother and baby. The placenta develops from the *chorion*. It is firmly attached to the lining of the woman's uterus and is connected to the baby by the *umbilical cord*. It is expelled shortly after the baby is born.

The placenta transfers oxygen and nutrients from the mother's circulation into the fetus's circulation, and removes waste products from the fetus's blood into the mother's blood for excretion by her lungs and kidneys. It also produces hormones such as *oestrogen*, *progesterone*, and *human chorionic gonadotrophin* (HCG). High levels of HCG appear in the woman's urine during early pregnancy, and detection of them in the urine forms the basis of *pregnancy tests*.

placental abruption Separation of all or part of the placenta from the wall of the uterus before the baby is delivered. The exact cause is not known, but placental abruption is more common in women with long-term *hypertension* and in those who have had the condition in a previous pregnancy or who have had several pregnancies. Smoking and high alcohol intake may also contribute to the risk of placental abruption.

Symptoms usually occur suddenly and depend on how much of the placenta has separated from the wall of the uterus. They include slight to heavy vaginal bleeding, which can be severe haemorrhaging in complete separation; cramps in the abdomen or backache; severe, constant abdominal pain; and reduced fetal movements. If the bleeding does not stop, or if it starts again, it may be necessary to induce labour (see *induction of labour*). A small placental abruption is usually treated with bed rest in hospital. In more severe cases of placental abruption, an emergency *caesarean section* is often necessary to save the life of the fetus. A *blood transfusion* is also sometimes required.

placenta praevia Implantation of the *placenta* in the lower part of the uterus, near or over the cervix. Placenta praevia occurs in about 1 in 200 pregnancies. It varies in severity from marginal placenta praevia, when the placenta reaches the edge of the cervical opening, to complete placental praevia, when the entire opening of the cervix is covered. Mild placenta praevia may have no adverse effect. More severe cases often cause painless vaginal bleeding in late pregnancy. If the bleeding is slight and the pregnancy has several weeks to run, bed rest in hospital may be all that is necessary. The baby will probably be delivered by *caesarean section* at the 38th week. If the bleeding is heavy or if the pregnancy

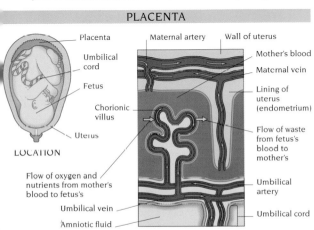

PLACENTA

Placenta

Umbilical cord

Fetus

Chorionic villus

Uterus

LOCATION

Flow of oxygen and nutrients from mother's blood to fetus's

Umbilical vein

Amniotic fluid

Maternal artery

Wall of uterus

Mother's blood

Maternal vein

Lining of uterus (endometrium)

Flow of waste from fetus's blood to mother's

Umbilical artery

Umbilical cord

PLACENTA PRAEVIA

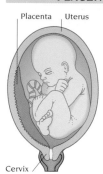

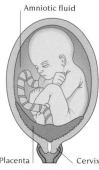

MARGINAL
PLACENTA PRAEVIA

COMPLETE
PLACENTA PRAEVIA

is near term, an immediate delivery is carried out.

placenta, tumours of See *choriocarcinoma; hydatidiform mole.*

plague A serious infectious disease caused by the bacterium YERSINIA PESTIS. It mainly affects rodents but can be transmitted to humans by flea bites. There are two main types. Bubonic plague is characterized by swollen lymph glands (called buboes). Symptoms usually start 2–5 days after infection, with fever, shivering, and severe headache. Soon, the smooth, red, intensely painful buboes appear, usually in the groin. There may be bleeding into the skin around the buboes, causing dark patches.

Pneumonic plague affects the lungs and can spread from person to person in infected droplets expelled during coughing. Symptoms are severe coughing that produces a bloody, frothy *sputum* and laboured breathing. Without early treatment, death is almost inevitable.

A sample of fluid from a bubo, or a sputum sample, is taken to confirm the diagnosis. Possible treatments include *streptomycin* and *tetracycline drugs.*

plantar fasciitis *Fasciitis* of the sole of the foot.

plantar wart See *wart, plantar.*

plants, poisonous Several species of plant, including foxglove, holly, deadly nightshade, and laburnum, are poisonous. Nettles, hogweed, poison ivy, and primula cause skin reactions, including rash and itching, on contact. Young children are the most commonly affected. Symptoms of poisoning vary according to the plant but may include abdominal pain, vomiting, flushing, breathing difficulties, *delirium,* and *coma* and require urgent medical advice. *Corticosteroid drugs* may be prescribed for severe reactions. Poisoning usually requires gastric *lavage.* Fatal poisoning is rare. (See also *mushroom poisoning.*)

plaque The term given to an area of *atherosclerosis.* The plaques are symptomless until they are large enough to reduce blood flow or until the surface of a plaque is disturbed, causing *thrombosis.* Plaques in coronary arteries cause *coronary artery disease.*

plaque, dental A rough, sticky coating on the teeth consisting of saliva by-products, food deposits, bacteria, and dead cells from the lining of the mouth. It is the chief cause of tooth decay (see *caries, dental*) and gingivitis, and forms the basis of a hard deposit (see *calculus, dental*). Some *microorganisms* in plaque, particularly STREPTOCOCCUS MUTANS, break down sugar in the remains of carbohydrate food that sticks to the mucus, creating an acid that can erode tooth enamel.

plasma The fluid part of *blood* that remains if the blood cells are removed.

plasmapheresis The removal or reduction in concentration of unwanted substances in the blood; also called plasma exchange. Blood is withdrawn from the body and the plasma portion is removed by machines called cell separators. The blood cells are then mixed with a plasma substitute and returned to the circulation. Plasmapheresis is used to remove damaging *antibodies* or antibody-antigen particles from the circulation in autoimmune disorders such as *myasthenia gravis* and *Goodpasture's syndrome.*

plasma proteins Proteins present in blood *plasma,* including *albumin, blood clotting* proteins, and *immunoglobulins.*

plasminogen activator See *tissue plasminogen activator.*

plaster cast See *cast*

plaster of Paris A white powder made of a calcium compound that, when mixed with water, produces a paste that can be shaped before it sets. Plaster of Paris is used for constructing *casts* and making dental models (see *impression, dental*).

plastic surgery Any operation carried out to repair or reconstruct skin and tissue that has been damaged or lost, is malformed, or has changed with aging. Plastic surgery is often performed after severe burns or injuries, cancer, or some operations, such as *mastectomy*. Congenital conditions that may require plastic surgery include *cleft lip and palate*, *hypospadias*, and imperforate anus (see *anus, imperforate*). Techniques include *skin grafts*, *skin flaps*, and *Z-plasty*; these may be combined with *implants* or a *bone graft*. *Microsurgery* allows transfer of tissue to other parts of the body. (See also *cosmetic surgery*.)

-plasty A suffix meaning shaping by surgery; performing *plastic surgery* on.

platelet The smallest type of *blood cell*, also called a *thrombocyte*. Platelets play a major role in *blood clotting*.

platyhelminth A flat or ribbon-shaped parasitic worm. (See *liver fluke, schistosomiasis, tapeworm*.)

play therapy A method used in the *psychoanalysis* of young children, based on the principle that all play has some symbolic significance. Watching a child at play helps a therapist diagnose the source of the child's problems; the child can then be helped to "act out" thoughts and feelings that are causing anxiety.

plethora A florid, bright-red, flushed complexion. It may be caused by dilation of blood vessels, or, less commonly, by *polycythaemia*.

plethysmography A way of estimating the blood flow in vessels by measuring changes in the size of a body part.

pleura A thin, two-layered membrane, one layer covering the outside of the lungs and the other lining the inside of the chest cavity. Fluid between the layers provides lubrication, allowing smooth movement of the lungs during breathing.

pleural effusion An accumulation of fluid between the layers of the *pleura*, making breathing difficult. Pleural effusion may be caused by *pneumonia*, *tuberculosis*, *heart failure*, *cancer*, *pulmonary embolism*, or *mesothelioma*.

Diagnosis is confirmed by *chest X-ray*. Some fluid may be removed with a nee-dle and syringe and examined to find the cause. A *biopsy* of the pleura may also be needed. The underlying cause is treated and fluid may be drained off to relieve breathing problems.

pleurisy Inflammation of the *pleura*. Causes include lung infections, such as *pneumonia*, or, more rarely, *pulmonary embolism*, *lung cancer*, and *rheumatoid arthritis*. Pleurisy causes a sharp chest pain, which is worse when breathing in. Treatment is of the underlying cause, along with *analgesic drugs*.

pleurodynia Pain in the chest caused by coxsackievirus B infection. Sometimes called Bornholm disease, it often occurs in epidemics and usually affects children. There is sudden severe pain in the lower chest or upper abdomen, with fever, sore throat, headache, and malaise. The disease usually clears up in 3–4 days without treatment.

plexus A network of interwoven nerves or blood vessels.

plication A surgical procedure in which tucks are taken in the walls of a hollow organ and then stitched to decrease the size of the organ.

Plummer–Vinson syndrome Difficulty in swallowing due to webs of tissue forming across the upper *oesophagus*. The syndrome often occurs with severe iron-deficiency *anaemia*.

plutonium A radioactive metallic element which occurs naturally only in *uranium* ores; it is produced artificially in breeder reactors.

P

PLEURA

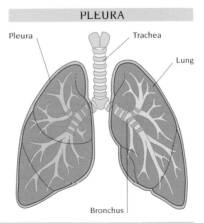

Pleura
Trachea
Lung
Bronchus

PMS The abbreviation for *premenstrual syndrome*.

PMT The abbreviation for premenstrual tension (an alternative name for *premenstrual syndrome*).

pneumaturia The presence of gas in the urine, usually indicating that a *fistula* has developed between the bladder and the intestine.

pneumo- A prefix meaning related to the lungs, to air, or to the breath.

pneumococcus A common name for *STREPTOCOCCUS PNEUMONIAE*, a bacterium that can cause various diseases, including *meningitis*, *pneumonia*, and *sinusitis*. Vaccination against pneumococcal infection is given at 2, 4, and 13 months as part of the childhood immunization schedule. Vaccination is also recommended for those over 65 and various groups at special risk, including those with chronic respiratory disease, chronic heart disease, chronic kidney disease, chronic liver disease, diabetes mellitus, a suppressed immune system, coeliac disease, some types of sickle cell disease, and people who have had their spleen removed or have a disorder of the spleen.

pneumoconiosis Any of a group of lung diseases caused by inhalation of certain mineral dusts. Only dust particles less than 0.005 mm across reach the alveoli (air sacs) in the lungs. The particles accumulate and may cause thickening and scarring. The main types of pneumoconiosis are asbestosis (see *asbestos-related diseases*), coal workers' pneumoconiosis, and silicosis, caused by silica dust. These diseases primarily affect workers aged over 50. However, the incidence is falling due to better preventive measures.

Pneumoconiosis is often detected by a *chest X-ray* before symptoms develop. The main symptom is shortness of breath. In severe cases, *cor pulmonale* or *emphysema* may develop. The risk of *tuberculosis* or *lung cancer* is increased following asbestos or haematite exposure. Diagnosis is based on a history of exposure to dusts, chest X-rays, medical examination, and *pulmonary function tests*. There is no treatment apart from treating any complications. Further exposure to dust must be avoided.

pneumocystis pneumonia An infection of the lungs caused by *PNEUMOCYSTIS CARINII*, a type of *protozoa*. Pneumocystis pneumonia is an *opportunistic infection* that is dangerous only to people with impaired resistance to infection. It is particularly common in those with *AIDS*. Symptoms include fever, dry cough, and shortness of breath lasting weeks to months. Diagnosis is made by examination of sputum or a lung *biopsy*. High doses of *antibiotic drugs* (commonly cotrimoxazole) may eradicate the infection; they may also be used over the long term to prevent infection in those people at increased risk.

pneumonectomy Surgery carried out to remove a lung.

pneumonia Inflammation of the lungs due to infection. There are two main types: lobar pneumonia and bronchopneumonia. Lobar pneumonia initially affects one lobe of a lung. In bronchopneumonia, inflammation initially starts in the bronchi and bronchioles (airways).

Pneumonia can be caused by any type of microorganism, but most cases are due to viruses, such as adenovirus, or bacteria, such as *STREPTOCOCCUS PNEUMONIAE*, *HAEMOPHILUS INFLUENZAE*, and *STAPHYLOCOCCUS AUREUS*. Symptoms are usually fever, chills, shortness of breath, and a cough that produces yellow-green *sputum* and occasionally blood. Potential complications include *pleural effusion*, *pleurisy*, and a lung *abscess*.

Diagnosis is made by physical examination, *chest X-ray*, and examining sputum and blood for microorganisms. Treatment depends on the cause, and may include *antibiotic drugs* or *antifungal drugs*. *Paracetamol* may be given to reduce fever, and, in severe cases, *oxygen therapy* and artificial *ventilation* may be needed. In most cases, recovery usually occurs within 2 weeks.

Vaccination against *influenza* and *pneumococcus* can help to prevent pneumonia, as can stopping smoking.

pneumonitis Inflammation of the lungs that may cause coughing, breathing difficulty, and wheezing. Causes include an allergic reaction to dust containing animal or plant material (see *alveolitis*) and exposure to radiation (see *radiation haz-*

P

ards). Pneumonitis may also occur as a side effect of drugs, such as *amiodarone* and *azathioprine*.

pneumothorax A condition in which air enters the pleural cavity (the space between the layers of the *pleura*). Symptoms are chest pain or shortness of breath. If air continues to leak, the pneumothorax may grow to produce a tension pneumothorax. This may be life-threatening. Diagnosis is confirmed by *chest X-ray*. A small pneumothorax may disappear in a few days without treatment. If not, treatment involves removing the air through a tube with a one-way valve.

pocket, gingival See *periodontitis*.

podiatry A paramedical specialty concerned with the feet (see *chiropody*).

podophyllin A drug used to treat genital warts (see *warts, genital*). It may cause irritation of the treated area and severe toxicity on excessive application.

poison A substance that, in relatively small amounts, disrupts the structure and/or function of cells. (See also *drug poisoning*; *poisoning*.)

poisoning *Poisons* may be swallowed, inhaled, absorbed through skin, or injected under the skin (as with an insect sting). Poisons may also originate in the body, as when bacteria produce *endotoxins*, or when *metabolic disorders* produce poisonous substances or allow them to build up. Poisoning may be acute (a large amount of poison over a short time) or chronic (gradual accumulation of poison that is not eliminated quickly).

Unintentional poisoning occurs mainly in young children. Adults may be poisoned by mistaking the dosage of a prescribed drug (see *drug poisoning*), by taking very high doses of vitamin or mineral supplements, by exposure to poisonous substances in industry, or by *drug abuse*. Poisoning may also be a deliberate attempt to commit *suicide*.

polio An abbreviation for *poliomyelitis*.

poliomyelitis An infectious viral disease, also called polio. It is usually mild, but in serious cases, it attacks the brain and spinal cord, sometimes causing paralysis or death. The virus is spread from the faeces of infected people to food. Airborne transmission also occurs. In countries with poor hygiene and sanitation, most children develop immunity through being infected early in life, when the infection rarely causes serious illness. In countries with better standards, this does not occur and, if children are not vaccinated, epidemics can occur. Because of the vaccination programme in the UK, there have been no cases of polio since 1993, and that case was in a person who contracted the disease abroad.

Most infected children have no symptoms. In others, there is a slight fever, sore throat, headache, and vomiting after a 3–5-day *incubation period*. Most children recover completely, but inflammation of the *meninges* may develop. Symptoms are fever, severe headache, stiff neck and back, and aching muscles, sometimes with widespread twitching. Often, extensive paralysis, usually of the legs and lower trunk, occurs in a few hours. If infection spreads to the *brainstem*, problems with, or total loss of, swallowing and breathing may result.

Diagnosis is made by *lumbar puncture*, throat *swab*, or a faeces sample. Characteristic paralysis with an acute feverish illness allows an immediate diagnosis. There is no effective drug treatment for polio. Nonparalytic patients usually need bed rest and *analgesic drugs*. In paralysis, *physiotherapy* and, in some cases, *catheterization*, *tracheostomy*, and artificial *ventilation* are needed.

Recovery from nonparalytic polio is complete. More than half of those with paralysis make a full recovery, fewer than a quarter are left with severe disability, and fewer than 1 in 10 dies.

In the UK, vaccination against polio is given at age 2, 3, and 4 months, with booster doses at 3–5 years and at 13–18 years (see *immunization*). The vaccine now in use contains inactivated polio virus, to minimize the risk of adverse reactions.

pollution Contamination of the environment by *poisons*, radioactive substances, *microorganisms*, or other wastes.

poly- A prefix meaning many or much.

polyarteritis nodosa An uncommon disease of medium-sized arteries, also called periarteritis nodosa. Areas of arterial wall become inflamed, weakened, and liable to *aneurysms*. The severity of the condition depends on the arteries that are affected and how much they are weakened. The cause seems to be an *immune system* disturbance, sometimes triggered by exposure to the *hepatitis B* virus. It is most common in adults and affects men more than women.

Early symptoms of polyarteritis nodosa include fever, aching muscles and joints, general malaise, loss of appetite and weight, and, sometimes, nerve pain. There is also *hypertension*, skin ulceration, and *gangrene*. If the coronary arteries are affected, *myocardial infarction* may occur. Many patients suffer abdominal pain, nausea, vomiting, diarrhoea, and blood in the faeces.

Diagnosis is made by *biopsy* and *angiography*. Large doses of *corticosteroids*, and in some cases *immunosuppressants*, may allow survival for at least 5 years. Without treatment, few patients survive for this length of time.

polycystic kidney See *kidney, polycystic.*

polycystic ovary syndrome (PCOS) See *ovary, polycystic.*

polycythaemia A condition in which increased production of red *blood cells* leads to an unusually large number of them in the blood. This condition is usually caused by another disorder or by *hypoxia*, and is called secondary polycythaemia. If it occurs for no apparent reason, it is called polycythaemia vera or primary polycythaemia.

Secondary polycythaemia occurs naturally at high altitudes due to the reduced oxygen level. It can also result from a disorder that impairs the oxygen supply to the blood, or can be secondary to *liver cancer* or some kidney disorders. Descending to sea level, or effective treatment of an underlying disorder, returns the blood to normal.

Polycythaemia vera is a rare disorder that mainly affects people over 40. The large number of red blood cells causes increased volume and thickening of the blood, which may lead to headaches, blurred vision, and *hypertension*. There may also be flushed skin, dizziness, night sweats, and widespread itching. The *spleen* is often enlarged. Possible complications include a tendency to bleed easily or to form blood clots; *stroke*; and *myelofibrosis* or acute leukaemia (see *leukaemia, acute*).

Diagnosis is made from a physical examination and *blood tests* and by ruling out other causes. Treatment is by *venesection*, sometimes in combination with *anticancer drugs*, radioactive phosphorus, or *interferon*. This enables most patients to survive for 10–15 years.

POLYCYTHAEMIA

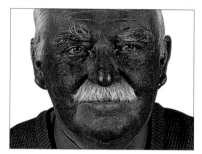

FLUSHED SKIN OF POLYCYTHAEMIA

polydactyly A birth defect in which there is an excessive number of fingers or toes. The extra digits may be fully formed or they may be fleshy stumps. Polydactyly often runs in otherwise normal families; however, it may also occur as part of *Laurence–Biedl–Moon syndrome* or other congenital syndromes.

polydipsia Persistent excessive thirst (see *thirst, excessive*).

polyhydramnios Excess *amniotic fluid* surrounding the fetus during pregnancy. It occurs in about 1 in 250 pregnancies and often has no known cause. The condition sometimes occurs if the fetus has a malformation that makes normal swallowing impossible, or if the pregnant woman has *diabetes mellitus*. The excess amniotic fluid usually accumulates in the second half of pregnancy, producing symptoms from about week 32. The main symptom is abdominal discomfort. Other possible symptoms are breathlessness and swelling of the legs. The uterus is larger than would usually be expected. Occasionally, fluid accumulates rapidly, causing abdominal pain, breathlessness, nausea, and vomiting, and leg swelling. Premature labour may result.

The condition is usually evident from a physical examination, but *ultrasound*

P

scanning may be needed. In mild cases, only rest is needed. In more severe cases, amniotic fluid may be withdrawn using a needle. In late pregnancy, *induction of labour* may be performed.

polymerase chain reaction (PCR) A method of rapidly copying *DNA* sequences so that they can be analysed.

polymyalgia rheumatica An uncommon disease of elderly people, marked by pain and stiffness in the muscles of the hips, thighs, shoulders, and neck. Symptoms are worse in the mornings. The cause is unknown, but the condition may be associated with *temporal arteritis*. It is unusual before the age of 50.

The diagnosis is based on the patient's history, a physical examination, and blood tests (including an *ESR*). If temporal arteritis is suspected, a *biopsy* may be performed on an artery at the side of the scalp. *Corticosteroid drugs* usually improve the condition within a few days.

polymyositis A rare disease in which the muscles are inflamed and weak.

polymyxins A group of *antibiotic drugs* derived from the bacterium BACILLUS POLYMYXA. Polymyxins, which include *colistin*, are commonly given to treat eye, ear, and skin infections.

polyp A growth that projects, usually on a stalk, from the lining of the nose, the cervix, the intestine, the larynx, or any other *mucous membrane*. Some types are liable to develop into cancer, and are surgically removed.

polypeptide A compound consisting of many *peptides*.

polypharmacy The practice of prescribing several drugs to one person at the same time.

polyposis, familial A rare, inherited disorder, also known as polyposis coli, in which many *polyps* are present throughout the gut, but mainly in the colon. If not treated, cancer of the colon (see *colon, cancer of*) is almost certain to develop. The polyps may appear from age 10. They may cause bleeding and diarrhoea; however, there are often no symptoms until cancer has developed. The polyps are detected by *colonoscopy*.

Since there is a 50 per cent chance that children of an affected person will inherit the disease, medical surveillance is nec-

essary from around the age of 12. Individual polyps may be cauterized (see *cauterization*). The high risk of developing cancer often means that a *colectomy* and an *ileostomy* are performed.

polyunsaturated fats Fats (see *fats and oils*) with relatively few hydrogen atoms in their chemical structure. These fats tend to protect against cardiovascular disease.

polyuria See *urination, excessive*.

PoM The abbreviation for *prescription-only medicine*.

pompholyx An acute form of *eczema* in which itchy blisters form on the palms and/or soles. The condition, also called dyshydrotic eczema, is sometimes due to an allergic response. Rarely, it is associated with *ringworm*. Treatment is with an astringent or with topical application of a *corticosteroid drug*.

pons The middle part of the *brainstem*

POP The abbreviation for *progestogen-only pill*, a type of *oral contraceptive*.

pore A tiny opening, usually in the skin.

porphyria Any of a group of uncommon and usually inherited disorders caused by the accumulation of substances called porphyrins. Sufferers often have a rash or blistering brought on by sunlight, and certain drugs may cause abdominal pain and nervous system disturbances. Porphyrins are formed in the body during the manufacture of haem (a component of *haemoglobin*). A block in this manufacture causes a build-up of porphyrins. Such blocks are the result of various *enzyme* deficiencies, which are *genetic disorders*. Porphyria may also be due to poisoning.

There are six types of porphyria. Acute intermittent porphyria usually appears in early adulthood, causing abdominal pain, and often limb cramps, muscle weakness, and psychiatric disturbances. The patient's urine turns red when left to stand. *Barbiturate drugs*, *phenytoin*, *oral contraceptives*, and *tetracyclines* precipitate attacks.

Variegate porphyria has similar effects but also causes blistering of sun-exposed skin. Hereditary coproporphyria also has similar effects and may cause additional skin symptoms.

Protoporphyria usually causes skin symptoms after exposure to sunlight, as does porphyria cutanea tarda. In this type, wounds are slow to heal, and urine

P

is sometimes pink or brown. Many cases are precipitated by liver disease.

The rarest and most serious form, congenital erythropoietic porphyria, causes red discoloration of urine and the teeth, excessive hair growth, severe skin blistering and ulceration, and haemolytic *anaemia*. Death may occur in childhood.

Diagnosis is made from abnormal levels of porphyrins in the urine and faeces. Treatment is difficult. Avoiding sunlight and/or precipitating drugs is the most important measure. Acute intermittent porphyria, variegate porphyria, and hereditary coproporphyria may be helped by administration of *glucose* or haematin. Cases of porphyria cutanea tarda may be helped by *venesection*.

portal hypertension Increased blood pressure in the portal vein, which carries blood from the stomach, intestine, and spleen to the liver. This causes *oesophageal varices*, which may rupture and cause internal bleeding, and *ascites*. The most common cause of portal hypertension is *cirrhosis*.

Diagnosis is usually made from the symptoms and signs. *Doppler ultrasound scanning* may be used to assess the pressure in the portal vein. Various treatments may be used to stop bleeding or prevent further bleeding. For example, ruptured blood vessels may be treated by *sclerotherapy*. A *shunt* is sometimes carried out to prevent further bleeding. Ascites is controlled by restriction of salt and with *diuretic drugs*.

port-wine stain A purple-red birthmark that is level with the skin's surface. It is a permanent type of *haemangioma*.

positron emission tomography See *PET scanning*.

posseting A term for the regurgitation of small quantities of milk by infants after they have been fed.

postcoital contraception See *contraception, emergency*.

posterior Relating to the back of the body, or referring to the rear part.

postherpetic neuralgia Burning pain caused by nerve irritation that occurs at the site of a previous attack of *herpes zoster* (shingles). See *neuralgia*.

postmaturity A condition in which a pregnancy persists for longer than 42 weeks; the average length of a normal pregnancy is 40 weeks (see *gestation*). Postmaturity may be associated with a family tendency to prolonged pregnancy, or it may be a sign that the baby is unable to descend properly (see *engagement*). The risk of fetal death increases after 42 weeks because the *placenta* becomes less efficient. Postmature infants tend to have dry skin and may be more susceptible to infection.

postmortem examination An alternative term for an *autopsy*.

postmyocardial infarction syndrome Another name for *Dressler's syndrome*.

postnasal drip A watery or sticky discharge from the back of the nose into the *nasopharynx*. The fluid may cause a cough, hoarseness, or the feeling of a foreign body. The usual cause is *rhinitis*.

postnatal care Care of the mother after *childbirth* until about 6 weeks later.

postnatal depression Depression in a woman after *childbirth*. The cause is probably a combination of sudden hormonal changes and psychological and environmental factors. The depression ranges from an extremely common and mild, shortlived episode ("baby blues") to a rare, severe depressive *psychosis*.

Most mothers first get the "blues" 4–5 days after childbirth and may feel miserable, irritable, and tearful. The cause is hormonal changes, perhaps coupled with a sense of anticlimax or an overwhelming sense of responsibility for the baby. With reassurance and support, the depression usually passes in 2–3 days. In about 10–15 per cent of women, the depression lasts for weeks and causes a constant feeling of tiredness, difficulty in sleeping, loss of appetite, and restlessness. The condition usually clears up of its own accord or is treated with *antidepressant drugs*.

Depressive psychosis usually starts 2–3 weeks after childbirth, causing severe mental confusion, feelings of worthlessness, threats of suicide or harm to the baby, and sometimes *delusions*. Hospital admission, ideally with the baby, and antidepressant drugs are often needed.

postpartum depression See *postnatal depression*.

postpartum haemorrhage Excessive blood loss after *childbirth*. It is more common after a long labour or after a multiple birth. The haemorrhage is usually due to excessive bleeding from where the *placenta* was attached to the uterus.

post-traumatic stress disorder A form of anxiety that develops after a stressful or traumatic event. Common causes include natural disasters, violence, rape, torture, serious physical injury, and military combat. Symptoms, which may develop many months after the event, include recurring memories or nightmares of the event, a sense of personal isolation, and disturbed sleep and concentration. There may be a deadening of feelings, or irritability and feelings of guilt, sometimes building up to *depression*. Most people recover, in time, with emotional support from family and friends. However, some people may require specialized trauma *counselling* or *cognitive-behavioural therapy*.

postural drainage A technique that enables sputum (phlegm) or other secretions to drain from a person's lungs in order to clear them. The person lies in a way that allows the secretions to drain by gravity into the *trachea*, from where they are coughed up. Tapping the person's chest with cupped hands can help to loosen sticky secretions.

postural hypotension See *hypotension*.

posture The relative position of different parts of the body at rest or during movement. Good posture consists of balancing the body weight around the body's centre of gravity in the lower spine and pelvis. Maintaining good posture helps prevent neck pain and back pain.

post-viral fatigue syndrome See *chronic fatigue syndrome*.

potassium A *mineral* needed to help maintain normal heart rhythm, regulate the body's water balance, conduct nerve impulses, and contract muscles. Dietary sources of potassium include lean meat, whole grains, green leafy vegetables, beans, and various fruits, such as apricots, dates, and peaches.

A low level of potassium in the blood is known as hypokalaemia. It is usually due to loss of fluids through diarrhoea and/or vomiting, and causes fatigue, drowsiness, dizziness, and muscle weakness. In severe cases, there may be abnormal heart rhythms and muscle paralysis.

Excess potassium in the blood is known as hyperkalaemia and is much less common than hypokalaemia. It may be due to excessive intake of potassium supplements, severe *kidney failure*, *Addison's disease*, or prolonged treatment with potassium-sparing *diuretics*. The effects of high potassium levels in the blood can include numbness and tingling, disturbances of the heart rhythm, and muscle paralysis. In severe cases, there may be *heart failure*.

potassium channel activators A class of drugs that are used in the prevention and long-term treatment of *angina*. Nicorandil is a potassium channel activator that acts in a similar way to *nitrates*, and widens both arteries and veins. Possible side effects may include flushing, headaches, nausea, vomiting, and dizziness.

potassium citrate A substance used to relieve discomfort in mild *urinary tract infections* by making the urine less acid.

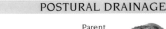

POSTURAL DRAINAGE

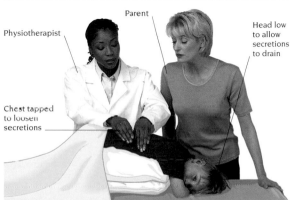

Parent

Head low to allow secretions to drain

Physiotherapist

Chest tapped to loosen secretions

POSTURAL DRAINAGE WITH CHEST PHYSIOTHERAPY

potassium permanganate A drug that has an *antiseptic* and *astringent* effect; and is useful in the treatment of *dermatitis*. It can occasionally cause irritation and can stain skin and clothing.

potency The ability of a man to perform *sexual intercourse*; or the ability of a drug to cause desired effects.

Pott's fracture A combined fracture and dislocation of the ankle caused by excessive or violent twisting. The *fibula* breaks just above the ankle; in addition, the *tibia* breaks or the *ligaments* tear, resulting in dislocation.

poultice A warm pack consisting of a soft, moist substance (such as *kaolin*) spread between layers of soft fabric.

pox Any of various infectious diseases characterized by blistery skin eruptions (for example *chickenpox*). Pox is sometimes used as a slang word for *syphilis*.

pravastatin A *lipid-lowering drug*.

praziquantel An *anthelmintic drug* used to treat *tapeworm infestation*. Adverse effects may include dizziness, drowsiness, and abdominal pain.

prazosin A *vasodilator drug* used to treat *hypertension, heart failure*, and *Raynaud's disease*. Prazosin is also used to treat urinary symptoms resulting from an enlarged prostate gland (see *prostate, enlarged*). Side effects include dizziness and fainting, nausea, headache, and dry mouth.

precancerous A term applied to any condition in which there is a tendency for cancer to develop. There are three types. In the first, no tumours are present but the condition carries an increased risk of cancer. In the second, there are noncancerous tumours that tend to become cancerous or are associated with development of cancerous tumours elsewhere. The third type comprises disorders which have irregular features from the beginning but do not always become fully cancerous.

precocious puberty The development of secondary *sexual characteristics* before age 8 in girls and 9 in boys. It is uncommon and may be caused by various disorders that can result in production of *sex hormones* at an abnormally early age. Possible underlying causes include a *brain tumour* or other brain abnormalities; abnormality of the adrenal glands (for example, congenital *adrenal hyperplasia*); *ovarian cysts*, and *tumours*, or a tumour in the testes. In some cases, no underlying cause can be identified.

The hormones may cause a premature growth spurt followed by early fusion of the bones. As a result, affected children may initially be tall but, if untreated, final height is often greatly reduced.

The child's pattern of pubertal development is assessed by a doctor. *Blood tests* are performed to measure hormone levels. *Ultrasound scanning* of the ovaries and testes, and *CT scanning* of the adrenal glands or brain, may also be carried out, depending on the underlying cause suspected.

Treatment is of the underlying cause, and hormone drugs may be given to delay puberty and increase final height.

predisposing factors Factors that lead to increased susceptibility to a disease.

prednisolone A *corticosteroid drug*.

pre-eclampsia A serious condition in which *hypertension, oedema*, and *proteinuria* develop in the last (third) trimester of pregnancy. If severe, symptoms may include headache, nausea and vomiting, abdominal pain, and visual disturbances. The condition, which is sometimes called pre-eclamptic toxaemia or PET, is more common in first pregnancies and if *diabetes mellitus*, hypertension, or kidney disease is present. Untreated pre-eclampsia may lead to *eclampsia*. For some cases of pre-eclampsia, treatment is bed rest and *antihypertensive drugs*. In late pregnancy, or if severe, *induction of labour* or *caesarean section* may be necessary.

pregnancy The period from *conception* to birth. Pregnancy begins with the *fertilization* of an ovum (egg) and its implantation. The egg develops into the *placenta* and the *embryo*, which grows to form the fetus. Most eggs implant into the uterus. Very occasionally, an egg implants into an abnormal site, such as a fallopian tube, resulting in an *ectopic pregnancy*.

A normal pregnancy lasts around 40 weeks from the first day of the woman's last menstrual period. It is divided into three stages (trimesters) of 3 months each. For the first 8 weeks of pregnancy, the developing baby is called an embryo; thereafter it is called a fetus.

PREGNANCY

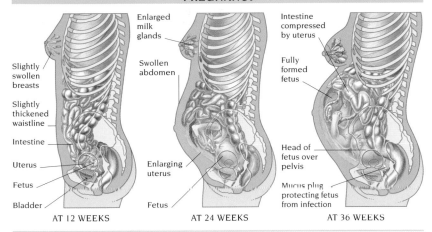

Enlarged milk glands

Slightly swollen breasts

Slightly thickened waistline

Intestine

Uterus

Fetus

Bladder

Swollen abdomen

Enlarging uterus

Fetus

Intestine compressed by uterus

Fully formed fetus

Head of fetus over pelvis

Mucus plug protecting fetus from infection

AT 12 WEEKS   AT 24 WEEKS   AT 36 WEEKS

In the first trimester the breasts start to swell and may become tender. Morning sickness (see *vomiting in pregnancy*) is common. The baby's major organs have developed by the end of this stage. During the second trimester, the mother's nipples enlarge and darken and weight rises rapidly. The baby is usually felt moving by 22 weeks. During the third trimester, stretch marks and *colostrum* may appear, and *Braxton Hick's contractions* may be felt. The baby's head engages at about 36 weeks.

Common, minor health problems during pregnancy include constipation, *haemorrhoids*, *heartburn*, *pica*, swollen ankles, and *varicose veins*. Other common disorders include *urinary tract infections*, stress incontinence (see *incontinence, urinary*), and *candidiasis*.

Complications of pregnancy and disorders that affect it include *antepartum haemorrhage*; *diabetic pregnancy*; *miscarriage*; *polyhydramnios*; *pre-eclampsia*; *prematurity*; and *Rhesus incompatibility*. (See also *childbirth*; *fetal heart monitoring*; *pregnancy, multiple*.)

pregnancy, drugs in Certain drugs taken during *pregnancy* may pass to the fetus through the *placenta* or interfere with fetal development. This may lead to *birth defects*. Although relatively few drugs have been proved to cause harm to a developing baby, no drug should be considered completely safe, especially during early pregnancy. For this reason, pregnant women should seek advice from their doctor or pharmacist before taking any drug, including over-the-counter preparations.

Problems may also be caused in a developing baby if a pregnant woman drinks *alcohol*, smokes (see *tobacco-smoking*), or takes drugs of abuse. The babies of women who use *heroin* during pregnancy tend to have a low birthweight and a higher death rate than normal during the first few weeks of life. Babies of women who abuse drugs intravenously are at high risk of *HIV* infection.

pregnancy, false An uncommon psychological disorder, medically known as pseudocyesis, in which a woman has physical signs of pregnancy, including morning sickness (see *vomiting in pregnancy*), *amenorrhoea* (absence of periods), enlarged breasts, and abdominal swelling, but is not pregnant. The woman is convinced that she is pregnant. Treatment for false pregnancy may involve *counselling* or *psychotherapy*. (See also *conversion disorder*.)

pregnancy, multiple The presence of more than one fetus in the uterus. Multiple pregnancy can occur if two or more ova (eggs) are fertilized at the same time, or if a single fertilized egg divides early in development.

P

Twins occur in about 1 in 80 pregnancies, triplets in about 1 in 8,000, and quadruplets in about 1 in 73,000. Multiple pregnancies are more common in women who are treated with *fertility drugs* or if a number of fertilized ova are implanted during *in vitro fertilization*.

PREGNANCY TEST

HOME PREGNANCY TEST

pregnancy tests Tests on urine or blood performed to determine whether or not a woman is pregnant. Pregnancy testing kits that are available from pharmacies allow testing to be carried out at home. All of the kits test for the presence of *human chorionic gonadotrophin* (HCG) in a sample of urine. This hormone is normally produced only by a developing placenta, and therefore the tests are extremely accurate (about 97 per cent accurate for a positive result and about 80 per cent accurate for a negative result), even in early pregnancy. Details for using a test vary with different brands; but all kits involve dipping a test stick that has been treated with a chemical that reacts with HCG into a sample of urine. Blood tests for detecting pregnancy produce a result from 9–12 days after conception.

premature ejaculation See *ejaculation, disorders of.*

prematurity Birth of a baby before 37 weeks' *gestation*. The premature infant may not be sufficiently developed to cope with independent life and needs special care. About 5–10 per cent of babies are born prematurely.

Some 40 per cent of premature deliveries occur for no known reason. The remainder are due to conditions such as *pre-eclampsia, hypertension, diabetes mellitus*, long-standing kidney disease, and heart disease. Other causes are *antepartum haemorrhage*, intrauterine infection, or premature rupture of membranes. A common cause is multiple pregnancy (see pregnancy, *multiple*).

A premature infant is smaller than a full-term baby, lacks subcutaneous fat, is covered with downy hair (*lanugo*), and has very thin skin. The baby's internal organs are also immature. The major complication is *respiratory distress syndrome*. There is increased risk of brain haemorrhage, *jaundice*, and *hypoglycaemia*. The baby has a limited ability to suck and maintain body temperature, and is prone to infection. The earlier a baby is born, the more likely it is to have such problems.

Premature infants are usually nursed in a special baby unit that provides intensive care. The baby is placed in an *incubator*, and may have artificial *ventilation* to assist breathing, artificial feeding through a stomach tube or into a vein, and treatment with *antibiotic drugs* and *iron* and *vitamin supplements*. With modern techniques, some infants survive even if they are born as early as 24 weeks' gestation.

premedication The term applied to drugs given, often by injection, 1–2 hours before an operation to prepare a person for surgery. Premedication usually contains a opioid *analgesic drug* and often an *anticholinergic drug*.

premenstrual syndrome The combination of physical and emotional symptoms that occurs in many women in the week or so before menstruation. Premenstrual syndrome (PMS) may be so severe that work and social relationships are seriously disrupted.

Theories for the cause of PMS include hormonal changes and vitamin or mineral deficiencies, but none have been confirmed. The most common emotional symptoms are irritability, tension, depression, and fatigue. Physical symptoms include breast tenderness, fluid retention, headache, backache, and lower abdominal pain.

No single treatment has proved completely successful. Treatments to relieve specific symptoms include *analgesic drugs* and relaxation techniques. Pyridoxine (vitamin B_6) may help some women. *Oral contraceptives* can relieve symptoms by suppressing the normal menstrual cycle.

premenstrual tension See *premenstrual syndrome*.

premolar One of eight permanent grinding teeth, two in the upper and two in the lower jaw on each side of the mouth, located between the canines and molars. (See also *permanent teeth*; *eruption of teeth*.)

prenatal The period of pregnancy before childbirth.

prepuce See *foreskin*.

presbyacusis The progressive loss of hearing that occurs with age. Presbyacusis is a form of sensorineural *deafness*, which makes sounds less clear and tones less audible. People with the condition often find it difficult to understand speech and cannot hear well when there is background noise. Presbyacusis may be exacerbated by exposure to high *noise* levels, diminished blood supply to the inner ear due to *atherosclerosis*, and damage to the inner ear from drugs such as *aminoglycoside drugs*. *Hearing-aids* help most people.

presbyopia The progressive loss of the power of adjusting the eye (see *accommodation*) for near vision. The focusing power of the eyes weakens with age. Presbyopia is usually noticed around age 45 when the eyes cannot accommodate to read small print at a normal distance. Reading *glasses* with convex lenses are used to correct presbyopia.

prescribed diseases A group of industrial diseases that give sufferers legal entitlement to financial benefit. A claimant has to have worked in an occupation recognized to increase the risk of developing a particular disease. Examples include asbestosis (see *asbestos-related diseases*), work-related asthma, work-related chronic bronchitis (see *bronchitis, chronic*), work-related deafness, and vibration white finger (see *Raynaud's phenomenon*). (See also *occupational disease and injury*.)

prescription An instruction written by a doctor, dentist or specially trained nurse that directs a pharmacist to dispense a particular drug in a specific dose. A prescription details how often the drug must be taken, how much is to be dispensed, and other relevant facts.

prescription-only medicine Drugs and medicines that are not available over the counter and can only be obtained by *prescription*. Prescription-only medicines are those whose safe use is difficult to ensure without medical supervision.

preservative A substance that inhibits growth of bacteria, yeasts, and moulds and so protects foods from putrefying and fermenting. Examples include sulphur dioxide, benzoic acid, salt, sugar, and nitrites. (See also *food additives*.)

pressure points Places on the body where arteries lie near the surface and pressure can be applied by hand to limit severe arterial bleeding (in which bright red blood is pumped out in regular spurts with the heartbeat). Major pressure points of the body include the brachial pressure point in the middle part of the upper arm and the carotid pressure point at the side of the neck, below the jaw.

pressure sores Ulcers that develop on the skin of patients who are unconscious or immobile. They are also known as decubitus ulcers or bedsores. Common sites include the shoulders, elbows, lower back, hips, buttocks, ankles, and heels. Pressure sores may develop following *stroke* or *spinal injuries* that result in a loss of sensation. *Incontinence*, if it results in constantly wet skin, may also be a contributory factor. Pressure sores start as red, painful areas that become purple before the skin breaks down. At this stage, the sores often become infected and are very slow to heal. Deep, chronic *ulcers* may require treatment with *antibiotic drugs* and, in some cases, possibly *plastic surgery*. Good nursing care, including changing the patient's position regularly, skin care, protection of vulnerable areas, and use of cushions and special mattresses, should prevent pressure sores from developing in most cases.

prevalence The total number of cases of a disease at any one time in a defined population. Prevalence is often expressed as the number of cases per 100,000 people. (See also *incidence*.)

preventive dentistry An aspect of dentistry concerned with the prevention of tooth decay and gum disease. It consists of the encouragement of good *oral hygiene*, *fluoride* treatment, and *scaling*.

preventive medicine The branch of medicine that deals with the prevention of disease by public health measures, such as the provision of pure water supplies; by health education; by specific preventive measures, such as *immunization* against infectious diseases; and by screening programmes to detect diseases before they cause symptoms.

priapism Persistent, painful *erection* of the *penis* without sexual arousal. Priapism occurs when blood does not drain from the spongy tissue of the penis, thus keeping the penis erect. This may be caused by clotting in the blood vessels due to a blood disorder or as a result of treatment for erectile dysfunction. Urgent treatment is needed in order to avoid permanent damage. The treatment may involve withdrawal of blood from the penis with a needle.

prickly heat An irritating skin rash that is associated with profuse sweating. The medical name is miliaria rubra. Multiple tiny, red, itchy spots cover the affected areas of skin and are accompanied by prickling sensations. The irritation tends to affect areas where sweat collects, such as the armpits. The cause is not fully known, but unevaporated sweat is an important factor. Sweat ducts become blocked with debris and leak sweat into the skin. Frequent cool showers and sponging of the affected areas relieve the itching.

primaquine A drug used to treat vivax and ovale *malaria*. It is often given after prophylactic treatment with *chloroquine* has failed to prevent infection.

Adverse effects include nausea, vomiting, and abdominal pain. In people with *G6PD deficiency*, primaquine may cause haemolytic *anaemia*.

primary A term applied to a disease that has originated within the organ or tissue affected, and is not derived from any other cause or source. The term primary is also applied to the first of several diseases to affect a tissue or organ in turn. Primary is also used to mean "of unknown cause".

primary care Health care provided by a general practitioner or other health-care professional who is the first contact for a patient seeking medical treatment.

primary teeth The first teeth (also known as milk teeth), which usually start to appear at age 6 months and are replaced by the *permanent teeth* from about age 6 years. There are 20 primary teeth, 10 in each jaw. (See also *teeth*; *eruption of teeth*; *teething*.)

primidone An *anticonvulsant drug* used to treat *epilepsy* and, occasionally, *tremor*. It is usually prescribed with another anticonvulsant. Adverse effects include drowsiness, clumsiness, and dizziness.

Prinzmetal's angina See *variant angina*.

prion A tiny, protein-based infectious particle. Prions transmit diseases, including *Creutzfeldt–Jakob disease* in humans and *bovine spongiform encephalopathy (BSE)* in cattle. Prions do not contain nucleic acids and are difficult to destroy. As yet, no treatment is available for prion diseases.

PRK The abbreviation for *photorefractive keratectomy*.

probenecid A drug used in the long-term treatment of *gout*. Probenecid also slows the excretion of some *antibiotic drugs* and so is occasionally prescribed with these drugs to boost their levels and thus their effects. It may cause nausea and vomiting. Other possible effects include flushing and dizziness.

probiotic bacteria Species of microorganisms that inhabit the digestive tract, guarding it against harmful bacteria, yeasts, and viruses.

procainamide An *antiarrhythmic drug* that is used to treat certain types of *tachycardia*. Procainamide may cause nausea, vomiting, loss of appetite, and, rarely, confusion. Prolonged treatment may induce *lupus erythematosus*.

procaine A local anaesthetic (see *anaesthesia, local*).

procarbazine An *anticancer drug* used most often in *Hodgkin's disease*. Side effects are typical of anticancer drugs.

prochlorperazine A *phenothiazine*-type *antipsychotic drug* used to relieve symptoms of certain psychiatric disorders, such as *schizophrenia* and *mania*. It is also used in small doses as an *antiemetic drug*. It may cause involuntary movements of the face and limbs, lethargy, dry mouth, blurred vision, and dizziness.

procidentia A medical term for severe *prolapse*, usually of the uterus.

proctalgia fugax A severe cramping pain in the *rectum* unconnected with any disease. It may be due to muscle spasm. The pain is of short duration and subsides without treatment.

proctitis Inflammation of the *rectum*, causing soreness and bleeding, sometimes with a mucus and pus discharge. Proctitis commonly occurs as a feature of *ulcerative colitis, Crohn's disease*, or *dysentery*. In cases where inflammation is confined to the rectum, the cause is often unknown. In male homosexuals, proctitis is sometimes due to *gonorrhoea* or another sexually transmitted infection. Rare causes include *tuberculosis, amoebiasis*, and *schistosomiasis*.

Diagnosis is made by *proctoscopy*. A *biopsy* is sometimes needed. Treatment depends on the underlying cause. When the cause is unknown, treatment is directed towards relieving symptoms.

proctoscopy Examination of the *anus* and *rectum* with a proctoscope (a rigid viewing instrument).

procyclidine An *anticholinergic drug* used to treat *Parkinson's disease* and minimize the side effects of some *antipsychotic drugs*. Possible adverse effects include dry mouth and blurred vision.

prodrome An early warning symptom of illness.

progeria Premature aging. There are two forms of progeria, and both are very rare. In Hutchinson–Gilford syndrome, the premature aging starts at about 4 years old, and many features of old age, including grey hair, balding, sagging skin, and *atherosclerosis*, have developed by age 10–12. Death usually occurs at puberty. Werner's syndrome (adult progeria) starts in adolescence or early adulthood and follows the same progression. The cause of progeria is unknown, although it is known that the cells in affected people reproduce far less frequently than those in healthy people.

progesterone hormone A female sex hormone essential for the functioning of the female reproductive system. Progesterone is made in the *ovaries*, and small amounts are produced by the *adrenal glands* and *testes*. During the menstrual cycle, changing progesterone levels cause thickening of the endometrium and menstruation. If pregnancy occurs, progesterone is produced by the *placenta*; a fall in its level helps to initiate *labour*. Progesterone also causes increased fat deposition and increased *sebum* production by glands in the skin.

progestogen drugs A group of drugs similar to *progesterone hormone*. The drugs are used in *oral contraceptives*, are prescribed to treat menstrual problems (see *menstruation, disorders of*), and are included in *hormone replacement therapy (HRT)*. Progestogen drugs are also used to treat *endometriosis*, and *hypogonadism*, and are sometimes used as *anticancer drugs*. Adverse effects include weight gain, *oedema*, headache, dizziness, rash, irregular periods, breast tenderness, and *ovarian cysts*.

progestogen-only pill (POP) Also known as the minipill, an *oral contraceptive* containing a *progestogen drug*. Various types are available. Most work by thickening the cervical mucus, making it difficult for sperm to penetrate, and by making the uterine lining thinner so that implantation of a fertilized ovum is less likely. A variety of POP containing *desogestrel* also inhibits ovulation. Possible adverse effects include irregular or absent periods, bleeding between periods, *ectopic pregnancy*, and *ovarian cysts*.

prognathism Abnormal protrusion of the lower jaw or both jaws.

prognosis An assessment of the probable course and outcome of a disease.

progressive A term used to describe a condition that becomes more severe and/or extensive over time.

progressive muscular atrophy A type of *motor neuron disease* in which the muscles of the hands, arms, and legs become weak and wasted and twitch involuntarily. The condition eventually spreads to other muscles.

proguanil An antimalarial drug used in the prevention of *malaria*. Side effects

P

are rare. Indigestion, nausea, or vomiting may occur but usually disappear as treatment continues.

prolactin A *hormone* produced by the *pituitary gland*. Prolactin helps to stimulate the development of the mammary glands (see *breast*), and to initiate and maintain milk production for *breast-feeding*. (See also *prolactinoma*.)

prolactinoma A noncancerous tumour of the *pituitary gland* that causes over-production of *prolactin*. In women, this may result in *galactorrhoea*, *amenor-rhoea*, or *infertility*. In men, it may cause *erectile dysfunction* and *gynaecomastia*. In either sex, it may cause headaches, *diabetes insipidus*, and, if the tumour presses on the optic nerves, loss of the outer *visual field*. Diagnosis is made from *blood tests* and *CT scanning* or *MRI* of the brain. Treatment may involve removal of the tumour, *radiotherapy*, or giving the drug *bromocriptine*.

prolapse Displacement of part or all of an organ or tissue from its normal position in the body (see *uterus, prolapse of*; *disc prolapse*).

promazine A *phenothiazine-type anti-psychotic drug* used as a sedative drug. Possible adverse effects include abnormal movements of the face and limbs, drowsiness, lethargy, dry mouth, constipation, and blurred vision. Long-term treatment may cause *parkinsonism*.

promethazine An *antihistamine drug* used to relieve itching in a variety of skin conditions, such as *eczema*. It is also used as an *antiemetic drug*, and sometimes as a *premedication*. Possible adverse effects include dry mouth, blurred vision, and drowsiness.

pronation The act of turning the body to a prone (facedown) position, or the hand to a palm backwards position.

propantheline An *antispasmodic drug* used to treat *irritable bowel syndrome* and forms of *urinary incontinence*. Possible adverse effects include dry mouth, blurred vision, and retention of urine.

prophylactic A drug, procedure, or piece of equipment used to prevent disease; also a *condom*.

propranolol A *beta-blocker drug* used to treat *hypertension*, *angina pectoris*, and cardiac *arrhythmias*. It may also be used to reduce the risk of further heart damage after *myocardial infarction*. It relieves symptoms of *hyperthyroidism* and *anxiety*, and can prevent *migraine* attacks. Possible adverse effects are typical of other beta-blocker drugs.

proprietary A term for a drug patented for production by one company.

proprioception The body's internal system for collecting information about its position and the state of contraction of its muscles. Information from proprioceptors (sensory nerve endings in the muscles, tendons, joints, and the inner ear) passes to the spinal cord and the brain. The information is used to make adjustments so that posture and balance are maintained.

proptosis A term for protrusion.

propylthiouracil A drug used to treat *hyperthyroidism* or to control its symptoms before a *thyroidectomy*. Possible adverse effects include itching, headache, rash, joint pain, and decreased production of white *blood cells*.

prostaglandin One of a group of *fatty acids* that is made naturally in the body and acts in a similar way to *hormones*. Prostaglandins cause pain and inflammation in damaged tissue, protect the lining of the stomach and duodenum against ulceration, lower blood pressure, and stimulate contractions in labour. (See also *prostaglandin drugs*.)

prostaglandin drugs Synthetically produced *prostaglandins*. Dinoprostone is used with *oxytocin* for *induction of labour*. Gemeprost softens and helps to dilate the cervix prior to inducing an *abortion*. Alprostadil is used to treat newborn infants awaiting surgery for some congenital heart diseases.

prostate, cancer of A cancerous growth in the *prostate gland*, of unknown cause. One of the most common cancers in men, it mainly occurs in elderly men.

An enlarged prostate (see *prostate, enlarged*) may cause symptoms including difficulty in starting to pass urine, poor urine flow, blood in the urine, and increased frequency of urination. Urine flow may eventually cease altogether. When there are no urinary symptoms, the first sign may be pain in the bones from secondary cancers.

Screening tests detect blood levels of a protein called *prostate specific antigen*; if above a certain level, it may indicate prostate cancer. *Rectal examination* allows a doctor to assess the size and hardness of the gland. *Ultrasound scanning* and a *biopsy* confirm the diagnosis. *Blood tests, CT scanning, MRI,* and a bone scan (see *radionuclide scanning*) may also be done. In an elderly man with a small prostate cancer that has not spread, no treatment may be recommended. For younger men, *prostatectomy, brachytherapy,* or external *radiotherapy* may be performed. Widespread disease is usually controllable for some years with *anticancer drugs* and/or hormone treatment.

prostatectomy An operation to remove part or all of the *prostate gland*. It is performed to treat enlargement of the gland (see *prostate, enlarged*), cancer of the prostate (see *prostate, cancer of*), or *prostatitis*. The most common method is transurethral prostatectomy, performed during *cystoscopy*. If the prostate gland is very enlarged, retropubic prostatectomy may be performed. An incision exposes the prostate and the tissue is removed. Transurethral prostatectomy rarely affects erectile function but about 8 in 10 men are infertile after the operation. Retropubic prostatectomy is more likely to affect erectile function and result in infertility. A newer method of prostatectomy using a laser may be more appropriate for some men.

prostate, enlarged An increase in the size of the inner zone of the *prostate gland*, also known as benign prostatic hyperplasia. It is most common in men over 50. The cause is unknown. The enlarging prostate compresses and distorts the *urethra*, impeding the flow of urine. Eventually the bladder is unable to expel all the urine (see *urine retention*) and becomes distended, causing abdominal swelling. There may also be *incontinence* and frequency of urination (see *urination, frequent*).

Prostate enlargement is detected by a *rectal examination*. Tests may include a blood test, *ultrasound scanning, urography,* and a recording of the strength of urine flow. Mild cases do not require treatment, but more severe ones usually

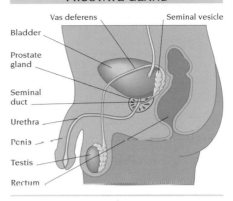

Vas deferens
Seminal vesicle
Bladder
Prostate gland
Seminal duct
Urethra
Penis
Testis
Rectum

require *prostatectomy*. Alternatively, drug treatment with *alpha-blocker drugs* or anti-androgen drugs may be given.

prostate gland A solid, chestnut-shaped organ that surrounds the first part of the male *urethra*, just below the *bladder*. It produces secretions that form part of the seminal fluid during *ejaculation*. The ejaculatory ducts from the seminal vesicles pass through the prostate gland to enter the urethra.

prostate specific antigen (PSA) An *enzyme* normally produced by the prostate gland. If produced in excess, it may indicate the presence of *prostate cancer*, although raised levels may also occur in benign prostatic hyperplasia (see *prostate, enlarged*). Conversely, a normal level of PSA does not exclude the possibility of prostate cancer.

prostatism Symptoms resulting from enlargement of the prostate gland (see *prostate, enlarged*).

prostatitis Inflammation of the prostate gland, usually affecting men aged 30–50. It is often caused by a bacterial infection that has spread from the *urethra*. A urinary *catheter* increases the risk. Prostatitis causes pain when passing urine and increased frequency of urination; it sometimes causes fever and a discharge from the *penis*. There may be pain in the lower abdomen, around the rectum, and in the lower back, and blood in the urine. Diagnosis is made by *rectal examination* and tests on urine samples and urethral secretions. Treatment is with *antibiotic*

P

drugs. The condition may be slow to clear up and tends to recur.

prosthesis An artificial replacement for a missing or diseased part of the body; for example, artificial limbs (see *limb, artificial*), heart valves (see *heart-valve surgery*), or glass eyes (see *eye, artificial*).

prosthetics, dental The branch of *dentistry* concerned with the replacement of missing teeth and their supporting structures. It includes *dentures*, overdentures (semipermanent fittings over existing teeth), crowns (see *crown, dental*), and bridges (see *bridge, dental*).

protease inhibitors A type of *antiviral drug* used to delay the progression of *HIV* infection (see *AIDS*).

proteins Large molecules consisting of hundreds or thousands of *amino acids* linked into long chains. Proteins may also contain sugars (glycoproteins) and *lipids* (lipoproteins). There are two main types of proteins. Fibrous proteins are insoluble and form the structural basis of many body tissues. Globular proteins are soluble and include all *enzymes*, many *hormones*, and some blood proteins, such as *haemoglobin*.

protein synthesis The formation of protein molecules through the joining of *amino acids*.

proteinuria The presence of *protein* in the *urine*. It may result from kidney disorders, including *glomerulonephritis* and *urinary tract infection*. Increased protein in the urine may also occur because of a generalized disorder that causes increased protein in the blood. Proteinuria is diagnosed by *urinalysis*.

proton pump inhibitors A type of *ulcer-healing drug* that is used to treat peptic ulcers.

protoplasm A term for the entire contents of a *cell*.

protozoa The simplest and most primitive type of animal, consisting of a single cell. All protozoa are bigger than *bacteria* but are still microscopic. About 30 types of protozoa are human parasites, including those that are responsible for *malaria, amoebiasis, giardiasis, sleeping sickness, trichomoniasis, toxoplasmosis,* and *leishmaniasis.*

proximal A term describing a part of the body nearer to a central point of reference, such as the trunk.

prurigo Thickening and *itching* of the *skin* due to repeated scratching.

pruritus The medical term for *itching.*

pruritus ani Itching of the anus. Causes may include an *anal fissure, haemorrhoids,* or *threadworm infestation.*

PSA An abbreviation for *prostate specific antigen.*

pseud-/pseudo- Prefixes meaning false.

pseudarthrosis A term meaning false joint, used to describe an operation in which the ends of the two opposing bones in a joint are removed and a piece of tissue is fixed in the gap as a cushion.

The term also describes a rare childhood condition in which congenital abnormality of the lower half of the *tibia* leads to spontaneous *fracture.*

pseudoacanthosis nigricans See *acanthosis nigricans.*

pseudocyesis See *pregnancy, false.*

pseudodementia Severe *depression* in elderly people that mimics *dementia.* Symptoms include intellectual impairment and loss of memory.

pseudoephedrine A *decongestant drug* used to relieve *nasal congestion.* High doses may cause anxiety, nausea, and dizziness. Occasionally, *hypertension,* headache, and *palpitations* occur.

pseudoepidemic An outbreak of an illness in a community or in an institution that is thought to be due to a form of *hysteria.* Typical symptoms are headache and a general feeling of sickness.

pseudogout A form of *arthritis* that results from the deposition of calcium pyrophosphate crystals in a joint. The underlying cause is unknown; in rare cases, it is a complication of *diabetes mellitus, hyperparathyroidism,* and *haemochromatosis.* Symptoms are similar to *gout.* Diagnosis is from a sample of

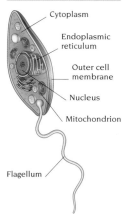

PROTOZOA

- Cytoplasm
- Endoplasmic reticulum
- Outer cell membrane
- Nucleus
- Mitochondrion

Flagellum

TYPICAL PROTOZOAN

joint fluid. Treatment is with *nonsteroidal anti-inflammatory drugs* (NSAIDs).

pseudohermaphroditism A *congenital* abnormality in which the external genitalia resemble those of the opposite sex, but ovarian or testicular tissue is present as normal. A female pseudohermaphrodite may have an enlarged *clitoris* resembling a *penis* and enlarged *labia* resembling a *scrotum*. A male may have a very small penis and a divided scrotum resembling labia. (See also *hermaphroditism; sex determination*.)

pseudomonas Species of rod-like *bacteria* that live in soil and decomposing matter. *PSEUDOMONAS AERUGINOSA* is capable of causing disease in humans and is present in pus from wounds.

psilocybin An *alkaloid* present in some mushrooms. It is a *hallucinogenic drug* with properties similar to those of *LSD*.

psittacosis A rare illness resembling *influenza* that is caused by the microorganism *CHLAMYDIA PSITTACI*. The disease is contracted by inhaling dust containing the droppings of infected birds, such as pigeons or poultry. Most cases occur among poultry farmers, pigeon owners, and people working in pet shops. Common symptoms are severe headache, fever, and cough, developing a week or more after infection. Other symptoms may include muscle pains, sore throat, nosebleed, lethargy, depression, and, in some cases, breathing difficulty.

A diagnosis is made by finding *antibodies* against *CHLAMYDIA PSITTACI* in the blood. Treatment is with *tetracycline* antibiotic drugs. With no treatment, death may result.

psoas muscle A muscle that bends the hip upwards towards the chest. There are two parts: psoas major and psoas minor. Psoas major acts to flex the hip and rotate the thigh inwards. Psoas minor bends the spine down to the pelvis.

psoralen drugs Drugs containing chemicals called psoralens, which occur in some plants and are present in some perfumes. When absorbed into the skin, psoralens react with *ultraviolet light* to cause skin darkening or inflammation. Psoralen drugs may be used in conjunction with ultraviolet light (a combination called *PUVA*) to treat *psoriasis* and

PSORIASIS

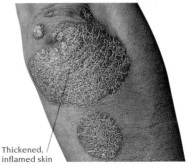

Thickened, inflamed skin

DISCOID PSORIASIS

vitiligo. Overexposure to ultraviolet light during treatment, or too high a dose of a psoralen drug, may cause redness and blistering of the skin. Psoralens in perfumes may cause *photosensitivity*.

psoriasis A common skin disease characterized by thickened patches of red, inflamed skin, often covered by silvery scales. It usually appears between ages 10 and 30, tends to run in families, and affects men and women equally.

The exact cause of psoriasis is unknown. New skin cells are made about 10 times faster than normal. The excess cells accumulate, forming thickened patches covered with dead, flaking skin. Sometimes, there is also a painful swelling and stiffness of the joints (see *arthritis*). Psoriasis tends to recur in attacks, which may be triggered by factors such as emotional stress, skin damage, and physical illness.

There are different forms of the disorder. The most common is discoid, or plaque, psoriasis, in which patches appear on the trunk, limbs, and scalp. Guttate psoriasis occurs most often in children, and consists of many small patches that develop over a wide area of skin. Pustular psoriasis is characterized by small *pustules*.

In most cases, psoriasis can be improved with topical treatments, such as those containing *corticosteroid drugs*, emollients, and coal tar. Other treatments include dithranol ointment; *PUVA; phototherapy* with UVB light; and

P

drugs such as *methotrexate*, vitamin D analogues (such as *calcipotriol*), and retinoids (such as *acitretin*). Psoriasis is usually a long-term condition.

psych- A prefix meaning mental processes or activities, as in psychology.

psyche A term meaning mind. (See also *psychoanalytic theory*.)

psychiatry The branch of medicine concerned with the study, prevention, and treatment of mental illness and emotional and behavioural problems. Psychiatrists usually conduct examinations of physical and mental state, and trace the patient's personal and family history. Treatment may include medication, *counselling, psychotherapy, psychoanalysis*, or *behaviour therapy*.

psychoanalysis A treatment based on *psychoanalytic theory* that can help people who have *neuroses* and *personality disorders*. A modified approach may also be used to treat *psychosis*. Psychoanalysis aims to help the patient to understand his or her emotional development and to make adjustments in particular situations. Interpretation of the patient's dreams is another aspect of the treatment (see *dream analysis*).

psychoanalytic theory A system of ideas developed by Sigmund Freud that explains personality and behaviour in terms of unconscious wishes and conflicts. The main emphasis was on sexuality. Freud believed that a child passes through three stages in the first 18 months of life: oral, anal, and genital. After this, the child develops a sexual attraction to the parent of the opposite sex and wants to eliminate the other parent (*Oedipus complex*). Sexual feelings become latent around age 5 but reemerge at puberty. Psychological problems may develop if *fixation* occurs at a primitive stage. Modern psychoanalysis has progressed from these ideas and is generally based on the observation that most emotional problems are caused by childhood experiences. Psychoanalysis attempts to free the individual from the past, helping him or her to become a real person in the present. Psychoanalytic theory is decreasing in influence.

psychodrama An aid to *psychotherapy* in which the patient acts out certain roles or incidents. Psychodrama is often carried out with a partner or in a group; music, dance, and mime are often used.

psychogenic A term for a symptom or disorder that is caused by psychological or emotional problems.

psychology The scientific study of mental processes. Psychology deals with all internal aspects of the mind, such as *memory*, feelings, *thought*, and *perception*, as well as external manifestations, such as *speech* and behaviour. Psychology is also concerned with *intelligence*, *learning*, and *personality* development.

psychometry The measurement of psychological functions using *intelligence tests, personality tests*, and tests for specific aptitudes, such as *memory*, logic, concentration, and speed of response.

psychoneurosis A term used interchangeably with *neurosis*.

psychopathology The study of abnormal mental processes. There are two main approaches: the descriptive, which aims to record symptoms that make up a diagnosis of mental illness; and the psychoanalytic, which is concerned with the unconscious feelings and motives of the individual.

psychopathy An outdated term for an *antisocial personality disorder*.

psychopharmacology The study of drugs that affect mental states, such as *antipsychotic drugs, antidepressant drugs*, and *anti-anxiety drugs*.

psychosexual disorders A range of disorders that are related to sexual function. Psychosexual disorders include *transsexualism, psychosexual dysfunction*, and sexual *deviation*.

psychosexual dysfunction A disorder in which there is interference with the sexual response for no physical cause.

psychosis A severe mental disorder in which the individual loses contact with reality. Three main categories of psychosis are recognized: *schizophrenia, bipolar disorder*, and organic brain syndrome (see *brain syndrome, organic*). The main feature of psychotic illnesses is that they cause a person to have a distorted view of life.

Symptoms include *delusions, hallucinations, thought disorders*, loss of *affect, mania*, and *depression*. The cause is most likely to be a disorder of brain function. *Antipsychotic drugs* are usually effective in controlling symptoms. Long-term treatment, *rehabilitation*, and support are often needed.

psychosomatic A term that describes physical disorders that seem to have been caused, or made worse, by psychological factors. Common examples of conditions that may in some cases be psychosomatic are headache, breathlessness, nausea, *asthma*, *irritable bowel syndrome*, *peptic ulcer*, and types of *eczema*. (See also *somatization disorder*.)

psychosurgery Any operation on the brain that is carried out as a treatment for serious mental illness. It is performed only as a last resort. Prefrontal *lobotomy* has now been largely replaced by types of *stereotaxic surgery*.

psychotherapy Treatment of mental and emotional problems by psychological methods. Patients talk to a therapist about their symptoms and problems, with the aim of learning about themselves, developing insights into relationships, and changing behaviour patterns.

psychotropic drugs Drugs that have an effect on the mind, including *hallucinogenic drugs*, *sedative drugs*, *sleeping drugs*, *tranquillizer drugs*, and *antipsychotic drugs*.

pterygium A wing-shaped thickening of the *conjunctiva* that extends from either side of the eye towards the centre. Pterygium is attributed to prolonged exposure to bright sunlight and is common in tropical areas. It is surgically removed if it threatens vision or causes discomfort.

ptosis Drooping of the upper eyelid. The condition may be *congenital*, occur spontaneously, or be due to injury or disease, such as *myasthenia gravis*. Ptosis is usually due to a weakness of the levator muscle of the upper eyelid or to interference with the nerve supply to the muscle. Severe congenital ptosis is corrected surgically to avoid the development of *amblyopia*.

ptyalism See *salivation, excessive*.

puberty The period when secondary *sexual characteristics* develop and the sexual organs mature. Puberty usually occurs between the ages of 10 and 15. (See also *precocious puberty*.)

pubes The pubic hair or the area of the body covered by this hair.

pubic bone The front part of the fused bones that form the *pelvis*.

pubic lice Small, wingless insects (*PHTHIRUS PUBIS*) that live in the pubic hair and feed on blood. Also called crab lice or crabs, they are usually spread by sexual contact. A louse has a flattened body, up to 2 mm across. Female lice lay eggs (nits) on the hair, where they hatch about 8 days later. On men, the lice may also be found in hair around the anus, on the legs, on the trunk, and even in facial hair. The bites sometimes cause itching. Children can become infested by transmission from parents, and the lice may live on the eyelids. An insecticide lotion kills the lice and eggs.

pudenda A term that refers to the external *genitalia*.

pudendal block A type of *nerve block* used to provide pain relief for a *forceps delivery*. A local anaesthetic (see *anaesthesia, local*) is injected into either side of the *vagina* near the pudendal nerve.

puerperal sepsis An infection that originates in the genital tract within 10 days after *childbirth*, *miscarriage*, or *abortion*. Once a common cause of death, it is now easily treated with *antibiotic drugs*.

puerperium The period of time after *childbirth* during which the woman's *uterus* and genitals return to their pre-pregnancy state.

pulmonary Relating to the lungs.

pulmonary disease, chronic obstructive A combination of chronic *bronchitis* and *emphysema*, in which there is persistent disruption of air flow into or out of the lungs. Patients are sometimes described as either pink puffers or blue bloaters, depending on their condition. Pink puffers maintain adequate oxygen in their bloodstream through an increase in their breathing rate, and remain "pink" despite damage to the lungs. However, they suffer from almost constant shortness of breath. Blue bloaters are cyanotic (have a bluish discoloration of the skin and mucous membranes) because of obesity, and sometimes *oedema*, mainly due to heart failure resulting from the lung damage.

pulmonary embolism Obstruction of the pulmonary artery or one of its branches in the lung by an *embolus*, usually after a deep vein thrombosis (see *thrombosis, deep vein*). If the embolus is large enough to block the main pulmonary artery, or if there are many clots, the condition is life-threatening. Pulmonary embolism is more likely after recent surgery, pregnancy, and immobility. It is also associated with using *oral contraceptives*, and there may be a family history of the condition. A massive embolus can cause sudden death. Smaller emboli may cause severe shortness of breath, rapid pulse, dizziness, chest pain made worse by breathing, and coughing up of blood. Tiny emboli may produce no symptoms, but, if recurrent, may eventually lead to *pulmonary hypertension*.

A diagnosis may be made by a *chest X-ray*, *radionuclide scanning*, blood tests, and pulmonary *angiography*. An *ECG*, *echocardiography*, and *venography* may also be performed. Treatment depends on the size and severity of the embolus. A small one gradually dissolves and *thrombolytic drugs* may be given to hasten this process. *Anticoagulant drugs* are given to reduce the chance of more clots. Surgery may be needed to remove larger clots.

pulmonary fibrosis Scarring and thickening of lung tissue, usually as a result of previous lung inflammation. It may be confined to an area of the lung affected by a condition such as *pneumonia* or *tuberculosis*, or it may be widespread through the lungs (see *fibrosing alveolitis*). Shortness of breath is a common symptom. Diagnosis is confirmed by *chest X-ray*. Treatment depends on the cause, but in most cases the fibrosis is irreversible and treatment aims to prevent the condition from progressing.

pulmonary function tests A group of procedures used to evaluate lung function, to confirm the presence of some lung disorders, and to ensure that planned surgery on the lungs will not disable the patient. The tests include *spirometry*, measurement of lung volume, assessment of the degree of *bronchospasm* with a *peak-flow meter*, and a test of *blood gases*.

pulmonary hypertension A disorder in which the blood pressure in the arteries supplying the lungs is abnormally high. Pulmonary hypertension develops in response to increased resistance to blood flow through the lungs. To maintain an adequate blood flow, the right side of the heart must contract more vigorously than before. Right-sided *heart failure* may later develop.

Causes of pulmonary hypertension may include chronic obstructive pulmonary disease (see *pulmonary disease, chronic obstructive*), a *pulmonary embolism*, *pulmonary fibrosis*, and some congenital heart diseases (see *heart disease, congenital*), but it can also develop without an obvious cause. Symptoms, which include enlarged veins in the neck, enlargement of the liver, and generalized *oedema*, only develop when heart failure occurs. Treatment is aimed at the underlying disorder (if known) and the relief of the heart failure. *Diuretic drugs* and *oxygen therapy* may be given.

pulmonary incompetence A rare defect of the pulmonary *valve* at the exit of the heart's right *ventricle*. The valve fails to close properly, allowing blood to leak back into the heart. The cause is usually *rheumatic fever*, *endocarditis*, or severe *pulmonary hypertension*.

pulmonary oedema Accumulation of fluid in the lungs, usually due to left-sided *heart failure*. It may also be due to chest infection, inhalation of irritant gases, or to any of the causes of generalized *oedema*. The main symptom is breathlessness, which is usually worse when lying flat and may disturb sleep. There may be a cough, producing frothy, sometimes pink, sputum. Breathing may sound bubbly or wheezy.

A diagnosis is made by a *physical examination* and by a *chest X-ray*. Treatment may include *morphine*, *diuretic drugs*, and *oxygen therapy*; artificial *ventilation* may also be given.

pulmonary stenosis A *heart* condition in which the outflow of blood from the right *ventricle* is obstructed, causing the heart to work harder to pump blood to the lungs. The obstruction may be caused by narrowing of the pulmonary *valve* at the exit of the *ventricle*; by narrowing of the pulmonary artery, which carries blood to the lungs; or by narrowing of the upper part of the ventricle.

Pulmonary stenosis is usually *congenital*, and may occur alone or with a set of heart defects called the *tetralogy of Fallot*. Rarely, the stenosis develops later in life, after *rheumatic fever*, and may cause symptoms of heart failure.

Diagnosis is made by a *chest X-ray*, *ECG*, *echocardiography*, and Doppler *ultrasound scanning*. A *balloon catheter* may relieve the narrowing. Otherwise, *heart-valve surgery* or other types of *open heart surgery* are often successful.

pulp, dental The soft tissue containing blood vessels and nerves in the middle of each tooth (see *teeth*).

pulpectomy The removal of the tooth *pulp*. It is part of *root-canal treatment*.

pulpotomy Removal of the coronal part of the *pulp* of a tooth after it has become inflamed, usually by infection. Infection is most often due to extensive tooth decay (see *caries, dental*). Pulpotomy prevents further degeneration of the pulp. If treatment is unsuccessful, *root-canal treatment* may be required.

pulse The rhythmic expansion and contraction of an artery as blood is forced through it, pumped by the heart.

pump, infusion A machine that is used for the administration of a continuous, controlled amount of a drug or other fluid. The fluid is delivered through a needle that is inserted into a vein or under the skin.

pump, insulin A type of infusion pump (see *pump, infusion*) used to administer a continuous dose of insulin to some patients with *diabetes mellitus*. The rate of flow is adjusted so that the level of blood glucose (sugar) is constant.

punch-drunk A condition that is characterized by slurred speech, impaired concentration, and slowed thought processes. It is caused by brain damage from several episodes of brief loss of consciousness due to head injury.

pupil The circular opening in the centre of the *iris*. In bright conditions, the pupil constricts; in dim light, it dilates.

purgative A term for a *laxative drug*.

purine Any of a group of nitrogen-containing compounds synthesized in the body or produced by the digestion of certain proteins. Increased levels of purine can cause *hyperuricaemia*, which may lead to *gout*. Foods that have a high purine content include sardines, liver, kidneys, pulses, and poultry.

purpura Any of a group of disorders characterized by purplish or reddish-brown areas or spots of discoloration, caused by bleeding within skin or mucous membranes. Purpura also refers to the discoloured areas themselves.

There are many different types and causes of purpura. Common (senile) purpura mostly affects middle-aged or elderly women. Large discoloured areas, caused by thinning of the tissues supporting blood vessels under the skin, appear on the thighs or the back of the hands and forearms. Henoch-Schönlein purpura is caused by inflammation of blood vessels beneath the skin. Purpura can occur as a result of *thrombocytopenia*. It can also be associated with *septicaemia* and can be seen with *meningitis* (see glass *test*).

purulent A term that means containing, producing, or consisting of *pus*.

pus A pale yellow or green, creamy fluid found at the site of bacterial infection. Pus is composed of millions of dead white *blood cells*, partly digested tissue, dead and living bacteria, and other substances. A collection of pus within solid tissue is called an *abscess*.

pustule A small skin *blister* that contains *pus*.

PUVA A type of *phototherapy* used to treat certain skin conditions, especially *psoriasis*. PUVA combines a *psoralen* drug and a controlled dose of long-wavelength *ultraviolet light*.

pyelitis See *pyelonephritis*.

pyelography See *urography*.

pyelolithotomy An operation performed to remove a kidney stone (see *calculus, urinary tract*). Pyelolithotomy has been largely replaced by other procedures, such as *lithotripsy*, which uses ultrasonic waves to break up the stones.

pyelonephritis Inflammation of the *kidney*, usually as a result of a bacterial infection. Pyelonephritis is more common in women and is more likely to occur during pregnancy. Symptoms of pyelonephritis include a high fever, chills, and back pain. *Septicaemia* is a possible complication. Pyelonephritis is treated with *antibiotic drugs*.

P

PYLORIC SPHINCTER

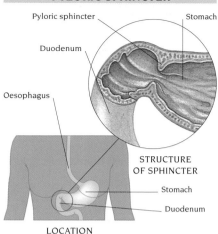

Pyloric sphincter   Stomach

Duodenum

Oesophagus

STRUCTURE
OF SPHINCTER

Stomach

Duodenum

LOCATION

pyloric sphincter The valve at the base of the *stomach* that controls movement of food into the *duodenum*.

pyloric stenosis Narrowing of the pylorus (the lower outlet from the stomach), which obstructs the passage of food into the *duodenum*. Pyloric stenosis occurs in babies due to thickening of the pyloric muscle, and in adults due to scarring from a *peptic ulcer* or *stomach cancer*. Babies start projectile vomiting (profuse vomiting in which the stomach contents may be ejected several feet) 2–5 weeks after birth. *Ultrasound scanning* is needed to confirm the diagnosis. In adults, diagnosis may be made by a *barium X-ray examination* and *gastroscopy*.

In infants, surgical treatment involves making an incision along the thickened muscle. In adults, surgery is carried out to correct the underlying cause.

pyloroplasty An operation in which the pylorus (the outlet from the stomach) is widened to allow free passage of food into the intestine. Pyloroplasty may be performed as part of the surgery for a *peptic ulcer*, or to prevent tightening of the pyloric muscles after *vagotomy*.

pyo- A prefix that denotes a relationship to *pus*. The prefix py- is also used.

pyoderma gangrenosum A rare condition characterized by ulcers, usually on the legs, that turn into hard, painful areas surrounded by discoloured skin. Pyoderma gangrenosum occurs as a rare complication in *ulcerative colitis*.

pyogenic granuloma A common, non-cancerous skin tumour that develops on exposed areas after minor injury. It can be removed surgically, by *electrocautery*, or by *cryosurgery*.

pyrazinamide A drug sometimes used to treat *tuberculosis*. Possible adverse effects are nausea, joint pains, *gout*, and liver damage.

pyrexia A medical term for *fever*.

pyrexia of uncertain origin Persistent fever with no apparent cause. The cause is usually an illness that is difficult to diagnose or a common disease that presents in an unusual way. These illnesses include various viral infections; *tuberculosis*; cancer, particularly *lymphoma*; and *collagen diseases*, such as systemic *lupus erythematosus* and *temporal arteritis*. Another possible cause is a *drug* reaction.

pyridoxine Vitamin B_6 (see *vitamin B complex*). Dietary deficiency of this vitamin is very rare but can be induced by some drugs. Pyridoxine is sometimes used to treat *premenstrual syndrome*. Long-term use of high-dose pyrodoxine has been associated with disorders of the peripheral nerves (see *neuropathy*).

pyrimethamine A drug that is used in combination with other drugs to treat resistant *malaria*.

pyrogen A substance that produces *fever*. The term is usually applied to proteins released by white *blood cells* in response to infections. The word is also sometimes used to refer to chemicals released by microorganisms.

pyromania A persistent impulse to start fires. The disorder is more often diagnosed in males, and may be associated with a low IQ, alcohol abuse, and a *psychosexual disorder*.

pyuria The presence of white *blood cells* in the *urine*, indicating infection of a *kidney* or *urinary tract infection* and inflammation.

P

Q

QALY A quality adjusted life year. QALY is used by health economists to compare costs and outcomes of treatment for various diseases. Each year of life saved or prolonged is adjusted by a factor, Q, which takes account of how close to normal is the individual's lifestyle before and after treatment.

Q fever An uncommon illness causing symptoms similar to *influenza*. Q fever occurs throughout the world. It is caused by the *rickettsia COXIELLI BURNETTI*, and may be contracted by inhaling dust contaminated with faeces, urine, or birth products from infected animals. Rarely, it may be spread by tick bites.

Symptoms develop with sudden onset about 20 days after infection, and include a high fever, severe headache, muscle and chest pains, and a cough. A form of *pneumonia* then occurs. In some cases *hepatitis* or *endocarditis* may develop. Less than 1 per cent of cases are fatal.

After diagnosis is confirmed by a *blood test*, treatment is with *antibiotic drugs*. There is an effective vaccine.

quackery A false claim to have the ability to diagnose and treat disease.

quadrantectomy A surgical procedure that involves the removal of tissue in one quadrant of a breast in order to treat *breast cancer*. (See also *lumpectomy*; *mastectomy*.).

quadriceps muscle A muscle with four distinct parts that is located at the front of the thigh and straightens the knee. The most common disorder of the quadriceps is a *haematoma* caused by a direct blow.

quadriparesis Weakness of the muscles in all four limbs and the trunk. (See also *quadriplegia*.).

quadriplegia *Paralysis* of all four limbs and the trunk. (See also *paraplegia*.).

quarantine The isolation of a person or animal recently exposed to a serious infectious disease. The aim is to prevent the spread of a disease by infected, but symptomless, people or animals.

Quarantine procedures are now less commonly necessary due to the reduced incidence of most serious infectious diseases and the availability of *vaccinations* for many of them.

quickening The first fetal movements felt by a pregnant woman, usually after about 18 weeks' gestation.

quinine The oldest drug treatment for *malaria*. Quinine is now used mainly to treat strains of malaria that are resistant to other antimalarial drugs. Large doses are needed, and there is a high risk of adverse effects, including headache, nausea, hearing loss, ringing in the ears, and blurred vision.

Quinine is commonly prescribed in low doses to help prevent leg cramps at night; adverse effects are rare.

quinolone drugs A group of *antibiotic drugs*, often called antibacterials, that are used to treat bacterial infections. Quinolone drugs are derived from chemicals, rather than living organisms. Examples include norfloxacin, *ciprofloxacin*, and *ofloxacin*.

Quinolones are used in the treatment of a wide range of conditions, including urinary tract infections, acute diarrhoeal diseases (such as that caused by *salmonella infections*), and enteric fever. Their absorption is reduced by antacids containing magnesium and aluminium.

Quinolones should be used with caution in patients with *epilepsy*, during pregnancy and breast-feeding, and in children and adolescents. Side effects include nausea, vomiting, diarrhoea, headache, sleep disorders, dizziness, rash, and blood disorders.

quinsy An abscess in the soft tissue around the tonsils, which is also known as a peritonsillar abscess. It is a possible complication of *tonsillitis*.

Q

R

rabies An acute viral infection of the nervous system, once known as hydrophobia, that primarily affects dogs but can be transmitted to humans by a bite or a lick over broken skin. The virus travels to the brain; once symptoms develop, rabies is usually fatal.

The average *incubation period* is 1–3 months, depending on where the bite is. The symptoms are slight fever and headache, leading to restlessness, hyperactivity, and, in some cases, hallucinations and paralysis. The victim develops convulsions, *arrhythmias*, and paralysis of the respiratory muscles and is often intensely thirsty, but drinking induces painful spasms of the throat. Death follows 10–14 days after the onset of symptoms.

Following an animal bite, the wound should be cleaned thoroughly and immediate medical advice should be sought. *Immunization* with human rabies *immunoglobulin* and a course of rabies vaccine is necessary; this may prevent rabies if given within 2 days. If symptoms appear, they are treated with sedative drugs and *analgesic drugs*. The main emphasis is on preventing the disease through *quarantine* regulations and human and animal immunization. (See also *bites, animal.*)

rachitic A term used to describe abnormalities associated with *rickets* or to refer to people or populations with rickets.

rad A unit of absorbed dose of ionizing radiation (see *radiation unit*), which has been superseded by the gray (Gy). "Rad" stands for radiation absorbed dose.

radial nerve A branch of the *brachial plexus*. The radial nerve, one of the main nerves of the arm, runs from the shoulder to the hand. It controls muscles which straighten the wrist, and conveys sensation from the back of the forearm; the thumb, second, and third fingers; and the base of the thumb. The nerve may be dam-

aged by a fracture of the *humerus* or by persistent pressure on the armpit.

radiation The emission of energy (as electromagnetic waves) or matter (as particles) from unstable atoms, which turns them into a more stable form. Some types of radiation are harmful to life; other types are essential (for example, light and heat energy radiated from the sun). Even harmful radiation may be used for beneficial purposes; for example, in treatment by *radiotherapy*, the biologically-damaging effects of radiation are used to destroy cancerous cells.

Four significant types of harmful radiation are gamma radiation, *X-rays*, alpha particles, and beta particles. Gamma radiation and X-rays are types of electromagnetic waves, and are similar to more energetic forms of light. All four types cause damage by ionization – the waves or particles knock out electrons from atoms in the matter that they pass through, turning them into highly reactive *ions*. In the case of living tissue, the ions formed cause biological damage.

Radioactive substances that emit any of these types of radiation constitute a health hazard. However, alpha particles cannot penetrate the skin, so sources of alpha radiation are only dangerous if ingested or inhaled. Gamma radiation can travel large distances through many substances, and even distant gamma sources can pose a risk to humans.

Most sources of ionizing radiation are natural, including cosmic rays from space and radioactive minerals. In some areas, the gas *radon*, found in soil, rocks, or building materials, is a major source. Artificial sources include X-ray machines, radioactive isotopes used in diagnosis and treatment (see *radionuclide scanning*), and nuclear reactors.

Less energetic types of radiation, such as *ultraviolet light*, may also cause biological damage by mechanisms other than ionization. Ultraviolet radiation from the sun does not penetrate the body deeply, but can damage genetic material in cells and may lead to skin cancer.

Other types of nonionizing radiation to which people are subjected are *ultrasound*, used in medicine for diagnosis and treatment, and radio waves that are generated during *MRI*. These techniques are not thought to have any adverse side effects. (See also *radiation hazards; radiation sickness; radiation units*.)

radiation hazards Hazards from *radiation* may arise from external sources of radiation or from radioactive materials taken into the body. The effects depend on the dose, the duration of exposure, and the organs exposed.

With some forms of radiation, damage occurs when the radiation dose exceeds a certain limit, usually 1 sievert (Sv) (see *radiation unit*). This damage may include radiation *dermatitis*, *cataracts*, organ failure (which may occur many years later), or *radiation sickness*.

For other types of radiation damage, the risk that damage will occur increases with increasing doses of radiation. *Cancer* caused by radiation-induced *mutation* is the major example of this type of damage. Radioactive leaks from nuclear reactors can cause a rise in mutation rates, which may lead to an increase in cancers, such as *leukaemias*; to *birth defects*; and to hereditary diseases. Cancer usually develops years after exposure.

Radiation damage can be controlled by limiting exposure. People exposed to radiation at work have their exposure closely monitored to ensure that it does not exceed safe limits. People of reproductive age or younger should have their reproductive organs shielded when having *X-rays* or *radiotherapy*.

There is no evidence of radiation hazards with visual display units (VDUs).

radiation sickness The term applied to the acute effects of ionizing *radiation* on the whole, or a major part, of the body when the dose is greater than 1 gray (1 Gy) of *X-rays* or gamma rays, or 1 sievert (1 Sv) of other types of radiation.

The effect of radiation depends on the dose and the exposure time. Total-body doses of less than 2 Gy are unlikely to be fatal to a healthy adult. At doses of 1–10 Gy, transient nausea and occasional vomiting may occur, but usually disappear rapidly and are often followed by a 2–3 week period of relative well-being. By the end of this period, the effects of radiation damage to the bone marrow and immune system begin to appear, with repeated

infections and petechiae (pinpoint spots of bleeding under the skin). Some people are successfully treated with a *stem cell* or *bone marrow transplant* or by isolation in a sterile environment until the bone marrow recovers.

With a dose of 10–30 Gy there is also an early onset of nausea and vomiting, which tends to disappear a few hours later. However, damage to the gastrointestinal tract, which causes severe and frequently bloody *diarrhoea* (called the gastrointestinal syndrome), and overwhelming infection due to damage to the *immune system* is likely to result in death 4–14 days after exposure.

Acute exposures of more than 30–100 Gy cause the rapid onset of nausea, vomiting, anxiety, and disorientation. Within hours, the victim usually dies due to *nervous system* damage and *oedema* of the brain; these effects are called the central nervous system syndrome.

radiation unit Several different internationally agreed units (called SI units) are used to measure ionizing *radiation*. For example, the roentgen (R) measures the amount of radiation in the air, and the becquerel is the SI unit of spontaneous activity of a radioactive source such as uranium. For medical purposes, the most commonly used units are the gray (Gy) and the sievert (Sv).

The gray is the SI unit of radiation that is actually absorbed by any *tissue* or substance as a result of exposure to radiation. 1 Gy is the absorption of 1 joule of energy (from gamma radiation or *X-rays*) per kilogram of irradiated matter. The gray supersedes an older unit called the rad (1 Gy = 100 rads).

Because some types of radiation affect biological organisms more than others, the sievert is used as a measure of the impact of an absorbed dose. It uses additional factors, such as the kind of radiation and its energy, to quantify the effects on the body of equivalent amounts of different types of absorbed energy. The sievert replaces an older unit, the rem (1 Sv=100 rems).

radical surgery Extensive surgery aimed at eliminating a major disease by removing affected tissue and surrounding tissues that might be diseased.

radiculopathy Damage to the nerve roots that enter or leave the *spinal cord*. Radiculopathy may be caused by *disc prolapse*, spinal *arthritis*, *diabetes mellitus*, or ingestion of heavy metals such as lead.

The symptoms are severe pain and, occasionally, numbness in the area supplied by the affected nerves, and weakness, *paralysis*, and wasting of muscles supplied by the nerves. If possible, the underlying cause is treated; otherwise, symptoms may be relieved by *analgesic drugs*, *physiotherapy*, or, in some cases, surgery.

radioactivity The emission of alpha particles, beta particles, and/or gamma radiation that occurs when the nuclei of unstable atoms spontaneously disintegrate. Many radioactive substances are naturally occurring – for example, uranium ores. (See also *radiation*.)

radiofrequency ablation A minimally invasive procedure in which radiofrequency alternating electric current is used to destroy diseased or abnormal tissue. The procedure may be carried out under local or general anaesthesia; the electric current is applied by electrodes inserted into the affected tissue. Radiofrequency ablation may be used to treat some tumours and certain abnormal heart rhythms.

radiography The use of *radiation*, such as *X-rays*, to image parts of the body. (See also *imaging techniques*; *radiology*.)

radioimmunoassay A sensitive laboratory technique that uses radioactive isotopes to measure the concentration of proteins such as hormones or antibodies in blood. (See also *immunoassay*.)

radioisotope scanning See *radionuclide scanning*.

radiology The medical speciality that makes use of *X-rays*, *ultrasound*, *MRI*, and *radionuclide scanning* for investigation, diagnosis, and treatment.

Radiological methods provide images of the body in a *noninvasive* way so that exploratory surgery is not needed. The techniques also enable instruments (such as needles and *catheters*) to be accurately guided into different parts of the body for diagnosis and treatment. This is called interventional radiology.

radiolucent A term for anything that is almost transparent to *radiation*, especially to *X-rays* and gamma radiation.

radionuclide scanning A diagnostic technique based on detection of *radiation* emitted by radioactive substances introduced into the body. Substances are taken up to different degrees by different tissues, allowing specific organs to be studied. For example, iodine is taken up mainly by the thyroid gland, so by "tagging" a sample of iodine with a radioactive marker (radionuclide), the uptake of iodine can be monitored to investigate the functioning of the gland.

A radionuclide is swallowed or injected into the blood and accumulates in the target organ. It emits radiation in the form of

R

RADIONUCLIDE SCANNING

Gamma camera counterbalance

Monitor displays image

Radiographer

Control panel

Gamma camera

Adjustable bed

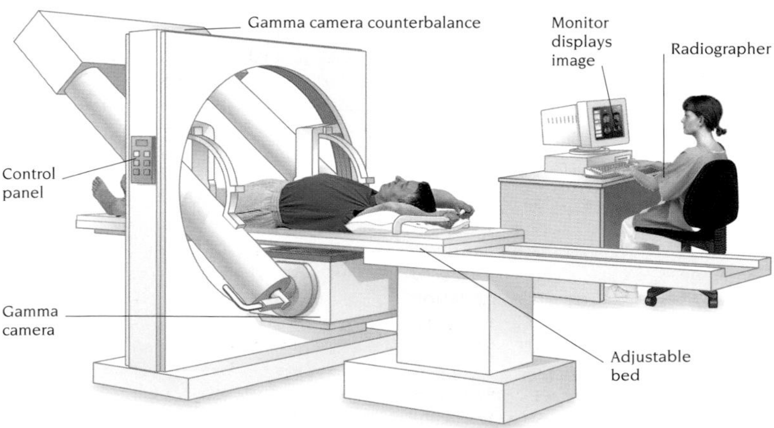

gamma radiation, which is detected by a gamma camera to produce an image. Cross-sectional images ("slices") can be obtained using a computer-controlled gamma camera that rotates around the patient. This specialized form of radionuclide scanning is known as SPECT (single photon emission computed tomography). Moving images can also be made using a computer to record a series of images. Radionuclide scan-

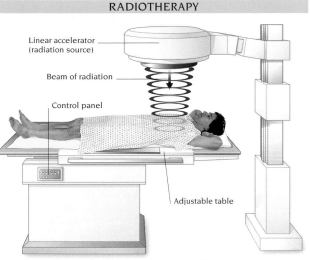

RADIOTHERAPY

Linear accelerator (radiation source)

Beam of radiation

Control panel

Adjustable table

EXTERNAL BEAM RADIOTHERAPY

ning can detect some disorders at an earlier stage than other imaging techniques because changes in the functioning of an organ often occur before the structure of the organ is affected. The technique is also used to detect disorders that affect only the function of organs. Moving images can provide information on blood flow, the movement of the heart walls, the flow of urine through the kidneys, and bile flow through the liver.

Radionuclide scanning is a safe procedure, requiring only minute doses of radiation that are excreted within hours. The radionuclides carry virtually no risk of toxicity or hypersensitivity.

radiopaque This term describes anything that blocks radiation, especially *X-rays* and gamma rays. As many body tissues are *radiolucent*, some X-ray imaging procedures require the introduction of radiopaque substances into the body to make organs stand out clearly.

radiotherapy Treatment of *cancer* and, occasionally, some noncancerous tumours, by *X-rays* or other radiation. Radioactive sources produce ionizing *radiation*, which destroys or slows down the development of abnormal cells. Normal cells suffer little or no long-term damage, but short-term damage is a side effect.

Radiotherapy may be used on its own to destroy all the abnormal cells in various types of cancer, such as *squamous cell carcinoma, Hodgkin's disease, breast cancer, prostate cancer*, cervical cancer (see *cervix, cancer of*), and laryngeal cancer (see *larynx, cancer of*), and to prevent recurrence of the cancer. Radiotherapy may also be used in conjunction with other cancer treatments. Surgical excision of a cancerous tumour is often followed by radiotherapy to destroy any remaining cancer cells. Radiotherapy may also be used to relieve symptoms of a cancer that is too far advanced to be cured. Total body irradiation is often given before a *stem cell* or *bone marrow transplant.*

If benefits outweigh risks, radiotherapy may be used to treat noncancerous diseases; for example, part of an overactive thyroid gland (see *thyrotoxicosis*) may be destroyed using radioactive iodine.

Radiotherapy is usually performed on an outpatient basis. *X-rays* (or sometimes electrons) produced by a machine called a linear accelerator are aimed at the tumour from many directions. This produces a large enough dose of radiation to destroy the tumour. Alternatively, a source of radiation, in the form of tiny pellets, is inserted into the tumour through a hollow

R

needle (see *interstitial radiotherapy*) or into a body cavity (see *intracavitary therapy*). Radioactive iodine used to treat thyrotoxicosis is given in liquid form and drunk through a straw.

There may be unpleasant side effects, including fatigue, nausea and vomiting, and hair loss from irradiated areas. Rarely, the skin may become red and blistered.

radium A rare, radioactive, metallic element that occurs naturally only as compounds in *uranium* ores.

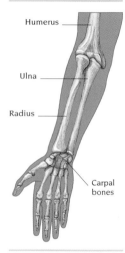

RADIUS

Humerus

Ulna

Radius

Carpal bones

radius The shorter of the two long bones of the forearm; the other is the ulna. The radius is the bone on the thumb side of the arm. It articulates with the humerus at the elbow and the carpal bones at the wrist. It takes most of the strain when weight is placed on the wrist and is a common site of fractures (see *radius, fracture of*; *Colles' fracture*).

radius, fracture of A common type of fracture that may affect any part of the *radius*. Fracture of the radius just above the wrist (see *Colles' fracture*) is the most common fracture in people over 40. Fracture of the head of the radius just below the elbow is one of the most common fractures in young adults. The bone is immobilized in a *cast* or surgically. Healing takes about 6 weeks.

radon A colourless, odourless, tasteless, radioactive gaseous element produced by the radioactive decay of *radium*.

raloxifene A drug prescribed to prevent and treat postmenopausal *osteoporosis*. It may increase the risk of deep vein thrombosis (see *thrombosis, deep vein*).

randomized controlled trials A form of *controlled trial* that evaluates the effectiveness of a drug, or other treatment, in which subjects are randomly allocated to one of the study groups.

This random allocation means individuals are equally likely to be selected for the particular treatment being investigated or for the control group of the trial.

ranitidine An *ulcer-healing drug* belonging to the H_2-receptor antagonist group. It is used to prevent and treat *peptic ulcers* and to treat *oesophagitis*. Side effects may include headache, skin rash, nausea, constipation, and lethargy.

ranula A *cyst* in the floor of the mouth, which produces a translucent, bluish swelling. Ranulas probably arise from damage to a *salivary gland*. They are removed surgically.

rape Sexual intercourse with an unwilling partner, which is achieved by the use or the threat of force or violence.

rash A group of spots or an area of red, inflamed skin. A rash is usually temporary and is only rarely a sign of a serious underlying problem. It may be accompanied by itching or fever.

Rashes are classified as localized (affecting a small area of skin) or generalized (covering the entire body), and by the type of spots. A bullous rash has large blisters, a vesicular rash has small blisters, and a pustular one has pus-filled blisters. A macular rash consists of spots level with the surrounding skin and discernible from it by a difference in colour or texture. Nodular and papular rashes consist of small, raised bumps.

Rashes are the main sign of many infectious diseases (such as *chickenpox*), and are a feature of many *skin disorders*, such as *eczema* and *psoriasis*. They may also indicate an underlying medical problem, such as the rashes of *scurvy* or *pellagra*, which are caused by vitamin deficiency. The rashes of *urticaria* or contact *dermatitis* may be caused by an allergic reaction. Drug reactions, particularly to *antibiotic drugs*, are a common cause of rashes.

A diagnosis is based on the appearance and distribution of the rash, the presence of any accompanying symptoms, and the possibility of allergy (for example, to drugs). Any underlying cause is treated if possible. An itching rash may be relieved by a lotion, such as *calamine*, or an *antihistamine drug*.

RAST An abbreviation for radioallergosorbent test. RAST is a type of *radio-*

R

immunoassay used to detect antibodies to specific *antigens*.

rats, diseases from Rats are rodents that live close to human habitation. They damage and contaminate crops and food stores and can spread disease.

The organisms responsible for *plague* and a type of *typhus* are transmitted to humans by the bites of rat fleas. *Leptospirosis* is caused by contact with anything contaminated by rat's urine.

Rat-bite fever is a rare infection transmitted by a rat bite. There are two types, caused by different bacteria. The symptoms include inflammation at the site and in nearby *lymph nodes* and vessels; bouts of fever; a rash; and, in one type, painful joint inflammation. Both types are treated with *antibiotic drugs*.

Rabies virus can be transmitted by the bites of infected rats. *Lassa fever*, also a viral disease, may be contracted from the urine of rats in West Africa. Rats also carry the viral infection lymphocytic choriomeningitis, as well as the bacterial infection *tularaemia*.

Raynaud's disease A disorder of blood vessels in which exposure to cold causes the small arteries supplying the fingers and toes to contract suddenly. This cuts off blood flow to the digits, which become pale. Fingers are more often affected than toes. The cause is unknown; but young women are most commonly affected.

On exposure to cold, the digits turn white due to lack of blood. As sluggish blood flow returns, the digits become blue; when they are warmed and normal blood flow returns, they turn red. During an attack, there is often tingling, numbness, or a burning feeling in the affected fingers or toes. In rare cases, the artery walls gradually thicken, permanently reducing blood flow. Eventually painful ulceration or even *gangrene* may develop at the tips of the affected digits.

Diagnosis is made from the patient's history. Treatment involves keeping the hands and feet as warm as possible. *Vasodilator drugs* or *calcium channel blockers* may be helpful in severe cases. (See also *Raynaud's phenomenon*.)

Raynaud's phenomenon A circulatory disorder affecting the fingers and toes that shares the mechanism, symptoms,

and signs of *Raynaud's disease* but results from a known underlying disorder. Possible causes include arterial diseases, such as *atherosclerosis*; connective tissue diseases, such as *rheumatoid arthritis*; and various drugs, such as *beta-blocker drugs*. The disorder is an occupational disorder (commonly known as vibration white finger) of people who use pneumatic drills, chain saws, or vibrating machinery; it is sometimes seen in typists, pianists, and others whose fingers suffer repeated trauma. Treatment is the same as for Raynaud's disease, along with treatment of the underlying disorder.

reactive arthritis Inflammation of the joints due to an abnormal immune response that occurs after an infection of the genital tract, such as *chlamydial infection*, or of the intestinal tract, such as *gastroenteritis*. If there is additional inflammation elsewhere in the body, such as in the eyes, the condition is known as *Reiter's syndrome*.

reagent A term for any chemical substance that takes part in a chemical reaction. The term usually refers to a chemical or mixture of chemicals used in chemical analysis or employed to detect a biological substance.

reboxetine An *antidepressant drug* that blocks the reuptake of *noradrenaline* (norepinephrine) within the nervous system. Side effects include insomnia, sweating, and dizziness on standing.

receding chin Underdevelopment of the lower jaw. The condition can be corrected by the use of *orthodontic appliances* during the growth spurt at adolescence or by *cosmetic surgery*.

receding gums Withdrawal of the gums from around the teeth, exposing part of the roots. The teeth may be sensitive to hot and cold substances, and the attachment of a tooth in the socket may weaken, causing the tooth to become loose. Severe cases are usually a sign of gum disease (see *periodontitis*; *gingivitis*).

receptor A general term for any sensory nerve cell (one that converts stimuli into nerve impulses). The term is also used to refer to structures on the surface of a cell that allow chemicals to bind with the cell.

recessive A term used in *genetics* to describe a *gene* that shows its effects only

R

when it is present in a double dose in the genotype: that is, when there is a pair of the recessive gene. If a recessive gene is not paired, its effects are overridden by the corresponding *dominant* gene. For example, the gene for blue eye colour is recessive and the gene for brown eyes is dominant; therefore if a child inherits the gene for brown eyes from one parent and the gene for blue eyes from the other, the "blue eye" gene is overridden by the "brown eye" gene and the child has brown eyes. The child must inherit two of the recessive blue eye genes, one from each parent, to have blue eyes. Many genetic disorders, such as *cystic fibrosis* and *sickle cell anaemia,* are determined by recessive genes. A child will only have the disease if he or she inherits the gene from both parents.

recombinant DNA A section of *DNA* from an organism that has been artificially spliced into the DNA of another organism. (See *genetic engineering.*)

reconstructive surgery See *arterial reconstructive surgery*; *plastic surgery.*

recovery position The position in which to place an unconscious, breathing casualty, while waiting for medical help. The body is placed on its side with the upper leg bent at a right angle; the lower leg is kept straight. The lower arm is bent at a right angle; the upper is bent with the palm of the hand placed against the lower cheek to support the head, which is tilted back to keep the airway open. Casualties with suspected spinal injuries should not be placed in the recovery position.

rectal bleeding The passage of blood from the *rectum* or *anus.* The blood may be red, dark brown, or black. It may be mixed with, or on the surface of, *faeces* or passed separately, and there may be pain.

Haemorrhoids are the most common cause of rectal bleeding. Small amounts of bright red blood appear on the surface of faeces or on toilet paper. *Anal fissure*, *anal fistula*, *proctitis*, or *rectal prolapse* may also cause rectal bleeding.

Cancer of the colon (see *colon, cancer of*) or the rectum (see *rectum, cancer of*) or *polyps* can also cause bleeding. Disorders of the colon such as *diverticular disease* may cause dark red faeces. Black faeces (*melaena*) may be due to bleeding high in the digestive tract. Bloody diarrhoea may be due to *ulcerative colitis, amoebiasis,* or *shigellosis.* Diagnosis may be made from a *rectal examination*, from *proctoscopy, sigmoidoscopy, colonoscopy,* or a double-contrast *barium X-ray examination.*

rectal examination Examination of the *anus* and *rectum*, performed as part of a general *physical examination*, to assess symptoms of pain or changes in bowel habits, and to check for the presence of *tumours* of the rectum or *prostate gland.*

rectal prolapse Protrusion outside the *anus* of the lining of the *rectum*, usually brought on by straining to defecate. The condition commonly causes discomfort, mucus discharge, and *rectal bleeding.*

Rectal prolapse is usually temporary in young children but is often permanent in elderly people. If the prolapse is large, leakage of faeces may occur.

Treatment is with a fibre-rich diet. Surgery may also be performed.

rectocele Bulging inwards and downwards of the back wall of the *vagina* as the *rectum* pushes against weakened tissues in the vaginal wall. A rectocele is usually associated with a *cystocele* or a prolapsed uterus (see *uterus, prolapse of*).

There may be no symptoms, or the rectocele may cause *constipation. Pelvic floor exercises* may help. If not, an operation to tighten the tissues at the back of the vagina may be recommended.

RECOVERY POSITION

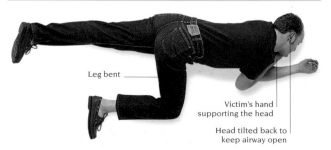

Leg bent

Victim's hand supporting the head

Head tilted back to keep airway open

rectum A short, muscular tube that forms the lowest part of the large intestine and connects it to the anus.

Rectal disorders are diagnosed by *rectal examination* and *proctoscopy* or by *sigmoidoscopy*.

rectum, cancer of A cancerous *tumour* in the *rectum*. The cause is unknown, but dietary factors and genetic factors are thought to play a part. It is more common between ages 50 and 70.

Early symptoms are *rectal bleeding* during defecation and diarrhoea or constipation. Later, pain may occur. Left untreated, the cancer may cause severe bleeding and pain and block the intestine. It may also spread to other organs.

The cancer may be detected by a *rectal examination* and confirmed with *proctoscopy* or *sigmoidoscopy* and *biopsy*. Screening for rectal cancer may be done with a faecal occult blood test (see *occult blood, faecal*).

Treatment is usually with surgery. For a tumour in the upper rectum, the affected area and the last part of the colon are removed and the two free ends of the intestine are sewn together. To promote healing, a temporary *colostomy* may be made. For a growth in the lower rectum, the entire rectum and anus are removed. Because there is no outlet for faeces, a permanent colostomy is created.

Radiotherapy and *anticancer drugs* may be used in addition to or instead of surgery. Up to 40 per cent of people treated for rectal cancer live for 10 years or more.

red-eye Another name for *conjunctivitis*.

reduction The process of manipulating a displaced part of the body back into its original position.

referred pain Pain felt in a part of the body at some distance from its cause. It occurs because some remote parts of the body are served by the same nerve or group of nerves. Nerve impulses that reach the brain from one of these areas may be misinterpreted as coming from another. A common example of referred pain is the pain down the left arm caused by a *myocardial infarction*.

reflex An action that occurs automatically and predictably in response to a particular stimulus, independent of the will of the individual.

In the simplest reflex, a sensory nerve cell reacts to a stimulus, such as heat or pressure, and sends a signal along its nerve fibre to the *central nervous system*. There, another nerve cell becomes stimulated and causes a muscle to contract or a gland to increase its secretory activity. The passage of the nerve signal from original sensation to final action is called a reflex arc.

Reflexes may be inborn or conditioned. Some inborn reflexes occur only in babies (see *reflex, primitive*). Inborn reflexes include those that control basic body functions, such as contraction of the bladder after it has filled beyond a certain point, and are managed by the *autonomic nervous system*. Conditioned reflexes are acquired through experience in a process called *conditioning*.

Several simple reflexes, such as the knee-jerk, are tested in a *physical examination*. Changes in the reflexes may indicate damage to the nervous system. The examination of vital reflexes controlled by the brainstem is the basis for diagnosing *brain death*.

reflexology A form of *complementary medicine* in which the practitioner massages parts of the patient's feet in an attempt to treat disorders affecting other areas of the body.

reflex, primitive An automatic movement in response to a stimulus that is present in newborn infants but disappears during the first few months after birth. Primitive reflexes are believed to represent actions that were important in earlier stages of human evolution. They include the grasp reflex when something is placed in the hand and the rooting reflex, in which the baby's head turns when his or her cheek is touched or stroked, enabling the baby to find the nipple. These reflexes are tested after birth to give an indication of the condition of the nervous system.

reflux An abnormal backflow of fluid in a body passage due to failure of the passage's exit to close fully. A common type of reflux is *regurgitation* of acid fluid from the stomach (see *gastro-oesophageal reflux disease*).

refraction The bending of light rays as they pass from one substance to another.

R

It is the mechanism by which images are focused on the *retina* in the eye.

regression A term used in *psychoanalytic theory* to describe the process of returning to a childhood level of behaviour, such as thumb-sucking.

regurgitation A backflow of fluid. In medicine, the term is used to describe the return of swallowed food or drink from the stomach into the *oesophagus* and mouth. The term is also used to describe the backflow of blood through a *heart valve* that does not close fully because of a disorder such as *mitral incompetence*. (See also *reflux*.)

rehabilitation Treatment aimed at enabling a person to live an independent life following injury, illness, *alcohol dependence*, or *drug dependence*. Treatment may include *physiotherapy*, *occupational therapy*, and *psychotherapy*.

rehydration, oral See *rehydration therapy*.

rehydration therapy The treatment of *dehydration* by administering fluids and salts by mouth (oral rehydration) or by *intravenous infusion*. The amount of fluid necessary depends on age, weight, and the degree of dehydration. Mild dehydration can usually be treated with oral solutions, which are available as effervescent tablet or powder to be made up at home. In severe dehydration, or if the patient cannot take fluids by mouth because of nausea or vomiting, an *intravenous infusion* of *saline* and/or *glucose* solution may be given in hospital.

reimplantation, dental Replacement of a *tooth* in its socket after an accident so that it can become reattached to supporting tissues. The front teeth are most commonly involved. The tooth needs to be reimplanted soon after the accident and is maintained with a splint (see *splinting, dental*) while it heals. Healing may take several weeks.

Reiter's syndrome A condition in which there is a combination of *urethritis*, *reactive arthritis*, and *conjunctivitis*. There may also be *uveitis*. Reiter's syndrome is more common in men.

The syndrome is caused by an *immune response* and usually develops only in people with a genetic predisposition. Most patients have the HLA-B27 tissue type (see *histocompatability antigens*).The syndrome's development is induced by infection: usually *nongonococcal urethritis*, but sometimes bacillary *dysentery*.

Reiter's syndrome usually starts with a urethral discharge, followed by conjunctivitis and then arthritis. The arthritis usually affects one or two joints (the knee and/or ankle) and is often associated with *fever* and *malaise*. Attacks can last for several months. *Tendons*, *ligaments*, and tissue in the soles of the feet may also become inflamed. Skin rashes are common.

Diagnosis is made from the symptoms. *Analgesic drugs* and *nonsteroidal anti-inflammatory drugs* relieve symptoms but may have to be taken for a long period. Relapses occur in about 1 in 3 cases.

rejection An *immune response* aimed at destroying organisms or substances that the body's *immune system* recognizes as foreign. Rejection commonly refers to the nonacceptance of tissue grafts or organ transplants. To avoid rejection, donor tissues are closely matched to the recipient (see *tissue-typing*). *Immunosuppressant drugs*, *corticosteroid drugs*, and *ciclosporin* are given to organ transplant recipients to suppress rejection. (See also *grafting*; *transplant surgery*.)

relapse The recurrence of a disease after an apparent recovery, or the return of symptoms after a *remission*.

relapsing fever An illness caused by infection with *spirochaetes*. Relapsing fever is transmitted to humans by *ticks* or *lice* and is characterized by high fever. It does not occur in the UK.

A high fever of up to 40°C suddenly develops, with shivering, headache, muscle pains, nausea, and vomiting. The symptoms persist for 3–6 days, culminating in a *crisis* with a risk of collapse and death. The person then apparently recovers but suffers another attack 7–10 days later. If tick-borne, there may be several such relapses, each progressively milder.

The spirochaetes can be seen in a *blood smear*, and they can be eliminated with *antibiotic drugs*.

relationship counselling Formerly known as marriage guidance, relationship counselling is a type of professional therapy for established partners aimed at resolving the problems within their relationship. The couple attends regular sessions together in which the counsellor promotes communication and attempts to help resolve differences between the partners. Relationship counselling is largely based on the ideas and methods of *behaviour therapy*. If some of the couple's problems are sexual, the counsellor may refer them for *sex therapy*.

relaxation techniques Methods of consciously releasing muscular tension to achieve mental calm. They can assist people with *anxiety* symptoms, help to reduce *hypertension*, and relieve stress, and may help pregnant women to cope with labour pains (see *childbirth, natural*).

Active relaxation consists of tensing and relaxing each of the muscles in turn. Passive relaxation involves clearing the mind and concentrating on a phrase or sound. *Breathing exercises* help to prevent *hyperventilation*, which often brings on or worsens anxiety. Traditional concentration methods, such as *yoga* and *meditation*, employ similar techniques.

releasing factors A group of *hormones*, produced by the *hypothalamus* in the brain, that stimulates the release of other hormones. *Luteinizing hormone-releasing hormone* is one such releasing factor.

rem An outdated unit of absorbed *radiation* dose, now superseded by the *sievert*. (See also *radiation units*.)

remission A temporary disappearance or reduction in the severity of the symptoms of a disease, or the period during which this occurs.

renal Related to the *kidney*.

renal biopsy See *kidney biopsy*.

renal cell carcinoma The most common type of *kidney cancer*.

renal colic Spasms of severe pain on one side of the back, usually caused by a kidney stone (see *calculus, urinary tract*) passing down the *ureter*. There may also be nausea, vomiting, sweating, and blood in the urine. Treatment is usually with bed rest, plenty of fluids, and injections of an *analgesic drug*, such as *pethidine*.

renal failure See *kidney failure*.

renal transplant Another term for *kidney transplant*.

renal tubular acidosis A condition in which the *kidneys* are unable to excrete normal amounts of acid made by the body. The blood is more acidic than normal, and the urine less acidic. Causes include kidney damage due to disease, drugs, or a *genetic disorder*; but in many cases the cause is unknown. The acidosis may result in *osteomalacia*, kidney stones (see *calculus, urinary tract*), nephrocalcinosis, and hypokalaemia (an abnormally low level of potassium in the blood).

renin An *enzyme* involved in the regulation of *blood pressure*. When the blood pressure falls, the *kidneys* release renin, which changes a substance called angiotensinogen into angiotensin I. This is rapidly converted into angiotensin II, which acts to increase blood pressure.

renography A technique that uses a radioactive substance to measure *kidney* function. Renography is quick and painless and is used when obstruction of the passage of *urine* is suspected.

The radioactive substance is injected into the bloodstream and passes through the kidneys into the urine. *Radiation* counts are taken continually throughout the procedure. Normally, the count rises and then falls as the substance passes into the bladder. If obstruction is present, the substance accumulates in the kidneys and the count continues to rise. (See also *kidney imaging*.)

repaglinide An oral *hypoglycaemic* drug used either alone or in combination with *metformin* in the treatment of type 2 *diabetes mellitus*. Repaglinide stimulates the release of *insulin*. Side effects may include abdominal pain, diarrhoea or constipation, nausea, and vomiting.

repetitive strain injury (RSI) An *overuse injury* that affects keyboard workers and musicians, causing weakness and pain in the wrists and fingers.

reproduction, sexual The process of creating offspring by the fusion of two cells from different individuals. This fusion (*fertilization*) occurs in humans when a *sperm* enters an *ovum* following *sexual intercourse* or *artificial insemination*.

reproductive system, female The female organs involved in *ovulation*, *sexual intercourse*, sustaining *pregnancy*, and *childbirth*. Apart from the *vulva*, which protects the opening of the *vagina*, these organs lie within the pelvic cavity.

R

REPRODUCTIVE SYSTEM, FEMALE

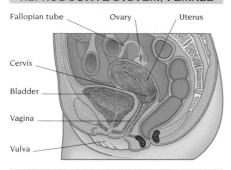

Ova (eggs) are released every month from the two *ovaries*, which also secrete *oestrogen hormone* and *progesterone hormones* to control the reproductive cycle. The ova travel through the *fallopian tubes* to the *uterus*. *Fertilization* takes place if a *sperm* released into the vagina during *sexual intercourse* travels through the *cervix* and uterus to penetrate an ovum while it is in the fallopian tube.

reproductive system, male The male organs involved in the production of *sperm* and in *sexual intercourse*. Sperm and male sex hormones (*androgen hormones*) are produced in the *testes*, which hang in the *scrotum*. From each testis, sperm pass into an *epididymis*, where they mature and are stored. Shortly before *ejaculation*, sperm are propelled into a duct called the *vas deferens*, which carries them to the two *seminal vesicles*. These sacs produce *seminal fluid*, which is added to the sperm to form *semen*.

REPRODUCTIVE SYSTEM, MALE

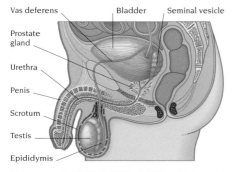

Semen travels along two ducts to the *urethra*. The ducts pass through the *prostate gland*, which produces secretions that are added to the semen. At *orgasm*, semen is ejaculated from the urethra through the erect *penis*, which is placed in the woman's *vagina* during sexual intercourse.

rescue breathing A form of *artificial respiration* in which air is supplied to a person's lungs by mouth-to-mouth or mouth-to-nose breaths. Rescue breathing is an emergency first aid measure, performed either alone or as part of *cardiopulmonary resuscitation* (CPR).

resection Surgical removal of all or part of a diseased or injured organ.

resistance Opposition to a physical or psychological process. Blood vessel walls exert a resistance to the flow of blood; increased resistance leads to raised blood pressure. In *psychoanalysis*, resistance is the blocking from consciousness of memories or emotions. "Resistance" may also refer to the body's ability to withstand attack from toxins, irritants, or *microorganisms*; resistance to infection is called *immunity*. The term "drug resistance" refers to the ability of some microorganisms to withstand attack from previously effective drug treatments.

resorption, dental Loss of substance from *teeth*. The loss may be external (affecting the surface of the root) or internal (affecting the wall of the pulp cavity). External resorption is part of the process by which *primary teeth* are lost. It occurs, to some degree, as part of aging, and may also be due to injury, inflammation of surrounding tissues, or pressure, for example from an impacted tooth. Internal resorption is rare, occurring in about 1 percent of adults.

respiration A term for the processes by which *oxygen* reaches body cells and is utilized by them, and by which *carbon dioxide* is eliminated. Air, containing oxygen, is breathed into the *lungs* and enters the *alveoli*. Oxygen diffuses into the blood, which carries it to cells in the body, where it is used to metabolize *glucose* to provide energy.

Carbon dioxide is produced as a waste product and passes into the blood from the body cells. It is transported to the lungs to be breathed out (see *respiratory system*).

respirator See *ventilator*.

respiratory arrest Sudden cessation of *breathing*, resulting from any process that severely depresses the function of the respiratory centre in the *brain*. Causes include prolonged *seizures*, an overdose of *opioid drugs*, *cardiac arrest*, *electrical injury*, serious *head injury*, *stroke*, or *respiratory failure*. Respiratory arrest leads to *anoxia* and, if untreated, cardiac arrest, brain damage, *coma*, and death.

respiratory distress syndrome An acute lung disorder that makes *breathing* difficult, resulting in a life-threatening deficiency of *oxygen* in the blood. There are two types of the syndrome. In premature babies, the lungs are stiff and do not inflate easily due to a lack of *surfactant*. In adults, it develops as a result of a severe injury or overwhelming infection. Treatment is for the underlying cause, and includes artificial *ventilation* and oxygen; inhaled surfactant is given to babies.

respiratory failure A condition in which there is a buildup of *carbon dioxide* and a fall in the level of *oxygen* in the blood (see *hypoxia*). Causes include lung disorders, such as severe *asthma*, *emphysema*, or chronic bronchitis (see *pulmonary disease, chronic obstructive*), or damage to the respiratory centre in the brain due to, for example, an overdose of *opioid drugs*, a *stroke*, or serious *head injury*.

Treatment is with *ventilation* and oxygen for the underlying cause.

respiratory function tests See *pulmonary function tests*.

respiratory system The organs responsible for carrying *oxygen* from the air to the blood and expelling *carbon dioxide*.

The upper part of the respiratory system consists of two nasal passages; the *pharynx*; the larynx (which contains the vocal cords); and the *trachea*. The lower part of the respiratory tract consists of two *lungs*, which are enclosed in a double membrane called the *pleura*, and the lower airways (the *bronchi* and smaller bronchioles). These structures are encased and protected by the bony ribcage. The airways terminate in millions of balloon-like sacs known as *alveoli*, where gas exchange with the tiny blood vessels surrounding them takes place. These small vessels feed into larger pulmonary vessels for blood transport to and from the heart.

Air is inhaled and exhaled (see *breathing*) by the action of the dome-shaped diaphragm and of abdominal and chest muscles including the intercostal muscles between the ribs.

respiratory tract infection Infection of the breathing passages, which extend from the *nose* to the *alveoli*. This type of infection is divided into upper and lower

RESPIRATORY SYSTEM

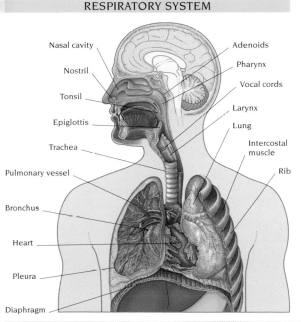

Nasal cavity
Nostril
Tonsil
Epiglottis
Trachea
Pulmonary vessel
Bronchus
Heart
Pleura
Diaphragm

Adenoids
Pharynx
Vocal cords
Larynx
Lung
Intercostal muscle
Rib

R

respiratory tract infections. Upper respiratory tract infections affect the *nose, throat, sinuses,* and *larynx.* They include the common *cold, pharyngitis, tonsillitis, sinusitis, laryngitis,* and *croup.* Lower respiratory tract infections, which affect the *trachea, bronchi,* and *lungs,* include acute *bronchitis,* acute *bronchiolitis,* and *pneumonia.*

restless legs A syndrome characterized by unpleasant tickling, burning, prickling, or aching sensations in the leg muscles. Symptoms tend to come on at night in bed; they may also be triggered by prolonged sitting. The condition tends to run in families and is common in middle-aged women, people with *rheumatoid arthritis* or *diabetes mellitus,* and during pregnancy. The cause is unknown, and there is no single cure; some patients benefit from cooling the legs, others from warming them. Treatment with *levodopa* and *calcium channel blockers* can sometimes help.

restoration, dental The reconstruction of part of a damaged tooth. Restoration also refers to the material or substitute part used to rebuild the tooth. Small repairs are usually made by *filling* the tooth. For extensive repairs, a dental *inlay* or a *crown* may be used. Chipped front teeth may be repaired by bonding (see *bonding, dental*).

restricted growth See *short stature.*

resuscitation See *artificial respiration; cardiopulmonary resuscitation.*

retardation See *learning difficulties.*

reticular formation A network of nerve cells scattered through the *brainstem.*

reticulocyte The medical term for a newly formed red *blood cell.* Reticulocytes are made in the bone marrow from *stem cells.* They remain in the bone marrow for 1–2 days and then pass into the bloodstream, where they mature into red blood cells.

reticulosarcoma See *lymphoma, non-Hodgkin's.*

retina The light-sensitive membrane that lines the back inner surface of the *eye,* and on which images are cast by the cornea and lens. The retina contains specialized nerve cells (rods and cones) that convert light energy into nerve impulses. The impulses travel from the rods and cones through other cells in the retina and along the *optic nerve* to the *brain.* The rods respond to very dim light and cones are responsible for *colour vision.*

The retina can be affected by congenital and genetic disorders, such as *colour vision deficiency* and *Tay–Sachs disease.* It can also be infected, injured (see *retinal detachment; retinal tear*), or affected by tumours such as *retinoblastoma.* Other disorders affecting the retina include *diabetes mellitus* and *retinal vein occlusion.*

retinal artery occlusion Blockage of an artery supplying blood to the *retina,* most commonly due to *thrombosis* or *embolism.* The disorder can result in permanent blindness or loss of part of the field of vision, depending on the artery affected and whether or not the condition can be treated quickly enough.

retinal detachment Separation of the *retina* from the outer layers at the back of the *eye.* Detachment may follow an eye injury but usually occurs spontaneously.

RETINA

| Lens | Retina | Nerve fibres carry impulses to brain | Direction of nerve impulse | Electrical signal from stimulated cell | Pigment cell |

Macula | Direction of light

Cornea | Optic nerve

LOCATION

Connecting nerve cells | Nerve fibre | Cone | Rod

STRUCTURE OF RETINA

It is usually preceded by a *retinal tear*, and is more common in highly myopic (shortsighted) people and in people who have had *cataract surgery*.

The detachment is painless. The first symptom is either bright flashes of light at the edge of the field of vision, accompanied by *floaters*, or a black "drape" obscuring vision.

Urgent treatment is required and usually involves surgical repair of the underlying tear. If the macula (site of central vision) has not been detached, the results can be excellent.

retinal haemorrhage Bleeding into the *retina* from one or more blood vessels, due to *diabetes mellitus, hypertension*, or *retinal vein occlusion*. When the macula (site of central vision) is involved, vision is severely impaired. Peripheral haemorrhages may be detected only when the eye is examined with an *ophthalmoscope*.

retinal tear The development of a split in the *retina*, usually caused by degeneration. A tear is more common in people with severe *myopia*. A retinal tear may also be caused by a severe eye injury. *Retinal detachment* usually follows a retinal tear. If a retinal tear is found before there is any detachment, the hole is sealed by *laser treatment* or cryopexy (application of extreme cold).

retinal vein occlusion Blockage of a vein carrying blood away from the retina. It usually results from *thrombosis* in the affected vein, and is more common in people who have *glaucoma*. Retinal vein occlusion may cause visual disturbances, glaucoma, or blindness.

retinitis Inflammation affecting the *retina*. (See also *retinopathy*.)

retinitis pigmentosa An inherited condition in which there is degeneration of the rods and cones of the *retina* at the back of both eyes.

The first symptoms appear during or after adolescence and include night blindness. Tests show a ring-shaped area of blindness which, over some years, extends to destroy an increasing area of the *visual field*, though central vision is retained, often for many years. Opthalmoscopy reveals several masses of black pigment corresponding to the

areas of visual loss. Affected individuals and their parents should have *genetic counselling*.

retinoblastoma A cancer of the *retina* that affects infants. The first indications of this disorder may be a *squint* caused by blindness in the affected eye or a visible whiteness in the pupil. Without early treatment, retinoblastoma can spread to the orbit (eye socket) and along the *optic nerve* to the brain.

Retinoblastoma has a genetic basis. People with this cancer lack part of one of the *chromosomes* in pair number 13. Newborn infants from affected families are given regular eye examinations, and prospective parents in affected families should have *genetic counselling*.

Treatment is by removing the eye, or by *radiotherapy*. If both eyes are involved, the one worse affected may be removed and the other given radiotherapy.

retinoids See *vitamin A*.

retinol The principal form of *vitamin A* found in the body.

retinopathy Disease of the *retina*, usually caused by *diabetes mellitus* or persistent *hypertension*.

In diabetic retinopathy, the capillaries in the retina are affected by *aneurysms*, leak fluid, and bleed into the retina. Abnormal capillaries then grow on the retinal surface. As these are fragile, *vitreous haemorrhage* may occur. Fibrous tissue may also grow into the *vitreous humour*. Treatment by laser surgery can often halt the progress of the condition.

In hypertensive retinopathy the retinal arteries become narrowed. Areas of retina may be destroyed, and bleeding and white deposits may occur in the retina. (See also *retrolental fibroplasia*.)

retinoscopy A type of *vision test* in which a beam of light is shone from an instrument called a retinoscope into each eye in turn. The effect of different lenses on the beam of light determines whether glasses are needed for various refractive errors, such as *hypermetropia*, *myopia*, or *astigmatism*. Retinoscopy is particularly useful for assessing babies or young children.

retractor A surgical instrument used to hold an incision open or to hold back surrounding tissue.

R

RETINOSCOPY

Retinoscope

Beam of light

Lens

retrobulbar neuritis A form of *optic neuritis* in which the *optic nerve* becomes inflamed behind the eyeball.

retrograde Moving backwards or in an opposite direction to normal. For example, in retrograde ejaculation, semen is forced into the bladder rather than out through the tip of the penis (see *ejaculation, disorders of*).

retrolental fibroplasia Also called retinopathy of prematurity, a condition that mainly affects the eyes of premature infants. The usual cause is high concentrations of *oxygen* being given as part of the treatment for *respiratory distress*. Excess oxygen causes the tissues at the margin of the *retina* to shut down their blood vessels. When oxygen concentrations return to normal, the affected tissues may send strands of new vessels and fibrous scar tissue into the *vitreous humour*. This may interfere with vision and cause *retinal detachment*. *Laser treatment* may be used.

retroperitoneal fibrosis Inflammation and scarring of tissues at the back of the abdominal cavity. The fibrosis often blocks the *ureters*, preventing urine flow from the kidneys. In severe cases, this results in *kidney failure*. Most cases occur in middle-aged men and are of unknown cause, but long-term treatment with the drug *methysergide* can cause the condition.

retrosternal pain Pain in the central region of the chest, behind the sternum. Causes include irritation of the *oesophagus*, *angina pectoris*, or *myocardial infarction*. (See also *chest pain*.)

retrovirus A type of virus whose genetic material is *RNA* rather than *DNA* and that uses an enzyme called reverse transcriptase to produce DNA from the RNA template. The DNA can then be incorporated into its host cells. A notable example of a retrovirus is *HIV* (human immunodeficiency virus).

Rett's syndrome A *brain* disorder, thought to be a *genetic disorder*, that only affects girls. Symptoms usually occur when the child is 12–18 months old. Acquired skills, such as walking and communication skills, disappear and the girl becomes progressively handicapped, perhaps with signs of *autism*. There are repetitive writhing movements of the limbs, and inappropriate outbursts of crying or laughter. There is no cure for Rett's syndrome and sufferers need constant care and attention. Parents of an affected child should receive *genetic counselling*.

reverse transcriptase inhibitors A class of drugs used in the treatment of diseases, including *HIV* infection, that are caused by retroviruses. The drugs affect the ability of the virus to reproduce by blocking reverse transcriptase, a key enzyme. Drugs include *lamivudine, zidovudine* (AZT), efavirenz, and stavudine.

Reye's syndrome A rare disorder in which brain and liver damage follow a viral *infection*. Children over 15 are rarely affected. The cause is unknown, but aspirin seems to be a predisposing factor and should therefore not be given to children under the age of 16 except on the advice of a doctor. The disorder starts as the child recovers from the infection. Symptoms include uncontrollable vomiting, lethargy, memory loss, and disorientation. Swelling of the brain may cause seizures, disturbances in heart rhythm, *coma*, and cessation of breathing.

Brain swelling may be controlled by *corticosteroid drugs* and by *intravenous* infusions of *mannitol*. *Dialysis* or *blood transfusions* may be needed. If breathing stops, a *ventilator* is used.

The death rate is around 10 per cent, and higher for those who have seizures, lapse into deep coma, and stop breathing. Permanent brain damage may occur.

rhabdomyolysis Destruction of muscle tissue accompanied by the release of *myoglobin* into the blood. The commonest cause is a severe, crushing muscle injury (see *crush syndrome*). Other causes include *polymyositis* and, rarely, excessive exercise. There is usually temporary *paralysis* or weakness of the affected muscle. Except in cases of severe injury, the condition clears up without treatment.

rhabdomyosarcoma A very rare cancerous *muscle tumour*. Treatment is by surgical removal, *radiotherapy*, and *anticancer drugs*.

rhesus immunoglobulin See *anti-D(Rh$_0$) immunoglobulin*.

rhesus incompatibility A mismatch between the blood group of a Rhesus (Rh)-negative pregnant woman and that of her baby. In certain circumstances, this mismatch leads to *haemolytic disease of the newborn*.

The Rh system is based on the presence or absence in the blood of several factors, the most important of which is a substance called D *antigen*. Rh-positive blood contains D antigen, whereas Rh-negative blood does not. The blood type is determined by genes.

Rhesus incompatibility results if a Rh-negative woman is exposed to the blood of her Rh-positive baby while it is being born. There are usually no problems during the first pregnancy with a Rh-positive baby. However, the woman may produce *antibodies* against the D antigen; in a subsequent pregnancy with a Rh-positive baby, these antibodies may cross the placenta and attack the red blood cells of the fetus. A Rh-negative woman can also be sensitized if she has had a *miscarriage*, *abortion*, or *amniocentesis*, in which fetal Rh-positive blood enters her circulation.

Rhesus incompatibility is now uncommon because injections of *anti-D(Rh$_0$) immunoglobulin* are given routinely to Rh-negative women during pregnancy and at delivery. They are also given after miscarriage, abortion, amniocentesis, or any procedure that might result in exposure of the mother to fetal blood cells.

rhesus isoimmunization The development of *antibodies* against Rhesus (Rh)-positive blood in a person who has Rh-negative blood (see *haemolytic disease of the newborn*; *rhesus incompatibility*).

rheumatic fever A disease that causes inflammation throughout the body, especially in the joints. Now rare in developed countries, it is an important cause of heart disease in developing countries. It is most common in children aged 5–15.

Rheumatic fever is believed to be an *autoimmune disorder* induced by certain strains of streptococcal bacteria, and always follows a throat infection. It can usually be prevented by *antibiotic drugs*.

The disease causes fever with pain, inflammation, and swelling of the larger joints. The *heart valves* may be scarred, leading to *mitral stenosis* or *mitral incompetence*. Involvement of the nervous system may cause *Sydenham's chorea*.

The condition may be suspected when arthritis moves from joint to joint but may be discovered only after development of *heart failure* or a *heart murmur*.

Treatment may include *penicillin drugs*, *aspirin*, and, in some cases, *corticosteroid drugs*.

rheumatism A popular term for any disorder that causes pain and stiffness in *muscles* and *joints*.

rheumatoid arthritis An inflammatory type of *arthritis* in which the *joints* in the fingers, wrists, knees, neck, toes, or elsewhere in the body become painful, swollen, stiff, and, in severe cases, deformed. Tissues outside the joints, such as the heart, can also be affected. Rheumatoid arthritis is an *autoimmune disorder* that usually starts in early adulthood or middle age but can also develop in children (see *juvenile chronic arthritis*) or elderly people. Women are

R

affected more often than men. There are usually recurrent attacks.

Symptoms are mild fever and aches followed by swelling, redness, pain, and stiffness in the joints. *Ligaments, tendons,* and *muscles* around the joint may also become inflamed. *Raynaud's phenomenon* may occur in the fingers, and swelling of the wrist may cause *carpal tunnel syndrome* and *tenosynovitis.* Complications caused by severe rheumatoid arthritis include *pericarditis, vasculitis, ulcers* on the hands and feet, *pleural effusion, pulmonary fibrosis,* and *Sjögren's syndrome.*

A diagnosis can be confirmed by *X-rays* and *blood tests.* Treatments include *nonsteroidal anti-inflammatory drugs* and *disease-modifying antirheumatic drugs* (DMARDs) such as sulfasalazine, methotrexate, azathioprine, gold, and penicillamine. DMARDs are usually started early in the condition as they relieve symptoms and also slow progression of the disease. Occasionally, *corticosteroid drugs* may also be injected into the joints.

Physiotherapy is needed to prevent or limit deformity or to help relieve symptoms and maintain mobility. People who are disabled by arthritis can be helped to cope with everyday tasks through *occupational therapy.*

In severe cases, surgery may be performed to replace damaged joints with artificial ones (see *arthroplasty*). Most sufferers must take drugs for life, but many can achieve a near-normal level of activity with effective control of symptoms.

rheumatoid spondylitis See *ankylosing spondylitis.*

rheumatology The branch of medicine concerned with the causes, development, diagnosis, and treatment of diseases that affect the *joints, muscles,* and *connective tissue.*

rhinitis Inflammation of the *mucous membrane* lining the nose, which may cause stuffiness, nasal discharge, and sneezing. The most common causes are the common cold (see *cold, common*), which leads to viral rhinitis, and *allergy,* which causes allergic rhinitis.

rhinitis, allergic Inflammation of the *mucous membrane* lining the nose due

to *allergy* to pollen, dust, or other airborne substances. Also called hay fever, it causes sneezing, a runny nose, nasal congestion, and itchy, watering eyes. Oral *antihistamine drugs* may help to relieve symptoms. To treat eye symptoms, antihistamine or *sodium cromoglicate* eye-drops may be used. Regular use throughout the pollen season of inhaled sodium cromoglicate or *corticosteroid drugs* may help prevent nasal symptoms.

rhinophyma Bulbous deformity and redness of the *nose* that occurs almost exclusively in elderly men. Rhinophyma is a complication of severe *rosacea.* The tissue of the nose thickens, small blood vessels enlarge, and the *sebaceous glands* become overactive, making the nose excessively oily. An operation can restore the nose to a satisfactory shape.

rhinoplasty An operation that alters the structure of the nose to improve its appearance or to correct a deformity. Incisions are made within the nose to avoid visible scars. The *septum* may be altered if breathing is blocked and the cartilage and bone are then reshaped. The nose is finally splinted in position for about 10 days. Rhinoplasty usually causes considerable bruising and swelling, and the results may not be clearly visible for weeks or months.

rhinorrhoea The discharge of watery mucus from the nose, usually due to *rhinitis.* Rarely, the discharge consists of cerebrospinal fluid and is the result of a head injury. (See also *nasal discharge.*)

rhythm method See *contraception, natural methods of.*

rib Any of the flat, curved bones that form a framework for the chest and a protective cage around the heart, lungs, and other underlying organs. There are 12 pairs of ribs, each joined at the back of the ribcage to a vertebra. The upper seven pairs, known as "true ribs", link directly to the *sternum* by flexible costal *cartilage.* The next two or three pairs of "false ribs" connect indirectly to the sternum by means of cartilage attached to the cartilage of the ribs above. Between and attached to the ribs are thin sheets of muscle (*intercostal muscles*) that act during *breathing.* The

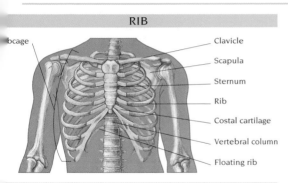

RIB

Clavicle
Scapula
Sternum
Rib
Costal cartilage
Vertebral column
Floating rib

bcage

spaces between the ribs also contain nerves and blood vessels.

ribavirin An *antiviral drug*, also called tribavirin, used to treat children with viral *bronchiolitis* caused by respiratory syncytial virus. It is also used in combination with other drugs in the treatment of chronic *hepatitis C*. Adverse effects are rare.

rib, fracture of *Fracture* of a rib may be caused by a fall or blow, or by stress on the ribcage, such as that produced by prolonged coughing. The fracture of a rib causes severe pain, which may be relieved by *analgesic drugs* or by injection of a local *anaesthetic*.

riboflavin The chemical name of vitamin B_2 (see *vitamin B complex*).

rickets A disease caused by nutritional deficiency that causes *bone* deformities in childhood. Bones become deformed because inadequate amounts of *calcium* and *phosphate* are incorporated into them as they grow. The most common cause is *vitamin D* deficiency. It also occasionally develops as a complication of *malabsorption* and may also occur in rare forms of kidney and liver disease.

Rickets due to dietary deficiency is treated with supplements. The deformities usually disappear as the child grows. Rickets occurring as a complication of a disorder is treated according to the cause.

rickettsia A type of small *bacteria* that can multiply only by invading other living cells. They are mainly parasites of arthropods such as ticks, lice, fleas, and mites. Human diseases caused by rickettsiae include *Q fever*, *Rocky Mountain spotted fever*, and *typhus*.

rifampicin An *antibacterial drug* used mainly to treat *tuberculosis*. It is also used to treat *leprosy* and *legionnaires' disease*. The drug is usually prescribed with other antibacterials because some strains of bacteria develop resistance if it is used alone.

Side effects include harmless, orange-red discoloration of the urine, saliva, and other body secretions, muscle pain, nausea, vomiting, diarrhoea, *jaundice*, flu-like symptoms, rash, and itching. The action of *oral contraceptives* is affected.

rigidity Increased tone in one or more *muscles*, causing them to feel tight; the affected part of the body becomes stiff and inflexible. Causes include muscle injury, *arthritis* in a nearby joint, a neurological disorder, or *stroke*. Rigidity of the abdominal muscles is a sign of *peritonitis*. (See also *spasticity*.)

rigor A violent attack of shivering, often associated with a fever. Rigor may also refer to stiffness or rigidity of body tissues, as in *rigor mortis*.

rigor mortis The stiffening of muscles that starts 3–4 hours after death. It is usually complete after about 12 hours; the stiffness then disappears over the next 48–60 hours. Physical exertion before death makes rigor mortis begin sooner. The sooner rigor mortis begins, the quicker it passes. These facts are used to help assess the time of death.

ringing in the ears See *tinnitus*.

ringworm A popular name for certain fungal skin infections. Ringworm causes ring-shaped, reddened, scaly, or blistery patches on the skin. (See also *tinea*.)

risperidone An *antipsychotic drug* used in the treatment of psychoses such as *schizophrenia* and *mania*. Possible side effects include weight gain, agitation, and dizziness. Risperidone is also associated with an increased risk of *stroke* in the elderly who have *dementia*.

ritodrine A drug used to prevent or delay premature labour. Side effects may include tremor, chest pain, *palpitations*, nausea, vomiting, and flushing.

R

ROOT-CANAL TREATMENT

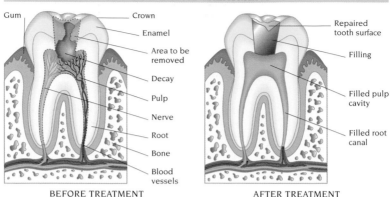

Gum · Crown · Enamel · Area to be removed · Decay · Pulp · Nerve · Root · Bone · Blood vessels

Repaired tooth surface · Filling · Filled pulp cavity · Filled root canal

BEFORE TREATMENT · AFTER TREATMENT

rivastigmine An *acetylcholinesterase inhibitor* drug used to treat mild to moderate *Alzheimer's disease*. It slows the progression of dementia and loss of mental abilities. Possible side effects include nausea, vomiting, dizziness, headaches, agitation, and difficulty in passing urine. Rivastigmine may also worsen the symptoms of *Parkinson's disease*.

river blindness See *onchocerciasis*.

RNA The abbreviation for ribonucleic acid. RNA and *DNA* carry inherited genetic instructions. In animal and plant cells, DNA carries the instructions and RNA helps decode them. In some *viruses* the instructions are held by RNA instead. (See also *nucleic acids*; *protein synthesis*.)

Rocky Mountain spotted fever A rare, infectious disease causing fever and a rash with spots that spread over the body, darken, enlarge, and bleed. The disease occurs in North and South America and is caused by a *rickettsia* transmitted from small mammals by *tick* bites. Treatment is with *antibiotic drugs*.

rod One of the two specialized types of nerve cell within the *retina* of the eye that convert light energy into nerve impulses. The rods are very sensitive and can respond to very dim light. (See also *cone*.)

rodent ulcer A common name for *basal cell carcinoma*.

role-playing The acting out of a role (the pattern of behaviour expected in a given situation). The phrase "sick role" describes the type of passive behaviour

expected and allowed of a patient; people with social or emotional problems may unconsciously adopt this role to gain sympathy and understanding.

root-canal treatment A dental procedure performed to save a tooth in which the pulp (see pulp, *dental*) has died or become untreatably diseased, usually as the result of extensive dental *caries*.

The pulp is removed through a hole drilled in the crown. An antibiotic paste and a temporary filling are packed in. A few days later, the filling is removed and the canals are checked for infection. When no infection is detected the cavity is filled and the roots are sealed with cement. If the cavity is not filled completely, *periodontitis* may occur.

Treated teeth may turn grey but their appearance can be restored by bonding (see *bonding, dental*), fitting an artificial crown (see *crown, dental*) or veneer, or by bleaching (see *bleaching, dental*).

Rorschach test A psychological test based on a person's responses to a set of ink-blot pictures. The test is now rarely used. (See also *personality tests*.)

rosacea A chronic *skin* disorder in which the nose and cheeks are abnormally red. The cause is usually unknown, but in some cases it results from overuse of *corticosteroid* creams. The disorder is most common among middle-aged women.

Rosacea may develop into permanent redness of the skin, sometimes with *acne*-like pustules. In elderly men, it may lead to *rhinophyma*. Treatment includes oral *tetracycline* or topical *metronidazole*. Rosacea tends to recur for 5–10 years before disappearing.

roseola infantum A common infectious disease, probably viral, that mainly affects children aged 6 months to 2 years. There is an abrupt onset of irritability and fever. The temperature drops to normal after 4–5 days and a rash appears on the trunk, often spreading to the neck, face, and limbs, before clearing up within 1–2 days. Other symptoms may include a sore throat and enlargement of *lymph nodes* in the neck. Convulsions may occur during the fever, but there are no serious effects. The only treatment is to keep the child cool and give *paracetamol*.

rosiglitazone An oral *hypoglycaemic* drug used in combination with other oral hypoglycaemics (either *metformin* or a sulphonylurea) in the treatment of type 2 *diabetes mellitus*. Rosiglitazone acts by reducing peripheral insulin resistance. Side effects may include gastrointestinal disturbances, weight gain, and *anaemia*.

rotator cuff A reinforcing structure around the shoulder *joint*, composed of four muscle tendons that merge with the fibrous capsule enclosing the joint.

rotavirus A type of virus that is one of the causes of *gastroenteritis*, especially in young children.

roughage See *fibre, dietary*.

roundworms Also known as nematodes, a class of worms, some of which are human *parasites* and usually inhabit the intestines. The only common roundworm disease in the UK is *threadworm infestation*; occasionally, *ascariasis*, *whipworm infestation*, *trichinosis*, and *toxocariasis* occur. Some people return from abroad with *hookworm infestation*. Treatment is usually with *anthelmintic drugs*.

RSI The abbreviation for *repetitive strain injury*, a type of *overuse injury*.

rubber dam A rubber sheet used to isolate one or more teeth during certain dental procedures. The dam acts as a barrier against saliva and prevents the inhalation of debris.

rubefacient A substance that causes redness of the skin by increasing blood flow to it. Rubefacients are sometimes included in ointments used to relieve muscular

aches and pains and work by creating a superficial feeling of heat or cold, which distracts the brain from the deeper muscular pain.

rubella A viral infection, also known as German measles. It is serious only if it affects a nonimmune woman in the early months of pregnancy, when there is a risk that the virus will cause severe *birth defects* in the fetus.

The rubella virus is spread by mother-to-baby transmission and in airborne droplets; it has an *incubation period* of 2–3 weeks. Infection usually occurs in children aged 6–12. A rash appears on the face, spreads to the trunk and limbs, then disappears after a few days. There may be slight fever and enlarged *lymph nodes* at the back of the neck.

The virus may be transmitted from a few days before symptoms appear until one day after they disappear. An unborn baby is at risk if the mother is infected during the first 4 months of pregnancy. The earlier the infection occurs, the more likely the infant is to be affected, and the more serious the abnormalities tend to be. The most common abnormalities are *deafness*, congenital *heart disease*, cataracts, *purpura*, *cerebral palsy*, and bone abnormalities. About 1 in 5 affected babies dies in early infancy.

There is no specific treatment, apart from *paracetamol* for fever. Treatment of rubella syndrome depends on the defects. Rubella vaccine provides immunity to the disease; it is given in the *MMR vaccine* to babies aged 12–15 months, with a booster at between 3 and 5 years old. Rubella infection also provides immunity. If a non-immune pregnant woman comes into contact with a person who has rubella, passive immunization by *immunoglobulin injection* may help prevent infection of the fetus.

rubeola Another name for *measles*.

running injuries Disorders resulting from the effects on the body of jogging or running. Common injuries include *tendinitis*, stress fractures, plantar *fasciitis*, torn *hamstring muscles*, back pain, tibial *compartment syndrome*, and *shin splints*.

rupture A common term for a *hernia*. The term also refers to a complete break in a structure, as in rupture of a *tendon*.

R

S

sac A bag-like organ or body structure.

saccharin An *artificial sweetener*.

sacralgia Pain in the *sacrum* caused by pressure on a spinal nerve, usually due to a *disc prolapse*. Rarely, it may caused by *bone cancer*. (See also *back pain*.)

sacralization Fusion of the 5th (lowest) lumbar *vertebra* with the upper *sacrum*. It may be present at birth, in which case there are usually no symptoms. Sacralization may also be produced deliberately to treat a *disc prolapse* or *spondylolisthesis*. (See also *spinal fusion*.)

sacroiliac joint One of a pair of rigid *joints* on each side of the body that form an interface between the *sacrum* and the *ilium*. They can be strained, usually by childbirth or overstriding, causing pain in the lower back and buttocks. They can also become inflamed (see *sacroiliitis*).

sacroiliitis Inflammation of a *sacroiliac joint*. Causes include *ankylosing spondylitis*, *rheumatoid arthritis*, *Reiter's syndrome* or arthritis associated with *psoriasis*. The main symptom is pain in the lower back, buttocks, groin, and back of the thigh. Treatment is with *nonsteroidal antiinflammatory drugs*.

sacrum The large triangular bone in the lower *spine*. The sacrum's broad upper part articulates with the 5th (lowest) lumbar *vertebra*, and its narrow lower part with the *coccyx*. The sides of the sacrum are connected by the *sacroiliac joints* to each *ilium*. The sacrum lies in the centre back of the *pelvis*. Disorders affecting the sacrum include *sacralgia*, *spondylolisthesis*, and *sacralization*. (See also *spine, disorders of*.)

sadism The tendency or practice of deriving pleasure, particularly sexual pleasure, from the infliction of suffering or pain on others. (See also *sadomasochism*.)

sadomasochism The tendency or practice of deriving sexual pleasure by inflicting pain (see *sadism*) and receiving abuse (see *masochism*); one trait usually predominates. The term also describes a relationship in which one partner is very dominant and one is submissive.

SADS The abbreviation for *seasonal affective disorder syndrome*.

safe period See *contraception, natural methods of*.

safer sex Preventive measures to reduce the risk of *sexually transmitted infections*; for example, maintaining a monogamous sexual relationship and using a *condom*.

salbutamol A *bronchodilator drug* used to treat *asthma*, chronic *bronchitis*, and *emphysema*. It is also occasionally used in the prevention of premature labour.

salicylic acid A *keratolytic drug* used to treat skin disorders, such as *dermatitis*, *eczema*, *psoriasis*, *dandruff*, *ichthyosis*, *acne*, *warts*, and callosities (see *callus, skin*), and also sometimes to treat *fungal infections*. Side effects are few and may include irritation and dryness of the skin.

saline A solution of salt (sodium chloride). "Normal saline" solution has the same concentration as body fluids and may be given by *intravenous infusion* to replace fluids lost in severe dehydration.

saliva The slightly alkaline fluid that is secreted into the mouth by the *salivary glands* and the *mucous membranes* lining the mouth. Saliva contains the enzyme amylase, which helps to break down carbohydrates (see *digestive system*). Saliva keeps the mouth moist, lubricates food to aid swallowing, and facilitates the sense of taste.

salivary glands Three pairs of glands that secrete *saliva*, via ducts, into the

SACRUM

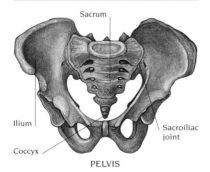

Sacrum

Ilium

Sacroiliac joint

Coccyx

PELVIS

SALIVARY GLANDS

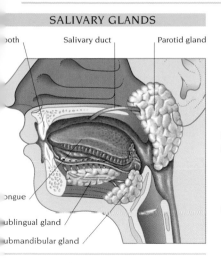

booth   Salivary duct   Parotid gland

ongue

ublingual gland

ubmandibular gland

Food poisoning symptoms, which usually develop suddenly, include nausea, headache, abdominal pain, diarrhoea, and sometimes fever. The symptoms usually last for 2–3 days; in severe cases, *dehydration* or *septicaemia* may develop.

Treatment is by *rehydration therapy*. In severe cases, fluid replacement by *intravenous infusion* may be needed.

salmon patch See *stork mark*.

salpingectomy Surgical removal of one or both *fallopian tubes*. Salpingectomy may be performed if the tube is infected (see *salpingitis*) or to treat *ectopic pregnancy*. (See also *salpingo-oophorectomy*.)

salpingitis Inflammation of a *fallopian tube*, commonly caused by infection spreading up from the vagina, cervix, or uterus. The infection is usually a sexually transmitted one, such as *gonorrhoea* or chlamydial infection. Salpingitis is also a feature of *pelvic inflammatory disease*.

Symptoms include severe abdominal pain and fever. Pus may collect in the tube, and a *pelvic abscess* may develop.

Diagnosis is by examination of vaginal discharge, or *laparoscopy*. Treatment is with *antibiotics*. Surgery may be needed if an abscess has formed.

If the infection damages the inside of the fallopian tubes, *infertility* or an increased risk of an *ectopic pregnancy* may result. In some cases, damage to a tube can be corrected surgically.

salpingo-oophorectomy Removal of one or both *fallopian tubes* and *ovaries*. This may be performed to treat a benign *ovarian cyst* or with a *hysterectomy* to treat cancer of the ovary (see *ovary, cancer of*) or uterus (see *uterus, cancer of*).

salt Commonly used to refer to *sodium chloride*, a substance formed when an acid and base react. (See also *saline*.)

salve A healing, soothing ointment.

sandfly bites Bites of small sandflies, which can transmit disease to humans. In tropical and subtropical areas they transmit *leishmaniasis*. In parts of Asia and the Mediterranean, they transmit sandfly fever, an influenza-like illness.

saphenous vein A major vein that runs the length of the leg. The saphenous vein is sometimes removed and used in *coronary artery bypass*.

mouth. The largest, the *parotid glands*, lie on each side of the jaw; the sublingual glands lie on the floor of the front of the mouth; and the submandibular glands lie near the back of the mouth.

The parotid glands are commonly infected with the *mumps* virus. Stones may form in a salivary duct or gland. Poor *oral hygiene* may allow bacterial infection of the glands, sometimes leading to an abscess. Salivary gland tumours are rare, except for a type of parotid tumour that is slow-growing, noncancerous, and painless. Insufficient salivation causes a dry mouth (see *mouth, dry*) and may be due to *dehydration* or *Sjögren's syndrome*, or occur as a side effect of certain drugs.

salivation, excessive The production of too much *saliva*. It sometimes occurs during pregnancy. Other causes include irritation of the mouth lining, *gingivitis*, *mouth ulcers*, *peptic ulcers*, *oesophagitis*, and *Parkinson's disease*. In some cases, it may be reduced by *anticholinergic drugs*.

salmeterol A *bronchodilator drug* used in the treatment of *asthma*. It is usually inhaled twice a day to prevent attacks.

salmonella infections Infections due to any of the salmonella group of bacteria. One type causes *typhoid fever*; others commonly cause bacterial *food poisoning*, usually via contamination of eggs or chicken. Infants and elderly or debilitated people are most susceptible.

S

sarcoidosis A rare disease of unknown cause in which there is inflammation of tissues throughout the body, especially the lymph nodes, lungs, skin, eyes, and liver. It occurs mainly in young adults.

Symptoms, which do not always occur, include fever, generalized aches, painful joints, and painful, bloodshot eyes. Breathlessness, enlarged lymph nodes, *erythema nodosum*, a purplish facial rash, and areas of numbness may also occur. Possible complications include *hypercalcaemia*, which may damage the kidneys, and *pulmonary fibrosis*.

Treatment is not always needed. Most people recover completely, with or without treatment, within 2 years, but some develop a persistent, chronic form of the disease. *Corticosteroids* are given to treat persistent fever or erythema nodosum, to prevent blindness in an affected eye, and to reduce the risk of lung damage.

sarcoma A cancer of *connective tissue*. Types are *osteosarcoma*, *Kaposi's sarcoma*, *chondrosarcoma*, and *fibrosarcoma*.

SARS The abbreviation for severe acute respiratory syndrome. SARS is a serious respiratory infection, sometimes causing pneumonia, that is thought to be due to a strain of coronavirus. Initial symptoms include fever and sometimes chills, aches, and headache. Later, a dry cough and shortness of breath may occur.

To exclude other causes of pneumonia, chest X-ray and sputum microscopy may be carried out. Supportive treatment includes oxygen therapy and, if necessary, artificial ventilation. Most people recover but in some cases the illness is fatal.

There is no vaccine or cure; control depends on wearing facemasks and gloves, and isolation.

saturated fats See *fats and oils*; *nutrition*.

scab A crust that forms on the skin or on a mucous membrane at the site of a healing wound or infected area.

scabies A skin infestation caused by the mite SARCOPTES SCABIEI, which burrows into the skin to lay eggs. Scabies is highly contagious by close physical contact and is most common in infants, children, and young adults.

The mite's burrows appear on the skin as grey, scaly swellings, usually between the fingers, on the wrists and genitals, and in the armpits. Later, reddish lumps may appear on the limbs and trunk. The infestation causes intense itching, particularly at night. Treatment is with an insecticide lotion.

scald A *burn* due to hot liquid or steam.

scaling, dental Removal of dental *calculi* (see *calculus, dental*) from the teeth to prevent or treat *periodontal disease*.

scalp The skin of the head, and its underlying tissue layers, that is normally covered with hair. Scalp skin is tougher than other skin and is attached to an underlying sheet of muscle that extends from the eyebrows, over the top of the head, to the nape of the neck. The scalp is richly supplied with blood vessels.

Disorders affecting the scalp include *dandruff*; *alopecia*; *sebaceous cysts*; *psoriasis*; fungal infections such as *tinea*; and parasitic infestations such as *lice*. *Cradle cap* is common in infants.

scalpel A surgical knife for cutting tissue.

scan An image produced by one of several *scanning techniques*.

scanning techniques Methods of producing images of organ structure (or sometimes function) using sound waves, radio waves, X-rays, or other forms of radiation. Techniques include *ultrasound*, *CT*, *radionuclide*, *MRI*, and *PET scanning*

scaphoid One of the *wrist* bones. It is the outermost bone on the thumb side of the hand, in the row of wrist bones nearest the elbow.

A fracture of the scaphoid is a common wrist injury usually caused by a fall on an outstretched hand. A characteristic symptom is tenderness in the space between the tendons at the base of the thumb on the back of the hand. Treatment is by immobilizing the wrist in a *cast*.

scapula One of a pair of wing-shaped bones, commonly called the shoulder-blades, which are situated over the upper ribs at the back. The scapula serves as an attachment for certain muscles and tendons of the arm, neck, chest, and back and is involved with movements of the arm and shoulder.

scar A mark left where damaged tissue has healed. The body repairs a lesion by increasing *collagen* production at the site of damage. If the edges of a lesion are brought together during *heal-*

S

ing, a narrow, pale scar forms; if the edges are left apart, more extensive scarring occurs.

A hypertrophic scar is a large, unsightly scar that sometimes develops at the site of an infected wound; some people have a family tendency to develop such scars. (See also *adhesion*; *keloid*.)

scarlatina Another name for *scarlet fever*.

scarlet fever An uncommon infectious disease, more often seen in childhood, that is caused by a strain of streptococcal bacteria. Symptoms include a severe sore throat, high fever, vomiting, and a rash of tiny red spots on the neck and upper trunk that spreads rapidly. The face is flushed, except around the mouth, and a white coating with red spots may develop on the tongue. This coating comes off after a few days to reveal a bright red colour. The fever then soon subsides, the rash fades, and the skin may peel.

As with other types of streptococcal infections, *rheumatic fever* or *glomerulonephritis* may rarely develop 6 weeks later. Treatment with *antibiotics* prevents this and promotes a rapid recovery.

schistosome A type of fluke. Three types of schistosome are parasites of humans, causing different forms of *schistosomiasis*.

schistosomiasis A parasitic tropical disease, caused by any of three species of flukes called schistosomes, and acquired from bathing in infested water. The larval form penetrates the bather's skin and develops in the body into adult flukes, which settle in the veins of the bladder and intestines. Eggs laid by adults provoke inflammatory reactions; there may be bleeding and ulceration in the bladder and intestinal walls, and the liver may also be affected.

The first symptom is usually tingling and an itchy rash where the flukes have penetrated the skin. An influenza-like illness may develop weeks later, when the adults produce eggs. Subsequent symptoms include blood in the urine or faeces, abdominal or lower back pain, and enlargement of the liver or spleen. Complications of long-term infestation include liver *cirrhosis*, *bladder tumours*, and *kidney failure*. Treatment is with the drug *praziquantel*.

schizoid personality disorder Inability to relate socially to other people. People with this trait, which is apparent from childhood, are often described as "loners" and have few, if any, friends. They are eccentric, seem to lack concern for others, and are apparently detached from normal day-to-day activities.

schizophrenia A general term for a group of psychotic illnesses that are characterized by disturbances in thinking, emotional reaction, and behaviour.

Onset can be at any age but is most common in late adolescence and the early 20s, and may be triggered by stress. No causes have been identified, but many have been implicated. It is likely that inheritance plays a role. Disruption of the activity of some neurotransmitters in the brain is a possible mechanism. Brain imaging techniques have revealed abnormalities of structure and function in people with schizophrenia.

Schizophrenia may begin insidiously, with the individual becoming slowly more withdrawn and losing motivation. In other cases, the illness comes on more suddenly, often in response to external stress. The main symptoms are various forms of *delusions* such as those of persecution (which are typical of paranoid schizophrenia); *hallucinations*, which are usually auditory (hearing voices), but which may also be visual or tactile; and thought disorder, leading to impaired concentration and thought processes. Disordered thinking is often reflected in

SCAPULA

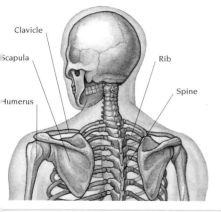

Clavicle

Scapula

Rib

Humerus

Spine

SCIATIC NERVE

Spinal cord

Spinal nerve root

Sciatic nerve

speech that is muddled and disjointed. Behaviour is eccentric, and self-neglect common. In a rare form of schizophrenia, catatonia may occur, in which rigid postures are adopted for prolonged periods, or there are outbursts of repeated movement.

Diagnosis of schizophrenia may take some time and, in some cases, it may be difficult to make a diagnosis at all.

Treatment is mainly with *antipsychotic drugs*, such as *phenothiazine drugs*, and new atypical antipsychotic drugs such as *risperidone*. In some cases, the drugs are given as monthly depot injections. Once the symptoms are controlled, community care, vocational opportunities, and family counselling can help to prevent a relapse.

Some people may make a complete recovery. However, the majority have relapses punctuated with partial or full recovery. A small proportion have a severe life-long disability.

sciatica Pain that radiates along the *sciatic nerve*. The pain usually affects the buttock and thigh, sometimes extending down the leg to the foot. In severe cases, the pain may be accompanied by numbness and/or weakness in the affected area.

The most common cause is a prolapsed intervertebral disc pressing on the nerve root (see *disc prolapse*). Other causes include a muscle spasm, sitting awkwardly for long periods, or, less commonly, pressure on the nerve from a tumour. Sometimes the cause is unknown.

Treatment of sciatica is with *analgesic drugs*. If the pain is severe, a short period of bed rest may be helpful, although prolonged rest may cause the condition to worsen. *Physiotherapy*, *osteopathy*, or *chiropractic* may help in some cases. It is important to maintain a healthy posture and weight.

sciatic nerve The main *nerve* in each leg and the largest nerve in the body. The sciatic nerves are formed from nerve roots in the spinal cord.

scintigraphy An alternative name for *radionuclide scanning*.

scirrhous A term that means hard and fibrous; usually applied to malignant tumours containing dense, fibrous tissue.

sclera The white fibrous outer coat that protects the *eye* from injury. The most common disorder of the sclera is *scleritis*. In *osteogenesis imperfecta*, the sclera is very thin.

scleritis Inflammation of the *sclera* that usually accompanies a *collagen disease* such as *rheumatoid arthritis*. Scleritis also occurs in *herpes zoster* ophthalmicus and *Wegener's granulomatosis*. It may lead to areas of thinning and perforation of the sclera. It is usually persistent but often responds to *corticosteroid* eye-drops.

scleroderma See *systemic sclerosis*.

scleromalacia Softening of the *sclera*, commonly a complication of *scleritis*, especially scleritis of *rheumatoid arthritis*.

sclerosing cholangitis A rare condition in which many of the bile ducts are narrowed, causing progressive liver damage for which the only treatment may be a *liver transplant*. (See also *cholangitis*.)

sclerosis A medical term for hardening of a body tissue, usually used to refer to hardening of blood vessels (as in *arteriosclerosis*) or of nerve tissue (as occurs in the later stages of *multiple sclerosis*).

sclerotherapy A method of treating *varicose veins*, especially in the legs; *haemorrhoids*; and *oesophageal varices*. The vein is injected with an irritant solution, which causes inflammation in the vessel lining, leading to scar tissue formation and the obliteration of the vein.

scoliosis A deformity in which the *spine* is bent to one side. The thoracic or lumbar regions are most commonly affected. Scoliosis usually starts in childhood or adolescence and becomes progressively more marked until growth stops. In many cases, another part of the spine curves to compensate, resulting in an S-shaped spine. The cause of juvenile scoliosis is unknown. Rarely, scoliosis is due to a congenital abnormality of the vertebrae.

S

In some cases, *physiotherapy* may be sufficient to control scoliosis. Progressive or severe scoliosis may require immobilization of the spine in a brace, followed by surgery (*spinal fusion*) to straighten it.

scorpion stings Injection of venom by a scorpion into a victim using a sting in its tail. Many species are not dangerous, but some in North Africa, southern US, South America, the Caribbean, and India are highly venomous. Some stings may cause only mild pain and tingling; but in more venomous species severe pain, restlessness, sweating, diarrhoea, and vomiting can occur. Stings are rarely fatal in adults but require prompt attention. If pain is the only symptom, *analgesics* and a cold compress may be enough. In severe cases, *antivenom* may be needed.

scotoma An area of abnormal vision within the *visual field*.

screening The testing of apparently healthy people with the aim of detecting disease at an early, treatable stage. (See also *blood spot screening tests; cancer screening; newborn screening tests*.)

scrofula *Tuberculosis* of the lymph nodes in the neck, often those just beneath the angle of the jaw. Scrofula is rare in developed countries. Antituberculous drugs clear up the condition in most cases.

scrotum The pouch that hangs behind the penis and contains the *testes*. It consists of an outer layer of thin, wrinkled skin over a layer of muscular tissue. Swelling of the scrotum may be due to an *inguinal hernia*, swollen testis, *hydrocele*, or fluid accumulation due to *heart failure*.

scuba-diving medicine A medical speciality concerned with the physiological hazards of diving with self-contained underwater breathing apparatus. Most hazards stem from the pressure increase with depth. Conditions treated include burst lung and *decompression sickness*.

scurvy A disease, now rare in developed countries, caused by inadequate *vitamin C* intake. Scurvy disturbs the production of *collagen*, a protein in *connective tissue*, causing weakness of small blood vessels and poor wound healing. Haemorrhages may occur anywhere in the body, including the brain. In the skin, haemorrhages result in bruising. Bleeding into the gums and loosening of teeth are common. Bleeding into muscles and joints causes pain. Scurvy is treated with large doses of vitamin C. Bleeding stops in 24 hours, healing resumes, and muscle and bone pain quickly disappear.

sealants, dental Plastic coatings that are applied to the crevices in chewing surfaces of the back *teeth* to help prevent decay.

seasickness A type of *motion sickness*.

seasonal affective disorder syndrome A form of *depression* in which mood changes occur with the seasons. Sufferers tend to become depressed in winter and feel better in spring. Exposure to bright light for 2–4 hours each morning seems to prevent occurrence in some people.

sebaceous cyst A harmless smooth nodule under the skin, most commonly on the scalp, face, ear, and genitals. The cyst contains a yellow, cheesy material and may become very large and infected by bacteria, making it painful. Large or infected cysts can be surgically removed.

sebaceous glands Glands in the *skin* that secrete a lubricating substance called *sebum*. Sebaceous glands either open into hair follicles or discharge directly on to the skin surface. They are most numerous on the scalp, face, and anus and are absent from the palms and soles of the feet. Sebum production is partly controlled by *androgen hormones*. Disorders of

SEBACEOUS GLANDS

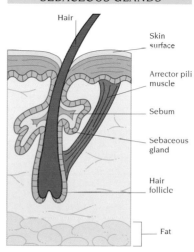

Hair
Skin surface
Arrector pili muscle
Sebum
Sebaceous gland
Hair follicle
Fat

S

the sebaceous glands may lead to *seborrhoea* or *acne* vulgaris.

seborrhoea Excessive secretion of *sebum*, causing oiliness of the face and a greasy scalp. The cause is unclear, but *androgen hormones* play a part. Seborrhoea is most common in adolescent boys; those affected are more likely to develop seborrhoeic *dermatitis* and *acne* vulgaris. The condition usually improves in adulthood without treatment.

seborrhoeic dermatitis See *dermatitis*.

sebum The oily secretion produced by the *sebaceous glands* of the *skin*. Sebum lubricates the skin, keeps it supple, and protects it from becoming waterlogged or dried out and cracked. It also protects the skin from invasion by bacteria and fungi. Oversecretion of sebum (see *seborrhoea*) causes greasy skin and may lead to seborrhoeic *dermatitis* or *acne*.

secondary A term applied to a disease or disorder that results from or follows another disease (the *primary* disease). It also refers to a malignant tumour that has spread from a primary cancer elsewhere in the body (see *metastasis*).

secretin A hormone produced by the *duodenum* when acidic food enters it from the stomach. Secretin stimulates the release of pancreatic juice, which contains bicarbonate to neutralize the acid, and bile from the liver.

secretion The manufacture and release by a cell, gland, or organ of substances, (such as *enzymes*) needed for metabolic processes elsewhere in the body.

secretory otitis media An alternative name for *glue ear*.

sectioning A commonly used term to describe the implementation of a section of the *Mental Health Act*.

security object A significant item, such as a favourite soft toy, that provides comfort and reassurance to a young child. Attachment to such an item is normal and usually diminishes by age 7 or 8.

sedation The use of a drug to calm a person. Sedation is used to reduce excessive *anxiety* and to control dangerously aggressive behaviour. It may also be used as part of *premedication*.

sedative drugs A group of drugs used to produce *sedation*. Sedative drugs include *sleeping drugs, antianxiety drugs,* *antipsychotic drugs,* and some *antidepressant drugs*. A sedative drug is often included in a *premedication*.

seizure A sudden episode of abnormal electrical activity in the *brain*. Recurrent seizures occur in *epilepsy*.

Seizures may be partial or generalized. In a partial seizure, the abnormal activity is confined to one area of the brain. Symptoms include tingling or twitching of a small area of the body, *hallucinations,* fear, or *déjà vu*. In a generalized seizure, the abnormal activity spreads through the brain, causing loss of consciousness.

Causes of seizures include *head injury, stroke, brain tumour,* infection, metabolic disturbances, withdrawal in *alcohol dependence,* or hereditary alcohol intolerance. In children, high fever may cause seizures (see *convulsion, febrile*). Anticonvulsant drugs can control seizures or reduce their frequency.

selective serotonin reuptake inhibitors (SSRIs) A group of drugs that are mainly used to treat *depression*, but may also be used in the treatment of *obsessive-compulsive disorder* and panic disorder. They work by blocking the reabsorption of the neurotransmitter serotonin following its release in the brain. The increased serotonin levels that result are associated with improved mood. Common drugs in this group include fluoxetine and *sertraline*. SSRIs are usually taken orally once a day; it may take 1–3 weeks for any noticeable improvement in symptoms. SSRIs usually produce fewer side effects than other types of antidepressant drug. However, they may cause diarrhoea, nausea, restlessness, and anxiety. Most SSRIs are not recommended for treating depression in those under 18.

selenium A *trace element* that may help to preserve the elasticity of body tissues. The richest sources are meat, fish, whole grains, and dairy products.

self-help organizations Organizations, usually set up by patients or their relatives, that provide people affected by particular conditions with information, support, and, sometimes, financial aid.

self-image A person's view of his or her own personality and abilities. Some neurotic disorders stem from an incongruity between self-image and how others see one. *Psychotherapy* treats neurosis by changing a person's self-image.

self-injury The act of deliberately injuring oneself. Self-mutilation most often occurs in young adults, many of whom are also drug or alcohol abusers, and is three times more common in women. It may take the form of cutting the wrists or burning the forearms with cigarettes. In some, it is a means of dealing with stress, such as that caused by child abuse.

More unusual forms of self-harm, such as mutilating the genitals, are usually due to *psychosis*. Self-destructive biting is a feature of Lesch–Nyhan syndrome, a rare *metabolic disorder*.

selegiline A drug used in the treatment of *Parkinson's disease*, either alone (in the disease's early stage) or with *levodopa*. Selegiline is also used to treat the symptoms of parkinsonism due, for example, to repeated head injury; it is not used if the symptoms are drug-induced, however. Side effects may include nausea, vomiting, diarrhoea or constipation, dry mouth, and sore throat.

semen Fluid produced by the male on *ejaculation*. It is composed of fluid from the *seminal vesicles*, fluid from the *prostate* and Cowper's glands, and *sperm*.

semen, blood in the A usually harmless condition in which a small amount of blood is present in the *semen*. Occasionally, there is an underlying cause (such as an infection or, very rarely, cancer) that requires treatment. Blood in the semen may also occur after a prostate *biopsy*.

semicircular canal A structure in the inner *ear* that plays a role in *balance*. There are three semicircular canals in each ear, at right angles to each other, and connected via a chamber called the vestibule. The fluid-filled canals contain small hairs that detect movement and acceleration, and transmit information to the brain via the vestibular nerve.

seminal fluid analysis Analysis of sperm concentration, shape, and motility (ability to move). It is used to investigate male *infertility* and is also done some weeks after *vasectomy* to ensure that the semen no longer contains sperm.

seminal vesicle One of a pair of sacs that lie behind the bladder in the male and produce seminal fluid, which is

SEMINAL VESICLE

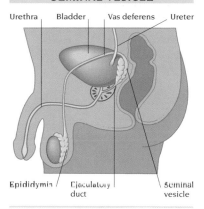

Urethra | Bladder | Vas deferens | Ureter

Epididymis / Ejaculatory duct \ Seminal vesicle

mixed with sperm to make up semen (see *reproductive system, male*).

seminoma See *testis, cancer of*.

senile dementia See *dementia*.

senile purpura A skin condition in which areas of the skin develop a purplish or reddish-brown appearance due to bleeding of small blood vessels underneath. Senile purpura is a disease of middle to old age and is more common in women.

senility A term meaning old age or, more commonly, the decline in mental ability that may occur in old age.

senna A *laxative drug* obtained from the leaves and pods of the Arabian shrubs *CASSIA ACUTIFOLIA* and *CASSIA ANGUSTIFOLIA*, which stimulates bowel contractions. It may colour the urine brown or red.

sensate-focus technique A method taught to couples who are experiencing sexual difficulties caused by psychological rather than physiological factors. The aim of the technique is to make both partners more aware of pleasurable bodily sensations, and to reduce anxiety about performance. It is particularly effective in treating loss of sexual desire (see *sexual desire, inhibited*), or inability to achieve orgasm (see *orgasm, lack of*), and in helping men to overcome *erectile dysfunction* or premature ejaculation (see *ejaculation, disorders of*).

sensation A feeling or impression that has entered consciousness. The senses convey information about the external

S

environment and about the body's internal state to the *central nervous system*.

Information is collected by millions of sense *receptors* found throughout body tissues and in special sense organs, such as the *eye*. Certain sensory information, mainly that from the special sense organs and skin receptors, enters the *sensory cortex* of the brain, where sensations are consciously perceived. Other types of sensory information, for example about body posture, are processed elsewhere and do not produce conscious sensation.

sensation, abnormal Dulled, unpleasant, or otherwise altered *sensations* in the absence of an obvious sensation.

Numbness and *pins-and-needles* are common abnormal sensations. The special senses can be impaired by damage to the relevant sensory apparatus (see *vision, disorders of*; *smell*; *deafness*; *tinnitus*). Other causes of abnormal sensation include peripheral nerve damage caused by *diabetes mellitus*, *herpes zoster* infection, or pressure from a tumour, and disruption of nerve pathways in the *brain* or *spinal cord* due to *spinal injury*, *head injury*, *stroke*, and *multiple sclerosis*.

Pressure on or damage to nerves can sometimes be relieved by surgery or by treatments for the cause. In other cases, distressing abnormal sensation can be relieved only by cutting the relevant nerve fibres or by giving injections to block the transmission of signals.

senses See *sensation*.

sensitization The initial exposure of a person to an allergen or other substance recognized as foreign by the *immune system*, which leads to an immune response. On subsequent exposures to the same substance, there is a much stronger and faster immune reaction. This forms the basis of allergy and other types of *hypersensitivity* reaction.

sensorineural deafness *Deafness* due to problems with the inner ear, nerves, or the brain's auditory area.

sensory cortex A region of the outer *cerebrum* of the *brain* in which sensory information comes to consciousness.

Pressure, pain, and temperature sensations from the skin, muscles, joints, and organs are perceived in the parietal lobes, as is taste. Visual sensations are perceived in the occipital lobes at the back of the cerebrum; sound is perceived in the temporal lobes at the sides.

sensory deprivation The removal of normal external stimuli, such as sight and sound, from a person's environment. Prolonged sensory deprivation can produce feelings of unreality, difficulty in thinking, and *hallucinations*.

separation anxiety The feelings of distress a young child experiences when parted from his or her parents or home. This is a normal aspect of infant behaviour and usually diminishes by age 3 or 4.

In separation anxiety disorder, the reaction to separation is greater than that expected for the child's level of development. The anxiety may manifest as physical symptoms. Separation anxiety disorder may be a feature of *depression*.

sepsis Infection of a wound or body tissues with bacteria that leads to the formation of *pus* or to the multiplication of the bacteria in the blood. (See also *bacteraemia*; *septicaemia*; *septic shock*.)

septal defect A congenital *heart* abnormality in which there is a hole in the septum between the left and right ventricles of the heart or, more rarely, between the left and right atria. Usually, the cause is unknown. The hole allows freshly oxygenated blood to mix with deoxygenated blood in the heart.

A small defect has little or no effect. A large ventricular hole may cause *heart failure* to develop 6–8 weeks after birth, causing breathlessness and feeding difficulties. A large atrial defect may never cause heart failure, but there may be fatigue on exertion. *Pulmonary hypertension* may develop in both types of defect.

Diagnosis may be aided by a *chest X-ray*, *ECG*, or *echocardiography*.

Atrial holes are repaired surgically if they cause symptoms or if complications develop. As the child grows, small ventricular holes often become smaller, or even close, on their own. A ventricular defect that is causing heart failure is treated with *diuretics* and *digitalis drugs*. If the hole does not close spontaneously, it may be repaired by *open heart surgery*.

septicaemia A potentially life-threatening condition in which there is rapid multiplication of bacteria and in which bacterial *toxins* are present in the blood. (See also *bacteraemia*.)

Septicaemia usually arises through escape of bacteria from a focus of infection, such as an *abscess*, and is more likely to occur in people with an *immunodeficiency disorder*, *cancer*, or *diabetes mellitus*; in those who take *immunosuppressant drugs*; and in drug addicts who inject.

Symptoms include a fever, chills, rapid breathing, headache, and clouding of consciousness. The sufferer may go into life-threatening *septic shock*.

Glucose and/or saline are given by *intravenous infusion*, and *antibiotics* by injection or infusion. Surgery may be necessary to remove the original infection. If treatment is given before septic shock develops, the outlook is good.

septic arthritis A type of *arthritis* caused by a bacterial infection entering a joint via an open wound. Symptoms of septic arthritis appear suddenly and may include swelling, tenderness, and fever. If pus builds up, the joint may be permanently damaged.

Fluid is taken from the joint and is analysed to determine the presence of infection (see *aspiration*), and pus may be drained to help relieve pain. Initially, treatment is with intravenous *antibiotic drugs*, followed by oral antibiotics for several weeks or months after that.

septic shock A life-threatening condition in which there is tissue damage and a dramatic drop in blood pressure as a result of *septicaemia*.

septum A thin dividing wall within or between parts of the body.

sequela A condition that results from or follows a disease, disorder, or injury. The term is usually used in plural (sequelae) to refer to the complications of a disease.

sequestration A portion of diseased or dead tissue separated from, or joined abnormally to, surrounding healthy tissue.

serology A branch of laboratory medicine concerned with analysis of blood *serum*. Applications of serological techniques include the diagnosis of infectious diseases by the identification of *antibodies*, the development of *antiserum* preparations for passive *immunization*, and the determination of *blood groups* in *paternity testing* and forensic investigations.

serotonin Also known by its chemical name 5-hydroxytryptamine (5HT), a substance found in many tissues, particularly blood platelets, the digestive tract lining, and the brain. Serotonin is released from platelets at the site of bleeding, where it constricts small blood vessels, reducing blood loss. In the digestive tract, it inhibits gastric secretion and stimulates smooth muscle of the intestine. In the brain, where it acts as a *neurotransmitter*, levels are reduced in people who are depressed; certain *antidepressants* raise the level.

serotonin agonists A group of drugs, also known as $5HT_1$ agonists, used to treat acute attacks of *migraine*. They work on the same receptors in the brain as 5-hydroxytryptamine (5HT, also known as serotonin), a *neurotransmitter* and *vasodilator*. Common serotonin agonists include naratriptan and *sumatriptan*. These drugs can cause chest pain, particularly in people with heart disease. They should be used with caution in those at increased risk of coronary artery disease. Other side effects include flushing, tingling, and nausea.

serotonin antagonists A group of drugs that oppose the effects of *serotonin* on the gastrointestinal tract and central nervous system and which are used to treat the nausea and vomiting caused by *radiotherapy* and *anticancer drugs*. They are also used to control nausea and vomiting following surgery. Common serotonin antagonists include granisetron and *ondansetron*.

sertraline A *selective serotonin reuptake inhibitor* drug used in the treatment of depression (see *antidepressants*).

serum The clear fluid that separates from *blood* when it clots. It contains salts, glucose, and proteins, including *antibodies*. Serum from the blood of a person who has been infected with a microorganism usually contains antibodies that can protect other people from that organism if injected into them. Such a preparation is called an *antiserum*; its use forms the basis of passive *immunization*.

serum sickness A type of *hypersensitivity* reaction that may develop about 10 days after injection with an *antiserum* of animal origin or after taking certain drugs such as *penicillins*.

S

Symptoms may include an itchy rash, joint pain, fever, and enlarged lymph nodes. In severe cases, a state similar to *shock* develops. Symptoms usually clear up in a few days; *antihistamine drugs* may hasten recovery. In severe cases, a *corticosteroid drug* may be prescribed.

severe acute respiratory syndrome See *SARS*.

sex Another term for gender and a commonly used term for *sexual intercourse*.

sex change Radical surgical procedures, usually combined with hormone therapy, that alter a person's anatomical gender. Sex-change operations are performed on transsexuals (see *transsexualism*) and on infants whose external sex organs are neither completely male nor female (see *genitalia, ambiguous*).

sex chromosomes A pair of *chromosomes* that determines an individual's sex. All human cells (except egg or sperm cells) contain a pair of sex chromosomes, together with 22 other pairs of chromosomes called autosomes. In women, there are two similar sex chromosomes called *X chromosomes*. Men have one X and one *Y chromosome*. The *genes* on the Y chromosome are concerned solely with *sex determination*; their presence ensures a male, their absence a female. The X chromosome carries genes vital to general development and functioning.

sex determination The factors that determine biological sex. The underlying determinants are the *sex chromosomes* which cause the differential development of the gonads in the embryo. In males, the testes then produce hormones that cause the male reproductive organs to form. In the absence of these hormones, a female reproductive tract develops. At *puberty*, another surge of hormones produces secondary *sexual characteristics*.

Chromosomal abnormalities or hormonal defects can lead to ambiguous sex (see *genitalia, ambiguous*), although true *hermaphroditism* is rare.

sex hormones Hormones that control the development of primary and secondary *sexual characteristics* and that regulate sex-related functions, such as the menstrual cycle. There are three main types: *androgen hormones*, *oestrogen hormones*, and *progesterone hormone*.

SEX CHROMOSOMES

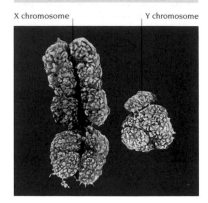

X chromosome   Y chromosome

sex-linked inheritance The passing on to the next generation of a trait or disorder determined by the *sex chromosomes*, or by the *genes* carried on them.

Disorders caused by an abnormal number of sex chromosomes include *Turner's syndrome* and *Klinefelter's syndrome*. Most other sex-linked traits or disorders are caused by *recessive* genes on the X chromosome (see *genetic disorders*).

sex therapy Counselling for and treatment of sexual difficulties not due to a physical cause. It may involve changing the attitude of the partners towards sex, increasing their understanding of sexual needs, and teaching techniques, such as the *sensate-focus technique,* for specific problems. Sex therapy is particularly successful in treating *vaginismus*, premature ejaculation (see *ejaculation, disorders of*), lack of orgasm (see *orgasm, lack of*), and *erectile dysfunction*.

sexual abuse The subjection of a person to sexual activity that has caused or is likely to cause physical or psychological harm. (See also *child abuse; rape*.)

sexual characteristics, secondary Physical features appearing at *puberty* that indicate the onset of adult reproductive life. In girls, breast enlargement is the first sign. Shortly afterwards, pubic and underarm hair appears, and body fat increases around the hips, stomach, and thighs to produce the female body shape. In boys, the first sign is enlargement of the testes, followed by thinning of the

S

scrotal skin and enlargement of the penis. Pubic, facial, axillary, and other body hair appears, the voice deepens, and muscle bulk and bone size increase.

sexual desire, inhibited Lack of sexual desire or of the ability to become physically aroused during sexual activity.

sexual deviation See *deviation, sexual.*

sexual dysfunction See *psychosexual dysfunction.*

sexual intercourse A term sometimes used to describe a variety of sexual activities, but which specifically refers to the insertion of the penis into the vagina.

sexuality A term describing the capacity for sexual feelings and behaviour, or an individual's sexual orientation or preference. *Heterosexuality* is sexuality directed towards the anatomically opposite sex; *homosexuality* is attraction to the same sex; and *bisexuality* is attraction to both sexes. (See also *gender identity.*)

sexually transmitted infections (STIs) Infections transmitted primarily, but not exclusively, by sexual intercourse. Common STIs include *chlamydial infections, genital herpes, pubic lice, genital warts, trichomoniasis, syphilis, gonorrhoea,* and *HIV* infection. *Antibiotics* can be used to treat most bacterial STIs. Confidential tracing and treatment of an affected person's partners is an essential part of the management of STIs (see *contact tracing*). Practising *safer sex* can help prevent STIs.

sexual problems Any difficulty associated with sexual performance or behaviour. Sexual problems are often psychological in origin (see *psychosexual dysfunction*). *Sex therapy* may help such problems. Some sexual problems are due to physical disease, such as a disorder affecting blood flow or a hormonal dysfunction. A disorder of the genitals may result in pain during intercourse (see *intercourse, painful*). Such problems are addressed by treating the cause, where possible.

Sézary syndrome A rare condition in which there is an abnormal overgrowth of *lymphocytes* in the skin, liver, spleen, and lymph nodes. It mainly affects middle-aged and elderly people. The first symptom is the appearance of red, scaly patches on the skin that spread to form an itchy, flaking rash. There may also be accumulation of fluid under the skin,

baldness, and distorted nail growth. Sézary syndrome is sometimes associated with *leukaemia*. Treatment includes *anticancer drugs* and *radiotherapy.*

shellfish poisoning See *food poisoning.*

shell shock See *post-traumatic stress disorder.*

shigellosis An acute infection of the intestine by bacteria of the genus SHI-GELLA. The source of the infection is the faeces of infected people; the bacteria are spread by poor hygiene. *Endemic* in some countries, shigellosis occurs in isolated outbreaks in the UK.

The disease usually starts suddenly, with diarrhoea, abdominal pain, nausea, vomiting, generalized aches, and fever. Persistent diarrhoea may cause *dehydration*, especially in babies and the elderly. Occasionally, *toxaemia* develops.

Shigellosis usually subsides after a week or so, but hospital treatment may be needed for severe cases. Dehydration is treated by *rehydration therapy*. *Antibiotics* may be given.

shingles See *herpes zoster.*

shin splints Pain in the front and sides of the lower leg that develops or worsens during exercise. There may also be tenderness and *oedema* in the affected area. Shin splints is a common problem in runners. It may be caused by various disorders, such as *compartment syndrome, tendinitis, myositis,* or *periostitis.*

In most cases, the pain disappears within 2 months. However, if it is severe or recurrent, a course of *non-steroidal anti-inflammatory drugs* or *corticosteroids* may be needed. Rarely, surgery is performed to alleviate excessive pressure in a muscle. Some people benefit from *physiotherapy.*

shivering Involuntary trembling of the entire body that is caused by rapid contraction and relaxation of muscles. Shivering is the body's normal automatic response to cold: contraction of muscles generates heat. Shivering also occurs in fever.

shock A dangerous reduction of blood flow throughout the body tissues, which may occur with severe injury or illness. Shock in this sense is physiological shock, as distinct from the mental distress that may follow a traumatic experience.

S

In most cases, reduced blood pressure is a major factor in causing shock and is one of its main features. Shock may develop in any situation in which blood volume is reduced, blood vessels are abnormally widened, the heart's action is weak, blood flow is obstructed, or there is a combination of these factors. Causes include severe *bleeding* or *burns,* persistent *vomiting* or *diarrhoea, myocardial infarction, pulmonary embolism, peritonitis,* and some types of *poisoning.*

Symptoms of shock include rapid, shallow breathing; cold, clammy skin; rapid, weak pulse; dizziness; weakness; and fainting. Untreated, shock can lead to collapse, coma, and death.

Emergency treatment is required. This involves an *intravenous infusion* of fluid, a blood transfusion, *oxygen therapy,* and, if necessary, *morphine* or similar powerful analgesics. Further treatment depends on the underlying cause. (See also *anaphylactic shock; septic shock; shock, electric; toxic shock syndrome.*)

shock, electric The sensation caused by an electric current passing through the body, and its effects. A current of sufficient size and duration can cause loss of consciousness, cardiac arrest, respiratory arrest, burns, and tissue damage. (See also *electrical injury.*)

shock therapy See *ECT.*

shortsightedness See *myopia.*

short sight, operations for See *LASIK; photorefractive keratectomy.*

short stature A height that is significantly below the normal range for a person's age. Short stature in children is often due to hereditary factors or slow bone growth. In most cases, growth eventually speeds up, resulting in normal adult height. Less commonly, it is due to a specific disorder such as bone disease (as in untreated *rickets* or *achondroplasia*) or to certain hormonal disorders such as *growth hormone* deficiency and *hypothyroidism. Emotional deprivation,* chronic malnutrition, and *malabsorption* can also limit growth. Certain chromosomal disorders cause short stature; stunting occurs in *Down's syndrome,* and the pubertal growth spurt is absent in *Turner's syndrome.* Other causes of restricted growth in children include prolonged use of *corticosteroids* and *anticancer* drugs. Severe untreated respiratory disease or congenital heart disease can also cause short stature.

An affected child's growth rate is monitored by regular measurement of height. *X-rays* and *blood tests* may help identify an underlying cause, which will then be treated. Growth hormone is given for hormone deficiency, and also to treat short stature due to disorders such as Turner's syndrome. (See also *growth, childhood.*)

shoulder The area of the body where the arm attaches to the trunk. Three bones meet here: the *scapula, clavicle,* and *humerus.* The ball-and-socket joint at the shoulder has a wide range of movement.

Common injuries include dislocation (see *shoulder, dislocation of*) and fractures of the clavicle or upper humerus. The shoulder may be affected by any *joint* disorder, which in severe cases may lead to *frozen shoulder.* Inflammation of a tendon or a bursa around a shoulder joint can cause *painful arc syndrome.*

shoulderblade The common name for the *scapula.*

shoulder, dislocation of Displacement of the head of the *humerus* out of the shoulder joint. The main symptom is pain in the shoulder and upper arm, made worse by movement. A forward dislocation often produces obvious deformity; a backward dislocation usually does not.

Diagnosis is by *X-rays.* The head of the humerus is repositioned in the joint socket. The shoulder is then immobilized in a sling for about 3 weeks.

Complications of shoulder dislocation include damage to nerves, causing temporary weakness and numbness in the shoulder; damage to an artery in the upper arm, causing pain and discoloration of the arm and hand; and damage to muscles that support the shoulder.

shoulder–hand syndrome Pain and stiffness affecting one shoulder and the hand on the same side; the hand may also become hot, sweaty, and swollen. Arm muscles may waste through lack of use (see *Sudeck's atrophy*). The cause of shoulder–hand syndrome is unknown, but it may occur as a complication of *myocardial infarction, stroke, herpes zoster,* or shoulder injury. Recovery usually occurs in about 2 years. This period may be shortened by *physiotherapy* and *corticosteroid drugs*. In rare cases, a cervical *sympathectomy* is performed.

shunt An abnormal or surgically created passage between two normally unconnected body parts.

Shy–Drager syndrome A rare degenerative disorder of unknown cause that progressively damages the *autonomic nervous system*. It begins gradually at age 60–70 and is more common in men. Symptoms include dizziness and fainting due to postural *hypotension*, urinary incontinence, *erectile dysfunction*, a reduced ability to sweat, and *parkinsonism*. The condition eventually leads to disability, and sometimes premature death. There is no cure or means of slowing degeneration, but many symptoms are relieved by drugs.

SIADH The abbreviation for syndrome of inappropriate antidiuretic hormone (secretion), associated with certain lung or brain disorders and some types of cancer.

Siamese twins See *twins, conjoined*.

sibling rivalry A term that describes the intense competition that sometimes occurs between siblings.

sibutramine A centrally acting *appetite suppressant* drug used to treat obesity in people who have not responded to other methods of weight loss, such as dieting. Common side effects include constipation, dry mouth, and *hypertension*. People taking this drug should have regular follow-ups and have their blood pressure and pulse monitored.

sick building syndrome A collection of symptoms reported by some workers in office buildings. Symptoms include loss of energy, headaches, and dry, itching eyes, nose, and throat. The cause is unknown, but various factors are involved, including air conditioning, passive smoking, lack of natural ventilation and light, and psychological factors.

sickle cell anaemia An inherited blood disease in which the red blood cells contain haemoglobin S, an abnormal type of *haemoglobin*. This crystallizes in the capillaries, making red cells sickle-shaped and fragile, and leading to haemolytic anaemia. The abnormal cells are unable to pass easily through tiny blood vessels.

The blood supply to organs is blocked intermittently, causing sickle cell crises. The disease affects mainly black people.

Symptoms usually appear after age 6 months, often beginning with painful swelling of the hands and feet. Chronic haemolytic anaemia causes fatigue, headaches, shortness of breath on exertion, pallor, and *jaundice*. Sickle cell crises start suddenly; they are sometimes brought on by an infection, cold weather, or dehydration, but may also occur for no apparent reason. The sufferer may experience pains (especially in the bones), blood in the urine (from kidney damage) or damage to the lungs or intestines. If the brain is affected, *seizures*, a *stroke*, or unconsciousness may result.

In some affected children, the *spleen* enlarges and traps red cells at a particularly high rate, causing a life-threatening form of anaemia. After adolescence, the spleen usually stops functioning, increasing the risk of infection in those affected.

Diagnosis is made from examination of a blood smear and *electrophoresis*. Babies may be screened for the condition shortly after birth (see *blood spot screening tests*). Supportive treatment may include *folic acid* supplements, and *penicillin* and immunization to protect against infection. Life-threatening crises are treated with *intravenous infusions* of fluids, *antibiotics*, *oxygen therapy*, and *analgesic drugs*. If the crisis still does not respond, an exchange *blood transfusion* may be performed. This may be done regularly for people who suffer frequent severe crises.

sick sinus syndrome Abnormal function of the heart's *sinoatrial node* that leads to episodes of *bradycardia* (slow heart-rate), alternating bradycardia and *tachycardia* (fast heart-rate), or very short episodes of *cardiac arrest*. The cause is usually *coronary artery disease*, but may be a *cardiomyopathy*. Symptoms may include lightheadedness, fainting, and palpitations. The diagnosis is confirmed by a 24-hour ECG recording. Treatment is usually by *antiarrhythmic drugs* and the fitting of an artificial *pacemaker*.

side effect A reaction or consequence of medication or therapy that is additional to the desired effect. The term usually refers to an unwanted or adverse effect,

S

SINUS, FACIAL

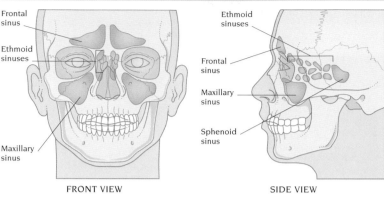

Frontal sinus

Ethmoid sinuses

Maxillary sinus

FRONT VIEW

Ethmoid sinuses

Frontal sinus

Maxillary sinus

Sphenoid sinus

SIDE VIEW

usually following a normal dose, rather than the toxic effects of a *drug* overdose.

siderosis Any of a variety of conditions in which there is too much iron in the body. (See also *haemosiderosis*.)

SIDS An abbreviation for *sudden infant death syndrome*.

sievert A unit for measuring doses of ionizing *radiation*. (See *radiation units*).

sight See *vision*.

sight, partial Loss of vision short of total *blindness*. Partial sight may involve loss of *visual acuity* and/or *visual field*.

sigmoid colon The S-shaped part of the *colon*, in the lower abdomen, extending from the brim of the pelvis, usually down to the third segment of the *sacrum*. It is connected to the descending colon above, and the rectum below.

sigmoidoscopy A form of *endoscopy* in which a viewing instrument is inserted through the anus to examine the *rectum* and *sigmoid colon*.

sign An objective indication of a disease or disorder (for example, jaundice) that is observed or detected by a doctor, as opposed to a *symptom* (for example, pain), which is noticed by the patient.

sildenafil Commonly known by its brand name Viagra, a drug used in the treatment of *erectile dysfunction*. Possible side effects include headaches, nasal congestion, flushing, indigestion, and *priapism*. Sildenafil should not be used by those taking *nitrate drugs* because of the possibility of a serious interaction.

silicone A long-chain, carbon-containing compound of silicon and oxygen. Synthetic silicones are sometimes used as implants in *cosmetic surgery*.

silicosis A lung disease caused by the inhalation of dusts containing silica. (See also *pneumoconiosis*.)

silver sulfadiazine An *antibacterial drug* applied as a cream to prevent infection after skin grafts or in burns, leg ulcers, and pressure sores. Side effects may include permanent grey skin discoloration, rashes, or itching.

simvastatin A *lipid-lowering drug* that acts on the liver enzymes that produce *cholesterol*. It may cause bowel upsets, headaches, and muscle pains.

sinew A nonmedical term for a *tendon*.

singer's nodes Small, greyish-white nodules that develop on the vocal cords as the result of constant voice strain. In acute cases, treatment consists of resting the voice. In chronic cases, surgical removal of the nodes may be necessary.

sinoatrial node The natural pacemaker of the *heart*. The sinoatrial node consists of a cluster of specialized muscle cells in the right atrial wall. These cells regularly emit electrical impulses, which initiate the contractions of the heart.

sinus A cavity in a bone, in particular one of the air-filled spaces in the bones surrounding the nose (see *sinus, facial*).

The term sinus also refers to any wide channel that contains blood, or to an abnormal, often infected, tract.

S

sinus bradycardia A slow, but regular heart-rate (less than 60 beats per minute) caused by reduced electrical activity in the *sinoatrial node*. Sinus bradycardia is normal in athletes, but in others it may be caused by *hypothyroidism*, a *myocardial infarction*, or by drugs such as *beta-blockers* or *digoxin*.

sinus, facial Any of the air-filled cavities in the bones surrounding the nose. These include two frontal sinuses in the lower forehead; two ethmoid sinuses between the eyes; two maxillary sinuses in the cheekbones; and the sphenoid sinuses in the skull behind the nose. Mucus drains from each sinus along a channel that opens into the nose. Infection of a sinus causes *sinusitis*.

sinusitis Inflammation of the membrane lining the facial *sinuses* caused by infection, usually spread from the nose. The maxillary and the ethmoid sinuses are most commonly affected.

Sinusitis may cause a feeling of fullness in the affected area, fever, a stuffy nose, and loss of the sense of smell. A common complication is the formation of pus in the affected sinuses, causing pain and nasal discharge.

Treatment of sinusitis is usually with *antibiotics* and a *decongestant*. *Steam inhalations* may also help. If sinusitis persists despite treatment, surgical drainage of the affected sinuses may be performed.

sinus tachycardia A fast, but regular, heart-rate (more than 100 beats per minute) caused by increased electrical activity in the *sinoatrial node*. Such a heartbeat is normal during sudden stressful moments or exercise. Persistent sinus tachycardia at rest may be caused by fever or *hyperthyroidism*.

situs inversus An unusual condition in which the internal organs are situated in the mirror image of their normal positions. No treatment is needed provided all the organs are functioning normally.

Sjögren's syndrome A condition in which the eyes and mouth are excessively dry. The nasal cavity, throat, and vagina may also be affected. The syndrome tends to occur with certain *autoimmune disorders*, such as *rheumatoid arthritis* and systemic *lupus erythematosus*. Most sufferers are middle-aged women.

SKELETON

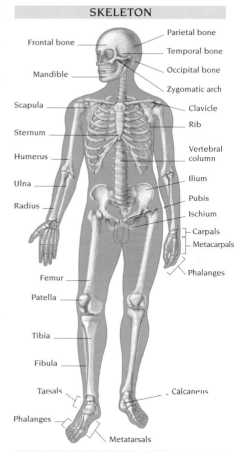

Frontal bone
Mandible
Scapula
Sternum
Humerus
Ulna
Radius
Femur
Patella
Tibia
Fibula
Tarsals
Phalanges

Parietal bone
Temporal bone
Occipital bone
Zygomatic arch
Clavicle
Rib
Vertebral column
Ilium
Pubis
Ischium
Carpals
Metacarpals
Phalanges
Calcaneus
Metatarsals

skeleton The framework of bones that gives the body shape and provides attachment points for muscles and underlying soft tissues. The average human adult skeleton has 213 *bones* (counting each of the 9 fused vertebrae of the sacrum and coccyx as individual bones) joined with *ligaments* and *tendons* at points called *joints*. The skeleton plays an indispensable role in movement as a strong, stable but mobile framework on which muscles can act. The skeleton also supports and protects internal body organs.

skin The outermost covering of body tissue, which protects internal organs from the environment. Skin has two layers: the outer epidermis, and the inner dermis.

S

SKIN

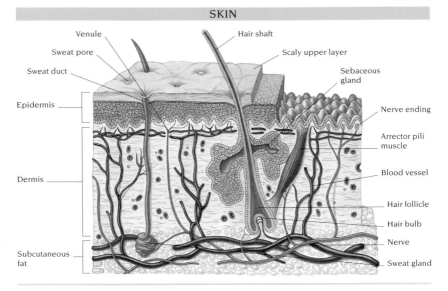

Venule
Hair shaft
Sweat pore
Scaly upper layer
Sweat duct
Sebaceous gland
Epidermis
Nerve ending
Arrector pili muscle
Dermis
Blood vessel
Hair follicle
Hair bulb
Nerve
Subcutaneous fat
Sweat gland

The outermost epidermis is composed of dead cells and the protein *keratin*. As these dead cells are worn away, they are replaced by new ones from the inner epidermis. Some epidermal cells produce the pigment *melanin*, which protects the body from *ultraviolet light* in sunlight.

The dermis is composed of *connective tissue* interspersed with *hair* follicles, *sweat glands, sebaceous glands*, blood and lymph vessels, and sensory receptors for pressure, temperature, and pain.

skin allergy Irritation of the skin following contact with a specific substance that provokes an inappropriate or exaggerated reaction from the *immune system*. There are two main types of allergic skin reaction. In contact allergic *dermatitis*, red, itchy patches develop a few hours to 2 days after contact with the allergen. In contact *urticaria*, red, raised areas appear a few minutes after skin contact. In some cases, *skin tests* are needed, to identify the allergen, for contact with it to be minimized. (See also *atopic eczema*.)

skin biopsy Removal of a portion of skin for laboratory analysis in order to diagnose a skin disorder.

skin cancer A malignant tumour in the *skin*. *Basal cell carcinoma, squamous cell carcinoma*, and *malignant melanoma* are common forms related to long-term exposure to sunlight. *Bowen's disease*, a rare disorder that can become cancerous, may also be related to sun exposure. Less common types include *Paget's disease of the nipple* and *mycosis fungoides*. *Kaposi's sarcoma* is a type usually found in people with *AIDS*. Most skin cancers can be cured if treated early.

skin, disorders of the The skin is vulnerable to various disorders, including *birthmarks* and other *naevi*; infections that may be viral (such as *cold sores* and *warts*), bacterial (for example, *cellulitis*), or fungal (such as *tinea*, which causes *athlete's foot*); *rashes* due to vitamin deficiency or the side effects of drugs; and tumours, both noncancerous and cancerous. *Acne* is common in adolescents and is partly related to the action of *androgen hormones*. Inflammation of the skin occurs in *dermatitis, eczema*, and *skin allergy*. The skin is also vulnerable to injuries such as *burns*, cuts, and bites (see *bites, animal; insect bites*).

skin flap A surgical technique in which a section of *skin* and underlying tissue, sometimes including muscle, is moved to cover an area from which skin and tissue have been lost or damaged by injury, disease, or surgery. Unlike a *skin graft*, a

S

skin flap retains its blood supply, either by remaining attached to the donor site or through reattachment to blood vessels at the recipient site by *microsurgery*, so skin flaps adhere well even where there is extensive loss of deep tissue.

skin graft A technique used to repair areas of lost or damaged *skin* that are too large to heal naturally, that are slow to heal, or that would leave tight or unsightly scars. A skin graft is often used in the treatment of burns or sometimes for nonhealing ulcers. A piece of healthy skin is detached from one part of the body and transferred to the affected area. New skin cells grow from the graft and cover the damaged area. In a meshed graft, donor skin is removed and made into a mesh by cutting. The mesh is stretched to fit the recipient site; new skin cells grow to fill the spaces in the mesh. In a pinch graft, multiple small areas of skin are pinched up and removed from the donor site. Placed on the recipient site, they gradually expand to form a new sheet of healthy skin. (See also *skin flap*.)

skin patch See *transdermal patch*.

skin peeling, chemical A cosmetic operation in which the outer layers of the skin are peeled away by the application of a caustic paste in order to remove freckles, acne scars, delicate wrinkles, or other skin blemishes.

skin tag A harmless, small, brown or flesh-coloured flap of skin that may appear spontaneously or as a result of poor healing of a wound.

skin tests Procedures for determining the body's reaction to various substances by injecting a small quantity of the substance under the skin or by applying it to the skin (usually on patches). Patch tests are used in the diagnosis of contact allergic *dermatitis*. Skin tests can also be used to test immunity to certain infectious diseases (such as in the *tuberculin test*).

skin tumours A growth on or in the *skin* that may be cancerous (see *skin cancer*) or noncancerous. *Keratoses* and squamous *papillomas* are common types of noncancerous tumour; other types include *sebaceous cysts*, cutaneous *horns*, *keratoacanthomas*, and *haemangiomas*.

skull The bony skeleton of the head, which rests on the 1st cervical vertebra. The skull protects the brain, houses the special sense organs, provides points of attachment for muscles, and forms part of the respiratory and digestive tracts.

The eight bones of the cranium encase the brain. The skull's facial skeleton includes the nasal and cheek bones, maxilla, and mandible. All except the mandible are fixed together by immovable joints.

skull, fracture of A break in one or more of the *skull* bones caused by a *head injury*. In most skull fractures, the broken bones are not displaced and there are no complications. Severe injury may result in bone fragments rupturing blood vessels in the *meninges*, or, more rarely, tearing the meninges, leading to brain damage.

A fracture without complications usually heals by itself; damage to brain structures often requires *neurosurgery*.

skull X-ray A technique for providing images of the *skull*. X-rays of the skull are usually taken after a *head injury* to look for a fracture or foreign body, or to evaluate disorders that affect the skull.

slapped cheek syndrome An alternative name for *fifth disease*.

SKIN GRAFT

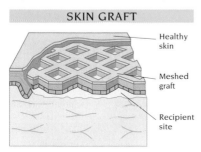

Healthy skin

Meshed graft

Recipient site

MESHED SKIN GRAFT

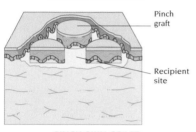

Pinch graft

Recipient site

PINCH SKIN GRAFT

S

SLE The abbreviation for the disorder systemic *lupus erythematosus*.

sleep The natural state of lowered consciousness and reduced *metabolism*.

There are two types of sleep: REM (rapid eye movement) and NREM (nonrapid eye movement) sleep, which alternate in cycles. NREM sleep consists of four stages of progressively greater "depth", with slowing of brain activity. In REM sleep, the brain becomes more active; the eyes move rapidly and *dreaming* occurs.

Sleep is a fundamental human need, although its purpose is not understood in detail. The need for sleep varies from person to person and decreases with age.

Sleep disorders include *insomnia*; difficulty in staying awake (see *narcolepsy*); disruption of sleep by *jet-lag* and *bedwetting*, *night terrors*, or *sleepwalking*. (See also *sleep apnoea*.)

sleep apnoea A disorder in which there are episodes of temporary cessation of breathing (lasting 10 seconds or longer) during sleep.

Obstructive sleep apnoea (OSA) is the most common type and may affect anyone, but more often middle-aged men, especially those who are overweight. The most common cause is over-relaxation of the muscles of the soft *palate*, which obstructs air flow. Obstruction may also be caused by enlarged *tonsils* or *adenoids*. The obstruction causes snoring. If complete blockage occurs, breathing stops. This triggers the brain to restart breathing, and the person may gasp and wake briefly.

People with OSA may not be aware of any problem at night but they may be sleepy during the day, with poor memory and concentration. They are also at increased risk of an accident due to tiredness. In addition, OSA may increase the risk of *hypertension*, *myocardial infarction*, or *stroke* occurring.

People who are overweight may find losing weight helps. Alcohol and sleeping drugs aggravate OSA. The condition may be treated by continuous positive airways pressure (CPAP), in which air at higher than normal pressure is breathed through a mask. *Tonsillectomy*, *adenoidectomy*, or surgery to shorten or stiffen the soft palate may be performed.

In central sleep apnoea (CSA), breathing stops because the chest and diaphragm muscles temporarily cease to work. It is usually due to disturbance in the nervous system's control of breathing, which may result from various causes, such as a disorder of the *brainstem* or *encephalitis*. CSA may also occur in people with certain neuromuscular disorders or *heart failure*. Treatment of CSA depends on the underlying cause.

sleep deprivation Insufficient *sleep*. Irritability and a shortened attention span may occur after a short night's sleep. Longer periods without sleep leave a person increasingly unable to concentrate or perform normal tasks. Three or more sleepless nights may lead to *hallucinations* and, in some cases, to *paranoia*.

sleeping drugs A group of drugs used to treat *insomnia*. They include *benzodiazepines*, *antihistamines*, *antidepressants*, and chloral hydrate. Sleeping drugs may cause drowsiness and impaired concentration on waking. Long-term use may induce *tolerance* and *dependence*.

sleeping sickness A serious infectious disease of tropical Africa caused by the protozoan parasite *TRYPANOSOMA BRUCEI*, which is transmitted to humans by the bites of tsetse flies.

One form of the disease, which occurs in West and Central Africa, causes bouts of fever and lymph node enlargement. After months or years, spread to the brain occurs, causing headaches, confusion, and, eventually, severe lassitude. Without treatment, coma and death follow. In the other, East African, form fever develops after a few weeks, and effects on the heart may be fatal before the disease has spread to the brain. Drugs can effect a cure, but there may be residual brain damage if the infection has already spread to the brain.

sleep paralysis The sensation of being unable to move at the moment of going to sleep or when waking up, usually lasting only a few seconds. It may be accompanied by *hallucinations*. Sleep paralysis most often occurs in people with *narcolepsy*. (See also *cataplexy*.)

sleep terror See *night terror*.

sleepwalking Walking while asleep. Sleepwalking is usually calm and aimless,

S

although it is sometimes more frantic when it occurs with *night terror*. Some people regularly sleepwalk. Sleepwalking in children is not normally a cause for concern and tends to disappear with age. In adults, it may be related to anxiety or the use of sleeping drugs.

slimming See *weight reduction*.

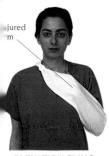

SLING

jured
m

ELEVATION SLING

sling A triangular bandage used to immobilize, support, or elevate an arm. The injured arm may be supported horizontally or held elevated, depending on the injury.

slipped disc See *disc prolapse*.

slipped femoral epiphysis See *femoral epiphysis, slipped*.

slit-lamp An illuminated type of microscope that is used to examine the internal structures of the front part of the eye and of the retina at the back. (See also *eye, examination of*.)

slough Dead tissue that has been shed from its original site.

small cell carcinoma One form of *lung cancer*.

smallpox A highly infectious viral disease that was declared eradicated in 1980 after a global vaccination campaign.

smear A specimen for microscopic examination prepared by spreading a thin film of cells on to a glass slide. (See also *blood film; cervical smear test*.)

smegma An accumulation of sebaceous gland secretions under the foreskin in an uncircumcised male, usually as a result of poor hygiene. Fungal or bacterial infection of smegma may cause *balanitis*.

smell One of the five senses. In the nose, hair-like projections from smell receptor cells lie in the mucous membrane. When the receptors are stimulated by certain molecules, they transmit impulses along the olfactory nerves to the smell centres in the *limbic system* and frontal lobes of the brain, where smell is perceived.

Possible causes of loss of the sense of smell include inflammation of the nasal membrane, as in a common *cold*; cigarette *smoking*; hypertrophic *rhinitis*, in which thickening of the mucous membrane obscures olfactory nerve endings; atrophic rhinitis, in which the nerves waste away; head injury that tears the nerves; or a tumour of the meninges or nasopharynx. The perception of illusory, unpleasant odours may be a feature of *depression, schizophrenia*, some forms of *epilepsy*, or alcohol withdrawal.

smelling salts A preparation of *ammonia* that was used in the past to revive a person who felt faint.

smoking Smoking *tobacco* in the form of cigarettes or cigars, or in pipes. Over 100,000 deaths per year in the UK are attributed to smoking. The main harmful effects of smoking are *lung cancer, bronchitis, emphysema, coronary artery disease*, and *peripheral vascular disease*. Smoking also increases the risk of *mouth cancer, lip cancer*, bladder cancer (see *bladder tumours*), and throat cancer (see *pharynx, cancer of*).

Smoking is extremely harmful during pregnancy. Babies of women who smoke are smaller and are less likely to survive than those of nonsmoking mothers. Children with parents who smoke are more likely to suffer from *asthma* or other respiratory diseases.

There is also evidence that *passive smokers* are at increased risk of tobacco-related disorders and also suffer discomfort in the form of coughing, wheezing, and sore eyes.

Tobacco contains many toxic chemicals. *Nicotine* is the substance that causes addiction to tobacco. It acts as a tranquillizer but also stimulates the release of *adrenaline* into the bloodstream. This can raise blood pressure. Tar in tobacco produces chronic irritation of the respiratory system and is thought to be a major cause of lung cancer. Carbon monoxide passes from the lungs into the bloodstream, where it easily combines with *haemoglobin* in red blood cells, interfering with oxygenation of tissues. In the long term, persistently high levels of carbon monoxide in the blood cause hardening of the arteries, which greatly increases the risk of *coronary thrombosis*.

S

snails and disease Snails act as host to various types of fluke that infest humans, such as *liver flukes*.

snake bites Most snake bites are by non-venomous species. Venomous snakes are found mainly in the tropics; the only species native to the UK is the adder.

The effects of a venomous bite depend on the species and size of the snake, the amount of venom injected, and the age and health of the victim. A bite from an adder or other viper typically causes immediate pain and swelling at the site, followed by dizziness and nausea, a drop in blood pressure, an increase in heart-rate, and internal bleeding.

Antibiotic drugs and *tetanus* antitoxin injections are given for all bites to prevent infection and tetanus. An injection of *antivenom* is also given for a venomous bite. With prompt treatment, most victims recover completely.

sneezing The involuntary expulsion of air through the nose and mouth as a result of irritation of the upper respiratory tract. This may be due to the common *cold*, allergic *rhinitis*, the presence of mucus, or inhaling an irritant substance.

Snellen chart A method of measuring *visual acuity* used during *vision tests*.

snoring Noisy breathing through the open mouth during sleep, produced by vibrations of the soft palate. Snoring is often caused by a condition that hinders breathing through the nose, such as a *cold*, allergic *rhinitis*, or enlarged *adenoids*. Snoring is more common when sleeping on the back. If the underlying cause can be treated, snoring may stop. Snoring is also a feature of *sleep apnoea*.

snow-blindness A common name for actinic *keratopathy*.

snuff A preparation of powdered *tobacco* (often with other substances) for inhalation. Snuff is addictive because it contains *nicotine*; it also irritates the nasal lining and increases the risk of cancer of the nose and throat.

social and communication disorders A collective term for disorders such as *Asperger's syndrome* and *autism*, which begin in childhood. Problems tend to persist throughout life.

social skills training A form of behaviour modification in which individuals are encouraged to improve their ability to communicate. This is an important part of *rehabilitation* for people with *learning difficulties* or those with chronic psychological disorders, such as *schizophrenia*. *Role-playing* is a commonly used technique in which various social situations are simulated in order to improve the individual's confidence and performance.

sociopathy An outdated term for *antisocial personality disorder*.

sodium A *mineral* that helps to regulate the body's water balance and maintain normal heart rhythm and is involved in conduction of nerve impulses and contraction of muscles. The level of sodium in the blood is controlled by the kidneys, which eliminate any excess in the urine.

Almost all foods contain sodium naturally or as an ingredient added during processing or cooking. Consequently, deficiency is rare and is usually the result of excessive loss of the mineral through persistent diarrhoea or vomiting, or profuse sweating. Symptoms include weakness, dizziness, and muscle cramps. In severe cases, there may be a drop in blood pressure, leading to confusion, fainting, and palpitations. Treatment is with supplements. In hot climates, sodium supplements may help to prevent *heat disorders* by compensating for sodium lost through heavy sweating.

Excessive sodium intake is thought to be a contributory factor in *hypertension*. Another adverse effect is fluid retention, which, in severe cases, may cause dizziness and swelling of the legs.

sodium aurothiomalate A *disease-modifying antirheumatic drug* (DMARD) used to treat active, progressive *rheumatoid arthritis*. A preparation of *gold*, sodium aurothiomalate is given by injection. It may have serious side effects, including gastrointestinal bleeding, and lung, liver, and kidney damage.

sodium bicarbonate An over-the-counter *antacid drug* used to relieve *indigestion*, *heartburn*, and pain caused by a *peptic ulcer*. It often causes belching and abdominal discomfort. Long-term use may cause swollen ankles, muscle cramps, tiredness, and nausea.

sodium cromoglicate A drug given by inhaler to control mild *asthma* in children

S

and allergic or exercise-induced asthma in adults; as a nasal spray to treat nasal symptoms of allergic *rhinitis*; in eye-drops for allergic *conjunctivitis* and to relieve eye symptoms of allergic rhinitis; and orally for *food allergy*. Side effects include coughing and throat irritation on inhalation.

sodium picosulfate A stimulant *laxative* drug used to treat *constipation* and to empty the bowel prior to procedures such as X-ray, *endoscopy*, and surgery on the intestines. Side effects may include abdominal cramps and diarrhoea. The drug should be avoided in cases of intestinal obstruction.

sodium valproate An *anticonvulsant* drug used to treat *epilepsy* and *mania*. Possible side effects include drowsiness, abdominal discomfort, temporary hair loss, weight gain, and rash. Sodium valproate may rarely cause liver damage and blood tests may sometimes be carried out while taking the drug to monitor liver function.

soft-tissue injury Damage to the tissues (see *ligament*; *tendon*; *muscle*) that surround bones and joints.

soiling Inappropriate passage of *faeces* after the age at which bowel control is achieved (usually at about 3 or 4 years). Causes include slowness in developing bowel control, longstanding *constipation*, poor *toilet-training*, and emotional stress. Soiling due to constipation is usually resolved with treatment. If there is no physical cause, *psychotherapy* may help.

Encopresis is a form of soiling in which children deliberately pass faeces in inappropriate places, such as behind furniture.

solar plexus The largest network of autonomic nerves in the body, located behind the stomach between the adrenal glands. The solar plexus incorporates branches of the *vagus nerve* and the splanchnic nerves, and sends branches into the stomach, intestines, and other abdominal organs.

solvent abuse Inhaling intoxicating fumes from solvents. Glue sniffing is the most common form.

Inhalation of solvent fumes produces a feeling of intoxication similar to that produced by alcohol. Solvent abuse can cause headache, vomiting, confusion, and coma. Death may occur due to a direct toxic effect on the heart, a fall, choking on vomit, or asphyxiation. Long-term effects include erosion of the lining of the nose and throat, and damage to the kidneys, liver, and nervous system.

Acute symptoms resulting from solvent abuse require urgent medical attention. Counselling may be helpful in discouraging the behaviour.

somatic A term meaning related to the body (soma), as opposed to the mind (psyche), or related to body cells, as opposed to germ cells (eggs and sperm). It also refers to the body wall, in contrast to visceral (of the internal organs).

somatization disorder A condition in which a person complains over a period of several years of various physical problems for which no organic cause can be found. The disorder, which is more common in women, usually begins before age 30 and leads to numerous tests by many doctors. Unnecessary surgery and other treatments may result. The condition is often associated with *anxiety*, *depression*, or substance abuse. (See also *conversion disorder*; *hypochondriasis*.)

somatostatin analogues Synthetic versions of the hormone somatostatin that acts on the *pituitary gland*, controlling the release of growth hormone. These drugs are used to treat *acromegaly* and symptoms associated with some other hormone-secreting tumours (particularly in *carcinoid syndrome*). *Octreotide* is a common somatostatin analogue.

somatotype A person's physical build.

somatropin A biosynthetic *growth hormone* given to children to treat *short stature* due to growth-hormone deficiency.

somnambulism See *sleepwalking*.

sore A term used nominally to describe any disrupted area of the skin or mucous membranes, or adjectivally to describe an area that is tender or painful.

sore throat A rough or raw feeling in the back of the throat that causes discomfort, especially when swallowing.

Sore throat is a common symptom, usually caused by *pharyngitis* and occasionally by *tonsillitis*. It is often the first symptom of the common *cold*, *influenza*, *laryngitis*, *infectious mononucleosis*, and many childhood viral illnesses, such as *chickenpox*, *measles*, and *mumps*.

S

A sore throat may be relieved by gargling with salt water. Sore throats due to bacterial infection are treated with *antibiotic drugs*. (See also *strep throat*.)

spasm An involuntary contraction of a *muscle*. Examples include *hiccups* and *tics*. Disorders characterized by spasm include *trigeminal neuralgia* and *tetanus*.

spasticity Increased rigidity in a group of *muscles*, causing stiffness and restriction of movement. Spasticity occurs in *Parkinson's disease*, *multiple sclerosis*, *cerebral palsy*, and *tetanus*.

spastic paralysis Inability to move a part of the body, accompanied by rigidity of the muscles. Causes of spastic paralysis include *stroke*, *cerebral palsy*, and *multiple sclerosis*. (See also *paralysis*.)

specific gravity The ratio of the *density* of a substance to that of water.

specific learning disability Difficulty in one or more areas of learning in a child of average or above average intelligence. Specific learning disabilities include *dyslexia* and dyscalculia, where there is a problem with mathematics.

specimen A sample of tissue, body fluids, waste products, or an infective organism taken for analysis, identification, and/or diagnosis. The sample may be prepared for examination under a *microscope*.

SPECT The abbreviation for single photon emission computed tomography, a type of *radionuclide scanning*.

spectacles See *glasses*.

speculum A device for holding open a body orifice to enable a doctor to perform an examination.

speech A system of sounds by which humans communicate. Children learn speech through listening to and imitating the speech of others.

Speech production originates in two regions of the cerebral cortex on each side of the *brain*. These regions are linked to the centre for language expression (Broca's area) in the dominant hemisphere. They send signals down nerve pathways to muscles controlling the larynx, tongue, and other parts involved in speech. The cerebellum plays a part in coordinating movements of these parts. Air from the lungs is vibrated through the vocal cords in the larynx. This produces a noise, which is amplified in the cavities of the throat, nose, and sinuses. The sound of the vibrated air is modified by movements of the tongue, mouth, and lips to produce speech sounds.

speech disorders Defects or disturbances in *speech* that lead to an inability to communicate effectively.

Damage to the language centres of the brain (usually due to a *stroke*, *head injury*, or *brain tumour*) leads to *aphasia*, which may impair speech.

Disorders of articulation may be caused by damage to nerves that go to muscles in the larynx, mouth or lips, due to stroke, head injury, *multiple sclerosis*, or *Parkinson's disease*. A structural abnormality of the mouth, such as a *cleft lip and palate*, can also be a cause.

Disorders of voice production include hoarseness and inappropriate pitch or loudness. In many cases, the cause is a disorder affecting closure of the vocal cords (see *larynx, disorders of*). A voice that is too high or low or too loud or soft may be caused by a hormonal or psychiatric disturbance or by hearing loss.

Disorders of fluency include *stuttering*, which is marked by hesitant speech and repetition of sounds.

Delayed speech development in a child may be due to hearing loss (see *deafness*), slow maturation of the nervous system, poor tongue and lip control, lack of stimulation, or emotional disturbance (see *developmental delay*).

Many people with speech disorders can be helped by *speech therapy*.

speech therapy A form of treatment for people who have a *speech disorder*. A speech therapist tests speech and *hearing* and devises exercises to improve the deficient aspect of speech.

sperm The male sex cell, which is responsible for *fertilization* of the female ovum. Inside the head of the sperm is genetic

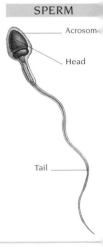

SPERM

Acrosome

Head

Tail

material, while the acrosome that caps the head contains enzymes that enable sperm to penetrate the ovum's outer covering. The tail of the sperm propels it.

Sperm are produced within the seminiferous tubules of the *testes* and mature in the *epididymis*. Production and development of sperm cells is dependent on *testosterone* and on *gonadotrophin hormones* secreted by the *pituitary gland*. Sperm production starts at *puberty*.

spermatic cord The structure in males that runs from the abdomen to the scrotum and contains the *vas deferens*. (See also *reproductive system, male*.)

spermatocele A harmless cyst of the *epididymis* containing fluid and sperm

spermatozoa See *sperm*.

spermicides Contraceptive preparations that kill *sperm*. They are usually recommended for use with a barrier device.

SPF Sun protection factor, the degree of protection a *sunscreen* provides against sunburn. It is a measure of the amount of UVB radiation a sunscreen absorbs: the higher the number, the more the protection.

sphenoid bone The bat-shaped bone in the centre of the base of the *cranium*.

spherocytosis, hereditary An inherited disorder in which there are a large number of unusually small, round red blood cells (spherocytes) in the circulation. These abnormal red cells are readily broken up when blood passes through the *spleen*. At times, the rate of red cell destruction exceeds the rate at which new cells can be made in the bone marrow, leading to symptoms of *anaemia*. Other symptoms include *jaundice* and enlargement of the spleen. Occasionally, crises occur (usually triggered by infection) in which all symptoms worsen. *Gallstones* are a frequent complication. *Splenectomy* usually leads to permanent improvement.

sphincter A ring of muscle around a natural opening or passage that acts as a valve, regulating inflow or outflow.

sphincter, artificial A surgically created valve or other device used to treat or prevent urinary or faecal *incontinence*.

sphincterotomy A surgical procedure that involves cutting the muscle that closes a body opening or that constricts the opening between body passages.

sphygmomanometer An instrument used for measuring *blood pressure*. A cuff attached to an electronic measuring device is wrapped around the person's arm. The cuff is inflated and then deflated. Readings of systolic and diastolic blood pressure are taken as the cuff deflates and the readings are displayed on a digital readout. Some sphygmomanometers also measure the pulse rate. Occasionally, mercury sphygmomanometers, which show the blood pressure readings on a mercury-filled glass column, are still used.

spider bites Nearly all spiders produce venom, which they use to kill their prey. However, only a few species, such as the black widow in North America, are harmful to humans. *Antivenoms* are available for many dangerous spider bites.

spider naevus A red, raised pinhead-sized dot, from which small blood vessels radiate, due to a dilated minor artery and its connecting capillaries. Small numbers of spider naevi are common in children and pregnant women, but in larger numbers, they may indicate liver disease. (See also *telangiectasia*.)

spina bifida A *congenital* defect that is a type of *neural tube defect* in which part of one or more *vertebrae* fails to develop completely. As a result, a portion of the *spinal cord* is left exposed.

spinal anaesthesia Injection of an anaesthetic into the cerebrospinal fluid in the spinal canal to block *pain* sensations before they reach the *central nervous system*. It is used mainly during surgery on the lower abdomen and legs. (See also *epidural anaesthesia*.)

spinal cord A cylinder of *nerve* tissue that runs from the *brain*, down the central canal in the *spine* to the 1st lumbar vertebra. Below that, the nerve roots continue within the canal as *cauda equina*.

Grey matter, the spinal cord's core, contains the cell bodies of nerve cells. Areas of white matter (tracts of nerve fibres running lengthwise) surround the grey matter. Sprouting from the cord on each side at regular intervals are the sensory and motor spinal nerve roots. The small nodule (ganglion) in each sensory root comprises nerve cell bodies. Nerve roots combine to form the *spinal nerves*

SPINAL CORD

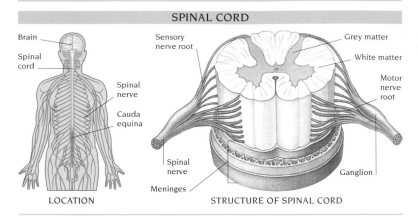

LOCATION | STRUCTURE OF SPINAL CORD

that link the spinal cord to all regions of the trunk and limbs. The entire spinal cord is bathed in *cerebrospinal fluid* and surrounded by the *meninges*.

The nerve tracts in the white matter act mainly as highways for sensory information passing up to the brain or motor signals passing down. However, the cord processes some sensory information itself and provides motor responses without involving the brain. Many *reflex* actions are controlled in this way.

The spinal cord may be injured by trauma (see *spinal injury*); spinal-cord infections such as *poliomyelitis* are rare but can cause serious damage.

spinal fusion Major surgery to join two or more adjacent *vertebrae*. It is performed if abnormal movement between adjacent vertebrae causes severe back pain or may damage the spinal cord.

spinal injury Damage to the *spine* and sometimes to the *spinal cord*. Spinal injury is most often the result of falling from a height or of a road traffic accident.

Damage to the *vertebrae* and their *ligaments* usually causes severe pain and swelling of the affected area. Damage to the spinal cord results in *paralysis* and/or loss of sensation below the site of injury.

X-rays of the spine are carried out to determine the extent of damage. If the bones are dislocated, surgery is needed to manipulate them back into position. Surgery may also be needed to remove any pressure on the cord, but damaged nerve tracts cannot be repaired. *Physio-*

therapy may stop joints locking and muscles contracting as the result of paralysis.

If there is no spinal-cord damage, recovery is usually complete. In cases of spinal-cord damage, some improvement may occur for up to 12 months.

spinal nerves A set of 31 pairs of *nerves* that connect to the *spinal cord*. Spinal nerves emerge in two rows from either side of the spinal cord and leave the *spine* through gaps between adjacent *vertebrae*. The nerves then branch out to supply all parts of the trunk, arms, and legs with sensory and motor nerve fibres. *Disc prolapse* may lead to pressure on a spinal nerve, causing pain. Injury to a nerve may lead to loss of sensation or movement in the area supplied by the nerve. (See also *nerve injury*; *neuropathy*.)

spinal tap See *lumbar puncture*.

spine The column of bones and cartilage that extends from the base of the skull to the pelvis, enclosing the *spinal cord* and supporting the trunk and head.

The spine is made up of 33 roughly cylindrical *vertebrae*. Each pair of adjacent vertebrae is connected by a facet *joint*, which stabilizes the vertebral column. Between each pair of vertebrae lies a disc-shaped pad of cartilage called an intervertebral disc (see *disc, intervertebral*). These discs cushion the vertebrae during movement. The vertebrae are bound together by two *ligaments* running the length of the spine and by smaller ligaments

SPINE

Cervical spine (7 vertebrae)

Thoracic spine (12 vertebrae)

Lumbar spine (5 vertebrae)

Sacrum (5 fused vertebrae)

Coccyx (4 fused vertebrae)

between each vertebra. Attached to the vertebrae are several groups of *muscles*, which control movement of, and help to support, the spine.

spine, disorders of Many disorders of the spine cause *back pain*. Spina bifida is a congenital disorder in which part of the spinal cord is exposed. Sometimes, the spine is abnormally curved (see *lordosis, kyphosis, scoliosis*). In *ankylosing spondylitis*, and in some cases of *rheumatoid arthritis*, spinal joints are affected; *osteoarthritis* affects the spinal joints of most people over 60. Other disorders affecting the spine are *spinal injuries*, *disc prolapse*, and *spondylolisthesis*.

spirochaete A spiral-shaped bacterium. Spirochaetes cause *syphilis, leptospirosis, relapsing fever*, and *Lyme disease*.

spirometry A *pulmonary function test* used to diagnose or assess a *lung* disorder or to monitor treatment. It records the rate at which a person exhales air from the lungs and the total volume exhaled.

spironolactone A potassium-sparing *diuretic drug*, which is given to treat *heart failure, oedema*, and *ascites*. Spironolactone may cause numbness, weakness, and nausea. Less common side effects include diarrhoea, lethargy, *erectile dysfunction*, rash, and irregular menstruation. High doses may cause abnormal breast enlargement in men.

spleen An organ that removes worn-out and defective red blood cells from the circulation and helps to fight infection by producing some of the *antibodies*, lym-

SPIROMETRY

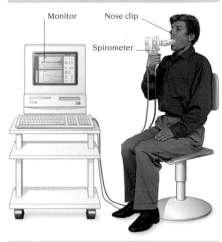

Monitor Nose clip Spirometer

phocytes, and *phagocytes* that destroy invading microorganisms. The spleen is a fist sized, spongy organ in the upper left abdomen behind the lower ribs.

The spleen enlarges in many diseases. These include infections such as *malaria* and *infectious mononucleosis*; blood disorders such as *leukaemia, thalassaemia*, and *sickle cell anaemia*; and tumours such as *lymphomas*. Enlargement of the spleen may be accompanied by *hypersplenism*. The spleen may be ruptured by a severe blow to the abdomen. This can cause potentially fatal haemorrhage, and an emergency *splenectomy* is needed.

splenectomy Surgical removal of the *spleen*. Splenectomy is performed after the spleen has been seriously injured or to treat *hypersplenism* or certain forms of *anaemia*. The absence of the spleen does not normally cause problems; its function is largely taken over by other parts of the *lymphatic system* and by the *liver*. People who have had a splenectomy are more susceptible to certain infections and are given pneumococcal vaccine (see *pneumococcus*) and long-term *antibiotics*.

splint A device used to immobilize a part of the body.

splinter haemorrhage Bleeding under the fingernails visible as tiny splinter-like marks. Usually due to trauma, it can also be a sign of infective *endocarditis*.

521

splinting The application of a *splint*, most often used to immobilize a fractured or otherwise injured limb or digit.

splinting, dental The mechanical joining of several teeth to hold them firmly in place while an injury heals or while *periodontal disease* is treated.

split personality A common term for *multiple personality*. It is also used, incorrectly, to describe *schizophrenia*.

spondylitis Inflammation of the joints between the vertebrae in the *spine*. It is usually caused by *osteoarthritis, rheumatoid arthritis*, or *ankylosing spondylitis*.

spondylolisthesis The slipping forwards (or occasionally backwards) of a *vertebra* over the one below it.

spondylolysis A disorder of the *spine* in which the arch of the 5th (or, rarely, the 4th) lumbar vertebra consists of soft fibrous tissue instead of normal bone. As a result, the arch is weak and prone to damage, which may produce *spondylolisthesis*. Otherwise, spondylolysis is usually symptomless. (See also *cervical spondylosis; cervical osteoarthritis*.)

sporotrichosis A chronic infection caused by the fungus SPOROTHRIX SCHENCKII, which grows on plants. The infection is most often contracted through a skin wound; gardeners are particularly vulnerable. An ulcer develops at the site of the wound, followed by the formation of nodules in lymph channels around the site. Potassium iodide solution taken orally usually clears up the infection. Rarely, in people with reduced immunity, sporotrichosis spreads to other parts of the body and requires treatment with an *antifungal drug*.

sport, drugs and Several types of drug are abused by athletes to enhance physical or mental condition. Stimulants such as *amphetamines* can prevent fatigue and increase confidence. Three types of hormone drugs may be abused: anabolic steroids (see *steroids, anabolic*) to speed muscle recovery after exercise; erythropoietin to boost the haemoglobin content of the blood, which may increase stamina; and *growth hormone* to stimulate muscle growth. *Analgesic drugs* may be used to mask the pain of an injury. *Beta-blockers* are taken to reduce tremor in sports that require a steady hand. *Diuretic drugs* may be used for temporary weight loss. Aside from the health risks associated with abuse of these drugs, their use is prohibited in many competitive sports.

sports injuries Any injury that arises during sports participation. Typical sports injuries include *fractures, head injury* (including *concussion*), muscle *strain* or *compartment syndrome*, ligament *sprain, tendinitis* or tendon rupture, and joint *dislocation* or *subluxation*. Some so-called sports injuries, such as *tennis elbow*, are in fact a type of *overuse injury*.

sports medicine The medical speciality concerned with assessment and improvement of *fitness* and the treatment and prevention of disorders related to sports.

spot A general term for a small lump, mark, or inflamed area on the skin.

spotting See *breakthrough bleeding*.

sprain Tearing or stretching of the *ligaments* that hold together the bone ends in a joint, caused by a sudden pull. The *ankle* is the most commonly sprained joint. A sprain causes painful swelling of the joint, which cannot be moved without increasing the pain. There may also be spasm of surrounding muscles.

Treatment consists of applying an *ice-pack*, wrapping the joint in a bandage, resting it in a raised position, and taking *analgesic drugs*. In severe cases, surgical repair may be necessary.

sprue An intestinal disorder causing failure to absorb nutrients from food. (See also *sprue, tropical; coeliac disease*.)

sprue, tropical A disease of the small intestine that causes failure to absorb nutrients from food. It occurs mainly in India, the Far East, and the Caribbean. Sprue leads to *malnutrition* and megaloblastic *anaemia*. It may be due to an intestinal infection. Symptoms include appetite and weight loss, an inflamed mouth, and fatty diarrhoea. Diagnosis is confirmed by *jejunal biopsy*. Sprue responds well to *antibiotic drug* treatment and vitamin and mineral supplements.

sputum Mucous material produced by cells lining the respiratory tract. Sputum production may be increased by *respiratory tract infection*, an allergic reaction (see *asthma*), or inhalation of irritants.

squamous cell carcinoma One of the most common types of *skin cancer*.

Squamous cell carcinoma is linked to long-term exposure to sunlight. It is most common in fair-skinned people over 60.

The tumour starts as a small, painless lump or patch (usually on the lip, ear, or back of the hand), which enlarges fairly rapidly, often resembling a wart or ulcer. Left untreated, the cancer may spread to other parts of the body and prove fatal.

Diagnosis is based on a *skin biopsy*. The tumour is removed surgically or destroyed by *radiotherapy*.

squint An abnormal deviation of one eye relative to the other. Many babies have a squint because the mechanism for aligning the eyes has not yet developed. A squint that starts later in childhood is usually due to breakdown of the alignment mechanism. Longsightedness is a common factor. In some cases, the brain suppresses the image from the deviating eye, leading to *amblyopia*.

In adults, squint may be a symptom of *stroke*, *diabetes mellitus*, *multiple sclerosis*, *hyperthyroidism*, or a tumour. A squint in adults causes double vision.

Treatment in children may include covering the normal eye with a patch to force the child to use the weak eye. Deviation of the squinting eye may be controlled by glasses and/or surgery. Sudden onset of a squint in adults may have a serious underlying cause and must be investigated promptly.

SSRIs See *selective serotonin reuptake inhibitors*.

stable A term used in medicine to describe a patient's condition that is neither deteriorating nor improving; a personality that is not susceptible to mental illness; or a chemical substance that is resistant to changes in its composition or physical state, or is not radioactive.

stage A term used in medicine to refer to a phase in the course of a disease, particularly in the progression of *cancer*.

staining The process of dyeing specimens of cells, tissues, or microorganisms in order for them to be clearly visible or easily identifiable under a *microscope*.

stammering See *stuttering*.

Stanford–Binet test A type of *intelligence test*.

stanozolol A type of anabolic steroid drug (see *steroids, anabolic*).

stapedectomy An operation on the *ear* to remove the *stapes* and replace it with an artificial substitute. It is used to treat *deafness* due to *otosclerosis*.

stapes The innermost of the three tiny, sound-conducting bones in the middle *ear*. The stapes is the smallest bone in the body. Its head articulates with the incus, and its base fits into the oval window in the wall of the inner ear.

In *otosclerosis*, the stapes becomes fixed and cannot transmit sound to the inner ear. Resultant hearing loss can be treated by *stapedectomy*.

staphylococcal infections Infections caused by *bacteria* of the genus STAPHYLOCOCCUS. Different types of taphylococci are responsible for a variety of disorders, including skin infections such as *pustules*, *boils*, and *abscesses*, and a rash in newborn babies (see *necrolysis, toxic epidermal*); *pneumonia*; *toxic shock syndrome* in menstruating

S

STAPEDECTOMY

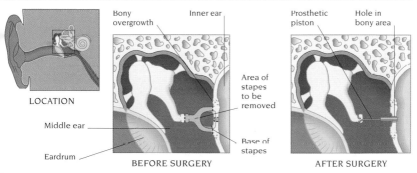

Bony overgrowth   Inner ear

Prosthetic piston   Hole in bony area

Area of stapes to be removed

LOCATION

Middle ear

Eardrum

Base of stapes

BEFORE SURGERY

AFTER SURGERY

women; *urinary tract infection*; *food poisoning*; and, if the bacteria enter the circulation, *septic shock*, infectious *arthritis*, *osteomyelitis*, or bacterial *endocarditis*. Some strains of STAPHYLO- COCCUS AUREUS have developed resistance to methicillin and many other antibiotics (see *MRSA*).

starch See *carbohydrates*.

starvation A condition caused by lack of food over a long period, resulting in weight loss, changes in *metabolism*, and extreme hunger. (See also *anorexia nervosa*; *fasting*; *nutritional disorders*.)

stasis Slowing down or cessation of flow.

statins A group of *lipid-lowering drugs* used to treat high blood levels of *cholesterol*. They are also used to lower blood lipid levels in people with *coronary artery disease* or those at risk of developing it, such as people with a family history of the disease, smokers, and those with *diabetes mellitus*. Possible side effects include headache, abdominal discomfort, vomiting, constipation, and diarrhoea. Rarely, *myositis* and liver damage may occur.

statistics, medical The collection and analysis of numerical data relating to medicine. Information on the *incidence* and *prevalence* of various conditions is an important aspect of medical statistics.

statistics, vital Assessment of a population's health that relies on the collection of data on birth and death rates and on the causes of death.

status asthmaticus A severe and prolonged attack of *asthma*. This is a potentially life-threatening condition that requires urgent treatment.

status epilepticus Prolonged or repeated epileptic seizures without recovery of consciousness between attacks. This is a medical emergency that may be fatal if not treated promptly. It is more likely to occur if *anticonvulsant drugs* are taken erratically or if they are withdrawn suddenly. (See also *epilepsy*.)

steam inhalation A method of relieving some of the symptoms of colds, sinusitis, and laryngitis by breathing in hot vapour from a bowl of hot water. The moisture loosens secretions in the nose and throat, making them easier to clear.

steatorrhoea The presence of excessive fat in the faeces. Steatorrhoea causes

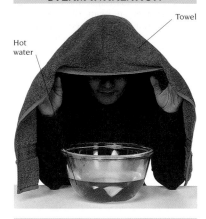

Towel

Hot water

offensive-smelling, bulky, loose, greasy, pale-coloured faeces, which float in the toilet. Steatorrhoea may occur in *pancreatitis* and *coeliac disease* and after the removal of substantial segments of small intestine. It is also a side effect of *orlistat* and some *lipid-lowering drugs*.

Stein-Leventhal syndrome See *ovary, polycystic*.

stem cell A basic cell in the body from which more specialized cells are formed. Stem cells within the *bone marrow* produce blood cells through a series of maturation steps. Stem cells are also found in the blood itself. Stem cell transplantation is increasingly used as an alternative to *bone marrow transplantation*. Stem cells for transplantation can be obtained from the blood or bone marrow of a donor sibling or a matched but unrelated donor, or from stored umbilical blood. Patients can also act as their own donors, with cells harvested and stored to be reinfused later after treatment has damaged their bone marrow. Stem cell transplantation does not carry the risk of rejection (known as *graft-versus-host disease*), which is a possibility with some types of bone marrow transplantation.

stenosis Narrowing of a duct, canal, passage, or tubular organ.

stent A rigid tube that is surgically inserted to open up or keep open any body canal that may have become narrowed or closed up due to disease. Stents are used to open narrowed coronary arteries in heart disease. Some arterial stents are coated with slow-release drugs to reduce the risk of arterial renarrowing. Stents are also used to relieve blockages caused by a tumour, for example in the *oesophagus* or *pancreas*.

sterculia A bulk-forming *laxative* used to treat constipation. It is especially useful when stools are small and hard. Sterculia should only be used if fibre intake cannot be increased; adequate fluid intake must be maintained to avoid intestinal obstruction. Side effects may include flatulence, bloating, and gastrointestinal obstruction or impaction.

stereotaxic surgery Brain operations carried out by inserting delicate instruments through a surgically created hole in the skull and guiding them, with the aid of *CT scanning*, to a specific area. Stereotaxic procedures can be used to treat *pituitary tumours*; for a brain *biopsy*; or to destroy small areas of the brain to treat disabling neurological disorders.

sterility The state either of being germ-free or of permanent *infertility*.

sterilization The complete destruction or removal of living organisms, usually to prevent spread of infection; any procedure that renders a person infertile (see *sterilization, female*; *vasectomy*).

sterilization, female A usually permanent method of *contraception* in which the fallopian tubes are sealed in order to prevent sperm reaching the ova.

Female sterilization is usually performed by *laparoscopy*, which involves two small incisions in the abdomen. Sometimes it is done by minilaparotomy, in which a single incision is made in the pubic area. The fallopian tubes are sealed using clips or by cutting and tying. The operations have a low failure rate. Fertility can sometimes be restored after sterilization using *microsurgery*.

sterilization, male See *vasectomy*.

sternum The long, narrow, flat plate of bone at the front of the chest. The sternum has three parts: an upper, triangular portion (manubrium); a long middle part (body); and, at the lower end, a small, leaf-shaped projection (xiphoid process). The upper manubrium articulates with the inner ends of the *clavicles*. The *ribs* are attached to the sides of the manubrium and body by cartilage. Between the manubrium and body is a *symphysis* joint, allowing slight movement when the ribs rise and fall during breathing.

Great force is required to fracture the sternum. The main danger of such an injury is the possibility that the broken bone may be driven inwards, damaging the heart, which lies behind the sternum.

steroid drugs A group of drugs including *corticosteroid drugs* and anabolic steroids (see *steroids, anabolic*).

steroids, anabolic Drugs that have an anabolic (protein-building) effect similar to *testosterone*. Anabolic steroids build tissue, promote muscle recovery after an injury, and strengthen bones. They are used to treat some types of *anaemia*. Anabolic steroids are often abused by athletes.

Possible adverse effects of the drugs include acne, *oedema*, damage to the liver and adrenal glands, infertility, *erectile dysfunction* in men, and *virilization* in women.

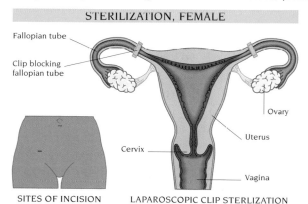

STERILIZATION, FEMALE

Fallopian tube

Clip blocking fallopian tube

Ovary

Uterus

Cervix

Vagina

SITES OF INCISION   LAPAROSCOPIC CLIP STERILIZATION

STETHOSCOPE

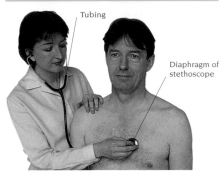

Tubing

Diaphragm of stethoscope

stethoscope An instrument that is used for listening to sounds in the body, particularly those made by the heart or lungs.

Stevens–Johnson syndrome A rare, life-threatening form of *erythema multiforme* characterized by severe blisters and bleeding in the mucous membranes of the eyes, mouth, nose, and genitals.

sticky eye One of the symptoms of *conjunctivitis* in which the eyelids become stuck together with discharge.

stiff neck A common symptom, usually due to spasm in muscles at the side or back of the neck. In most cases, it occurs suddenly and for no apparent reason. It may result from a neck injury, such as a ligament sprain, *disc prolapse*, or *whiplash injury*. A rare cause is *meningitis*.

Mild stiffness may be relieved by massage, warming, and use of a *liniment*. Severe or persistent stiffness requires medical attention. (See also *torticollis*.)

stiffness A term used to describe difficulty in moving a joint or stretching a muscle.

stilboestrol A drug that mimics the natural oestrogen hormone *estradiol*. It is occasionally used to treat *breast cancer* and *prostate cancer*. Side effects are those of oestrogens.

stillbirth Delivery of a dead fetus after the 24th week of *pregnancy*. The cause is unknown in many cases. Some stillborn babies have severe malformations, such as *anencephaly*, *spina bifida*, or *hydrocephalus*. Other possible causes include a maternal disorder, such as *antepartum haemorrhage* or *hypertension*, or severe *rhesus incompatibility*. The risk of stillbirth is increased if the mother has a severe infection during pregnancy.

Still's disease See *rheumatoid arthritis, juvenile*.

stimulant drugs Drugs that increase *brain* activity by initiating the release of noradrenaline (norepinephrine). Stimulants are of two types: central nervous system stimulants (for example, *amphetamines*), which increase alertness; and respiratory stimulants (see *analeptic drugs*), which encourage breathing.

stimulus Anything that directly results in a change in the activities of the body as a whole or of any individual part.

stings Stinging animals include scorpions, some insects, jellyfish, and some fish (see *venomous bites and stings*). Stinging plants may cause an allergic skin reaction. (See also *poisonous plants*.)

STIs See *sexually transmitted infections*.

stitch A temporary, sudden, sharp pain in the abdomen or side that occurs during severe or unaccustomed exercise. Stitch is also the common name for a suture (see *suturing*) to close a wound.

St. John's wort A herbal remedy derived from the plant HYPERICUM PERFORTUM. Capsules or infusions taken orally are effective in treating mild depression. St. John's wort is also used in creams for burns, wounds, and joint problems. It should not be used during pregnancy nor while breast-feeding. St. John's wort also interacts with a wide variety of medications and should not be taken without first consulting a doctor or pharmacist if other medications are being taken.

Stokes–Adams syndrome Recurrent episodes of temporary loss of consciousness caused by insufficient blood flow to the brain due to a cardiac *arrhythmia* or complete *heart block*.

Most people with the syndrome are fitted with a *pacemaker* to prevent attacks.

stoma A term meaning mouth or orifice. A stoma can be created surgically in the abdominal wall (see *colostomy*; *ileostomy*) to allow the intestine to empty into a bag or pouch on the surface of the skin.

stomach A hollow, bag-like organ of the *digestive system* located in the left side of the abdomen under the diaphragm. Food enters the stomach from the oesophagus and exits into the duodenum.

S

STOMACH

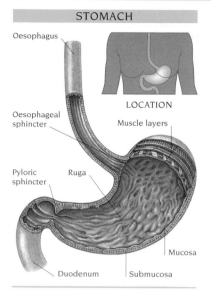

Oesophagus

LOCATION

Oesophageal sphincter

Muscle layers

Pyloric sphincter

Ruga

Mucosa

Duodenum

Submucosa

The sight and smell of food, and its arrival in the stomach, stimulate gastric secretion from the stomach lining. Gastric juice contains pepsin, an enzyme that breaks down protein; hydrochloric acid, which kills bacteria and creates the optimum *pH* for pepsin activity; and intrinsic factor, which is essential for absorption of vitamin B_{12} in the small intestine. The gastric lining also secretes mucus to stop the stomach digesting itself.

The muscular stomach wall produces rhythmic contractions that churn the food and gastric juice to aid digestion. Partly digested food is squirted into the duodenum at regular intervals by stomach contractions and by relaxation of the ring of muscle at the stomach outlet.

stomachache Discomfort in the upper abdomen. (See also *indigestion*.)

stomach cancer A malignant tumour that arises from the lining of the *stomach*. The exact cause is unknown, but *HELICO-BACTER PYLORI* infection is thought to be linked to increased incidence. Other likely factors include smoking and alcohol intake; diet may also play a part, in particular eating large amounts of salted or pickled foods. Pernicious *anaemia*, a partial *gastrectomy*, and belonging to blood group A also seem to increase the risk.

Stomach cancer rarely affects people under 40 and is more common in men. Symptoms may include weight loss, loss of appetite, and difficulty swallowing. There may also be other symptoms indistinguishable from those of *peptic ulcer*.

Diagnosis is usually made by *gastroscopy* or by a *barium X-ray examination*. The only effective treatment is total gastrectomy. In advanced cases in which the tumour has spread, *anticancer drugs* may prolong life.

stomach, disorders of the The stomach may be affected by various disorders, including gastrointestinal infections, *peptic ulcers*, *gastritis*, *pyloric stenosis*, *volvulus*, *polyps*, and *stomach cancer*.

stomach imaging See *barium X-ray examinations*.

stomach pump See *lavage, gastric*.

stomach ulcer A type of *peptic ulcer*.

stomatitis Any form of inflammation or ulceration of the mouth.

stones Small, hard collections of solid material within the body. (See also *calculus, urinary tract*; *gallstones*.)

stool Another word for *faeces*.

stork mark A small, flat, harmless, pinkish-red skin blemish found in many newborn babies. Such marks, which may be temporary, are a type of *haemangioma* and are usually found around the eyes and at the nape of the neck.

strabismus See *squint*.

strain Tearing or stretching of *muscle* fibres as a result of suddenly pulling them too far. There is bleeding into the damaged area of muscle, causing pain, swelling, muscle spasm, and bruising.

Treatment may include applying an ice-pack, resting the affected part, taking *analgesic drugs*, and *physiotherapy*.

strangulation The constriction, usually by twisting or compression, of a tube or passage in the body, blocking blood flow and interfering with the function of the affected organ. Strangulation may occur with a *hernia*, for example.

Strangulation of the neck causes compression of the *jugular veins*, preventing blood from flowing out of the brain, and compression of the windpipe, which restricts breathing. The victim loses consciousness, and brain damage and death from lack of oxygen follow.

S

strangury A symptom characterized by a painful and frequent desire to empty the bladder, although only a few drops of urine can be passed. Causes include *prostatitis, cystitis,* bladder cancer (see *bladder tumours*), and bladder stones (see *calculus, urinary tract*).

strapping The application of adhesive tape to part of the body to exert pressure and hold a structure in place.

strawberry naevus A bright red, raised spot which appears in early infancy. It is a type of *haemangioma.*

strep throat A *streptococcal infection* of the throat. It is most common in children. The bacteria are spread in droplets coughed or breathed into the air.

In some people, the bacteria cause no symptoms, but others suffer a sore throat, fever, and enlarged lymph nodes in the neck. In some cases, the bacterial toxins produce a rash (see *scarlet fever*).

Treatment may include *antibiotic drugs* and/or *analgesic drugs*. Very rarely, untreated strep throat may lead to *glomerulonephritis* or *rheumatic fever*.

streptococcal infections Infections caused by *bacteria* of the STREPTOCOCCUS group. A particular group, haemolytic streptococci, can cause *tonsillitis, strep throat, scarlet fever, otitis media, pneumonia, erysipelas,* and wound infections. Another type is often responsible for *urinary tract infection,* and another can cause bacterial *endocarditis* if it enters the bloodstream.

streptokinase A *thrombolytic drug* used to dissolve blood clots following a *myocardial infarction* or *pulmonary embolism.* Side effects include nausea, rash, and cardiac *arrhythmias.*

streptomycin An *antibiotic drug* used to treat a number of uncommon infections, including *tularaemia, plague, brucellosis,* and *glanders.* It may damage nerves in the inner ear, disturbing balance and causing dizziness, tinnitus, or deafness. Other side effects are facial numbness, tingling in the hands, and headache.

stress Any interference that disturbs a person's mental and physical well-being. Stress may be experienced in response to a range of physical and emotional stimuli. When faced with stressful situations, the body responds by increasing production of the hormones *adrenaline* (epinephrine) and *cortisol,* which produce changes in heart-rate, blood pressure, and metabolism to improve performance. However, at a certain level, they disrupt a person's ability to cope. Continued exposure to stress often leads to mental and physical symptoms, such as *anxiety* and *depression, indigestion,* palpitations, and muscular aches and pains. *Post-traumatic stress disorder* is a direct response to a specific stressful event. (See also *relaxation techniques*.)

stress fracture A *fracture* that occurs as a result of repetitive jarring of a bone. Common sites include the metatarsal bones in the foot (see *march fracture*), the tibia or fibula, the neck of the femur, and the lumbar spine. The main symptoms are pain and tenderness at the fracture site. Diagnosis is by *bone imaging.* Treatment consists of resting the affected area for 4–6 weeks. The fracture may be immobilized in a *cast.*

stress ulcer An acute *peptic ulcer* that develops after *shock,* severe burns or injuries, or during a major illness. Stress ulcers are usually multiple and are most common in the stomach. The exact cause is unknown. Drugs are often given to severely ill patients in hospital to prevent the development of stress ulcers.

stretcher A frame covered with fabric that is used in first aid for carrying the sick, injured, or deceased.

stretch-mark Another name for *stria.*

stria Also called a stretch-mark, a line on the *skin* caused by thinning and loss of elasticity in the dermis. Striae first appear as red, raised lines. Later they become purple, eventually fading to shiny streaks.

Striae often develop on the hips and thighs during the adolescent growth spurt, especially in athletic girls. They are a common feature of pregnancy, occurring on the breasts, thighs, and lower abdomen. Purple striae are a characteristic feature of *Cushing's syndrome.*

Striae are thought to be caused by an excess of *corticosteroid hormones.* There is no means of prevention, but in some cases laser treatment may be used.

stricture Narrowing of a duct, canal, or other passage in the body.

stridor An abnormal breathing sound caused by narrowing or obstruction of the *larynx* or *trachea*. Stridor is most common in young children. It usually occurs in *croup*. Other causes include *epiglottitis*, an inhaled *foreign body*, *hypocalcaemia*, and some larynx disorders.

stroke Damage to part of the *brain* caused by an interruption to its blood supply. The interruption is most often due to the blockage of a cerebral artery by a blood clot, which may have formed within the artery (see *thrombosis*), or may have been carried into the artery in the circulation from a clot elsewhere in the body (see *embolism*). Stroke may also result from localized haemorrhage due to rupture of a blood vessel in or near the brain.

The incidence of stroke rises with age and is higher in men. Certain factors increase the risk. The most important are *hypertension* and *atherosclerosis* (and, by association, factors such as *smoking* that contribute to these disorders). Other risk factors are *atrial fibrillation*, a damaged *heart valve*, and a recent *myocardial infarction*; these can cause clots in the heart which may migrate to the brain.

Symptoms usually develop abruptly and, depending on the site, cause, and extent of brain damage, may include headache, dizziness, visual disturbance, and difficulty in swallowing. Sensation, movement, or function controlled by the damaged area of the brain is impaired. Weakness or paralysis on one side of the body, called *hemiplegia*, is a common effect of a serious stroke. A stroke that affects the dominant cerebral hemisphere may cause disturbance of language (see *aphasia*). About a third of major strokes are fatal, a third result in some disability, and a third have no lasting ill effects (see *transient ischaemic attack*).

In some cases, urgent treatment may improve the chances of recovery. *ECG*, *CT scanning*, *chest X-rays*, *blood tests*, *angiography*, and *MRI* may be used to investigate the cause and extent of brain damage. If a stroke is proven by scan to be due to thrombosis, *thrombolytic drugs* may be given. *Anticoagulants* may be given if there is an obvious source of an embolism, such as atrial fibrillation. In some cases, antiplatelet agents such as *aspirin* are given. In most cases, attention to hydration and pressure areas, and good nursing care, are important influences on outcome. *Physiotherapy* may restore lost movement or sensation; *speech therapy* may help language disturbances. Any underlying risk factors, such as hypertension, diabetes mellitus, and high blood cholesterol, should be treated, and it is also important to stop smoking.

stroma The tissue that forms an organ's framework, as distinct from the functional tissue (the *parenchyma*) and the fibrous outer layer that holds the organ together.

strongyloidiasis An infestation of the intestines by the parasitic worm STRONGYLOIDES STERCORALIS. It is widespread in the tropics. Strongyloidiasis is contracted in affected areas by walking barefoot on soil contaminated with faeces. Larvae penetrate the soles, migrating via the lungs and throat to the intestine. Here they develop into adults and produce larvae. Most larvae are passed in the faeces, but some enter the skin around the anus to begin a new cycle. A person may be infested for more than 40 years.

The larvae cause itching and red weals where they enter the skin. In the lungs they may cause *asthma* or *pneumonia*. Heavy intestinal infestation may cause swelling of the abdomen and diarrhoea. Occasionally, an infected person with reduced immunity dies of complications, such as *septicaemia* or *meningitis*.

Treatment with an *anthelmintic drug*, usually *tiabendazole*, kills the worms.

strontium A metallic element occurring in various compounds in certain minerals, seawater, and marine plants. A compound of strontium, strontium ranalate, is used in the treatment of *osteoporosis* in postmenopausal women.

A radioactive variety of strontium, strontium 90, is produced during nuclear reactions and may be present in nuclear fallout. Strontium 90 accumulates in bone, where the *radiation* it emits may cause *leukaemia* and/or *bone tumours*. Other forms of radioactive strontium have been used to diagnose and treat bone tumours.

strychnine poisoning Strychnine is a poisonous chemical found in the seeds

S

of *STRYCHNOS* species (tropical trees and shrubs). Its main use is as an ingredient in some rodent poisons; most cases of strychnine poisoning occur in children who accidentally eat such poisons.

Symptoms begin soon after ingestion and include restlessness, stiffness of the face and neck, increased sensitivity of hearing, taste, and smell, and *photosensitivity*, followed by alternating episodes of seizures and floppiness. Death may occur from *respiratory arrest*.

The victim is given intravenous injections of a *tranquillizer* or a *barbiturate*, with a *muscle-relaxant drug* if needed. Breathing may be maintained by a *ventilator*. With prompt treatment, recovery usually occurs in about 24 hours.

stuffy nose See *nasal congestion*.

stump The end portion of a limb that remains after *amputation*.

stupor A state of almost complete *unconsciousness* from which a person can be aroused only briefly and by vigorous external stimulation. (See also *coma*.)

Sturge–Weber syndrome A rare, congenital condition that affects the skin and the brain. Characteristically, a large purple birthmark (port-wine stain) extends over one side of the face, including the eye. Malformation of cerebral blood vessels may cause weakness on one side of the body, progressive *learning difficulties*, and *epilepsy*. *Glaucoma* may develop in the affected eye, leading to loss of vision.

Seizures can usually be controlled with *anticonvulsant drugs*. In severe cases, brain surgery may be necessary.

stuttering A speech disorder in which there is repeated hesitation and delay in uttering words, unusual prolongation of sounds, and repetition of word elements. Stuttering usually starts before the age of 8 and may continue into adult life. It is more common in males, twins, and left-handed people, and may occur with *tics* or *tremors*. The severity may be related to social circumstances. The exact cause is unknown, although it tends to run in families. *Speech therapy* often helps.

stye A small, pus-filled *abscess* at the base of an eyelash, caused by infection.

subacute A term used for a disease that runs a course between *acute* and *chronic*.

subarachnoid haemorrhage A type of *brain haemorrhage* in which a blood vessel ruptures into the *cerebrospinal fluid* that surrounds the brain and spinal cord. It usually occurs spontaneously but may follow unaccustomed exercise. It is most common in people between 35 and 60. The most common cause is a burst aneurysm (see *berry aneurysm*).

An attack may cause loss of consciousness, sometimes preceded by a sudden violent headache. If the person remains conscious, symptoms such as *photophobia*, nausea, drowsiness, and stiffness of the neck may develop. Even unconscious patients may recover, but further attacks are common and often fatal.

Diagnosis is by *CT scanning* and *angiography*. Treatment includes life-support procedures and control of blood pressure to prevent recurrence. Burst or leaking aneurysms are usually treated by surgery. About half of those people affected survive; some recover completely, whereas others have residual disability such as paralysis.

subclavian steal syndrome Recurrent attacks of blurred or double vision, loss of coordination, or dizziness caused by reduced blood flow to the base of the brain when one arm (usually the left) is moved. The cause is narrowing of the arteries that carry blood to the arms, usually due to *atherosclerosis*. Treatment is by *arterial reconstructive surgery*.

subclinical A term applied to a disorder that produces no symptoms or signs because it is either mild or in the early stages of development.

subconjunctival haemorrhage Bleeding under the *conjunctiva* that is usually harmless and disappears in a few days without treatment.

subconscious A term describing mental events (such as thoughts) of which one is temporarily unaware but which can be recalled under the right circumstances.

subcutaneous Beneath the skin.

subdural haemorrhage Bleeding into the space between the outer and middle layers of the *meninges*, usually following *head injury*. The trapped blood slowly forms a large clot within the skull that presses on brain tissue. The symptoms, which tend to fluctuate, may include

S

SUBDURAL HAEMORRHAGE

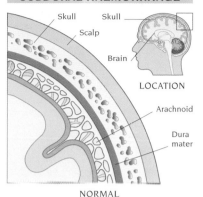

LOCATION

NORMAL

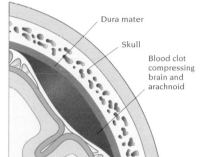

SUBDURAL HAEMORRHAGE

headache, confusion, drowsiness, and one-sided weakness or *paralysis*. The interval between the injury and the start of symptoms varies from days to months.

Diagnosis is by *CT scanning* or *MRI*. In many cases, surgical treatment is needed. This involves drilling burr holes in the skull (see *craniotomy*), so that the blood can be drained out and damaged blood vessels repaired. If treatment is carried out at an early enough stage, the person usually makes a full recovery. A subdural haemorrhage that is small and produces few symptoms may not require any treatment. The affected person is usually monitored with regular scans, and the clot may clear up on its own. (See also *extradural haemorrhage*.)

sublimation In *psychoanalytic theory*, the unconscious process by which primitive, unacceptable impulses are redirected into to socially acceptable forms of behaviour.

sublingual A term meaning under the tongue. Drugs taken sublingually, either as tablets or spray, are rapidly absorbed into the bloodstream via the lining of the mouth. For example, nitrate tablets are given sublingually to provide rapid relief of an angina attack.

subluxated tooth A tooth displaced in its socket as the result of an accident. The upper front teeth are the most vulnerable. A subluxated tooth can usually be manipulated back into position, and is then immobilized (see *splinting, dental*). If the tooth's blood vessels are torn, *root-canal treatment* is required.

subluxation Incomplete *dislocation* of a *joint*, in which the surfaces of the bones remain in partial contact.

submucous resection An operation to correct a *deviated nasal septum*.

subphrenic abscess An *abscess* under the diaphragm.

substance abuse Use of drugs such as stimulant drugs, or other substances such as glue and solvents, for a purpose other than that which is normally recommended. Problems may arise due to adverse effects or the substance's habit-forming potential. (See also *drug abuse*.)

substrate A substance on which an *enzyme* acts.

sucking chest wound An open wound in the chest wall through which air passes, causing the lung on that side to collapse. Severe breathlessness and a life-threatening lack of oxygen result.

sucralfate An *ulcer-healing drug* used to treat *peptic ulcer*. Possible side effects are constipation and abdominal pain.

suction The removal of unwanted fluid or semi-fluid material from the body with a syringe and hollow needle or with an intestinal tube and a mechanical pump.

suction lipectomy A cosmetic procedure, also called *liposuction*, that is used in *body contour surgery*.

sudden death See *death, sudden*.

sudden infant death syndrome (SIDS) The sudden, unexpected death of an infant that cannot be explained. Possible risk factors include laying the baby face-down to sleep; overheating; parental smoking before and after the birth; *prematurity* and

S

low birth weight; and the baby sleeping in the parent's bed. Preventive measures include ensuring the baby sleeps on his or her back at the foot of the cot; making sure the baby does not overheat; not sharing a bed with the baby but keeping the baby's cot in the parent's room for the first 6 months; and stopping smoking.

Sudeck's atrophy Swelling and loss of use of a hand or foot after a *fracture* or other injury. Treatment includes elevation, gentle exercise, and *heat treatment*. Full recovery is usual within 4 months.

suffocation A condition in which there is a lack of oxygen due to obstruction to the passage of air into the lungs. (See also *asphyxia; choking; strangulation.*)

sugar See *carbohydrates.*

suicide The act of intentionally killing oneself. Suicide results from a person's reaction to a perceivedly overwhelming problem, for example, social isolation, a stressful event such as death of a loved one, serious physical illness, or financial problems. It is often associated with a psychiatric illness, such as severe *depression* or *schizophrenia,* or dependency on drugs or alcohol.

Suicide is most common among young men. More men than women commit suicide, although women attempt it more often (see *suicide, attempted*). The most common methods among men are hanging and suffocation; drug overdose is the most common method among women.

suicide, attempted Any deliberate act of self-harm that is or is believed to be life-threatening but that in effect proves nonfatal. Attempted suicide is more common in women and most common in the 15–30 age group. The rate is highest in people with personality disorders and in those who live in deprived urban areas or have alcohol or drug problems. Common precipitating factors include the death of a loved one, financial worries, or severe loss of any kind that results in *depression*. The most common method is drug overdose.

Urgent treatment is needed for *drug poisoning*. Longer-term therapy aims to provide support and treat depression.

sulfasalazine An *immunosuppressant drug* that is used to relieve inflammation in *Crohn's disease* and *ulcerative colitis*. It is also a *disease-modifying antirheumatic drug* (DMARD) used to treat *rheumatoid arthritis* and psoriatic arthritis (see *psoriasis*). Possible side effects include nausea, headache, fever, and loss of appetite.

sulfinpyrazone A drug that reduces the frequency of attacks of *gout*. Side effects include nausea and abdominal pain.

sulindac A *nonsteroidal anti-inflammatory drug* (NSAID) used to relieve joint pain and stiffness in various types of *arthritis* and acute *gout*. Side effects are as for other NSAIDs.

sulphasalazine See *sulfasalazine.*

sulphinpyrazone See *sulfinpyrazone.*

sulphonamide drugs A group of *antibacterial drugs* that has largely been superseded by more effective and less toxic alternatives.

sulphur A mineral that is a constituent of vitamin B_1 (see *vitamin B complex*) and several essential *amino acids*. In the body, it is needed for the manufacture of *collagen* and is a constituent of *keratin*. It is used in the form of a cream to treat *acne*.

sulpiride An *antipsychotic drug* used in the treatment of *schizophrenia* and *Gilles de la Tourette's syndrome*.

sumatriptan A *serotonin agonist* drug that relieves acute attacks of *migraine*, especially those that have not responded to *analgesics*; it is particularly effective in treating *cluster headaches*. Sumatriptan may cause chest pain and tightness, flushing, dizziness, and weakness.

sunburn Inflammation of the *skin* caused by overexposure to the sun. The *ultraviolet light* in sunlight may destroy cells in the outer layer of the skin and damage tiny blood vessels beneath.

Fair-skinned people are most susceptible. The affected skin turns red and tender and may become blistered. The dead skin cells are later shed by peeling. *Calamine* lotion soothes the burned skin. *Analgesic drugs* may be taken to relieve discomfort. A high protection factor *sunscreen* helps to prevent sunburn. Severe sunburn in childhood increases the risk of *skin cancer* in later life.

sunlight, adverse effects of Problems resulting from overexposure to sunlight. Fair-skinned people are more susceptible. Short-term overexposure causes

S

sunburn and, in intense heat, can result in *heat exhaustion* or *heatstroke*. Repeated overexposure over a long period can cause premature aging of the skin and solar *keratoses*. It increases the risk of *skin cancer*. Protection of the skin with *sunscreens* helps to prevent sun damage. *Photosensitivity* is an abnormal sensitivity to sunlight, resulting in a rash.

Exposure to sunlight can affect the eyes, causing irritation of the conjunctiva, actinic *keratopathy*, or *pterygium*. Good sunglasses help to prevent eye problems.

sunscreens Preparations that help to protect the skin from the harmful effects of sunlight.

sunstroke A common form of *heatstroke*.

suntan Darkening of the *skin* after exposure to sunlight. Specialized cells in the epidermis respond to *ultraviolet light* by producing the pigment *melanin*. (See also *sunlight, adverse effects of*; *sunburn*.)

superego The part of the personality, as described in *psychoanalytic theory*, that is responsible for maintaining a person's standards of behaviour. Popularly termed the "conscience", the superego arises as a result of a child adopting the moral views of those in authority (usually parents).

superficial Situated near the surface.

superinfection A second *infection* that occurs during the course of an existing infection. The term usually refers to an infection by a microorganism that is resistant to drugs being used against the original infection.

superiority complex An individual's exaggerated and unrealistic belief that he or she is better than other people. In modern *psychoanalytic theory*, a superiority complex is considered to be a compensation for unconscious feelings of inadequacy or low self-esteem.

supernumerary A term meaning more than the normal number.

supernumerary teeth One or more *teeth* in excess of the usual number. These teeth are usually extracted.

supination The act of turning the body to a supine position (lying on the back with the face upward) or of turning the hand to a palm forward position. The opposite of supination is *pronation*.

suppository A solid medical preparation, of cone or bullet shape, designed to be placed in the rectum to dissolve. Suppositories are used to treat rectal disorders such as *haemorrhoids* or *proctitis*. They may also be used to soften faeces and stimulate defaecation. In addition, suppositories may be used to administer drugs into the general circulation, via blood vessels in the rectum, if vomiting is likely to prevent absorption after oral administration or if the drug would cause irritation of the stomach.

suppuration The formation or discharge of *pus*.

suprarenal glands Another name for the *adrenal glands*.

supraspinatus syndrome See *painful arc syndrome*.

supraventricular tachycardia An abnormally fast but regular heart-rate that occurs in episodes lasting for several hours or days. Supraventricular tachycardia occurs when abnormal electrical impulses that arise in the atria of the *heart* take control of the heartbeat from the *sinoatrial node*. Symptoms include palpitations, breathlessness, chest pain, or fainting (see *Stokes–Adams syndrome*).

Diagnosis is by an *ECG*. An attack can sometimes be terminated by *Valsalva's manoeuvre* or by drinking cold water. Recurrent attacks are treated with *antiarrhythmic drugs*. Rarely, the condition may require application of an electric shock to the heart (see *defibrillation*).

surfactant A substance, such as a soap or emulsifier, that reduces surface tension. Pulmonary surfactant is secreted by the alveoli in the lungs, preventing them from collapsing during exhalation, and is absent in babies who are born born significantly prematurely. This deficiency causes breathing difficulties, and the infant needs *artificial ventilation* and the administration of an artificial surfactant.

surfer's nodules Multiple bony outgrowths on the foot bones and on the bony prominence just below the knee.

surgery The treatment of disease, injury, or other disorders by direct physical intervention, or those aspects of medicine that deal with the study, diagnosis, and management of disorders treated in this way.

surgical spirit A liquid preparation, consisting mainly of ethyl alcohol, that

S

SUTURING

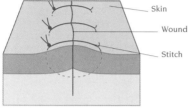

SUBCUTICULAR STITCH

INTERRUPTED STITCHES

has a soothing and hardening effect when applied to the skin. It may be used before injections as an *antiseptic*.

surrogacy The agreement by a woman to become pregnant and give birth to a child with the understanding that she will surrender the child after birth to the contractual parents. Surrogacy may be accomplished by *artificial insemination* or by *in vitro fertilization*.

susceptibility A total or partial vulnerability to an infection or disorder.

suture A type of *joint*, found only between the bones of the skull, in which the adjacent bones are mobile during birth but then become so closely and firmly joined by a layer of connective tissue that movement between them is impossible.

The term suture is also used to refer to a surgical stitch (see *suturing*).

suturing The closing of a surgical incision or a wound by sutures (stitches) to promote healing. This may be done by means of a single stitch under the skin (subcuticular) or by using individual stitches (interrupted). Some materials used in suturing, such as catgut, eventually dissolve in the body; skin sutures made of other materials are removed about 1–2 weeks after insertion.

swab A wad of absorbent material used to apply antiseptics or soak up body fluids during surgery, or to obtain a sample of bacteria from an infected patient.

swallowing The process by which food or liquid is conveyed from the mouth to the stomach via the oesophagus. Once food has been chewed and mixed with saliva to form a bolus, the tongue pushes the bolus to the back of the mouth and the voluntary muscles in the palate push it into the throat. The rest of the swallowing process occurs by a series of *reflexes*. Entry of food into the throat causes the epiglottis to tilt down to seal the trachea and the soft palate to move back in order to close off the nasal cavity. The throat muscles push the food into the oesophagus. Waves of contraction (peristalsis) along the oesophagus propel the food towards the stomach.

swallowing difficulty A common symptom with various possible causes, including a foreign object in the throat; insufficient production of saliva (see *mouth, dry*); a disorder of the oesophagus such as *oesophageal stricture*; pressure

SWALLOWING

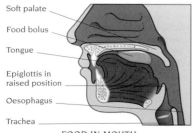

Soft palate
Food bolus
Tongue
Epiglottis in raised position
Oesophagus
Trachea

FOOD IN MOUTH

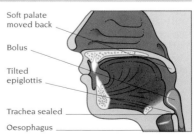

Soft palate moved back
Bolus
Tilted epiglottis
Trachea sealed
Oesophagus

FOOD IN THROAT

on the oesophagus, for example from a *goitre*; or tumour (see *oesophagus, cancer of*); a nervous system disorder such as *myasthenia gravis* or *stroke*; or a psychological problem such as *globus hystericus*.

Investigations of swallowing difficulty may include *oesophagoscopy* or barium swallow (see *barium X-ray examinations*). Treatment depends on the cause.

swamp fever Another name for *leptospirosis*. The term is also sometimes applied to *malaria*.

sweat glands Structures deep within the *skin* that produce sweat, which is mainly water with some dissolved substances, including salt. There are two types of sweat glands: eccrine glands, which are most numerous and open directly on to the skin surface, and apocrine glands, which develop at puberty. Apocrine glands, which open into a hair follicle, occur only in hairy areas, particularly the armpits, pubic region, and around the anus.

SWEAT GLANDS

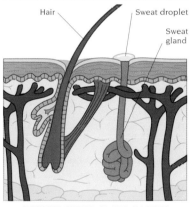

Hair — Sweat droplet

Sweat gland

ECCRINE SWEAT GLAND IN SKIN

The sweat glands are controlled by the *autonomic nervous system*. The glands are usually stimulated to keep the body cool, but anxiety or fear can also cause sweating. Sweat is odourless until bacteria act upon it, producing *body odour*.

A common disorder of the sweat glands is *prickly heat*. Other disorders include *hyperhidrosis* and *hypohidrosis*.

sweating The process by which the body cools itself. (See also *sweat glands*.)

sweeteners, artificial See *artificial sweeteners*.

swimmer's ear A common name for *otitis externa*.

sycosis barbae Inflammation of the beard area due to infection of the hair follicles, usually with STAPHYLOCOCCUS AUREUS bacteria contracted from infected razors or towels. Pus-filled blisters appear around the follicles. Treatment is usually with *antibiotic drugs*.

Sydenham's chorea A rare childhood disorder of the *central nervous system* that causes involuntary jerky movements of the head, face, limbs, and fingers. Voluntary movements are clumsy, and the limbs become floppy. The disorder usually follows an attack of *rheumatic fever*.

Sydenham's chorea usually clears up after 2–3 months and has no long-term adverse effects.

sympathectomy An operation in which the ganglia (nerve terminals) of sympathetic nerves are destroyed to interrupt the nerve pathway. This may be performed to improve blood supply to a limb (as a treatment for *peripheral vascular disease*) or to relieve chronic pain.

sympathetic nervous system One of the two divisions of the *autonomic nervous system*. In conjunction with the other division (the parasympathetic nervous system), this system controls many of the involuntary activities of the body's glands and organs.

symphysis A type of *joint* in which two bones are firmly joined by tough cartilage. Such joints occur between the *vertebrae*; between the pubic bones at the front of the *pelvis*; and between the upper and middle parts of the *sternum*.

symptom An indication of a disease or disorder that is noticed by the sufferer. By contrast, the indications that a doctor notes are called signs.

symptothermal method See *contraception, natural methods of*.

synaesthesia A condition in which stimulation of one of the senses (by a sound, for example) produces an additional response, such as the appearance of a colour in addition to the normal perception associated with that stimulus.

synapse A junction between two *neurons* across which a signal can pass. At a synapse, the two neurons do not connect but are separated by a gap called the synaptic cleft. When an electrical signal passing along a neuron reaches a synapse, it causes the release of a chemical called a *neurotransmitter*. The neurotransmitter travels across the synaptic cleft to the surface membrane of the next neuron, where it changes the electrical potential of the membrane. Signals can be transmitted across a synapse in one direction only.

Most drugs affecting the nervous system work as a result of their effects on synapses. Such drugs may affect the release of neurotransmitters, or they may modify their effects.

syncope The medical term for *fainting*.

syndactyly A *congenital* defect in which two or more fingers or toes are joined. Syndactyly is often inherited and is more common in males. In mild cases, the affected fingers or toes are joined only by a web of skin. In more serious cases, the bones of adjacent digits are fused. Surgery to separate the affected digits may be performed in early childhood.

syndrome A group of symptoms and/or signs that, occurring together, constitutes a particular disorder.

synovectomy Surgical removal of the membrane lining a joint capsule to treat recurrent or persistent *synovitis*, usually due to severe *rheumatoid arthritis*.

synovitis Inflammation of the membrane lining a joint capsule. The condition may be *acute*, in which case it is usually caused by an attack of arthritis, injury, or infection; or *chronic*, as in a disorder such as *rheumatoid arthritis*. The affected joint becomes swollen, painful, and often warm and red. To find the cause, joint aspiration or *biopsy* may be needed.

Symptoms are relieved by rest, supporting the joint with a splint or cast, *analgesics, nonsteroidal anti-inflammatory drugs*, and, occasionally, a *corticosteroid* injection. Chronic synovitis may be treated by *synovectomy*.

synovium A membrane that lines the capsule surrounding a movable *joint*. The synovium also forms a sheath for certain tendons of the hands and feet. The membrane secretes synovial fluid, which lubricates the joint or tendon. The

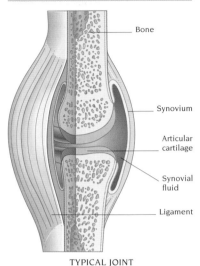

SYNOVIUM

Bone

Synovium

Articular cartilage

Synovial fluid

Ligament

TYPICAL JOINT

synovium can become inflamed; in a joint this is known as *synovitis*, in a tendon sheath it is known as *tenosynovitis*.

syphilis An infection caused by *TREPONEMA PALLIDUM* bacteria and spread through sexual intercourse or other intimate body contact, or, less commonly, from mother to fetus during pregnancy.

Following sexual infection, the organism spreads rapidly via the bloodstream and lymphatic system. The first symptom is a sore (chancre) that appears on the genitals, anus, rectum, lips, throat, or fingers and heals in 4–8 weeks. A rash then develops, which may be transient, recurrent, or may last for months. Other possible symptoms include lymph node enlargement, headache, bone pain, loss of appetite, fever, and fatigue. Thickened, grey or pink patches may develop on moist areas of skin and are highly infectious. *Meningitis* may also develop.

Following this symptomatic phase, the disease becomes latent for a few years, or sometimes indefinitely. A few untreated cases proceed, eventually, to a final stage characterized by widespread tissue destruction. This may be accompanied by cardiovascular syphilis, which affects the aorta and leads to *aneurysm* and *heart-valve* disease; *neurosyphilis*, with progressive brain damage and paralysis; and *tabes dorsalis* of the spinal cord.

Signs of congenital infection include a rash, persistent snuffles, bone abnormalities, jaundice, and enlargement of the liver and spleen. *Keratitis*, *arthritis*, a characteristic flat face, peg-shaped teeth, and learning difficulties may appear later in childhood.

Diagnosis is by examination of chancre serum or by blood tests. All forms of syphilis are treated with *antibacterial drugs*. Organ damage already caused by the disease cannot be reversed.

Practising *safer sex* can help to prevent syphilis infection. People with syphilis are infectious in the early stages but not in the latent and final stages.

syphilis, nonvenereal An infection due to TREPONEMA PALLIDUM bacteria that is spread by nonsexual means, such as through broken skin or saliva. It occurs mainly in the Middle East and Africa. Treatment is with *antibacterial drugs*.

syringe An instrument that is commonly used with a needle for injecting fluid into, or withdrawing fluid from, a body cavity, blood vessel, or tissue.

syringe driver A portable device used to provide continuous pain relief in conditions such as cancer. The *syringe* driver delivers a certain amount of an *analgesic* (painkiller) over a set period of time. It is attached to a syringe, which pumps the drug, via a tube, through a needle inserted into the skin.

syringing of ears The flushing out of excess *earwax* or a foreign body from the outer ear canal by introducing water from a syringe into the ear canal.

syringomyelia A rare, progressive condition, usually congenital, in which a cavity forms in the *brainstem* or in the *spinal cord* at neck level and gradually expands, filling with *cerebrospinal fluid*. Symptoms usually appear in early adulthood and include lack of temperature or pain sensation, wasting of muscles in the neck, shoulders, arms, and hands, and some loss of the sense of touch. Later, there is difficulty in moving the legs and controlling the bladder and bowel.

There is no drug treatment. Surgery can relieve pressure in the central cavity to prevent further enlargement, or alternatively, decompress the distended spinal cord (see *decompression, spinal canal*).

system A group of interconnected or interdependent organs with a common function, as in the *digestive system*.

systemic A term applied to something that affects the whole body rather than a specific part of it. For example, fever is a systemic symptom, whereas swelling is a localized symptom. The term systemic is also applied to the part of the blood circulation that supplies all parts of the body except the lungs.

systemic lupus erythematosus See *lupus erythematosus*.

systemic sclerosis Also known as scleroderma, a rare *autoimmune disorder* that can affect many organs and tissues, particularly the skin, arteries, kidneys, lungs, heart, gastrointestinal tract, and joints. The condition is three times as common in women and is most likely to appear between the age of 30 and 50.

The number and severity of symptoms varies. The most common symptom is *Raynaud's phenomenon*. Also common are changes in the skin, especially of the face and fingers, which becomes shiny, tight, and thickened, leading to difficulty with movements. Other parts of the body may also be affected, leading to difficulty in swallowing, shortness of breath, palpitations, high blood pressure, joint pain, or muscle weakness. Progression of scleroderma is often rapid in the first few years and then slows down or even stops. In a minority of people, degeneration is rapid, and leads to death from *heart failure*, *respiratory failure*, or *kidney failure*.

There is no cure for scleroderma, but many of the symptoms can be relieved.

systole A period of muscular contraction of a chamber of the *heart* that alternates with a resting period known as *diastole*.

S

T

tabes dorsalis A rare complication of untreated *syphilis* that appears years after infection. The condition causes abnormalities of sensation, sharp pains, incoordination, and incontinence.

tachycardia An adult heart rate of over 100 beats per minute. The average heart rate is 72–78 beats per minute. Tachycardia occurs in healthy people during exercise. At rest, it may be due to *fever*, *anxiety*, *hyperthyroidism*, *coronary artery disease*, high *caffeine* intake, or treatment involving *anticholinergic* or *diuretic drugs*. There are various types of tachycardia, which originate in different areas of the heart; the types include *atrial fibrillation*, *sinus tachycardia*, *supraventricular tachycardia*, and *ventricular tachycardia*.

tachypnoea An abnormally fast rate of breathing, which may be caused by exercise, anxiety, or lung or cardiac disorders.

tadalafil A drug used in the treatment of *erectile dysfunction*. It is similar to *sildenafil* but is longer-acting. Possible side effects of tadalafil include headaches, nasal congestion, flushing, indigestion, and *priapism*. Tadalafil should not be used by those taking *nitrate drugs* because of the possibility of a serious interaction.

T'ai chi A Chinese exercise system based on a series of over 100 postures between which slow, continuous movements are made. The aim is to exercise the muscles and integrate mind and body.

talipes A *birth defect* (commonly called club-foot) in which the foot is twisted out of shape or position. The cause may be pressure on the feet from the mother's uterus, or a genetic factor. The most common form is an equinovarus deformity, in which the heel turns inwards and the rest of the foot bends down and inwards. It is treated by repeated manipulation of the foot and ankle, starting soon after birth. A plaster *cast*, *splint*, or *strapping* may be used to hold the foot in position. If this is not successful, surgery will be needed.

talus The square-shaped foot bone that forms the ankle joint together with the *tibia* and *fibula*.

tamoxifen An *anticancer drug* that is used to treat certain forms of *breast cancer*, and, sometimes, to treat some types of female *infertility*. It may cause nausea, vomiting, hot flushes, swollen ankles, and irregular vaginal bleeding.

tampon A plug of absorbent material inserted into a wound or body opening to soak up blood or other secretions. The term commonly refers to a vaginal tampon, used to absorb menstrual blood.

tamponade Compression of the heart by fluid within the *pericardium*, which may cause breathlessness and collapse. Causes include *pericarditis*, complications after heart surgery, or a chest injury. A diagnosis is made by *echocardiography*, and the fluid is removed through a needle.

tamsulosin An *alpha-blocker drug* used for the treatment of urinary symptoms due to an enlarged prostate gland (see *prostate, enlarged*). Side effects include low blood pressure, drowsiness, dry mouth, and gastrointestinal disturbances.

tan See *suntan*.

tannin Also known as tannic acid, a chemical that occurs in many plants, particularly tea. It may cause constipation, and large amounts cause liver damage.

tantrum An outburst of bad behaviour, common in toddlers, usually indicating frustration and anger.

tapeworm infestation Tapeworms (cestodes) are ribbon-shaped worms that infest the intestines of humans and animals. They are usually acquired by eating undercooked meat or fish. Tapeworms from beef, pork, and fish usually only cause mild abdominal discomfort or diarrhoea. However, if eggs of pork worms are ingested, the hatched larvae burrow into tissues to form cysts. This leads to cysticercosis, the symptoms of which are muscle pain and convulsions. Rarely, fish tapeworms cause *anaemia*. Dwarf tapeworms, common in the tropics, can cause diarrhoea and abdominal discomfort. Tapeworms acquired from dogs cause *hydatid disease*. A diagnosis is made from the presence of worm segments or eggs in the faeces. Treatment is with *anthelmintic drugs*.

tardive dyskinesia Abnormal, uncontrolled movements, mainly of the face, tongue, mouth, and neck. Tardive dyskinesia may be caused by prolonged use of *antipsychotic drugs*, and is distinct from *parkinsonism*.

tarsalgia Pain in the rear part of the foot, usually associated with *flat-feet*.

tarsorrhaphy Surgery in which the upper and lower eyelids are sewn together. It may be used to protect the corneas of people unable to close their eyes or with *exophthalmos*. The eyelids are later cut apart and allowed to open.

tarsus The seven bones that make up the back of the foot and the ankle.

tartar See *calculus, dental*.

taste One of the five senses. There are generally thought to be five basic tastes, sweet, salty, sour, bitter, and umami (a savoury, meaty taste), although, in combination with the sense of *smell*, many different flavours can be distinguished. Tastes are detected by *taste buds*, most of which are on the tongue.

taste bud One of 10,000 specialized structures located on the *tongue*, with some at the back of the throat and on the palate. Each bud has about 25 sensory receptor cells, with tiny taste hairs that respond to food and drink. Taste buds on the tongue sense the five basic *tastes*: sweet, sour, salty, bitter, and umami (a savoury taste).

taste, loss of Loss of the sense of *taste*, usually as a result of the loss of the sense of *smell*. The most common cause is inflammation of the nasal passages. Other causes of loss of taste include any condition that causes a dry mouth (see *mouth, dry*); natural degeneration of the *taste buds*; damage to the taste buds from *stomatitis*, *mouth cancer*, or *radiotherapy* to the mouth; or damage to nerves that carry taste sensations.

tattooing The introduction of permanent colours under the skin surface, usually to create a picture. Tattooing equipment must be sterile to reduce the risk of infection. Small tattoos can be removed by cutting out the tattoo and stitching the wound edges together. Larger tattoos can sometimes be removed by *dermabrasion* or by *laser treatment*.

taxanes A group of *anticancer drugs* used to treat certain cancers, such as ovarian cancer (see *ovary, cancer of*) and *breast cancer*. They work by preventing the growth of cancer cells. Common taxane drugs include *paclitaxel* and docetaxel.

Tay-Sachs disease A serious inherited metabolic disorder (see *metabolism, inborn errors of*) that causes premature death. The cause is deficiency of the enzyme hexosaminidase A, which results in a buildup in the brain of a harmful substance. Symptoms usually appear after age 6 months and include blindness, paralysis, and seizures leading to death. Diagnosis is made by enzyme analysis of white blood cells. It is now largely prevented by *genetic counselling* of high-risk groups.

TB An abbreviation for *tuberculosis*.

T-cell A class of *lymphocyte*.

tears The watery, salty secretion that is produced by the lacrimal glands, part of the *lacrimal apparatus* of the eye. Tears keep the *cornea* and *conjunctiva* moist to maintain transpar-

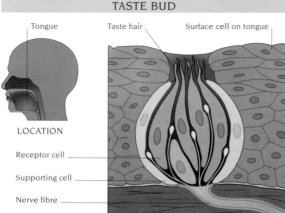

TASTE BUD

Tongue

Taste hair

Surface cell on tongue

LOCATION

Receptor cell

Supporting cell

Nerve fibre

ency of the cornea and prevent ulcers; aid blinking; and wash away foreign particles. Tear production increases in response to eye irritation and emotion.

tears, artificial Preparations to supplement tear production in disorders that cause dry eye, such as *keratoconjunctivitis sicca*, and to relieve irritation.

technetium A radioactive element used in *radionuclide scanning*.

TEETH

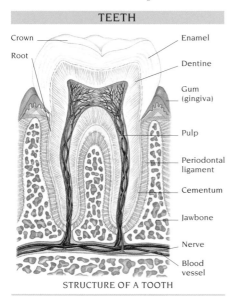

Crown

Root

Enamel

Dentine

Gum (gingiva)

Pulp

Periodontal ligament

Cementum

Jawbone

Nerve

Blood vessel

STRUCTURE OF A TOOTH

teeth Hard, bone-like projections set in the jaws and surrounded by the gums. The teeth are used for *mastication*, help to form speech, and give shape to the face. At the centre of each tooth is the pulp, which contains blood vessels and nerves and is surrounded by hard dentine. The part of the tooth above the gum, the crown, is covered by enamel, the hardest substance in the body. The roots of the tooth, which fit into the jawbone, are covered by bone-like cementum. Humans have 32 *permanent teeth*, which erupt after the *primary teeth* are lost. These teeth comprise chisel-shaped, biting incisors; sharp, pointed canines; grinding premolars; and larger grinding molars.

teeth, care of See *oral hygiene*.

teething The period when a baby cuts his or her *primary teeth* (see *eruption of teeth*). While teething, a baby may be irritable, fretful, clingy, have difficulty sleeping, and may cry more than usual. Symptoms may be relieved by the use of painkilling gels that are rubbed on the gums, or liquid preparations.

telangiectasia An increase in the size of small blood vessels beneath the surface of an area of skin, causing redness and a "broken veins" appearance. It is most common on the nose and cheeks. There may be no obvious cause, or the condition may be due to many years of excessive alcohol consumption, *rosacea*, overexposure to sunlight, or a connective tissue disease such as *dermatomyositis*.

Telangiectasia is not a cause for concern, but the veins can be removed in some cases by electrodesiccation (electrical destruction of the upper layers of the skin) or laser surgery. (See also *spider naevus*.)

temazepam A *benzodiazepine drug* that is used to treat *insomnia* and also as a drug of abuse.

temperature The degree of hotness of a body or substance. In the human body, the temperature must be maintained at around 37°C for optimum functioning. Body temperature is maintained by the *hypothalamus*, which monitors blood temperature and activates mechanisms to compensate for changes. When body temperature falls, *shivering* creates heat by muscle activity, and constriction of blood vessels in the skin minimizes heat loss. When the body temperature rises, *sweating* results in cooling, and dilation of blood vessels in the skin increases heat loss.

temperature method See *contraception, natural methods of.*

temporal A medical term meaning of or near the temples or a temple.

temporal arteritis An uncommon disease of older people in which the walls of the arteries in the scalp over the temples become inflamed. Other arteries in the body may also be affected. The cause is unknown, but the condition is often associated with *polymyalgia rheumatica*. Symptoms may include severe headache on one or both sides, scalp tenderness, a low fever, and poor appetite. In about

T

half of the cases, the arteries supplying the eyes are affected, which may cause sudden blindness if left untreated.

Diagnosis of temporal arteritis is made by *blood tests* (including *ESR*) and, in some cases, by a *biopsy* of the temporal artery. Treatment involves the use of a *corticosteroid drug*. If this is not successful, *immunosuppressants* may be given. The disease usually clears up within 2 years.

temporal lobe epilepsy A form of *epilepsy* in which abnormal electrical discharges occur in the temporal lobe (most of the lower side of each half of the *cerebrum*) in the *brain*. The usual cause is damage to the temporal lobe, which may be due to a *birth injury, head injury, brain tumour, brain abscess,* or *stroke*. Attacks of this form of epilepsy cause dreamlike states, unpleasant *hallucinations* of smell or taste, the perception of an illusory scene, or déja vu. There may also be grimacing, rotation of the head and eyes, and sucking and chewing movements. The affected person may have no memory of activities during an attack, which can last for minutes or hours. Sometimes, the seizure develops into a *grand mal* seizure. Diagnosis and drug treatment is the same as for other forms of epilepsy.

temporomandibular joint The joint between the mandible (lower jaw bone) and the *skull*.

temporomandibular joint syndrome Pain and other symptoms affecting the head, jaw, and face, thought to result when the *temporomandibular joints* and the muscles and ligaments attached to them do not work together correctly. Causes include spasm of the chewing muscles, an incorrect bite (see *malocclusion*), jaw, head, or neck injuries, or *osteoarthritis*. Common symptoms include headaches, tenderness of the jaw muscles, and aching facial pain. Treatment of temporomandibular joint syndrome involves correction of any underlying abnormality, *analgesic drugs*, and, in some cases, injection of *corticosteroid drugs* into the joint.

tenderness Pain or abnormal sensitivity in a part of the body when it is pressed or touched.

tendinitis Inflammation of a tendon, usually caused by injury or overuse. Symptoms of tendinitis include pain, tenderness, and restricted movement. Treatment is with *nonsteroidal antiinflammatory drugs* (NSAIDs), *ultrasound treatment*, or injection of a *corticosteroid drug* around the tendon.

tendolysis An operation performed to free a *tendon* from *adhesions* that limit its movement. The adhesions are usually caused by *tenosynovitis*.

tendon A fibrous cord that joins muscle to bone or muscle to muscle. Tendons are strong and flexible, but inelastic. Those in the hands, wrists, and feet are enclosed in synovial sheaths (fibrous capsules) that secrete a lubricating fluid.

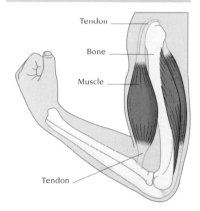

TENDON

Tendon

Bone

Muscle

Tendon

tendon release See *tendolysis*.

tendon repair Surgery to join the cut or torn ends of, or to replace, a *tendon*.

tendon rupture A complete tear in a *tendon*. A tendon may rupture when the muscle to which it is attached contracts suddenly and powerfully, such as during vigorous exercise. Rupture may also be due to an injury or joint disorder such as *rheumatoid arthritis*. Symptoms include a snapping sensation, impaired movement, pain, and swelling. Diagnosis is usually obvious from the symptoms. Surgery to repair the tendon may be needed. In some cases, the tendon may heal if immobilized in a plaster *cast*.

tendon transfer Surgery to reposition a *tendon* so that it makes a muscle perform a different function. The tendon is cut from its original point of attachment and reattached elsewhere, making the muscle lie in a different position. The procedure may be used to treat *talipes* or permanent muscle injury or paralysis.

tenesmus A feeling of incomplete emptying of the bowel in which an urge to pass *faeces* accompanies ineffective straining. It may be a symptom of inflammation or a tumour (see *colon, cancer of*).

tennis elbow Pain and tenderness on the outside of the elbow and in the back of the forearm. Commonly called epicondylitis, it is caused by inflammation of the *tendon* that attaches the muscles that straighten the fingers and wrist to the *humerus*. Treatment consists of resting the arm, and taking *analgesic drugs* or *nonsteroidal anti-inflammatory drugs* (NSAIDs). *Ultrasound treatment*, injection of a *corticosteroid drug*, or surgery are sometimes needed.

tenosynovitis Inflammation of the lining of the sheath that surrounds a *tendon*. The usual cause is excessive friction caused by repetitive movements; bacterial infection is a rare cause. The hands and wrists are most often affected. Symptoms include pain, tenderness, and swelling over the tendon. Treatment is with *nonsteroidal anti-inflammatory drugs* (NSAIDs) or a local injection of a *corticosteroid drug*. However, if infection is the cause, *antibiotic drugs* are prescribed. A *splint* to immobilize the joint, or surgery, may also be needed.

tenovaginitis Inflammation or thickening of the fibrous wall of the sheath that surrounds a *tendon*.

TENS Abbreviation for transcutaneous electrical nerve stimulation, a method of pain relief. Minute electrical impulses, which block pain messages to the brain, are relayed from an impulse generator to electrodes attached to the skin in the area of the pain. TENS can help relieve chronic pain not controlled by *analgesic drugs* and may be used in *childbirth*.

tension A feeling of mental and physical strain associated with *anxiety*. Muscle tension may cause headaches and stiffness in muscles. Persistent tension is related to generalized anxiety disorder. (See also *stress*.)

teratogen A physical, chemical, or biological agent, such as radiation, the drug *thalidomide*, and the *rubella* virus, that causes abnormalities in a developing *embryo* or *fetus*.

teratoma A primary *tumour* consisting of cells totally unlike those normally found in that part of the body.

terbinafine An *antifungal drug* used to treat fungal nail or skin infections. Side effects are rare with topical use but may include local irritation. Taken as tablets, the drug may cause nausea, abdominal pain, and, occasionally, a rash.

terbutaline A *bronchodilator drug* used to treat *asthma* and chronic obstructive *pulmonary disease*, and also to prevent premature labour. Possible adverse effects include nervousness, restlessness, tremor, nausea, and palpitations.

terminal care See *dying, care of the*.

termination of pregnancy See *abortion, induced*.

testicle See *testis*.

testicular feminization syndrome A rare inherited condition in which a genetic male with internal *testes* has the external appearance of a female. The syndrome is a form of *intersex* and is the most common form of male *pseudohermaphroditism*. The cause is a defective response of the body tissues to *testosterone*. The causative genes are carried on

TENS

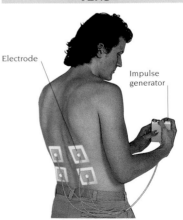

Electrode

Impulse generator

TESTIS

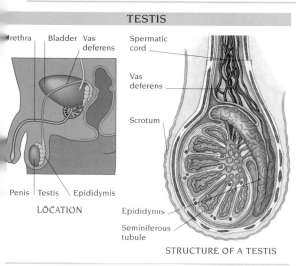

Urethra | Bladder | Vas deferens

Penis | Testis | Epididymis

LOCATION

Spermatic cord

Vas deferens

Scrotum

Epididymis

Seminiferous tubule

STRUCTURE OF A TESTIS

aged men, and the risk increases in individuals with a history of unde-scended testis (see *testis, undescended*). The most common types of testicular cancer are seminomas, which are made up of only one type of cell, and *terato-mas*. The cancer usually appears as a firm, pain-less swelling of one testis. There may also be pain and inflamma-tion. *Biopsy*, followed by *orchidectomy*, is the usual treatment, and may be combined with *chemotherapy*. The tu-mours usually respond well to treatment.

the X chromosome, and so females can be carriers. Affected individuals appear to be girls throughout childhood, and most develop female secondary *sexual characteristics* at *puberty*; but *amenor-rhoea* occurs, and a diagnosis is usually made during investigations to find its cause. *Chromosome analysis* shows the presence of male chromosomes and blood tests show male levels of testoster-one. Treatment of testicular feminization syndrome involves surgical removal of the testes, to prevent cancerous change in later life, and therapy with *oestrogen drugs*. An affected person is not fertile but can live a normal life as a woman.

testis One of two male sexual organs, also called testicles, that produce *sperm* and the hormone *testosterone*. The testes develop in the fetus within the abdomen and usually descend into the *scrotum* by birth or within the next few months. Each testis contains seminiferous tubules that produce sperm. Cells between the seminiferous tubules produce testosterone. Each testis is suspended by the *spermatic cord*, composed of the *vas deferens*, blood vessels, and nerves. (See also *testis, undescended*.)

testis, cancer of A rare, cancerous tumour of the *testis*. Testicular cancer is most common in young to middle-

testis, ectopic A *testis* that is absent from the *scrotum* because it has descen-ded into an abnormal position, usually in the groin or at the base of the penis. The condition is most often discovered soon after birth during a routine physical examination. It is treated by *orchidopexy*. (See also *testis, undescended*.)

testis, pain in the Pain in a *testis* may be caused by mild injury, a tear in the wall of the testis due to a direct blow, *orchitis, epididymo-orchitis*, and torsion of the testis (see *testis, torsion of*). Some-times, no cause is found and the pain disappears without treatment. If the wall of the testis is torn, an operation to repair it may be needed.

testis, retractile A *testis* that is drawn up high into the groin by a pronounced muscle reflex in response to cold or touch. A retractile testis is normal in young children, but it usually disap-pears by *puberty*.

testis, swollen Swelling of the *testis* or the surrounding tissues in the *scrotum*. Harmless and painless swellings include *epididymal cysts, hydroceles, varicoceles*, and *spermatoceles*. Cancer of the testis (see *testis, cancer of*) is rare but may be a cause of painless swelling. Swelling that is painful may be caused by a direct blow, torsion of the testis (see *testis, tor-sion of*), *orchitis, epididymo-orchitis*, or,

T

in very rare cases, cancer of the testis. Any swelling of the testes should be assessed promptly by a doctor.

testis, torsion of Twisting of the *spermatic cord* that causes severe pain and swelling of the *testis*. The pain develops rapidly and is sometimes accompanied by abdominal pain and nausea. The testis becomes swollen and very tender, and the skin of the *scrotum* becomes discoloured. Unless the torsion is treated within a few hours, permanent damage to the testis results. The condition is most common around puberty. It is more likely to occur if the testis is unusually mobile within the scrotum.

TESTIS, TORSION OF

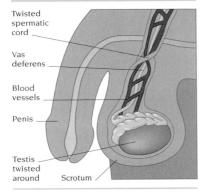

Twisted spermatic cord

Vas deferens

Blood vessels

Penis

Testis twisted around   Scrotum

Diagnosis is by physical examination. Surgery is performed to untwist the testis and anchor it in the scrotum with small stitches to prevent recurrence. If irreversible damage has occurred, *orchidectomy* is performed. In either case, the other testis is anchored to the scrotum to prevent torsion on that side. With prompt treatment, recovery of the testis is complete.

testis, undescended A testis that has failed to descend from the abdomen to the *scrotum*. The condition usually affects only one testis and occurs in about 1 per cent of full-term and 10 per cent of premature male babies. An undescended testis often descends within months of birth but rarely descends after this time.

An undescended testis does not develop normally, is incapable of normal sperm production, and is at increased risk of developing testicular cancer (see

testis, cancer of). If both testes are undescended, *infertility* results.

A diagnosis is made during a physical examination after birth or later in infancy. Treatment is by *orchidopexy*, which usually reduces the risk of later infertility or testicular cancer (see *testis, cancer of*). A poorly developed undescended testis may be removed if the other is normal.

testosterone The main *androgen hormone* (male sex hormone). It stimulates bone and muscle growth and sexual development. It is produced by the *testes* and, in very small amounts, the *ovaries*. Synthetic or animal testosterone is used to stimulate delayed *puberty* or treat some forms of male *infertility*.

tests, medical Tests may be performed to investigate the cause of symptoms and establish a diagnosis, to monitor the course of a disease, or to assess response to treatment. A medical testing programme carried out on apparently healthy people to find disease at an early stage is known as *screening*.

The accuracy of a test is based on its sensitivity (ability to correctly identify diseased subjects), specificity (ability to correctly identify healthy subjects), and predictive value. The predictive value is determined by a mathematical formula that involves the number of accurate test results and the total number of tests performed. The best tests have both high specificity and high sensitivity, and therefore high predictive value.

tetanus A serious, sometimes fatal, disease of the *central nervous system* caused by infection of a wound with spores of the bacterium CLOSTRIDIUM TETANI. The spores live mainly in soil and manure but are also found elsewhere, including in the human intestine. When the spores infect poorly oxygenated tissues they multiply and produce a *toxin* that acts on the nerves controlling muscle activity. The most common symptom of this is *trismus* (commonly known as lockjaw). Other symptoms include stiffness of the abdominal and back muscles, and contraction of facial muscles, producing a fixed grimace. There may also be a fast pulse, slight fever, and profuse sweating. Painful muscle spasms then develop, and may result in *asphyxia* if they affect the

T

larynx or chest wall. The spasms usually subside after 10 to 14 days.

About half a million cases of tetanus occur worldwide each year, but fewer than 20 occur in the UK. The diagnosis is made from the symptoms and signs, and a course of tetanus *antitoxin* injections is started. Most people recover completely if treated promptly.

In the UK tetanus is prevented by routine immunization, with three doses during the first year (at 2, 3, and 4 months of age), a booster at 3–5 years, and another booster at 13–18 years. Generally, five doses of vaccine provide lifelong immunity, although further boosters may be required after a dirty wound or if travelling to an area with poor medical services.

tetany Spasms and twitching of the muscles, most commonly in the hands and feet, although the muscles of the face, *larynx*, or spine may also be affected. The spasms are caused by a biochemical disturbance and are painless at first; if the condition persists, the spasms tend to become increasingly painful. Muscle damage may result if the underlying cause is not treated. The most common underlying cause is *hypocalcaemia*. Other causes include *hypokalaemia*, *hyperventilation* during a panic attack, or, more rarely, *hypoparathyroidism*.

tetracosactide A drug used to test the functioning of the *adrenal glands*. Tetracosactide is a chemical analogue of the natural hormone corticotrophin (*ACTH*). ACTH stimulates the cortices of the adrenal glands to secrete hormones such as *cortisol*. To diagnose a disorder of the adrenal glands, a tetracosactide injection is given and the blood cortisol level measured. Failure of the level to rise indicates an abnormality.

tetracycline drugs A group of *antibiotic drugs* used to treat *bronchitis*, *acne*, *syphilis*, *gonorrhoea*, *nongonococcal urethritis*, and certain types of *pneumonia*. If taken with milk, tetracyclines are not absorbed effectively into the intestines. Possible side effects include nausea, vomiting, diarrhoea, worsening of kidney disorders, rash, and itching. Tetracyclines may discolour developing teeth and are therefore not usually prescribed for children under age 12 or pregnant or breast-feeding women.

tetralogy of Fallot A form of congenital *heart disease* in which the heart has four coexisting anomalies: displacement of the aorta, narrowing of the pulmonary valve, a hole in the ventricular septum, and thickening of the right ventricle wall. These cause poor oxygenation of the blood pumped to the body, resulting in *cyanosis* and breathlessness. Tetralogy of Fallot occurs in about 1 in 1,000 infants.

Affected infants appear normal at birth. Severely affected infants may become cyanosed and breathless early in life. Other symptoms include failure to gain weight and poor development.

An *ECG*, echocardiogram (see *echocardiography*), and sometimes cardiac *catheterization* are performed to confirm the diagnosis and assess the severity of the condition. The disorder is corrected by *open heart surgery*.

tetraplegia An alternative term for the condition *quadriplegia*.

thalamus One of two structures within the *brain* consisting of a walnut-sized mass of nerve tissue. The thalami sit at the top of the *brainstem* and are connected to all parts of the brain.

Each thalamus relays sensory information flowing into the brain. Some basic sensations, such as pain, may reach consciousness within the thalamus. Other types of sensory information are processed and relayed to parts of the cerebral cortex (outer layer of the brain), where sensations are perceived.

The thalamus seems to act as a filter by selecting only information of particular importance. Certain centres in the thalamus may also play a part in long-term memory.

thalassaemia A group of inherited *blood* disorders in which there is a fault in the production of *haemoglobin*. Many of the red *blood cells* become fragile and haemolyse (break up), leading to anaemia (see *anaemia, haemolytic*). Thalassaemia is prevalent in the Mediterranean, the Middle East, and Southeast Asia, and in families originating from these areas.

Normal adult haemoglobin contains two pairs of globins (protein chains):

alpha and beta. In thalassaemia, a recessive defective *gene* results in reduced synthesis of one of the chains. Usually beta-chain production is disturbed (beta-thalassaemia). Beta-thalassaemia minor (thalassaemia trait), which is never severe, is caused by one defective gene. The presence of two defective genes causes beta-thalassaemia major (Cooley's anaemia). The much rarer disorder alpha-thalassaemia varies in severity; alpha-thalassaemia major usually results in fetal death.

Symptoms of beta-thalassaemia major appear 3–6 months after birth. If untreated, bone marrow cavities expand, leading to a characteristic enlargement of the skull and facial bones.

Beta-thalassaemia major is diagnosed from microscopic examination of the blood, and from other *blood tests*. Babies may be screened for the condition shortly after birth (see *blood spot screening tests*). Treatment is with *blood transfusions* and, sometimes, *splenectomy*. However, successive *blood transfusions* cause a buildup of iron in the body (see *haemosiderosis*). *Chelating agents* are given by continuous infusion to help the body excrete the excess iron. A *stem cell* or *bone marrow transplant* may offer a cure for the disease.

Genetic counselling is advised for parents or other close relatives of a child with thalassaemia, and also for any person with thalassaemia trait.

thalidomide A drug that was withdrawn in the UK in 1961 after it was found to cause limb deformities in many babies born to women given the drug during pregnancy. Thalidomide is still used to treat certain forms of *Hansen's disease* (leprosy) and *multiple myeloma*.

thallium A rare metallic element that is present as compounds in some zinc and lead ores. Poisoning over a prolonged period causes loss of hair, disorders of the nerves in the limbs, and disturbance of the stomach and intestines. Thallium-201 (an artificial radioactive isotope) is sometimes used in *radionuclide scanning* of the heart.

THC The abbreviation for tetrahydrocannabinol, the active ingredient in *marijuana*.

theophylline A *bronchodilator drug* sometimes used to treat severe *asthma* in cases that have failed to respond to other treatments. Theophylline is usually given orally but can be given intravenously as emergency treatment. Possible adverse effects include dizziness, nausea, vomiting, diarrhoea, *palpitations*, and *seizures*.

therapeutic A term meaning related to treatment. The therapeutic dose of a drug is the amount required to have the greatest beneficial effect.

therapeutic community A method of treating *drug dependence* and *alcohol dependence*, and some *personality disorders*, that entails patients living together as a group in a nonhospital environment, usually under supervision. (See also *social skills training*.)

therapy The treatment of any disease or abnormal physical or mental condition.

thermometer An instrument used to measure *temperature*. A traditional clinical thermometer consists of a glass capillary tube (a tube with a very fine bore) that is sealed at one end and has a mercury-filled bulb at the other.

Modern versions of the clinical thermometer include an electronic probe connected to a digital display, and an aural thermometer, which measures the temperature of the *eardrum*. Both versions give an almost instant reading. There are also disposable skin thermometers that employ heat-sensitive chemicals, which change colour at specific temperatures. These are not as reliable, however. Clinical

THERMOMETER

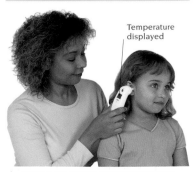

Temperature displayed

USING AN AURAL THERMOMETER

thermometers may be calibrated in degrees Celsius (centigrade), degrees Fahrenheit, or sometimes both.

thiabendazole See *tiabendazole*.

thiamine See *vitamin B complex*.

thiazides A type of *diuretic drug*.

thiopental A *barbiturate drug* that is widely used as a general anaesthetic (see *anaesthesia, general*). Thiopental is given by intravenous injection.

thirst The desire to drink. Thirst is one means by which the amount of water in the body is controlled (the other is the volume of urine excreted).

Thirst is stimulated by an increased concentration of salt, sugar, or certain other substances in the blood. As the blood passes through the *hypothalamus* in the brain, special nerve receptors are stimulated, inducing the sensation of thirst. Thirst is also stimulated if blood volume decreases as a result of sweating, vomiting, diarrhoea, severe bleeding, or extensive burns. Thirst may also be caused by a dry mouth.

thirst, excessive A strong and persistent need to drink, most commonly due to *dehydration*. Other causes include untreated *diabetes mellitus* and *diabetes insipidus*, kidney failure, treatment with phenothiazine drugs, and severe blood loss. Abnormal thirst may also be due to a psychological condition known as psychogenic polydipsia.

thoracic outlet syndrome A condition in which pressure on the *brachial plexus* causes pain in the arms and shoulders, pins-and-needles sensation in the fingers, and weakness of grip and other hand movements. Severe symptoms are usually caused by a *cervical rib*. Thoracic outlet syndrome may also be caused by drooping of the shoulders, an enlarged scalenus muscle in the neck, or a tumour. The condition is made worse by lifting and carrying heavy loads or by increases in body weight.

Treatment of thoracic outlet syndrome consists of exercises to improve posture, sometimes together with *nonsteroidal anti-inflammatory drugs* and *muscle relaxant drugs*. Severe cases may be treated by surgical removal of the first rib.

thoracic surgery A surgical speciality concerned with operations on organs within the chest cavity. Sometimes, thoracic surgery is combined with heart surgery, in which case it is known as cardiothoracic surgery.

thoracotomy An operation in which the chest is opened to provide access to organs in the chest cavity.

There are two types of thoracotomy: lateral and anterior. In a lateral thoracotomy the chest is opened between two ribs to provide access to the *lungs*, major blood vessels, and the *oesophagus*. In an anterior thoracotomy, an incision down the sternum (breastbone) provides access to the *heart* and the *coronary arteries*.

thorax The medical name for the chest. The thorax extends from the base of the neck to the *diaphragm muscle*.

thought The mental activity that enables humans to reason, form judgments, and solve problems. The essential features of thought include the substitution of symbols (in the form of words, numbers, or images) for objects, the formation of symbols into ideas, and the arrangement of ideas into a certain order in the mind. (See also *thought disorders*.)

thought disorders Abnormalities in the structure or content of *thought*, as reflected in a person's speech, writing, or behaviour. *Schizophrenia* causes several thought disorders, including loss of logical connections between associations, the invention of new words (see *neologisms*), thought blocking (sudden interruption in the train of thought), the feeling that thoughts are being inserted into or withdrawn from the mind, and auditory *hallucinations*.

Incoherent thoughts occur in all types of *confusion*, including *dementia* and delirium. Rapidly jumping from one idea to another occurs in *hypomania* and *mania*. In *depression*, thinking becomes slow, there is a lack of association, and a tendency to dwell in great detail on trivial subjects. In *obsessive–compulsive disorder*, recurrent ideas seem to come into a person's mind involuntarily. *Delusions*, which occur in schizophrenia and other psychotic illnesses, may be an expression of distorted thinking.

threadworm infestation A common infestation with a small worm, *ENTEROBIUS*

VERMICULARIS (pinworm), that lives in the intestines. Threadworms primarily affect children. The female adult threadworms are white and about 1 cm long (large enough to see). They lay eggs in the skin around the anus, and their movements cause tickling or itching in the anal region, often at night. Eggs are transferred from the fingers to the mouth to cause reinfestation or are carried on toys or blankets to other children. Swallowed eggs hatch in the intestine and the worms reach maturity after a period of 2–6 weeks. Diagnosis is made by seeing the worms or by applying a piece of sticky tape to the anal area to collect the worms or eggs. Treatment is with an *anthelmintic drug.*

thrill A vibrating sensation felt when the flat of the hand is held against an area of the body. Thrill is caused by turbulent blood flow in an *artery* or the *heart.* The term is also used to describe the feeling produced by fluid within the abdominal cavity in *ascites.*

throat A popular term for the *pharynx.* The term is also sometimes used to refer to the front of the neck.

throat cancer See *pharynx, cancer of; larynx, cancer of.*

thrombectomy The removal of a *thrombus* that is blocking a blood vessel. It is performed as an emergency procedure if a major artery is blocked, or as a precautionary measure if there is a risk of an *embolus* breaking off. Before surgery, the site of the thrombus is established by *angiography* and the patient may be given *anticoagulant drugs.*

thromboangiitis obliterans Another name for *Buerger's disease.*

thrombocyte An alternative name for a *platelet.*

thrombocytopenia A reduction in the number of *platelets* in the blood, resulting in a tendency to bleed. Sometimes thrombocytopenic *purpura* (abnormal bleeding into the skin) develops. The cause may be a reduced rate of platelet production or fast rate of platelet destruction. Thrombocytopenia can be a feature of *leukaemia, lymphoma,* systemic *lupus erythematosus, HIV* infection, megaloblastic *anaemia,* or *hypersplenism.* It can also be caused by exposure to *radiation,* excessive alcohol intake, or, more

often, by an adverse reaction to a prescribed drug such as a thiazide *diuretic. Idiopathic thrombocytopenic purpura* (ITP) is of unknown cause, but it may be an *autoimmune disorder.*

Thrombocytopenia is confirmed by a *blood count;* a bone marrow test may also be performed. Any underlying disease is treated if possible. Children with ITP may not need treatment but adults are usually given *corticosteroid drugs.* In some cases of severe, acute bleeding, a transfusion of platelets may be given. Persistent thrombocytopenia may be treated with a *splenectomy.*

thromboembolism The blockage of a blood vessel by a piece of a blood clot (embolus) that has broken off from a *thrombus* elsewhere in the circulation. (See also *thrombosis; embolism*).

thrombolytic drugs Sometimes called fibrinolytic drugs, this group of drugs is used to treat *thrombosis, embolism,* and *myocardial infarction.* Thrombolytic drugs act within blood vessels to dissolve clots. Possible adverse effects include abnormal bleeding and an allergic reaction.

thrombophilia A tendency for blood to clot too readily due to an inherited abnormality in proteins such as *factor V.* It may not be recognized until specific circumstances such as injury or air travel cause symptoms or signs. (See also *thrombosis, deep vein.*)

thrombophlebitis Inflammation of a section of vein, usually just under the skin, with clot formation in the affected part. This can occur after minor injury to the vein or as a complication of *varicose veins* or *Buerger's disease.* The affected blood vessel is swollen, red, and tender, and feels hard. Fever and malaise may occur. A blood clot may develop. Treatment includes support with a bandage, *nonsteroidal anti-inflammatory drugs,* and sometimes *antibiotic drugs.* The condition usually clears up in 10–14 days.

thrombosis The formation of a *thrombus* (blood clot) in an undamaged blood vessel. A thrombus that forms within an artery supplying the heart muscle (coronary thrombosis) is the usual cause of *myocardial infarction.* A thrombus in an artery of the brain (cerebral thrombosis) is a common cause of *stroke.* Thrombi sometimes form in veins, either just below the skin or in deeper veins (see *thrombosis, deep vein*).

In arteries, thrombus formation may be encouraged by *atherosclerosis*, smoking, *hypertension*, and damage to blood vessel walls from *arteritis* and *phlebitis*. An increased clotting tendency may occur in *pregnancy*, when using *oral contraceptives*, or through prolonged immobility.

An arterial thrombosis may cause no symptoms until blood flow is impaired. Then, there is reduced tissue or organ function and sometimes severe pain. Venous thrombosis may also cause pain and swelling. Diagnosis is made by Doppler *ultrasound*. In some cases, *angiography* or *venography* may also be used. Treatment may include *anticoagulant drugs* or *thrombolytic drugs, nonsteroidal anti-inflammatory drugs*, and *antibiotic drugs*. In life-threatening cases, *thrombectomy* may be needed.

thrombosis, deep vein The formation of a *thrombus* within deep-lying veins in the leg. The cause is usually a combination of slow blood flow through one part of the body (such as when sitting for long periods or when the tissues are compressed, as occurs in long-haul flights) and an increase in the clotting tendency of the blood, which occurs with dehydration, after surgery or injury, during pregnancy, and in women taking *oral contraceptives*. Deep vein thrombosis may also be caused by *polycythaemia*. Deep vein thrombosis is common in people with *heart failure* and those who have had a *stroke* or who have been immobile for long periods. Clots in the leg veins may cause pain, tenderness, swelling, discoloration, and ulceration of the skin, but they can be symptomless. A deep vein thrombosis is not necessarily serious in itself, but part of the clot may break off and travel in the bloodstream to the lungs. This is known as a *pulmonary embolism*.

A diagnosis is made by Doppler *ultrasound scanning*. Treatment depends on the site and extent of the clots. Small clots may not need treatment if they are confined to the calf and the patient is mobile. Otherwise, *anticoagulant drugs* or *thrombolytic drugs* are given. If there

is a high risk of a pulmonary embolism, *thrombectomy* may be performed.

thrombus A blood clot that has formed inside an intact blood vessel. A thrombus is life-threatening if it obstructs the blood supply to an organ such as the heart or brain. A thrombus may also lead to *gangrene* in an organ or extremity, or to *embolism*. (See also *blood clotting; thrombosis*.)

thrush A common name for the fungal infection *candidiasis*.

thumb-sucking A common habit in young children, which provides comfort, oral gratification, amusement when bored, and reassurance. Thumb-sucking tends to decrease after age 3, and most children grow out of it by age 7. In most cases, it is not harmful. However, *malocclusion* of the permanent teeth may develop if the habit continues past age 7. This is usually temporary, if not, an *orthodontic appliance* may be needed.

thymoma A rare *tumour* of the *thymus gland*. The tumour can arise from any of the cell types in the thymus gland and can be cancerous or noncancerous.

thymoxamine See *moxisylyte*.

thymus A gland that forms part of the *immune system*. The thymus lies behind the *sternum* and consists of two lobes that join in front of the *trachea*. Each lobe is made of lymphoid tissue consisting of *lymphocytes, epithelium*, and fat. The thymus conditions lymphocytes to become *T-cells*. It plays a part in the immune response until *puberty*, gradually enlarging during this time. After puberty, it shrinks, but some glandular tissue remains until middle-age.

thyroglossal disorders A set of congenital defects caused by failure of the thyroglossal duct to disappear during embryonic development. In *embryos*, this duct runs from the base of the tongue to the *thyroid gland*. Abnormal development may cause the duct to persist in its entirety or partly as a cyst. A cyst usually becomes infected and swollen, which may lead to formation of a *fistula*. The cyst and any remaining parts of the duct are removed.

thyroid cancer Rare *tumours* of the *thyroid gland*. In most cases the cause is unknown, although exposure to radioactive

T

fallout increases the risk of developing the condition. There are several types, depending on the type of cells involved. In all of them, however, the first sign is a firm nodule in the neck, which may grow slowly or rapidly. In many cases, the cancer is painless and symptoms such as difficulty swallowing, and hoarseness or loss of voice, only develop when the tumour presses on other structures. A diagnosis is made by *thyroid scanning* and needle *aspiration* or a *biopsy*. A *thyroidectomy* is usually followed by treatment with radioactive *iodine* or external *radiotherapy* to destroy any residual cancer. Cure rates depend on the cell type and on the size and spread of the tumour when diagnosed. Patients need to take *thyroxine* replacement therapy for the rest of their lives.

thyroidectomy Surgical removal of all or part of the *thyroid gland*, performed to treat *thyroid cancer*, some cases of *hyperthyroidism*, *goitre*, or a noncancerous tumour of the thyroid gland.

thyroid-function tests A group of blood tests used to evaluate the function of the *thyroid gland* and to detect or confirm any thyroid disorder. The thyroid hormones T_3 and T_4 are measured, as well as thyroid-stimulating hormone (TSH), the *pituitary gland* hormone that stimulates the thyroid gland.

thyroid gland One of the main *endocrine glands*, which helps to regulate the rate of all the body's internal processes. The thyroid gland is situated in the front of the neck, just below the *larynx* (voice box). It consists of two lobes, one on each side of the *trachea* (windpipe), joined by a portion of tissue called the isthmus. Thyroid tissue is composed of follicular cells, which secrete the iodine-containing hormones thyroxine (T_4) and triiodothyronine (T_3), and parafollicular cells (or C cells), which secrete the hormone *calcitonin*. T_4 and T_3 are important in controlling the body's metabolism. Calcitonin helps to regulate calcium balance in the body. (See also *thyroid gland, disorders of*; *thyroid hormones*.)

thyroid gland, disorders of Disorders of the thyroid gland may cause *hyperthyroidism*, *hypothyroidism*, or enlargement or distortion of the gland. *Myxoedema*, *Graves' disease*, and *Hashimoto's thyroiditis* are common disorders. *Goitre* may sometimes occur with no accompanying abnormality of thyroid function. In rare cases, the gland is absent at birth, producing severe *cretinism*. Sometimes it develops in an abnormal position in the neck, causing, in rare cases, difficulty in swallowing or breathing.

THYROID GLAND

LOCATION

Thyroid cartilage

Thyroid gland

Trachea

A genetic disorder may impair the thyroid's ability to secrete hormones and goitre may result. Thyroid infection is uncommon and leads to *thyroiditis*. Viral infection can cause extreme pain and temporary hyperthyroidism. Hormonal changes during puberty or pregnancy may cause a degree of goitre temporarily. Hyperthyroidism due to excessive production of TSH by the pituitary gland is rare but can occur as a result of a *pituitary tumour*.

Because iodine is necessary for the production of thyroid hormone, its deficiency may lead to goitre. Severe iodine deficiency in children may cause myxoedema. (See also *thyroid cancer*.)

thyroid hormones The three hormones produced by the *thyroid gland* are thyroxine (T_4) and triiodothyronine (T_3), which regulate metabolism, and *calcitonin*, which helps to regulate calcium levels in the body.

thyroiditis Inflammation of the *thyroid gland*. Thyroiditis occurs in several different forms. The most common is *Hashimoto's thyroiditis*, an *autoimmune* *disorder* that results in *hypothyroidism*. Less commonly, the inflammation is associated with a viral infection, or it may occur temporarily soon after childbirth; in both these cases, long-term damage to the gland is uncommon.

thyroid scanning Techniques, such as *radionuclide scanning* and *ultrasound scanning*, that are used to provide information about the location, anatomy, and function of the *thyroid gland*.

thyrotoxicosis Overactivity of the thyroid gland, also called *hyperthyroidism*.

thyroxine The most important *thyroid hormone*. Thyroxine is represented by the symbol T_4.

TIA The abbreviation for *transient ischaemic attack*.

tiabendazole An *anthelmintic drug* used to treat *worm infestations*, including *strongyloidiasis*.

tibia Also called the shin, the inner and thicker of the two long bones in the lower leg. The tibia runs parallel to the *fibula*, the narrower bone to which it is attached by *ligaments*. The upper end articulates with the *femur* to form the *knee* joint; the lower end articulates with the *talus* to form part of the *ankle* joint. On the inside of the ankle, the tibia is widened and forms a bony prominence called the medial malleolus.

TIBIA

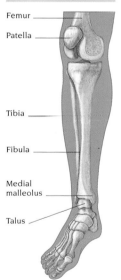

Femur
Patella
Tibia
Fibula
Medial malleolus
Talus

tibolone A drug used for short-term treatment of symptoms during the *menopause*. Tibolone combines the actions of *oestrogen drugs* and *progestogen drugs*. Possible side effects include irregular vaginal bleeding, changes in weight, ankle *oedema*, dizziness, skin reactions, headache, *migraine*, growth of facial hair, *depression*, and *myalgia*. Tibolone is also used to treat *osteoporosis* (although it is not recommended as a first-line treatment).

tic A repeated, uncontrolled, purposeless contraction of a *muscle* or group of muscles, most commonly in the face, arms, or shoulders. Typical tics include blinking, mouth twitching, and shrugging. Tics usually develop in childhood and may be associated with stress. They usually stop within a year of onset but in some cases persist into adult life. (See also *Gilles de la Tourette's syndrome*.)

tic douloureux An alternative name for *trigeminal neuralgia*.

ticks and disease Small, eight-legged animals that feed on blood and sometimes transmit diseases to humans via their bites. Ticks are about 3 mm long before feeding and become larger when bloated with blood. Ticks may be picked up in long grass, scrub, woodland, or caves.

In the UK, the only disease known to be transmitted to humans by ticks is *Lyme disease*. Others transmitted in various parts of the world include *relapsing fever*, *Rocky Mountain spotted fever*, *Q fever*, *tularaemia*, and certain types of viral *encephalitis*. The prolonged bite of certain female ticks can cause tick paralysis, in which a toxin in the tick saliva affects the nerves that control movement. In extreme cases, this can be fatal.

Tietze's syndrome Chest pain localized to an area on the front of the chest wall, usually made worse by movement of the arms or trunk or by pressure on the chest wall. The syndrome is caused by inflammation of one or several rib cartilages and symptoms may persist for months. Treatment is with *analgesics*, *nonsteroidal anti-inflammatory drugs*, or local injections of *corticosteroid drugs* into the cartilage.

timolol A *beta-blocker drug* used to treat *hypertension* and *angina pectoris*. Timolol may also be given after a *myocardial infarction*. It is used as eye-drops to treat *glaucoma*. Possible side effects, such as cold hands and feet, are typical of other beta-blockers. Eye-drops may cause irritation, blurred vision, and headache.

tinea Any of a group of common *fungal infections* of the skin, hair, or nails. Most are caused by fungi called dermatophytes. The infections may be acquired from another person, an animal, soil, the floors of showers, or from household objects, such as chairs or carpets.

The most common type of tinea infection is tinea pedis (*athlete's foot*). Tinea corporis causes itchy, usually circular, patches on the body. Tinea cruris (jock itch) produces a reddened, itchy area spreading from the genitals over the inside of the thighs. Tinea capitis causes round, itchy, patches of hair loss on the scalp; it occurs mainly in children. Ringworm of the nails (tinea unguium) is often accompanied by scaling of the soles or palms. The nails become thick and turn white or yellow.

Most types are diagnosed by appearance and by culturing the organisms in a laboratory. Treatment is usually with either topical or oral *antifungal drugs*.

tingling See *pins-and-needles*.

tinidazole An *antibacterial* drug that is particularly useful in treating *anaerobic* infections. Side effects may include nausea, vomiting, gastrointestinal disturbances, headache, and dizziness.

tinnitus A ringing, buzzing, whistling, hissing, or other noise heard in the ear or ears in the absence of a noise in the environment. Tinnitus is almost always associated with hearing loss, particularly that due to *presbyacusis* and exposure to loud noise. It can also occur as a symptom of ear disorders such as *labyrinthitis*, *Ménière's disease*, *otitis media*, *otosclerosis*, *ototoxicity*, and blockage of the ear canal with earwax. It may also be caused by certain drugs, such as *aspirin* or *quinine*, or may follow a *head injury*.

Any underlying disorder is treated if possible. Many sufferers make use of a radio, television, cassette player, or headphones to block out the noise in their ears. A tinnitus masker, a hearing-aid type device that plays white noise (a random mixture of sounds at a wide range of frequencies), may be effective.

tinzaparin A type of low molecular weight *heparin* that may be injected once daily in the treatment or prevention of deep vein thrombosis (see *thrombosis, deep vein*).

tiredness A common complaint that is usually the result of overwork or poor quality, or insufficient sleep. Persistent tiredness may be caused by a number of conditions, including *depression, anxiety, anaemia*, and *diabetes*.

tissue A collection of *cells* specialized to perform a particular function.

tissue fluid The watery liquid present in the tiny gaps between body cells, also known as interstitial fluid.

tissue-plasminogen activator A substance produced by body tissues that prevents abnormal *blood clotting*. Also called TPA, it is produced by the inner lining of blood vessels. TPA can be prepared artificially for use as a *thrombolytic drug*, which is called alteplase. This is used in the treatment of acute *myocardial infarction, pulmonary embolism*, and acute *stroke*. Possible side effects include bleeding or the formation of a *haematoma* at the injection site and an allergic reaction. (See also *fibrinolysis*.)

tissue-typing The classification of certain characteristics of the *tissues* of prospective organ donors and recipients (see *transplant surgery*). This minimizes the risk of *rejection* of a donor organ by the recipient's *immune system*.

A person's tissue type is classified in terms of their *histocompatibility antigens*, the most important of which are the human leukocyte antigens (HLAs), on the surface of cells. A person's set of HLAs is inherited and unique (except for identical twins, who have the same set). Nevertheless, close relatives often have closely matching HLA types. A person's tissue-type is established by laboratory tests on cells from a blood sample. In one method, an antiserum containing *antibodies* to a particular HLA is added to the test specimen. If the HLA is present, it is detected by an observable colour or other change.

titanium dental implants See *implants, dental*.

TMJ syndrome See *temporomandibular joint syndrome*.

toadstool poisoning See *mushroom poisoning*.

tobacco The dried leaf of the plant NICOTIANA TABACUM. Tobacco is used for *smoking*, chewing, or as snuff by billions of people. It contains a variable percentage of *nicotine*, and several carcinogenic substances. There is a direct proportion between the amount of tobacco used, the period over which it is used, and the likelihood of *cancer*. Smokers are at increased risk of several types of cancer, including *lung cancer, bladder cancer, kidney cancer,* and pancreatic cancer (see *pancreas, cancer of*). Smoking also increases the risk of *coronary artery disease, stroke, emphysema,* and chronic *bronchitis,* and it exacerbates *asthma* and *Raynaud's phenomenon.* In addition, children living with smokers have an increased risk of most respiratory disorders and *sudden infant death syndrome.* All tobacco users have an increased risk of cancers of the oral cavity (see *mouth cancer*), pharynx (see *pharynx, cancer of*), larynx (see *larynx, cancer of*) and oesophagus (see *oesophagus, cancer of*).

tobacco-smoking See *smoking.*

tobramycin An *antibiotic drug* used to treat serious infections such as *peritonitis, meningitis,* and severe infections of the lungs, skin, bones, and joints. In eye-drop form, it is sometimes used to treat *conjunctivitis* and *blepharitis.* High doses of injected tobramycin may cause kidney damage, deafness, nausea, vomiting, and headache. Any preparation of tobramycin may cause rash and itching.

tocography An obstetric procedure for recording muscular contractions of the uterus during *childbirth.* It is usually combined with *fetal heart monitoring* (see *cardiotocography*).

tocopherol A constituent of *vitamin E.* Four tocopherols (alpha, beta, gamma, and delta) and several tocopherol derivatives together make up the vitamin.

toddler's diarrhoea A common condition affecting some children for a period after the introduction of an adult diet. It occurs because the child is unable to digest food properly, perhaps because of inadequate chewing; the diarrhoea contains recognizable pieces of food. This diarrhoea is no cause for concern, and no treatment is needed.

Todd's paralysis Weakness in part of the body following some types of epileptic seizure (see *epilepsy*). The weakness may last for minutes, hours, or even days, but there is no lasting effect. The cause is thought to be temporary damage to the motor cortex (the area of the *brain* that controls movement).

toe One of the digits of the foot. Each toe has three *phalanges* (bones), except for the *hallux* (big toe), which has two. The phalanges join at hinge joints. An artery, vein, and nerve run down each side of the toe, and the whole structure is enclosed in skin with a nail at the top. The main function of the toes is to maintain balance during walking. *Congenital* disorders include toes missing at birth. (See also *polydactyly; syndactyly; webbing.*)

toenail, ingrowing A painful condition of a toe (usually the big toe) in which one or both edges of the *nail* press into the adjacent skin, leading to infection and inflammation. The cause is usually incorrect cutting of the nail or wearing tight shoes. Temporary pain relief can be obtained by bathing the foot once or twice daily in a warm, strong salt solution, then covering the nail with a dry gauze dressing. *Antibiotics* may be prescribed. In some cases, the edge of the nail is removed and the nail bed obliterated to prevent recurrence.

toilet-training The process of teaching a young child to acquire complete bowel and bladder control. A child is unlikely to be completely toilet-trained before age 3 and may normally take much longer to remain dry at night (see *enuresis*).

tolbutamide An oral hypoglycaemic drug (see *hypoglycaemics, oral*) used in the treatment of type 2 *diabetes mellitus.*

tolerance The need to take increasingly higher doses of a *drug* to obtain the same physical or mental effect. Tolerance develops after taking a drug over a period of time and usually results either from the liver becoming more efficient at breaking the drug down or from body tissues becoming less sensitive to it.

tolnaftate An *antifungal drug* applied to the skin to treat, and sometimes prevent, recurrent *tinea* infections, including *athlete's foot.* In rare cases, tolnaftate may cause skin irritation or a rash.

tomography An *imaging technique* that produces a cross-sectional image ("slice") of an organ or part of the body. Most tomography today is performed using *CT scanning* and *MRI,* which produce accurate and detailed images.

-tomy A suffix denoting the operation of cutting or making an incision.

tone, muscle The natural tension in the *muscle* fibres. At rest, all muscle fibres are kept in a state of partial contraction by nerve impulses from the spinal cord. Abnormally high muscle tone causes an increased resistance to movement, *spasticity*, and rigidity. Abnormally low muscle tone causes floppiness (see *hypotonia*; *hypotonia in infants*).

tongue A muscular, flexible organ in the floor of the *mouth* that is composed of a mass of muscles covered by a *mucous membrane*. The muscles are attached to the *mandible* (lower jaw) and *hyoid* bone above the *larynx*. Tiny nodules called papillae stick out from the tongue's upper surface, giving it a rough texture. Most of the tongue's *taste buds* are located on the papillae. Taste signals are picked up by nerve fibres from one of four *cranial nerves*, and impulses then travel to the brain. The tongue plays an essential part in *mastication*, *swallowing*, and *speech*.

tongue cancer The most serious type of *mouth cancer* due to its rapid spread. It mainly affects people over 40 and is associated with *smoking*, heavy alcohol consumption, and poor oral hygiene. The edge of the tongue is most commonly affected. The first sign may be a small ulcer with a raised margin, a *leukoplakia*, a fissure, or a raised, hard mass.

Diagnosis of tongue cancer is made by a *biopsy*. Small tumours, especially those occurring at the tip of the tongue, are usually removed surgically. Larger tumours or those that have spread often require *radiotherapy*.

tongue depressor A flat wooden or metal instrument used to hold the tongue on the floor of the mouth to allow examination of the throat.

tongue-tie A minor *mouth* defect, also known as ankyloglossia, in which the frenulum (the band of tissue attaching the underside of the tongue to the floor of the mouth) is too short and extends forwards to the tip of the tongue. There are usually no symptoms apart from limited movement of the tongue. Rarely, the condition causes a speech defect, and a minor operation is required to divide the frenulum.

tonic One of a diverse group of remedies intended to relieve symptoms such as malaise, lethargy, and loss of appetite. Evidence suggests that tonics mainly have a *placebo* effect. The term tonic is also used adjectivally to relate to muscle tone (see *tone, muscle*), as in the tonic neck reflex, one of the primitive *reflexes* found in newborn infants.

tonometry The procedure for measuring the pressure of the fluid within the *eye*, usually performed by an ophthalmologist during an eye examination (see *eye, examination of*). Tonometry is useful in diagnosing *glaucoma*.

tonsil One of a pair of oval tissue masses at the back of the throat on either side. The tonsils are made up of lymphoid tissue and form part of the *lymphatic system*. Along with the *adenoids*, at the base of the tongue, the tonsils protect against upper respiratory tract infections. The tonsils gradually enlarge from birth until the age of 7, after which time they shrink substantially. *Tonsillitis* is a common childhood infection.

TONSIL

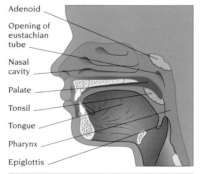

Adenoid
Opening of eustachian tube
Nasal cavity
Palate
Tonsil
Tongue
Pharynx
Epiglottis

tonsillectomy Surgical removal of the *tonsils*, which is now performed only if a child suffers frequent, recurrent attacks of severe *tonsillitis*. The operation is also carried out to treat *quinsy* (an abscess around the tonsil).

tonsillitis Inflammation of the *tonsils* as a result of infection. Tonsillitis mainly occurs in children under age 9. Sometimes the tonsils become repeatedly infected by the microorganisms they are supposed to protect against. The main symptoms are a sore throat and difficulty in swallowing. The throat is visibly inflamed. Other common symptoms are fever, headache, earache, enlarged and tender *lymph nodes* in the neck, and bad breath. Occasionally, there may be temporary deafness or *quinsy* (an abscess around the tonsil).

Tonsillitis is treated with plenty of fluids and an *analgesic drug* such as paracetamol; in some cases *antibiotic drugs* may also be prescribed.

tooth See *teeth.*

tooth abscess See *abscess, dental.*

toothache Pain in one or more *teeth* and sometimes the *gums.* Causes include dental *caries*, a tooth fracture (see *fracture, dental*), a deep, unlined filling (see *filling, dental*), *periodontitis*, a dental abscess (see *abscess, dental*), a blow to a tooth, or referred pain from *sinusitis. Analgesic drugs* may provide temporary relief. Treatment depends on the cause.

toothbrushing Cleaning of the *teeth* with a brush to remove *plaque* and food particles from tooth surfaces and to stimulate the gums. Toothbrushing should be carried out twice a day using a fluoride *dentifrice* (usually toothpaste).

tooth decay See *caries, dental.*

tooth extraction See *extraction, dental.*

toothpaste See *dentifrice.*

tophus A collection of *uric acid* crystals deposited in tissues, especially around joints, but occasionally in other places such as the ear. It is a sign of *hyperuricaemia*, which accompanies *gout.*

topical A term describing a *drug* that is applied to the surface of the body, not swallowed or injected.

torsion A term that means twisting, often applied to the intestine or *testis.*

torticollis Twisting of the neck, causing the head to be tilted and fixed in an abnormal position (wry neck). There is often neck pain and stiffness. The cause is usually a minor neck injury that irritates *cervical* nerves, leading to *muscle spasm.* Other causes are sleeping in an awkward position, a neck-muscle injury at birth, and a burn or injury that has caused heavy scarring.

Torticollis due to muscle spasm may be treated with *nonsteroidal anti-inflammatory drugs, heat treatment, ultrasound treatment*, or *physiotherapy.* In severe cases, torticollis may be treated with injections of *botulinum toxin.* When the cause is an injury arising from birth, the muscle is gently stretched several times a day; occasionally, an operation is necessary.

touch The sense by which certain characteristics of objects, such as their size, shape, temperature, and surface texture, can be ascertained by physical contact.

TOUCH

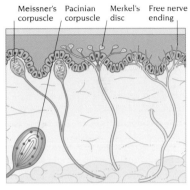

TOUCH RECEPTORS IN SKIN

The skin has many types of touch *receptors*, including Merkel's discs and Meissner's corpuscles to detect light touch, and Pacinian corpuscles to sense deep pressure and vibration. Signals from these receptors pass, via sensory nerves, to the spinal cord, from there to the *thalamus* in the brain, and on to the *sensory cortex*, where touch sensations are perceived and interpreted.

The various parts of the body differ in their sensitivity to painful stimuli and in touch discrimination. For example, the cornea is several hundred times more sensitive to painful stimuli than the soles of the feet. (See also *sensation.*)

Tourette's syndrome See *Gilles de la Tourette's syndrome.*

tourniquet A device placed around a limb to compress blood vessels. A tourniquet may be used to help locate a vein for an intravenous injection or for the withdrawal of blood. An inflatable tourniquet, called an *Esmarch's bandage*, is used to control blood flow in some limb operations. The use of a tourniquet as a first-aid measure to stop severe bleeding can cause *gangrene*.

toxaemia Presence in the bloodstream of *toxins* produced by *bacteria*. (See also *pre-eclampsia*; *toxic shock syndrome*.)

toxaemia of pregnancy See *pre-eclampsia*.

toxicity The property of being toxic (poisonous). Toxicity also refers to the severity of adverse effects or illness produced by a *toxin*, a *poison*, or a drug overdose.

toxicology The study of *poisons*. (See also *poisoning*.)

toxic shock syndrome An uncommon, severe illness caused by a *toxin* produced by the bacterium STAPHYLOCOCCUS AUREUS. Many cases occur in women using vaginal tampons. Other cases have been linked to use of a contraceptive cap or diaphragm (see *contraception*), or to skin wounds or infections by the bacterium elsewhere in the body. A high fever, vomiting, diarrhoea, headache, muscle aches and pains, dizziness, and disorientation develop suddenly. A widespread skin rash that resembles sunburn and also affects the palms and soles, develops. Blood pressure may fall dangerously low, and *shock* may develop. Other complications include *kidney failure* and *liver failure*. Treatment in an intensive care unit may be needed.

toxin A poisonous protein produced by pathogenic (disease-causing) bacteria, various animals, or some plants. Bacterial toxins are sometimes subdivided into three categories: *endotoxins*, which are released from dead bacteria; *exotoxins*, which are released from live bacteria; and *enterotoxins*, which inflame the intestine. (See also *poison*; *poisoning*; *toxaemia*.)

toxocariasis An infestation of humans, usually children, with the larvae of TOXOCARA CANIS: a small, threadlike worm that lives in the intestines of dogs. Children who play with an infested dog or soil contaminated with dog faeces, and who then put their fingers in their mouths, may swallow some of the worm eggs. The eggs hatch in the intestines, and the released larvae migrate to organs such as the liver, lungs, brain, and eyes. Usually, infestation causes mild fever and *malaise*, which soon clears up; but heavy infestation may lead to *pneumonia* and *seizures*. Loss of vision may occur if larvae enter the eye and die there.

A diagnosis is made from sputum analysis, and by a *liver biopsy*. Severe cases require treatment in hospital with an *anthelmintic drug* and an *anticonvulsant drug*.

toxoid An inactivated bacterial *toxin*. Certain toxoids are used to immunize against specific diseases, such as *tetanus*.

toxoplasmosis An infection caused by the *protozoan* TOXOPLASMA GONDII that is often caused by eating undercooked meat from infected animals, or by handling faeces from infected cats. In most cases there are no symptoms, but sometimes there may be a feverish illness that resembles infectious *mononucleosis*. Retinitis (inflammation of the retina) and *choroiditis* may also develop. In people with an *immunodeficiency disorder* toxoplasmosis may cause lung and heart damage and severe *encephalitis*.

Toxoplasmosis contracted by a pregnant woman is transmitted to the fetus in about a third of cases. It may result in *miscarriage* or *stillbirth*, or the infant may have an enlarged liver and spleen, blindness, *hydrocephalus*, learning difficulties, or may die during infancy. Infection in late pregnancy usually has no ill effects.

The diagnosis is made from *blood tests*. Treatment (with *pyrimethamine* and a *sulphonamide drug*) is necessary only in pregnant women, in children with severe symptoms, in people with an immune system deficiency, and in cases of retinitis or choroiditis.

TPA The abbreviation used for *tissue-plasminogen activator*.

trabeculectomy A surgical procedure to control *glaucoma* by allowing the fluid from the front chamber of the eye to drain out under the conjunctiva.

trace elements *Minerals* necessary in minute amounts in the diet to maintain health. Examples are *chromium*, *copper*, *zinc*, and *selenium*. (See also *nutrition*.)

tracer A radioactive substance that is introduced into the body so that its distribution, processing, and elimination from the body can be monitored.

trachea The air passage, also called the windpipe, that runs from immediately below the *larynx* to behind the

TRACHEA

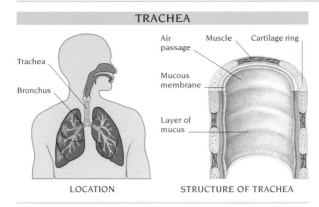

Air passage   Muscle   Cartilage ring

Trachea

Bronchus

Mucous membrane

Layer of mucus

LOCATION   STRUCTURE OF TRACHEA

upper part of the *sternum*, where it divides to form the *bronchi*. The trachea is made of fibrous and elastic tissue and smooth muscle. It also contains about 20 rings of *cartilage*, which keep it open. The lining of the trachea has cells (goblet cells) that secrete mucus and cells with *cilia*, which beat the mucus upwards to help keep the lungs and airways clear.

tracheitis Inflammation of the *trachea*. Tracheitis is usually caused by a viral infection and is aggravated by inhaled fumes, especially tobacco smoke. It often occurs with *laryngitis* and *bronchitis* in a condition known as laryngotracheobronchitis. Symptoms include a painful dry cough and hoarseness. In most cases, no treatment is needed.

tracheoesophageal fistula A rare birth defect in which an abnormal passage connects the *trachea* with the *oesophagus*. About 3 babies per 10,000 are born with this *fistula*.

The condition is often discovered soon after birth; diagnosis may be confirmed by *X-rays*. Treatment consists of an operation to close the fistula and connect the trachea and oesophagus correctly.

tracheostomy An operation in which an opening is made in the *trachea* and a tube is inserted to maintain an effective airway. A tracheostomy is used for the emergency treatment of airway problems involving the *larynx*. A planned tracheostomy is most commonly performed on a person who has lost the ability to breathe naturally and is undergoing long-term *ventilation* or who is unable to keep saliva and other secretions out of the trachea. Permanent tracheostomy is needed after a *laryngectomy*.

tracheotomy Cutting of the *trachea*. (See also *tracheostomy*.)

trachoma A persistent infectious disease of the *cornea* and *conjunctiva*. Trachoma is caused by CHLAMYDIA TRACHOMATIS and is spread by direct contact and possibly by flies (see *chlamydial infections*). It is uncommon in the UK, but, worldwide, is the most common cause of blindness.

tract Any one of a group of organs that form a common pathway to perform a particular function. The term also refers to a bundle of nerve fibres that have a common function.

traction A procedure in which part of the body is placed under tension to correct the alignment of two adjoining structures or to hold them in position. Traction is most commonly used to treat a *fracture* in which muscles around the bone ends are pulling the bones out of alignment.

training A programme of exercises that is undertaken to prepare for a particular sport. Training may be concentrated on improving skills or on improving physical *fitness*. Fitness training should include both *aerobic* and anaerobic exercises, which together build up strength, flexibility, and endurance. Interval training is a type of fitness programme in which a particular exercise is repeated several times with a rest period between. Circuit training consists of performing a set number of different exercises.

trait Any characteristic or condition that is inherited (determined by one or more *genes*). Blue or brown eye colour, dark or light skin, body proportions, and nose shape are examples of genetic traits. The term trait is also sometimes used to describe a mild form of a recessive *genetic disorder*.

tramadol An *opioid drug* used to relieve severe pain following a heart attack, surgery, or serious illness. It is less likely to cause dependence with long-term use than most opioids. Possible side effects include nausea, vomiting, drowsiness, confusion, and impaired consciousness.

trance A sleeplike state in which consciousness is reduced, voluntary actions lessened or absent, and body functions diminished. Trances are claimed to be induced by *hypnosis* and have been reported as part of a group experience. Trances may be a feature of *catalepsy*, *automatism*, and petit mal *epilepsy*.

tranexamic acid An antifibrinolytic drug that promotes *blood clotting*. It is used to treat *menorrhagia*. Possible side effects include diarrhoea, nausea, and vomiting.

tranquillizer drugs Drugs that have a sedative effect. Tranquillizers are divided into two types: major tranquillizers (see *antipsychotic drugs*) and minor tranquillizers (see *antianxiety drugs*).

transcutaneous electrical nerve stimulation See *TENS*

transdermal patch A method of administering a drug through the skin. The drug is released from the patch over a period of time and is absorbed by the skin.

TRANSDERMAL PATCH

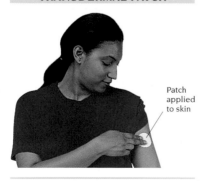

Patch applied to skin

transference The unconscious displacement of emotions from people who were important during one's childhood, such as parents, to other people during adulthood. (See also *psychoanalysis*.)

transfusion See *blood transfusion*.

transfusion, autologous See *blood transfusion, autologous*.

transient ischaemic attack (TIA) A brief interruption of the blood supply to part of the brain, which causes temporary impairment of vision, speech, sensation, or movement. The episode typically lasts for a few minutes or a few hours but symptoms disappear completely within 24 hours. TIAs are sometimes described as mini strokes, and they can be the prelude to a *stroke*.

TIAs may be caused by a blood clot (see *embolism*) temporarily blocking an artery that supplies the brain, or by narrowing of an artery as a result of *atherosclerosis*.

After a TIA, tests such as *CT scanning*, *blood tests*, *ultrasound scanning*, or *angiography* may be needed to determine a cause. In some cases, the heart is studied as a possible source of blood clots. Treatment is aimed at preventing stroke, which occurs within 1 year in up to 10 per cent of patients with TIA. Treatments include *endarterectomy*, *anticoagulant drugs*, or *aspirin*. It is also important to treat any risk factors, such as *hypertension* and high blood cholesterol. Stopping smoking is essential.

transillumination A procedure that is sometimes carried out during physical examination of a lump or swelling. Light from a small torch is shone on one side of the lump; if it can be seen on the other side, the lump contains clear fluid.

translocation A rearrangement of the *chromosomes* inside a person's cells; it is a type of *mutation*. Sections of chromosomes may be exchanged or the main parts of two chromosomes may be joined. A translocation may be inherited or acquired as the result of a new mutation.

A translocation often has no obvious effect, and causes no abnormality. However, in some cases, it can mean that some of the affected person's egg or sperm cells carry too much or too little chromosomal material, which may cause a *chromosomal abnormality*, such as *Down's syndrome*, in his or her children.

transmissible A term meaning capable of being passed from one person, or one organism, to another.

transplant surgery Replacement of a diseased organ or tissue with a healthy, living substitute. The organ is usually taken from a person who has just died. Some kidneys are transplanted from a patient's living relatives (see *organ donation*). The results of surgery have also been improved by testing for *histocompatibility antigens* and *tissue-typing*.

Rejection is a major problem. Every patient who undergoes an organ transplant operation must take *immunosuppressant drugs* indefinitely. (See also *heart transplant*; *heart–lung transplant*; *liver transplant*; *kidney transplant*.)

transposition of the great vessels A serious form of congenital *heart disease* in which the *aorta* and pulmonary artery are transposed. *Open heart surgery* is needed to correct the defect.

transsexualism A rare disorder in which a person wishes to live as a member of the opposite sex. Transsexuals commonly seek hormonal or surgical treatment to bring about a physical *sex change*. A psychiatric evaluation and a physical examination are necessary before such treatment is undertaken.

transvestism Also called cross-dressing, a persistent desire by a man to dress in women's clothing.

tranylcypromine An *antidepressant drug* that belongs to the *monoamine oxidase inhibitor* (MAOI) group and is used mainly in patients with severe depression.

trapezius muscle A large, diamond-shaped *muscle* extending from the back of the skull to the lower part of the spine in the chest and across the width of the shoulders. It is attached to the top and back of the shoulderblade and to the outermost part of the collarbone. The trapezius helps support the neck and spine and is involved in moving the arm.

trapped nerve See *nerve, trapped*.

trastuzumab More commonly known by its brand name Herceptin, a monoclonal antibody (see *antibody, monoclonal*) used to treat some cases of advanced *breast cancer* in which the cancer has metastasized. It may be used alone or with *chemotherapy*. Possible side effects include headache, diarrhoea, gastrointestinal disturbances, breathing problems, rash, and heart damage.

trauma A physical injury or severe emotional shock. (See also *post-traumatic stress disorder*.)

trauma surgery See *traumatology*.

traumatology Emergency treatment of patients suffering from acute trauma (such as severe and/or multiple injuries).

travel immunization Anyone planning to travel abroad may need *immunizations* before departure. Although few immunizations are compulsory for international travel, some are recommended for the traveller's protection.

Travel agents and tour operators often include information about which immunizations may be needed, but travellers should consult a doctor or qualified nurse about individual requirements. Some vaccines must be given in 2–3 doses several weeks apart. Therefore, a doctor or nurse should be consulted at least 3 months before departure. Children under 1 year, and people with a compromised immune system or serious underlying disorder may not be able to have some vaccinations, such as those for yellow fever and tuberculosis (BCG).

traveller's diarrhoea A disorder occurring in people who are visiting foreign countries. Episodes of diarrhoea range in severity and are due to *gastroenteritis*. Attention to hygiene, drinking bottled water, and avoiding ice in drinks can prevent a large proportion of episodes.

travel sickness See *motion sickness*.

trazodone An *antidepressant drug* with a strong sedative effect that is used to treat *depression* accompanied by *anxiety* or *insomnia*. Possible side effects include drowsiness, constipation, dry mouth, dizziness, and, rarely, *priapism*.

treatment Any measure that is taken to prevent or cure a disease or disorder or to relieve symptoms.

trematode The scientific name for any *fluke* or *schistosome*.

trembling See *tremor*.

tremor An involuntary, rhythmic, oscillating movement in the *muscles* of part of the body, most commonly those of the hands, feet, jaw, tongue, or head. Tremor is the result of rapidly alternating muscle contraction and relaxation. Occasional tremors are experienced by most people and are due to increased production of the hormone *adrenaline* (epinephrine). A slight, persistent tremor is common in elderly people.

Essential tremor, which runs in families, is a slight-to-moderate tremor that may be temporarily relieved by consuming a small amount of alcohol or by taking *beta-blocker drugs.*

Coarse tremor (4–5 muscle movements per second), which is present at rest but reduced during movement, is often a sign of *Parkinson's disease.* An intention tremor (tremor that is worse on movement of the affected part) may be a sign of *cerebellar ataxia.* Tremor may also be caused by *multiple sclerosis, Wilson's disease, mercury poisoning, thyrotoxicosis,* or hepatic *encephalopathy;* drugs, such as *amphetamines* and *caffeine;* and withdrawal from drugs, including *alcohol.*

trench fever An infectious disease that is now rare or unknown in most parts of the world. The disease is caused by *rickettsiae* spread by body *lice.* Symptoms include headache, muscle pains, and fever, which may occur in bouts. Treatment is with *antibiotic drugs.*

trench foot See *immersion foot.*

trench mouth See *gingivitis, acute ulcerative.*

trephine A hollow, cylindrical instrument with a saw-toothed edge used for cutting a circular hole, usually in bone.

tretinoin A *topical* drug that is chemically related to *vitamin A* and is mainly used to treat *acne.* Tretinoin may aggravate acne in the first few weeks of treatment but usually improves the condition within 3–4 months. Possible side effects include irritation, peeling, and discoloration of the skin. Exposure of the skin to sunlight while using tretinoin may aggravate irritation and can lead to *sunburn.*

trial, clinical A test on human volunteers of the effectiveness and safety of a drug. A trial can also involve systematic comparison of alternative forms of medical or surgical treatment for a particular disorder. Patients involved in clinical trials have to give their consent, and the trials are approved and supervised by an ethics committee.

triamcinolone A *corticosteroid drug* that is used to treat inflammation of the mouth, gums, skin, and joints; *asthma;* allergic rhinitis (see *rhinitis, allergic*); and certain blood disorders, such as *thrombocytopenia* and *leukaemia.*

triamterene A *diuretic drug* used to treat *hypertension* and *oedema.* Possible adverse effects include nausea, vomiting, weakness, and rash.

tribavirin see *ribavirin.*

triceps muscle The *muscle* at the back of the upper arm. At the upper end of the triceps are three "heads"; one is attached to the outer edge of the *scapula* (shoulderblade), and the other two to either side of the *humerus* (upper-arm bone). The lower part of the triceps is attached to the olecranon process of the ulna (the bony prominence on the elbow). Contraction of the muscle straightens the arm. (See also *biceps muscle.*)

trichiasis An alteration in the direction of eyelash growth, in which the lashes grow inwards towards the eyeball. They can rub against the eye, causing severe discomfort and sometimes damage to the *cornea. Trachoma* is a cause.

trichinosis An infestation with the larvae of the TRICHINELLA SPIRALIS worm, usually acquired by eating undercooked pork. Trichinosis is rare in the UK. Thorough cooking of all pork products, and freezing meat to a temperature below −18°C for 24 hours, helps to avoid infection. Slight infestation usually causes no symptoms. However, heavy infestation may cause diarrhoea and vomiting within a day or two of eating the infected meat, followed by fever, swelling around the eyelids, and severe muscle pains, which may last for several weeks. Trichinosis may be suspected from the symptoms, and the diagnosis is confirmed by *blood tests,* or by a muscle *biopsy.* Treatment of the infestation is with an *anthelmintic drug.*

trichomoniasis An infection caused by the *protozoan* TRICHOMONAS VAGINALIS. Trichomoniasis is a common cause of *vaginitis.* In some cases, the infection is sexually transmitted.

In women, the causative organism may inhabit the *vagina* for years without causing symptoms. If symptoms occur, they include painful inflammation of the vagina and *vulva*, and a greenish, frothy, offensive-smelling discharge. Men usually have no symptoms.

The diagnosis is made from examination of a sample of the discharge. Diagnosis is usually difficult in men. Treatment is with *metronidazole*. The sexual partner or partners of an infected person should be treated at the same time to prevent reinfection.

trichotillomania The habit of constantly pulling out one's hair. It can be associated with severe *learning difficulties* or with a psychotic illness. It may also occur in psychologically disturbed children. The sufferer typically pulls, twists, and breaks off chunks of hair from the scalp, leaving bald patches; occasionally, pubic hair is pulled out. Children sometimes eat the removed hair, which may form a hairball in the stomach, known medically as a trichobezoar (see *bezoar*). Treatment depends on the cause, and may consist of *psychotherapy* or *antipsychotic drugs*.

trichuriasis A parasitic infestation with the tropical worm TRICHURIS TRICHURIA (whipworm). Children are most commonly affected. Infestation occurs when eggs are ingested and develop into adult worms in the intestines. Severe infestation may cause bloody diarrhoea, abdominal pain, and weight loss. Treatment is with *anthelmintic drugs*.

triclosan An *antiseptic*.

tricuspid incompetence Failure of the *tricuspid valve* to close fully, allowing blood to leak back into the right atrium when the right ventricle contracts. The condition, which is also known as tricuspid insufficiency, reduces the pumping efficiency of the heart. The usual cause is *pulmonary hypertension*, but more rarely, it follows *rheumatic fever*, or, in intravenous drug users, a bacterial infection of the heart.

Tricuspid incompetence results in symptoms of right-sided *heart failure*, notably *oedema* of the ankles and abdomen. The liver is swollen and tender, and veins in the neck are distended.

A diagnosis is made from the symptoms, from hearing a heart *murmur* through a stethoscope, and by tests that may include an *ECG, chest X-rays*, echo-cardiography, and cardiac *catheterization*. Treatment with *diuretic drugs* and *ACE inhibitors* often relieves the symptoms. In severe cases, surgery may be recommended.

tricuspid stenosis Narrowing of the opening of the *tricuspid valve*, usually caused by a previous attack of *rheumatic fever*. Tricuspid stenosis is uncommon and often occurs with another heart-valve disorder. For example, *tricuspid incompetence* may also occur in intravenous drug users who have a bacterial infection of the heart. Tricuspid stenosis causes enlargement of the right atrium. The symptoms and diagnosis are similar to those of tricuspid incompetence. Treatment of tricuspid stenosis is carried out with *diuretic drugs* and sometimes a *digitalis drug*. Heart valve surgery is sometimes needed.

tricuspid valve A valve in the *heart* consisting of three flaps that lies between the right atrium and the right ventricle. It ensures that blood flow from the atrium to the ventricle is in one direction only.

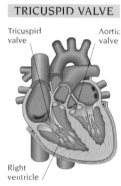

TRICUSPID VALVE

Tricuspid valve

Aortic valve

Right ventricle

STRUCTURE OF HEART

tricyclic antidepressants A type of *antidepressant drug*. Tricyclic antidepressants prevent *neurotransmitters* in the brain from being reabsorbed, thereby increasing their level. Examples are *amitriptyline, clomipramine*, and *imipramine*.

trifluoperazine An *antipsychotic drug* used to treat *schizophrenia*.

trigeminal nerve The 5th *cranial nerve*. The trigeminal nerves, one on each side of the face, arise from the *brainstem*. Both nerves divide into three branches that supply sensation to the face, scalp, nose, teeth, lining of the mouth, upper eyelid, *sinuses*, and the front portion of the tongue. They stimulate *saliva* and *tear* production and contraction of *jaw* muscles for chewing.

trigeminal neuralgia A disorder of the *trigeminal nerve* in which brief episodes of severe, stabbing pain affect the cheek, lips, gums, or chin on one side of the face. The disorder usually occurs over age 50. Pain may come in bouts that last for weeks at a time. The cause is uncertain, and pain is often brought on by touching the face, eating, drinking, or talking. *Analgesic drugs* may be tried, but often, *carbamazepine* is more effective. If this fails, surgery may help.

trigger finger Locking of one or several fingers in a bent position due to inflammation of the sheath enclosing the *tendon* of the affected finger. The finger is usually tender at the base and slightly swollen over the tendon. Treatment involves local injection of a *corticosteroid drug* or, if this is unsuccessful, surgery.

triglyceride A type of simple fat (see *fats and oils*) made up of a molecule of *glycerol* and three molecules of fatty acids. Triglycerides are the main type of fat found in stores of body fat.

trimeprazine Also called alimemazine. An *antihistamine drug* used to relieve itching in allergic conditions, and as a *premedication* in children. Side effects are typical of antihistamines.

trimester A period of 3 months; human *pregnancy* is conventionally divided into three trimesters.

trimethoprim An *antibacterial drug* used to treat a range of infections, most commonly those of the urinary tract. Possible side effects include rash, itching, nausea, vomiting, diarrhoea, and a sore tongue.

trimipramine A tricyclic *antidepressant drug* used to treat *depression* accompanied by *anxiety* or *insomnia*. Possible side effects of trimipramine include dry mouth, blurred vision, dizziness, constipation, and nausea.

triprolidine An *antihistamine drug* that is used to treat *allergy*, as an ingredient of cough and cold remedies, and to treat or prevent allergic reactions to certain foods or *blood transfusions*. Possible side effects of triprolidine include dry mouth, dizziness, difficulty in passing urine, and *hyperactivity*.

trismus Involuntary contraction of the jaw muscles, which causes the mouth to become tightly closed. Commonly known as lockjaw, it may occur as a symptom of *tetanus*, *tonsillitis*, *mumps*, or acute ulcerative *gingivitis* and other dental problems affecting the back teeth. Treatment is of the underlying cause.

trisomy The presence of an extra *chromosome* within a person's cells, making three of a particular chromosome instead of the usual two. A fault during *meiosis* to form egg or sperm cells leaves an egg or sperm with an extra chromosome. When the egg or sperm takes part in fertilization, the resulting embryo inherits an extra chromosome in each of its cells.

The most common trisomy is of chromosome 21 (*Down's syndrome*). Trisomy 18 (Edward's syndrome) and trisomy 13 (Patau's syndrome) are less common; trisomy 8 and trisomy 22 are very rare. Partial trisomy, with only part of a chromosome in triplicate, also occurs. Full trisomies cause abnormalities such as skeletal and heart defects and *learning difficulties*. Except in Down's syndrome, babies usually die in early infancy. The effects of partial trisomies depend on the amount of extra chromosomal material present.

Diagnosis is made by *chromosome analysis* of cells, which may be obtained from the fetus by *amniocentesis* or after the birth. There is no specific treatment. Parents of an affected child should seek *genetic counselling*.

trisomy 21 syndrome Another name for *Down's syndrome*.

trochlear nerve The 4th *cranial nerve*. The two trochlear nerves arise in the *brainstem*, one on each side of the midbrain, and enter the eye sockets through gaps in the skull bones. Each trochlear nerve controls one of the two superior oblique muscles, which rotate the eyes downwards and outwards.

trophoblastic tumour A growth arising from the tissues that develop into the *placenta*. The most common type of trophoblastic tumour is a *hydatidiform mole*. (See also *choriocarcinoma*.)

tropical diseases Diseases prevalent in the tropics because of living conditions and diet include *malnutrition*, *measles*, *diphtheria*, *tuberculosis*, *typhoid* fever, shigellosis, cholera, amoebiasis, and *tapeworm infestation*. Diseases spread through the tropics by insects include *malaria, yellow fever, sleeping sickness*, and *leishmaniasis*. Exposure to strong sunlight in the tropics causes an increased tendency to *skin cancer*, and may lead to *pinguecula* and *pterygium*.

tropical ulcer An area of persistent skin and tissue loss caused by infection with one or more organisms. The condition is most common in malnourished people living in the tropics. Treatment is cleaning and dressing of the ulcer, a course of *antibiotic drugs*, and a high protein diet. The ulcer usually heals but may scar.

tropicamide A drug used to dilate the *pupil*. Adverse effects of the drug include blurred vision, increased sensitivity to light, stinging, and, rarely, dry mouth, flushing, and *glaucoma*.

trunk The central part of the body, comprising the chest and abdomen. The term also refers to any large blood vessel or nerve, from which smaller vessels or nerves branch off.

truss An elastic, canvas, or padded metal appliance used to hold an abdominal *hernia* in place. Trusses are only used if corrective surgery cannot be undertaken.

trypanosomiasis A tropical disease caused by *TRYPANOSOMA* parasites. (See also *sleeping sickness; Chagas'disease*.)

tsetse fly bites The bites of tsetse flies, which are found in Africa, can be painful. The flies, resembling brown houseflies, spread *sleeping sickness*.

T-tube cholangiography An *imaging technique* performed to check that there are no *gallstones* left in the bile duct after a *cholecystectomy*. A T-shaped rubber tube is inserted into the bile duct during the surgery. A week or so later, *contrast medium* is inserted into the tube and *X-rays* are taken.

tubal ligation See *sterilization, female*.

tubal pregnancy See *ectopic pregnancy*

tubercle A grey, nodular mass found in tissues affected by *tuberculosis*. The term also refers to a small rounded protrusion on the surface of a bone.

tuberculin tests Skin tests used to determine whether or not a person has been exposed to the bacterium that causes *tuberculosis*. Tuberculin tests are

carried out for diagnosis of tuberculosis, and before *BCG vaccination*. A small amount of tuberculin (purified protein from the bacteria) is injected into the skin. A few days later, the skin reaction, if any, is noted. A reaction indicates previous exposure.

tuberculosis An infectious notifiable disease, commonly called TB, caused in humans by the bacterium *MYCOBACTERIUM TUBERCULOSIS*. TB is usually transmitted in airborne droplets expelled when an infected person coughs or sneezes. An inhaled droplet enters the lungs and the bacteria begin multiplying. The immune system usually seals off the infection at this point, but in about 5 per cent of cases the infection spreads to the *lymph nodes*. It may also spread to other organs through the bloodstream, which may lead to miliary tuberculosis, a potentially fatal form of the disease.

In about another 5 per cent of cases, bacteria held in a dormant state by the immune system become reactivated months, or even years, later. The infection may then progressively damage the lungs, forming cavities.

The primary infection is usually without symptoms. Progressive infection in the lungs causes coughing (sometimes bringing up blood), chest pain, shortness of breath, fever and sweating, poor appetite, and weight loss. *Pleural effusion* or *pneumothorax* may develop. The lung damage may be fatal.

A diagnosis is made from the symptoms and signs, from a *chest X-ray*, and from tests on the sputum. Alternatively, a *bronchoscopy* may also be carried out to obtain samples for culture.

Treatment is usually with a course of four drugs, taken daily for 2 months, followed by daily doses of *isoniazid* and *rifampicin* for 4 months. However, TB bacteria are increasingly resistant to the drugs used in treatment, and others may have to be used and treatment carried out for a longer period. If the full course of drugs is taken, most patients recover. TB is a notifiable disease and any contacts of an infected person are traced and examined, and, if infected, are treated early to reduce the risk of the infection spreading.

TB can be prevented by *BCG vaccination*, which is offered to people at risk of contracting the disease.

tuberosity A prominent area on a *bone* to which *tendons* are attached.

tuberous sclerosis An inherited disorder that affects the skin and *nervous system*. An acne-like condition of the face, *epilepsy*, and *learning difficulties* often occur. Noncancerous tumours of the brain, kidney, retina, and heart may also develop. There is no cure, and treatment aims only to relieve symptoms. In serious cases, death occurs before the age of 30. *Genetic counselling* is recommended for affected families.

tuboplasty Surgery in which a damaged *fallopian tube* is repaired to treat *infertility*. It may be performed by *microsurgery*.

tularaemia A bacterial infection of wild animals that is sometimes transmitted to humans. Tularaemia does not occur in the UK but is seen in North America. It may result from contact with an infected animal or carcass, or a tick, flea, fly, or louse bite. A diagnosis is made by blood tests. Treatment is with *antibiotic drugs*. Tularaemia is fatal in 5 per cent of untreated cases.

tumbu fly bites A cause of *myiasis*.

tumour A term that describes any swelling but which is generally used to refer to an abnormal mass of tissue that forms when cells in a specific area reproduce at an increased rate. Tumours can be cancerous or noncancerous.

tumour-specific antigen A substance secreted by a specific type of *tumour* that can be detected in the blood and may be used to help monitor a patient's response to therapy. *Alpha-fetoprotein* is an example of a tumour-specific antigen.

tuning fork tests *Hearing tests* carried out to diagnose conductive *deafness*. In the Weber test, a vibrating tuning fork is held against the forehead. If there is conductive hearing loss, the sound seems louder in the affected ear. In the Rinne test, a vibrating tuning fork is held first near the ear, and then against the bone behind it. If it sounds louder when held against the bone, there is conductive hearing loss.

tunnel vision Loss of the peripheral *visual field* to the extent that only objects straight ahead can be seen clearly. Tunnel vision is most commonly caused by chronic *glaucoma*. *Retinitis pigmentosa* is another possible cause.

Turner's syndrome A disorder caused by a *chromosomal abnormality* that only affects females. The abnormality may arise in one of three ways: affected females may have only one X *chromosome* instead of two; they may have one normal and one defective X chromosome; or they may have a mixture of cells (see *mosaicism*), in which some of the cells are missing an X chromosome, some have extra chromosomes, and others have the normal complement of chromosomes. Turner's syndrome causes short stature; webbing of the skin of the neck; absence or retarded development of sexual characteristics; *amenorrhea, coarctation of the aorta*, and abnormalities of the eyes and the bones.

Treatment with *growth hormone* from infancy helps girls with Turner's syndrome to achieve near normal height. Coarctation of the aorta is treated surgically. Treatment with *oestrogen drugs* induces menstruation, but it does not make affected girls fertile.

TURP The abbreviation for transurethral resection of the prostate. TURP is a surgical procedure in which the central part of an enlarged *prostate gland* is removed (see *prostate, enlarged*). A viewing instrument called a resectoscope is passed along the *urethra* until it reaches the prostate. A heated wire loop, or sometimes a cutting edge, is inserted through the resectoscope and used to cut away excess prostate tissue.

twins Two offspring resulting from one pregnancy. Monozygotic, or identical, twins develop when a single fertilized egg divides at an early stage of development. Incomplete division of the egg results in conjoined twins (see *twins, conjoined*). Monozygotic twins share the same *placenta*. Dizygotic twins develop when two eggs are fertilized at the same time. They each have a placenta and may be of different sexes. Twins occur in about 1 in 80 pregnancies. (See also *pregnancy, multiple*.)

TWINS

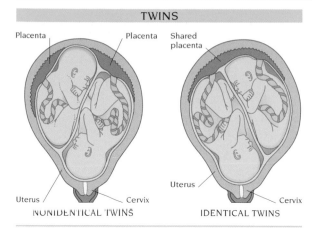

NONIDENTICAL TWINS

IDENTICAL TWINS

Placenta — *Placenta* — Shared placenta — Uterus — Cervix — Uterus — Cervix

twins, conjoined Identical *twins* physically joined due to a failure to separate during development from a single fertilized egg. Also called Siamese twins.

twitch See *fasciculation*; *tic*.

tympanic membrane The medical term for the *eardrum*.

tympanometry A type of *hearing test* used to establish the cause of conductive *deafness*. During the test, a probe that contains a tone generator, a microphone, and an air pump is introduced into the outer-ear canal. The air pressure in the ear is varied and tones are played into it. The tone pattern reflected from the *eardrum* and received by the microphone reveals whether the eardrum is moving normally. The test is particularly useful in children because it does not rely on a response from the person being tested.

tympanoplasty An operation on the *ear* to treat conductive *deafness* by repairing a hole in the eardrum (see *myringoplasty*) or by repositioning or reconstructing diseased *ossicles*.

typhoid fever An infectious disease contracted by eating food or drinking water contaminated with the bacterium *SALMONELLA TYPHI*. Typhoid fever is spread by drinking water contaminated with sewage, by flies carrying the bacteria from faeces to food, or by infected people handling food.

The first symptom, severe headache, occurs 7–14 days after infection and is followed by fever, loss of appetite, *malaise*, abdominal tenderness, constipation, and often delirium. Diarrhoea soon develops. In the 2nd week of illness, pink spots develop on the chest and abdomen, and the liver and *spleen* enlarge. Diagnosis is confirmed by a *blood test* or by obtaining a *culture* of typhoid bacteria from blood, faeces, or urine. Treatment is with *antibiotic drugs*. In rare cases, the bacterium continues to be excreted after recovery has taken place. Vaccination is recommended for travellers to areas with poor sanitation.

typhus Any of a group of infectious diseases with similar symptoms that are caused by *rickettsiae* and are spread by insects or similar animals.

Except in some highland areas of tropical Africa and South America, epidemic typhus is rare today. Endemic typhus, also called murine typhus, is a disease of rats that is occasionally spread to humans by fleas; sporadic cases occur in North and Central America. Scrub typhus is spread by mites and occurs in India and Southeast Asia.

The symptoms and complications of all types of typhus are similar. Severe headache, back and limb pain, coughing, and constipation develop suddenly and are followed by high fever, a measles-like rash, confusion, and prostration. Left untreated, the condition may be fatal, especially in elderly or debilitated people.

A diagnosis is made by *blood tests*, and treatment is with *antibiotic drugs* and supportive treatment.

typing A general term for procedures by which blood or tissues are classified (see *blood groups*; *tissue-typing*).

U

ulcer An open sore appearing on the skin or on a *mucous membrane* that results from the destruction of surface tissue. Ulcers may be shallow, or deep and crater-shaped, and they are usually inflamed and painful.

Skin ulcers most commonly occur on the leg (see *leg ulcer*), usually as the result of inadequate blood supply to, or drainage from, the limb. In some cases skin cancers, particularly *basal cell carcinomas* or *squamous cell carcinomas*, may be ulcerated. Rarely, a cancer may develop in the skin at the edge of a longstanding ulcer.

The most common types of ulcers of the mucous membranes are *mouth ulcers*, *peptic ulcers*, and those that occur in *ulcerative colitis*.

Ulcers may also affect the skin or mucous membranes of the genitalia (see *genital ulcer*). Most genital ulcers are caused by sexually transmitted infections. Examples of this type of ulcer are hard chancres (see *chancre, hard*), which develop during the first stage of *syphilis*, and soft chancres (see *chancroid*). In addition, ulcers may develop on the cornea (see *corneal ulcers*).

ulcer, aphthous A small, painful *ulcer* that occurs, alone or in a group, on the inside of the cheek or lip or underneath the tongue. Aphthous ulcers are most common between the ages of 10 and 40 and affect more women than men. The most severely affected people have continuously recurring ulcers; others have just one or two ulcers each year.

Each ulcer is usually small and oval, with a grey centre and a surrounding red, inflamed halo. The ulcer, which usually lasts for 1–2 weeks, may be a hypersensitive reaction to haemolytic streptococcus *bacteria*. Other factors commonly associated with the occurrence of these ulcers are minor injuries (such as at an injection site or from a toothbrush), acute stress, or allergies (such as allergic *rhinitis*). In women, aphthous ulcers are most common during the premenstrual period. They may also be more likely if other family members suffer from recurrent ulceration.

Analgesic mouth gels or mouthwashes may ease the pain of an aphthous ulcer. Some ointments form a waterproof covering that protects the ulcer while it is healing. Ulcers heal by themselves, but a doctor may prescribe a paste containing a *corticosteroid drug*.

ulceration The formation or presence of one or more *ulcers*.

ulcerative colitis Chronic inflammation and ulceration of the lining of the *colon* and *rectum*, or, especially at the start of the condition, of the rectum alone. The cause of ulcerative colitis is unknown, but the condition is most common in young and middle-aged adults.

The main symptom of ulcerative colitis is bloody diarrhoea; and the faeces may also contain mucus. In severe cases, the diarrhoea and bleeding are extensive, and there may be abdominal pain and tenderness, fever, and general malaise. The incidence of attacks varies considerably. Most commonly, the attacks occur at intervals of a few months. However, in some cases, there may be only a single episode.

Ulcerative colitis may lead to *anaemia*, caused by blood loss. Other complications include a toxic form of *megacolon*, which may become life-threatening; rashes; aphthous *ulcers*; arthritis; conjunctivitis; or uveitis. There is also an increased risk of cancer of the colon developing (see *colon, cancer of*).

A diagnosis is based on examination of the rectum and lower colon (see *sigmoidoscopy*) or the entire colon (see *colonoscopy*). During sigmoidoscopy or colonoscopy, a *biopsy* may be performed. Samples of faeces may be taken for laboratory analysis in order to exclude the possibility of infection by bacteria or parasites. *Blood tests* may also be needed.

Medical treatments of ulcerative colitis include *corticosteroid drugs* and *mesalazine* and its derivatives. *Colectomy* may be required for a severe attack that fails to respond to other treatments, or to avoid colon cancer in those people who are at high risk.

ulcer-healing drugs A group of drugs that are used to treat or prevent *peptic ulcers*. The eradication of HELICOBACTER PYLORI infection by treatment with *antibiotic drugs* and a drug to reduce acid secretion is now the preferred treatment for peptic ulceration.

Ulcer-healing drugs work in several ways. H_2-*receptor antagonists* function by blocking the effects of histamine, an action that reduces acid secretion in the stomach, thereby promoting the healing of ulcers. Taking *antacid drugs* regularly may be effective in healing duodenal ulcers because the drugs neutralize excess acid. *Misoprostol* and *proton pump inhibitors* such as *omeprazole* work by reducing acid secretion. Other ulcer-healing drugs, such as *sucralfate*, are believed to form a protective barrier over the ulcer, allowing healing of the underlying tissues to take place.

ulna The longer of the two bones of the forearm; the other is the *radius*. With the arms straight at the sides, palm forwards, the ulna is the inner bone (that is, nearer the trunk) running down the forearm on the side of the little finger.

The upper end of the ulna articulates with the radius and extends into a rounded projection (known as the *olecranon* process) that fits around the lower end of the humerus to form part of the *elbow* joint. The lower end of the ulna articulates with the carpals (*wrist* bones) and lower part of the radius.

ulna, fracture of A fracture of the *ulna*, one of the two bones of the forearm. Ulnar fractures typically occur across the shaft of the bone or at the *olecranon* process (at the elbow).

A fracture to the shaft usually results from a blow to the forearm or a fall onto the hand. Sometimes the radius is fractured at the same time (see *radius, fracture of*). Surgery is usually needed to reposition the broken bone ends and fix them together using either a plate and screws or a long nail down the centre of the bone. The arm is immobilized in a *cast*, with the elbow at a right-angle, until the fracture heals.

A fracture of the olecranon process is usually the result of a fall onto the *elbow*. If the bone ends are not displaced, the arm is immobilized in a cast that holds the elbow at a right-angle. If the bone ends are displaced, however, they are fitted together and fixed with a metal screw.

ulnar nerve One of the principal *nerves* of the arm. The ulnar nerve, a branch of the *brachial plexus*, runs down the full length of the arm and into the hand. The ulnar nerve controls muscles that move the thumb and fingers. It also conveys sensation from the fifth finger, part of the fourth finger, and the palm.

A blow to the olecranon process, over which the ulnar nerve passes, causes a pins-and-needles sensation and pain in the forearm and fourth and fifth fingers. Persistent numbness and weakness in areas controlled by the ulnar nerve may be caused by an abnormal bony outgrowth from the *humerus*. This may be due to *osteoarthritis* or a fracture of the humerus, and surgery is needed to relieve the pressure on the nerve. Permanent damage to the ulnar nerve can result in *claw-hand*.

ultrasound Sound with a frequency that is greater than the human ear's upper limit of perception: that is, higher than 20,000 hertz (cycles per second). Ultrasound used in medicine for diagnosis or treatment is typically in the range of 1–15 million hertz (see *ultrasound scanning*; *ultrasound treatment*).

ultrasound scanning A diagnostic technique in which very high frequency sound waves are passed into the body and the reflected echoes analysed to build a picture of the internal organs or of a fetus in the uterus. The procedure is painless and considered safe.

Ultrasonic waves are emitted by a transducer, which is placed on the skin over the part of the body to be viewed. The transducer contains a crystal that converts an electric current into sound waves. These pass readily through soft tissues and fluids, making this procedure useful for examining fluid-filled or soft organs.

One of the most common uses of ultrasound is to view the uterus and fetus, at any time during *pregnancy*, but often at

ULTRASOUND SCANNING

Radiographer | Gel | Monitor | Ultrasound transducer

ULTRASOUND SCANNING IN PREGNANCY

18–20 weeks. The age, size, and growth rate of the fetus can be determined; multiple pregnancies detected; and certain problems, such as *neural tube defects*, diagnosed. Scans may be taken early in pregnancy if problems, such as an *ectopic pregnancy*, are suspected.

Ultrasound scanning can also be used in newborn babies to examine the brain through a gap in the skull (for example, to investigate *hydrocephalus*). Ultrasound can help to diagnose disorders such as *cirrhosis*, *gallstones*, *hydronephrosis*, and *pancreatitis*, as well as problems in the thyroid gland, breasts, bladder, testes, ovaries, spleen, and eyes. The technique is also used during needle *biopsy* to help guide the needle.

Doppler ultrasound is a modified form of ultrasound that uses the *Doppler effect* to investigate moving objects. This can be used to examine the fetal heartbeat and to obtain information about the rate of blood flow in vessels.

ultrasound treatment The use of *ultrasound* to treat soft-tissue injuries (such as injuries to ligaments, muscles, and tendons). Ultrasound treatment reduces inflammation and speeds up healing. It is thought to work by improving blood flow in tissues under the skin.

ultraviolet light Invisible light from the part of the electromagnetic spectrum immediately beyond the violet end of the visible light spectrum. Long wavelength ultraviolet light is termed UVA, intermediate UVB, and short UVC.

Ultraviolet light occurs in sunlight, but much of it is absorbed by the *ozone* layer. The ultraviolet light (mainly UVA) that reaches the earth's surface causes the tanning effects of sunlight and the production of *vitamin D* in the skin. It can have harmful effects, such as *skin cancer* (see *sunlight, adverse effects of*).

Ultraviolet light is sometimes used in *phototherapy*. A mercury-vapour lamp (Wood's light) can also produce ultraviolet light. This is used to diagnose skin conditions such as *tinea* because it causes the infected area to fluoresce.

umbilical cord The ropelike structure connecting the *fetus* to the *placenta* that supplies the fetus with oxygen and nutrients from the mother's circulation. The umbilical cord is usually 40–60 cm long and contains two arteries and a vein.

umbilical hernia A soft swelling at the *umbilicus* due to protrusion of the abdominal contents through a weak area of abdominal wall. Umbilical hernias are quite common in newborn babies and occur twice as often in boys as in girls. The swelling increases in size when the baby cries, and it may cause discomfort. Umbilical hernias usually disappear without treatment by age 2. If a hernia is still present at age 4, surgery may be needed.

Umbilical hernias sometimes develop in adults, especially in women after *childbirth*. Surgery may be necessary for a large, persistent, or disfiguring hernia.

umbilicus The scar on the abdomen that marks the site of attachment of the *umbilical cord* to the *fetus*. It is commonly called the navel.

U

unconscious A specific part of the mind in which ideas, memories, perceptions, or feelings that a person is not currently aware of are stored and processed. The contents of the unconscious mind are not easily retrieved, in contrast to those of the *subconscious*. (See also *Freudian theory*; *Jungian theory*.)

unconsciousness An abnormal loss of awareness of self and one's surroundings due to a reduced level of activity in the reticular formation of the *brainstem*. An unconscious person can be roused only with difficulty or not at all. Unconsciousness may be brief and light, as in *fainting*, or deep and prolonged (see *coma*).

underbite See *prognathism*

unsaturated fats See *fats and oils*.

unstable bladder Another name for *irritable bladder*

uraemia The presence of excess *urea* and other chemical waste products in the blood, caused by *kidney failure*.

uranium A radioactive metallic element that does not occur naturally in its pure form but is widely found in ores such as pitchblende, carnotite, and uraninite. Radioactive decay of uranium yields a series of radioactive products, including *radium* and *radon*. During the various decay stages, *radiation* is emitted. Uranium is also poisonous.

urea A waste product of the breakdown of proteins by the liver that is transported to the kidneys and eliminated in the urine. Urea is also formed in the body from the breakdown of cell proteins. *Kidney failure* impairs the kidneys' ability to eliminate urea and leads to uraemia; measurement of blood levels of urea is a routine kidney function test. Urea is used in various creams and ointments to treat skin disorders such as *psoriasis*.

ureter One of the two tubes that carry urine from the *kidneys* to the *bladder*. Each ureter is 25–30 cm long. There are three layers in the walls of the ureters: a fibrous outer layer; muscular middle layer; and inner watertight layer. Each ureter is supplied by blood vessels and nerves. Urine flows down the ureters partly from gravity but mainly as a result of *peristalsis*.

Some people are born with double ureters, on one or both sides of the body. This sometimes causes *reflux* of urine, *incontinence*, or infection.

ureteric colic See *renal colic*.

ureterolithotomy The surgical removal of a stone (see *calculus, urinary tract*) stuck in a *ureter*. It is not commonly needed because *lithotripsy* and *cystoscopy* can be used to deal with stones.

urethra The tube through which *urine* is excreted from the *bladder*. In females, it is short and opens to the outside in front of the vagina. In males, it is much longer, is surrounded by the prostate gland at its upper end, and forms a channel through the length of the penis.

urethral dilatation The procedure in which a *urethral stricture* in a male is widened by inserting a slim, round-tipped instrument through the opening of the *urethra* at the tip of the *penis*.

urethral discharge A fluid that flows from the *urethra* in some cases of *urethritis* caused by infection.

urethral stricture A rare condition in which the male *urethra* becomes narrowed and sometimes shortened as a result of shrinkage of scar tissue within its walls. Scar tissue may form after injury to the urethra or after persistent *urethritis*. The stricture may make passing urine or ejaculation difficult or painful, and it may cause some deformation of the penis when erect. Treatment is usually by *urethral dilatation*.

urethral syndrome, acute A set of symptoms, usually affecting women, that are very similar to *cystitis* but which occur in the absence of infection.

urethritis Inflammation of the *urethra*, usually due to an infection but sometimes having other causes.

Urethritis may be caused by various infectious organisms, including the bacterium that causes *gonorrhoea*. *Nongonococcal urethritis* may be caused by any of a large number of different types of microorganisms. Urethritis may also be caused by damage from an accident or from a *catheter* or *cystoscope*. Other possible causes include irritant chemicals, such as antiseptics and some spermicidal preparations. Treatment of infection is with *antibiotic drugs*.

urethrocele An anatomical abnormality in females caused by a weakness in the tissues in the front wall of the *vagina*. The urethra bulges backwards and downwards into the vagina. A urethrocele may be *congenital* but more commonly develops after *childbirth*.

-uria A suffix relating to *urine*.

uric acid A waste product of the breakdown of *nucleic acids* in body cells. A small amount is also produced by the digestion of foods rich in nucleic acids, such as liver, kidney, and other offal. Most uric acid produced in the body passes to the kidneys, which excrete it in the *urine*, but some passes into the intestine, where it is broken down into chemicals excreted in the *faeces*.

When uric acid excretion is disrupted, for example by kidney disease, it may result in *hyperuricaemia*, kidney stones (see *calculus, urinary tract*), or *gout*.

urinal A container for *urine*, useful for bedridden men (women use a *bedpan*).

urinalysis Tests on *urine*, including measurements of its physical characteristics (such as colour, cloudiness, and concentration), microscopic examination, and chemical testing such as dipstick urinalysis. This involves dipping a test stick into a urine sample; chemically impregnated squares on the stick change colour in the presence of test substances. The intensity of colour change shows the amount of the substance present in the urine. Urinalysis can be used to check kidney function, and to help detect and diagnose urinary tract and other disorders.

urinary diversion Any surgical procedure (temporary or permanent) that allows urine flow when the outlet channel of the urinary tract, via the bladder and urethra, is obstructed or cannot be used, or the bladder has been surgically removed.

Temporary urinary diversion is sometimes needed when urine passage is blocked by *prostate gland* enlargement or by *urethral stricture*. A tube is passed directly into the bladder through a small opening in the abdomen (see *catheterization, urinary*). Temporary diversion is also required after some urinary tract operations; a small tube is introduced into the kidney and brought to the abdominal surface.

Permanent diversion is needed when the bladder has been surgically removed, when neurological bladder control is severely disturbed, such as after severe spinal injury, or if there is an irreparable *fistula* between a female patient's bladder or urethra and her vagina. A section of the *ileum* is removed to create a substitute bladder, into one end of which the surgeon implants the ureters. The other end of the substitute bladder is then brought out through an incision in the abdominal wall. The patient wears a bag attached to the skin to collect urine.

urinary retention Inability to empty the *bladder* or difficulty in doing so. Urinary retention may be complete (urine cannot be passed voluntarily at all) or incomplete (the bladder fails to empty completely). In males, causes include *phimosis*, *urethral stricture*, *prostatitis*, a stone in the bladder (see *calculus, urinary tract*), and enlargement or tumour of the prostate (see *prostate, enlarged*; *prostate, cancer of*). In females, causes include

URINALYSIS

Test stick is dipped in urine sample

Colour chart

Urine sample

Squares on test stick are matched to colour chart

DIPSTICK URINALYSIS

URINARY TRACT

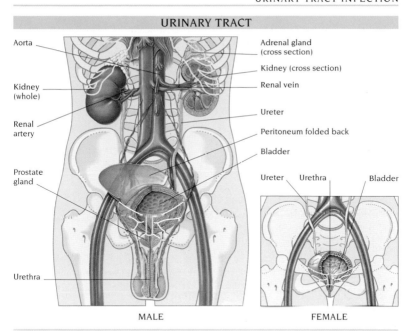

Aorta

Adrenal gland
(cross section)

Kidney (cross section)

Renal vein

Kidney
(whole)

Renal
artery

Ureter

Peritoneum folded back

Bladder

Prostate
gland

Ureter   Urethra   Bladder

Urethra

MALE   FEMALE

pressure on the urethra from uterine *fibroids* or from a *fetus*. In either sex, the cause may be a bladder tumour.

Retention may also be due to defective functioning of the nerve pathways supplying the bladder as a result of general or spinal *anaesthesia*, drugs affecting the bladder, surgery, injury to the nerve pathways, or disease of the spinal cord.

Complete retention causes discomfort and lower abdominal pain, except when nerve pathways are defective. The full bladder can be felt above the pubic bone. However, chronic or partial retention may not cause any serious symptoms. Retention can lead to kidney damage and, often, a urinary tract infection.

Treatment of retention is by catheterization (see *catheterization, urinary*). The cause is then investigated. Obstruction can usually be treated; if nerve damage is the cause, permanent or intermittent catheterization is sometimes necessary.

urinary system See *urinary tract*.

urinary tract The part of the body concerned with the formation and excretion of *urine*. The urinary tract consists of the *kidneys* (with their blood and nerve

supplies), the renal pelvises (funnel-shaped ducts that channel urine from the kidneys), the *ureters*, the *bladder*, and the *urethra*.

The kidneys make urine by filtering blood. The urine collects in the renal pelvises and is then passed down the ureters into the bladder by the actions of gravity and *peristalsis*. Urine is stored in the bladder until there is a sufficient amount present to stimulate *micturition*. When the bladder contracts, the urine is expelled through the urethra.

urinary tract infection An infection anywhere in the *urinary tract*. It has differing symptoms, depending on the area affected. *Urethritis* causes a burning sensation when urine is being passed. *Cystitis* causes a frequent urge to pass urine, lower abdominal pain, *haematuria*, and, often, general malaise with a mild fever. *Pyelonephritis* causes fever and pain in the back under the ribs. Cystitis and pyelonephritis are almost always the result of a bacterial infection. Urethritis is often due to a *sexually transmitted infection*, such as gonorrhoea, but may have other causes.

Urethral infections are more common in men. Infections further up the urinary tract are more common in women. In men, there is often a predisposing factor, such as an enlarged prostate gland (see *prostate, enlarged*). In women, pregnancy is a risk factor.

In both sexes, causes of urinary tract infections include stones (see *calculus, urinary tract*), *bladder tumours*, *congenital* abnormalities of the urinary tract, or defective bladder emptying as a result of *spina bifida* or a *spinal injury*. The risks of developing a urinary tract infection can be reduced by strict personal hygiene, drinking lots of fluids, and regularly emptying the bladder.

Urethritis can lead to the formation of a *urethral stricture*. Cystitis usually only causes complications if the infection spreads to the *kidneys*. Pyelonephritis, if it is left untreated, can lead to permanent kidney damage, *septicaemia*, and *septic shock*.

The infection is diagnosed by the examination of a urine *culture*. Further investigations using *urography* or *ultrasound scanning* may be necessary. Most infections of the urinary tract are treated with *antibiotic drugs*.

urination, excessive The production of more than 2.5 litres of *urine* per day. The medical term is polyuria.

Causes include psychiatric problems, which may cause a person to drink compulsively; *diabetes mellitus*; disorders of the kidney known as salt-losing states; and central *diabetes insipidus*. Any person who passes large quantities of urine should consult a doctor.

urination, frequent Also known as urinary frequency, the passing of urine more often than the average of 4–6 times daily. Causes of frequent urination include excessive production of urine (see *urination, excessive*), *cystitis*, anxiety, stones in the bladder (see *calculus, urinary tract*), enlargement of the prostate gland (see *prostate, enlarged*) in men, and, rarely, a *bladder tumour*. Some people who are suffering from *kidney failure* pass urine more frequently, especially during the night. Treatment of frequent urination is always of the underlying cause.

urination, painful Pain or discomfort that occurs when urine is being passed. Painful urination is known medically as dysuria. The pain is often described as burning; sometimes it is preceded by difficulty in starting urine flow. Pain after the flow has ceased, with a strong desire to continue, is called strangury.

The most common cause, especially in women, is *cystitis*. Other causes include a *bladder tumour*, bladder stone (see *calculus, urinary tract*), *urethritis*, *balanitis*, *prostatitis*, vaginal *candidiasis* (thrush), or allergy to vaginal deodorants. Strangury is usually caused by spasm of an inflamed bladder wall, but it may be due to bladder stones. Mild discomfort when passing urine may be caused by highly concentrated urine.

Dysuria may be investigated by physical examination, *urinalysis*, *urography*, or *cystoscopy*. (See also *urethral syndrome, acute*.)

urine The pale yellow fluid produced by the *kidneys* and excreted from the body via the *ureters*, *bladder*, and *urethra*. Urine is produced when blood is filtered through the *kidneys* to remove waste products and excess water or chemical substances. The main component is *urea*.

A healthy adult produces between 0.5 and 2 litres of urine per day. The minimum volume of urine needed to remove all waste products is about 0.5 litres. A high fluid intake increases the amount of urine produced; high fluid loss from sweating, vomiting, or diarrhoea leads to reduced production.

urine, abnormal *Urine* may be produced in abnormal amounts or have an abnormal appearance or composition.

Conditions of abnormal production of urine include excessive production (see *urination, excessive*), *oliguria*, and *anuria*. Abnormal appearances of urine include cloudiness (which may be caused by a *urinary tract infection*, a *calculus*, or the presence of salts); *haematuria*; discoloration from certain foods or drugs; and frothiness (which may be caused by an excess of *protein*).

Abnormal composition of the urine may occur in *diabetes mellitus*, *kidney failure*, and sometimes *glomerulonephritis*

U

and *nephrotic syndrome*, as well as in other kidney disorders such as *Fanconi's syndrome* and *renal tubular acidosis*.

urine tests See *urinalysis*.

urodynamics A group of tests carried out to investigate problems with *bladder* control, such as *incontinence*. Urodynamic studies involve the insertion of probes into the *urethra*, bladder, and *rectum* or *vagina* in order to monitor pressure changes while the bladder is being filled and emptied.

In *X-ray* monitoring, the patient stands against an upright table while his or her bladder is filled with a *contrast medium* through a *catheter* and is then emptied again. The shape and functioning of the bladder, and the functioning of the urethra, can then be viewed on an X-ray monitor. At the same time, a continuous recording of pressure changes within the bladder is made on a paper trace. As the bladder is being filled, the patient is asked to cough. This action increases the pressure in and around the bladder, and if it causes leakage of urine onto an electronic absorbent pad, the patient has stress incontinence (see *incontinence, urinary*).

urography See *intravenous urography*.

urology A branch of medicine concerned with the structure, functioning, and disorders of the *urinary tract* in males and females, and of the *reproductive system* in males. Investigative techniques that are used in urology include *urography*, *cystoscopy, ultrasound scanning, cystometry*, and *urinalysis*.

ursodeoxycholic acid A drug used to dissolve *gallstones*. It is only suitable if the stones are made exclusively of *cholesterol* and if the gallbladder is functioning normally. Side effects of the drug are rare but can include diarrhoea, indigestion, and a rash. Drug treatment is less commonly used since the introduction of *minimally invasive surgery*.

urticaria A skin condition, also known as nettle rash or hives, that is characterized by the development of itchy weals, usually on the limbs and trunk. Large weals may merge to form irregular, raised patches.

Urticaria is generally harmless and usually lasts only a few hours. Sometimes a persistent or recurrent form develops. *Dermographism* is a less common form of urticaria in which weals form after the

URODYNAMICS

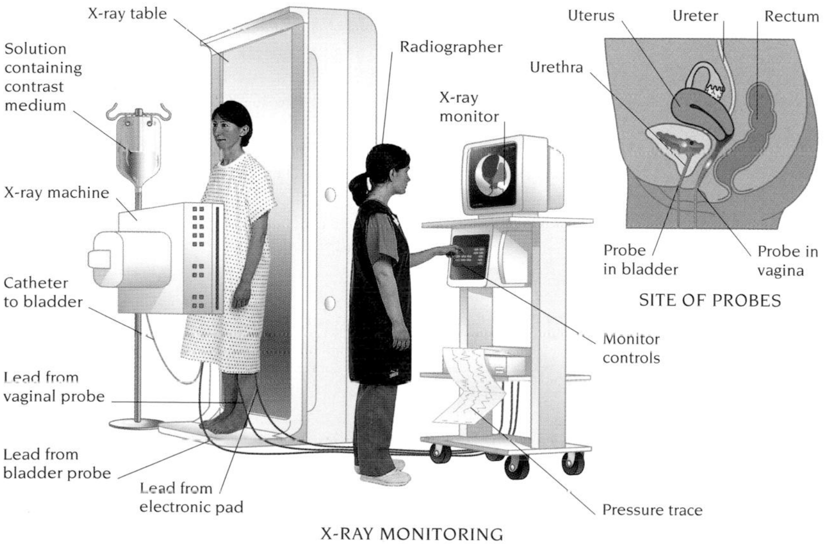

X-ray table
Solution containing contrast medium
Radiographer
Uterus   Ureter   Rectum
Urethra
X-ray monitor
X-ray machine
Catheter to bladder
Probe in bladder
Probe in vagina
SITE OF PROBES
Lead from vaginal probe
Monitor controls
Lead from bladder probe
Lead from electronic pad
Pressure trace

X-RAY MONITORING

U

skin is stroked. Urticaria sometimes occurs with *angioedema*.

The cause of urticaria is often unknown. The most common known cause is an allergic reaction (see *allergy*), often to a particular food, food additive, or drug. Urticaria may also be caused by exposure to heat, cold, or sunlight. Less commonly, it may be associated with another disorder, such as *vasculitis*, systemic *lupus erythematosus*, or *cancer*.

Itching can be relieved by applying *calamine lotion* or by taking *antihistamine drugs*. More severe cases may require *corticosteroid drugs*. Identifying and avoiding known trigger factors can help prevent future reactions. A tendency to urticaria often disappears in time without treatment.

urticaria, neonatal A very common, harmless skin condition, also known as erythema neonatorum or toxic erythema, that affects newborn infants. A blotchy rash, in which raised white or yellow lumps are surrounded by ill-defined red areas of inflammation, forms, mainly affecting the face, chest, arms, and thighs. The cause of neonatal urticaria is unknown. The rash usually clears up without treatment.

uterine muscle relaxants Drugs that are used to delay the premature delivery of a *fetus*. Beta$_2$-adrenoceptor stimulants, such as *salbutamol*, relax the muscle of the *uterus* and may postpone labour for days or weeks in at-risk pregnancies of 24–33 weeks' gestation. Delay of premature labour for up to 48 hours allows time for *corticosteroid drugs* to be given to the mother to help the fetal lungs to mature.

uterovaginal prolapse See *uterus, prolapse of*.

uterus The hollow, muscular organ of the female reproductive system in which the fertilized *ovum* (egg) normally becomes embedded and in which the *embryo* and *fetus* develop. The uterus is commonly known as the womb. It is situated in the pelvic cavity, behind the *bladder* and in front of the intestines.

In a nonpregnant woman, the uterus is 7.5–10 cm long and weighs 60–90 g. The lower part opens into the *vagina* at the *cervix*; the upper part opens into

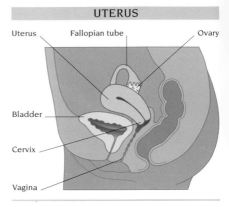

UTERUS

Uterus Fallopian tube Ovary

Bladder

Cervix

Vagina

the *fallopian tubes*. The inside is lined with *endometrium*. The uterus expands in size during pregnancy to accommodate the growing baby. At full-term, the powerful uterine muscles expel the baby via the birth canal (see *childbirth*). After the *menopause*, the endometrium atrophies (becomes thinner) and the uterine muscle and connective tissue are reduced.

Conditions that affect the uterus include *congenital* disorders, such as malformation or absence of the uterus; tumours, including *polyps*, *fibroids*, and cancer of the endometrium (see *uterus, cancer of*); infections, causing *endometritis*; and hormonal disorders. (See also *uterus, prolapse of*; *uterus, retroverted*.)

uterus, cancer of A malignant growth in the tissues of the *uterus*. Cancer of the uterus mainly affects the cervix (see *cervix, cancer of*) and *endometrium*. In rare cases, the uterine muscle is affected by a type of cancer called a leiomyosarcoma. The term uterine cancer usually refers to cancer of the endometrium.

Risk factors for endometrial cancer include anything that may raise oestrogen levels in the body, such as *obesity*, a history of failure to ovulate, or taking *oestrogen hormones* long term if these are not balanced with *progestogen drugs*. It is also more common in women who have had few or no children.

Before the *menopause*, the first symptom of cancer of the uterus may be *menorrhagia* or bleeding between periods or after sexual intercourse; after the menopause, it is usually a blood-stained vaginal discharge. Diagnosis is made by *hysteroscopy* or *biopsy*.

Very early endometrial cancer is usually treated by *hysterectomy* and removal of the fallopian tubes and ovaries. If the cancer has spread, *radiotherapy* and *anticancer drug* treatment may also be used.

uterus, prolapse of A condition in which the *uterus* descends from its normal position into the *vagina*. The degree of prolapse varies from 1st-degree prolapse, in which there is only slight displacement of the uterus, to 3rd-degree prolapse (procidentia), in which the uterus can be seen outside the *vulva*.

Stretching of the ligaments supporting the uterus (during *childbirth*, for example) is the most common cause. Prolapse is aggravated by obesity.

There are often no symptoms, but sometimes there is a dragging feeling in the pelvis. Diagnosis is made by physical examination.

Pelvic floor exercises strengthen the muscles of the vagina and thus reduce the risk of a prolapse, especially following childbirth. Treatment usually involves surgery (*hysterectomy*). Rarely, if surgery is not wanted or is not recommended, a plastic ring-shaped pessary may be inserted into the vagina to hold the uterus in position. (See also *cystocele*; *rectocele*; *urethrocele*.)

uterus, retroverted A normal variation in which the uterus inclines backwards rather than forwards. A retroverted uterus rarely causes problems unless it is combined with a *pelvic infection*

uvea Part of the *eye*, comprising the *iris*, the *ciliary body* and its muscle that focuses the *lens*, and the *choroid*.

uveitis Inflammation of the *uvea*, which may seriously affect vision. Uveitis may affect any part of the uvea, including the *iris* (when it is called iritis), the *ciliary body* (when it is known as cyclitis), or the *choroid* (when it is called *choroiditis*). The most common cause is an *autoimmune disorder*. Other causes include infections such as *tuberculosis* and *syphilis*. Treatment is with *corticosteroid drugs* and eye-drops containing an *atropine*-related substance. The inflammation is monitored with a *slit-lamp*. Various other drugs may be prescribed if the cause is an infection.

uvula The small, fleshy protuberance that hangs from the middle of the lower edge of the soft *palate*.

UTERUS, RETROVERTED

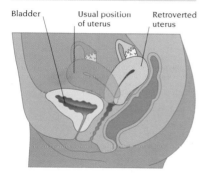

Bladder | Usual position of uterus | Retroverted uterus

V

vaccination A form of *immunization* in which killed or weakened *micro-organisms*, or inactivated bacterial *toxins*, are introduced into the body, usually by injection, to sensitize the *immune system* (see *vaccine*). If disease-causing organisms or toxins of the same type later enter the body, the sensitized immune system rapidly produces *anti-bodies* that destroy them.

vaccine A preparation given to induce *immunity* against an infectious disease. Most vaccines contain the organisms (or parts of the organisms) against which protection is sought.

Vaccines are usually given by injection. Some require several doses spaced weeks apart whereas others require only a single dose. Boosters may also be required, the interval depending on the original vaccine given.

vacuum extraction An obstetric procedure to facilitate the delivery of a baby. It may be used if the second stage of labour (see *childbirth*) is prolonged, if the mother becomes exhausted, or if the baby shows signs of *fetal distress*. Vacuum suction techniques are also used to perform early *abortions*.

The vacuum extraction instrument consists of a suction cup connected to a vacuum bottle. The suction cup is placed on the baby's head in the birth canal, and the vacuum machine sucks the baby's scalp into the cup. The obstetrician draws the baby out of the mother's vagina by gently pulling on the cup with each uterine contraction.

The baby is born with a swelling on the scalp, but this disappears after a few days, usually without treatment.

vagina The muscular passage, forming part of the female *reproductive system*, between the *cervix* and the external genitalia. The vagina has muscular walls, which are highly elastic to allow *sexual intercourse* and *childbirth* and are richly supplied with blood vessels.

vaginal bleeding Bleeding, via the *vagina*, that may come from the *uterus*, the *cervix*, or from the vagina itself.

The most common source of bleeding is the uterus and the most likely reason for it is *menstruation*. From puberty to the menopause, menstrual bleeding usually occurs at regular intervals. However, problems may occur with either the character or the timing of the bleeding (see *menstruation, disorders of*).

Nonmenstrual bleeding from the uterus may be due to a variety of causes. Hormonal drugs, such as *oral contraceptives*, can cause spotting. Other possible causes include *endometritis*, endometrial cancer (see *uterus, cancer of*), and *fibroids*. In early pregnancy, bleeding may be a sign of threatened *miscarriage*. Later in pregnancy, it may indicate *placenta praevia* or placental abruption (see *antepartum haemorrhage*).

Bleeding from the cervix may be due to *cervical ectopy*, in which case it may occur after intercourse. *Cervicitis* and *polyps* may also cause bleeding. More seriously, bleeding may be a sign of cervical cancer (see *cervix, cancer of*).

A possible cause of bleeding from the vagina is injury during intercourse, especially following the menopause, when the walls of the vagina become thinner and more fragile. Occasionally, severe *vaginitis* causes bleeding. Rarely, vaginal bleeding is caused by cancer of the vagina.

vaginal discharge The emission of secretions from the *vagina*. Some mucous secretion from the vaginal walls and from the cervix is normal in the reproductive years; its amount and nature vary from woman to woman and at different times in the menstrual cycle (see *menstruation*). *Oral contraceptives* can increase or decrease the discharge. Secretions tend to be greater during pregnancy. Sexual stimulation also produces increased vaginal discharge.

Discharge may be abnormal if it is excessive, offensive-smelling, yellow or green, or if it causes itching. Abnormal discharge often accompanies *vaginitis*, and may be the result of infection, as in candidiasis or trichomoniasis, or may be due to a foreign body, such as a forgotten tampon, in the vagina.

vaginal itching Irritation in the *vagina*, often associated with *vulval itching*. In many cases, it is a symptom of *vaginitis*, which may be caused by infection or an allergic reaction to hygiene or spermicidal products. Vaginal itching is common after the *menopause*, when it is caused by low oestrogen levels. Depending on the cause, treatment may be with *antibiotic drugs* or hormones.

vaginal repair An operation to correct prolapse of the vaginal wall. This may be accompanied by a vaginal *hysterectomy* if the uterus is also prolapsed (see *uterus, prolapse of*).

vaginismus Painful, involuntary spasm of the muscles surrounding the entrance to the *vagina*, interfering with *sexual intercourse* and sometimes also medical vaginal examinations. (See also *intercourse, painful*; *psychosexual dysfunction*.)

vaginitis Inflammation of the *vagina* that may be caused by infection, commonly by the fungus CANDIDA ALBICANS (see *candidiasis*), the parasite TRICHOMONAS VAGINALIS (see *trichomoniasis*), or bacteria. After the *menopause* the vaginal lining becomes fragile and prone to inflammation. This is called atrophic vaginitis and is due to a reduction in the production of *oestrogen hormones*.

Infections are treated with *antibiotics* or *antifungal drugs*. In cases of allergy, irritants should be avoided. Any foreign body is removed. Atrophic vaginitis is usually treated with topical *oestrogen*. (See also *vulvitis*; *vulvovaginitis*.)

vagotomy An operation in which the *vagus nerve*, which controls production of digestive acid by the stomach wall, is cut. Once widely used to treat some cases of *peptic ulcer*, it has now largely been replaced by drug treatment.

vagus nerve The 10th *cranial nerve* and principal component of the parasympathetic division of the *autonomic nervous system*. The vagus nerve passes from the medulla oblongata (in the *brainstem*) through the neck and chest to the abdomen, and has branches to most major organs, including the larynx, pharynx, trachea, lungs, heart, and digestive system.

valgus The medical term for outward displacement of a part of the body.

valproate See *sodium valproate*.

Valsalva's manoeuvre A forcible attempt to breathe out when the airway is closed. The manoeuvre occurs naturally when an attempt is made to breathe out while holding the *vocal cords* tightly together. This happens, for example, at the beginning of a sneeze. When performed deliberately by pinching the nose and holding the mouth closed, the manoeuvre can prevent pressure damage to the eardrums (see *barotrauma*).

valve A structure that allows fluid or semi-fluid material to flow in one direction through a tube or passageway but closes to prevent reflux in the opposite direction. The valves at the exits from the *heart* chambers and in the *veins* are essential to the *circulatory system*. There are also small valves in the vessels of the *lymphatic system*.

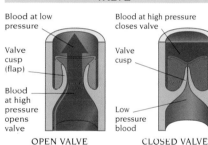

VALVE

Blood at low pressure

Valve cusp (flap)

Blood at high pressure opens valve

OPEN VALVE

Blood at high pressure closes valve

Valve cusp

Low pressure blood

CLOSED VALVE

valve replacement A surgical operation to replace a defective or diseased heart valve. (See also *heart-valve surgery*.)

valvotomy An operation that is performed to correct a narrowed *heart valve*. Cuts are made, or pressure is applied, to separate the flaps of the valve where they have joined, thereby reducing the degree of narrowing. Valvotomy is performed either by opening the heart up (see *heart-valve surgery*) or by balloon *valvuloplasty*.

valvular heart disease A defect of one or more of the *heart valves*.

valvuloplasty Reconstructive or repair surgery on a defective heart valve (see *heart-valve surgery*). Valvuloplasty may be performed as *open heart surgery*. However, the technique of balloon valvuloplasty makes it possible to treat a narrowed valve without opening the chest. A *balloon catheter* is passed through the skin into a blood vessel and from there to the heart. Inflation of the balloon via the catheter then separates the flaps of a narrowed valve.

vancomycin A glycopeptide *antibiotic drug* given by injection to treat serious bacterial infections such as *endocarditis* and *MRSA*. Given by mouth, it may be used to treat a form of *colitis* induced by antibiotic drugs. Possible side effects include rash, nausea, kidney damage, and hearing damage.

vaporizer A device for converting a drug or water into a fine spray so that medication can be taken by inhalation or so that inhaled air can be moistened.

variant angina A form of *angina* that causes chest pain at rest, often during sleep. The pain may occur with breathlessness, fainting, and *palpitations*. The cause is thought to be narrowing of the *coronary arteries* by muscular spasm in their walls. Treatment with *calcium channel blockers* or *nitrates* is usually effective.

varicella Another name for *chickenpox*.

varicella-zoster The virus that causes *chickenpox* and *shingles*.

varices Enlarged, tortuous, or twisted sections of vessels, usually veins. Varices is the plural of varix. A vein affected by varices is called a *varicose vein*.

varicocele *Varicose veins* surrounding a *testis*. Varicocele is a common condition. It almost exclusively affects the left testis and is usually harmless, although there may be aching in the *scrotum* or an abnormally low sperm count (see *infertility*). Aching may be relieved by supportive underwear. Surgery to divide and tie off the swollen veins may be performed if the sperm count is low.

varicose veins Enlarged, tortuous *veins* just beneath the skin. Varicose veins most often occur in the legs but can also occur in the anus (see *haemorrhoids*), oesophagus (see *oesophageal varices*), and scrotum (see *varicocele*).

A defect of the *valves* in the leg veins causes blood to pool in the veins near the surface of the skin, causing them to become varicose. Contributing factors include *obesity*, hormonal changes and pressure on the pelvic veins during *pregnancy*, hormonal changes occurring at the *menopause*, and standing for long periods of time. Varicose veins are common, tend to run in families, and affect more women than men.

Varicose veins may not cause any problems but may ache severely; swollen feet and ankles and persistent itching may occur. These symptoms may worsen during the day and can be relieved only by sitting with the legs raised. In women, symptoms are often worse just before menstruation. In severe cases, *leg ulcers* may occur. *Thrombophlebitis* may be associated with varicose veins.

Usually, support stockings, regular walking, and sitting with the feet up as much as possible are the only measures required. In more severe cases *sclerotherapy* may be carried out or the varicose veins may be removed surgically. Other treatment options include microwave or laser therapy, in which the varicose veins are obliterated using instruments inserted into the veins.

variola Another name for *smallpox*.

varus The medical term for an inward displacement of part of the body.

vascular Relating to the blood vessels (see *circulatory system*).

vasculitis Inflammation of blood vessels. Vasculitis usually leads to damage to the lining of vessels, with narrowing or blockage, that restricts or stops blood flow. As a result, the body tissues supplied by the affected vessels are damaged or destroyed by *ischaemia*.

Vasculitis is thought to be caused in most cases by the presence of minute bodies, called immune complexes, in the circulating blood. Immune complexes (consisting of *antigens* bound to *antibodies*) are normally destroyed by white blood cells, but sometimes adhere to the walls of blood vessels, where they cause inflammation. In some cases, the antigens are *viruses*. Vasculitis is the basic disease process in a number of disorders, including *polyarteritis nodosa*, *erythema nodosum*, *Henoch–Schönlein purpura*, *serum sickness*, *temporal arteritis*, and *Buerger's disease*.

V

VASECTOMY

SITES OF
INCISIONS

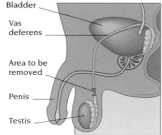

Bladder

Vas
deferens

Area to be
removed

Penis

Testis

BEFORE THE PROCEDURE

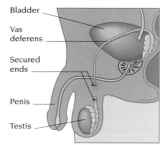

Bladder

Vas
deferens

Secured
ends

Penis

Testis

AFTER THE PROCEDURE

vas deferens Either of a pair of tubes that convey *sperm* from each *testis* and *epididymis* to the *urethra*. The plural form is vasa deferentia.

vasectomy The operation of male sterilization. Vasectomy is a minor surgical procedure, performed under local anaesthetic (see *anaesthesia, local*), that consists of cutting out a short length of each *vas deferens*. After vasectomy, the man continues to achieve orgasm and ejaculate as normal, but the *semen* no longer contains *sperm*, which are reabsorbed in the testes. Male sterilization is a safe and effective method of *contraception*. However, rarely, the severed ends of a vas deferens reunite, and sperm appear in the ejaculate. If this occurs, the man can safely undergo another vasectomy. Some operations to restore fertility after vasectomy are successful, but the process should be regarded as irreversible.

vasoconstriction Narrowing of blood vessels, causing reduced blood flow to a part of the body. Vasoconstriction under the skin occurs in response to the cold and reduces heat loss from the body.

vasodilation Widening of blood vessels, causing increased blood flow to a part of the body. Vasodilation under the skin occurs in response to hot weather and increases heat loss from the body.

vasodilator drugs A group of drugs that widen blood vessels. Vasodilator drugs include *ACE inhibitors, alphablockers, calcium channel blockers, nitrate drugs,* and sympatholytic drugs. They are used to treat disorders in which

abnormal narrowing of blood vessels reduces blood flow through tissues, impairing the supply of oxygen. Such disorders include *angina pectoris* and *peripheral vascular disease*. Vasodilators are also used to treat *hypertension* and *heart failure*. All vasodilator drugs may cause flushing, headaches, dizziness, fainting, and swollen ankles.

vasopressin Another name for *ADH*.

vasovagal attack Temporary loss of consciousness due to sudden slowing of the heartbeat, usually brought on by severe pain, stress, shock, or fear. A vasovagal attack, a common cause of *fainting* in healthy people, results from overstimulation of the *vagus nerve*.

VD The abbreviation for venereal disease, an outdated term for *sexually transmitted infections*.

vector An animal that transmits a particular *infectious disease*. A vector picks up disease-causing organisms from a source of infection (such as an infected person's or animal's blood or faeces), carries them in or on its body, and later deposits them where they infect a new host, directly or indirectly. Mosquitoes, fleas, lice, ticks, and flies are the most important vectors of disease to humans.

veganism The adoption of a diet that excludes all meat and fish and all animal products, including milk and eggs. A vegan diet may result in *vitamin B_{12}* or *calcium* deficiency. Supplements are essential during pregnancy.

vegetarianism Eating a diet that excludes meat and fish, and sometimes all other animal products. Humans do not need to eat meat or animal products to maintain health as long as the nutrients supplied by plant foods provide a balanced diet (see *nutrition*). However, people who exclude all animal products (vegans) need to plan their diet carefully or take supplements to avoid *vitamin B$_{12}$* or *calcium* deficiency.

Vegetarian diets are relatively rich in *fibre*, which may help protect against *diverticular disease* and cancer of the intestine (see *colon, cancer of*; *rectum, cancer of*). Vegetarian diets are low in *fats*, especially saturated fats (which may contribute to *coronary artery disease* and possibly some forms of cancer). These diets are also likely to contain less *sodium* and more *potassium*.

vegetative state A term that is sometimes used to describe a type of indefinite deep *coma*. Although the eyes may be open and occasional random movements of the head and limbs may occur, there are no other signs of consciousness, and there is no responsiveness to stimuli. Only the basic functions, such as breathing and heartbeat, are maintained.

vein A vessel that returns blood towards the *heart* from the various organs and tissues of the body. The walls of veins, like those of arteries, consist of a smooth inner lining, a muscular middle layer, and a fibrous outer covering. However, blood pressure in veins is lower than in arteries, and the walls of veins are thinner, less elastic, less muscular, and weaker than those of arteries. The linings of many veins contain folds, which act as valves, ensuring that blood flows only towards the heart. Blood is helped on its way through the veins by pressure on the vessel walls from the contraction of surrounding muscles. (See also *circulatory system*.)

veins, disorders of Common disorders affecting *veins* include *varicose veins*, deep vein thrombosis (see *thrombosis, deep vein*), and *thrombophlebitis*.

VENA CAVA

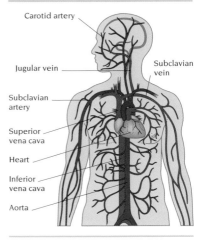

Carotid artery
Jugular vein
Subclavian vein
Subclavian artery
Superior vena cava
Heart
Inferior vena cava
Aorta

vena cava Either of two large *veins* into which all circulating (deoxygenated) blood drains. The venae cavae (superior and inferior) deliver blood to the right atrium of the *heart* for pumping to the lungs.

The superior vena cava starts at the top of the chest, close to the *sternum*, and passes down through the *pericardium* before connecting to the right atrium. It collects blood from the upper trunk, head, neck, and arms. The inferior vena cava starts in the lower abdomen and travels upwards in front of the spine, behind the liver, and through the *diaphragm* before joining the right atrium. It collects blood from the legs, pelvic organs, liver, and kidneys.

venepuncture A common procedure in which a *vein*, usually in the forearm, is pierced with a needle to inject fluid or withdraw blood. A *tourniquet* is used to

VEIN

Outer layer
Inner lining
Muscle laye
Valve flap

STRUCTURE OF A VEIN

V

VENEPUNCTURE

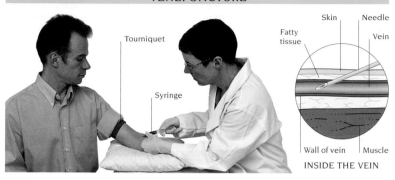

Tourniquet

Syringe

Skin | Needle

Fatty tissue | Vein

Wall of vein | Muscle

INSIDE THE VEIN

swell the veins, and a sterile needle is inserted. A syringe is attached to the needle if blood is to be taken or medication injected. For *intravenous infusion*, a cannula (tube) is inserted via the needle. After the fluid has been injected or withdrawn, the needle or cannula is removed. The area is then covered and pressure applied to stop any bleeding. The procedure is not usually painful but may cause some discomfort.

venereal diseases See *sexually transmitted infections*.

venereology The medical discipline concerned with the study and treatment of *sexually transmitted infections*.

venesection The process of withdrawing blood from a *vein* for *blood donation* or therapeutic bloodletting. Regular bloodletting is performed in the treatment of *polycythaemia* and *haemochromatosis*.

venlafaxine A serotonin and noradrenaline reuptake inhibitor (SNRI) drug used in the treatment of *depression*. Venlafaxine combines the effects of *selective serotonin reuptake inhibitors* and *tricyclic antidepressants* to produce fewer side effects than other types of antidepressant. Side effects may include nausea, dry mouth, and constipation.

venography A diagnostic procedure that enables *veins* to be seen on an *X-ray* film after they have been injected with a substance opaque to X-rays. It is used to detect abnormalities or diseases of the veins, such as narrowing or blockage from *thrombosis*.

venomous bites and stings The injection of venom by certain animals via their mouthparts (bites) or other injecting apparatus (stings). Venoms are often carried to discourage predators, and are sometimes used to kill or immobilize prey. It is rare for a venomous animal to attack a person unless it has been provoked or disturbed. Specific *antivenoms* are available to treat many, though not all, types of animal venom. (See also *insect stings*; *jellyfish stings*; *scorpion stings*; *snake bites*; *spider bites*.)

ventilation The use of a machine called a *ventilator* to take over or assist *breathing*. Arrested or severely impaired breathing may be due to *head injury*, brain disease, an overdose of *opioid drugs*, chest injury, respiratory disease, a nerve or muscle disorder, or major chest or abdominal surgery. Ventilation may be needed if a muscle relaxant has been given during an operation as part of general *anaesthesia*. Premature babies with *respiratory distress syndrome* may also need ventilation for a period until their lungs develop sufficiently. Positive pressure ventilation (continuous pumping of air under high pressure) may be used in the home in the treatment of *sleep apnoea*.

ventilator A device used for the artificial *ventilation* of a person who is unable to breathe naturally. A ventilator is an electrical pump connected to an air supply that works like bellows. Air is directed through a tube passed down the windpipe to inflate the lungs. The air is then expelled by the natural elasticity of the lungs and ribcage. A valve on the ventilator prevents the expelled air from re-entering the lungs.

ventilatory failure A life-threatening condition in which the amount of carbon dioxide in the blood rises, and the amount of oxygen falls, due to disruption of the normal exchange of gases between the air in the lungs and the blood. Ventilatory failure may be due to brain damage or to depression of the respiratory centres by excessive doses of drugs such as *morphine*. Treatment may involve artificial *ventilation* or, in some cases, the use of respiratory stimulant drugs. (See also *respiratory failure*.)

ventouse See *vacuum extraction*.

ventral Relating to the front of the body, or describing the lowermost part of a body structure when a person is lying face-down. The opposite is *dorsal*

ventricle A cavity or chamber. Both the *heart* and *brain* have anatomical parts known as ventricles.

The brain has four ventricles: one in each of the two cerebral hemispheres; a third at the centre of the brain, above the brainstem; and a fourth between the brainstem and cerebellum. These cavities are filled with *cerebrospinal fluid*.

The ventricles of the heart are its two lower chambers, which receive blood from each *atrium* and pump it to the lungs and to the rest of the body.

ventricular ectopic beat A type of cardiac *arrhythmia* in which abnormal heartbeats are initiated from electrical impulses in the *ventricles* of the *heart*. In a normal heart, beats are initiated by the *sinoatrial node* in the right atrium.

Ventricular ectopic beats may be detected on an *ECG*. If there are frequent abnormal beats that cause symptoms, or beats that arise from more than one site in the ventricles, treatment with an *antiarrhythmic drug* may be required.

ventricular fibrillation One of the two life-threatening cardiac *arrhythmias* that occur in *cardiac arrest*. The *heart* has rapid, uncoordinated, ineffective contractions and does not pump blood. The problem is due to abnormal heartbeats initiated by electrical activity in the ven-

tricles. It is a common complication of *myocardial infarction* and may also be caused by electrocution or drowning.

The diagnosis is confirmed by *ECG*. Emergency treatment is with *defibrillation* and *antiarrhythmic drugs*.

ventricular septal defect The medical term meaning a hole between the lower two chambers of the heart. The abnormality is present from birth and in many cases is small and closes without treatment. Surgery may be performed for larger defects, usually with good results.

VENTRICULAR SEPTAL DEFECT

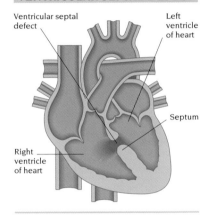

Ventricular septal defect

Left ventricle of heart

Septum

Right ventricle of heart

ventricular tachycardia A serious cardiac *arrhythmia* in which each heartbeat is initiated from electrical activity in the *ventricles* rather than from the *sinoatrial node* in the right atrium. It is caused by an abnormally fast heart-rate due to serious heart disease, such as *myocardial infarction* or *cardiomyopathy*. It may last for a few seconds or for several days. Diagnosis is confirmed by *ECG*. Emergency treatment is with *defibrillation* and an *antiarrhythmic drug*.

verapamil A drug that acts as a *calcium channel blocker* to treat *hypertension*, *angina pectoris*, and certain *arrhythmias*. Possible side effects include headache, flushing, dizziness, and ankle swelling.

vernix The white, cheese-like substance covering a newborn baby. Vernix comprises fatty secretions and dead cells. It protects the skin, insulates against heat loss before birth, and lubricates the baby's passage down the birth canal.

verruca The Latin name for a *wart*, commonly applied to warts on the soles.

version A change in the direction in which a *fetus* lies so that a *malpresentation*, most often a breech (bottom-down) presentation, replaces the normal head-down presentation.

vertebra Any of the 33 approximately cylindrical bones that form the *spine*. There are 7 vertebrae in the cervical spine; 12 vertebrae in the thoracic spine; 5 vertebrae in the lumbar spine; 5 fused vertebrae in the *sacrum*; and 4 fused vertebrae in the *coccyx*. The top 24 vertebrae are separated by discs of cartilage (see *disc, intervertebral*). Each vertebra has a hole in the centre through which the *spinal cord* runs, and processes to which muscles are attached.

VERTEBRA

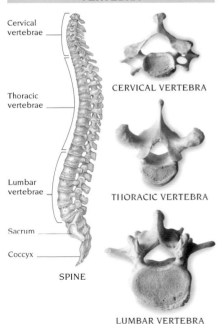

Cervical vertebrae

Thoracic vertebrae

CERVICAL VERTEBRA

Lumbar vertebrae

THORACIC VERTEBRA

Sacrum

Coccyx

SPINE

LUMBAR VERTEBRA

vertebrobasilar insufficiency Intermittent episodes of dizziness, double vision, weakness, and difficulty in speaking caused by reduced blood flow to

parts of the *brain*. It is usually due to *atherosclerosis* of the basilar and vertebral arteries and other arteries in the base of the brain. Vertebrobasilar insufficiency sometimes precedes a *stroke*.

vertigo An illusion that one or one's surroundings are spinning. Vertigo is due to a disturbance of the *semicircular canals* in the inner ear or the nerve tracts leading from them. Sudden-onset vertigo is treated with rest and *antihistamine drugs*, which, in some cases, are also given to prevent recurrent attacks.

vesicle A small *blister*, usually filled with clear fluid, that forms at a site of skin damage. The term is also used to refer to any small sac-like structure in the body.

vestibule A chamber. The vestibule in the inner ear is a hollow chamber that connects the three *semicircular canals*.

vestibulitis Inflammation of the nasal vestibule (the part of the nasal cavity just inside the nostril), usually as a result of bacterial infection.

vestibulocochlear nerve The 8th *cranial nerve*. It consists of two branches: the vestibular nerve (concerned with balance) and the cochlear nerve (concerned with hearing). Each vestibulocochlear nerve (one on each side) carries sensory impulses from the inner *ear* to the *brain*, which it enters between the pons and medulla oblongata (in the *brainstem*).

A tumour of the cells that surround the vestibulocochlear nerve (see *acoustic neuroma*) may cause loss of balance, *tinnitus*, and *deafness*. Deafness may also result from damage to the nerve, which may be due to an infection, such as *meningitis* or *encephalitis*, or to a reaction to a drug such as *streptomycin*.

viability The capability of independent survival and development.

vibration white finger See *Raynaud's phenomenon*.

villus A minute finger-like projection from a membranous surface. Millions of villi are present on the mucous lining of the small *intestine*. Each intestinal villus contains a small *lymph* vessel and a network of *capillaries*. Its surface is covered with hundreds of hairlike structures (microvilli). The villi and microvilli provide a large surface area for absorption of food

VILLUS

Capillary network

Villus

Mucus-producing cell

Lymph vessel

Artery

Vein

VILLI OF SMALL INTESTINE

molecules from the intestine into the blood and the lymphatic system.

vinca alkaloids A group of substances derived from the periwinkle plant (*VINCA ROSEA*) that are used to treat *leukaemias*, *lymphomas*, and some solid tumours, such as *breast cancer* and *lung cancer*. All vinca alkaloids can cause neurological toxicity, which appears as *neuropathy*. Other side effects may include abdominal pain, constipation, and reversible *alopecia*. Common vinca alkaloids are vinblastine, vindesine, and *vincristine*.

Vincent's disease A severe form of gingivitis in which bacterial infection causes painful ulceration of the gums. (See also *gingivitis, acute ulcerative*.)

vincristine A *vinca alkaloid* used to treat certain cancers. One particular side effect of vincristine is peripheral or autonomic *neuropathy*; but, unlike the other vinca alkaloids, it causes very little reduction in blood-cell production by the bone marrow. Other side effects may include abdominal pain, constipation, and reversible *alopecia*.

viraemia The presence of *virus* particles in the blood. Viraemia can occur at certain stages in a variety of viral infections. Some viruses, such as those responsible for viral *hepatitis*, *yellow fever*, and *poliomyelitis*, are transported in the bloodstream. Others, such as the *rubella* virus and *HIV*, multiply in, and spread

via, certain white blood cells. If viraemia is a feature of a viral infection, there is a risk that the infection may be transmitted to other people in blood or blood products, or by insects that feed on blood.

viral haemorrhagic fever Diseases that are prevalent in Africa and cause severe bleeding. There are several types, including Ebola fever, Lassa fever, Hantavirus, and Marburg fever. The diseases are fatal in a large percentage of cases, but Lassa fever may respond to *antiviral drugs* if given in the first week.

virginity The physical state of not having experienced sexual intercourse.

virilism The presence in a woman of masculine characteristics. Virilism is caused by excessive levels of *androgen hormones*. Androgens are male sex hormones which, in women, are normally secreted in small amounts by the adrenal glands and ovaries. Raised levels induce various changes in women, including *hirsutism*; male-pattern baldness; disruption or cessation of *menstruation*; enlargement of the *clitoris*; loss of normal fat deposits around the hips; development of the arm and shoulder muscles; and deepening of the voice.

virility A term used to describe the quality of maleness, especially in sexual characteristics and performance.

virilization The development in a woman of male characteristics as a result of overproduction of *androgen hormones* by the adrenal glands and/or ovaries. This may be due to various conditions such as certain *adrenal tumours*, polycystic ovary (see *ovary, polycystic*) and some other *ovarian cysts*, or congenital *adrenal hyperplasia*.

virion A single, complete, *virus* particle.

virology The study of *viruses* and the *epidemiology* and treatment of diseases caused by viruses. In a more restricted sense, virology also refers to the isola-tion and identification of viruses to diagnose specific viral infections. Depending on the type of virus, this may involve growing viruses in cultures of human or animal cells, *staining* or microscopic examination of specimens containing viruses, *immunoassay* techniques, or sequencing viral genomes.

V

virulence The ability of a microorganism to cause disease. This can be assessed by measuring what proportion of the population exposed to the microorganism develops symptoms of disease, how rapidly the infection spreads through the body, or the mortality from the infection.

viruses Extremely small infectious agents. It is debatable whether viruses are truly living organisms or just collections of molecules capable of self-replication under specific conditions. Their sole activity is to invade the cells of other organisms, which they then take over to make copies of themselves. Outside living cells, viruses are inert.

VIRUSES

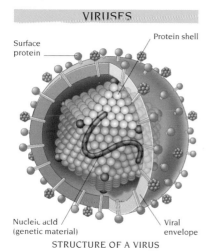

Surface protein

Protein shell

Nucleic acid (genetic material)

Viral envelope

STRUCTURE OF A VIRUS

A single virus particle (virion) consists of an inner core of *nucleic acid*, which may be either *DNA* or *RNA*, covered by one or two protective protein shells (capsids). Surrounding the outer capsid may be another layer, the viral envelope, which consists mainly of protein. The nucleic acid consists of a string of *genes* that have coded instructions for making copies of the virus.

Common viral diseases include the common *cold*, *influenza*, and *chickenpox* (caused by the varicella-zoster virus). *AIDS* is caused by the human immunodeficiency virus (*HIV*).

viscera A collective term used to describe the internal organs.

viscosity The resistance to flow of a fluid; its "stickiness". The viscosity of blood affects its ability to flow through small vessels. An increase in the viscosity of blood increases the risk of *thrombosis*.

vision The faculty of sight. When light-rays reach the *eye*, most of the focusing is done by the *cornea*, but the eye also has an automatic fine-focusing facility, *accommodation*, that operates by altering the curvature of the *lens*. Together, these systems form an image on the *retina*. The light-sensitive rod and cone cells in the retina convert the elements of this image into nerve impulses that pass into the visual cortex of the *brain* via the *optic nerves*. The rods, which are more concentrated at the periphery of the retina, are highly sensitive to light but not to colour. The colour-sensitive cones are concentrated more at the centre of the retina (see *colour vision*).

The brain coordinates the motor nerve impulses to the six tiny muscles that move each eye to achieve alignment of the eyes. Accurate alignment allows the brain to fuse the images from each eye, but because each eye has a slightly different view of a given object, the brain obtains information that is interpreted as solidity or depth. This stereoscopic vision is important in judging distance.

vision, disorders of The most common visual disorders are refractive errors, such as *myopia*, *hypermetropia*, and *astigmatism*, which can almost always be corrected by *glasses* or *contact lenses*. Other disorders include *amblyopia*; *double vision*; and disorders of the eye (see *eye, disorders of*) or *optic nerve*, of the nerve pathways connecting the optic nerves to the *brain*, and of the brain itself.

The eye may lose its transparency through corneal opacities, *cataract*, or *vitreous haemorrhage*. Defects near the centre of the retina cause loss of the corresponding parts of the *visual field* (see *macular degeneration*). *Floaters*, which are usually insignificant, may indicate a *retinal tear* or haemorrhage, or they may herald a *retinal detachment*. *Optic neuritis* can cause a blind spot in the centre of the visual field

Damage to the brain (for example, from a *stroke*) may cause visual impairment such as *hemianopia*, *agnosia*, visual perseveration (in which a scene continues to be perceived after the direction of gaze has shifted), and visual hallucinations.

vision, loss of Inability to see. This may develop slowly or suddenly and may be temporary or permanent, depending on the cause. Vision loss may affect one or both eyes. It can cause complete *blindness* or may affect only peripheral, or only central, vision.

Progressive loss of visual clarity is common with advancing age and may be due to a number of disorders (see *vision, disorders of*).

Sudden loss of vision may be caused by disorders such as *hyphaema*, severe *uveitis*, *vitreous haemorrhage*, or *retinal haemorrhage*. *Optic neuritis* can reduce vision in one eye. Damage to the nerve connections between the eyes and brain, or to the visual area of the brain, can cause loss of peripheral vision and may be a result of *embolism*, *ischaemia*, tumour, inflammation, or injury. (See also *eye, disorders of*.)

vision tests The part of an *eye examination* that determines whether there is any reduction in the ability to see. Most vision tests (for example the *Snellen chart*) are tests of *visual acuity*.

In visual acuity tests, a device called a phoropter is used to hold different lenses in front of each eye. The lenses in the phoropter are changed until the letters near the bottom of the Snellen chart can be read. Tests of *visual field* may also be performed to assess disorders of the eye and the nervous system. Refraction tests can detect *hypermetropia*, *myopia*, or *astigmatism*; the effect of lenses on movements of light reflected from the eye is observed to calculate the corrective *glasses* or *contact lenses* needed. If *presbyopia* is suspected, close-reading tests are used to assess *accommodation*.

visual acuity Sharpness of central *vision*. Refractive errors, such as *myopia*, *hypermetropia* and *astigmatism*, are the most common causes of poor visual acuity. Poor visual acuity for near objects occurs in *presbyopia*.

visual field The total area in which visual perception is possible while a person is looking straight ahead. The visual fields normally extend outwards over an angle of about 90 degrees on either side of the midline of the face, but are more restricted above and below, especially if the eyes are deep-set or the eyebrows are prominent. The visual fields of the two eyes overlap to a large extent, giving binocular vision. Partial loss of the visual field may occur in *glaucoma* or *stroke*.

vital sign An indication that a person is still alive. Vital signs include chest movements caused by breathing, the presence of a pulse, and the constriction of the *pupil* of the eye when it is exposed to a bright light.

vitamin Any of a group of complex organic substances that are essential in small amounts for the normal functioning of the body. There are 13 vitamins: A, C, D, E, K, B_{12}, and 7 grouped under the *vitamin B complex*. Apart from the B vitamin niacin and vitamin D, which the body can synthesize itself, vitamins must be obtained from the diet. A varied diet is likely to contain adequate amounts of all the vitamins, but *vitamin supplements* may be helpful for some people, such as young children, women who are pregnant or breast-feeding, or those taking drugs that interfere with vitamin function.

Vitamins can be categorized as fat-soluble or water-soluble.

VISION TESTS

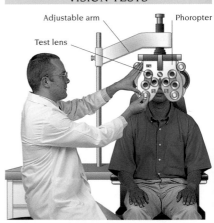

Adjustable arm

Phoropter

Test lens

The fat-soluble vitamins (A, D, E, and K) are absorbed with fats from the intestine into the bloodstream and then stored in fatty tissue (mainly in the liver). Body reserves of some of these vitamins last for several years, so a daily intake is not usually necessary. Deficiency of a fat-soluble vitamin is usually due to a disorder in which intestinal absorption of fats is impaired (see *malabsorption*) or to a prolonged poor diet.

Vitamin C, B_{12}, and those of the B complex are water-soluble. Vitamin C and B complex vitamins can be stored in the body in only limited amounts and are excreted in the urine if taken in greater amounts than needed. A regular intake is therefore essential to prevent deficiency. However, vitamin B_{12} is stored in the liver; these stores may last for years.

The role of all the vitamins in the body is not fully understood. Most vitamins have several important actions on one or more body systems, and many are involved in the activities of *enzymes*.

vitamin A A fat-soluble *vitamin* essential for normal growth, for the formation of bones and teeth, for cell structure, for night vision, and for protecting the linings of the respiratory, digestive, and urinary tracts against infection.

Vitamin A is absorbed by the body in the form of retinol. This is found in liver, fish-liver oils, egg yolk, dairy produce, and is added to margarines. *Carotene*, which the body converts into retinol, is found in various vegetables and fruits.

Vitamin A deficiency is rare in developed countries. In most cases, it is due to *malabsorption*. Vitamin A deficiency may also result from long-term treatment with certain *lipid-lowering drugs*. Deficiency is common in some developing countries due to poor diet. The first symptom of deficiency is night blindness, followed by dryness and inflammation of the eyes (see *xerophthalmia*), *keratomalacia*, and eventually blindness. Deficiency also causes reduced resistance to infection, dry skin, and, in children, stunted growth.

Prolonged excessive intake of vitamin A can cause headache, nausea, loss of appetite, skin peeling, hair loss, and irregular menstruation. In severe cases,

the liver and spleen become enlarged. Excess vitamin A, particularly in the form of retinol, has been linked with an increased risk of bone fractures. Excessive intake during pregnancy may cause birth defects. In infants, excessive intake may cause skull deformities, which disappear if the diet is corrected.

Retinoid drugs are derivatives of vitamin A that are principally used to treat skin conditions. For example, *tretinoin* and *isotretinoin* are used to treat severe *acne*, and *acitretin* is used to treat severe *psoriasis* and *ichthyosis*.

vitamin B See *vitamin B_{12}*; *vitamin B complex*.

vitamin B_{12} A water-soluble *vitamin* that plays a vital role in the activities of several *enzymes* in the body. Vitamin B_{12} is important in the production of the genetic material of cells (and thus in growth and development), the production of red blood cells in bone marrow, the utilization of folic acid and carbohydrates in the diet, and the functioning of the nervous system. Foods rich in vitamin B_{12} include liver, kidney, chicken, beef, pork, fish, eggs, and dairy products.

Deficiency is almost always due to inability of the intestine to absorb vitamin B_{12}, usually because of pernicious anaemia (see *anaemia, megaloblastic*). Less commonly, deficiency may result from *gastrectomy*, *malabsorption*, or *veganism*. The effects of vitamin B_{12} deficiency are megaloblastic anaemia, a sore mouth and tongue, and symptoms caused by damage to the *spinal cord*, such as numbness and tingling in the limbs. There may also be depression and memory loss. A high intake of vitamin B_{12} has no known harmful effects.

vitamin B complex A group of water-soluble *vitamins* comprising thiamine (vitamin B_1), riboflavin (vitamin B_2), niacin, pantothenic acid, pyridoxine (vitamin B_6), biotin (vitamin H), and folic acid. *Vitamin B_{12}* is discussed above.

Thiamine plays a role in the activities of various *enzymes* involved in the utilization of *carbohydrates* and thus in the functioning of nerves, muscles, and the heart. Sources include whole-grain cereals, wholemeal breads, brown rice, pasta, liver, kidney, pork, fish, beans, nuts, and eggs. Those susceptible to deficiency include elderly people on a poor diet, and people with *hyperthyroidism*, *malabsorption*, or severe *alcohol dependence*. Deficiency may also occur as a result of severe illness, surgery, or injury. Mild deficiency may cause tiredness, irritability, and appetite loss. Severe deficiency may cause abdominal pain, constipation, depression, memory impairment, and *beriberi*; in alcoholics, it may cause *Wernicke–Korsakoff syndrome*. Severe allergic reactions may occur when thiamine is given by intravenous injection.

Riboflavin is necessary for the activities of various enzymes involved in the breakdown and utilization of carbohydrates, fats, and proteins; the production of energy in cells; the utilization of other B vitamins; and hormone production by the adrenal glands. Liver, whole grains, milk, eggs, and brewer's yeast are good sources. People who are susceptible to riboflavin deficiency include those taking phenothiazine *antipsychotic drugs*, tricyclic *antidepressant drugs*, or oestrogen-containing *oral contraceptives*, and those with malabsorption or severe alcohol dependence. Riboflavin deficiency may also occur as a result of serious illness, surgery, or injury. Prolonged deficiency may cause soreness of the tongue and the corners of the mouth, and eye disorders such as *amblyopia* and *photophobia*. Excessive intake of riboflavin is not known to have any harmful effects.

Niacin plays an essential role in the activities of various enzymes involved in the metabolism of carbohydrates and fats, the functioning of the nervous and digestive systems, the manufacture of sex hormones, and the maintenance of healthy skin. The main dietary sources are liver, lean meat, fish, nuts, and dried beans. Niacin can be made in the body from tryptophan (an *amino acid*). Most cases of deficiency are due to malabsorption disorders or to severe alcohol dependence. Prolonged niacin deficiency causes *pellagra*. Excessive intake is not known to cause harmful effects.

Pantothenic acid is essential for the activities of various enzymes involved in the metabolism of carbohydrates and fats, the manufacture of *corticosteroids* and *sex hormones*, the utilization of other vitamins, the functioning of the nervous system and *adrenal glands*, and growth and development. It is present in almost all vegetables, cereals, and animal foods. Deficiency of pantothenic acid usually occurs as a result of malabsorption or alcoholism, but may also occur after severe illness, surgery, or injury. The effects include fatigue, headache, nausea, abdominal pain, numbness and tingling, muscle cramps, and susceptibility to respiratory infections. In severe cases, a *peptic ulcer* may develop. Excessive intake has no known harmful effects.

Pyridoxine aids the activities of various enzymes and hormones involved in the utilization of carbohydrates, fats, and proteins, in the manufacture of red blood cells and antibodies, in the functioning of the digestive and nervous systems, and in the maintenance of healthy skin. Dietary sources are liver, chicken, pork, fish, whole grains, wheatgerm, bananas, potatoes, and dried beans. Pyridoxine is also manufactured by intestinal bacteria. People who are susceptible to pyridoxine deficiency include elderly people who have a poor diet, those with malabsorption or severe alcohol dependence, or those who are taking certain drugs (including *penicillamine* and *isoniazid*). Deficiency may cause weakness, irritability, depression, skin disorders, inflammation of the mouth and tongue, *anaemia*, and, in infants, *seizures*. Long-term use of high-dose pyridoxine has been associated with peripheral nerve disorders (see *neuropathy*).

Biotin is essential for the activities of various enzymes involved in the breakdown of fatty acids and carbohydrates and for the excretion of the waste products of protein breakdown. It is present in many foods, especially liver, peanuts, dried beans, egg yolk, mushrooms, bananas, grapefruit, and watermelon. Biotin is also manufactured by bacteria in the intestines. Deficiency may occur during prolonged treatment with *antibiotics* or *sulphonamide drugs*. Symptoms are weakness, tiredness, poor appetite,

V

hair loss, depression, inflammation of the tongue, and eczema. Excessive intake has no known harmful effects.

Folic acid is vital for various enzymes involved in the manufacture of *nucleic acids* and consequently for growth and reproduction, the production of red blood cells, and the functioning of the nervous system. Sources include green vegetables, mushrooms, liver, nuts, dried beans, peas, egg yolk, and whole-meal bread. Mild deficiency is common, but can usually be corrected by increasing dietary intake. More severe deficiency may occur during pregnancy or breast-feeding, in premature or low-birthweight infants, in people undergoing *dialysis*, in people with certain blood disorders, *psoriasis*, malabsorption, or alcohol dependence, and in people taking certain drugs. The main effects include anaemia, sores around the mouth, and, in children, poor growth. During pregnancy folic acid is important for fetal growth and development, and folic acid supplements help prevent *neural tube defects* such as *spina bifida*. Women who are planning a pregnancy should take the recommended dose of folic acid supplement before conceiving and then during the first 12 weeks of pregnancy. If there is a family history of neural tube defects, a higher dose of supplement is recommended.

vitamin C A water-soluble *vitamin* that plays an essential role in the activities of various *enzymes*. Vitamin C is important for the growth and maintenance of healthy bones, teeth, gums, ligaments, and blood vessels; in the production of certain *neurotransmitters* and adrenal gland hormones; in the response of the *immune system* to infection; in wound healing; and in the absorption of *iron*.

The main dietary sources are fruits and vegetables. Considerable amounts of vitamin C are lost when foods are processed, cooked, or kept warm.

Mild deficiency of vitamin C may result from a serious injury or burn, major surgery, the use of *oral contraceptives*, fever, or continual inhalation of carbon monoxide (from traffic fumes or tobacco smoke). It may cause weakness, general aches, swollen gums, and *nosebleeds*.

More serious deficiency is usually caused by a very restricted diet. Severe deficiency leads to *scurvy* and *anaemia*.

If the daily dose of vitamin C exceeds about 1g, it may cause nausea, stomach cramps, and diarrhoea.

vitamin D The collective term for a group of substances that help to regulate the balance of *phosphate* and *calcium* in the body, aid calcium absorption in the intestine, and promote strong bones and teeth.

Good sources include oily fish, liver, and egg yolk; vitamin D is also added to margarines. In the body, vitamin D is synthesized by the action of ultraviolet light on a particular chemical in the skin.

Deficiency may occur in people with a poor diet, in premature infants, and in those deprived of sunlight. It can also result from *malabsorption*. Other causes include liver or kidney disorders and some genetic defects. Prolonged use of certain drugs, such as *phenytoin*, may also lead to deficiency. Deficiency in young children causes *rickets*, long-term deficiency in adults leads to *osteomalacia*.

Excessive intake of vitamin D may lead to *hypercalcaemia* and abnormal calcium deposits in the soft tissues, kidneys, and blood vessel walls. In children, it may cause growth retardation.

vitamin E The collective term for a group of substances that are essential for normal cell structure, for maintaining the activities of certain *enzymes*, and for the formation of red blood cells. Vitamin E also protects the lungs and other tissues from damage by pollutants and is believed to slow aging of cells. Sources include vegetable oils, nuts, meat, green vegetables, cereals, and egg yolk.

Dietary deficiency is rare; deficiency is most common in people with *malabsorption*, certain liver disorders, and in premature infants. It leads to the destruction of red blood cells, which eventually leads to *anaemia*. In infants, deficiency causes irritability and *oedema*.

Prolonged excessive intake of vitamin E may cause abdominal pain, nausea, and diarrhoea. It may also reduce intestinal absorption of vitamins A, D, and K.

vitamin K A fat-soluble *vitamin* that is essential for the formation in the liver of substances that promote blood clotting. Good sources are green vegetables, vegetable oils, egg yolk, cheese, pork, and liver. Vitamin K is also manufactured by bacteria in the intestine.

Dietary deficiency rarely occurs. Deficiency may develop in people with *malabsorption*, certain liver disorders, or chronic diarrhoea. It may also result from prolonged treatment with *antibiotics*. Newborns lack the intestinal bacteria that produce vitamin K and are routinely given supplements to prevent deficiency. Vitamin K deficiency may cause nosebleeds and bleeding from the gums, intestine, and urinary tract. In rare, severe cases, brain haemorrhage may result. Excessive intake of vitamin K is not known to cause harmful effects.

vitamin supplements A group of dietary preparations containing one or more *vitamins*. Most healthy people who have a balanced diet do not need them and excessive intake of some vitamins may be harmful. Supplements are used to treat diagnosed vitamin deficiency. They may also be recommended for certain groups, such as those with increased requirements (for example, women who are pregnant or breast-feeding); infants (see *feeding, infant*); those who follow a restricted diet (in *veganism*, for example); those with severe *alcohol dependence*; and people who have *malabsorption*, *liver disorders*, *kidney disorders*, or another serious illness or injury. In addition, vitamins are used to treat certain disorders. For example, vitamin D is used to treat *osteomalacia*, and vitamin A derivatives may be given for severe *acne*.

vitiligo A common disorder of *skin* pigmentation in which patches of skin, most commonly on the face, hands, armpits, and groin, lose their colour. Vitiligo is thought to be an *autoimmune disorder*. It may occur at any age but usually develops in early adulthood.

Spontaneous repigmentation occurs in some cases. A course of *phototherapy* using *PUVA* can also induce repigmentation of the skin, and creams containing *corticosteroid drugs* may help.

vitreous haemorrhage Bleeding into the *vitreous humour*. Common causes include a blow to the eye, diabetic *retin-*

opathy, and a blocked retinal vein (see *retinal vein occlusion*). A vitreous haemorrhage often affects vision and may even cause sudden loss of vision; it requires immediate medical assessment. Treatment depends on the underlying cause.

vitreous humour The transparent, gel-like body that fills the rear compartment of the *eye*. The vitreous humour consists almost entirely of water.

vivisection The performance of a surgical operation on a live animal. (See also *animal experimentation*.)

vocal cords Two fibrous sheets of tissue in the *larynx* that are responsible for voice production. The vocal cords are attached at the front to the thyroid cartilage and at the rear to the arytenoid cartilages. To produce sound, the vocal cords, which normally form a V-shaped opening, close and vibrate as air expelled from the lungs passes between them. Alterations in cord tension produce sounds of different pitch, which are modified by the tongue, mouth, and lips to form *speech*.

VOCAL CORDS

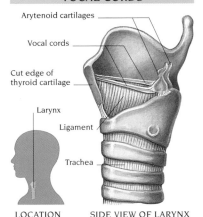

Arytenoid cartilages

Vocal cords

Cut edge of thyroid cartilage

Larynx

Ligament

Trachea

LOCATION   SIDE VIEW OF LARYNX

voice-box See *larynx*.

voice, loss of Inability to speak normally. Temporary partial loss of voice commonly results from straining of the muscles of the *larynx* through overuse of the voice or from inflammation of the *vocal cords* in *laryngitis*. Persistent or recurrent voice loss may be due to *polyps* on the vocal cords, thickening of the cords in *hypothyroidism*, or interference with the nerve supply to the larynx muscles due to cancer of the larynx, *thyroid gland*, or *oesophagus*. Total loss of voice is rare and is usually of psychological origin. (See also *hoarseness; larynx, disorders of.*)

Volkmann's contracture A disorder in which the wrist and fingers become permanently fixed in a bent position. It occurs because of an inadequate blood supply to the forearm muscles that control the wrist and fingers as a result of an injury. Initially, the fingers become cold, numb, and white or blue. Finger movements are weak and painful, and there is no pulse at the wrist. Unless treatment is started within a few hours, wrist and finger deformity develops.

Treatment is by manipulation back into position of any displaced bones, followed, if necessary, by surgical restoration of blood flow in the forearm. If there is permanent deformity, *physiotherapy* may help to restore function.

volvulus Twisting of a loop of *intestine* or, in rare cases, of the *stomach*. Volvulus is a serious condition that causes obstruction of the passage of intestinal contents (see *intestine, obstruction of*) and a risk of *strangulation*. If strangulation occurs, blockage of blood flow to the affected area leads to potentially fatal *gangrene*. The symptoms of volvulus are severe episodes of abdominal pain followed by vomiting. Volvulus may be present from birth or may be a result of *adhesions*. It requires emergency treatment, usually by surgery.

vomiting Involuntary forcible expulsion of stomach contents through the mouth. Vomiting may be preceded by nausea, pallor, sweating, excessive salivation, and slowed heart-rate. It occurs when the vomiting centre in the *brainstem* is activated by signals from one of three places in the body: the digestive tract; the balancing mechanism of the inner ear; or the brain, either due to thoughts and emotions or via the part of the brain that responds to poisons in the body. The vomiting centre sends messages to both the *diaphragm*, which

presses down on the stomach, and the abdominal wall, which presses inwards, thereby expelling the stomach contents upwards through the *oesophagus*.

Vomiting may be due to overindulgence in food or alcohol, is a common side effect of many drugs, and may follow general *anaesthesia*. Vomiting is also common in gastrointestinal disorders such as *peptic ulcer*, acute *appendicitis*, *gastroenteritis*, and *food poisoning*. Less commonly, it is due to obstruction (see *pyloric stenosis; intussusception*) or a tumour of the digestive tract. It may also be due to inflammation (see *hepatitis; pancreatitis; cholecystitis*).

Other possible causes are pressure on the skull (see *encephalitis; hydrocephalus; brain tumour; head injury; migraine*), conditions affecting the ear's balancing mechanism (see *Ménière's disease; labyrinthitis; motion sickness*), and hormonal disorders (see *Addison's disease*).

Vomiting may be a symptom of ketoacidosis in poorly controlled *diabetes mellitus*. It may also be a symptom of an emotional problem or be part of the disorders *anorexia nervosa* or *bulimia*.

Persistent vomiting requires medical investigation. Treatment depends on the cause. *Antiemetics* may be given. (See also *vomiting blood, vomiting in pregnancy.*)

vomiting blood A symptom of bleeding from within the digestive tract. Vomiting blood may be caused by a tear in the lower oesophagus (see *Mallory–Weiss syndrome*), bleeding from *oesophageal varices*, erosive *gastritis*, *peptic ulcer*, or, rarely, *stomach cancer*. Blood can also be vomited if it is swallowed during a nosebleed. Vomited blood may be dark red, brown, black, or may resemble coffee grounds. Vomiting of blood is often accompanied by the passing of black, tarry faeces.

The cause of vomiting blood is investigated by *endoscopy* of the oesophagus and stomach, or by *barium X-ray examinations*. If blood loss is severe, *blood transfusion*, and possibly surgery to stop the bleeding, may be required.

vomiting in pregnancy Nausea and vomiting in early *pregnancy* are common and are most likely to be caused by changes in the hormone levels.

Vomiting occurs most frequently in the morning, but it may occur at any time. It is sometimes precipitated by stress, travelling, or food.

In rare cases, the vomiting becomes severe and prolonged. This can cause dehydration, nutritional deficiency, alterations in blood acidity, and weight loss. Immediate hospital admission is then required to replace lost fluids and chemicals by *intravenous infusion*, to rule out any serious underlying disorder, and to control the vomiting.

von Recklinghausen's disease Another name for *neurofibromatosis*.

von Willebrand's disease An inherited lifelong *bleeding disorder* similar to *haemophilia*. People with the condition have a reduced concentration in their blood of a substance called von Willebrand factor, which helps *platelets* in the blood to plug injured blood vessel walls and forms part of *factor VIII* (a substance vital to blood coagulation). Symptoms of deficiency of this factor include excessive bleeding from the gums and from cuts and nosebleeds. Women may have heavy menstrual bleeding. In severe cases, bleeding into joints and muscles may occur.

The disease is diagnosed by *blood-clotting tests* and measurement of blood levels of von Willebrand factor. Bleeding episodes can be prevented or controlled by desmopressin (a substance resembling *ADH*). Factor VIII or concentrated von Willebrand factor may also be used to treat bleeding.

voyeurism The observation, on a regular basis, of unsuspecting people who may be naked, getting undressed, or engaged in sexual activity, in order to achieve sexual arousal.

VSD The abbreviation for *ventricular septal defect*.

vulva The external part of the female genitalia, comprising the *clitoris* and two pairs of skin folds called *labia*.

The most common symptom affecting the vulva is *vulval itching*. Various skin disorders, such as *dermatitis*, may affect the vulva. Specific vulval conditions include genital *warts*, *vulvitis*, *vulvo-vaginitis*, and cancer (*vulva, cancer of*).

vulva, cancer of A rare disorder that most commonly affects postmenopausal women. Cancer of the vulva may be preceded by vulval itching, but in many cases the first symptom is a lump or painful ulcer on the vulva.

A diagnosis of vulval cancer is made by *biopsy*. Treatment is by surgical removal of the affected area. The outlook depends on how soon the cancer is diagnosed and treated.

vulval itching Irritation of the *vulva*. Most commonly, vulval itching is due to an allergic reaction to chemicals in spermicidal or hygiene products. Itching is also common after the *menopause*, when it is due to low levels of *oestrogen*. In addition, vulval itching may be caused by a vaginal discharge due to infection (see *vaginitis*) or by vulval skin changes (see *vulvitis*). Rarely, vulval itching may be an early symptom of *vulval cancer*. Treatment of vulval itching depends on the cause.

vulvitis Inflammation of the *vulva*. Infections that may cause vulvitis are *candidiasis*, genital herpes (see *herpes, genital*), and warts (see *warts, genital*). Infestations with *pubic lice* or *scabies* are other possible causes. Vulvitis may also occur as a result of changes in the vulval skin. These changes tend to affect women after the *menopause*, although there is no apparent trigger. They may take the form of red or white patches and/or thickened or thinned areas that may be inflamed. Other possible causes of vulvitis include allergic reactions to hygiene products, excessive vaginal discharge, or urinary *incontinence*.

Treatment depends on the cause. A combination of drugs applied to the vulva and good hygiene is usually recommended. A *biopsy* may be taken, if there are skin changes, to exclude the slight possibility of vulval cancer. (See also *vulvovaginitis*; *vaginitis*.)

vulvovaginitis Inflammation of the *vulva* and *vagina*. Vulvovaginitis is often provoked as a result of the infections *candidiasis* or *trichomoniasis*. (See also *vaginitis*; *vulvitis*.)

V

W

walking Movement of the body by lifting the feet alternately and bringing one foot into contact with the ground before the other starts to leave it. A person's gait is determined by body shape, size, and posture. The age at which children first walk varies enormously.

Walking is controlled by nerve signals from the brain's motor cortex (see *cerebrum*), *basal ganglia*, and *cerebellum* that travel via the spinal cord to the muscles.

Abnormal gait may be caused by joint stiffness, muscle weakness (sometimes due to conditions such as *poliomyelitis* or *muscular dystrophy*), or skeletal abnormalities (see, for example, *talipes*; *developmental dysplasia of the hip*; *scoliosis*; *bone tumour*; *arthritis*). Children may develop *knock-knee* or *bowleg*; *synovitis* of the hip and *Perthes' disease* are also common. Adolescents may develop a painful limp due to a slipped epiphysis (see *femoral epiphysis, slipped*) or to fracture or disease of the *tibia*, *fibula* or *femur*.

Abnormal gait may also be the result of neurological disorders such as *stroke* (commonly resulting in *hemiplegia*), *parkinsonism*, peripheral neuritis, multiple sclerosis, various forms of *myelitis*, and *chorea*. *Ménière's disease* may cause severe loss of balance and instability.

walking aids Equipment for increasing the mobility of people who have a disorder that affects their ability to *walk*. Aids include walking sticks, crutches, and walking frames.

walking, delayed Most children walk by around 15 months of age. Delayed walking may be suspected if the child is unable to walk unassisted by 18 months (see *developmental delay*).

warfarin An *anticoagulant drug* used to treat and prevent abnormal *blood clotting*. Warfarin is used to treat deep vein *thrombosis*, *pulmonary embolism*, and people with *atrial fibrillation* who are at risk of an *embolism*. It is also prescribed to prevent emboli from developing on replacement valves (see *heart-valve surgery*). A faster-acting anticoagulant, such as *heparin*, may also be prescribed for the first few days following a deep vein thrombosis or pulmonary embolism.

Warfarin may cause abnormal bleeding in different parts of the body, so regular tests are carried out to allow careful regulation of dosage. Warfarin may also cause nausea, diarrhoea and a rash.

wart A common, contagious, harmless growth that occurs on the skin or mucous membranes. Only the topmost layer of skin is affected. An overgrowth of cells in this layer causes a visible lump to develop. Warts are caused by the human papillomavirus, of which at least 50 different types are known. These cause different types of warts at various sites, such as on the hands or genitals.

WART

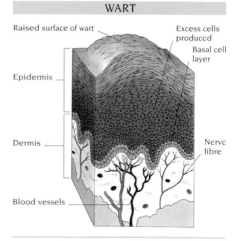

Raised surface of wart — Excess cells produced — Basal cell layer — Epidermis — Dermis — Nerve fibre — Blood vessels

Flat warts are flesh-coloured, sometimes itchy lumps with flat tops that occur mainly on the wrists, backs of hands, and face. About 50 per cent of warts disappear in 6–12 months without treatment. However, genital warts should be treated promptly. Common, flat, and plantar warts can sometimes be destroyed using a wart-removing liquid or special plaster. Several treatments may be necessary, and sometimes the wart returns. Warts are commonly treated by *cryosurgery*.

W

wart, plantar A hard, horny, and rough-surfaced area on the sole of the foot caused by a virus called a papillomavirus. Plantar warts, also known as verrucas, may occur singly or in clusters. The wart is flattened and forced into the skin and may cause discomfort or pain when walking. Infection can be acquired from contaminated floors in swimming pools and communal showers.

Many plantar warts disappear without treatment, but some persist for years or recur. They can be removed by *cryosurgery* or by applying plasters or gel containing *salicylic acid*.

warts, genital Fleshy, painless, usually soft lumps that grow in and around the entrance of the vagina, around the anus, and on the penis. Genital warts are transmitted by sexual contact and are caused by some forms of *human papillomavirus* (HPV). The warts appear from a few weeks to 18 months after infection. They may be removed by *cryosurgery* or by the application of the drug *podophyllin*, but tend to recur.

Genital warts due to some types of human papillomavirus are linked wih the development of cervical cancer (see *cervix, cancer of*).

wasp stings See *insect stings*.

water A simple compound that is essential for all life. Its molecular structure is H_2O (two atoms of hydrogen bonded to one of oxygen). Water is the most common substance in the body, accounting for about 99 per cent of all molecules, but a smaller percentage of total body weight. Approximately two-thirds of the body's water content is contained within the body cells, and the remaining third is extracellular (found, for example, in the blood plasma, lymph, and cerebrospinal and *tissue fluid*).

Water provides the medium in which all metabolic reactions take place (see *metabolism*), and transports substances around the body. The blood plasma carries water to all body tissues, and excess water from tissues for elimination via the *liver*, *kidneys*, *lungs*, and *skin*. The passage of water in the tissue fluid into and out of cells takes place by *osmosis*.

Water is taken into the body in food and drink and is lost in *urine* and *faeces*, as exhaled water vapour, and by sweating (see *dehydration*). The amount of water excreted in urine is regulated by the kidneys (see also *ADH*). Extra water is needed to excrete excess amounts of substances, such as sugar or salt, in the blood, and high water intake is essential in hot climates where a large amount of water is lost in sweat.

In some disorders, such as *kidney failure* or *heart failure*, insufficient water is excreted in the urine, resulting in *oedema*.

water-borne infection A disease caused by infective or parasitic organisms transmitted via water. Infections can be contracted if infected water is drunk, if it contaminates food, or if individuals swim or wade in it. Worldwide, contamination of drinking water is an important mode of transmission for various diseases including *hepatitis A*, many viral and bacterial causes of *diarrhoea*, *typhoid fever*, *cholera*, *amoebiasis*, and some types of *worm infestation*.

Swimming in polluted water should be avoided because, if swallowed, there is a risk of contracting disease. In addition, a form of *leptospirosis* is caused by contact with water contaminated by rat's urine. In tropical countries, there is also a risk of contracting *schistosomiasis* (bilharzia), which is a serious disease caused by a fluke that can burrow through the swimmer's skin.

waterbrash The sudden filling of the mouth with tasteless saliva. It is normally accompanied by other symptoms, and usually indicates a disorder of the upper gastrointestinal tract.

Waterhouse–Friderichsen syndrome A serious condition caused by infection of the bloodstream by bacteria of the meningococcus group. The main features are bleeding into the skin, low blood pressure, and *shock*. Without urgent medical treatment, coma and death follow in a few hours. The syndrome is often associated with *meningitis*.

watering eye An increase in volume of the tear film, usually producing epiphora (overflow of *tears*). Watering may be caused by excess tear production due to emotion, conjunctival or corneal irritation, or an obstruction to the channel that drains tears from the eye. (See also *lacrimal apparatus*.)

water intoxication A condition that is caused by excessive water retention in the brain. The principal symptoms are headaches, dizziness, nausea, confusion, and, in severe cases, seizures and unconsciousness.

Various disorders can disrupt the water balance in the body, leading to accumulation of water in the tissues. Examples include *kidney failure*, liver *cirrhosis*, severe *heart failure*, diseases of the *adrenal glands*, and certain lung or ovarian tumours producing a substance similar to *ADH* (antidiuretic hormone). Water intoxication is also seen in association with the use of *Ecstasy* (MDMA), during which excessive amounts of water are drunk. There is also a risk of water intoxication after surgery, caused by increased ADH production.

water on the brain A nonmedical term for *hydrocephalus*.

water on the knee A popular term for accumulation of fluid within or around the knee joint. The most common cause is *bursitis*. (See also *effusion, joint*.)

water retention Accumulation of fluid in body tissues (see *oedema*).

water tablets A nonmedical term for *diuretic drugs*.

wax bath A type of *heat treatment* in which hot liquid wax is applied to a part of the body to relieve pain and stiffness in inflamed or injured joints. Wax baths may be used to treat the hands of people with *rheumatoid arthritis*.

weakness A term used to describe a lack of vigour or strength. This is a common symptom of a wide range of conditions, including *anaemia*, emotional problems, and various disorders affecting the heart, nervous system, bones, joints, and muscles. When associated with emotional disorders, weakness may represent a lack of desire or ambition, rather than loss of muscle strength.

More specifically, the term describes loss of power in particular muscle groups, which may be accompanied by muscle wasting and loss of sensation. (See also *paralysis*.)

weal A raised bump on the skin that is paler than the adjacent tissue and which may be surrounded by an area of red inflammation. Weals are characteristic of *urticaria*.

weaning The gradual substitution of solid foods for milk or milk formula in an infant's diet (see *feeding, infant*).

webbing A flap of skin, such as might occur between adjacent fingers or toes. Webbing is a common congenital abnormality that often runs in families and which may affect two or more digits. Mild webbing is completely harmless, but surgical correction may be performed for cosmetic reasons. In severe cases, adjacent digits may be completely fused (see *syndactyly*). Webbing of the neck is a feature of *Turner's syndrome*.

Wegener's granulomatosis A rare disorder in which *granulomas* (nodular collections of abnormal cells), associated with areas of chronic tissue inflammation due to *vasculitis*, develop in the nasal passages, lungs, and kidneys. It is thought that the condition is an *autoimmune disorder* (in which the body's natural defences attack its own tissues).

Principal symptoms include a bloody nasal discharge, coughing (which sometimes produces bloodstained sputum), breathing difficulty, chest pain, and blood in the urine. There may also be loss of appetite, weight loss, weakness, fatigue, and joint pains.

Treatment is with *immunosuppressant drugs*, such as *cyclophosphamide* or *azathioprine*, combined with *corticosteroids* to alleviate symptoms and attempt to bring about a remission. With prompt treatment, most people recover completely within about a year, although *kidney failure* occasionally develops. Without treatment, complications may occur, including perforation of the nasal septum, causing deformity of the nose; inflammation of the eyes; a rash, nodules, or ulcers on the skin; and damage to the heart muscle, which may be fatal.

weight The heaviness of a person or object. In children, weight is routinely used as an index of growth. In healthy adults, weight remains more or less stable as dietary energy intake matches energy expenditure (see *metabolism*) *Weight loss* or weight gain occurs if the net balance is disturbed.

The standard method of assessing weight is the *body mass index* (BMI), which is obtained by dividing weight in (kilograms) by the square of the height (in metres). A BMI of 18.4 or less is classed as underweight; a BMI of 18.5–24.9 is classed as an ideal weight; a BMI of 25–29.9 is classed as overweight; a BMI of 30–39.9 is classed as obese; and a BMI over 40 is classed as very obese. However, these figures are general ones that apply to most healthy adults under the age of 60. They are not applicable to children or people over 60; people with chronic health problems; pregnant or breast-feeding women; or athletes, weight-trainers, or similar groups of people with a high proportion of body muscle.

weight loss This occurs any time there is a decrease in energy intake compared with energy expenditure. The decrease may be due to deliberate *weight reduction* or a change in diet or activity level. It may also be a symptom of a disorder. Unexplained weight loss should always be investigated by a doctor.

Many diseases disrupt the appetite, which may lead to weight loss. *Depression* reduces the motivation to eat, *peptic ulcer* causes pain and possible food avoidance, and some kidney disorders cause loss of appetite due to the effect of *uraemia*. In *anorexia nervosa* and *bulimia*, complex psychological factors affect an individual's eating pattern.

Digestive disorders, such as *gastroenteritis*, lead to weight loss through vomiting. Cancer of the oesophagus (see *oesophagus, cancer of*) and *stomach cancer* cause loss of weight, as does *malabsorption* of nutrients in certain disorders of the intestine or pancreas.

Some disorders cause weight loss by increasing the rate of metabolic activity in cells. Examples are any type of *cancer*, chronic infection such as *tuberculosis*, and *hyperthyroidism*. Untreated *diabetes mellitus* also causes weight loss due to a number of factors.

weight reduction The process of losing excess body fat. A person who is severely overweight (see *obesity*) is more at risk of various illnesses, such as *diabetes mellitus*, *hypertension* (high blood pressure), and heart disease.

The most efficient way to lose weight is to eat 500–1,000 kcal (2,100–4,200 kJ) a day less than the body's total energy requirements. Exercise also forms an extremely important part of a reducing regime, burning excess energy and improving muscle tone.

In most circumstances, drugs play little part in a weight loss programme. However, *sibutramine* and *orlistat* may be useful adjuncts to a reducing diet and may be appropriate for some people with a high BMI (see *body mass index*), especially if they also have other health risk factors, such as *diabetes mellitus* or a raised blood cholesterol level. *Appetite suppressants* related to *amphetamines* are not recommended. Surgery may be considered for people who are very obese (with a BMI over 40).

Weil's disease Another name for *leptospirosis*.

welder's eye Acute *conjunctivitis* and *keratopathy* (corneal damage) caused by the intense *ultraviolet light* emitted by an electric welding arc. Welder's eye, which is also known as arc eye, results from the failure to wear adequate eye protection while welding.

wen A name for a *sebaceous cyst*.

Werdnig–Hoffmann disease A very rare inherited disorder of the *nervous system* that affects infants. Also known as infantile spinal muscular atrophy, Werdnig–Hoffmann disease is a type of *motor neuron disease*, affecting the nerve cells in the spinal cord that control muscle movement.

Marked floppiness and paralysis occur during the first few months, and affected children rarely survive beyond age 3.

There is no cure for the disease. Treatment aims to keep the affected infant as comfortable as possible.

Wernicke–Korsakoff syndrome An uncommon *brain* disorder almost always related to malnutrition occurring in chronic *alcohol dependence*, but occasionally due to that which occurs in other conditions, such as *cancer*. Wernicke–Korsakoff syndrome is caused by deficiency of thiamine (see *vitamin B complex*), which affects the brain and nervous system.

W

The disease consists of two stages: Wernicke's encephalopathy and Korsakoff's psychosis. Wernicke's encephalopathy usually develops suddenly and produces *nystagmus* (abnormal, jerky eye movements), *ataxia* (difficulty in coordinating body movements), slowness, and confusion. Sufferers usually have signs of *neuropathy*, such as loss of sensation, pins-and-needles, or impaired reflexes. The level of consciousness falls progressively and may lead to coma and death unless treated. The condition is a medical emergency. Treatment with high doses of intravenous thiamine often reverses most of the symptoms, sometimes within a few hours.

Korsakoff's psychosis may follow Wernicke's encephalopathy if treatment is not begun promptly enough. Symptoms consist of severe *amnesia*, apathy, and disorientation. Korsakoff's psychosis is usually irreversible.

Wernicke's area An area of the cerebral cortex in the brain that is involved in the interpretation of spoken and written language.

Wernicke's encephalopathy See *Wernicke–Korsakoff syndrome.*

West Nile virus A virus transmitted from infected animals or birds to humans by a mosquito bite. In most cases, there are either no symptoms or a flu-like illness. Rarely, a serious and potentially fatal illness, in which the virus infects the brain, can develop. The virus is found in Africa, Eastern Europe, West Asia, the Middle East, and, since 1999, the East coast of the US.

wet dream Ejaculation that occurs during sleep. See also *nocturnal emission.*

wheelchair A chair mounted on wheels used to provide mobility for a person unable to walk. Manual wheelchairs are designed so that the hand-rims can be easily gripped by a disabled person. They can also be pushed by a helper. Powered wheelchairs use batteries and are controlled electronically by finger or chin pressure, or breath control.

wheeze A high-pitched, whistling sound produced in the chest during breathing, caused by narrowing of the airways. It is a feature of *asthma, bronchitis, bronchiolitis,* and *pulmonary oedema.* Inhalation of a foreign body may also be a cause (See also *breathing difficulty.*)

whiplash injury An injury to the soft tissues, *ligaments*, and spinal joints of the neck caused by a forcible and violent bending of the neck backwards (hyperextension) and then forwards (flexion), or vice versa. Such injury most commonly results from sudden acceleration or deceleration, as occurs in a car collision.

Damage to the spine usually involves minor *sprain* of a neck ligament, or *subluxation* (partial dislocation) of a cervical joint. Occasionally, a ligament may rupture or a cervical vertebra may fracture (see *spinal injury*). Characteristically, pain and stiffness in the neck are much worse 24 hours after the injury.

Treatment may include early mobilization, exercises, and *analgesic drugs.* It may take a few weeks before full pain-free movement is possible.

WHIPLASH INJURY

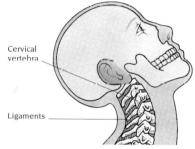

BACKWARD FORCE (HYPEREXTENSION)

Cervical vertebra
Ligaments

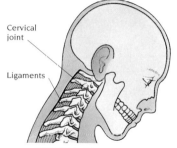

FORWARD FORCE (FLEXION)

Cervical joint
Ligaments

Whipple's disease A rare disorder, also called intestinal lipodystrophy, that can affect many organs. Symptoms include *steatorrhoea* as a result of *malabsorption*, abdominal pain, joint pains, progressive weight loss, swollen lymph nodes, *anaemia*, and fever. The heart, lungs, and brain can also be affected. The condition is most common in middle-aged men.

The cause is thought to be bacterial; affected tissues are found to contain macrophages (a type of scavenging cell) containing rod-shaped bacteria. Treatment is with *antibiotic drugs* for at least a year. Dietary supplements are used to correct nutritional deficiencies occurring as a result of malabsorption.

Whipple's operation A type of *pancreatectomy* in which the head of the pancreas and the loop of the duodenum are surgically removed.

whipworm infestation Small, cylindrical whip-like worms, 2.5–5 cm long, that live in the human large intestine. Infestation occurs worldwide but is most common in the tropics. Light infestation causes no symptoms; heavy infestation can cause abdominal pain, diarrhoea, and, sometimes, *anaemia*, since a small amount of the host's blood is consumed every day.

Diagnosis is through the identification of whipworm eggs in the faeces. Treatment is with *anthelmintic drugs*, such as *mebendazole*. A heavy infestation may require more than one course of treatment.

whitehead A very common type of skin blemish (see *milia*).

white matter Tissue in the nervous system composed of nerve fibres (*axons*). White matter makes up the bulk of the cerebrum (the two large hemispheres of the *brain*) and continues down into the *spinal cord*; its main role is to transmit nerve impulses. (See also *grey matter*.)

whitlow An abscess on the fingertip or toe, causing the finger to swell and become extremely painful and sensitive to pressure and touch. It most commonly develops from acute *paronychia*. A whitlow may be due to the virus that causes *herpes simplex* or to a bacterial infection. In some cases, it may be necessary to drain pus from the abscess.

WHO The commonly used abbreviation for the *World Health Organization*.

whooping cough See *pertussis*.

will, living See *living will*.

Wilms' tumour A type of *kidney cancer*, also called nephroblastoma, that occurs mainly in children.

Wilson's disease A rare, inherited disorder in which copper accumulates in the liver, resulting in conditions such as *hepatitis* and *cirrhosis*. Copper is slowly released into other body parts, damaging the brain, causing mild intellectual impairment, and leading to debilitating rigidity, tremor, and dementia. Symptoms usually appear in adolescence but can occur much earlier or later. Lifelong treatment with *penicillamine* is needed and, if begun soon enough, can sometimes produce some improvement. If the disease is discovered before the onset of symptoms, the drug may prevent them from developing.

wind A common name for gas in the gastrointestinal tract, which may be expelled through the mouth (see *belching*) or passed through the anus (see *flatus*).

Babies often swallow air during feeding which, unless the baby is "winded", can accumulate in the stomach and cause discomfort.

windpipe Another name for the *trachea*.

wiring of the jaws Immobilization of the jaws by means of metal wires to allow a fracture of the jaw to heal or as part of a treatment for *obesity*.

When a fracture is being treated, the jaws are kept wired in a fixed position for about 6 weeks. For promoting weight

WHITE MATTER

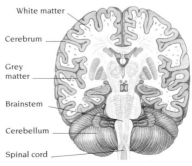

White matter

Cerebrum

Grey matter

Brainstem

Cerebellum

Spinal cord

SECTION THROUGH BRAIN

loss, the jaws are wired for as long as a year. In both cases, the person is unable to chew and can take only a liquid or semi-liquid diet. This form of diet treatment often fails because the person resumes previous eating habits following removal of the wires.

wisdom tooth One of the four rearmost *teeth*, also known as 3rd molars. The wisdom teeth normally erupt between the ages of 17 and 21, but in some people, one or more fails to develop or erupt. In many cases, wisdom teeth are unable to emerge fully from the gum as a result of overcrowding (see *impaction, dental*).

witches' milk A thin, white discharge from the nipple of a newborn infant, caused by maternal hormones that entered the fetus's circulation through the placenta. Witches' milk occurs quite commonly. It is usually accompanied by enlargement of one or both of the baby's breasts. The condition is harmless and usually disappears spontaneously within a few weeks.

withdrawal The process of retreating from society and from relationships with others; usually indicated by aloofness, lack of interest in social activities, preoccupation with one's own concerns, and difficulty in communicating.

The term is also applied to the psychological and physical symptoms that develop on discontinuing use of a substance on which a person is dependent (see *withdrawal syndrome*).

withdrawal bleeding Vaginal blood loss that occurs when the body's level of *oestrogen* or *progesterone hormones* or *progestogen drugs* drops suddenly.

The withdrawal bleeding that occurs at the end of each month's supply of combined *oral contraceptive pills* mimics menstruation but is usually shorter and lighter. Discontinuation of a progestogen-only preparation also produces bleeding, which may differ from normal menstruation in its amount and duration.

withdrawal method See *coitus interruptus*.

withdrawal syndrome Unpleasant mental and physical symptoms experienced when a person stops using a drug on which he or she is dependent (see *drug dependence*). Withdrawal syndrome most commonly occurs in those with *alcohol dependence* or *dependence* on *opioids*, in smokers, and in people addicted to *tranquillizers, amphetamines, cocaine, marijuana*, and *caffeine*.

Alcohol withdrawal symptoms start 6–8 hours after cessation of intake and may last up to 7 days. They include trembling of the hands, nausea, vomiting, sweating, cramps, anxiety, and, sometimes, seizures. (See also *confusion, delirium tremens*, and *hallucinations*.)

Opioid withdrawal symptoms start after 8–12 hours and may last for 7–10 days. Symptoms include restlessness, sweating, runny eyes and nose, yawning, diarrhoea, vomiting, abdominal cramps, dilated pupils, loss of appetite, irritability, weakness, tremor, and depression.

Withdrawal symptoms from *barbiturate drugs* and *meprobamate* start after 12–24 hours, beginning with tremor, anxiety, restlessness, and weakness, sometimes followed by delirium, hallucinations, and, occasionally, seizures. A period of prolonged sleep occurs 3–8 days after onset. Withdrawal from *benzodiazepine drugs* may begin much more slowly and can be life-threatening.

Withdrawal symptoms from *nicotine* develop gradually over 24–48 hours and include irritability, concentration problems, frustration, headaches, and anxiety.

Discontinuation of cocaine or amphetamines results in extreme tiredness, lethargy, and dizziness. Cocaine withdrawal may also lead to tremor, severe depression, and sweating.

Withdrawal symptoms from marijuana include tremor, nausea, vomiting, diarrhoea, sweating, irritability, and sleep problems. Caffeine withdrawal may lead to tiredness, headaches, and irritability.

Severe withdrawal syndromes require medical treatment. Symptoms may be suppressed by giving the patient small quantities of the drug he or she had been taking. More commonly, a substitute drug is given, such as *methadone* for opioid drugs or a benzodiazepine for alcohol. The dose of the drug is then gradually reduced.

wobble board A balancing board used during *physiotherapy* to improve muscle strength and coordination in the feet, ankles, and legs. A wobble board is sometimes used after an ankle sprain.

womb See *uterus*.

word blindness See *alexia; dyslexia*.

World Health Organization (WHO) An international organization established in 1948 as an agency of the United Nations with responsibilities for international health matters and public health. The WHO headquarters are in Geneva, Switzerland.

The WHO has campaigned effectively against some infectious diseases, most notably smallpox, tuberculosis, and malaria. Other functions include sponsoring medical research programmes, organizing a network of collaborating national laboratories, and providing expert advice and specific targets to its 192 member states with regard to health matters.

worm infestation Several types of worm, or their larvae, existing as parasites of humans. They may live in the intestines, blood, lymphatic system, bile ducts, or in organs such as the liver. In many cases, they cause few or no symptoms, but some can cause chronic illness. There are two main classes: *roundworms* and *platyhelminths*, which are subdivided into cestodes (tapeworms) and trematodes (flukes).

Worm diseases found in developed countries include *threadworm infestation, ascariasis, whipworm infestation, toxocariasis,* liver-fluke infestation, and various *tapeworm infestations.*

WORM INFESTATION

Threadworm egg   Larva inside egg

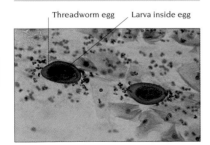

MICROSCOPIC VIEW OF WORM EGGS

Those occurring in tropical regions include *hookworm infestation, filariasis, guinea worm disease,* and *schistosomiasis.*

Worms may be acquired by eating undercooked, infected meat, by contact with soil or water containing worm larvae, or by accidental ingestion of worm eggs from soil contaminated by infected faeces. Most infestations can be easily eradicated with *anthelmintic drugs.*

wound Any damage to the skin and/or underlying tissues caused by an accident, act of violence, or surgery. Wounds in which the skin or mucous membrane is broken are called open; those in which they remain intact are termed closed.

Wounds can be divided into the following categories: an incised wound; an abrasion (or graze); a *laceration*; a penetrating wound; and a *contusion*.

wound infection Any type of *wound* is susceptible to the entry of bacteria; the resultant infection can delay healing, result in disability, and may even cause death. Infection of a wound is indicated by redness, swelling, warmth, pain, and sometimes by the presence of pus or the formation of an *abscess*. Infection may spread locally to adjacent organs or tissue, or to more distant parts of the body via the blood.

The type of infection depends upon how the wound occurred. For example, wounds brought into contact with soil can result in *tetanus*. *STAPHYLOCOCCI*, including *MRSA*, are also common wound infections.

Once infection is discovered, a sample of blood or pus is taken and the patient is given an antibiotic drug. Any abscess should be drained surgically.

wrinkle A furrow in the *skin*. Wrinkling is a natural feature of aging and is caused by a loss of skin elasticity. Premature deep wrinkling is usually due to overexposure to the ultraviolet rays in sunlight, and to smoking.

No treatment can permanently restore skin elasticity, although some *vitamin A* derivatives are believed to reduce wrinkling. A *face-lift* smoothes out wrinkles by stretching the skin; the effects may last up to 10 years.

WRIST

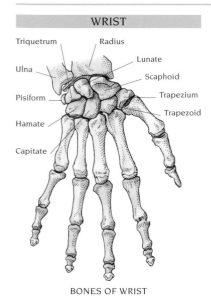

Triquetrum
Radius
Lunate
Ulna
Scaphoid
Pisiform
Trapezium
Trapezoid
Hamate
Capitate

BONES OF WRIST

wrist The joint between the *hand* and the arm that allows the hand to be bent forward and backward relative to the arm and also to be moved side to side.

The wrist contains eight bones (known collectively as the carpus) arranged in two rows, one articulating with the bones of the forearm, and the other connecting to the bones of the palm. Tendons connect the forearm muscles to the fingers and thumb, and arteries and nerves supply the muscles, bones, and skin of the hand and fingers.

Wrist injuries may lead to serious disability by limiting hand movement. A common injury in adults is *Colles' fracture*, in which the lower end of the radius is fractured and the wrist and hand are displaced backwards. In young children, similar displacement results from a fracture through the epiphysis (growing end) of the radius A *sprain* can affect ligaments at the wrist joint, but most wrist sprains are not severe. (See also *carpal tunnel syndrome*; *wrist-drop*; *tenosynovitis*; *osteoarthritis*.)

wrist-drop Inability to straighten the *wrist*, so that the back of the hand cannot be brought into line with the back of the forearm. This causes weakness of grip because the hand muscles can function efficiently only when the wrist is held straight.

Wrist-drop is caused by damage to the *radial nerve*, either by prolonged pressure in the armpit (see *crutch palsy*) or by fracture of the humerus (see *humerus, fracture of*). Treatment involves holding the wrist straight. This may be achieved by means of a splint, but if damage to the radial nerve is permanent, the usual treatment is *arthrodesis* (surgical fusion) of the wrist bones in a straight position.

writer's cramp See *cramp, writer's.*

wry neck Abnormal tilting and twisting of the head. It may be due to injury to, or spasm of, the muscles on one side of the neck (see *torticollis*), among other factors.

X

xanthelasma A yellowish deposit of fatty material that is visible in the skin around the eyes. Xanthelasmas are common in elderly people and are usually of no more than cosmetic importance. However, in younger people they may be associated with *hyperlipidaemias*, in which there is excess fat in the blood. Xanthelasmas may be removed, if necessary, by a simple surgical procedure under a local anaesthetic. Any associated hyperlipidaemia must also be treated. (See also *xanthomatosis*.)

xanthoma A yellowish deposit of fatty material in the skin, often on the elbow or buttock. They may be associated with *hyperlipidaemias* (see *xanthomatosis*).

xanthomatosis A condition in which deposits of yellowish, fatty material develop in various parts of the body, particularly in the skin, internal organs, corneas of the eyes, brain, and tendons. The deposits may occur only in the eyelids (see *xanthelasma*). A key feature of xanthomatosis is the tendency for fatty material to be deposited in the linings of blood vessels, leading to generalized *atherosclerosis*. Xanthomatosis is often associated with *hyperlipidaemias*.

Treatment aims to lower the levels of fats in the blood by means of a diet that is low in cholesterol and high in polyunsaturated fat, and by drug treatment.

X chromosome A *sex chromosome*, of which every normal female body cell has a pair. Male body cells have one X and one *Y chromosome*; each sperm carries either an X or a Y chromosome. Abnormal genes located on X chromosomes cause *X-linked disorders*.

xeroderma pigmentosum A rare, inherited skin disease. The skin is normal at birth, but *photosensitivity* (extreme sensitivity to sunlight) causes it to become dry, wrinkled, freckled, and

prematurely aged by about the age of 5. Noncancerous skin tumours and *skin cancers* also develop. Xeroderma pigmentosum is often accompanied by related eye problems, such as *photophobia* and *conjunctivitis*.

Treatment of the condition consists of protecting the skin from sunlight. Skin cancers are usually treated surgically or with *radiotherapy*.

xerophthalmia An *eye* disorder in which *vitamin A* deficiency causes the conjunctiva and cornea to become abnormally dry. Without treatment, xerophthalmia may progress to *keratomalacia*, a condition in which severe damage is caused to the cornea.

xerostomia Abnormal dryness of the mouth, which can cause bad breath and may predispose the sufferer towards tooth decay (see *caries, dental*). Xerostomia is sometimes a symptom of *Sjögren's syndrome*. (See also *mouth, dry*.)

xipamide A thiazide *diuretic* drug used to treat *oedema* (accumulation of fluid in tissues) and high blood pressure. Side effects may include dizziness and mild gastrointestinal disturbances.

xiphisternum An alternative name for the xiphoid process, the small, leaf-shaped projection that forms the lowest of the three parts of the *sternum*.

X-linked disorders Sex-linked *genetic disorders* in which the abnormal gene or genes (the causative factors) are located on the X chromosome. Almost all affected people are males. *Haemophilia*, *fragile X syndrome*, and *colour vision deficiency* are examples.

X-rays A form of electromagnetic radiation of short wavelength and high energy. X-rays are widely used in medicine for diagnosis and treatment.

X-rays are produced artificially by bombarding a heavy metal tungsten target with electrons, in a device known as an X-ray tube. Low doses of the X-rays that are emitted are passed through body tissue and form images on film or a fluorescent screen. The X-ray image, also known as a radiograph or roentgenogram, shows the internal structure of the area that is being examined. Dense structures, such as bone, absorb X-rays well and appear white on an X-

X-RAY

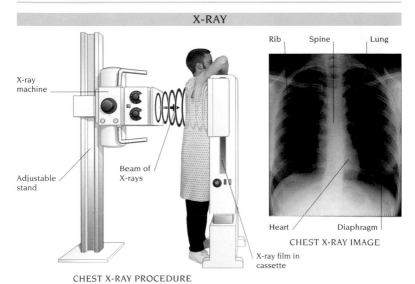

X-ray machine

Adjustable stand

Beam of X-rays

X-ray film in cassette

CHEST X-RAY PROCEDURE

Rib | Spine | Lung

Heart | Diaphragm

CHEST X-RAY IMAGE

ray image. Soft tissues, such as muscle, absorb less and appear grey.

Because X-rays can damage living cells, especially those that are dividing rapidly, high doses of radiation are used for treating cancer (see *radiotherapy*).

Hollow or fluid-filled parts of the body often do not show up well on X-ray film unless they first have a contrast medium (a substance that is opaque to X-rays) introduced into them. Contrast-medium X-ray techniques are used to image the gallbladder (see *cholecystography*), bile ducts (see *cholangiography*), the urinary tract (see *urography*), the gastrointestinal tract (see *barium X-ray examinations*), blood vessels (see *angiography*; *venography*), and the spinal cord (see *myelography*).

X-rays can be used to obtain an image of a "slice" through an organ or part of the body by using a technique known as *tomography*. More detailed images of a body slice are produced by combining tomography with the capabilities of a computer (see *CT scanning*).

Large doses of X-rays can be extremely hazardous, and even small doses carry some risk (see *radiation hazards*). Modern X-ray film, equipment, and

techniques produce high-quality images with the lowest possible radiation exposure to the patient. The possibility of genetic damage can be minimized by using a lead shield to protect the patient's reproductive organs from X-rays. Radiographers and radiologists wear a *film badge* to monitor their exposure to radiation. (See also *imaging techniques*; *radiography*; *radiology*.)

X-rays, dental See *dental X-rays*.

xylitol A naturally occurring carbohydrate that is only partially absorbed by the body and is sometimes used as a sweetener by people with diabetes. Xylitol chewing gum has been shown to reduce recurrent ear infections in some children. Excess xylitol may lead to abdominal discomfort and flatulence.

xylometazoline A *decongestant* drug used in the form of a spray or drops to relieve nasal congestion caused by a common *cold*, *sinusitis*, or hay fever (see *rhinitis, allergic*). Xylometazoline is also used as an ingredient of eye drops in the treatment of allergic *conjunctivitis*.

Excessive use of xylometazoline may cause headache, palpitations, or drowsiness. Long-term use of the drug may cause nasal congestion to worsen when treatment is stopped.

Y

yawning An involuntary act, or reflex action, usually associated with drowsiness or boredom. The mouth is opened wide and a slow, deep breath is taken through it in order to draw air into the lungs. The air is then slowly released. Yawning is accompanied by a momentary increase in the heart-rate, and, in many cases, watering of the eyes.

The purpose of yawning is unknown, but one theory suggests it is triggered by raised levels of carbon dioxide in the blood; thus, its purpose could be to reduce the level of carbon dioxide and increase that of oxygen in the blood.

yaws An infectious disease that tends to be found throughout poorer subtropical and tropical areas of the world. Yaws is caused by a *spirochaete* (a spiral-shaped bacterium), and it spreads principally in conditions of poor hygiene. The infection is almost always acquired in childhood, and it mainly affects the skin and bones.

The bacteria enter the body through abrasions in the skin. Three or four weeks after infection, an itchy, raspberry-like growth appears at the site of infection, sometimes preceded by fever and pains. Scratching spreads the infection and causes more growths to develop elsewhere on the skin. Without treatment, the growths heal slowly over the course of about 6 months, but recurrence is common. In about 10 per cent of untreated cases, widespread tissue loss eventually occurs. This may eventually lead to gross destruction of the skin, bones, and joints of the legs, nose, palate and upper jaw.

Yaws can be cured by a single large dose of a *penicillin drug* given as an injection into muscle.

Y chromosome A *sex chromosome* that is present in every normal male body cell. It is paired with an *X chromosome* and is absent in every female body cell. Each sperm carries either a single X or a single Y chromosome.

Unlike the X chromosome, the Y chromosome carries little genetic material. Its major function is to stimulate the development of the *testes* in the *embryo*. There are no significant diseases related to abnormalities of the Y chromosome, but hairy ears is a trait thought to be determined by a Y-linked gene.

yeasts Types of *fungi* in which the body of the fungus comprises individual cells that occur either singly, in pairs, or in longer chains. Certain yeasts can cause infections of the skin or mucous membranes; the most important of these disease-causing yeasts is *CANDIDA ALBICANS*, which causes *candidiasis*.

YEASTS

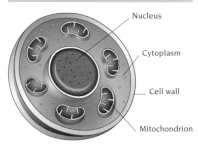

YEAST CELL

yellow fever An infectious disease of short duration and variable severity that is caused by a virus transmitted by mosquitoes. In severe cases, the skin yellows due to *jaundice*, from which the name yellow fever derives. The infection may be spread from monkeys to humans in forest areas through various species of mosquito; and in urban areas it can be transmitted between humans by *AEDES AEGYPTI* mosquitoes.

Today, yellow fever is contracted only in Central America, parts of South America, and a large area of Africa. Eradication of the causative mosquito from populated areas has greatly reduced its incidence.

Yellow fever is characterized by a sudden onset of fever and headache, often with nausea and nosebleeds and, despite the high fever, a very low heart-rate. In more serious cases, the fever is higher and there is severe headache and pain in the neck, back, and legs. Damage may occur rapidly to the liver and kidneys, causing jaundice and *kidney failure*. This may be followed by *meningitis*, severe agitation and delirium, leading to coma and death.

Vaccination confers long-lasting immunity and should always be obtained before travel to affected areas. A single injection of the vaccine gives protection for at least 10 years. Serious reactions to the vaccine are rare. Children under the age of 9 months are not usually vaccinated unless there is an unavoidable risk of infection.

During yellow fever epidemics, diagnosis is simple. A diagnosis can be confirmed by carrying out blood tests to isolate the causative virus or to find *antibodies* to the virus.

No drug is effective against the yellow fever virus; treatment is directed at maintaining the blood volume. Transfusion of fluids is often necessary. Many patients recover in about 3 days and, in mild to moderate cases, complications are few. Relapses do not occur and one attack confers lifelong immunity. However, despite treatment the disease is fatal in some cases.

Yersinia A class of bacteria containing the organism responsible for the bubonic plague (*YERSINIA PESTIS*). In other forms, *YERSINIA* is responsible for a variety of infections, such as *gastroenteritis*, particularly in young children, and *arthritis* and *septicaemia* in adults.

yin and yang The two opposing and interdependent principles that are fundamental to traditional *Chinese medicine* and philosophy. Yin is associated with the female, darkness, coldness, and quiescence; yang embodies qualities of maleness, brightness, heat, and activity. In a healthy body, yin and yang are in balance. The concepts of yin and yang are also central to the theoretical basis of *macrobiotics*.

yoga A system of Hindu philosophy and physical discipline that is becoming increasingly popular throughout the world. The main form of yoga that is practised in the West is hatha-yoga, in which the follower adopts a series of poses, called asanas, and uses a special breathing technique. The practice of yoga maintains flexibility of the body, teaches both physical and mental control, and is a useful *relaxation technique*.

If attempted by people in poor health, or practised incorrectly, yoga may pose certain health hazards, such as back disorders, *hypertension* (high blood pressure), and *glaucoma* (increased pressure in the eye).

yolk sac The membranous sac, otherwise known as the vitelline sac, that lies against, and is attached to, the front of the *embryo* during the early stages of its existence. During development, the sac decreases proportionately in size to the body, reducing finally to a narrow duct that passes through the *umbilicus*. The yolk sac is believed to assist in the transportation of nutrients from the mother to the early embryo.

yttrium A very rare metal that, in its radioactive form, is sometimes used in cancer therapy and to treat joints affected by arthritis.

Z

zanamivir An *antiviral drug* used to treat infection with the *influenza* A and B viruses, particularly in people who are at a high risk of developing complications from influenza, such as those with *diabetes mellitus* or chronic chest problems. To be effective, the drug should be taken within 48 hours of the onset of flu symptoms. Possible side effects of zanamivir include nausea, vomiting, and diarrhoea. Occasionally, it may cause breathing problems or worsen asthma.

zidovudine An *antiretroviral drug*, formerly known as azidothymidine or *AZT*, that is used in combination with other antiretroviral drugs to slow the progression of *AIDS*. The principal aim of antiretrovirals is to keep viral replication to as low a level as possible for as long as possible; they do not constitute a cure. Zidovudine was the first drug to be introduced to combat *HIV* infection.

Possible side effects of zidovudine include *anaemia*, which may be severe enough to require a blood transfusion, nausea, loss of appetite, and headache.

ZIFT See *zygote intrafallopian transfer*.

zinc A *trace element* that is essential for normal growth, the development of the reproductive organs, normal functioning of the prostate gland, healing of wounds, and the manufacture of *proteins* and *nucleic acids* in the body. Zinc also controls the activities of more than 100 enzymes and is involved in the functioning of the hormone *insulin*.

Particularly rich sources of zinc include lean meat, wholemeal breads, whole grain cereals, dried beans, and seafood.

Zinc deficiency is rare. Most cases occur in people who are generally malnourished. Deficiency may also be caused by any disorder that causes *malabsorption*; *acrodermatitis enteropathica*; or by increased zinc requirements due to cell damage (for example, as a result of a burn or in *sickle cell anaemia*). Symptoms of deficiency include impairment of taste and loss of appetite; there may also be hair loss and inflammation of the skin, mouth, tongue, and eyelids. In children, zinc deficiency impairs growth and delays sexual development.

Prolonged excessive intake of zinc may interfere with the intestinal absorption of *iron* and *copper*, leading to a deficiency of these minerals.

Zinc compounds, such as *zinc oxide*, are included in many preparations for treating skin and scalp disorders.

zinc oxide An ingredient of many skin preparations that has a mild *astringent* action and a soothing effect. Zinc oxide is used to treat painful, itchy, or moist skin conditions and to ease the pain caused by haemorrhoids and insect bites or stings. It also blocks the ultraviolet rays of the sun (see *sunscreens*).

Zollinger–Ellison syndrome A rare condition characterized by severe and recurrent *peptic ulcers* in the stomach, duodenum, and jejunum (the second part of the small intestine). Zollinger–Ellison syndrome is caused by one or more tumours in the *pancreas* that secrete the hormone gastrin. Gastrin stimulates production of large quantities of acid by the stomach, which leads to ulceration. The high levels of acid in the digestive tract often also cause diarrhoea.

The tumours are cancerous, but of a slow-growing type. If possible, they are removed surgically. *Proton pump inhibitor* drugs are given to treat the ulcers.

zolpidem A drug used in the short-term treatment of *insomnia*. Zolpidem has a brief duration of action and causes little hangover effect. Side effects include diarrhoea, nausea, and dizziness.

zona pellucida The thick, transparent, noncellular layer that surrounds a developing egg cell in the ovarian follicle. At *fertilization*, the zona pellucida is penetrated by at least one sperm.

zoonosis Any infectious or parasitic disease of animals that can be transmitted to humans. Unlike many disease organisms, zoonotic organisms are flexible and can adapt themselves to many different species.

Zoonoses are usually caught from animals closely associated with humans, either as pets, food sources, or scavenging parasites, such as rats. Examples include *toxocariasis, cat-scratch fever*, some *fungal infections, psittacosis, brucellosis, trichinosis*, and *leptospirosis. Rabies* can infect virtually any mammal, but dog bites are a common cause of human infection worldwide.

Other zoonoses are transmitted from animals less obviously associated with humans, usually by insect *vectors*. For example, *yellow fever* is transmitted by mosquito bites. (See also *dogs, diseases from; cats, diseases from; rats, diseases from, insects and disease*.)

zopiclone A drug used in the short-term treatment of *insomnia*. It has a brief duration of action and causes little hangover effect. Side effects include a bitter metallic taste, nausea, and dry mouth.

Z-plasty A technique that is used in *plastic surgery* to change the direction of a pre-existing scar so that it can be hidden in natural skin creases, or to relieve skin tension caused by the *contracture* of a scar. Z-plasty is especially useful for revising unsightly scars on the face and for releasing scarring across those joints, such as on the fingers or in the armpits, that may restrict normal movement or cause deformity.

zygomatic arch The arch of bone, commonly known as the cheek bone, on either side of the *skull* just below the eye socket. The zygomatic arch is formed of the zygomatic and temporal bones.

zygote The cell that is produced when a *sperm* fertilizes an *ovum*. A zygote, measuring about 0.1 mm in diameter in humans, contains all the genetic material for a new individual. The zygote is surrounded by a protein-rich layer known as the *zona pellucida*.

ZYGOTE

Zona pellucida   Zygote

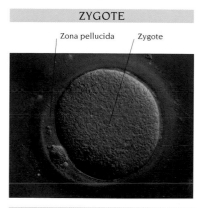

The zygote travels down one of the woman's *fallopian tubes*, dividing as it does so. After about a week, the mass of cells (now called a blastocyst) implants into the lining of the uterus, and the next stage of embryological growth begins. (See also *embryo; fertilization*.)

zygote intrafallopian transfer A type of *in vitro fertilization*, also referred to as ZIFT, in which *ova* are fertilized outside the body and returned to a *fallopian tube* rather than to the *uterus*.

ZYGOMATIC ARCH

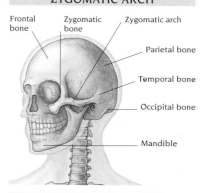

Frontal bone
Zygomatic bone
Zygomatic arch
Parietal bone
Temporal bone
Occipital bone
Mandible

Z

ACKNOWLEDGMENTS

PICTURE CREDITS

Dr D.A.Burns: 374 cl, 469tr; Professor Terry Hamblin, The Royal Bournemouth
Hospital Medical Illustration Department: 456cr; Dr N. R. Patel: 185cr; Science
Photo Library: 600bl; Biophoto Associates 506tr; CNRI 129tcr, 250tr; Dr P. Marazzi 67bl,
218br; Eye of Science 284bcr; John Radcliffe Hospital 293tr; National Institute
of Health 444br; Professor P. Motta/Department of Anatomy/University "La Sapienza",
Rome 424bcl; National Meningitis Trust: 252bl; St John's Institute of Dermatology:
302br, 361tr; The Wellcome Institute Library, London: 255br, 257bl, 325bcl

All other images copyright © Dorling Kindersley.
For further information see: www.dkimages.com

ILLUSTRATORS

Evi Antoniou, Joanna Cameron, Mick Gillah, Tony Graham, Mark Iley,
Deborah Maizels, Patrick Mulrey, Peter Ruane, Richard Tibbitts,
Halli Verrinder, Philip Wilson, Deborah Woodward,

PHOTOGRAPHERS

Andy Crawford, Steve Gorton, Gary Ombler, Tim Ridley,
Spike Walker (microphotography)

Every effort has been made to acknowledge those individuals, organizations, and
corporations that have helped with this book and to trace copyright holders.
DK apologizes in advance if any omission has occurred. If an omission does come
to light, the company will be pleased to insert the appropriate acknowledgment
in any subsequent editions of this book.

PREVIOUS EDITION

BMA Consulting Medical Editor Dr Michael Peters
Medical Consultants Dr Sue Davidson, Dr Penny Preston, Dr Frances Williams

Category Publisher Jackie Douglas
Senior Managing Editor Martyn Page
Editorial Manager Andrea Bagg
Project Editors Jolyon Goddard, Teresa Pritlove
Editors Joanna Benwell, Katie John, Alyson Lacewing, Janet Mohun,
Mukul Patel, Hazel Richardson, Esther Ripley
Additional Editorial Assistance Nina Blackett, Edda Bohnsack
Managing Art Editor Louise Dick
Senior Art Editor Marianne Markham
Design Assistant Iona Hoyle
Additional Design Assistance Tessa Bindloss, Gadi Farfour, Sara Freeman
DTP Designer Julian Dams
Picture Researcher Sarah Duncan
Picture Librarian Melanie Simmonds
Production Rita Sinha